Cyrus Khojasteh

# DRUG SAFETY EVALUATION

# DRUG SAFETY EVALUATION

SHAYNE C. GAD

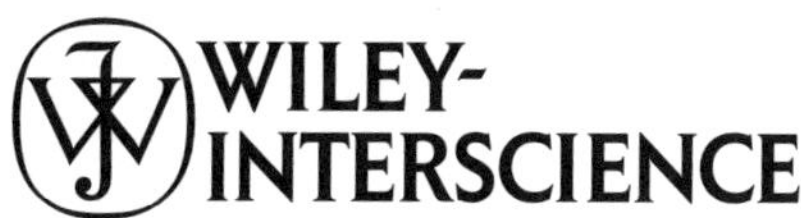

A John Wiley & Sons, Inc., Publication

*Library of Congress Cataloging-in-Publication Data:*

Gad, Shayne C., 1848-
   Drug Safetey evaluation/Shayne C. Gad.
      p. cm.
   Includes index.
   ISBN 0-471-40727-5 (cloth: alk. paper)
   1. Drugs—Toxicology. 2. Drugs—Testing. I. Title.
RA1238. G334 2002
615′.19—dc21
Printed in the United States of America.

10  9  8  7  6  5  4  3  2  1

*To Spunky Dustmop, who always listens
so well and is always there.*

# CONTENTS

# PREFACE

*Drug Safety Evaluation* has been written with the central objective of presenting an all-inclusive practical guide for those who are responsible for ensuring the safety of drugs and biologics to patients, health care providers, those involved in the manufacture of medicinal products, and all those who need to understand how the safety of these products is evaluated.

This practical guide presents a road map for safety assessment as an integral part of the development of new drugs and therapeutics. Individual chapters also address specific approaches to evaluating hazards, including problems that are encountered and their solutions. Also covered are the scientific and philosophical bases for evaluation of specific concerns (e.g., carcinogenicity, development toxicity, etc.) to provide both understanding and guidance for approaching new problems. *Drug Safety Evaluation* is aimed specifically at the pharmaceutical and biotechnology industries. It is hoped that the approaches and methodologies presented here will show a utilitarian yet scientifically valid path to the everyday challenge of safety evaluation and the problem-solving that is required in drug discovery and development.

Shayne C. Gad
*Cary, North Carolina*

# ABOUT THE AUTHOR

Shayne C. Gad, Ph.D. (Texas, 1977), DABT, ATS, has been the Principal of Gad Consulting Services since 1994. He has more than 25 years of broad based experience in toxicology, drug and device development, document preparation, statistics and risk assessment, having previously been Director of Toxicology and Pharmacology for Synergen (Boulder, CO), Director of Medical Affairs Technical Support Services for Becton Dickinson (RTP, NC) and Senior Director of Product Safety and Pharmacokinetics for G.D. Searle (Skokie, IL). He is a past president and council member of the American College of Toxicology and the President of the Roundtable of Toxicology Consultants. He has previously served the Society of Toxicology on the placement, animals in research [twice each], and nominations committees, as well as president of two SOT specialty sections (Occupational Health and Regulatory Toxicology) and officer of a third (Reproductive and Developmental Toxicity). He is also a member of the Teratology Society, Biometrics Society, and the American Statistical Association. Dr. Gad has previously published 24 books, and more than 300 chapters, papers and abstracts in the above fields. He has also organized and taught numerous courses, workshops and symposia both in the United States and internationally.

# DRUG SAFETY
# EVALUATION

# 1

# STRATEGY AND PHASING FOR DRUG SAFETY EVALUATION IN THE DISCOVERY AND DEVELOPMENT OF PHARMACEUTICALS

## 1.1. INTRODUCTION

The preclinical assessment of the safety of potential new pharmaceuticals represents a special case of the general practice of toxicology (Gad, 1996, 2000; Meyer, 1989), possessing its own peculiarities and special considerations, and differing in several ways from the practice of toxicology in other fields—for some significant reasons. Because of the economics involved and the essential close interactions with other activities, (e.g., clinical trials, chemical process optimization, formulation development, regulatory reviews, etc.), the development and execution of a crisp, timely and flexible, yet scientifically sound, program is a prerequisite for success. The ultimate aim of preclinical assessment also makes it different. A good pharmaceutical safety assessment program seeks to efficiently and effectively move safe, potential therapeutic agents into, and support them through, the clinical evaluation, then to registration, and, finally, to market. This requires the quick identification of those agents that are not safe. At the same time, the very biological activity which makes a drug efficacious also acts to complicate the design and interpretation of safety studies.

Pharmaceuticals, unlike industrial chemicals, agricultural chemicals, and environmental agents, are intended to have human exposure and biological activity. And, unlike these materials and food additives, pharmaceuticals are intended to have biological effects on the people that receive them. Frequently, the interpretation of results and the formulation of decisions about the continued development and

1

eventual use of a drug are based on an understanding of both the potential adverse effects of the agent (its safety) and its likely benefits, as well as the dose separation between these two (the "therapeutic index"). This makes a clear understanding of dose-response relationships critical, so that the actual risk/benefit ratio can be identified. It is also essential that the pharmacokinetics be understood and that "doses" (plasma tissue levels) at target organ sites be known (Scheuplein et al., 1990). Integral evaluation of pharmacokinetics are essential to any effective safety evaluation program.

The development and safety evaluation of pharmaceuticals have many aspects specified by regulatory agencies, and this has also tended to make the process more complex [until recently, as ICH (International Conference on Harmonization) has tended to take hold] as markets have truly become global. An extensive set of safety evaluations is absolutely required before a product is ever approved for market. Regulatory agencies have increasingly come to require not only the establishment of a "clean dose" in two species with adequate safety factors to cover potential differences between species, but also an elucidation of the mechanisms underlying such adverse effects as are seen at higher doses and are not well understood. These regulatory requirements are compelling for the pharmaceutical toxicologist (Traina, 1983; Smith, 1992). There is not, however, a set menu of what must be done. Rather, much (particularly in terms of the timing of testing) is open to professional judgment and is tailored for the specific agent involved and its therapeutic claim.

The discovery, development, and registration of a pharmaceutical is an immensely expensive operation, and represents a rather unique challenge (Zbinden, 1992). For every 9000 to 10,000 compounds specifically synthesized or isolated as potential therapeutics, one (on average) will actually reach the market. This process is illustrated diagrammatically in Figure 1.1. Each successive stage in the process is more expensive, making it of great interest to identify as early as possible those agents that are not likely to go the entire distance, allowing a concentration of effort on the compounds that have the highest probability of reaching the market. Compounds "drop out" of the process primarily for three reasons:

1. Toxicity or (lack of) tolerance.
2. (lack of) efficacy.
3. (lack of) bioavailability of the active moiety in man.

Early identification of poor or noncompetitive candidates in each of these three categories is thus extremely important (Fishlock, 1990), forming the basis for the use of screening in pharmaceutical discovery and development. How much and which resources to invest in screening, and each successive step in support of the development of a potential drug, are matters of strategy and phasing that are detailed in a later section of this chapter. *In vitro* methods are increasingly providing new tools for use in both early screening and the understanding of mechanisms of observed toxicity in preclinical and clinical studies (Gad, 1989b, 2001), particularly with the growing capabilities and influence of genomic and proteomic technologies.

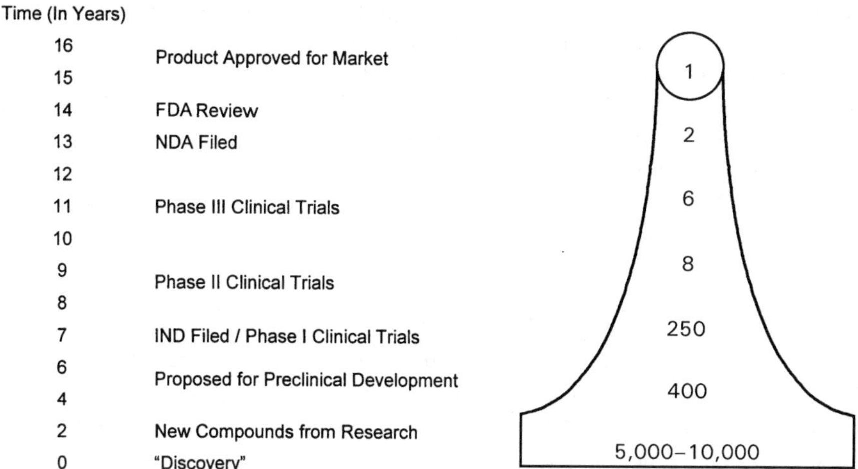



**FIGURE 1.1.** Attrition during the development of new molecules with a promise of therapeutic potential. Over the course of taking a new molecular entity through scale-up, safety and efficacy testing, and, finally, to market, typically only one out of every 9000 to 10,000 will go to the marketplace.

This is increasingly important as the societal concern over drug prices has grown (Littlehales, 1999). Additionally, the marketplace for new drugs is exceedingly competitive. The rewards for being either early (first or second) into the marketplace or achieving a significant therapeutic advantage are enormous in terms of eventual market share. Additionally, the first drug approved sets agency expectations for those drugs which follow. In mid-2001, there are 182 pharmaceutical products awaiting approval (41 of these are biotech products), the "oldest" having been in review seven years and some 1700 additional agents in the IND stage (Bryostowsi, 2001). Not all of these (particularly the oldest) will be economically successful.

The successful operation of a safety assessment program in the pharmaceutical industry requires that four different phases of the product-related operation be simultaneously supported. These four phases of pharmaceutical product support [discovery support, investigation new drug (IND) support, clinical and registration support, and product support] constitute the vast majority of what is done by the safety assessment groups in the pharmaceutical industry. The constant adjustment of balance of resources between these four areas is the greatest management challenge in pharmaceutical safety assessment. An additional area, occupational toxicology, is conducted in a manner similar to that for industrial environments and is the subject of Chapter 14 of this volume. In most companies, occupational toxicology is the responsibility of a separate group.

The usual way in which transition (or "flow") between the different phases is handled in safety assessment is to use a tiered testing approach. Each tier generates more specific data (and costs more to do so) and draws on the information generated in earlier tiers to refine the design of new studies. Different tiers are keyed to the support of successive decision points (go/no-go points) in the development process, with the intent of reducing risks as early as possible.

The first real critical decisions concerning the potential use of a compound in humans are the most difficult. They require an understanding of how well particular animal models work in predicting adverse effects in humans (usually very well, but there are notable lapses; for example, giving false positives and false negatives), and an understanding of what initial clinical trials are intended to do. Though an approved IND grants one entry into limited evaluations of drug effects in man, flexibility in the execution and analysis of these studies offers a significant opportunity to also investigate efficacy (O'Grady and Linet, 1990).

Once past the discovery and initial development stages, the safety assessment aspects of the process become extremely tightly connected with the other aspects of the development of a compound, particularly the clinical aspects. These interconnections are coordinated by project management systems. At many times during the early years of the development process, safety assessment constitutes the rate-limiting step; it is, in the language of project management, on the critical path.

Another way in which pharmaceutical safety assessment varies from toxicology as practiced in other industries is that it is a much more multidisciplinary and integrated process. This particularly stands out in the incorporation of the evaluation of ADME (absorption, distribution, metabolism and excretion) aspects in the safety evaluation process. These pharmacokinetic–metabolism (PKM) aspects are evaluated for each of the animal model species (most commonly the rat and dog or primate) utilized to evaluate the preclinical systemic toxicity of a potential drug prior to evaluation in man. Frequently, *in vitro* characterizations of metabolism for model (or potential model) species and man are performed to allow optimal model selection and understanding of findings. This allows for an early appreciation of both the potential bioavailability of active drug moieties and the relative predictive values of the various animal models. Such data early on are also very useful (in fact, sometimes essential) in setting dose levels for later animal studies and in projecting safe dose levels for clinical use. Unlike most other areas of industrial toxicology, one is not limited to extrapolating the relationships between administered dose and systemic effects. Rather, one has significant information on systemic levels of the therapeutic moiety; typically, total area under the curve (AUC), peak plasma levels ($C_{max}$), and plasma half-lives, at a minimum. Chapter 18 looks at these aspects in detail.

The state of the art for preclinical safety assessment has now developed to the point where the resulting products of the effort (reports, IND/NDA summaries, and the overall professional assessment of them) are expected to reflect and integrate the best effort of all the available scientific disciplines. Actual data and discussion should thus come from toxicology, pharmacology, pathology, and metabolism, at a minimum. The success of current premarket efforts to develop and ensure that only safe drugs make it to market are generally good, but clearly not perfect. This is reflected in popular (Arnst, 1998; Raeburn, 1999) and professional (Moore, et al., 1998; Lazarou et al., 1998) articles looking at both the number of recent marketed drug withdrawals for safety (summarized in Table 1.1) and at rates of drug-related

**TABLE 1.1. Post-approval Adverse Side Effects and Related Drug Withdrawals Since 1990**

- 51% of approval Drugs had serious post-approval identified side effects
- FDAMA passed in 1997

| Year | Drug | Indication/Class | Causative Side Effect |
|---|---|---|---|
| 1991 | Enkaid<br>(4 years on market) | Antiarrhythmic | Cardiovascular<br>(sudden cardiac death) |
| 1992 | Temafloxacin | Antibiotic | Blood & Kidney |
| 1997 | Fenfuramine*/Dexafluramine<br>(Combo used since 1984)<br>(*24 years on market) | Diet pill | Heart Valve Abnormalities |
| 1998 | Posicor (Midefradil)<br>(1 year on market) | Ca$^{++}$ Channel Blocker | Lethal Drug Interactions<br>(Inhibited Liver Enzymes) |
| | Duract (Bronfemic Sodium)<br>(Early preapproval warnings of liver enzymes) | Pain Relief | Liver Damage |
| 1999 | Tronan<br>(use severely restricted) | Antibiotic | Liver/Kidney Damage |
| | Raxar | Quinolone antibiotic | QT internal prolongation/<br>ventricular arrhythmias (deaths) |
| | Hismanal | Antihistamine | Drug-drug interactions |
| | Rotashield | Rotavirus Vaccine | Bowel Obstruction |
| 2000 | Renzulin<br>(Approved Dec 1996) | Type II Diabetes | Liver Damage |
| | Propulsid | Heartburn | Cardiovascular Irregularities/Deaths |
| | Lotonex | Irritable Bowel Syndrome | Ischemic colitis/death |
| 2001 | Phenylpropanolamine (PPA) | OTC ingredient | Hemorrhagic stroke |
| | Baychlor | Cholesterol reducing (satin) | Rhabdomyolysis (muscle-<br>weakening) (deaths) |

AALAC certified laboratory. In-housing testing included acute, subacute, and subchronic oral, dermal and inhalation studies and specialty reproductive, behavioural, haematological and renal function toxicity studies. Preparation of risk assessment, submissions and presentations to regulatory agencies and trade association.

adverse drug events and deaths in hospital patients. It is hoped that this system can be improved, and there are a lot of efforts to improve or optimize drug candidate selection and development (Lesko, et al., 2000).

## 1.2. REGULATORY REQUIREMENTS

Minimum standards and requirements for safety assessment of new pharmaceuticals are established by the need to meet regulatory requirements for developing, and eventually gaining approval to market, the agent. Determining what these requirements are is complicated by (1) the need to compete in a global market, which means gaining regulatory approval in multiple countries that do not have the same standards or requirements, and (2) the fact that the requirements are documented as guidelines, the interpretation of which is subject to change as experience alters judgments. The ICH process has much improved this situation, as detailed in Chapter 2.

Standards for the performance of studies (which is one part of regulatory requirements) have as their most important component good laboratory practices (GLPs). Good laboratory practices largely dictate the logistics of safety assessment: training, adherence to other regulations (such as those governing the requirements for animal care), and (most of all) the documentation and record-keeping that are involved in the process. There are multiple sets of GLP regulations (in the United States alone, agencies such as the FDA and EPA each have their own) that are not identical; however, adherence to U.S. Food and Drug Administration GLPs (FDA, 1987a) will rarely lead one astray.

Not all studies that are done to assess the preclinical safety of a new pharmaceutical need be done in strict adherence to GLPs. Those studies that are "meant to support the safety of a new agent" (i.e., are *required* by regulatory guidelines) must be so conducted or run a significant risk of rejection. However, there are also many other studies of an exploratory nature (such as range finders and studies done to understand the mechanisms of toxicity) that are not required by the FDA, and which may be done without strict adherence to GLPs. A common example are those studies performed early on to support research in selecting candidate agents. Such studies do not meet the requirements for having a validated analytical method to verify the identity, composition, and stability of materials being assayed, yet they are essential to the processes of discovery and development of new drugs. All such studies must eventually be reported to the FDA if an IND application is filed, but the FDA does not in practice "reject" such studies (and therefore the IND) because they are "non-GLP."

There is a second set of "standards" of study conduct that are less well defined. These are "generally accepted practice," and though not written down in regulation, are just as important as GLPs for studies to be accepted by the FDA and the scientific community. These standards, which are set by what is generally accepted as good science by the scientific community, include techniques, instruments utilized, and interpretation of results. Most of the chapters in this book will reflect these generally accepted practices in one form or another.

Guidelines establish which studies must be done for each step in the process of development. Though guidelines supposedly are suggestion (and not requirements), they are in fact generally treated as minimums by the promulgating agency. The exceptions to this are special cases where a drug is to meet some significant need (a life-threatening disease such as AIDS) or where there are real technological limitations as to what can be done (as with many of the new biologically derived [or biotechnology] agents, where limitations on compound availability and biological responses make traditional approaches inappropriate).

There are some significant differences in guideline requirements between the major countries [see Alder and Zbinden (1988) for an excellent country-by-country review of requirements], though this source is now becoming dated. The core of what studies are generally done are those studies conducted to meet U.S. FDA requirements. These are presented in Table 1.2. As will be discussed in Chapter 2, these guidelines are giving way to the ICH guidelines. However, while the length and details of studies have changed, the nature and order of studies remain the same.

The major variations in requirements for other countries still tend to be in the area of special studies. The United States does not formally require any genotoxicity studies, but common practice for U.S. drug registration is to perform at least a bacterial gene mutation assay (Ames test), a mammalian cell mutation assay and a clastogenicity assay, while Japan requires specific tests, including a gene mutation assay in Escherichia coli. Likewise, the European Economic Community (EEC) has a specified set of requirements, while individual countries have additional special requirements (Italy, for example, requires a mutagenicity assay in yeast). As detailed in Chapter 6, the new ICH genotoxicity guidelines have come to meet multinational requirements. Japan maintains a special requirement for an antigenicity assay in guinea pigs. The new safety pharmacology requirements are likely to be adopted over a period of time by different adherents.

It is possible to interact with the various regulatory agencies (particularly the FDA) when peculiarities of science or technology leave one with an unclear understanding of what testing is required. It is best if such discussions directly involve the scientists who understand the problems, and it is essential that the scientists at the FDA be approached with a course of action (along with its rationale) that has been proposed to the agency in advance.

The actual submissions to a regulatory agency that request permission either to initiate (or advance) clinical trials of a drug, or to market a drug, are not just bundles of reports on studies. Rather, they take the form of summaries that meet mandated requirements for format, accompanied by the reports discussed in these summaries (Guarino, 1987). In the United States, these summaries are the appropriate section of the IND and the New Drug Application (NDA). The formats for these documents have recently been revised (FDA, 1987b). The EEC equivalent is the expert report, as presented in EEC Directive 75/319. Similar approaches are required by other countries. In each of these cases, textual summaries are accompanied by tables that also serve to summarize significant points of study design and of study findings.

All of these approaches have in common that they are to present integrated evaluations of the preclinical safety data that are available on a potential new drug.

**TABLE 1.2. Synopsis of General Guidelines for Animal Toxicity Studies (U.S. FDA)**

| Category | Duration of human administration[a] | Phase[b] | Subacute or chronic toxicity[c] | Special studies |
|---|---|---|---|---|
| Oral or parenteral | Several days (up to 3)<br>Up to 2 weeks | I, II, III, NDA<br>I<br>II<br>III, NDA | 2 species: 2 weeks<br>2 species: 4 weeks<br>2 species: up to 4 weeks<br>2 species: up to 3 months | For parenterally administered drugs; compatibility with blood and local tolerance at injection site where applicable. |
| | Up to 3 months | I, II<br>III<br>NDA | 2 species: 4 weeks<br>2 species: 3 months<br>2 species: up to 6 months | |
| | 6 months to unlimited | I, II<br>III<br><br>NDA | 2 species: 3 months<br>2 species: 6 months or longer<br>2 species: 12 months in rodents, 9 months in nonrodents + 2 rodent species for CA; 18 months (mouse)—may be met by use of a transgenic model 24 months (rat) | |

| Route | Phase | Duration | Special studies |
|---|---|---|---|
| Inhalation (general anesthetics) | Single administration | I, II, III, NDA | 4 species: 5 days (3 h/day) | |
| Dermal | Single application | I | 1 species: single 24-h exposure followed by 2-week observation | Sensitization |
| | Single or short-term application | II | 1 species: 20-day repeated exposure (intact and abraded skin) | |
| | Short-term application | III | As above | |
| | Unlimited application | NDA | As above, but intact skin study extended up to 6 months | |
| Ophthalmic | Single application | I | | Eye irritation tests with graded doses |
| | Multiple application | I, II, III | 1 species: 3 weeks, daily applications, as in clinical use | |
| | | NDA | 1 species: duration commensurate with period of drug administration | |
| Vaginal or rectal | Single application | I | | Local and systematic toxicity after vaginal or rectal application in 2 species |
| | Multiple application | I, II, III, NDA | 2 species: duration and number of applications determined by proposed use | |

(*continued*)

**TABLE 1.2.** (*continued*)

| Category | Duration of human administration[a] | Phase[b] | Subacute or chronic toxicity[c] | Special studies |
|---|---|---|---|---|
| Drug combinations[d] | I | | | |
| | II, III, NDA | 2 species: up to 3 months | | Lethality by appropriate route, compared to components run concurrently in 1 species |

[a] Phase I dosing of females if childbearing potential requires a Segment II study in at least one species; Phase III dosing of this population requires a Segment I study and both Segment II studies.

[b] Phase I, II, and III are defined in Section 130.0 of the New Drug Regulations.

[c] Acute toxicity should be determined in three species; subacute or chronic studies should be by the route to be used clinically. Suitable mutagenicity studies should also be performed.

Observations:

| | | |
|---|---|---|
| Body weights | Food consumption | Behavior |
| Metabolic studies | Ophthalmologic examination | Fasting blood sugar |
| Gross and microscopic examination | Hemogram | Liver and kidney function tests |
| Coagulation tests | Others as appropriate | |

[d] Where toxicity data are available on each drug individually

The individual studies and reports are to be tied together to present a single, cohesive overview of what is known about the safety of a drug.

Lever (1987) presents an excellent overview of the regulatory process involved in FDA oversight of drug development, and gives the historical perspective for the evolution of the conservative process that is designed to ensure that any new pharmaceutical is both safe and efficacious.

There are other regulatory, legal and ethical safety assessment requirements beyond those involved in the selection and marketing of a drug as a product entity. The actual drug product must be manufactured and transported in a safe manner, and any waste associated with this manufacture disposed of properly. Chapter 14 of this volume specifically addresses this often overlooked aspect of safety assessment programs.


## 1.3. ESSENTIAL ELEMENTS OF PROJECT MANAGEMENT

It is important to keep in mind that safety assessment is only one of many components involved in the discovery and development of new pharmaceuticals. The entire process has become enormously expensive, and completing the transit of a new drug from discovery to market has to be as efficient and expeditious a process as possible. Even the narrow part of this process (safety assessment) is dependent on many separate efforts. Compounds must be made, analytical and bioanalytical methods developed, and dosage formulations developed, to name a few. One needs only to refer to Beyer (1978), Hamner (1982), Matoren (1984), Sneader (1986) (a good short overview), Zbinden, (1992) or Spilker (1994) for more details on this entire process and all of its components.

The coordination of this entire complex process is the province of project management, the objective of which is to ensure that all the necessary parts and components of a project mate up. This discipline in its modern form was first developed for the Polaris missile project in the 1960s. Its major tool that is familiar to pharmaceutical scientists is the "network" or PERT (Program Evaluation Review Technique) chart, as illustrated in Figure 1.2. This chart is a tool that allows one to see and coordinate the relationships between the different components of a project. One outcome of the development of such a network is identification of the rate-limiting steps, which, in aggregate, comprise the critical path (see Table 1.3 for a lexicon of the terms used in project management).

A second graphic tool from project management is the Gantt chart, as illustrated in Figure 1.3. This chart allows one to visualize the efforts underway in any one area, such as safety assessment, for all projects that are currently being worked on.

Figure 1.4 is a hybrid from of the PERT and Gantt charts, designed to allow one to visualize all the resources involved in any one project.

An understanding of the key concepts of project management and their implications are critical for strategic planning and thinking for safety assessment. Kliem (1986) and Knutson (1980) offer excellent further reading in the area of project management.

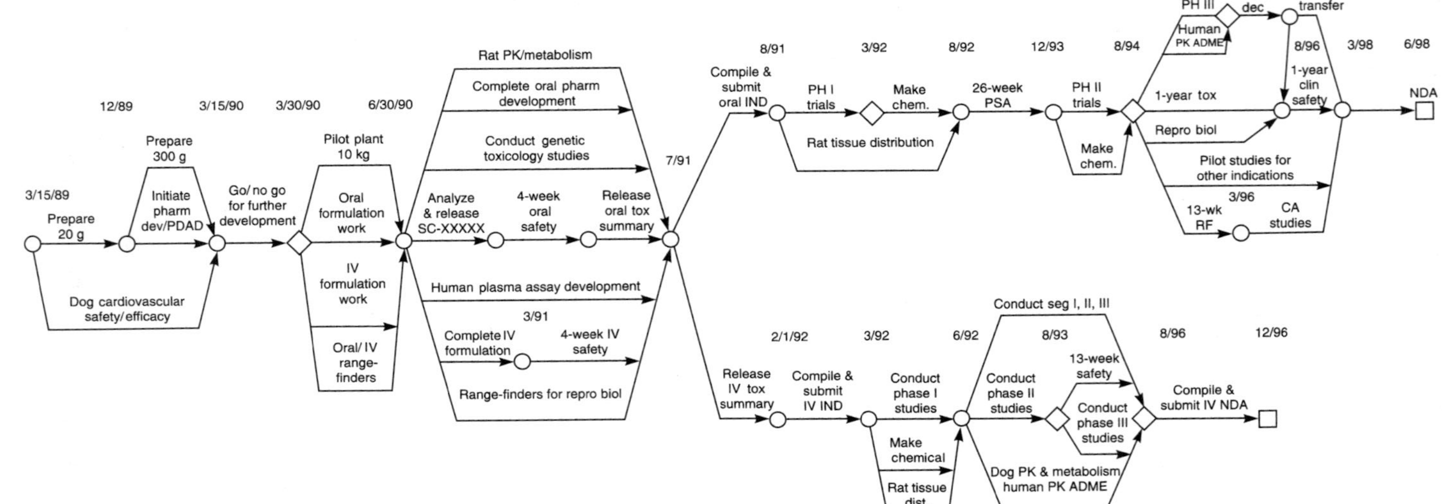



**FIGURE 1.2.** An example PERT (Program Evaluation Review Technique) chart of the development of a new pharmaceutical through to the filing of an NDA (New Drug Application). Circles are "nodes" indicating completion of activities. Diamonds are initiation points for tasks that have starting points independent of others. This "network" serves to illustrate the relationships between different activities and to evaluate effects of changes on project timing.

**TABLE 1.3. Glossary of Project Management Terms**

| | |
|---|---|
| Activity | The work or effort needed to complete a particular event. It consumes time and resources. |
| Average daily resource requirement | The likely amount of resources required to complete an activity or several activities on any workday during a project. The average daily labor requirement is one example. |
| CPM | Acronym for Critical Path Method. A network diagramming technique that places emphasis on time, cost, and the completion of events. |
| Critical path | The longest route through a network that contains activities absolutely crucial to the completion of the project. |
| Dummy arrow | A dashed line indicating an activity that uses no time or resources. |
| Duration | The time it takes to complete an activity. |
| Earliest finish | The earliest time an activity can be completed. |
| Earliest start | The earliest an activity can begin if all activities before it are finished. It is the earliest time that an activity leaves its initiation node. |
| Event | A synonym for node. A point in time that indicates the accomplishment of a milestone. It consumes neither time nor resources and is indicated whenever two or more arrows intersect. |
| Free float | The amount of time that an activity can be delayed without affecting succeeding activities. |
| Gantt chart | A bar chart indicating the time interval for each of the major phases of a project. |
| Histogram | A synonym for bar chart. |
| Latest finish | The latest time an activity can be completed without extending the length of a project. |
| Latest start | The latest time an activity can begin without lengthening a project. |
| Leveling | The process of "smoothing" out labor, material and equipment requirements to facilitate resource allocation. The project manager accomplishes this by "rescheduling" noncritical activities so that the total resource requirements for a particular day match the average daily resource requirements. |
| Most likely time | Used in PERT diagramming. The most realistic time estimate for completing an activity or project under normal conditions. |
| Node | A synonym for event. |
| Optimistic time | Used in PERT diagramming. The time the firm can complete an activity or project under the most ideal conditions. |
| PERT | Acronym for Program Evaluation and Review Technique. A network diagramming technique that places emphasis on the completion of events rather than cost or time. |
| Pessimistic time | Used in PERT diagramming. The time the firm can complete an activity or project under the worst conditions. |
| Project | The overall work or effort being planned. It has only one beginning node and ending node. Between those nodes are countless activities and their respective nodes. |
| Project phase | A major component, or segment, of a project. It is determined by the process known as project breakdown structuring. |
| Total float | The total amount of flexibility in scheduling activities on a noncritical path. Hence, it provides the time an activity could be prolonged without extending a project's final completion date. |

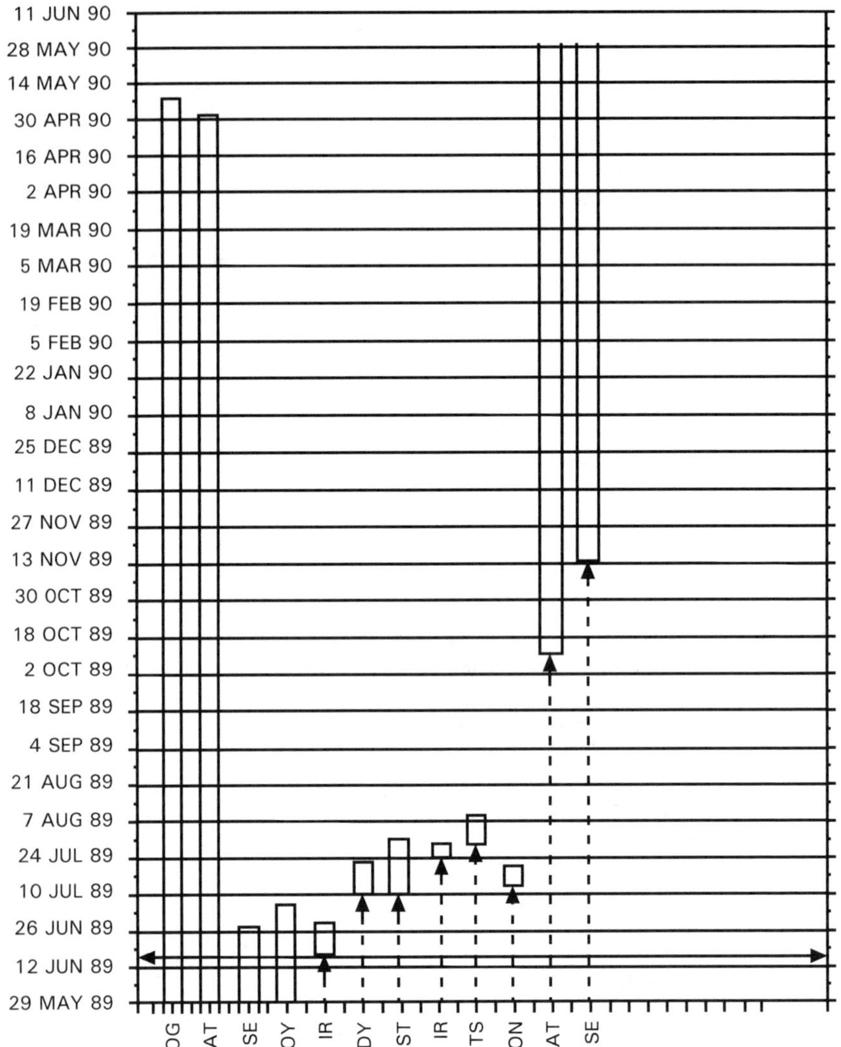


**FIGURE 1.3.** A GANTT or bar chart showing scheduling of the major safety assessment activities (studies) involved in a pharmaceutical development project.

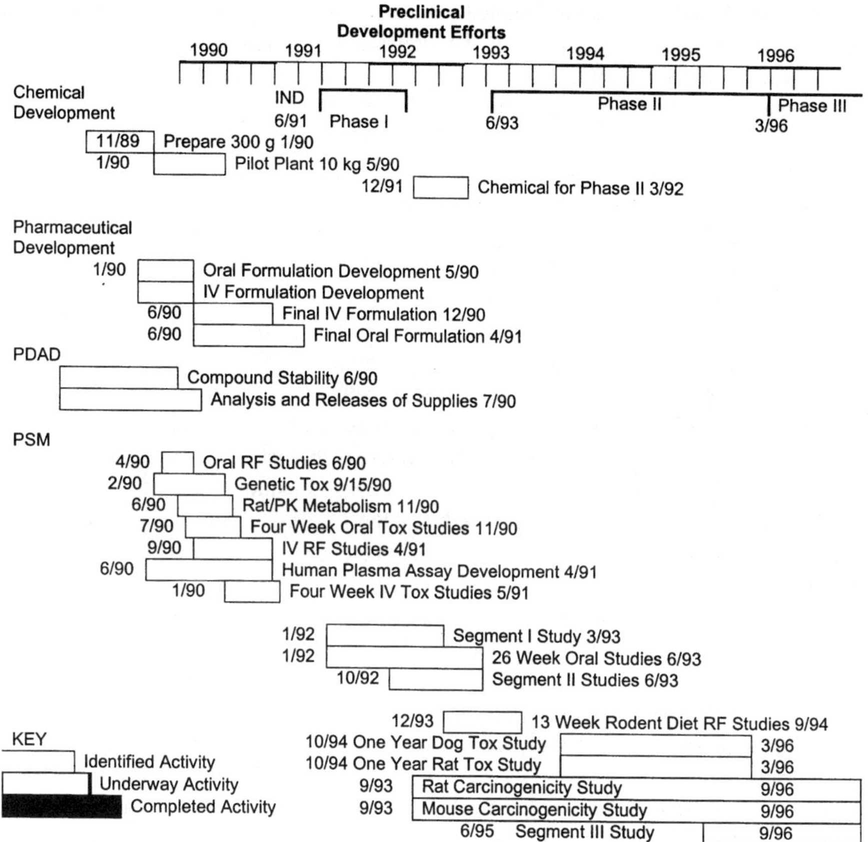


**FIGURE 1.4.** A hybrid project GANTT chart, which identifies the work of each of the development functions ("line operations") in the development of a new compound and how it matches the phase of development.

## 1.4. SCREENS: THEIR USE AND INTERPRETATION IN SAFETY ASSESSMENT

Much (perhaps even most) of what is performed in safety assessment can be considered screening, trying to determine if some effect is or is not (to an acceptable level of confidence) present (Zbinden et al., 1984). The general concepts of such screens are familiar to toxicologists in the pharmaceutical industry because the approach is a major part of the activities of the pharmacologists involved in the discovery of new compounds. But the principles underlying screening are not generally well recognized or understood. And such understanding is essential to the proper use, design, and analysis of screens (Gad, 1988a, 1989a). Screens are the biological equivalent of exploratory data analysis, or EDA (Tukey, 1977).

Each test or assay has an associated activity criterion, that is, a level above which the activity of interest is judged to be present. If the result for a particular test compound meets this criterion, the compound may pass to the next stage. This criterion could be based on statistical significance (e.g., all compounds with observed activities significantly greater than the control at the 5% level could be tagged). However, for early screens, such a formal criterion may be too strict, resulting in few compounds being identified as "active."

A useful indicator of the efficacy of an assay series is the frequency of discovery of truly active compounds. The frequency is related to the probability of discovery and to the degree of risk (hazard to health) associated with an active compound passing a screen undetected. These two factors in turn depend on the distribution of activities in the series of compounds being tested, and the chances of rejecting or accepting compounds with given activities at each stage.

Statistical modeling of the assay system may lead to the improvement of the design of the system by reducing the interval between discoveries of active compounds. The objectives behind a screen and considerations of (1) costs for producing compounds and testing and (2) the degree of uncertainly about test performance will determine desired performance characteristics of specific cases. In the most common case of early toxicity screens performed to remove possible problem compounds, preliminary results suggest that it may be beneficial to increase the number of compounds tested, decrease the numbers of animals per group, and increase the range and number of doses. The result will be less information on more structure, but there will be an overall increase in the frequency of discovery of active compounds (assuming that truly active compounds are entering the system at a steady rate).

The methods described here are well-suited to analyzing screening data when the interest is truly in detecting the absence of an effect with little chance of false negatives. There are many forms of graphical analysis methods available, including some newer forms that are particularly well-suited to multivariate data (the type that are common in more complicated screening test designs). It is intended that these aspects of analysis will be focused on in a later publication.

The design of each assay and the choice of the activity criterion should, therefore, be adjusted, bearing in mind the relative costs of retaining false positives and rejecting false negatives. Decreasing the group sizes in the early assays reduces the chance of obtaining significance at any particular level (such as 5%), so the activity criterion must be relaxed, in a statistical sense, to allow more compounds through. At some stage, however, it becomes too expensive to continue screening many false positives, and the criteria must be tightened accordingly. Where the criteria are set depends on what acceptable noise levels are in a screening system.

### 1.4.1. Characteristics of Screens

An excellent introduction to the characteristics of screens is Redman's (1981) interesting approach, which identifies four characteristics of an assay. Redman assumes that a compound is either active or inactive and that the proportion of activities in a compound can be estimated from past experience. After testing, a compound will be classified as positive or negative (i.e., possessing or lacking activity). It is then possible to design the assay so as to optimize the following characteristics.

1. Sensitivity: the ratio of true positives to total activities;
2. Specificity: the ratio of true negatives to total inactives;
3. Positive accuracy: the ratio of true to observed positives;
4. Negative accuracy: the ratio of true to observed negatives;
5. Capacity: the number of compounds that can be evaluated;
6. Reproducibility: the probability that a screen will produce the same result at another time (and, perhaps, in some other lab).

An advantage of testing many compounds is that it gives the opportunity to average activity evidence over structural classes or to study quantitative structure-activity relationships (QSARs). Quantitative structure-activity relationships can be used to predict the activity of new compounds and thus reduce the chance of *in vivo* testing on negative compounds. The use of QSARs can increase the proportion of truly active compounds passing through the system.

To simplify this presentation, datasets drawn only from neuromuscular screening activity were used. However, the evaluation and approaches should be valid for all similar screening datasets, regardless of source. The methods are not sensitive to the biases introduced by the degree of interdependence found in many screening batteries that use multiple measures (such as the neurobehavioral screen).

1. Screens almost always focus on detecting a single endpoint of effect (such as mutagenicity, lethality, neurotoxicity, or development toxicity), and have a particular set of operating characteristics in common.
2. A large number of compounds are evaluated, so ease and speed of performance (which may also be considered efficiency) are very desirable characteristics.
3. The screen must be very sensitive in its detection of potential effective agents. An absolute minimum of active agents should escape detection; that is, there should be very few false negatives (in other words, the type II error rate or beta level should be low). Stated yet another way, the signal gain should be way up.
4. It is desirable that the number of false positives be small (i.e., there should be a low type I error rate or alpha level).
5. Items (2)–(4), which are all to some degree contradictory, require the involved researchers to agree on a set of compromises, starting with the acceptance of a relatively high alpha level (0.10 or more), that is, an increased noise level.

6. In an effort to better serve item (2), safety assessment screens are frequently performed in batteries so that multiple endpoints are measured in the same operation. Additionally, such measurements may be repeated over a period of time in each model as a means of supporting item (3).

7. This screen should use small amounts of compound to make item (1) possible and should allow evaluation of materials that have limited availability (such as novel compounds) early on in development.

8. Any screening system should be validated initially using a set of blind (positive and negative) controls. These blind controls should also be evaluated in the screening system on a regular basis to ensure continuing proper operation of the screen. As such, the analysis techniques used here can then be used to ensure the quality or modify the performance of a screening system.

9. The more that is known about the activity of interest, the more specific the form of screen that can be employed. As specificity increases, so should sensitivity.

10. Sample (group) sizes are generally small.

11. The data tend to be imprecisely gathered (often because researchers are unsure of what they are looking for), and therefore possess extreme within-group variability. Control and historical data are not used to adjust for variability or modify test performance.

12. Proper dose selection is essential for effective and efficient screen design and conduct. If insufficient data are available, a suitably broad range of doses must be evaluated (however, this technique is undesirable on multiple grounds, as has already been pointed out).

The design, use and analysis of screens is covered in detail in Chapter 4 of this volume.

## 1.5. STRATEGY AND PHASING

Regulatory requirements and our understanding of the pharmacology, marketing, and clinical objectives for a potential product provide a framework of requirements for the safety assessment of potential new pharmaceuticals. How one meets these requirements is not fixed, however. Rather, exactly what is done and when activities are performed are reflections of the philosophy and managerial climate of the organization that is doing the discovery and development. It should be kept in mind that establishing and maintaining an excellent information base on the biological basis for a compound's expected therapeutic activity and safety is essential but often left undone. This subject is addressed in Chapter 2 of this volume.

There are multiple phases involved in the safety assessment portion of the discovery, development and marketing process. The actual conduct of the studies in each phase forms the basis of the bulk of the chapters in this book. However, unless the pieces are coordinated well and utilized effectively (and completed at the right times), success of the safety assessment program is unlikely or very expensive.

First, support needs to be given to basic research (also called discovery, biology, or pharmacology in different organizations) so that it can efficiently produce a stream of potential new product compounds with as few overt toxicity concerns as possible. This means that there must be early and regular interaction between the individuals involved, and that safety assessment must provide screening services to rank the specific safety concerns of the compounds. These screens may be *in vitro* (both for genetic and nongenetic endpoints) or *in vivo* (designed on purpose for a single endpoint, such as effects on reproductive performance, promotion activity, etc.). There must also be ongoing work to elucidate the mechanisms and structure-activity relationships behind those toxicities that are identified (Gad, 1989b).

Second is the traditional core of safety assessment that is viewed as development. Development includes providing the studies to support compounds getting into the clinic (an IND application being filed and accepted), evaluating a compound to the point at which it is considered safe, able to be absorbed, and effective (clinical phase II), and, finally, registration (filing an NDA and having it approved). Various organizations break this process up differently. Judgements are generally made on the likelihood of compounds failing ("dying") at different stages in the clinical development process, and the phasing of preclinical support is selected and or adjusted accordingly. If an organization has a history of many compounds failing early in the clinic (such as in the initial phase I tolerance trials, where there may be only three to ten days of human dosing), then initial "pivotal" preclinical studies are likely to be only four-week-long studies. If compounds tend to fail only in longer efficacy trials, then it is more efficient to run longer initial preclinical trials. Figure 1.5 shows several variations on these approaches. Additionally, the degree of risk involved in study design (particularly in dose selection) is also an organizational characteristic. Pivotal studies can fail on two counts associated with dose selection. Either they cannot identify a "safe" (no-effect) dose or they can neglect to find a dose that demonstrates a toxic effect (and therefore allows identification of potential target organs). Therefore, picking the doses for such studies is an art that has been risky because, traditionally, only three different dose groups have been used, and before clinical trials are conducted there is at best a guess as to what clinical dose will need to be cleared. The use of four (or five) dose groups only marginally increases study cost, and, in those cases where the uncertainty around dose selection is great, provides a low-cost alternative to repeating the study.

Pivotal studies can also be called shotgun tests, because it is unknown in advance what endpoints are being aimed at. Rather, the purpose of the study is to identify and quantitate all potential systemic effects resulting from a single exposure to a compound. Once known, specific target organ effects can then be studied in detail if so desired. Accordingly, the generalized design of these studies is to expose groups of animals to controlled amounts or concentrations of the material of interest, and then to observe for and measure as many parameters as practical over a period past or during the exposure. Further classification of tests within this category would be the route by which test animals are exposed/dosed or by the length of dosing.

**PLAN 1:  Clinical Decision Point** Is Short Term Tolerance Or Human Pharmacokinetics**

| Range Finder | Pivotal Study | Phase I | | Phase II |
|---|---|---|---|---|
| "Pyramid" or "rolling acute" (see Chapter 4) | → Two or four weeks in two species by the intended route | → Tolerance and pharmacokinetics (PK) with up to 3 to 14 days human dosing | → DELAY*** → | → |

**PLAN 2:  Clinical Decision Point Is An Indication Of Efficacy In Man**

| Range Finder | Pivotal Study | Phase I/II | | Phase II/III |
|---|---|---|---|---|
| "Pyramid" or "rolling acute" and/or two or four week study | → Thirteen weeks in two species | → Tolerance, PK and efficacy with human dosing up to one month in length | → DELAY*** → | → |

**PLAN 3:  Plan For Success Or Resources Are Not A Constraint**

| Range Finder | Pivotal Study | Phase I/II | Phase III | | |
|---|---|---|---|---|---|
| | | **Preclinical** | **Preclinical** | | |
| "Pyramid" or "rolling acute: and/or two week study | Four weeks in two species | Thirteen weeks in two species | One year in two species | Carcinogenicity in two rodents (if required) | |

**FIGURE 1.5.** Three different approaches to matching preclinical safety efforts to support the clinical development of a new drug. Which is the best one for any specific case depends on considerations of resource availability and organizational tolerance of "risk." In Plan 1, little effort will be "wasted" on projects that fail during early (phase I) clinical trials—but if phase I trials are successful, there will be major delays. In Plan 3, clinical development will never be held up waiting for more safety work, but a lot of effort will go into projects that never get past Phase I. Plan 2 is a compromise. Delays are to allow additional preclinical (animal safety) studies to support longer clinical trials in accordance with FDA or other applicable guidelines.

"Acute," for example, implies a single exposure interval (of 24 h or less) or dose of test material. Using the second scheme (length of dosing), the objectives of the successive sets of pivotal studies could be defined as follows:

Acute studies:

1. Set doses for next studies.
2. Identify very or unusually toxic agents.
3. Estimate lethality potential.
4. Identify organ system affected.

Two-week studies:

1. Set doses for next studies.
2. Identify organ toxicity.

3. Identify very or unusually toxic agents.
4. Estimate lethality potential.
5. Evaluate potential for accumulation of effects.
6. Get estimate of kinetic properties (blood sampling/urine sampling).

Four-week studies:

1. Set doses for next studies.
2. Identify organ toxicity.
3. Identify very or unusually toxic agents.
4. Estimate lethality potential.
5. Evaluate potential for accumulation of effects.
6. Get estimate of kinetic properties (blood sampling/urine sampling).
7. Elucidate nature of specific types of target organ toxicities induced by repeated exposure.

Thirteen-week studies:

1. Set doses for next studies.
2. Identify organ toxicity.
3. Identify very or unusually toxic agents.
4. Evaluate potential for accumulation of effects.
5. Evaluate pharmacokinetic properties.
6. Elucidate nature of specific types of target organ toxicities induced by repeated exposure.
7. Evaluate reversibility of toxic effects.

Chronic studies:

1. Elucidate nature of specific types of target organ toxicities induced by prolonged repeated exposure.
2. Identify potential carcinogens.

The problems of scheduling and sequencing toxicology studies and entire testing programs have been minimally addressed in print. Though there are several books and many articles available that address the question of scheduling multiple tasks in a service organization (French, 1982), and an extremely large literature on project management (as briefly overviewed earlier in this chapter), no literature specific to a research testing organization exists.

For all the literature on project management, however, a review will quickly establish that it does not address the rather numerous details that affect study/program scheduling and management. There is, in fact, to my knowledge, only a single article (Levy et al., 1977) in the literature that addresses scheduling, and it describes a computerized scheduling system for single studies.

There are commercial computer packages available for handling the network construction, interactions, and calculations involved in what, as will be shown below, is a complicated process. These packages are available for use on both mainframe and microcomputer systems.

Scheduling for the single study case is relatively simple. One should begin with the length of the actual study and then factor in the time needed before the study is started to secure the following resources:

- Animals must be on hand and properly acclimated (usually for at least two weeks prior to the start of the study).
- Vivarium space, caging, and animal care support must be available.
- Technical support for any special measurements such as necropsy, hematology, urinalysis, and clinical chemistry must be available on the dates specified in the protocol.
- Necessary and sufficient test material must be on hand.
- A formal written protocol suitable to fill regulatory requirements must be on hand and signed.

The actual study (from first dosing or exposure of animals to the last observation and termination of the animals) is called the in-life phase, and many people assume the length of the in-life phase defines the length of a study. Rather, a study is not truly completed until any samples (blood, urine, and tissue) are analyzed, slides are prepared and microscopically evaluated, data are statistically analyzed, and a report is written, proofed, and signed off. Roll all of this together, and if you are conducting a single study under contract in an outside laboratory, an estimate of the least time involved in its completion should be equal to (other than in the case of an acute or single and point study) no more than

$$L + 6 \text{ weeks} + \tfrac{1}{2}L,$$

where L is the length of the study. If the study is a single endpoint study and does not involve pathology, then the least time can be shortened to $L + 6$ weeks. In general, the best that can be done is $L + 10$ weeks.

When one is scheduling out an entire testing program on contract, it should be noted that, if multiple tiers of tests are to be performed (such as acute, two-week, thirteen-week, and lifetime studies), then these must be conducted sequentially, as the answer from each study in the series defines the design and sets the doses for the subsequent study.

If, instead of contracting out, one is concerned with managing a testing laboratory, then the situation is considerably more complex. The factors and activities involved are outlined below. Within these steps are rate-limiting factors that are invariably due to some critical point or pathway. Identification of such critical factors is one of the first steps for a manager to take to establish effective control over either a facility or program.

Before any study is actually initiated, a number of prestudy activities must occur (and, therefore, these activities are currently underway, to one extent or another, for the studies not yet underway but already authorized or planned for this year for any laboratory).

- Test material procurement and characterization.
- Development of formulation and dosage forms for study.
- If inhalation study, development of generation and analysis methodology, chamber trials, and verification of proper chamber distribution.
- Development and implementation of necessary safety steps to protect involved laboratory personnel.
- Arrangement for waste disposal.
- Scheduling to assure availability of animal rooms, manpower, equipment, and support services (pathology and clinical).
- Preparation of protocols.
- Animal procurement, health surveillance, and quarantine.
- Preparation of data forms and books.
- Conduct of prestudy measurements on study animals to set baseline rates of body weight gain and clinical chemistry values.

After completion of the in-life phase (i.e., the period during which live animals are used) of any study, significant additional effort is still required to complete the research. This effort includes the following.

- Preparation of data forms and books. Preparation of tissue slides and microscopic evaluation of these slides;
- Preparation of data tables;
- Statistical analysis of data;
- Preparation of reports.

There are a number of devices available to a manager to help improve the performance of a laboratory involved in these activities. One such device (cross-training) is generally applicable enough to be particularly attractive.

Identification of rate-limiting steps in a toxicology laboratory over a period of time usually reveals that at least some of these are variable (almost with the season). At times, there is too much work of one kind (say, inhalation studies) and too little of another (say, dietary studies). The available staff for inhalation studies cannot handle this peak load and since the skills of these two groups are somewhat different, the dietary staff (which is now not fully occupied) cannot simply relocate down the hall and help out. However, if, early on, one identifies low- and medium-skill aspects of the work involved in inhalation studies, one could cross-train the dietary staff at a convenient time so that it could be redeployed to meet peak loads.

It should be kept in mind that there are a number of common mistakes (in both the design and conduct of studies and in how information from studies is used) that have led to unfortunate results, ranging from losses in time and money and the discarding of perfectly good potential products to serious threats to people's health. Such outcomes are indeed the great disasters in product safety assessment, especially since many of them are avoidable if attention is paid to a few basic principles.

It is quite possible to design a study for failure. Common shortfalls include

1. Using the wrong animal model.
2. Using the wrong route or dosing regimen.
3. Using the wrong vehicle or formulation of test material.
4. Using the wrong dose level. In studies where several dose levels are studied, the worst outcome is to have an effect at the lowest dose level tested (i.e., the safe dosage in animals remains unknown). The next worst outcome is to have no effect at the highest dose tested (generally meaning that the signs of toxicity remain unknown, invalidating the study in the eyes of many regulatory agencies).
5. Making leaps of faith. An example is to set dosage levels based on others' data and to then dose all test animals. At the end of the day, all animals in all dose levels are dead. The study is over; the problem remains.
6. Using the wrong concentration of test materials in a study. Many effects (including both dermal and gastrointestinal irritation, for example) are very concentration dependent.
7. Failing to include a recovery (or rebound) group. If one finds an effect in a 90-day study (say, gastric hyperplasia), how does one interpret it? How does one respond to the regulatory question, "Will it progress to cancer?" If an additional group of animals were included in dosing, then were maintained for a month after dosing had been completed, recovery (reversibility) could be both evaluated and (if present) demonstrated.

Additionally, there are specialized studies designed to address endpoints of concern for almost all drugs (carcinogenicity, reproductive or developmental toxicity) or concerns specific to a compound or family of compounds (local irritation, neurotoxicity, or immunotoxicity, for example). When these are done, timing also requires careful consideration. It must always be kept in mind that the intention is to ensure the safety of people in whom the drug is to be evaluated (clinical trials) or used therapeutically. An understanding of special concerns for both populations should be considered essential.

Safety evaluation does not cease being an essential element in the success of the pharmaceutical industry once a product is on the market. It is also essential to support marketed products and ensure that their use is not only effective but also safe and unclouded by unfounded perceptions of safety problems. This requires not only that clinical trials be monitored during development (Spector et al., 1988), but also that experience in the marketplace be monitored.

The design and conduct of safety assessment studies and programs also require an understanding of some basic concepts:

1. The studies are performed to establish or deny the safety of a compound, rather than to characterize the toxicity of a compound.

2. Because pharmaceuticals are intended to affect the functioning of biological systems, and safety assessment characterizes the effects of higher-than-therapeutic doses of compounds, it is essential that one be able to differentiate between hyperpharmacology and true (undesirable) adverse effects.

3. Focus of the development process for a new pharmaceutical is an essential aspect of success, but is also difficult to maintain. Clinical research units generally desire to pursue as many or as broad claims as possible for a new agent, and frequently also apply pressure for the development of multiple forms for administration by different routes. These forces must be resisted because they vastly increase the work involved in safety assessment, and they may also produce results (in one route) that cloud evaluation [and impede Institutional Review Board (IRB) and regulatory approval] of the route of main interest.

## 1.6. CRITICAL CONSIDERATIONS

In general, what the management of a pharmaceutical development enterprise wants to know at the beginning of a project are three things: what are the risks (and how big are they), how long will it take, and how much (money and test compound) will it take?

The risks question is beyond the scope of this volume. The time question was addressed earlier in this chapter. How much money is also beyond the scope of this volume. But calculating projected compound needs for studies is a fine challenge in the design and conduct of a safety evaluation program. The basic calculation is simple. The amount needed for a study is equal to

$$N \, W \, I \, L \, D,$$

where

$N =$ the number of animals per group.
$W =$ the mean weight per animal during the course of the study (in kg).
$\phantom{}I =$ the total number of doses to be delivered (such as in a 28-day study, 28 consecutive doses).

L = a loss or efficiency factor (to allow for losses in formulation and dose delivery, a 10% factor is commonly employed, meaning a value of 1.1 is utilized).

D = the total dose factor. This is the sum of all the dose levels. For example, if the groups are to receive 1000, 300, 100, 30 and 30 mg/kg, then the total dose factor is $1000 + 300 + 100 + 30$ or 1430 mg/kg.

As an example, let's take a 28-day study in rats where there are 10 males and 10 females per group and the dose levels employed at 1000, 3000, 100 and 30 mg/kg. Over the course of the 28 days the average weight of the rats is likely to be 300 g (or 0.3 kg). This means our values are

N = 20
W = 0.3 kg
 I = 28
 L = 1.1
 D = 1430 mg/kg

and therefore our total compound needs will be $(20)(0.3)(28)(1.1)(1430\,\text{mg}) =$ 2642.64 mg or 0.264 kg. This is the simplest case, but shows the principles.

A governing principle of pharmaceutical safety assessment is the determination of safety factors: the ratio between the therapeutic dose (that which achieves the desired therapeutic effect) and the highest dose which evokes no toxicity. This grows yet more complex (but has less uncertainty) if one bases these ratios on plasma levels rather than administered doses. Traditionally based on beliefs as to differences of species sensitivity, it has been held that a minimum of a five-fold (5X) safety factor should be observed based on toxicity findings in nonrodents and a ten-fold (10X) based on rodents.

The desire to achieve at least such minimal therapeutic indices and to also identify levels associated with toxicity (and the associated toxic effects) form the basis of dose selection for systemic (and most other *in vivo*) toxicity studies.

## 1.7. SPECIAL CASES IN SAFETY ASSESSMENT

It may seem that the course of preclinical safety assessment (and of other aspects of development) of a pharmaceutical is a relatively linear and well-marked route, within some limits. This is generally the case, but not always. There are a number of special cases where the pattern and phasing of development (and of what is required for safety assessment) do not fit the usual pattern. Four of these cases are

1. When the drug is intended to treat a life-threatening disease, such as acquired immunodeficiency syndrome (AIDS).
2. When the drug is actually a combination of two previously existing drug entities.
3. When the drug actually consists of two or more isomers.
4. When the drug is a peptide produced by a biotechnology process.

Drugs intended to treat a life-threatening disease for which there is no effective treatment are generally evaluated against less rigorous standards of safety when making decisions about advancing them into and through clinical testing. This acceptance of increased risk (moderated by the fact that the individuals involved will die if not treated at all) is balanced against the potential benefit. These changes in standards usually mean that the phasing of testing is shifted: animal safety studies may be done in parallel or (in the case of chronic and carcinogenicity studies) after clinical trials and commercialization. But the same work must still be performed eventually.

Combination drugs, at least in terms of safety studies up to carcinogenicity studies, are considered by regulatory agencies as new drug entities and must be so evaluated. The accordingly required safety tests must be performed on a mixture with the same ratio of components as is to be a product. Any significant change in ratios of active components means one is again evaluating, in regulatory eyes, a new drug entity.

Now that it is possible to produce drugs that have multiple isomers in the form of single isomers (as opposed to racemic mixtures), for good historical reasons, regulatory agencies are requiring at least some data to support any decision to develop the mixture as opposed to a single isomer. One must, at a minimum, establish that the isomers are of generally equivalent therapeutic activity, and, if there is therapeutic equivalence, that any undesirable biological activity is not present to a greater degree in one isomer or another.

## 1.8. SUMMARY

It is the belief of this author that the entire safety assessment process that supports pharmaceutical research and development is a multistage process of which no single element is overwhelmingly complex. These elements must be coordinated and their timing and employment carefully considered on a repeated basis. Focus on the objectives of the process, including a clear definition of the questions being addressed by each study, is essential, as is the full integration of the technical talents of each of the many disciplines involved. A firm understanding of the planned clinical development of the drug is essential. To stay competitive requires that new technologies be identified and incorporated effectively into safety assessment programs as they become available. It is hoped that this volume will provide the essential knowledge of the key elements to allow these goals to be realized.

## REFERENCES


Alder, S. and Zbinden, G. (1988). *National and International Drug Safety Guidelines*. MTC Verlag, Zollikon, Switzerland.

Arnst, C. (1998). Danger: Read the label. *Business Week*, May 11, p. 100.

Beyer, K. (1978). Discovery, Development and Delivery of New Drugs. *Monographs in Pharmacology and Physiology*, No. 12. Spectrum, New York.

Bryostowski, M. (2001). On the horizon. *R&D Directions*, May 2001, pp. 30–44.

FDA (Food and Drug Administration). (1987a). *Good Laboratory Practice Regulations: Final Rule*. 21 CFR Part 58, *Federal Register*, September 4, 1987.

FDA (Food and Drug Administration). (1987b). New drug, antibiotic, and biologic drug produce regulations. 21 CFR Parts 312, 314, 511, and 514, *Federal Register*, 52(53) 8798–8857.

Fishlock, D. (1990, April 24). Survival of the fittest drugs. *Financial Times*, pp. 16–17.

French, S. (1982). *Sequencing and Scheduling*. Halsted Press, New York.

Gad, S.C. (1988a). An approach to the design and analysis of screening studies in toxicology, *J. Am. Coll.Toxicol.* 7(2): 127–138.

Gad, S.C. (1989a). Principles of screening in toxicology: with special emphasis on applications to neurotoxicology. *J. Am. Coll. Toxicol.* 8(1): 21–27.

Gad, S.C. (1989b). A tier testing strategy incorporating in vitro testing methods for pharmaceutical safety assessment. *Humane Innovations and Alternatives in Animal Experimentation* 3: 75–79.

Gad, S.C. (1996). Preclinical toxicity testing in the development of new therapeutic agents, *Scand. J. Lab Anim. Sci.* 23: 299–314.

Gad, S.C. (2000). *Product Safety Evaluation Handbook*, 2nd ed. Marcel Dekker, New York.

Gad, S.C. (2001). *In Vitro Toxicology*, 2nd ed. Taylor and Francis, Philadelphia. PA.

Guarino, R.A. (1987). *New Drug Approval Process*. Marcel Dekker, New York.

Hamner, C.E. (1982). *Drug Development*. CRC Press, Boca Raton, FL, pp. 53–80.

Kliem, R.L. (1986). *The Secrets of Successful Project Management*. Wiley, New York.

Knutson, J.R. (1980). *How to Be a Successful Project Manager*. American Management Associations, New York.

Lazarou, J., Parmeranz, B.H. and Corey, P.N. (1998). Incidence of Adverse Drug Reactions in Hospitilized Patients. *JAMA*, 279: 1200–1209.

Leber, P. (1987). FDA: The federal regulations of drug development. In: *Psychopharmacology: The Third Generation of Progress* (Meltzer, H.Y., ed.). Raven Press, New York, pp. 1675–1683.

Lesko, L.J., Rowland, M., Peck, C.C., and Blaschke, T.F. (2000). Optimizing the science of drug development: opportunities for better candidate selection and accelerated evaluation in humans, *Pharmaceutical Research* 17: 1335–1344.

Levy, A.E., Simon, R.C., Beerman, T.H., and Fold, R.M. (1977). Scheduling of toxicology protocol studies. *Comput. Biomed. Res.* 10: 139–151.

Littlehales, C. (1999). The price of a pill. *Modern Drug Discovery*, Jan/Feb 1999, pp. 21–30.

Matoren, G.M. (1984). *The Clinical Process in the Pharmaceutical Industry*. Marcel Dekker, New York, pp. 273–284.

Meyer, D.S. (1989). Safety evaluation of new drugs. In: *Modern Drug Research* (Martin, Y.C., Kutter, E., and Austel, V., Eds). Marcel Dekker, New York, pp. 355–399.

Moore, T.J., Patsy, D. and Furnberg, J. (1998). Time to act on drug safety, *JAMA* 279: 1971–1976.

O'Grady, J. and Linet, O.I. (1990). *Early Phase Drug Evaluation in Man*. CRC Press, Boca Raton, FL.

Raeburn, P. (1999). Drug safety needs a second opinion. *Business Week*, Sept. 20, pp. 72–74.

Redman, C. (1981). Screening compounds for clinically active drugs. In: *Statistics in the Pharmaceutical Industry*. (C.R. Buncher and J. Tsay, Eds.). Marcel Dekker, New York, pp. 19–42.

Scheuplein, R.J., Shoal, S.E., and Brown, R.N. (1990). Role of pharmacokinetics in safety evaluation and regulatory considerations. *Ann. Rev. Pharamcol. Toxicol.* 30: 197–218.

Smith, Charles G. (1992). *The Process of New Drug Discovery and Development*. CRC Press, Boca Raton, FL.

Sneader, W. (1986). *Drug Development: From Laboratory to Clinic*. Wiley, New York.

Spector, R., Park, G.D., Johnson, G.F., and Vessell, E.S. (1988). Therapeutic drug monitoring, *Clin. Pharmacol. Therapeu.* 43: 345–353.

Spilker, B. (1994). *Multinational Drug Companies*, 2nd ed. Raven Press, New York.

Traina, V.M. (1983). The role of toxicology in drug research and development. *Med. Res. Rev.* 3: 43–72.

Tukey, J.W. (1977). *Exploratory Data Analysis*. Addison-Wesley, Reading, MA.

Zbinden, G. (1992). *The Source of the River Po*. Haag and Herschen, Frankfurt, Germany.

Zbinden, G., Elsner, J., and Boelsterli, U.A. (1984). Toxicological screening. *Reg. Toxicol. Pharamcol.* 4: 275–286.

# 2

# REGULATION OF HUMAN PHARMACEUTICAL SAFETY

## 2.1. INTRODUCTION

The safety of pharmaceutical agents, medical devices, and food additives are the toxicology issues of the most obvious and longest-standing concern to the public. A common factor among the three is that any risk associated with a lack of safety of these agents is likely to affect a very broad part of the population, with those at risk having little or no option as to undertaking this risk. Modern drugs are essential for life in our modern society, yet there is a consistent high level of concern about their safety.

This chapter examines the regulations which establish how the safety of human pharmaceutical products are evaluated and established in the United States and the other major international markets. As a starting place, the history of this regulation will be reviewed. The organizational structure of the Food and Drug Administration (FDA) will be briefly reviewed, along with the other quasi-governmental bodies that also influence the regulatory processes. The current structure and context of the regulations in the United States and overseas will also be presented. From this point the general case of regulatory product development and approval will be presented. Toxicity assessment study designs will be presented. The broad special case of biotechnology-derived therapeutic products and environmental concerns associated with the production of pharmaceuticals will be briefly addressed. The significant changes in regulation brought about by harmonization (ICH 1997, 2000) are also reflected.

As an aid to the reader, appendices are provided at the end of this book: a codex of acronyms that are used in this field, followed by a glossary which defines some key terms.

## 2.2. BRIEF HISTORY OF U.S. PHARMACEUTICAL LAW

A synopsis of the history of U.S. drug legislation is presented in Table 2.1. Here we will review the history of the three major legislative acts covering pharmaceuticals.

### 2.2.1. Pure Food and Drug Act 1906

As so eloquently discussed by Temin (1980), the history of health product legislation in the United States largely involved the passage of bills in Congress which were primarily in response to the public demand. In 1902, for example, Congress passed the Biologics Act in response to a tragedy in St. Louis where ten children died after being given contaminated diphtheria toxins. Interestingly, the background that led to the passage of the first Pure Food and Drug Act in 1906 had more to do with food processing than drugs. The conversion from an agrarian to an urban society fostered the growth of a food-processing industry that was rife with poor practices. Tainted and adulterated foods were commonly sold. These practices were sensationalized by the muckraking press, including books such as *The Jungle* by Upton Sinclair.

In the early debates in Congress on the Pure Food and Drug Act passed in 1906, there was little mention of toxicity testing. When Harvey Wiley, chief of the Bureau of Chemistry, Department of Agriculture and driving force in the enactment of this early law, did his pioneering work (beginning in 1904) on the effects of various food preservatives on health, he did so using only human subjects and with no prior experiments in animals (Anderson, 1958). Ironically, work that led to the establishment of the FDA would probably not have been permitted under the current guidelines of the agency. Wiley's studies were not double-blinded, so it is also doubtful that his conclusions would have been accepted by the present agency or the modern scientific community. Legislation in place in 1906 consisted strictly of a labeling law prohibiting the sale of processed food or drugs that were misbranded. No approval process was involved and enforcement relied on post-marketing criminal charges. Efficacy was not a consideration until 1911, when the Sherley Amendment outlawed fraudulent therapeutic claims.

### 2.2.2. Food, Drug and Cosmetic Act 1938

The present regulations are largely shaped by the law passed in 1938. It will, therefore, be discussed in some detail. The story of the 1938 Food, Drug and Cosmetic Act (FDCA) actually started in 1933. Franklin D. Roosevelt had just won his first election and installed his first cabinet. Walter Campbell was the Chief of the FDA, reporting to Rexford Tugwell, the Undersecretary of Agriculture. The country was in the depths of its greatest economic depression. This was before the therapeutic revolution wrought by antibiotics in the 1940s, and medicine and pharmacy as we know it in the 1990s were not practiced. Most medicines were, in fact, self-prescribed. Only a relatively small number of drugs were sold via physicians' prescription. The use of so-called patent (because the ingredients were kept secret) preparations was rife, as was fraudulent advertising. Today, for example,

**TABLE 2.1. Important Dates in U.S. Federal Drug Law[a]**

| Year | Event |
| --- | --- |
| 1902 | Passage of the Virus Act, regulating therapeutic serums and antitoxins. Enforcement by the Hygienic Laboratory (later to become the National Institute of Health), Treasury Department. |
| 1906 | Passage of Pure Food Act, including provisions for the regulations of drugs to prevent the sale of misbranded and adulterated products. Enforcement by the Chemistry Laboratory, Agriculture. |
| 1912 | Passage of the Sherley Amendment. Specifically outlawed any false label claims as to curative effect. |
| 1927 | Bureau of Chemistry renamed the Food, Drug and Insecticide Administration. |
| 1931 | Renamed again to Food and Drug Administration. |
| 1938 | Passage of the Food, Drug and Cosmetic Act. Superseded the law of 1906. Required evidence of safety, e.g., studies in animals. Included coverage of cosmetics and medical devices. Specifically excluded biologics. |
| 1944 | Administrative Procedures Act, codifying Public Health Laws: included provision that for a biological license to be granted, a product must meet standards for safety, purity, and potency. NIH also given the responsibility for developing biologics not developed by the private sector. |
| 1945 | Amendment to the 1936 Act requiring that the FDA examine and certify for release each batch of penicillin. Subsequently amended to include other antibiotics. |
| 1949 | Publication of the first set of criteria for animal safety studies. Following several revisions, guidelines published in 1959 as Appraisals Handbook. |
| 1951 | Passage of Durham-Humphrey Amendment. Provided the means for manufacturers to classify drugs as over-the-counter (not requiring prescription). |
| 1953 | Transfer of FDA to the Department of Health, Education and Welfare from Agriculture (now the Department of Health and Human Services). |
| 1962 | Passage of major amendments (the Kefauver Bill) to the 1938 FDCA, which required proof of safety and effectiveness (efficacy) before granting approval of New Drugs Applications. Required affirmative FDA approval. |
| 1968 | FDA placed under the Public Health Service of HEW. |
| 1970 | Controlled Substance Act and Controlled Substances Import and Export Act. Removed regulation of drug abuse from FDA (transferred to the Drug Enforcement Agency) and provided for stringent regulation of pharmaceuticals with abuse potential. |
| 1972 | Transfer of authority to regulate biologics transferred from NIH to FDA. The NIH retained the responsibility of developing biologics. |
| 1973 | Consumer Product Safety Act, leading to the formation of separate Consumer Product Safety Commission, which assumes responsibilities once handled by the FDA's Bureau of Product Safety. |
| 1976 | Medical Device Amendment to the FDCA requiring for devices that not only effectiveness be proven, but also safety. |
| 1979 | Passage of the Good Laboratory Practices Act. |
| 1983 | Passage of the first Orphan Drug Amendment to encourage development of drugs for small markets. |

**TABLE 2.1.  (*continued*)**

| Year | Event |
| --- | --- |
| 1984 | Drug Price Competition and Patent Term Restoration Act intended to allow companies to recover some of the useful patent life of a novel drug lost due to the time it takes the FDA to review and approve. Also permits the marketing of generic copies of approved drugs. |
| 1985 | The "NDA rewrite" final rule. An administrative action streamlining and clarifying the New Drug Application process. Now embodied in 21 CFR 314. |
| 1986 | The United States Drug Export Amendment Act of 1986. Permitted the export of drugs outside the U.S. prior to approval for the U.S. market. |
| 1987 | The "IND rewrite" final rule. "...to encourage innovation and drug development while continuing to assure the safety of (clinical) test subjects." Federal Register 52:8798, 1987. Now embodied in 21 CFR 312. |
| 1990 | Safe Medical Device Act, providing additional authority to the FDA for regulation of medical devices. |
| 1992 | Safe Medical Device Amendments, requiring more extensive testing of devices. |
| 1992 | Prescription Drug User Fee Act. Established the payment of fees for the filing of applications (e.g., IND, NDA, PLA, etc.) |
| 1994 | Orphan Drug Amendment. |
| 1997 | The Food and Drug Administration Modernization Act: to streamline the drug and device review and approval process. |

[a]Laws and amendments that have covered other aspects of FDA law, such as those governing food additives (e.g., FQPA), are not included in this table.

it is difficult to believe that in the early 1930s a preparation such as Radithor (nothing more than a solution of radium) was advertised for treatment of 160 diseases. It is in this environment that one day in the winter of 1933, Campbell delivered a memo to Tugwell on an action level of an insecticide (lead arsenite) used on fruits. Tugwell briskly asked why, if the chemical was so toxic, was it not banned outright. He was amazed to find out from Campbell that the Agency had no power to do so.

The 1906 law was designed to control blatantly misbranded and/or adulterated foods and drugs that relied on post-facto criminal charges for enforcement. Safety and efficacy were not an issue so long as the product was not misbranded with regard to content. Premarketing review of a drug was an unknown practice. Thus, attempts at rewriting the old 1906 law to include control of bogus therapeutic claims and dangerous preparations proved to be unsatisfactory. Paul Dunbar of the FDA suggested to Campbell that an entirely new law was needed. A committee of FDA professionals and outside academic consultants drafted a new bill, which immediately ran into trouble because no one in Congress was willing to sponsor it. After peddling the bill up and down the halls of Congress, Campbell and Tugwell persuaded Senator Royal Copeland of New York to sponsor the bill. Unknowingly at the time, Copeland put himself in the eye of a hurricane that would last for five years.

The forces that swirled around Copeland and the Tugwell Bill (Senate Bill S.1944) were many. First was the immediate and fierce opposition from the patent medicine lobby. Flyers decried S.1944 as everything from a communist plot to being un-American, stating it "would deny the sacred right of self-medication." In opposition to the patent trade organizations were two separate but unlikely allies: a variety of consumer advocacy and women's groups (such as the American Association of University Women, whose unfaltering support for the bill eventually proved critical to passage) and the mainline professional organizations. Interestingly, many of these organizations at first opposed the bill because it was not stringent enough. There were also the mainline professional pharmacy and medical organizations [such as the American Medical Association (AMA) and the American Association of Colleges of Pharmacy] whose support for the bill ranged from neutral to tepid, but did grow over the years from 1933 to 1938.

Second, there was the basic mistrust on the part of Congress toward Tugwell and other "New Dealers." At the same time, Roosevelt gave the measure only lukewarm support at best (tradition has it that if it had not been for the First Lady, Eleanor, he would have given it no support at all) because of his political differences with Royal Copeland.

Third, there was a considerable bureaucratic turf war over the control of pharmaceutical advertising. Finally, despite the efforts of the various lobbying groups, there was no popular interest or support for the bill. By the end of the congressional period, S.1944 had died for lack of passage.

The next five years would see the introductions of new bills, amendments, competing measures, committee meetings and hearings, lobbying, and House/ Senate conferences. The details of this parliamentary infighting make for fascinating history, but are outside the scope of this book. The reader is referred to the excellent history of this period by Jackson (1970).

The FDA was surprised by the force and depth of the opposition to the bill. The proposed law contained a then novel idea that a drug was misbranded if its labeling made any therapeutic claim which was contrary to general medical practice and opinion. The definition of a drug was broadened to include devices used for medical purposes.* *Adulteration* was defined as any drug product dangerous to health when used according to label directions. The patent manufacturers charged that the bill granted too much discretionary power to a federal agency, that no manufacturer could stay in business except by the grace of the Department of Agriculture, a charge that may have been correct. In response to the patent trade lobbying effort, the FDA launched its own educational drive of radio spots, displays (such as the sensationalized Chamber of Horrors exhibition, in which the toxicity of a variety of useless medicines was clearly displayed), mimeographed circulars, speaking engagements, posters, and so on.

Ruth Lamb, FDA information officer at the time, was perhaps one of the hardest working and most quotable of the FDA staffers working the street at the time. For example, in reference to one of the counter-bills that had language similar to the original Copeland bill, but with extremely complicated enforcement provisions,

---

*The use of a broad definition of what constitutes a drug for regulatory purposes is a precedent that remains in place today. For example, the computer software used in diagnostic systems is considered to be a pharmaceutical for purposes of regulation.

Ruth Lamb called it "an opus for the relief of indigent and unemployed lawyers." She once described the Bailey amendment, which would have made proprietary drugs virtually immune to multiple seizures, as permitting the "sale of colored tap water as a cure for cancer...unless arsenic was added to each dose making [it] immediately dangerous." After 1934, however, the educational efforts of the FDA were greatly attenuated by federal laws prohibiting lobbying by federal agencies (Grabowski and Vernon, 1983).

The fall of 1937 witnessed the beginning of the often-told Elixir of Sulfanilamide incident, which remains one of the nation's worst drug tragedies. The Massengil Company was not one of the industry giants, but neither was it a "snake oil peddler." The company's chief chemist, Harold Watkins, was simply trying to develop a product and, in fact, did so in a manner consistent with the norms of the time. There was a perceived need for a liquid form of sulfanilamide, but it was difficult to dissolve. Watkins hit upon diethylene glycol. No toxicity tests were performed on the finished product, although the product did pass through the "control lab" where it was checked for appearance, fragrance, and consistency.

The first reports of human toxicity occurred in October 1937 when Dr. James Stevenson of Tulsa requested some information from the AMA because of the six deaths in his area that were attributable to the elixir. At the time, no product of Massengil stood accepted by the Council on Pharmacy and Chemistry, and the Council recognized no solution of sulfanilamide. The AMA telegraphed Massengil, requesting samples of the preparation for testing. Massengil complied. The test revealed the diethylene glycol to be the toxic agent and the AMA issued a general warning to the public on October 18, 1937. In the meantime, the FDA had become aware of the deaths and launched an investigation through its Kansas City station. By October 20, when at least 14 people had died, Massengil wired the AMA to request an antidote for their own product. By the end of October, at least 73 people had died and another 20 suspicious deaths were linked to the drug. Had it not been for the response of the FDA, more deaths may have occurred. The Agency put its full force of field investigators (239 members) on the problem and eventually recovered and accounted for 99.2% of the elixir produced. Massengil fully cooperated with the investigation and in November published a public letter expressing regret over the matter, but further stating that no law had been broken. In fact, the company was eventually convicted on a long list of misbranding charges and fined a total of $26,000 (the largest fine ever levied under the 1906 law).

The Massengil incident made the limits of the 1906 law quite clear. Because there were no provisions against dangerous drugs, the FDA could move only on the technicality of misbranding. The term *elixir* was defined by the U.S. Pharmacopoeia (USP) as "a preparation containing alcohol," which Elixir of Sulfanilamide was not. It was only this technicality that permitted the FDA to declare the "Elixir" misbranded, to seize the inventory, and to stop the sale of this preparation. If it had been called *Solution of Sulfanilamide*, no charges could have been brought.

The extensive press coverage of the disaster became part of the national dialogue. Letters poured in to congressmen demanding action to prevent another such tragedy. Medical and pharmacy groups and journals insisted that a new law was required. Congress was in special session in November 1937, and did not need to be told about the tragedy. Copeland and Representative Chapman (of Kentucky) pressed resolutions calling for a report from the FDA on the tragedy. When issued, the FDA report stunned Congress, not only because of the human disaster, but also because it made apparent that even had the bill then before Congress been law, the entire tragedy would still have occurred because there were no provisions for toxicity testing before new drugs entered the market. By December 1937 a new bill, S.3037, was introduced which stated that manufacturers seeking to place new drugs on the market would be required to supply records of testing, lists of components, descriptions of each manufacturing process, and sample labels. Drugs would require certification by the FDA before sale was permitted. A similar bill was introduced in the House by Chapman, although the issues of which agency was to control advertising of drugs was still festering in the House. In January 1938, debate started on the Wheeler–Lea Bill, which would ensure that all controls over drug advertising would remain in the Federal Trade Commission (FTC). Despite strong opposition by the FDA, the Wheeler–Lea Bill was signed into law March 1938. While the loss of advertising control was a blow to the FDA, the Wheeler–Lea Bill did facilitate the passage of the new Food and Drug Law.

With the issue of advertising controls settled, the Copeland–Chapman Bill faced one last hurdle. Section 701, which had been added in committee, provided for appeal suits that could be entered in any federal district court to enjoin the agency from enforcing new regulations promulgated as a result of the Act. Interestingly, this issue had more to do with foods than drugs, as its major focus was with acceptable tolerance limits for insecticides in food. The new bill defined an *adulterated food* as one containing any poison. However, because efforts to remove insecticides from fresh fruits and vegetables had never been completely successful, the Secretary of Agriculture needed this power to set tolerance levels. Allies of food producers tried to introduce provisions in the new bill that provided methods for stalling a tolerance regulation with rounds of appeals. The bill passed the House despite such provisions (Section 701) and despite the resistance of consumer groups and the FDA, and went into joint committee. Roosevelt, in one of his rare efforts to support the FDA, made it clear that he would not accept the bill with such a cumbersome appeals process. The resulting compromise was an appeals process which limited the new evidence that could be introduced into one of the ten circuit courts. Other provisions regarding labeling were also rectified in joint committee. In May, 1938, S.3073 passed by unanimous vote. Both chambers ratified the joint committee report, and Franklin Delano Roosevelt signed it into law in June, 1938.

A historical note to this story was that Royal Copeland did not live to see his measure passed. In May, 1938, he collapsed on the Senate floor. His death occurred one month before President Roosevelt signed his bill into law.

### 2.2.3. Major Amendment 1962

The 1938 law very much changed the manner in which Americans purchased pharmaceutical agents. In effect, it changed the pharmaceutical industry from a traditional consumer product industry to one in which purchases were made as directed by a third party (the physician). In 1929, ethical pharmaceuticals (prescription drugs) comprised only 32% of all medicines, while by 1969 this was up to 83% (Temin, 1980). This led to a peculiar lack of competition in the ethical market. In 1959, Senator Estes Kefauver initiated his now-famous hearings on the drug industry. Interestingly, almost 30 years later, Senator Edward Kennedy had hearings on exactly the same matter. In 1961, Kefauver submitted a proposed legislation to amend the 1938 Act in such a way as to increase FDA oversight of the drug industry. The proposed amendment contained two novel propositions. The first was compulsory licensing, which would have required, for example, company A (with a royalty of no greater than 8% of sales) to license company B to market a drug patented by company A. Company A would have only three years' exclusivity with its patent. The second novel provision was that new drugs had to be not only "safe," but also "efficacious." There was not a ground swell of support for this legislation. When it was reported out of committee, it had been rewritten (including the removal of the licensing requirement) to the point that even Kefauver refused to support it. The Kennedy administration wanted new legislation but did not specifically support the Kefauver Bill; rather it introduced its own legislation, sponsored by Representative Orren Harris of Arkansas. It also had little support.

As in 1938, a tragic incident would intercede in the legislative process: 1961 would see the development of the thalidomide tragedy. An antianxiety agent marketed in Europe, thalidomide, was prescribed for pregnancy-related depression and taken by countless numbers of women. At about the same time, phocomelia, a birth defect marked by the imperfect development of arms and legs, appeared in Europe. Thalidomide was eventually determined to be the causative teratogen in 1961 and subsequently taken off the market in Europe. The William S. Merrill Company had applied for a New Drug Application (NDA) for thalidomide in the United States in 1960. It was never approved because the FDA examiner, Dr. Frances Kelsey, had returned the application for lack of sufficient information. Eventually, the company withdrew the application. Senator Kefauver's staff had uncovered the thalidomide story as it was unfolding and had turned its findings over to the *Washington Post*. The *Post* reported the episode under the headline "Heroine of the FDA Keeps Bad Drug off the Market" in July 1962, three days after the Kefauver Bill was reported out of committee. Needless to say, the news created public support for the bill, which was sent back to committee and reported out again with new language in August 1962. The Kefauver–Harris bill was signed into law in October, 1962. It was demonstrated after the fact that thalidomide was teratogenic in the rabbit; out of the episode grew the current practice that new human pharmaceuticals are tested for teratogenicity in two species, one generally being the rabbit.

The 1962 Drug Amendment made three major changes in the manner in which new drugs could be approved (Merrill, 1994). First, and perhaps the most important, was that it introduced the concept of effectiveness into the approval process. An NDA had to contain evidence that the drug was not only safe, but also effective. The 1938 law contained no such specification. The effectiveness requirement necessitated that a drug company had to do more extensive clinical trials. The new law required that companies apply to the FDA for approval of its clinical testing plan under an Investigational New Drug Application (INDA). No response from the FDA was deemed to be acceptance. As each level of clinical testing came to require FDA review and approval, the new law made the FDA an active partner in the development of all drugs.

The second major change enacted under the 1962 amendment was the change in the approval process from premarket notification to a premarket approval system. Under the terms of the 1938 law, an NDA would take effect automatically if the FDA did not respond. For example, the only reason thalidomide was not approved was because Dr. Kelsey returned the application to the sponsor with a request for more information. In contrast, the 1962 law required affirmative FDA action before a drug could be put on the market. Under the terms of the 1962 amendments, the FDA was also empowered to withdraw NDA approval and remove the drug from the market for a variety of reasons, including new evidence that the product was unsafe or that the sponsor had misrepresented or under-reported data.

The third major change enlarged the FDA's authority over clinical testing of new drugs. Thus, not only was evidence of effectiveness required, but Section 505(d) of the act specified the types of studies required. "Substantial evidence consisting of adequate and well-controlled investigations, including clinical investigations by qualified expert." In its role of meeting the statutory requirement for setting standards of clinical evidence, the FDA has become highly influential in the design of drug testing regimens (Merrill, 1994). Interestingly, discussed in detail by Hutt (1987), the FDA was initially quite unprepared for this new level of responsibility. It was not until 1973 that audited regulations on the determination of safety and effectiveness were put into place (these were, in fact, approved by the Supreme Court). While there have been several procedural changes [e.g., the 1985 Investigational New Drug (IND) rewrite] and additions (e.g., the 1988 IND procedures for life-threatening disease treatment), there have actually been no major changes in the law through 2001, despite procedural changes in 1992 with PDUFA and 1997 with FDAMA.

We must interject an interesting historical sidelight at this point. Despite its reputation, thalidomide made a bit of a comeback in the 1990s (Blakeslee, 1994). Among other properties, thalidomide has been shown to have good anti-inflammatory properties, because it apparently decreases the synthesis and/or release of tissue necrosis factor.

### 2.2.4. PDUFA and FDAMA 1992 and 1997

The history of pharmaceutical regulations has been dominated by two often opposing schools of thought: the need to provide the citizenry with effective medicaments, and the need to protect the consumer from unsafe and misbranded products. The reader is referred to Peter B. Hutt's in-depth reviews (1983a, b) on the subject. For example, the very first federal drug legislation in the United States was the Vaccine Act of 1813, which mandated the provision of the smallpox vaccine to the general public. In the modern era, legislative debate could be further defined as the constant swing back and forth on these two issues (see Hutt, 1983a, b), that is, safety versus development costs. In 1963, for example, Senator Hubert Humphrey presided over hearings on the FDA's implementation of the Drug Amendment of 1962. The FDA came under substantial criticism for failure to take strong action to protect the public from dangerous drugs. Eleven years later (1974), Senator Edward Kennedy conducted hearings addressing exactly the same issue. Commissioner Schmidt pressed the point that the FDA is under constant scrutiny regarding the approval of "dangerous" drugs, but no hearing had ever been conducted (up to that time) on the failure of the FDA to approve an important new therapy.

The next decade and a half saw a proliferation of work that analyzed the impact of regulation on competitiveness and the introduction of new therapies (see Hutt, 1983(b) for a complete review). This included, for example, Grabowski and Vernon's work (1983), which concluded that regulation had significant adverse effects on pharmaceutical innovation. This examination of the cost of regulation continued into the 1990s. In a meticulous and well researched study, DiMasi et al. (1994), reported that throughout the 1980s the number of Investigational New Drug applications were decreasing while the new drug application success rate was also dropping, and the length of time between discovery and approval was increasing. Clearly this was a situation that could not go on forever. The cost of new drug development rose from $54 million (U.S.) in 1976 to $359 million (U.S.) in 1990 (Anon., 1998a). Members of the pharmaceutical industry and the biotechnology industry were becoming increasingly alarmed by the negative synergy caused by increased costs and increased time to market. In 1991, Dranove published an editorial examining the increased costs and decreased product flow that resulted from the 1962 amendment. He made the observation that European requirements are less stringent than those of the United States, yet the Europeans did not seem to be afflicted by a greater number of dangerous drugs (see Table 1.2). Yet, if one looks at an analysis of worldwide withdrawals for safety from 1960 to 1999 (Fung, et. al., 2001), one sees that of 121 products identified, 42.1% were withdrawn from European markets alone, 5% from North America, 3.3% from Asia Pacific, and 49.6% from multiple markets. The top five safety reasons for withdrawal were hepatic (26.2%), hemotologic (10.5%), cardiovascular (8.7%), dermatologic (6.3%) and carcinogenic (6.3%) issue.

In an age of decreasing regulatory recourses, the FDA as well as Congress were under increasing pressure to review and release drugs more quickly. In response, Congress passed the 1992 Prescription Drug Users Fee Act (PDUFA). Under the terms of this act, companies would pay a fee to the agency to defray costs associated with application review. They would supposedly provide the FDA with the resources available to decrease application review time. In return, companies were guaranteed a more rapid review time. By all accounts, PDUFA has been successful. In 1992, the year PDUFA was passed, 26 NDAs were approved, requiring on average 29.9 months for data review; while in 1996, 53 new drug (or biological) products were approved, each requiring an average of 17.8 months of review time. PDUFA has been successful in decreasing review times, but has not really streamlined the procedures (Hegg, 1999).

The AIDS activist community was particularly vocal and effective in demanding more rapid approvals and increased access to therapies. There was also demand for

**TABLE 2.2. Summary of the Contents of the 1997 Food and Drug Administration Modernization Act**

| Title and Subtitle<br>I. Improving Regulatory<br>Drugs | Section<br>Number | Section Name |
| --- | --- | --- |
| A. Fees Relating to Drugs | 101 | Findings |
| | 102 | Definitions |
| | 103 | Authority to assess and use drug fees |
| | 104 | Annual reports |
| | 105 | Savings |
| | 106 | Effective date |
| | 107 | Termination of effectiveness |
| B. Other Improvements | 111 | Pediatric studies of drugs |
| | 112 | Expanding study and approval of fasttrack drugs |
| | 113 | Information program on trials for serious disease |
| | 114 | Healthcare economic information |
| | 115 | Manufacturing changes for drugs |
| | 116 | Streamlining clinical research for drugs |
| | 118 | Data requirements for drugs and biologics |
| | 119 | Content and review of applications |
| | 120 | Scientific advisory panels |
| | 121 | Positron emission tomography |
| | 122 | Requirements for radiopharmaceuticals |
| | 123 | Modernization of regulation |
| | 124 | Pilot and small scale manufacture |
| | 125 | Insulin and antibiotics |
| | 126 | Elimination of certain labeling requirements |
| | 127 | Application of federal law to pharmacy compounding |
| | 128 | Reauthorization of clinical pharmacology program |
| | 129 | Regulation of sunscreen products |
| | 130 | Report of postmarketing approval studies |
| | 131 | Notification of discontinuance of a life-saving product |
| II. Improving Regulation<br>of Devices | 201 | Investigational device exemptions |
| | 202 | Special review for certain devices |
| | 203 | Expanding humanitarian use of devices |
| | 204 | Device standards |
| | 205 | Collaborative determinations of device data requirements |
| | 206 | Premarket notification |
| | 207 | Evaluation of automatic Class III designation |
| | 208 | Classification panels |
| | 209 | Certainty of review time frames |
| | 210 | Accreditation of person for review of premarket notification reports |
| | 211 | Device tracking |
| | 212 | Postmarket notification |

**TABLE 2.2.** (*continued*)

| Title and Subtitle<br>I. Improving Regulatory<br>Drugs | Section<br>Number | Section Name |
|---|---|---|
| | 213 | Reports |
| | 214 | Practice of medicine |
| | 215 | Noninvasive blood glucose meter |
| | 216 | Data relating to premarket approval: product development protocol |
| | 217 | Number of required clinical investigations for approval |
| III. Improving Regulation of Food | 301 | Flexibility for regarding claims |
| | 302 | Petitions for claims |
| | 303 | Health claims for food products |
| | 304 | Nutrient content claims |
| | 305 | Referral statements |
| | 306 | Disclosure of radiation |
| | 307 | Irradiation petition |
| | 308 | Glass and ceramic ware |
| | 309 | Food contact substance |
| IV. General Provisions | 401 | Dissemination of information new uses |
| | 402 | Expanded access of investigational therapies and diagnostics |
| | 403 | Approval of supplemental applications for approved products |
| | 404 | Dispute resolution |
| | 405 | Informal agency statements |
| | 406 | FDA mission and annual report |
| | 407 | Information system |
| | 408 | Education and training |
| | 409 | Centers for education and research on therapeutics |
| | 410 | Mutual recognition of agreements and global harmonization |
| | 411 | Environmental impact review |
| | 412 | National uniformity for nonprescription drugs and cosmetics |
| | 413 | FDA study of mercury in drugs and foods |
| | 414 | Interagency collaboration |
| | 415 | Contracts for expert review |
| | 416 | Product classification |
| | 417 | Registration of foreign establishments |
| | 418 | Clarification of seizure authority |
| | 419 | Interstate commerce |
| | 420 | Safety report disclaimers |
| | 421 | Labeling and advertising compliance with statutory requirements |
| | 422 | Rule of construction |
| Title V. Effective Date | 501 | Effective date |

FDA reform on a number of other fronts (e.g., medical devices, pediatric claims, women and minority considerations, manufacturing changes, etc.). In 1993 the House Commerce Committee on Oversight and Investigations, chaired by John Dingel (D-MI) released a comprehensive investigation and evaluation of the FDA entitled, *Less than the Sum of its Parts*. The report was highly critical of the FDA, and made a number of recommendations (Pilot and Wladerman, 1998). The mid-1990s also saw the reinventing of government initiatives (RIGO) chaired by Vice-President Al Gore. Under RIGO, the FDA sought to identify and implement administrative reform. The RIGO report issued was entitled *Reinventing Regulation of Drugs and Medical Devices*. The 104th Congress started hearings on FDA reform again in the winter of 1995. Two bills were introduced that provided the essential outline of what would become FDAMA. Senator Nancy Kassebaum (R-KS), chair of the Senate Committee on Labor and Human Resources, introduced S.1477. The second was H.R.3201, introduced by Rep. Joe Barton (R-TX). Other bills were introduced by Senator Paul Wellstone (D-MN) and Rep. Ron Weyden (D-OR), which focused more on medical devices but still paved the way for bipartisan support of FDA reform (Pilot and Waldermann, 1998). Eventually, the 105th Congress passed the Food and Drug Administration Modernization Act (FDAMA), which was signed into law by President Clinton in November, 1997. The various sections of FDAMA are listed in Table 2.2. By any measure, it was a very broad and complex, if not overdeep, piece of legislation. In 1998, Marwick (1998) observed, "a measure of the extent of the task is that implementation of the act will require 42 new regulations, . . . , 23 new guidance notices, and 45 reports and other tasks." The FDA has identified the various tasks, regulations and guidances necessary for the implementation of FDAMA. FDA's FDAMA Implementation Chart is available at http://www.fda.gov/po/modact97.html, and the reader is urged to explore this site. There is a FDAMA icon on the FDA home page, and both CBER and CDER have issued various guidance documents. Some of the more interesting sections of the Act that may be of interest to toxicologists include

- Renewal of PDUFA for another five years.
- Fast track for breakthrough products.
- Change in the fashion biologicals regulated (elimination of the Establishment and Product licenses, both replaced with a Biological License Application or BLA).
- Change in the fashion antibiotics developed and regulated.
- Incentives for the development of pediatric claims.
- Companies permitted to disseminate information about approved uses for their products.
- FDAMA requires that FDA establish a clinical trials database for drugs used to treat serious and life-threatening diseases, other than AIDS and cancers (data bases for these diseases already established).

The full impact of FDAMA in the pharmaceutical industry in general, and on toxicology within this industry in particular, remains to be established.

While it is not possible to review the history of regulations worldwide, it is possible to point out some differences. We will highlight specific differences where appropriate throughout the remainder of the text.

The strength of the U.S. regulatory system was highlighted at the BioEurope 1993 Conference. David Holtzman stated: "...the main subject of the conference was regulation, and the United States was perceived to have the superior regulatory agency. It may be more difficult to satisfy but it is more predictable and scientifically based." (Holtzman, 1994) This predictability has not stultified the growth of biotechnology industry in the United States, and has, in fact, made the United States a more inciting target for investment than Europe. It is also a system that, while not perfect, has permitted very few unsafe products on the market.


## 2.3. FDAMA SUMMARY: CONSEQUENCES AND OTHER REGULATIONS

In summary, federal regulation of the safety of drugs has had three major objectives:

- Requiring testing to establish safety and efficacy.
- Establishing guidelines as to which tests are required and how they are designed.
- Promulgating requirements of data recording and reporting.

The first of these objectives was served by the 1906 Act, which required that agents be labeled appropriately. This was amended in 1938, in response to the tragedies associated with Elixir of Sulfanilamide and Lash Lure, to require that drugs and marketed formulations of drugs be shown to be safe when used as intended. In the aftermath of the thalidomide tragedy, the 1962 Kefauver–Harris Amendment significantly tightened requirements for preclinical testing (the INDA) and premarket approval (the NDA) of new drugs. The regulations pertaining to INDAs and NDAs have been modified (most recently in 1988), but essentially remain as the backbone of regulations of the toxicity evaluation of new human pharmaceutical agents. The Good Laboratories Practice (GLP) Act, which specifies standards for study planning, personnel training, data recording, and reporting, came out in 1978 in response to perceived shoddy practices of the operations of laboratories involved in the conduct of preclinical safety studies. It was revised in 1985 and 1988 (FDA, 1988).

The final major regulatory initiative on how drugs will be preclinically evaluated for safety arose out of the acquired immune deficiency syndrome (AIDS) crisis. To that point, the process of drug review and approval had very generally been perceived as slowing down, the FDA pursuing a conservative approach to requiring proof of safety and efficacy before allowing new drugs to become generally available. In response to AIDS, in 1988 the Expedited Delivery of Drugs for Life-Threatening Diseases Act established a basis for less rigorous standards (and more rapid drug development) in some limited cases.

In the United Kingdom, the Committee on Safety of Medicines (reporting to the Minister of Health) regulates drug safety and development under the Medicines Act of 1968 (which has replaced the Therapeutic Substances Act of 1925). Details on differences in drug safety regulations in the international marketplace can be found in Alder and Zbinden (1988), but key points are presented in this chapter. Other major markets are also addressed in Currie (1999), Evers (1985), Cadden (1999) and Yakuji Nippo, (1991).

## 2.4. OVERVIEW OF U.S. REGULATIONS

### 2.4.1. Regulations: General Considerations

The U.S. federal regulations that govern the testing, manufacture, and sale of pharmaceutical agents and medical devices are covered in Chapter 1, Title 21 of the Code of Federal Regulations (21 CFR). These comprise nine six-inch by eight-inch volumes (printing on both sides of the pages) which stack eight inches high. This title also covers foods, veterinary products, and cosmetics. As these topics will be discussed elsewhere in this book, here we will briefly review those parts of 21 CFR that are applicable to human health products and medicinal devices.

Of most interest to a toxicologist working in this arena would be Chapter 1, Subchapter A (parts 1–78), which cover general provisions, organization, and so on. The GLPs are codified in 21 CFR 58.

General regulations that apply to drugs are in Subchapter C (parts 200–299). This covers topics such as labeling, advertising, commercial registration, manufacture, and distribution. Of most interest to a toxicologist would be a section on labeling (Part 201, Subparts A–G, which covers Sections 201.1 through 201.317 of the regulations) because much of the toxicological research on a human prescription drug goes toward supporting a label claim. For example, specific requirements on content and format of labeling for human prescription drugs are covered in section 201.57. Directions for what should be included under the "Precautions" section of a label are listed in 201.57(f). This included 201.57(f)(6), which covers categorization of pregnancy risk, and the reliance upon animal reproduction studies in making these categorizations are made quite clear. For example, a drug is given a Pregnancy category B if "animal reproduction studies have failed to demonstrate a risk to the fetus." The point here is not to give the impression that the law is most concerned with pregnancy risk. Rather, we wish to emphasize that much basic toxicological information must be summarized on the drug label (or package insert). This section of the law is quite detailed as to what information is to be presented and the format of the presentation. Toxicologists working in the pharmaceutical arena should be familiar with this section of the CFR.

### 2.4.2. Regulations: Human Pharmaceuticals

The regulations specifically applicable to human drugs are covered in Subchapter D, Parts 300–399. The definition of a new drug is

A new drug substance means any substance that when used in the manufacture, processing or packaging of a drug causes that drug to be a new drug but does not include intermediates used in the synthesis of such substances—21 CFR Chapter 1, sub chapter D, Part 310(g).

The regulation then goes on to discuss "newness with regard to new formulations, indications, or in combinations." For toxicologists, the meat of the regulations can be found in Section 312 (INDA) and Section 314 (applications for approval to market a new drug or antibiotic drug or NDA). The major focus for a toxicologist working in the pharmaceutical industry is on preparing the correct toxicology "packages" to be included to "support" these two types of applications. (The exact nature of these packages will be covered below.)

In a nutshell, the law requires solid scientific evidence of safety and efficacy before a new drug will be permitted in clinical trials or (later) on the market. The INDA (covered in 21 CFR 310) is for permission to proceed with clinical trials on human subjects. Once clinical trials have been completed, the manufacturer or "sponsor" can then proceed to file an NDA (covered in 21 CFR 314) for permission to market the new drug.

As stated in 321.21, "A sponsor shall submit an IND if the sponsor intends to conduct a clinical investigation with a new drug...[and] shall not begin a clinical investigation until...an IND...is in effect." [Similar procedures are in place in other major countries. In the United Kingdom, for example, a Clinical Trials Certificate (CTC) must be filed or a CTX (clinical trial exemption) obtained before clinical trials may proceed.] Clinical trials are divided into three phases, as described in 21 CFR 312.21. Phase I trials are initial introductions into healthy volunteers primarily for the purposes of establishing tolerance (side effects), bioavailability, and metabolism. Phase II clinical trials are "controlled studies...to evaluate effectiveness of the drug for a particular indication or disease." The secondary objective is to determine common short-term side effects; hence the subjects are closely monitored. Phase III studies are expanded clinical trials. It is during this phase that the definitive, large-scale, double-blind studies are performed.

The toxicologist's main responsibilities in the IND process are to design, conduct, and interpret appropriate toxicology studies (or "packages") to support the initial IND and then design the appropriate studies necessary to support each additional phase of investigation. Exactly what may constitute appropriate studies are covered elsewhere in this chapter. The toxicologist's second responsibility is to prepare the toxicology summaries for the (clinical) investigator's brochure [described in 312.23(a)(8)(ii)]. This is an integrated summary of the toxicological effects of the drug in animals and *in vitro*. The FDA has prepared numerous guidance documents covering the content and format of INDs. It is of interest that in the Guidance for Industry (Lumpkin, 1996) an in-depth description of the expected contents of the Pharmacology and Toxicology sections was presented. The document contains the following self-explanatory passage:

Therefore, if final, fully quality-assured individual study reports are not available at the time of IND submission, an integrated summary report of toxicological findings based on the unaudited draft toxicologic reports of the completed animal studies may be submitted—Lumpkin (1996).

If unfinalized reports are used in an initial IND, the finalized report must be submitted within 120 days of the start of the clinical trial. The sponsor must also prepare a document identifying any differences between the preliminary and final reports, and the impact (if any) on interpretation.

Thus, while the submission of fully audited reports is preferable, the agency does allow for the use of incomplete reports.

Once an IND or CTC/X is opened, the toxicologists may have several additional responsibilities. First, to design, conduct, and report the additional tests necessary to support a new clinical protocol or an amendment to the current clinical protocol (Section 312.20). Secondly, to bring to the sponsor's attention any finding in an ongoing toxicology study in animals "suggesting a significant risk to human subjects, including any finding of mutagenicity, teratogenicity or carcinogenicity," as described in 21 CFR 312.32. The sponsor has a legal obligation to report such findings within 10 working days. Third, to prepare a "list of the preclinical studies...completed or in progress during the past year" and a summary of the major preclinical findings. The sponsor is required (under Section 312.23) to file an annual report (within 60 days of the IND anniversary date) describing the progress of the investigation. INDs are never "approved" in the strict sense of the word. Once filed, an IND can be opened 30 days after submission, unless the FDA informs the sponsor otherwise. The structure of an IND is outlined in Table 2.3.

If the clinical trials conducted under an IND are successful in demonstrating safety and effectiveness [often established at a Pre-NDA meeting, described in 21 CFR 312.47(b)(2)], the sponsor can then submit an NDA. Unlike an IND, the NDA must be specifically approved by the Agency. The toxicologist's responsibility in the

**TABLE 2.3. Composition of Standard Investigational New Drug Application**[a]

1. IND cover sheets (Form FDA-1571)
2. Table of contents
3. General (clinical) investigation plan
4. (Reserved)
5. (Clinical) investigators brochure
6. (Proposed) clinical protocol(s)
7. Chemistry, manufacturing, and control information
8. Pharmacology and toxicology information (includes metabolism and pharmacokinetic assessments done in animals)
9. Previous human experience with the investigational drug
10. Additional information
11. Other relevant information

[a]Complete and thorough reports on all pivotal toxicological studies must be provided with the application.

NDA/Marketing Authorization Application (MAA) process is to prepare an integrated summary of all the toxicology and/or safety studies performed and be in a position to present and review the toxicology findings to the FDA or its advisory bodies. The approval process can be exhausting, including many meetings, hearings, appeals, and so on. The ground rules for all of these are described in Part A of the law. For example, all NDAs are reviewed by an "independent" (persons not connected with either the sponsor or the Agency) scientific advisory panel which will review the findings and make recommendations as to approval. MAAs must be reviewed by and reported on by an expert recognized by the cognizant regulatory authority. Final statutory approval in the United States lies with the Commissioner of the FDA. It is hoped that few additional studies will be requested during the NDA review and approval process. When an NDA is approved, the Agency will send the sponsor an approval letter and will issue a Summary Basis of Approval (SBA) (312.30), which is designed and intended to provide a public record on the Agency's reasoning for approving the NDA while not revealing any proprietary information. The SBA can be obtained through Freedom of Information, and can provide insights into the precedents for which types of toxicology studies are used to support specific types of claims.

### 2.4.3. Regulations: Environmental Impact

Environmental Impact Statements, while once important only for animal drugs, must now accompany all NDAs. This assessment must also be included in the Drug Master File (DMF). The procedures, formats, and requirements are described in 21 CFR 2531. This requirement has grown in response to the National Environmental Policy Act, the heart of which required that federal agencies evaluate every major action that could effect the quality of the environment. In the INDs, this statement can be a relatively short section claiming that relatively small amounts will pose little risk to the environment. The EEC has similar requirements for drug entities in Europe, though data requirements are more strenuous. With NDAs, this statement must be more substantial, detailing any manufacturing and/or distribution process that may result in release into the environment. Environmental fate (e.g., photo-hydrolysis) and toxicity (e.g., fish, daphnia, and algae) studies will be required. While not mammalian toxicology in the tradition of pharmaceutical testing, preparing an environmental impact statement will clearly require toxicological input. The FDA has published a technical bulletin covering the tests it may require (FDA, 1987).

### 2.4.4. Regulations: Antibiotics

The NDA law (safety and effectiveness) applies to all drugs, but antibiotic drugs were treated differently until the passage of FDAMA in 1997. Antibiotic drugs had been treated differently by the FDA since the development of penicillin revolutionized medicine during World War II. The laws applicable to antibiotic drugs were covered in 21 CFR 430 and 431. Antibiotics such as penicillin or doxorubicin are drugs derived (in whole or in part) from natural sources (such as molds or plants) which have cytotoxic or cytostatic properties. They were treated differently from other drugs; the applicable laws required a batch-to-batch certification process. Originally passed into law in 1945 specifically for penicillin, this certification process was expanded by the 1962 amendment (under Section 507 of the Food, Drug, and Cosmetic Act) to require certification of all antibiotic drugs, meaning that the FDA would assay each lot of antibiotic for purity, potency, and safety. The actual regulations were covered in 21 CFR Subchapter D, Parts 430–460 (over 600 pages), which describes the standards and methods used for certification for all approved antibiotics. Section 507 was repealed by FDAMA (Section 125). As a result of this repeal, the FDA is no longer required to publish antibiotic monographs. In addition, the testing, filing, and reviewing of antibiotic applications are now handled under Section 505 of the Act like any other new therapeutic agent. The FDA has published a guidance document to which the reader is referred for more details. (Anon., 1998a, b).

### 2.4.5. Regulations: Biologics

Biological products are covered in Subchapter F, parts 600–680. As described in 21 CFR 600.3(h), "biological product means any virus, therapeutic serum, toxin, antitoxin or analogous product applicable to the prevention, treatment or cure of diseases or injuries of man." In other words, these are vaccines and other protein products derived from animal sources. Clearly the toxicological concerns with such products are vastly different than those involved with low-molecular-weight synthetic molecules. There is little rational basis, for example, for conducting a one-year, repeated dose toxicity study with a vaccine or a human blood product. The FDA definition for safety with regard to these products is found in 21 CFR 603.1(p): "Relative freedom from harmful effect to persons affected, directly or indirectly, by a product when prudently administered." Such a safety consideration has more to do with purity, sterility, and adherence to good manufacturing standards than with the toxicity of the therapeutic molecule itself. The testing required to show safety is stated in the licensing procedures 21 CFR 601.25(d)(1): "Proof of safety shall consist of adequate test methods reasonably applicable to show the biological product is safe under the prescribed conditions." Once a license is granted, each batch or lot of biological product must be tested for safety, and the methods of doing so are written into the law. A general test for safety (i.e., required in addition to other safety tests) is prescribed using guinea pigs as described in 610.11. Additional tests are often applied to specific products. For example, 21 CFR 630.35 describes the safety tests required for measles vaccines, which includes tests in mice and *in vitro* assays with tissue culture. Many new therapeutic entities produced by biotechnology are seeking approval as biologics with the results being FDA approval of a Product License Application (PLA) (Buesing, 1999). Table 2.4 presents general guidance for the basis of deciding if an individual entity falls under the Center for Drug Evaluation and Research (CDER) or the Center for Biologic Evaluation and Research (CBER) authority for review.

**TABLE 2.4. Product Class Review Responsibilities**

*Center for Drug Evaluation and Review*
Natural products purified from plant or mineral sources
Products produced from solid tissue sources (excluding procoagulants, venoms, blood
   products, etc.)
Antibiotics, regardless of method of manufacture
Certain substances produced by fermentation
   Disaccharidase inhibitors
   HMG-CoA inhibitors
Synthetic chemicals
   Traditional chemical synthesis
   Synthesized mononuclear or polynuclear products including antisense chemicals
Hormone products

Center for Biologics Evaluation and Review
Vaccines, regardless of manufacturing method
*In vivo* diagnostic allergenic products
Human blood products
Protein, peptide, and/or carbohydrate products produced by cell culture
   (other than antibiotics and hormones)
Immunoglobulin products
Products containing intact cells or microorganisms
Proteins secreted into fluids by transgenic animals
Animal venoms
Synthetic allergens
Blood banking and infusion adjuncts

---

The International Conferences on Harmonization has published its document S6, Preclincial Safety Evaluation of Biotechnology-Derived Pharmaceuticals. The FDA (the Center for Drug Evaluation and Research, and the Center for Biologics Evaluation and Research jointly) has published the document as a Guidance for Industry (Anon., 1997a, b; FDA, 1989, Hayes and Reyffel, 1999).

A current list of regulatory documents available by e-mail (including the most recent PTCs, or points to consider) can be found at DOC_LIST@A1.FDA.GOV.

### 2.4.6. Regulations versus Law

A note of caution must be inserted here. The law (the document passed by Congress) and the regulations (the documents written by the regulatory authorities to enforce the laws) are separate documents. The sections in the law do not necessarily have numerical correspondence. For example, the regulations on the NDA process is described in 21 CFR 312, but the law describing the requirement for an NDA process is in Section 505 of the FDCA. Because the regulations rather than the laws themselves have a greater impact on toxicological practice, greater emphasis is placed on regulation in this chapter. For a complete review of FDA law, the reader is referred to the monograph by the Food and Drug Law Institute (FDLI) 1999.

Laws authorize the activities and responsibilities of the various federal agencies. All proposed laws before Congress are referred to committees for review and approval. The committees responsible for FDA oversight are summarized in Table 2.5. This table also highlights the fact that authorizations and appropriations (the funding necessary to execute authorizations) are handled by different committees.

## 2.5. ORGANIZATIONS REGULATING DRUG AND DEVICE SAFETY IN THE U.S.

The agency formally charged with overseeing the safety of drugs in the United States is the FDA. It is headed by a commissioner who reports to the Secretary of the Department of Health and Human Services (DHHS) and has a tremendous range of responsibilities. Drugs are overseen primarily by the CDER (though some therapeutic or health care entities are considered biologics and are overseen by the corresponding CBER). Figure 2.1 presents the organization of CDER. The organization of CBER is shown in Figure 2.2.

Most of the regulatory interactions of toxicologists are with the five offices of Drug Evaluation (I–V) which have under them a set of groups focused on areas of therapeutic claim (cardiorenal, neuropharmacological, gastrointestinal and coagulation, oncology and pulmonary, metabolism and endocrine, antiinfective and antiviral). Within each of these are chemists, pharmacologists/toxicologists, statisticians, and clinicians. When an INDA is submitted to the offices of Drug Evaluation, it is assigned to one of the therapeutic groups based on its area of therapeutic claim. Generally, it will remain with that group throughout its regulatory approval "life." INDs, when allowed, grant investigators the ability to go forward into clinical (human) trials with their drug candidate in a predefined manner, advancing through various steps of evaluation in human (and in additional

**TABLE 2.5. Congressional Committees Responsible for FDA Oversight**

*Authorization*

Senate   All public health service agencies are under the jurisdiction of the Labor and Human Resources Committee

House   Most public health agencies are under the jurisdiction of the Health and the Environmental Subcommittee of the House Energy and Commerce Committee

*Appropriation*

Senate   Unlike most other public health agencies, the FDA is under the jurisdiction of the Agriculture, Rural Development, and Related Agencies Subcommittee of the Senate Appropriations Committee

House   Under the jurisdiction of the Agriculture, Rural Development, and Related Agencies Subcommittee of the House Appropriations Committee

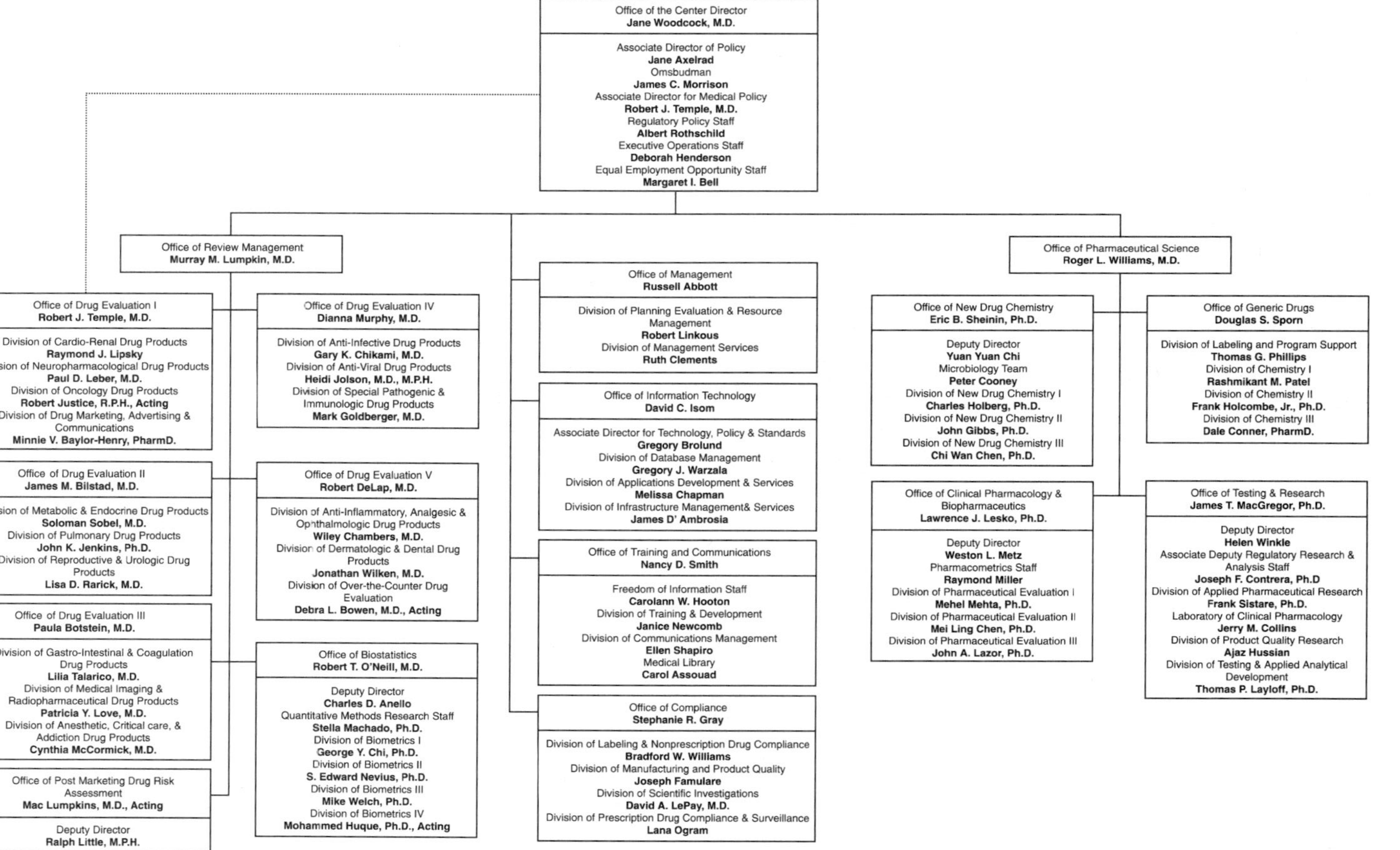


**FIGURE 2.1.** Organizational chart of CDER.

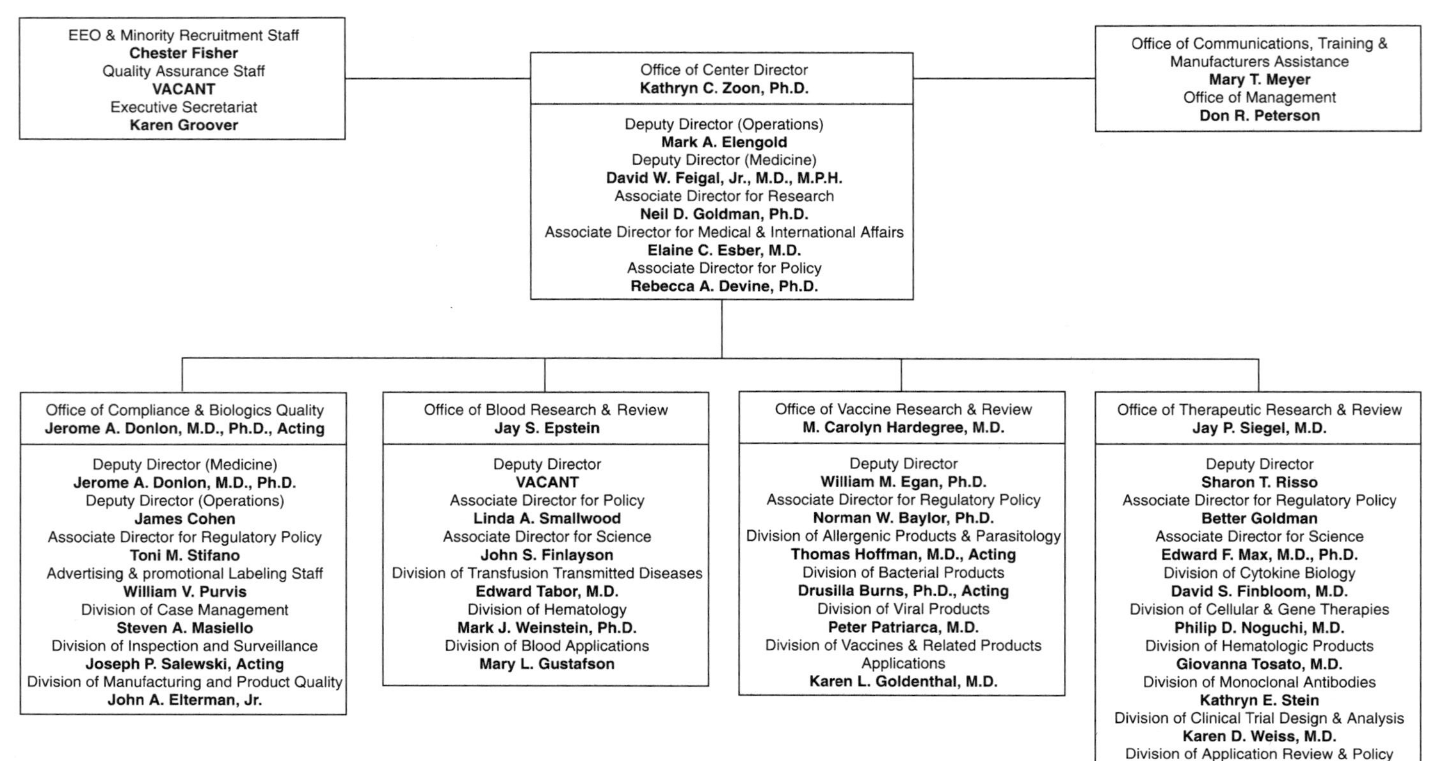


**FIGURE 2.2.** Organizational chart of CBER.

preclinical or animal studies) until an NDA can be supported, developed, and submitted. Likewise for biological products, the PLA or other applications (INDA, IND) are handled by the offices of Biological Products Review of the CBER.

For drugs, there is at least one nongovernmental body which must review and approve various aspects: the USP (United States Pharmacopeia, established in 1820), which maintains (and revises) the compendia of the same name, as well as the National Formulary which sets drug composition standards (Ember, 2001). This volume sets forth standards for purity of products in which residues may be present and tests for determining various characteristics of drugs, devices, and biologics. The USP also contains significant "guidance" for the evaluation of safety for devices (USP, 2000).

## 2.6. PROCESS OF PHARMACEUTICAL PRODUCT DEVELOPMENT AND APPROVAL

Except for a very few special cases (treatments for life-threatening diseases such as cancer or AIDS), the safety assessment of new drugs as mandated by regulations proceeds in a rather fixed manner. The IND is filed to support this clinical testing. An initial set of studies [typically, studies of appropriate length by the route intended for humans are performed in both a rodent (typically rat) and a nonrodent (usually a dog or a primate)] are required to support Phase I clinical testing. Such Phase I testing is intended to evaluate the safety ("tolerance" in clinical subjects), pharmacokinetics, and general biological effects of a new drug, and is conducted in normal volunteers (almost always males).

Successful completion of Phase I testing allows, with the approval of the FDA, progression into Phase II clinical testing. Here, selected patients are enrolled to evaluate therapeutic efficacy, dose ranging, and more details about the pharmacokinetics and metabolism. Longer-term systemic toxicity studies must be in conformity with the guidelines that are presented in the next section. Once a sufficient understanding of the actions, therapeutic dose response, and potential risk/benefit ratio of the drug is in hand (once again, with FDA approval), trials move to Phase III testing.

Phase III tests are large, long, and expensive. They are conducted using large samples of selected patients and are intended to produce proof of safety and efficacy of the drug. Two studies providing statistically significant proof of the claimed therapeutic benefit must be provided. All the resulting data from preclinical and clinical animal studies are organized in a specified format in the form of an NDA, which is submitted to the FDA.

By the time Phase III testing is completed, some additional preclinical safety tests must also generally be in hand. These include the three separate reproductive and developmental toxicity studies (Segments I and III in the rat, and Segment II in the rat and rabbit) and carcinogenicity studies in both rats and mice (unless the period of therapeutic usage is intended to be very short). Some assessment of genetic toxicity will also be expected.

The ultimate product of the pharmaceutical toxicologist will thus generally be the toxicology summaries of the IND and NDA (or PLA). For medical devices, the equivalents are the IDE and Product Development Notification (PDN). Data required to support each of these documents is specified in a series of guidelines, as will be discussed below.

Acceptance of these applications is contingent not only upon adherence to guidelines and good science, but also adherence to GLPs.

## 2.7.  TESTING GUIDELINES

### 2.7.1.  Toxicity Testing: Traditional Pharmaceuticals

Although the 1938 Act required safety assessment studies, no consistent guidelines were available. Guidelines were first proposed in 1949 and published in the *Food, Drug and Cosmetic Law Journal* that year (Burns, 1982). Following several revisions, these guidelines were issued as *The Appraisal Handbook* in 1959. While never formally called a guideline, it set the standard for preclinical toxicity test design for several years. The current basic guidelines for testing required for safety assessment in support of the phases of clinical development of drugs were first outlined by Goldenthal (1968) and later incorporated into a 1971 FDA publication entitled *FDA Introduction to Total Drug Quality*.

### 2.7.2.  General or Systematic Toxicity Assessment

Table 2.6 presents an overview of the current FDA toxicity testing guidelines for human drugs. Table 2.7 presents the parallel ICH guidance (ICH 2000) which are now largely supplanting the FDA guidelines. They are misleading in their apparent simplicity, however. First, each of the systemic toxicity studies in these guidelines must be designed and executed in a satisfactory manner. Sufficient animals must be used to have confidence in finding and characterizing any adverse drug actions that may be present. In practice, as the duration of the study increases, small doses are administered and larger numbers of animals must be employed per group. These two features—dosage level and group size—are critical to study designs. Table 2.8 presents general guidance on the number of animals to be used in systemic studies. These and other technical considerations for the safety assessment of pharmaceuticals are present in detail in Gad (1994).

The protocols discussed thus far have focused on general or systemic toxicity assessment. The agency and, indeed, the lay public have a special set of concerns with reproductive toxicity, fetal/embryo toxicity, and developmental toxicity (also called teratogenicity). Collectively, these concerns often go by the acronyms DART (Developmental and Reproductive Toxicity) or RTF (Reproduction, Teratogenicity, Fertility). Segment II studies are designed more to detect developmental toxicity. Only pregnant females are dosed during the critical period of organogenesis. Generally, the first protocol DART test (exclusive of range-finding studies) is a

Segment I study of rats in fertility and general reproductive performance. This is generally done while the drug is in Phase II clinical trials. Alternatively, many companies are now performing the Segment II teratology study in rats before the Segment I study because the former is less time- and resource-intensive. One or both should be completed before including women of child-bearing potential in clinical trials. The FDA requires teratogenicity testing in two species: a rodent (rat or mouse) and the rabbit. The use of the rabbit was instituted as a result of the finding that thalidomide was a positive teratogen in the rabbit but not in the rat. On occasion, when a test article is not compatible with the rabbit, teratogenicity data in the mouse may be substituted. There are also some specific classes of therapeutics (the quinalone antibiotics, for example) where Segment II studies in primates are effectively required prior to product approval. Both should be completed before entering Phase III clinical trials. The most complicated of the DART protocols— Segment III—is generally commenced during Phase III trials and should be part of the NDA. There are differences in the different national guidelines (as discussed later with international considerations) regarding the conduct of these studies. The large multinational drug companies try to design their protocols to be in compliance with as many of the guidelines as possible to avoid duplication of testing while allowing the broadest possible approval and marketing of therapeutics.

### 2.7.3. Genetic Toxicity Assessment

Genetic toxicity testing generally focuses on the potential of a new drug to cause mutations (in single-cell systems) or other forms of genetic damage. The tests, generally short in duration, often rely on *in vitro* systems and generally have a single endpoint of effect (point mutations, chromosomal damage, etc.). For a complete review of protocols, technology, and so on, the reader is referred to Brusick (1987). It is of interest that the FDA has no standard or statutory requirement for genetic toxicity testing but generally expects to see at least some such tests performed and will ask for them if the issue is not addressed. If one performs such a study, any data collected, of course, must be sent to the Agency as part of any INDA, PLA, or NDA. These studies have yet to gain favor with the FDA (or other national regulatory agencies) as substitutes for *in vivo* carcinogenicity testing. However, even with completed negative carcinogenicity tests, at least some genetic toxicity assays are generally required. Generally, pharmaceuticals in the United States are evaluated for mutagenic potential (e.g., the Ame's Assay) or for chromosomal damage (e.g., the *In Vivo* Mouse Micronucleus Test). In general, in the United States, pharmaceutical companies apply genetic toxicity testing in the following fashion.

- *As a Screen.* An agent that is positive in one or more genetic toxicity tests may be more likely than one that is negative to be carcinogenic and, therefore, may not warrant further development.
- *As an Adjunct.* An agent that is negative in carcinogenicity testing in two species and also negative in a genetic toxicity battery is more likely than not to be noncarcinogenic in human beings.

**TABLE 2.6. Synopsis of General Guidelines for Animal Toxicity Studies for Drugs**

| Category | Duration of Human Administration | Clinical Phase | Subacute or Chronic Toxicity | Special Studies |
|---|---|---|---|---|
| Oral or parenteral | Several days | I, II, III, NDA | 2 species; 2 weeks | For parentally administered drugs |
| | Up to 2 weeks | I | 2 species; 4 weeks | |
| | | II | 2 species; up to 4 weeks | |
| | | III, NDA | 2 species; up to 3 months | Compatibility with blood where applicable |
| | Up to 3 months | I, II | 2 species; 4 weeks | |
| | | III | 2 species; 3 months | |
| | | NDA | 2 species; up to 6 months | |
| | 6 Months to Unlimited | I, II | 2 species; 3 months | |
| | | III | 2 species; 6 months or longer | |
| | | NDA | 2 species; 9 months (nonrodent) and 12 months (rodent) +2 rodent species for CA; 18 months (mouse). May be replaced with an allowable transgenic mouse study 24 months (rat) | |
| Inhalation (General anesthetics) | | I, II, III, NDA | 4 species; 5 days (3 hours/day) | |
| Dermal | Single application | I | 1 species; single 24-hour exposure followed by 2-week observation | Sensitization |

| | | | | |
|---|---|---|---|---|
| | Single or short-term application | II | 1 species; 20-day repeated exposure (intact and abraded skin) | |
| | Short-term application | III | As above | |
| | Unlimited application | NDA | As above, but intact skin study extended up to 6 months | |
| Ophthalmic | Single application | I | | Eye irritation tests with graded doses |
| | Multiple application | I, II, III | 1 species; 3 weeks daily applications, as in clinical use | |
| | | NDA | 1 species; duration commensurate with period of drug administration | |
| Vaginal or Rectal | Single application | I | | Local and systematic toxicity after vaginal or rectal application in 2 species |
| | Multiple application | I, II, III, NDA | 2 species; duration and number of applications determined by proposed use | |
| Drug Combinations | (4) | I | | Lethality by appropriate route, compared to components run concurrently in 1 species |
| | | II, III, NDA | species; up to 3 months | |

**TABLE 2.7. Duration of Repeated Dose Toxicity Studies to Support Clinical Trials and Marketing[a]**

| Duration of clinical trials | Minimum duration of repeated dose toxicity studies[c] | | Duration of clinical trials | Minimum duration of repeated dose toxicity studies[d,e] | |
| --- | --- | --- | --- | --- | --- |
| | Rodents | Nonrodents | | Rodents | Nonrodents |
| Single dose | 2 weeks[b] | 2 weeks | Up to 2 weeks | 1 month | 1 month |
| Up to 2 weeks | 2 weeks[b] | 2 weeks | Up to 1 month | 3 months | 3 months |
| Up to 1 month | 1 month | 1 month | Up to 3 months | 6 months | 3 months |
| Up to 6 months | 6 months | 6 months[c] | More than 3 months | 6 months | Chronic[b] |
| More than 6 months | 6 months | Chronic[c] | | | |

[a]In Japan, if there are no Phase II clinical trials of equivalent duration to the planned Phase III trials, conduct of longer duration toxicity studies is recommended as given in Table 2.

[b]In the US, as an alternative to 2-week studies, single dose toxicity studies with extended examinations can support single-dose human trials (4).

[c]Data from 6 months of administration in nonrodents should be available before the initiation of clinical trials longer than 3 months. Alternatively, if applicable, data from a 9-month nonrodent study should be available before the treatment duration exceeds that which is supported by the available toxicity studies.

[d]To support Phase I and II Trials in the EU AND Phase I, II and III Trials in the U.S. and Japan.

[e]The above table also reflects the marketing recommendations in the 3 regions except that a chronic nonrodent study is recommended for clinical use longer than 1 month.

**TABLE 2.8. Numbers of Animals per Dosage Group in Systemic Toxicity Studies**

| Study Duration (per sex) | Rodents (per sex) | Nonrodents |
| --- | --- | --- |
| 2–4 weeks | 5 | 3 |
| 13 weeks | 20[a] | 6 |
| 26 weeks | 30 | 8 |
| Chronic | 50 | 10 |
| Carcinogenicity | 60[b] | Applies only to contraceptives |
| Bioassays | | Applies only to contraceptives |

[a]Starting with 13-week studies, one should consider adding animals (particularly to the high dose) to allow evaluation of reversal of effects.

[b]In recent years there have been decreasing levels of survival in rats on two-year studies. What is required is that at least 20–25 animals/sex/group survive at the end of the study. Accordingly, practice is beginning to use 70 or 75 animals per sex, per group.

- *To Provide Mechanistic Insight.* For example, if an agent is negative in a wide range of genetic toxicity screens, but still produces tumors in animals, then one could hypothesize that an epigenetic mechanism was involved.

While not officially required, the FDA does have the authority to request, on a case-by-case basis, specific tests it feels may be necessary to address a point of concern. A genetic toxicity test could be part of such a request. In general, therefore, companies deal with genetic toxicity (after "screening") on a case-by-case basis, dictated by good science. If more than a single administration is intended, common practice is to perform the tests prior to submitting an IND.

### 2.7.4. Toxicity Testing: Biotechnology Products

As mentioned, the regulation of traditional pharmaceuticals (small molecules such as aspirin or digitalis) and biologicals (proteins such as vaccines and antitoxins derived from animal sources) have very different histories. See the discussion on biologics earlier in this chapter. Until 1972, the NIH (or its forerunning agency, the Hygienic Laboratory of the Department of the Treasury) was charged with the responsibilities of administering the Virus Act of 1902. With the passage of the Food and Drug Laws of 1906, 1938, and 1962, there was recurring debate about whether these laws applied or should apply to biologicals (Wessinger, 1989). This debate was resolved when the authority for the regulation of biologics was transferred to the FDA's new Bureau of Biologics (now the CBER) in 1972. Since then, there appears to have been little difference in the matter of regulation for biologics and pharmaceuticals. The FDA essentially regulates biologics as described under the 1902 act, but then uses the rule-making authority granted under the Food and Drug Act to "fill in the gaps."

The Bureau of Biologics was once a relatively "sleepy" agency, primarily concerned with the regulation of human blood products and vaccines used for mass immunization programs. The authors of the 1902 law could hardly have foreseen the explosion in biotechnology that occurred in the 1980s. New technology created a welter of new biological products, such as recombinant-DNA-produced proteins (e.g., tissue plasminogen activator), biological response modifiers (cytokinins and colony-stimulating factors), monoclonal antibodies, antisense oligonucleotides, and self-directed vaccines (raising an immune response to self-proteins such as gastrin for therapeutic reasons). The new products raised a variety of new questions on the appropriateness of traditional methods of evaluating drug toxicity that generated several points-to-consider documents. For the sake of brevity, this discussion will focus on the recombinant DNA proteins. Some of the safety issues that have been raised over the years:

- The appropriateness of testing a human-specific peptide hormone in nonhuman species;
- The potential that the peptide could break down due to nonspecific metabolism, resulting in products that had no therapeutic value or even be a toxic fragment;
- The potential sequelae to an immune response (formation of neutralizing antibodies, provoking an autoimmune or a hypersensitivity response), and pathology due to immune precipitation, and so on;
- The presence of contamination with oncogenic virus DNA (depending on whether a bacterial or mammalian system was used on the synthesizing agent) or endotoxins;
- The difficulty of interpreting the scientific relevance of response to supraphysiological systemic doses of potent biological response modifiers.

The last few years have shown that some of these concerns were more relevant than others. The "toxic peptide fragment" concern, for example, has been shown to be without merit. The presence of potentially oncogenic virus DNA and endotoxins is a quality assurance concern and is not truly a toxicological problem. Regardless of the type of synthetic pathway, all proteins must be synthesized in compliance with Good Manufacturing Practices. Products must be as pure as possible, not only free of rDNA but also free of other types of cell debris (endotoxin). Batch-to-batch consistency with regard to molecular structure must also be demonstrated using appropriate methods (e.g., amino acid). Regulatory thinking and experience over the last 15 years has come together in the document, "S6 Preclincial Safety Evaluation of Biotechnology-Derived Pharmaceuticals" prepared by the International Conferences on Harmonization. The FDA (both the Center for Drug Evaluation and Research, and the Center for Biologics Evaluation and Research jointly) has published the document as a *Guidance for Industry* and a *Point to Consider*, respectively (Anon. 1997a, b). The document was intended to provide basic guidance for the preclinical evaluation of biotechnology derived products, including proteins and peptides, either produced by cell culture or using rDNA technology (FDA, 1993), but did not cover antibiotics, allergenic extracts, heparin, vitamins, cellular drug products, vaccines, or other products regulated as biologics. Items covered are summarized as follows.

*Test Article Specifications.* In general, the product that is used in the definitive pharmacology and toxicology studies should be comparable to the product proposed for the initial clinical studies.

*Animal Species/Model Selection.* Safety evaluation should include the use of relevant species, in which the test article is pharmacologically active due, for example, to the expression of the appropriate receptor molecule. These can be screened with *in vitro* rector binding assays. Safety evaluation should normally include two appropriate species, if possible and/or feasible. The potential utility of gene knockout and/or transgenic animals in safety assessment is discussed.

*Group Size.* No specific numbers are given, but it does state that a small sample size may lead to failure to observe toxic events.

*Administration.* The route and frequency should be as close as possible to that proposed for clinical use. Other routes can be used when scientifically warranted.

*Immunogenicity.* It has also been clearly demonstrated in the testing of rDNA protein products that animals will develop antibodies to foreign proteins. This response has been shown to neutralize (rapidly remove from circulation) the protein, but no pathological conditions have been shown to occur as a sequelae to the immune response. Bear in mind, however, that interleukins have powerful effects on immune response, but these are due to their physiological activity and not due to an antigen–antibody response. The first has to do with "neutralizing antibodies"; that is, is the immune response so great that the test article is being removed from circulation as fast as it is being added? If this is the case, does long-term testing of such a chemical make sense? In many cases, it does not. The safety testing of any large molecule should include the appropriate assays for determining whether the test system has developed a neutralizing antibody response. Depending on the species, route of administration, intended therapeutic use, and development of neutralizing antibodies (which generally takes about two weeks), it is rare for a toxicity test on an rDNA protein to be longer than four weeks' duration. However, if the course of therapy in humans is to be longer than two weeks, formation of neutralizing antibodies must be demonstrated or longer-term testing performed. The second antigen–antibody formation concern is that a hypersensitivity response will be elicited. Traditional preclinical safety assays are generally adequate to guard against this if they are two weeks or longer in duration and the relevant endpoints are evaluated.

*Safety Pharmacology.* It is important to investigate the potential for unwanted pharmacological activity in appropriate animal models and to incorporate monitoring for these activities in the toxicity studies.

*Exposure Assessment.* Single and multiple dose pharmacokinetics, toxicokinetics and tissue distribution studies in relevant species are useful. Proteins are not given orally; demonstrating absorption and mass balance is not typically a primary consideration. Rather, this segment of the test should be designed to determine half-life (and other appropriate pharmacokinetic descriptor parameters), the plasma concentration associated with biological effects, and potential changes due to the development of neutralizing antibodies.

*Reproductive Performance and Developmental Toxicity Studies.* These will be dictated by the product, clinical indication and intended patient population.

*Genotoxicity Studies.* The S6 document states that the battery of genotoxicity studies routinely conducted for traditional pharmaceuticals are not appropriate for biotechnology-derived pharmaceuticals. In contrast to small molecules, genotoxicity testing with a battery of *in vitro* and *in vivo* techniques of protein molecules has not become common U.S. industry practice. Such tests are not formally required by the FDA but, if performed, have to be reported. They are required by European and Japanese regulatory authorities. This has sparked a debate as to whether or not genotoxicity testing is necessary or appropriate for rDNA protein molecules. It is the author's opinion that such testing is, scientifically, of little value. First, large protein molecules will not easily penetrate the cell wall of bacteria or yeast, and (depending on size, charge, lipophilicity, etc.) penetration across the plasma lemma of mammalian cells will be highly variable. Second, if one considers the well-established mechanism(s) of genotoxicity of small molecules, it is difficult to conceive how a protein can act in the same fashion. For example, proteins will not be metabolized to be electrophilic active intermediates that will crosslink guanine residues. In general, therefore, genotoxicity testing with rDNA proteins is a waste of resources. It is conceivable, however, that some proteins, because of their biological mechanism of action, may stimulate the proliferation of transformed cells. For example, it is a feasible hypothesis that a colony-stimulating factor could stimulate the proliferation of leukemic cells (it should be emphasized that this is a hypothetical situation, presented here for illustrative purposes). Again, this is a question of a specific pharmacological property, and such considerations should be tested on a case-by-case basis.

*Carcinogenicity Studies.* These are generally inappropriate for biotechnology-derived pharmaceuticals; however, some products may have the potential to support or induce proliferation of transformed cells...possibly leading to neoplasia. When this concern is present, further studies in relevant animal models may be needed.

These items are covered in greater detail in the S6 guidance document and in a review by Ryffel (1997)

So, given the above discussion, what should the toxicology testing package of a typical rDNA protein resemble? Based on the products that have successfully wound their way through the regulatory process, the following generalizations can be drawn:

- The safety tests look remarkably similar to those for traditional tests. Most have been done on three species: the rat, the dog, or the monkey. The big difference has to do with the length of the test. It is rare for a safety test on a protein to be more than 13 weeks long.

- The dosing regimens can be quite variable and at times very technique-intensive. These chemicals are almost always administered by a parenteral route of administration; normally intravenously or subcutaneously. Dosing regimens have run the range from once every two weeks for an antihormone "vaccine" to continuous infusion for a short-lived protein.

- As reviewed by Ryffel (1996) most side effects in humans of a therapy with rDNA therapy may be predicted by data from experimental toxicology studies, but there are exceptions. IL-6 for example, induced a sustained increase in blood platelets and acute phase proteins, with no increase in body temperature. In human trials, however, there were increases in temperature.

- The S6 document also mentions monoclonal antibody products. Indeed, many of the considerations for rDNA products are also applicable to monoclonal antibodies (including hybridized antibodies). With monoclonal antibodies, there is the additional concern of crossreactivity with nontarget molecules.

As mentioned, the rapid development in the biotechnology industry has created some confusion as to what arm of the FDA is responsible for such products. In October 1992, the two major reviewing groups, CBER and CDER, reached a series of agreements to explain and organize the FDA's position on products that did not easily fall into its traditional classification schemes. CDER will continue to have responsibility for traditional chemically synthesized molecules as well as those purified from mineral or plant sources (except allergenics), antibiotics, hormones (including insulin, growth hormone, etc.), most fungal or bacterial products (disaccharidase inhibitors), and most products from animal or solid human tissue sources. CBER will have responsibility for products subject to licensure (BLA), including all vaccines, human blood or blood-derived products (as well as drugs used for blood banking and transfusion), immunoglobulin products, products containing intact cells, fungi, viruses, proteins produced by cell culture or transgenic animals, and synthetic allergenic products. This situation was further simplified by the introduction of the concept of "well-characterized" biologics. When introduced during the debate on FDA reform in 1996, the proposed section of S.1447 stated that "Biological products that the secretary determines to be well-characterized shall be regulated solely under the Federal Food, Drug and Cosmetic Act." Under this concept, highly purified, well-characterized therapeutic rDNA proteins would be regulated by CDER, regardless of therapeutic target (Anon. 1996).

### 2.7.5. Toxicity/Safety Testing: Cellular and Gene Therapy Products

Human clinical trials of cellular and gene therapies involve administration to patients of materials considered investigational biological, drug or device products. Somatic cell therapy refers to the administration to humans of autologous, allogeneic or xenogenic cells which have been manipulated or processed *ex vivo*. Gene therapy refers to the introduction into the human body of genes or cells containing genes foreign to the body for the purposes of prevention, treatment, diagnosing or curing disease.

Sponsors of cellular or gene therapy clinical trials must file an Investigational New Drug Application (IND) or in certain cases an Investigational Device Exemption (IDE) with the FDA before initiation of studies in humans. It is the responsibility of the Center of Biologics Evaluation and Research (CBER) to review the application and determine if the submitted data and the investigational product meet applicable standards. The critical parameters of identity, purity, potency, stability, consistency, safety and efficacy relevant to biological products are also relevant to cellular and gene therapy products.

In 1991, FDA first published a Points to Consider document on human somatic cell and gene therapy. At this time virtually all gene therapies were retroviral and were prepared as *ex vivo* somatic cell therapies. This was subsequently reviewed by Kessler et al. (1993). While the data for certain categories of information such as the data regarding the molecular biology were defined in previous guidance documents relating to recombinant DNA products, the standards for preclinical and clinical development were less well-defined. Over the past five years, the field has advanced to include not only new vectors but also novel routs of administration. The *Points to Consider on Human Somatic Cell and Gene Therapy* (1996) has thus been recently amended to reflect both the advancements in product development and more important, the accumulation of safety information over the past five years.

FDA regulations state that the sponsor must submit, in the IND, adequate information about pharmacological and toxicological studies of the drug including laboratory animals or *in vitro* studies on the basis of which the sponsor has considered that it is reasonably safe to conduct the proposed clinical investigation. For cellular and gene therapies, designing and conducting relevant preclinical safety testing has been a challenge to both FDA and the sponsor. For genes delivered using viral vectors, the safety of the vector system per se must be considered and evaluated.

The preclinical knowledge base is initially developed by designing studies to answer fundamental questions. The development of this knowledge base is generally applicable to most pharmaceuticals as well as biopharmaceuticals, and include data to support (1) the relationship of the dose to the biological activity, (2) the relationship of the dose to the toxicity, (3) the effect of route and/or schedule on activity or toxicity and (4) identification of the potential risks for subsequent clinical studies. These questions are considered in the context of indication and/or disease state. In addition there are often unique concerns related to the specific category or product class.

For cellular therapies safety concerns may include development of a data base from studies specifically designed to answer questions relating to growth factor dependence, tumorigenicity, local and systemic toxicity, and effects on host immune responses including immune activation and altered susceptibility to disease. For viral-mediated gene therapies, specific questions may relate to the potential for overexpression of the transduced gene, transduction of normal cells and tissues, genetic transfer to germ cells and subsequent alterations to the genome, recombination or rescue with endogenous virus, reconstitutions of replication competence, potential for insertional mutagenesis or malignant transformation, altered susceptibility to disease, and/or potential risk(s) to the environment.

To date, cellular and gene therapy products submitted to FDA have included clinical studies indicated for bone marrow marking, cancer, cystic fibrosis, AIDS, and inborn errors of metabolism and infectious diseases. Of the current active INDs approximately 78% have been sponsored by individual investigators or academic institutions and 22% have also been industry sponsored. In addition to the variety of clinical indications the cell types have also been varied. Examples include tumor infiltrating lymphocytes (TIL) and lymphocyte activated killer (LAK) cells, selected cells from bone marrow and peripheral blood lymphocytes, for example, stem cells, myoblasts, tumor cells and encapsulated cells (e.g., islet cells and adrenal chromaffin cells).

***Cellular Therapies.*** Since 1984 CBER has reviewed close to 300 somatic cell therapy protocols. Examples of the specific categories include manipulation, selection, mobilization, tumor vaccines and other.

*Manipulation.* Autologous, allogenic, or xenogenic cells which have been expanded, propagated, manipulated or had their biological characteristics altered *ex vivo* (e.g., TIL or LAK cells; islet cells housed in a membrane).

*Selection.* Products designed for positive or negative selection of autologous or allogenic cells intended for therapy (e.g., purging of tumor from bone marrow, selection of CD34+ cells).

*Mobilization. In vivo* mobilization of autologous stem cells intended for transplantation.

*Tumor Vaccines.* Autologous or allogenic tumor cells which are administered as vaccine (e.g., tumor cell lines; tumor cell lysates; primary explant). This group also includes autologous antigen presenting cells pulsed with tumor specific peptides or tumor cell lysates.

*Other.* Autologous, allogenic, and xenogenic cells which do not specifically fit above. This group includes cellular therapies such as extracorporeal liver assist devices.

***Gene Therapies.*** The types of vectors that have been used, or proposed, for gene transduction include retrovirus, adenovirus, adeno-associated viruses, other viruses (e.g., herpes, vaccinia, etc.), and plasmid DNA. Methods for gene introduction include *ex vivo* replacement, drug delivery, marker studies, and others and *in vivo*, viral vectors, plasmid vectors, and vector producer cells.

*Ex vivo*

*Replacement.* Cells transduced with a vector expressing a normal gene in order to correct or replace the function of a defective gene.

*Drug Delivery.* Cells transduced with a vector expressing a gene encoding a therapeutic molecule which can be novel or native to the host.

*Marker Studies.* Cells (e.g., bone marrow, stem cells) transduced with a vector expressing a marker or reporter gene used to distinguish it from other similar host tissues.

*Other.* Products that do not specifically fit under the above (e.g., tumor vaccines in which cells are cultured or transduced *ex vivo* with a vector).

*In vivo*

*Viral Vectors.* The direct administration of a viral vector (e.g., retrovirus, adenovirus, adeno-associated virus, herpes, vaccinia) to patients.

*Plasmid Vectors.* The direct administration of plasmid vectors with or without other vehicles (e.g., lipids) to patients.

*Vector Producer Cells.* The direct administration of retroviral vector producer cells (e.g., murine cells producing HTK vector) to patients.

***Preclinical Safety Evaluation.*** The goal of preclinical safety evaluation includes recommendation of an initial safe starting dose and safe dose-escalation scheme in humans, identification of potential target organ(s) of toxicity, identification of appropriate parameters for clinical monitoring and identification of "at risk" patient population(s). Therefore, when feasible, toxicity studies should be performed in relevant species to assess a dose-limiting toxicity. General considerations in study design include selection of the model (e.g., species, alternative model, animal model or disease), dose (e.g., route, frequency and duration) and study endpoint (e.g., activity and/or toxicity).

The approach to preclinical safety evaluation of biotechnology-derived products, including novel cellular and gene therapies, has been referred to as the "case-by case" approach. This approach is science-based, data-driven and flexible. The major distinction from past practices with traditional pharmaceuticals is that the focus is directed at asking specific questions across various product categories. Additionally, there is a consistent re-evaluation of the knowledge base to reassess real or theoretical safety concerns and hence re-evaluation of the need to answer the same questions across all product categories. In some cases there may even be conditions which may not need specific toxicity studies, for example, when there is a strong efficacy model which is rationally designed to answer specific questions and/or there is previous human experience with a similar product with respect to dose and regimen.

***Basic Principles for Preclinical Safety Evaluation of Cellular and Gene Therapies.*** For biotechnology-derived products in general

- Use of product in animal studies that is comparable or the same as the product proposed for clinical trial(s);
- Adherence to basic principles of GLP to ensure quality of the study including a detailed protocol prepared prospectively.
- Use of the same or similar route and method of administration as proposed for clinical trials (whenever possible).

- Determination of appropriate doses delivered based upon preliminary activity obtained from both *in vitro* and *in vivo* studies (i.e., finding a dose likely to be effective yet not dangerous, no observed adverse effect level, and a dose causing dose-limiting toxicity).
- Selection of one or more species sensitive to the endpoint being measured, for example, infections or pathologic sequelae and/or biological activity or receptor binding.
- Consideration of animal model(s) of disease may be better to assess the contribution of changes in physiologic or underlying physiology to safety and efficacy.
- Determination of effect on host immune response.
- Localization/distribution studies: evaluation of target tissue, normal surrounding tissue and distal tissue sites and any alteration in normal or expected distribution.
- Local reactogenicity.

*Additional Considerations for Cellular Therapies*

- Evaluation of cytopathogenicity.
- Evaluation of signs of cell transformation/growth factor dependence-effect on animal cells, normal human cells and cells prone to transform easily.
- Determination of alteration in cell phenotype, altered cell products and/or function.
- Tumorigenicity.

*Additional Considerations for Gene Therapies*

- Determination of phenotype/activation state of effector cells.
- Determination of vector/transgene toxicity.
- Determination of potential transfer to germ line.
- *In vitro* challenge studies: evaluation of recombination or complementation, potential for "rescue" for subsequent infection with wild-type virus.
- Determination of persistence of cells/vector.
- Determination of potential for insertional mutagenesis (malignant transformation).
- Determination of environmental spread (e.g., viral shedding).

## 2.8. TOXICITY TESTING: SPECIAL CASES

On paper, the general case guidelines for the evaluation of the safety of drugs are relatively straightforward and well understood. However, there are also a number of special case situations under which either special rules apply or some additional requirements are relevant. The more common of these are summarized below.

### 2.8.1. Oral Contraceptives

Oral contraceptives are subject to special testing requirements. These have recently been modified so that in addition to those preclinical safety tests generally required, the following are also required (Berliner, 1974):

Three-year carcinogenicity study in beagles (this is a 1987 modification in practice from earlier FDA requirements and the 1974 publication).

A rat reproductive (Segment I) study including a demonstration of return to fertility.

### 2.8.2. Life-Threatening Diseases (Compassionate Use)

Drugs to treat life-threatening diseases are not strictly held to the sequence of testing requirements as put forth in Table 2.3 because the potential benefit on any effective therapy in these situations is so high. In the early 1990s, this situation applied to AIDS-associated diseases and cancer. The development of more effective HIV therapies (protease inhibitors) has now made cancer therapy more the focus of these considerations. Though the requirements for safety testing prior to initial human trials are unchanged, subsequent requirements are flexible and subject to negotiation and close consultation with FDA's Division of Oncology (within CDER) (FDA, 1988). This also led to modification of the early operative restrictions on drug exports (Young et al., 1959). The more recent thinking on anticancer agents has been reviewed by DeGeorge et al. (1994). The preclinical studies that will be required to support clinical trials and marketing of new anticancer agents will depend on the mechanism of action and the target clinical population. Toxicity studies in animals will be required to support initial clinical trials. These studies have multiple goals: to determine a starting dose for clinical trials, to identify target organ toxicity and assess recovery, and to assist in the design of clinical dosing regimens.

The studies should generally confirm to the protocols recommended by the National Cancer Institute as discussed by Greishaber (1991). In general, it can be assumed that most antineoplastic cytotoxic agents will be highly toxic. Two studies are essential to support initial clinical trials (IND phase) in patients with advanced disease. These are studies of 5 to 14 days in length, but with longer recovery periods. A study in rodents is required that identifies those doses that produce either life-threatening or nonlife-threatening toxicity. Using the information from this first study, a second study in nonrodents (generally the dog) is conducted to determine if the tolerable dose in rodents produces life-threatening toxicity. Doses are compared on a mg/m$^2$ basis. The starting dose in initial clinical trails is generally one-tenth of that required to produce severe toxicity in rodents (STD10) or one-tenth the highest dose in nonrodents that does not cause severe irreversible toxicity. While not required, information on pharmacokinetic parameters, especially data comparing the plasma concentration associated with toxicity in both species, is very highly regarded. Special attention is paid to organs with high cell-division rates: bone marrow, testes, lymphoid tissue testing, and GI tract. As these agents are almost always given intravenously, special attention needs to be given relatively early in development to intravenous irritation and blood compatibility study. Subsequent studies to support the New Drug Application will be highly tailored, depending on the following.

- Therapeutic indication and mechanism of action.
- The results of the initial clinical trials.
- The nature of the toxicity.
- Proposed clinical regimen.

Even at the NDA stage, toxicity studies with more than 28 days of dosing are rarely required. While not required for the IND, assessment of genotoxicity and developmental toxicity will need to be addressed. For genotoxicity, it will be important to establish the ratio between cytotoxicity and mutagenicity. *In vivo* models, for example, the mouse micronucleus test, can be particularly important in demonstrating the lack of genotoxicity at otherwise subtoxic doses. For developmental toxicity, ICH stage C-D studies (traditionally known as Segment II studies for teratogenicity in rat and rabbits) will also be necessary.

The emphasis of this discussion has been on purely cytotoxic neoplastic agents. Additional consideration must be given to cytotoxic agents that are administered under special circumstances: those that are photo-activated, delivered as liposomal emulsions, or delivered as antibody conjugates. These types of agents will require additional studies. For example, a liposomal agent will need to be compared to the free agent and a blank liposomal preparation. There are also studies that may be required for a particular class of agents. For example, anthracylcines are known to be cardiotoxic, so comparison of a new anthracylcine agent to previously marketed anthracylines will be expected.

In addition to antineoplastic, cytotoxic agents, there are cancer therapeutic or preventative drugs that are intended to be given on a chronic basis. This includes chemopreventatives, hormonal agents, immunomodulators, and so on. The toxicity assessment studies on these will more closely resemble those of more traditional pharmaceutical agents. Chronic toxicity, carcinogenicity, and full developmental toxicity (ICH A-B, C-D, E-F) assessments will be required. For a more complete review, the reader is referred to DeGeorge et al. (1998).

### 2.8.3. Optical Isomers

The FDA (and similar regulatory agencies, as reviewed by Daniels et al., 1997) has become increasingly concerned with the safety of stereoisomeric or chiral drugs. Stereoisomers are molecules that are identical to one another in terms of atomic formula and covalent bonding, but differ in the three-dimensional projections of the atoms. Within this class are those molecules that are nonsuperimposable mirror images of one another. These are called enantiomers (normally designated as R- or S-). Enantiometric pairs of a molecule have identical physical and chemical characteristics except for the rotation of polarized light. Drugs have generally been mixtures of optical isomers (enantiomers), because of the difficulties in separating the isomers. It has become apparent in recent years, however, that these different isomers may have different degrees of both desirable therapeutic and undesirable toxicologic effects. Technology has also improved to the extent that it is now possible to perform chiral specific syntheses, separations, and/or analyses. It is now highly desirable from a regulatory (FDA, 1988; Anon., 1992a) basis to develop a single isomer unless all isomers have equivalent pharmacological and toxicologic activity. The FDA has divided enantiometric mixtures into the following categories.

- Both isomers have similar pharmacologic activity, which could be identical, or they could differ in the degrees of efficacy.
- One isomer is pharmacologically active, while the other is inactive.
- Each isomer has completely different activity.

During preclinical assessment of an enantiometric mixture, it may be important to determine to which of these three classes it belongs. The pharmacological and toxicological properties of the individual isomers should be characterized. The pharmacokinetic profile of each isomer should be characterized in animal models with regard to disposition and interconversion. It is not at all unusual for each enantiomer to have a completely different pharmacokinetic behavior.

If the test article is an enantiomer isolated from a mixture that is already well characterized (e.g., already on the market), then appropriate bridging guides need to be performed which compare the toxicity of the isomer to that of the racemic mixture. The most common approach would be to conduct a subchronic (three months) and a Sement II-type teratology study with an appropriate "positive" control group which received the racemate. In most instances no additional studies would be required if the enantiomer and the racemate did not differ in toxicity profile. If, on the other hand, differences are identified, that the reasons for this difference need to be investigated and the potential implications for human subjects need to be considered.

### 2.8.4. Special Populations: Pediatric and Geriatric Claims

Relatively few drugs marketed in the United States (approximately 20%) have pediatric dosing information available. Clinical trials had rarely been done specifically on pediatric patients. Traditionally, dosing regimens for children have been derived empirically by extrapolating on the basis of body weight or surface area. This approach assumes that the pediatric patient is a young adult, which simply may not be the case. There are many examples of how adults and children differ qualitatively in metabolic and/or pharmacodynamic responses to pharmaceutical agents. In their review, Schacter and DeSantis state

> The benefit of having appropriate usage information in the product label is that health care practitioners are given the information necessary to administer drugs and biologics in a manner that maximizes safety, minimizes unexpected adverse events, and optimizes treatment efficacy. Without specific knowledge of potential drug effects, children may be placed at risk. In addition, the absence of appropriate proscribing information, drugs and biologics that represent new therapeutic advances may not be administered to the pediatric population in a timely manner—Schacter and Desartis (1998).

In response to the need for pediatric information, the FDA developed a pediatric plan. This two-phase plan called first for the development of pediatric information on marketed drugs. The second phase focused on new drugs. The implementation of the plan was to be coordinated by the Pediatric Subcommittee of the Medical Policy Coordinating Committee of CDER. The Pediatric Use Labeling Rule was a direct result of phase 1 in 1994. (Anon., 1998b). Phase 2 resulted in 1997 from a proposed rule entitled Pediatric Patients; Regulations Requiring Manufacturers to Assess the Safety and Effectiveness of New Drugs and Biologics. Soon after this rule was proposed, the FDA Modernization Act of 1997 was passed. FDAMA contained provisions that specifically addressed the needs and requirements for the development of drugs for the pediatric population.

The FDAMA bill essentially codified and expanded several regulatory actions initiated by the FDA during the 1990s. Among the incentives offered by the bill, companies will be offered an additional six months of patent protection for performing pediatric studies (clinical trials) on already approved products. In fact, the FDA was mandated by FDAMA to develop a list of over 500 drugs for which additional information would produce benefits for pediatric patients. The FDA is supposed to provide a written request for pediatric studies to the manufacturers (Hart, 1999).

In response to the pediatric initiatives, the FDA has published policies and guidelines and conducted a variety of meetings. CDER has established a web site (http//www.fda.gov/cder/pediatric) which lists three pages of such information. Interestingly, the focus has been on clinical trials, and almost no attention has been given to the preclinical toxicology studies that may be necessary to support such trials. There are three pages of documents on the pediatric web site. None appear to address the issue of appropriate testing. This is a situation that is just now being addressed and is in a great deal of flux.

In the absence of any guidelines from the Agency for testing drugs in young or "pediatric" animals, one must fall back on the maxim of designing a program that makes the most scientific sense. As a guide, the FDA designated levels of post-natal human development and the approximate equivalent ages (in the author's considered opinion) in various animal models are given in Table 2.9. The table is somewhat

**TABLE 2.9. Comparison of Postnatal Development Stages**

| Stage | Human | Rat | Dog | Pig |
|---|---|---|---|---|
| Neonate | Birth to 1 month | Birth–1 week | Birth–3 weeks | Birth–2 weeks |
| Infant | 1 month to 2 years | 1 week–3 weeks | 3 weeks–6 weeks | 2 weeks–4 weeks |
| Child | 2 years to 12 years | 3 weeks– 9 weeks | 6 weeks– 5 months | 4 weeks to 4 months |
| Adolescent | 12 years to 16 years | 9 weeks– 13 weeks | 5 months– 9 months | 4 months– 7 months |
| Adult | Over 16 years | Over 13 weeks | Over 9 months | Over 7 months |

inaccurate, however, because of difference in the stages of development at birth. A rat is born quite underdeveloped when compared to a human being. A one-day old rat is not equivalent to a one-day old full-term human infant. A four-day old rat would be more appropriate. In terms of development, the pig may be the best model of those listed; however, one should bear in mind that different organs have different developmental schedules in different species.

Table 2.9 can be used as a rough guide in designing toxicity assessment experiments in developing animals. In designing of the treatment period, one needs to consider, not only the dose and the proposed course of clinical treatment, but also the proposed age of the patient, and whether or not an equivalent dosing period in the selected animal model covers more than one developmental stage. For example, if the proposed patient population is human infants, initiating a toxicity study of the new pharmaceutical agent in three-day-old rats is not appropriate. Furthermore, if the proposed course of treatment in adult children is two weeks, it is unlikely that this would crossover into a different developmental stage. A two-week treatment initiated in puppies, however, might easily span two developmental stages. Thus, in designing an experiment in young animals, one must carefully consider the length of the treatment period balancing the developmental age of the animal model and the proposed length of clinical treatment. Where appropriate (infant animals), one needs to also assess changes in standard developmental landmarks, (e.g., eye opening, pinae eruption, external genitalia development, etc.) as well as the more standard indicators of target organ toxicity. The need for maintaining the experimental animals past the dosing period, perhaps into sexual maturity, to assess recovery or delayed effects needs also to be carefully considered.

To summarize, the current status of assessment of toxicity in postnatal mammals, in response to the pediatric initiatives covered in FDAMA, is an extremely fluid situation. One needs to carefully consider a variety of factors in designing the study and should discuss proposed testing programs with the appropriate office at CDER.

Drugs intended for use in the elderly, like those intended for the very young, may also have special requirements for safety evaluation, but geriatric issues were not addressed in the FDAMA of 1997. The FDA has published a separate guidance document for geriatric labeling. As was the case with pediatric guidance, this document does not address preclinical testing. With the elderly, the toxicological concerns are quite different than the developmental concerns associated with pediatric patients: One must be concerned with the possible interactions between the test article and compromised organ function. The FDA had previously issued a guidance for clinically examining clinical safety of new pharmaceutical agents in patients with compromised renal and/or hepatic function (CDER, 1989). The equivalent ICH Guideline (S5A) was issued in 1994. Whether this type of emphasis will require toxicity testing in animal models with specifically induced organ insufficiency remains to be seen. In the interim, we must realize that there is tacit evaluation of test article-related toxicity in geriatric rodents for those agents that undergo two-year carcinogenicity testing. As the graying of America continues, labeling for geriatric use may become more of an issue in the future.

### 2.8.5. Orphan Drugs

The development of sophisticated technologies, coupled with the rigors and time required for clinical and preclinical testing has made pharmaceutical development very expensive. In order to recoup such expenses, pharmaceutical companies have tended to focus on therapeutic agents with large potential markets. Treatment for rare but life-threatening diseases have been "orphaned" as a result. An orphan product is defined as one targeted at a disease which affects 200,000 or fewer individuals in the United States. Alternatively, the therapy may be targeted for more than 200,000 but the developer would have no hope of recovering the initial investment without exclusivity. The Orphan Drug Act of 1983 was passed in an attempt to address this state of affairs. Currently applicable regulations were put in place in 1992 (Anon, 1992). In 1994, there was an attempt in Congress to amend the Act, but it failed to be passed into law. The current regulations are administered by the office of Orphan Product Development (OPD). The act offers the following incentives to encourage the development of products to treat rare diseases.

- Seven years exclusive market following the approval of a product for an orphan disease.
- Written protocol assistance from the FDA.
- Tax credits for up 50% of qualified clinical research expenses.
- Available grant to support pivotal clinical trials.

As reviewed by Haffner (1998), other developed countries have similar regulations.

The ODA did not change the requirements of testing drug products. The nonclinical testing programs are similar to those used for more conventional products. They will undergo the same FDA review process. A major difference, however, is the involvement of the OPD. A sponsor must request OPD review. Once OPD determines that a drug meets the criteria for orphan drug status it will work with the sponsor to provide the assistance required under the Act. The ODA does not review a product for approval. The IND/NDA process is still handled by the appropriate reviewing division (e.g., Cardiovascular) for formal review. The Act does not waive the necessity for submission of an IND, nor for the responsibility of toxicological assessment. As always, in cases where there is ambiguity, a sponsor may be well-served to request a pre-IND meeting at the appropriate Division to discuss the acceptability of a toxicology assessment plan.

### 2.8.6. Botanical Drug Products

There is an old saying, "what goes around, comes around" and so it is with botanicals. At the beginning of the twentieth century, most marketed pharmaceutical agents were botanical in origin. For example, aspirin was first isolated from willow bark. These led the way in the middle part of the century, for reasons having to do with patentability, manufacturing costs, standardization, selectivity, and potency. The dawning of the twenty-first century has seen a grass roots return to botanical preparations (also sold as herbals or dietary supplements). These preparations are being marketed to the lay public as "natural" supplements to the nasty synthetic chemicals now proscribed as pharmaceutical products. In 1994, the Dietary Supplement Health and Education Act was passed which permitted the marketing of dietary supplements (including botanicals) with limited submissions to the FDA. (Wu et al., 2000). If a producer makes a claim that a herbal preparation is beneficial to a specific part of the body (e.g., enhanced memory), then it may be marketed after a 75-day period of FDA review but without formal approval. On the other hand, if any curative properties are claimed, then the botanical will be regulated as a drug and producers will be required to follow the IND/NDA process. In 1997 and 1998 combined, some 26 INDs were filed for botanical products. (Wu et al., 2000).

The weakness in the current regulation has to do with its ambiguity. The line between a beneficial claim and a curative claim is sometimes difficult to draw. What is the difference, for example, between an agent that enhances memory and one that prevents memory loss? Given the number of products and claims hitting the shelves every day, this situation will probably demand increased regulatory scrutiny in the future.

### 2.9. INTERNATIONAL PHARMACEUTICAL REGULATION AND REGISTRATION

### 2.9.1. International Conference on Harmonization

The International Conference on Harmonization (ICH) of Technical Requirements for Registration of Pharmaceuticals for Human Use was established to make the drug-regulatory process more efficient in the United States, Europe, and Japan. The U.S. involvement grew out of the fact that the United States is party to the General Agreement on Tariffs and Trade, which included the Agreement on Technical Barriers to Trade, negotiated in the 1970s, to encourage reduction of nontariff barriers to trade. (Barton, 1998). The main purpose of ICH is, through harmonization, to make new medicines available to patients with a minimum of delay. More recently, the need to harmonize regulation has been driven, according to ICH, by the

**TABLE 2.10. ICH Representation[a]**

| Country/Region | Regulatory | Industry |
|---|---|---|
| European Union | European Commission (2) | European Federation of Pharmaceutical Industries Associations (2) |
| Japan | Ministry of Health and Welfare (2) | Japanese Pharmaceutical Manufactures Association (2) |
| United States | Food and Drug Administration (2) | Pharmaceutical Research and Manufacturers of America (2) |
| Observing organizations | World Health Organization, European Free Trade Area, Canadian Health Protection Branch | International Federation of Pharmaceutical Manufactures Associations (2): also provides the secretariat. |

[a]( ) = number of representatives on the ICH steering Committee.

escalation of the cost of R&D. The regulatory systems in all countries have the same fundamental concerns about safety, efficacy, and quality, yet sponsors had to repeat many time-consuming and expensive technical tests to meet country-specific requirements. Secondarily, there was a legitimate concern over the unnecessary use of animals. Conference participants include representatives from the drug-regulatory bodies and research-based pharmaceutical industrial organizations of three regions; the European Union, the United States and Japan were over 90% of the world's pharmaceutical industry. Representation is summarized on Table 2.10. The biennial conference has met four times, beginning in 1991, rotating between sites in the United States, Europe, and Japan.

The ICH meets its objectives by issuing guidelines for the manufacturing, development, and testing of new pharmaceutical agents that are acceptable to all three major parties. For each new guideline, the ICH Steering Committee establishes an expert working group with representation from each of the six major participatory ICH bodies. Each new draft guideline goes through the five various steps of review and revision summarized in Table 2.11. So far, ICH has proposed or adopted over 40 safety, efficacy, and quality guidelines (listed in Table 2.12) for use by the drug-

**TABLE 2.11. Steps in ICH Guideline Development and Implementation**

| Step | Action |
|---|---|
| 1 | Building scientific consensus in joint regulatory/industry expert working groups |
| 2 | Agreement by the steering committee to release the draft consensus text for wider consultation |
| 3 | Regulatory consultation in the three regions. Consolidation of the comments |
| 4 | Agreement on a harmonized ICH guideline; adopted by the regulators |
| 5 | Implementation in the three ICH regions |

**TABLE 2.12. International Conference on Harmonization Guidelines**

| Ref. | Guideline | Date |
|---|---|---|
| E1 | The extent of population exposure to assess clinical safety | Oct 94 |
| E2A | Clinical safety data management: Definitions and standards for expedited reporting | Oct 94 |
| E2B | Guideline on Clinical Safety Data Management; Notice | Jan 98 |
| E2C | Clinical safety data management: Periodic safety update reports for marketed drugs | May 97 |
| E3 | Structure and content of clinical study reports | Nov 95 |
| E4 | Dose response information to support drug registration | Mar 94 |
| E5 | Ethnic factors in the acceptability of foreign clinical data | Feb 98 |
| E6 | Good Clinical Practice: Consolidated Guideline; Notice of Availability | May 97 |
| E6A | GCP Addendum on investigator's brochure | Mar 95 |
| E6B | GCP: Addendum on essential documents for the conduct of a clinical trial | Oct 94 |
| E7 | Studies in support of special populations: geriatrics | Jun 93 |
| E8 | Guidance on General Considerations for Clinical Trials; Notice | Dec. 97 |
| E9 | Draft Guideline on Statistical Principles for Clinical Trials; Notice of Availability | May 97 |
| M3 | Guidance on Nonclinical Safety Studies for the Conduct of Human Clinical Trials for Pharmaceuticals; Notice | Nov 97 |
| Q1A | Stability testing of new drug substances and products | Oct 93 |
| Q1B | Stability testing | |
| Q1C | Stability testing | |
| Q2A | Validation of analytical procedures: definitions and terminology | Oct 94 |
| Q2B | Validation of analytical procedures: methodology | |
| Q3A | Guideline on Impurities in New Drug Substances | Mar 95 |
| Q3B | Guideline on Impurities in New Drug Products; Availability; Notice | May 97 |
| Q3C | Guideline on Impurities: Residual Solvents; Availability; Notice | Dec 97 |
| Q5A | Quality of biotechnological products. Viral safety evaluation of biotechnology products derived from cell lines of human or animal origin | |
| Q5B | Quality of biotechnology products, analysis of the expression construct in cells used for production of r-DNA derived protein product | Nov 95 |
| Q5C | Quality of biotechnological products: stability testing of biotechnological/Biology products | Nov 95 |
| Q5D | Availability of Draft Guideline on Quality of Biotechnological/Biological Products: Derivation and Characterization of Cell Substrates Used for Production of Biotechnological/Biological Products; Notice | May 97 |
| Q6A | Draft Guidance on Specifications: Test Procedures and Acceptance Criteria for New Drug Substances and New Drug Products: Chemical Substances; Notice | Nov 97 |

**TABLE 2.12.** (*continued*)

| Q6B | Specifications: Test Procedures and Acceptance Criteria for Biotechnology Products | Feb 98 |
|---|---|---|
| S1A | Guidance on the need for carcinogenicity studies of pharmaceuticals | Nov 95 |
| S1B | Draft Guideline on Testing for Carcinogenicity of Pharmaceuticals; Notice | Nov 98 |
| S1C | Dose selection for carcinogenicity studies of pharmaceuticals | Oct 94 |
| S1Ca | Guidance on Dose Selection for Carcinogenicity Studies of Pharmaceuticals: Addendum on a Limit Dose and Related Notes; Availability; Notice | Dec 97 |
| S2A | Genotoxicity: Guidance on specific aspects of regulatory genotoxicity tests for pharmaceuticals | Jul 95 |
| S2B | Guidance on Genotoxicity: A Standard Battery for Genotoxicity Testing of Pharmaceuticals; Availability; Notice | Nov 97 |
| S3A | Toxicokinetics: Guidance on the assessment of systemic exposure in toxicity studies | Oct 94 |
| S3B | Pharmacokinetics: Guidance for repeated dose tissue distribution studies | Oct 94 |
| S4 | Single Dose Acute Toxicity Testing for Pharmaceuticals; Revised Guidance; Availability; Notice | Aug 96 |
| S4A | Draft Guidance on the Duration of Chronic Toxicity Testing in Animals (Rodent and Nonrodent Toxicity Testing); Availability; Notice | Nov 97 |
| S5A | Detection of toxicity to reproduction for medicinal products | Jun 93 |
| S5B | Reproductive toxicity to male fertility | |
| S6A | Guidance on Preclinical Safety Evaluation of Biotechnology-Derived Pharmaceuticals; Availability | Nov 97 |

regulatory agencies in the United States, Europe, and Japan. The guidelines are organized under broad categories: the "E" series having to do with clinical trials, the "Q" series having to do with quality (including chemical manufacturing and control as well as traditional GLP issues), and the "S" series having to do with safety. Guidelines may be obtained from the ICH secretariat, c/o IFPMA, 30 rue de St.-Jean, PO Box 9, 1211 Geneva 18, Switzerland, or may be down-loaded from a website set up by Ms. Nancy McClure (http://www.mcclurenet.com/index.html). They are also published in the *Federal Register*. The guidelines of the "S" series will have the most impact on toxicologists. The biggest changes having to do with toxicological assessment are summarized as follows.

*Carcinogenicity Studies.* Carcinogenicity studies are covered in Guidelines S1A, S1B, and S1C. The guidelines are almost more philosophical than they are technical. In comparison to the EPA guidelines for example, the ICH guidelines contain little in the way on concrete study criteria (e.g., the number of animals, the necessity for clinical chemistry, etc.). There is discussion on when carcinogenicity studies should be done, whether two species are more appropriate than one, and how to set dosages on the basis of human clinical PK data. The major changes being wrought by these guidelines are

- Only one two-year carcinogenicity study should be generally required. Ideally, the species chosen should be the one most like man in terms of metabolic transformations of the test article.
- The traditional second long-term carcinogenicity study can be replaced by a shorter-term alternative model. In practical terms, this guideline is beginning to result in sponsors conducting a two-year study in the rat and a six-month study in an alternative mouse model, such as the P53 or the TG.AC genetically manipulated mouse strains.
- In the absence of target organ toxicity with which to set the high dose at the maximally tolerated dose, the high dose can be set at the dose that produces an area under the curve (AUC). This is 25-fold higher than that obtained in human subjects.

*Chronic Toxicity.* Traditionally, chronic toxicity of new pharmaceuticals in the United States was assessed in studies of one-year duration in both the rodent and the nonrodent species of choice. The European view was that studies of six months are generally sufficient. The resulting guideline (S4A) was a compromise. Studies of six months duration were recommended for the rodent, as rodents would also be examined in two-year studies. For the nonrodent (dog, nonhuman primate, and pig) studies of nine months duration were recommended.

*Developmental and Reproductive Toxicity.* This was an area in which there was considerable international disagreement and the area in which ICH has promulgated the most technically detailed guidelines (S5A and S5B). Some of the major changes include:

- The traditional Segment I, II, and III nomenclature has been replaced with different nomenclature, as summarized in Table 2.13.
- The dosing period of the pregnant animals during studies on embryonic development (traditional Segment II studies) has been standardized.
- New guidelines for fertility assessment (traditional Segment I) studies that have shortened the premating dosing schedule (for example, in male rats from 10 weeks to 4 weeks). There has been an increased interest in assessment of spermatogenesis and sperm function.
- The new guidelines allow for a combination of studies in which the endpoint typically assessed in the traditional Segment II and Segment III studies are now examined under a single protocol.

For a more complete review of the various study designs, the reader is refereed to the review by Manson (1994).

While they were not quite as sweeping in approach as the aforementioned guidelines, a toxicologist working in pharmaceutical safety assessment should become familiar with the all the other ICH Guidelines in the S series.

In an interesting recent article, Ohno (1998) discussed not only the harmonization of nonclinical guidelines, but also the need to harmonize the timing of nonclinical tests in relation to the conduct of clinical trials. For example, there are regional differences in the inclusion of women of childbearing potential in clinical trials. In the United States including woman in such trials is becoming more important, and therefore evaluation of embryo and fetal development will occur earlier in the drug development process than in Japan. Whether or not such timing or staging of nonclinical tests becomes part of an ICH guideline in the near future remains to be established.

### 2.9.2. Other International Considerations

The United States is the single largest pharmaceutical market in the world. But the rest of the world (particularly, but not limited to the second and third largest markets, Japan and the European Union) represents in aggregate a much larger market, so no one develops a new pharmaceutical for marketing in just the United States. The effort at harmonization (exemplified by the International Conference on Harmonization, or ICH) has significantly reduced differences in requirements for these other countries, but certainly not obliterated them. Though a detailed understanding of their regulatory schemes is beyond this volume, the bare bones and differences in toxicology requirements are not.

***European Union.*** The standard European Union toxicology and pharmacologic data requirements for a pharmaceutical include

Single-dose toxicity;

Repeat-dose toxicity (subacute and chronic trials);

Reproduction studies (fertility and general reproductive performance, embryotoxicity and peri/postnatal toxicity);

Mutagenic potential (*in vitro* and *in vivo*);

Carcinogenicity;

Pharmacodynamics:

Effects related to proposed drug indication;

General pharmacodynamics;

Drug interactions;

Pharmacokinetics:

Single dose;

Repeat dose;

**TABLE 2.13. Comparison of Traditional and ICH Guidelines for Reproductive and Developmental Toxicology**

| Traditional protocol | Stages covered | ICH Protocol | Dosing regimen |
| --- | --- | --- | --- |
| Segment I (rats) | A. Premating to conception | Fertility and early embryonic development, including implantation | Males: 4 weeks pre-mating, mating (1–3 weeks) plus 3 weeks post-mating |
| | B. Conception to implantation | | Females: 2 weeks premating, mating through day 7 of gestation |
| Segment II (rabbits) | C. Implantation to closure of hard palate | Embryo-fetal development | Female Rabbits: Day 6 to Day 20 of pregnancy |
| | D. Closure of hard palate to the end of pregnancy | | |

| Study Title | Termination | Endpoints: In-life | Endpoints: postmortem |
| --- | --- | --- | --- |
| Fertility and early embryonic development, including implantation | Females: Day 13 to 15 of pregnancy<br>Males: Day after completion of dosing | Clinical signs and mortality<br>Body weights and feed intake<br>Vaginal cytology | Macroscopic exam + histo on gross lesions<br>Collection of reproductive organs for possible histology<br>Quantitation of corpa lutea and implantation sites<br>Seminology (ocunt, motility and morphology) |

| Embryo-fetal development | Clinical signs and mortality | Macroscopic exam + histo on gross lesions |
| | | Quantitation of corpa lutea and implantation sites |
| | | Fetal body weights |
| | | Fetal abnormalities |
| Pre- and post-natal development, including maternal function | Clinical signs and mortality | Macroscopic exam + histo on gross lesions |
| | Body weights and changes | Implantation |
| | Feed intake | Abnormalities (including terata) |
| | Duration of pregnancy | Live/dead offspring at birth |
| | Parturition | Pre-and post-weaning survival and growth $(F_1)$ |
| | | Physical development $(F_1)$ |
| | | Sensory functions and reflexes $(F_1)$ |
| | | Behavior $(F_1)$ |

Distribution in normal and pregnant animals;

Biotransformation;

Local tissue tolerance;

Environmental toxicity.

In general, the registration process in the EU allows one to either apply to an overall medicines authority or to an individual national authority. Either of these steps is supposed to lead to mutual recognition by all the individual members.

***Japan.*** In Japan, the Koseisho is the national regulatory body for new drugs.

The standard $LD_{50}$ test is no longer a regulatory requirement for new medicines in the United States, the European Union, or Japan. The Japanese guidelines were the first to be amended in accordance with this agreement, with the revised guidelines becoming effective in August 1993. The Japanese may still anticipate that single dose (acute) toxicity studies should be conducted in at least two species, one rodent and one nonrodent (the rabbit is not accepted as a nonrodent). Both males and females should be included from at least one of the species selected: if the rodent, then a minimum of 5 per sex; if the nonrodent, at least two per sex. In nonrodents, both the oral and parenteral routes should be used, and normally the clinical route of administration should be employed. In nonrodents, only the intended route of administration need be employed; if the intended route of administration in humans is intravenous, then use of this route in both species is acceptable. An appropriate number of doses should be employed to obtain a complete toxicity profile and to establish any dose-response relationship. The severity, onset, progression, and reversibility of toxicity should be studied during a 14-day follow-up period, with all animals being necropsied. When macroscopic changes are noted, the tissue must be subjected to histological examination.

Chronic and subchronic toxicity studies are conducted to define the dose level, when given repeatedly, that cause toxicity, and the dose level that does not lead to toxic findings. In Japan, such studies are referred to as repeated-dose toxicity studies. As with single-dose studies, at least two animal species should be used, one rodent and one nonrodent (rabbit not acceptable). In rodent studies, each group should consist of at least 10 males and 10 females; in nonrodent species, 3 of each sex are deemed adequate. Where interim examinations are planned, however, the numbers of animals employed should be increased accordingly. The planned route of administration in human subjects is normally explored. The duration of the study will be dictated by the planned duration of clinical use (Table 2.14).

At least three different dose groups should be included, with the goals of demonstrating an overtly toxic dose and a no-effect dose, and establishing any dose-response relationship. The establishment of a nontoxic dose within the framework of these studies is more rigorously adhered to in Japan than elsewhere in the world. All surviving animals should also be necropsied, either at the completion of the study or during its extension recovery period, to assess reversal of toxicity and the possible appearance of delayed toxicity. Full histological examination is

**TABLE 2.14. Planned Duration of Clinical Use**

| Duration of Dosing in Toxicity Study | Duration of Human Exposure |
| --- | --- |
| 1 month | Single dose or repeated dosage not exceeding 1 week |
| 3 months | Repeated dosing exceeding 1 week and to a maximum of 4 weeks |
| 6 months | Repeated dosing exceeding 4 weeks and to a maximum of 6 months |
| 12 months[a] | Repeated dosing exceeding 6 months or where this is deemed to be appropriate |

[a]Where carcinogenicity studies are to be conducted, the Koseisho had agreed to forego chronic dosage beyond six months.
*Source:* New Drugs Division Notification No. 43, June 1992.

mandated on all nonrodent animals used in a chronic toxicity study; at a minimum, the highest-dose and control groups of rodents must be submitted to a full histological examination.

While the value of repeated-dose testing beyond six months has been questioned (Lumley and Walker, 1992), such testing is a regulatory requirement for a number of agencies, including the U.S. FDA and the Koseisho. In Japan, repeated-dose testing for 12 months is required only for new medicines expected to be administered to humans for periods in excess of six months (Yakuji Nippo, 1994). At the First International Conference on Harmonization held in Brussels, the consensus was that 12-month toxicity studies in rodents could be reduced to six months where carcinogenicity studies are required. While not yet adopted in the Japanese guidelines, six-month repeated-dose toxicity studies have been accepted by the agencies of all three regions. Japan, like the European Union, accepts a six-month duration if accompanied by a carcinogenicity study. The United States still requires a nine-month nonrodent study.

With regard to reproductive toxicology, as a consequence of the first ICH, the United States, the European Union, and Japan agreed to recommend mutual recognition of their respective current guidelines. A tripartite, harmonized guideline on reproductive toxicology has achieved ICH Step 4 status and should be incorporated into the local regulations of all three regions soon. This agreement represents a very significant achievement that should eliminate many obstacles to drug registration.

*Preclinical Male Fertility Studies.* Before conducting a single-dose male volunteer study in Japan, it is usually necessary to have completed a preclinical male fertility study (Segment 1) that has an in-life phase of 10 or more weeks (i.e., 10 weeks of dosing, plus follow-up). Although government guidelines do not require this study to be completed before Phase 1 trials begin, the responsible Institutional Review Board or the investigator usually imposes this condition. Japanese regulatory authorities are aware that the Segment 1 male fertility study is of poor predictive value. The rat, which is used in this study, produces a marked excess of sperm. Many scientists therefore believe that the test is less sensitive than the evaluation of testicular weight and histology that constitute part of the routine toxicology assessment.

*Female Reproductive Studies.* Before entering a female into a clinical study, it is necessary to have completed the entire reproductive toxicology program, which consists of the following studies.

Segment 1: Fertility studies in the rat or mouse species used in the segment 2 program;

Segment 2: Teratology studies in the rat or mouse, and the rabbit;

Segment 3: Late gestation and lactation studies in a species used in the Segment 2 studies.

Such studies usually take approximately two years. Although the U.S. regulations state the need for completion of Segments 1 and 2, and the demonstration of efficacy in male patients, where appropriate, before entering females into a clinical program, the current trend in the United States is toward relaxation of the requirements to encourage investigation of the drug both earlier and in a larger number of females during product development. Growing pressure for the earlier inclusion of women in drug testing may encourage selection of this issue as a future ICH topic. The trend in the United States and the European Union toward including women earlier in the critical program has not yet been embraced in Japan, however.

The three tests required in Japan for genotoxicity evaluation are a bacterial gene mutation test, *in vitro* cytogenetics, and *in vivo* tests for genetic damage. The Japanese regulations state these tests to be the minimum requirement and encourage additional tests. Currently, Japanese guidelines do not require a mammalian cell gene mutation assay. Harmonization will likely be achieved by the Koseisho recommending all four tests, which will match requirements in the United States and the European Union; at present, this topic is at Step 1 in the ICH harmonization process. The mutagenicity studies should be completed before the commencement of Phase 2 clinical studies.

Guidelines presented at the second ICH are likely to alter the preclinical requirements for registration in Japan; they cover toxicokinetics and when to conduct repeated-dose tissue distribution studies. The former document may improve the ability of animal toxicology studies to predict possible adverse events in humans; currently, there are no toxicokinetic requirements in Japan, and their relevance is questioned by many there. Although there is general agreement on the registration requirement for single-dose tissue distribution studies, implementation of the repeated-dose study requirement has been inconsistent across the three ICH parties.

### 2.9.3. Safety Pharmacology

Japan was the first major country to require extensive pharmacological profiling on all new pharmaceutical agents as part of the safety assessment profile. Prior to commencement of initial clinical studies, the drug's pharmacology must be characterized in animal models. In the United States and Europe, these studies have been collectively called safety pharmacology studies. For a good general review of the issues surrounding safety pharmacology, the reader is referred to Hite (1997). The Japanese guidelines for such characterizations were published in 1991.* They include

- Effects on general activity and behavior;
- Effects on the central nervous system;
- Effects on the autonomic nervous system and smooth muscle;
- Effects on the respiratory and cardiovascular systems;
- Effects on the digestive system;
- Effects on water and electrolyte metabolism;
- Other important pharmacological effects.

In the United States, pharmacological studies in demonstration of efficacy have always been required, but specific safety pharmacological studies have never been required. Special situational or mechanistic data would be requested on a case-by-case basis. This is a situation that is changing. In the United States the activities of the Safety Pharmacology Discussion Group, for example, have helped bring attention to the utility and issues surrounding safety pharmacology data. In 1999 and 2000, the major toxicological and pharmacological societal meetings had symposia on safety pharmacological testing. Many major U.S. pharmaceutical companies are in the process of implementing programs in safety pharmacology. The issue has been taken up by ICH and the draft guideline is currently at the initial stages of review. This initial draft (Guideline S7) includes core tests in the assessment of CNS, cardiovascular and respiratory function. Studies will be expected to be performed under GLP guidelines.


## 2.10. COMBINATION PRODUCTS

Recent years have seen a vast increase in the number of new therapeutic products which are not purely drug, device, or biologic, but rather a combination of two or more of these. This leads to a problem of deciding which of the three centers shall have ultimate jurisdiction.

The Center for Devices and Radiological Health is designated the center for major policy development and for the promulgation and interpretation of procedural regulations for medical devices under the Act. The Center for Devices and Radiological Health regulates all medical devices inclusive of radiation-related devices that are not assigned categorically or specifically to CDER. In addition,

*Source:* New Drugs Division Notification No. 4, January 1991.

CDRH will independently administer the following activities (references to "Sections" here are the provisions of the Act).

1. A. Small business assistance programs under Section 10 of the amendments (See PL 94-295). Both CDER and CDRH will identify any unique problems relating to medical device regulation for small business;

   B. Registration and listing under Section 510 including some CDER administered device applications. The Center for Drug Evaluation and Research will receive printouts and other assistance, as requested;

   C. Color additives under Section 706, with review by CDER, as appropriate;

   D. Good Manufacturing Practices (GMPs) Advisory Committee. Under Section 520(f) (3), CDER will regularly receive notices of all meetings, with participation by CDER, as appropriate;

   E. Medical Device Reporting. The manufacturers, distributors, importers, and users of all devices, including those regulated by CDER, shall report to CDRH under Section 519 of the Act as required. The Center for Devices and Radiological Health will provide monthly reports and special reports as needed to CDER for investigation and follow-up of those medical devices regulated by CDER.

### 2.10.1. Device Programs that CDER and CBRH Each Will Administer

Both CDER and CDRH will administer and, as appropriate, enforce the following activities for medical devices assigned to their respective Centers (References to "Sections" are the provisions of the Act):

1. A. Surveillance and compliance actions involving general controls violations, such as misbranded or adulterated devices, under Sections 301, 501, and 502.

   B. Warning letters, seizures, injunctions, and prosecutions under Sections 302, 303, and 304.

   C. Civil penalties under Section 303(f) and administrative restraint under Section 304(g).

   D. Nonregulatory activities, such as educational programs directed at users, participation in voluntary standards organizations, and so on.

   E. Promulgation of performance standards and applications of special controls under Section 514.

   F. Premarket Notification, Investigational Device exemptions including Humanitarian Exemptions, Premarket Approval, Product Development Protocols, Classification, Device Tracking, Petitions for Reclassification, postmarket surveillance under Sections 510(k), 513, 515, 519, 520(g) and (m), and 522, and the advisory committees necessary to support these activities.

G. Banned devices under Section 516.

H. FDA-requested and firm-initiated recalls whether under Section 518 or another authority and other Section 518 remedies such as recall orders.

I. Exemptions, variances and applications of CGMP regulations under Section 520(f).

J. Government-Wide Quality Assurance Program.

K. Requests for export approval under Sections 801(e) and 802.

### 2.10.2. Coordination

The Centers will coordinate their activities in order to assure that manufacturers do not have to independently secure authorization to market their product from both Centers unless this requirement is specified in Section VII.

### 2.10.3. Submissions

Submissions should be made to the appropriate center, as specified herein, at the addresses provided:

Food and Drug Administration
Center for Drug Evaluation and Research
Central Document Room (Room 2-14)
12420 Parklawn Drive
Rockville, Maryland 20852

or

Food and Drug Administration
Center for Devices and Radiological Health
Document Mail Center (HFZ-401)
1390 Piccard Drive
Rockville, Maryland 20850

For submissions involving medical devices and/or drugs that are not clearly addressed in this agreement, sponsors arc referred to the product jurisdiction regulations (21 CFR Part 3). These regulations have been promulgated to facilitate the determination of regulatory jurisdiction but do not exclude the possibility for a collaborative review between the centers.

### 2.10.4. Center Jurisdiction

The following subsections provide details concerning status, market approval authority, special label/regulatory considerations, investigational options, and intercenter consultations for the categories of products specified. Section VII provides the general criteria that CDRH and CDER will apply in reaching decisions as to which center will regulate a product.

> A. 1 (a)  Device with primary purpose of delivering or aiding in the delivery of a drug that is distributed without a drug (i.e., unfilled).

EXAMPLES

Devices that calculate drug dosages.

Drug delivery pump and/or catheter infusion pump for implantation iontophoreses device.

Medical or surgical kit (e.g., tray) with reference in instructions for use with specific drug (e.g., local anesthetic).

Nebulizer.

Small particle aerosol generator (SPAG) for administering drug to ventilated patient.

Splitter block for mixing nitrous oxide and oxygen.

Syringe; jet injector; storage and dispensing equipment.

*Status:* Device and drug, as separate entities.

*Market Approval Authority:* CDRH and CDER, respectively, unless the intended use of the two products, through labeling, creates a combination product.

*Special label/regulatory considerations:* The following specific procedures will apply depending on the status of the drug delivery device and drugs that will be delivered with the device.

> (i)  It may be determined during the design or conduct of clinical trials for a new drug that it is not possible to develop adequate performance specifications data on those characteristics of the device that are required for the safe and effective use of the drug. If this is the case, then drug labeling cannot be written to contain information that makes it possible for the user to substitute a generic, marketed device for the device used during developments to use with the marketed drug. In these situation, CDER will be the lead center for regulation of the device under the device authorities.

> (ii)  For a device intended for use with a category of drugs that are on the market, CDRH will be the lead center for regulation for the device under the device authorities. The effects of the device use on drug stability must be addressed in the device submission, when relevant. An additional showing of clinical effectiveness of the drug when delivered by the specific device will generally not be required. The device and drug labeling must be mutually conforming with respect to indication, general mode of delivery (e.g., topical, IV), and drug dosage/schedule equivalents.

(iii) For a drug delivery device and drug that are developed for marketing to be used together as a system, a lead center will be designated to be the contact point with the manufacturer(s). If a drug has been developed and marketed and the development and studying of device technology predominates, the principle mode of action will be deemed to be that of the device, and CDRH would have the lead. If a device has been developed and marketed and the development and studying of drug predominates then, correspondingly, CDER would have the lead. If neither the drug nor the device is on the market, the lead center will be determined on a case-by-case basis.

*Investigation options:* IDE or IND, as appropriate.

*Intercenter consultation:* CDER, when lead Center, will consult with CDRH if CDER determines that a specific device is required as part of the NDA process. CDRH as lead center will consult with CDER if the device is intended for use with a marketed drug and the device creates a significant change in the intended use, mode of delivery (e.g., topical, IV), or dose/schedule of the drug.

(b) Device with primary purpose of delivering or aiding in the delivery of a drug and distributed containing a drug (i.e., "prefilled delivery system").

EXAMPLES

Nebulizer

Oxygen tank for therapy and OTC emergency use.

Prefilled syringe.

Transdermal patch.

*Status:* Combination product.

*Market approval authority:* CDER using drug authorities and device authorities, as necessary.

*Special label/regulatory considerations:* None.

*Investigation options:* IND.

*Intercenter consultations:* Optional.

2. Device incorporating a drug component with the combination product having the primary intended purpose of fulfilling a device function.

EXAMPLES

Bone cement containing antimicrobial agent.

Cardiac pacemaker lead with steroid-coated tip.

Condom, diaphragm, or cervical cap with contraceptive or antimicrobial agent (including virucidal) agent.

Dental device with fluoride.

Dental wood wedge with hemostatic agent.

Percutaneous cuff (e.g., for a catheter or orthopedic pin) coated/impregnated with antimicrobial agent.

Skin closure or bandage with antimicrobial agent.

Surgical or barrier drape with antimicrobial agent.

Tissue graft with antimicrobial or other drug agent.

Urinary and vascular catheter coated/impregnated with antimicrobial agent.

Wound dressing with antimicrobial agent.

*Status:* Combination product.

*Market approval authority:* CDRH using device authorities.

*Special label/regulatory considerations:* These products have a drug component that is present to augment the safety and/or efficacy of the device.

*Investigation options:* IDE.

*Intercenter consultation:* Required if a drug or the chemical form of the drug has not been legally marketed in the United States as a human drug for the intended effect.

3. Drug incorporating a device component with the combination product having the primary intended purpose of fulfilling a drug function.

EXAMPLES

Skin-prep pads with antimicrobial agent.

Surgical scrub brush with antimicrobial agent.

*Status:* Combination product.

*Market approval authority:* CDER using drug authorities and, as necessary, device authorities.

*Special label/regulatory considerations:* Marketing of such a device requires a submission of an NDA with safety and efficacy data on the drug component or it meets monograph specifications as generally recognized as safe (GRAS) and generally recognized as effective (GRAE). Drug requirements, for example, CGMPs, registration and listing, experience reporting, apply to products.

*Investigation options:* IND.

*Intercenter consultation:* Optional.

4. (a) Device used in the production of a drug either to deliver directly to a patient or for the use in the producing medical facility (excluding use in a registered drug manufacturing facility).

EXAMPLES

Oxygen concentrators (home or hospital).

Oxygen generator (chemical).

Ozone generator.

*Status:* Device.

*Market approval authority:* CDER, applying both drug and device authorities.

*Special Label/Regulatory Consideration:* May also require an NDA if the drug produced is a new drug. Device requirements, for example, CGMPs, registration and listing, experience reporting will apply to products.

*Investigation options:* IDA or NDA, as appropriate.

*Intercenter consultation:* Optional.

4. (b) Drug/device combination product intended to process a drug into a finished package form.

EXAMPLES

Device that uses drug concentrates to prepare large volume parenterals.

Oxygen concentrator (hospital) output used to fill oxygen tanks for use within that medical facility.

*Status:* Combination product.

*Market approval authority:* CDER, applying both drug and device authorities.

*Special label/regulatory considerations:* Respective drug and device requirements, for example, CGMPs, registration and listing, experience reporting will apply.

*Investigation options:* IDE or NDA, as appropriate.

*Intercenter consultation:* Optional, but will be routinely obtained.

B. Device used concomitantly with a drug to directly activate or to augment drug effectiveness.

EXAMPLES

Biliary lithotriptor used in conjunction with dissolution agent.

Cancer hyperthermia used in conjunction with chemotherapy.

Current generator used in conjunction with an implanted silver electrode (drug) that produces silver ions for an antimicrobial purpose.

Materials for blocking blood flow temporarily to restrict chemotherapy drug to the intended site of action.

UV and/or laser activation of oxsoralen for psoriasis or cutaneous T-Cell lymphoma.

*Status:* Device and drug, as separate entities.

*Market approval authority:* CDRH and CDER, respectively.

*Special label/regulatory considerations:* The device and drug labeling must be mutually conforming with respect to indications, general mode of delivery (e.g., topical, IV), and drug dosage/schedule equivalence. A lead center will be designated to be the contact point with the manufacturer. If a drug has been developed and approved for another use and the development and studying of device technology predominates, then CDRH would have lead. If a device has been developed and marketed for another use and the development and studying of drug action predominates, then CDER would have lead. If neither the drug nor the device is on the market, the lead center will be determined on a case-by-case basis. If the labeling of the drug and device creates a combination product, as defined in the combination product regulations, then the designation of the lead Center for both applications will be based upon a determination of the product's primary mode of action.

*Investigation options:* IDE or IND, as appropriate.

*Intercenter consultations:* Required.

2. Device kits labeled for use with drugs that include both device(s) and drug(s) as separate entities in one package with the overall primary intended purpose of the kit fulfilling a device function.

EXAMPLES

Medical or surgical kit (e.g., tray) with drug component.
*Status:* Combination product.

*Market approval authority:* CDRH, using device authorities is responsible for the kit if the manufacturer is repackaging a market drug. Responsibility for overall packaging resides with CDRH. CDER will be consulted as necessary on the use of drug authorities for the repackaged drug component.

*Special label/regulatory consideration:* Device requirements, for example, CGMPs, registration and listing, experience reporting apply to kits. Device manufacturers must assure that manufacturing steps do not adversely affect drug components of the kit. If the manufacturing steps do affect the marketed drug (e.g., the kit is sterilized by irradiation), an ANDA or NDA would also be required with CDRH as lead center.

*Investigation options:* IDA or IND, as appropriate.

*Intercenter consultation:* Optional if ANDA or NDA not required.

C. Liquids, gases or solids intended for use as devices (e.g., implanted, or components, parts, or accessories to devices).

EXAMPLES

Dye for tissues used in conjunction with laser surgery, to enhance absorption of laser light in target tissue.

Gas mixtures for pulmonary function testing devices.

Gases used to provide "physical effects."

Hemodialysis fluids.

Hemostatic devices and dressings.

Injectable silicon, collagen, and Teflon.

Liquids functioning through physical action applied to the body to cool or freeze tissues for therapeutic purposes.

Liquids intended to inflate, flush, or moisten (lubricate) indwelling device (in or on the body).

Lubricants and lubricating jellies.

Ophthalmic solutions for contact lenses.

Organ/tissue transport and/or perfusion fluid with antimicrobial or other drug agent, that is, preservation solutions.

Powders for lubricating surgical gloves.

Sodium hyaluronate or hyaluronic acid for use as a surgical aid.

Solution for use with dental "chemical drill".

Spray on dressings not containing a drug component.

*Status:* Device.
*Market approval authority:* CDRH.
*Special label/regulatory considerations:* None.
*Investigation options:* IDE.
*Intercenter consultation:* Required if the device has direct contact with the body and the drug or the chemical form of the drug has not been legally marketed as a human drug.

D. Products regulated as drugs.

EXAMPLES

Irrigation solutions;

Purified water or saline in prefilled nebulizers for use in inhalation therapy;

Skin protectants (intended for use on intact skin);

Sun screens;

Topical/internal analgesic-antipyretic.

*Status:* Drug;
*Market approval authority:* CDER;
*Special label/regulatory considerations:* None.
*Investigation options:* IND.
*Intercenter consultations:* Optional.

E. Ad hoc jurisdictional decisions.

EXAMPLES

Motility marker constructed of radiopaque plastic; (a CDRH regulated device)

Brachytherapy capsules, needles, and so on, that are radioactive and may be removed from the body after radiation therapy has been administered; (a CDRH regulated device)

Skin markers. (a CDRH regulated device)

*Status:* Device or drug;
*Market approval authority:* CDRH or CDER as indicated;
*Special label/regulatory considerations:* None;
*Investigation options:* IDE or IND, as appropriate;
*Intercenter consultation:* Required to assure agreement on drug/device status.

### 2.10.5. General Criteria Affecting Drug and Device Determination

The following represent the general criteria that will apply in making device/drug determinations.

A. Device criteria:

1. A liquid, powder, or other similar formulation intended only to serve as a component, part, or accessory to a device with a primary mode of action that is physical in nature will be regulated as a device by CDRH.

2. A product that has the physical attributes described in 201(h) (e.g., instrument, apparatus) of the Act and does not achieve its primary intended purpose through chemical action within or on the body, or by being metabolized, will be regulated as a device by CDRH.

3. The phrase "within or on the body" as used in 201(h) of the Act does not include extra corporeal systems or the solutions used in conjunction with such equipment. Such equipment and solutions will be regulated as devices by CDRH.

4. An implant, including an injectable material, placed in the body for primarily a structural purpose even though such an implant may be absorbed or metabolized by the body after it has achieved its primary purpose will be regulated as a device by CDRH.

5. A device containing a drug substance as a component with the primary purpose of the combination being to fulfill a device function is a combination product and will be regulated as a device by CDRH.

6. A device (e.g., machine or equipment) marketed to the user, pharmacy, or licensed practitioner that produces a drug will be regulated as a device or combination product by CDER. This does not include equipment marketed to a registered drug manufacturer.

7. A device whose labeling or promotional materials make reference to a specific drug or generic class of drugs unless it is prefilled with a drug ordinarily remains a device regulated by CDRH. It may, however, also be subject to the combination products regulation.

B. Drug Criteria

1. A liquid, powder, tablet, or other similar formulation that achieves its primary intended purpose through chemical action within or on the body,

or by being metabolized, unless it meets one of the specified device criteria, will as regulated as a drug by CDER.

2. A device that serves as a container for a drug or a device that is a drug delivery system attached to the drug container where the drug is present in the container is a combination product that will be regulated as a drug by CDER.

3. A device containing a drug substance as a component with the primary purpose of the combination product being to fulfill a drug purpose is a combination product and will be regulated as a drug by CDER.

4. A drug whose labeling or promotional materials makes reference to a specific device or generic class of devices ordinarily remains a drug regulated by CDER. It may, however, also be subject to the combination products regulation.

## 2.11. CONCLUSIONS

We have touched upon the regulations that currently control the types of preclinical toxicity testing done on potential human pharmaceuticals and medical device products. We have reviewed the history, the law, the regulations themselves, the guidelines, and common practices employed to meet regulatory standards. Types of toxicity testing were discussed, as were the special cases pertaining to, for example, biotechnology products.

## REFERENCES AND SUGGESTED READINGS


Alder, S. and Zbinden G. (1988). *National and International Drug Safety Guidelines*. (MTC Verlag, Zoblikon, Switzerland.

Anderson, O. (1958). *The Health of a Nation; Harvey Wiley and the Fight for Pure Food*. University of Chicago Press.

Anon. (1992a). FDA's Policy Statement for the Development of New Stereoisomeric Drugs. http://www.fda.gov/cder/guidance/stereo.htm

Anon. (1992b). Orphan Drug Regulations 21 CFR PART 316. http://www.fda.gov/orphan/about/odreg.htm

Anon. (1996). Well-characterized biologics would be regulated under FD&C Act by Kassebaum FDA Reform Bill: *F-D-C Reports (pink sheets)* 58: 11–12.

Anon. (1997a). *Guidance for Industry and Reviewers:* Repeal of Section 507 of the Federal Food, Drug and Cosmetic Act. http://www.fda.gov/cder/guidance/index.htm

Anon. (1997b). *Points to Consider in the Manufacture* and *Testing of Monoclonal Antibody Products for Human Use*. http://www.fda.gov/cber/cberftp.html

Anon. (1998a). *Annual Report of the Pharmaceutical Research and Manufacturer's Association*. (Priority #2: Improved FDA Regulation of Drug Development).

Anon. (1998b) *Guidance for Industry: Content and Format for Geriatic Labeling* (Draft guidance). http://www.fda.gov/cder/guidance/2527dft.pdf

Barton, B. (1998). International Conference on Harmonization: good clinical practices update. *Drug Information J.* 32; 1143–1147.

Berliner, V.R. (1974). U.S. Food and Drug Administration requirements for toxicity testing of contraceptive products. In: Briggs, M.H. and Diczbalusy, E., eds. Pharmacological models in contraceptive development. *Acta Endocrinol (Copenhagen)* supp. 185: 240–253.

Blakeslee, D. (1994). Thalidomide, a background briefing. JAMA HIV/AIDS Information Center Newsline. http://www.ama-assn.org/special/hiv/newsline/briefing/briefing.htm

Brusick, D. (1987) *Principles of Genetic Toxicology*, 2nd ed., Plenum Press, New York.

Buesing, Mary McSweegan. (1999). Submitting biologics applications to the center for biologics evaluation and research electronically. *Drug Information J.* 33: 1–15.

Burns, J. (1982). Overview of safety regulations governing food, drug and cosmetics. In: *The United States in Safety and Evaluation and Regulation of Chemicals 3: Interface between Law and Science* (Homberger F., Ed.) Karger, New York.

Cadden, S. (1999). *New Drug Approval in Canada.* Parexel, Waltham, MA.

CDER. (1989). Guideline for the study of drugs likely to be used in the elderly. *FDA,* November 1989.

Currie, W.J.C. (1995). *New Drug Approval in Japan.* Parexel, Waltham, MA.

Daniels, J., Nestmann, E., and Kerr, A. (1997). Development of stereoisomeric (chiral) drugs: A brief review of the scientific and regulatory considerations. *Drug Information J.* 639–646.

DeGeorge, J., Ahn, C., Andrews, P., Bower, M., Giorgio, D., Goheer, M., Lee-Yam, D., McGuinn, W., Schmidt, W., Sun, C., and Tripathi, S. (1998). Regulatory considerations for the preclinical development of anticancer drugs. *Cancer Chemother. Pharmacol.* 41: 173–185.

DiMasi, J., Seibring, M. and Lasagna, L. (1994). New drug development in the United States from 1963 to 1992. *Clin. Pharmacol. Ther.* 55: 609–622.

Ember, L.F. (2001). Raising the bar for quality of drugs, *C&EN* March 19, 26–30.

Evers, P.T. (1985). *New Drug Approval in the European Union.* Parexel, Waltham, MA.

FDA. (1971). *FDA Introduction to Total Drug Quality.* U.S. Government Printing Office, Washington, D.C.

FDA. (1987). *Environmental Assessment Technical Assistance Handbook.* NTIS No. PB87-175345.

FDA. (1988). Good Laboratory Practices, CFR 21 Part 58, April 1988.

FDA. (1988). Investigational new drug, antibiotic, and biological drug product regulations, procedures for drug intended to treat life-threatening and severely debilitating illnesses. *Federal Register* 53 No. 204, 1988; 41516–41524.

FDA. (1988). FDA Perspective on development of stereoisomers. AAPS, May 16, 1988.

FDA. (1996). *Points to Consider in Human Somatic Cell Therapy and Gene Therapy.*

FDA. (1993). *Points to Consider in the Characterization of Cell Lines Used to Produce Biologicals.*

FDA. (1985). *Points to Consider in the Production and Testing of New Drugs and Biologicals Produced by Recombinant DNA Technology.*

FDLI. (1999). *Compilation of Food and Drug Laws, Vol I & II*, Food and Drug Law Institute, Washington.

Fung, M., Thornton, A., Mybeck, K., Ksiao-Hui, J., Hornbuckle, K. and Muniz, E. (2001). Evaluation of the characteristics of safety withdrawal of prescription drugs from worldwide pharmaceutical markets: 1960 to 1999, *Drug Information J.* 35: 293–317.

Gad, S.C. (1994). *Safety Assessment for Pharmaceuticals*. Van Nostrand Reinhold, New York.

Goldenthal, E. (1968). Current view on safety evaluation of drugs. *FDA Papers*, May 1968; 13–18.

Grabowski, H.G. and Vernon, J.M. (1983). *The Regulation of Pharmaceuticals*. American Enterprise Institute, Washington, D.C.

Grieshaber, C. (1991). Prediction of human toxicity of new antineoplastic drugs from studies in animals. In: *The Toxicity of Anticancer Drugs*. Powis, G. and Hacker, M. Eds. Pergamon Press, New York, pp. 10–24.

Haffner, M. (1998). Orphan drug development—International program and study design issues. *Drug Information J.* 32: 93–99.

Hart, C. (1999). Getting past the politics and paperwork of pediatric drug studies. *Modern Drug Discovery* 2: 15–16.

Hayes, T. and Ryffel, B. (1997). Symposium in writing: Safety considerations of recombinant protein therapy; Introductory comments. *Clinical Immunology and Immunotherapy* 83: 1–4.

Hess, G. (1999). FDA accelerates its approval of new drugs. *Chem. Market Newsletter* 255: 21.

Hite, M. (1997). Safety pharmacology approaches. *Int. J. Toxicology* 16: 23–31.

Holtzman, D.C. (1994) European biotech firms invest in US facilities, *Bioworld Today*, June 2, 1994.

Hutt, P.B. (1987). Progress in new drug regulation. *Clin. Res. Prac. Reg. Affairs* 5 (1987), 307–318.

Hutt, P.B. (1983a). Investigations and reports respecting FDA regulations of new drugs. *Clin. Pharmacol. Ther.* 33, 1983a, 537–548.

Hutt, P.B. (1983b). Investigations and reports respecting FDA regulations of new drugs. *Clin. Pharmacol. Ther.* 33: 1983(b) 174–187.

ICH. (2000). *Non-Clinical Safety Studies for the Conduct of Human Clinical Trials for Pharmaceuticals.*

ICH. (1997). *International Conference on Harmonization Safety Steps 4/5 Documents.* Interpharm Press, Inc., Buffalo Grove, IL.

Jackson, S. (1970). Evolution of the regulation of ethical drugs, *American Economic Review* 60: 107–124.

Kessler, D., Siegel, J., Noguchi, P., Zoon, K., Feidon, K. and Woodcock, J. (1993). Regulation of somatic-cell therapy and gene therapy by the food and Drug Administration. *New Engl. J. Med.* 329: 1169–1173.

Lumley, C. E., and Walker, S. E. (1992). An international appraisal of the minimum duration of chronic animal toxicity studies. *Hum. Exp. Toxicology*, 11: 155–162.

Lumpkin, M. (1996). *Guidance for Industry*: Content and Format of Investigational New Drug Applications (INDs) for Phase 1 Studies of Drugs, Including well-characterized, therapeutic, and biotechnology-derived products. http://www.fda.gov/cder/guidance/phase1.pdf

Manson, J. (1994). *Testing of Pharmaceutical Agents for Reproductive Toxicity in Developmental Toxicology* (Kimmel, C. and Buelke-Sam, J., Eds.) Raven Press, New York, pp. 379–402.

Marwick, C. (1998). Implementing the FDA modernization act (Medical News and Perspectives). *JAMA* 279: 815–816.

Merrill, R. (1994). Regulation of drugs and devices: An evolution. *Health Affairs* 13: 47–69.

Ohno, Y. (1998). Harmonization of the timing of the non-clinical tests in relation to the conduct of clinical trials. *J. Controlled Release* 62: 57–63.

Pilot, L. and Waldemann, D. (1998). Food and Drug Modernization Act of 1997: Medical device provisions. *Food and Drug Law J.* 53: 267–295.

Ryffel, B. (1996). Unanticipated human toxicology of recombinant proteins. *Arch. Toxicol. Suppl.* 18: 333–341.

Ryffel, B. (1996). Safety of human recombinant proteins. *Biomed. Environ. Sciences* 10: 65–71.

Schacter, E. and DeSantis, P. (1998). Labeling of drug and biologic products for pediatric use. *Drug Information J.* 32: 299–303.

Temen, P. (1980) Regulation and Choice of Prescription Drugs, *American Economic Review*, 70: 301–305.

USP (2000). *United States Pharmacopeia XXIV and National Formulary 19*, Philadelphia, PA.

Wessinger, J. (1989). Pharmacologic and toxicologic considerations for evaluating biologic products. *Reg. Tox. Pharmacol* 10: 255–263.

Wu, K.-M., DeGeorge, J., Atrachi, A., Barry, E., Bigger, A., Chen, C.,. Du, T., Freed, L., Geyer, H., Goheer, A., Jacobs, A., Jean, D., Rhee, H., Osterburg, R., Schmidt, W., and Farrelly, J. (2000). Regulatory science: A special update from the United States Food and Drug Administration. Preclinical issues and status of investigations of botanical drug products in the United States. *Toxicol. Lett.* 111: 199–202.

Yakuji Nippo, Ltd. (1991). *Drug Registration Requirements in Japan*. Yakuji Nippo, Ltd., Tokyo, Japan.

Yakuji Nippo, Ltd. (1994). *Guidelines for Toxicity Study of Drugs Manual*. Yakuji Nippo Ltd., Tokyo, Japan.

Young, F., Nightingale, S., Mitchell, W., and Beaver, L. (1989). The United States Drug Export Amendment Act of 1986: Perspectives from the Food and Drug Administration. *International Digest of Health Legislation* 40: 246–252.

# 3

# INFORMATION SOURCES: BUILDING AND MAINTAINING DATA FILES

## 3.1. TRADITIONAL INFORMATION SOURCES

The appropriate starting place for the safety assessment of any new chemical entity, particularly a potential new drug, is to first determine what is already known about the material and whether there are any close structural or pharmacological analogues (pharmacological analogues being agents with assumed similar pharmacological mechanisms). Such a determination requires complete access to the available literature. This chapter focuses on the full range of approaches. In using this information, one must keep in mind that there is both an initial requirement to build a data file or base and a need to update such a store on a regular basis. Updating a data base requires not merely adding to what is already there, but also discarding out-of-date (i.e., now known to be incorrect) information and reviewing the entire structure for connections and organization.

## 3.1.1. Claims

Claims are what is said in labeling and advertising, and may be either of a positive (therapeutic or beneficial) or negative (lack of an adverse effect) nature. The positive or efficacy claims are not usually the direct concern of the toxicologist though it must be kept in mind that such claims both must be proved and can easily exceed the limits of the statutory definition of a device, turning the product into a drug or combination product.

Negative claims such as "nonirritating" or "hypoallergenic" also must be proved and it is generally the responsibility of the product safety professional to provide proof for them. There are special tests for such claims.

### 3.1.2. Time and Economies

The final factors of influence or arbitrator of test conduct and timing are the requirements of the marketplace, the resources of the organization, and the economic worth of the product. Plans for filings with regulatory agencies and for market launches are typically set before actual testing (or final stage development) is undertaken, as the need to be in the marketplace in a certain time-frame is critical. Such timing and economic issues are beyond the scope of this volume, but must be considered.

### 3.1.3. Prior Knowledge

The appropriate starting place for the safety assessment of any new chemical entity, is to determine what is already known about the material and whether there are any close structural or pharmacological analogues (pharmacological analogues being agents with assumed similar pharmacological mechanisms).

The first step in any new literature review is to obtain as much of the following information as possible:

1. Correct chemical identity including molecular formula, Chemical Abstracts Service (CAS) Registry number, common synonyms, trade names, and a structural diagram. Gosselin et al. (1984) and Ash and Ash (1994, 1995) are excellent sources of information on existing commercial products, their components and uses;
2. Chemical composition (if a mixture) and major impurities;
3. Production and use information;
4. Chemical and physical properties (physical state, vapor pressure, pH, solubility, chemical reactivity, and so on;
5. Any structurally related chemical substances that are already on the market or in production;
6. Known or presumed pharmacologic properties.

Collection of the above information is not only important for hazard assessment (high vapor pressure would indicate high inhalation potential, just as high and low pH would indicate high irritation potential), but the prior identification of all intended use and exposure patterns may provide leads to alternative information sources; for example, drugs to be used as antineoplastics or antibiotics may already have extensive toxicology data obtainable from government or private sources. A great deal of the existing toxicity information (particularly information on acute toxicity) is not available in the published or electronic literature because of concerns about the proprietary nature of this information and the widespread opinion that it does not have enough intrinsic scholarly value to merit publication. This unavailability is unfortunate, because it leads to a lot of replication of effort and expenditure of resources that could be better used elsewhere. It also means that an experienced toxicologist must use an informal search of the unpublished literature of his colleagues as a supplement to searches of the published and electronic literature.

There are now numerous published texts that should be considered for use in literature-reviewing activities. An alphabetic listing of 24 of the more commonly used hard copy sources for safety assessment data is provided in Table 3.1. Obviously, this is not a complete listing and consists of only the general multipurpose texts that have a wider range of applicability for toxicology. Texts dealing with specialized classes of agents (e.g., disinfectants) or with specific target organ toxicity (neurotoxins and teratogens) are generally beyond the scope of this text. Parker (1987) should be consulted for details on the use of these texts. Wexler (2000), Parker (1987), and Sidhu et al. (1989) should be consulted for more extensive listings of the literature and computerized data bases. Such sources can be off direct (free) Internet sources (where one must beware of GIGO: garbage in,

**TABLE 3.1. Published Information Sources for Safety Assessment**

| Title | Author, date |
| --- | --- |
| *Acute Toxicology* | Gad and Chengelis, 1998 |
| *Annual Report on Carcinogens* | National Toxicology Program, 2000 |
| *Burger's Medicinal Chemistry* | Wolff, 1997 |
| *Carcinogenically Active Chemicals* | Lewis, 1991 |
| *Catalog of Teratogenic Agents* | Shepard, 1998 |
| *Chemical Hazards of the Workplace* | Proctor and Hughes, 1978 |
| *Chemically Induced Birth Defects* | Schardein, 1999 |
| *Clinical Toxicology of Commercial Products* | Gossellin et al., 1984 |
| *Contact Dermatitis* | Cronin, 1980 |
| *Criteria Documents* | NIOSH, various |
| *Current Intelligence Bulletins* | NIOSH, various |
| *Dangerous Properties of Industrial Materials* | Sax., 2000 |
| *Documentation of the Threshold Limit Values for Substances in Workroom Air* | AGGIH, 1986 |
| *Encyclopedia of Toxicology* | Wexler, 1998 |
| *Handbook of Toxic and Hazardous Chemicals* | Sittig, 1985 |
| *Hygienic Guide Series* | AIHA, 1980 |
| *Hamilton and Hardy's Industrial Toxicology* | Finkel, 1983 |
| *Medical Toxicology* | Ellenhorn, 1997 |
| *Merck Index* | Budavari, 1989 |
| *NIOSH/OSHA Occupational Health Guidelines for Chemical Hazards* | Mackison, 1981 |
| *Patty's Toxicology* | Bingham et al., 2001 |
| *Physician's Desk Reference* | Barnhart, 1999 |
| *Registry of Toxic Effects of Chemical Substances (RTECS)* | NIOSH, 1984 |
| *Casarett and Doull's Toxicology: The Basic Science of Poisons* | Klassen, 2001 |
| *Toxicology of the Eye* | Grant, 1993 |

garbage out), commercial databases, and package products, to mention just the major categories. Appendix C provides addresses for major free Internet sources.

### 3.1.4. Miscellaneous Reference Sources

There are some excellent published information sources covering some specific classes of chemicals, for example, heavy metals, plastics, resins, or petroleum hydrocarbons. The National Academy of Science series *Medical and Biologic Effects of Environment Pollutants* covers 10–15 substances considered to be environmental pollutants. *CRC Critical Reviews in Toxicology* is a well-known scientific journal that over the years has compiled over 20 volumes of extensive literature reviews of a wide variety of chemical substances. A photocopy of this journal's topical index will prevent one from overlooking information that may be contained in this important source. Trade organizations such as the Fragrance Industry Manufacturers Association and the Chemical Manufacturers Association have extensive toxicology data bases from their research programs that are readily available to toxicologists of member companies. Texts that deal with specific target organ toxicity—neurotoxicity, hepatotoxicity, or hematotoxicity—often contain detailed information on a wide range of chemical structures. Published information sources like the *Target of Organ Toxicity* series published by (Taylor & Francis, now halfway through revision) offer examples of the types of publications that often contain important information on many industrial chemicals that may be useful either directly or by analogy. The discovery that the material one is evaluating may possess target organ toxicity, warrants a cursory review of these types of texts.

In the last decade, for many toxicologists the on-line literature search has changed from an occasional, sporadic activity to a semicontinuous need. Usually, nontoxicology-related search capabilities are already in place in many companies. Therefore, all that is needed is to expand the information source to include some of the data bases that cover the types of toxicology information one desires. However, if no capabilities exist within an organization, one can approach a university, consultant, or a private contract laboratory and utilize their on-line system at a reasonable rate. It is even possible to access most of these sources from home using a personal computer. The major available on-line data bases are described in the following.

***National Library of Medicine.*** The National Library of Medicine (NLM) information retrieval service contains the well-known and frequently used Medline, Toxline, and Cancerlit data bases. Data bases commonly used by toxicologists for acute data in the NLM service are the following:

1. Toxline (Toxicology Information Online) is a bibliographic data base covering the pharmacological, biochemical, physiological, environmental, and toxicological effects of drugs and other chemicals. It contains approximately 1.7 million citations, most of which are complete with abstract, index terms, and CAS Registry numbers. Toxline citations have publication dates of 1981 to the present. Older information is on Toxline 65 (pre-1965 through 1980).

2. Medline (Medical Information Online) is a data base containing approximately 7 million references to biomedical journal articles published since 1966. These articles, usually with an English abstract, are from over 3000 journals. Coverage of previous years (back to 1966) is provided by back files, searchable on-line, that total some 3.5 million references.

3. Toxnet (Toxicology Data Network) is a computerized network of toxicologically oriented data banks. Toxnet offers a sophisticated search and retrieval package that accesses the following three subfiles:

   a. Hazardous Substances Data Bank (HSDB) is a scientifically reviewed and edited data bank containing toxicological information enhanced with additional data related to the environment, emergency situations, and regulatory issues. Data are derived from a variety of sources including government documents and special reports. This data base contains records for over 4100 chemical substances.

   b. Toxicology Data Bank (TDB) is a peer-reviewed data bank focusing on toxicological and pharmacological data, environmental and occupational information, manufacturing and use data, and chemical and physical properties. References have been extracted from a selected list of standard source documents.

   c. Chemical Carcinogenesis Research Information System (CCRIS) is a National Cancer Institute-sponsored data base derived from both short- and long-term bioassays on 2379 chemical substances. Studies cover carcinogenicity, mutagenicity, promotion, and cocarcinogenicity.

4. Registry of Toxic Effects of Chemical Substances (RTECS) is the NLM's online version of the National Institute for Occupational Safety and Health's (NIOSH) annual compilation of substances with toxic activity. The original collection of data was derived from the 1971 Toxic Substances Lists. RTECS data contains threshold limit values, aquatic toxicity ratings, air standards, National Toxicology Program carcinogenesis bioassay information, and toxicological/carcinogenic review information. The National Institute for Occupational Safety and Health is responsible for the file content in RTECS, and for providing quarterly updates to NLM: RTECS currently covers toxicity data on more than 106,000 substances.

***The Merck Index.*** *The Merck Index* is now available on-line for up-to-the minute access to new chemical entities.

### 3.1.5. Search Procedure

As mentioned earlier, chemical composition and identification information should already have been obtained before the chemical is to be searched. With most information retrieval systems this is a relatively straightforward procedure. Citations on a given subject may be retrieved by entering the desired free text terms as they appear in titles, key words, and abstracts of articles. The search is then initiated by entering the chemical CAS number and/or synonyms. If you are only interested in a specific target organ effect—for instance, carcinogenicity—or specific publication years, searches can be limited to a finite number of abstracts before requesting the printout.

Often it is unnecessary to request a full printout (author, title, abstract). You may choose to review just the author and title listing before selecting out the abstracts of interest. In the long run, this approach may save you computer time, especially if the number of citations being searched is large.

Once you have reviewed the abstracts, the last step is to request photocopies of the articles of interest. Extreme caution should be used in making any final health hazard determination based solely on an abstract or nonprimary literature source.

### 3.1.6. Monitoring Published Literature and Other Research in Progress

Although there are a few other publications offering similar services, the *Life Sciences* edition of *Current Contents* is the publication most widely used by toxicologists for monitoring the published literature. *Current Contents* monitors over 1180 major journals and provides a weekly listing by title and author. Selecting out those journals you wish to monitor is one means of selectively monitoring the major toxicology journals.

Aids available to the toxicologist for monitoring research in progress are quite variable. The National Toxicology Program's (NTP) *Annual Plan for Fiscal Year 1999* highlights all the accomplishments of the previous year and outlines the research plans for the coming year. The Annual Plan contains all projects in the President's proposed fiscal year budget that occur within the National Cancer Institute/National Institutes of Health, National Institute of Environmental Health Sciences/National Institutes of Health, National Center for Toxicological Research/Food and Drug Administration, and National Institute for Occupational Safety and Health/Centers for Disease Control. This report includes a list of all the chemicals selected for testing in research areas that include but are not limited to mutagenicity, immunotoxicity, developmental/reproductive toxicology, neurotoxicity, pharmacokinetics, subchronic toxicity, and chronic toxicity/carcinogenicity.

The Annual Plan also contains a bibliography of NTP publications from the previous year. A companion publication is the 1999 NTP *Review of Current DHHS, DOE, and EPA Research Related to Toxicology*. Similar to the Annual Plan, this document provides detailed summaries of both proposed and ongoing research.

Another mechanism for monitoring research in progress is by reviewing abstracts presented at the annual meetings of professional societies such as the Society of Toxicology, Teratology Society, Environmental Mutagen Society, and American College of Toxicology. These societies usually have their abstracts prepared in printed form; for example, the current *Toxicologist* contains over 1700 abstracts presented at the annual meeting. Copies of the titles and authors of these abstracts are usually listed in the societies' respective journals, which, in many cases, would be reproduced and could be reviewed through *Current Contents*.

## 3.2.  NEW SOURCES

Scientists today are more aware than ever before of the existence of what has been called the "Information Revolution". At no other time in recent history has so much information become available from so many different "traditional" resources—including books, reviews, journals, and meetings—as well as personal computer-based materials such as data bases, alerting services, optical-disk-based information, and news media.

The good news for toxicologists interested in the safety of chemical entities of all types is that numerous new computer-based information products are available that can be extremely useful additions to current safety and toxicology libraries. These tools enable one to save considerable time, effort, and money while evaluating the safety of chemical entities.

The primary focus of this section is on the description and applications of the recent innovations of newly emerging information services based on the personal computer (PC).

### 3.2.1.  Kinds of Information

The kinds of information described here are found on three types of PC media: floppy, CD-ROM, and laser disks. The products run the gamut of allowing one to assess current developments on a weekly basis, as well as to carry out more traditional reviews of historical information. The general types of information one can cover include basic pharmacology, preclinical toxicology, competitive products, and clinical safety.

The specific products discussed are as follows: two floppy disk-based products called Current Contents on Diskette and Focus On: Global Change; five CD-ROM products called Toxic Release Inventory, Material Safety Data Sheets, CCINFOdisk, Pollution/Toxicology, and Medline Ondisk; and a laser disk product entitled the Veterinary Pathology Slide Bank. We provide a brief synopsis of the major features of each as well as a description of their integration into a functional, PC-based Toxicology Information Center (TIC).

When such a TIC is established, one will find that some unusual benefits accrue. One now has immediate and uninterrupted access to libraries of valuable and comprehensive scientific data. This access is free of "on-line" constraints and designed to be user friendly, with readily retrievable information available 24 hours a day, 7 days a week. The retrieved information can also usually be manipulated in electronic form, so one can use it in reports and/or store it in machine-readable form as ASCII files.

The minimal hardware requirements, which are certainly adequate for all items discussed here, are an IBM or IBM-compatible PC equipped with at least 640 K RAM, a single floppy disk drive, at least a 40-Mbyte hard disk drive, a CD-ROM drive, a VGA color monitor, and a printer. The basic point here is that hardware requirements are minimal and readily available. In the case of the laser disk products, a laser disk drive and high resolution (VGA) monitor are also required.

***PC-Based Information Products: Floppy Disk Based.*** We currently have ready access to a rapidly growing variety of relevant information resources. From a current awareness perspective, an excellent source of weekly information is the floppy disk-based product called Current Contents on Diskette (CCOD). Several versions are available; however, the Life Sciences version is most appropriate for this review because of its coverage, on a weekly basis, of over 1200 journals describing work in the biological sciences. One will note that the product has several useful features, including very quick retrieval of article citations as well as several output options (including either hard copy or electronic storage of references as well as reprint requests).

***PC-Based Information Products: CD-ROM Media.*** The gradual emergence of this technology during the past several years has recently blossomed with the introduction of several CD-ROM products that deal with safety issues surrounding the toxicology and safety of chemicals. CD-ROM media with such information can generally be characterized by two major advantages: they are relatively easy to use and are amazingly quick in retrieving data of interest.

*Toxic Release Inventory (TRI).* Before a discussion of products describing health, toxicology, and safety issues, attention should be called to a new, pilot CD-ROM version of the Environmental Protection Agency's (EPA) 1987 Toxic Chemical Release Inventory and Hazardous Substances Fact Sheets. This TRI resource, which contains information regarding the annual inventory of hundreds of named toxic chemicals from certain facilities (since 1987), as well as the toxicological and ecological effects of chemicals, is available from the National Technical Information Service (NTIS), U.S. Department of Commerce, Springfield, Virginia 22161.

The list of toxic chemicals subject to reporting was originally derived from those designed for similar purposes by the states of Maryland and New Jersey. As such, over 300 chemicals and categories are noted. (After appropriate rule making, modifications to the list can be made by the EPA.) The inventory is designed to inform the public and government officials about routine and accidental releases of toxic chemicals to the environment.

The CD-ROM version of the data base can be efficiently searched with a menu-driven type of software called Search Express. It allows one to search with Boolean expressions as well as individual words and/or frequency of "hits" as a function of the number of documents retrieved on a given topic. Numerous searchable fields have been included, allowing one to retrieve information by a variety of means, for example, the compound name; the chemical registry number, the amount of material released into the air, water, or land; the location of the site of release; and the SIC code of the releasing party. One can also employ ranging methods with available numeric fields and sorting of output.

It is hoped that this shared information will help to increase the awareness, concern, and actions of individuals to ensure a clean and safe environment. The TRI data base is a significant contribution to that effort and the CD-ROM version is a superb medium with which to widely publicize and make accessible the findings.

*Material Safety Data Sheets (MSDS).*  The MSDS CD-ROM is a useful resource that contains over 33,000 MSDS on chemicals submitted to the Occupational Safety and Health Administration (OSHA) by chemical manufacturers. This resource contains complete Material Safety Data Sheet (MSDS) information as well as other important information such as the chemical formula, structure, physical properties, synonyms, registry number, and safety information.

Users can easily search the CD-ROM by employing the Aldrich catalog number, Chemical Abstracts Service (CAS) number, chemical name, or molecular formula. One can also export the chemical structures to some supported software for subsequent inclusion into word processing programs. The product is available from Aldrich Chemical Company, Inc., 940 West St. Paul Ave., Milwaukee, WI 54233.

*Canadian Centre for Occupational Health and Safety (CCINFO).*  This set of four CD-ROM disks contains several valuable data bases of information that are updated on a quarterly basis: MSDS, CHEM Data, OHS Source, and OHS Data. The MSDS component currently contains over 60,000 MSDS supplied by chemical manufacturers and distributors. It also contains several other data bases [RIPP, RIPA, Pest Management Research Information System (PRIS)], one of which (PRIS) even includes information on pest management products, including their presence and allowable limits in food.

A second disk in the series (CHEM Data) contains comprehensive information from the CHEMINFO, Registry of Toxic Effects of Chemical Substances (RTECS), and Chemical Evaluation Search and Retrieval System (CESARS) data bases, as well as recommendations on Transport of Dangerous Goods (TDG)/Hazardous Materials (49 CFR).

The third and fourth disks include Occupational Health and Safety (OHS) information. These disks contain data bases on Resource Organizations, Resource People, Case Law, Jurisprudence, Fatalities, Mining Incidents, and ADISCAN. Furthermore, information on Noise Levels, National Institute for Occupational Safety and Health (NIOSHTEC) Non-Ionizing Radiation Levels, and a Document Information Directory System is readily retrievable. These CD-ROM materials are available from the Canadian Center for Occupational Health and Safety, 250 Main Street East, Hamilton, Ontario L8N 1H6.

*Pollution and Toxicology (POLTOX).*  This CD-ROM library also focuses our attention on environmental health and safety concerns. Scientists working in any industry or capacity that deals with toxic or potentially toxic chemicals will find it very useful. It allows one access to seven major data bases in this field in a single search through its use of "linking" features in its software. The distributors of this product have provided us with a spectrum of information dealing with toxic substances and environmental health.

The collection of these data bases include five that are available exclusively from Cambridge Scientific Abstracts (CSA): Pollution Abstracts, Toxicology Abstracts, Ecology Abstracts, Health and Safety Science Abstracts, and Aquatic Pollution and

Environmental Quality. The abstracts come from journals or digests published by CSA on important issues including environmental pollution, toxicological studies of industrial chemicals, ecological impacts of biologically active chemicals, as well as health, safety, and risk management in occupational situations. The POLTOX CD-ROM contains over 200,000 records from these sources since 1981.

POLTOX also contains two other useful data bases: Toxline (described earlier) and the Food Science and Technology Abstracts (FSTA) libraries. The FSTA component is a reasonably comprehensive collection of information regarding toxicological aspects of compounds found in food, including contamination, poison, and carcinogenic properties. The CD-ROM product is available from Compact Cambridge, 7200 Wisconsin Avenue, Bethesda, MD 20814.

*Medline.* The Medline data base, which comes from the National Library of Medicine, is a superb, indispensable reference library that is particularly strong in its wide coverage of research activities in the biomedical literature. It also encompasses the areas of clinical medicine, health policy, and health care services. Each year, over 300,000 articles are reviewed and indexed into the data base. The full bibliographic citations of these articles, usually including the abstract of the published work, are available from numerous vendors in CD-ROM format and are usually updated on a monthly basis.

Information can be accessed from Medline in a variety of ways: by author, title, subject, Chemical Abstracts Service registration number, keyword, publication year, and journal title. Medline Ondisk is the CD-ROM product we employ (from Dialog Information Services, Inc., 3460 Hillview Ave., Palo Alto, CA 94304). It allows one access to the full Medline files back to 1984. Each year from that time until 1988 is covered on a single CD-ROM disk; starting in 1989, each disk covers only a six-month time period. The information is accessed through either an easily employed "menu-driven" system or a more standard on-line type of "command language."

Gower Publishing (Brookfield, VT) has published a series of "electronic hand-books" providing approved ingredient information on materials used in cosmetics, personal care additives, food additives, and pharmaceuticals. Academic Press, through its Sci-Vision branch, has just (2000) launched an ambitious service of CD-ROM-based toxicity database products which are structure and substructure searchable.

It is worth nothing that the CD-ROM-based system has been seamlessly integrated with (proprietary) both record-keeping and communications software so that one can optionally monitor the use of the on-line services and easily continue searching in the Dialog "on-line" environment after using the CD-ROM-based Medline library. Another very useful feature includes the storage of one's search logic so that repetitive types of searches, over time, for example, can be done very easily.

### PC-Based Information Products: Laser Disk

*International Veterinary Pathology Slide Bank (IVPSB).* This application represents an important complementary approach toward training and awareness using laser disk technology. The IVPSB provides a quality collection of transparencies, laser videodisks, and interactive computer/videodisk training programs. In particular, the videodisk contains over 21,000 slides from over 60 contributors representing 37 institutions from 6 countries. These slides are accessible almost instantaneously because of the tremendous storage capacity and rapid random search capabilities of the videodisk through the interactive flexibility of the computer. The information available is of particular interest to toxicologists and pathologists because the visuals illustrate examples of gross lesions of infectious diseases, regional diseases, clinical signs or external microscopy, histopathology, normal histology, cytology and hematology, and parasitology.

The laser disk, a catalog of the entrees, a computer data base, and selected interactive programs can be obtained from Dr. Wayne Crowell, Dept. of Veterinary Pathology, University of Georgia, Athens, GA 30602.

## 3.3.  CONCLUSION

This brief overview of some of the readily available PC-based information resources will, hopefully, encourage more widespread use of this type of technology. Toxicologists and pathologists, in particular, can avail themselves of these useful resources in a way that was simply not possible just a few years ago. The information one needs to make decisions is now far more accessible to many more of us for relatively reasonable expenditures of money for software and hardware.

An effective approach to provide maximal access to these resources is to set up a "Toxicology Information Center (TIC)," which consists of the earlier noted PC hardware and single, centrally available copies of the noted floppy disk, CD-ROM-based, and laser disk products. By employing a menu-based system (available commercially or by shareware) to access the respective products, one can usually provide entry into each of the products discussed here with a single keystroke.

As time goes on, one can grow with the system by considering networking the CD-ROM-based resources and/or setting up other, strategically located TICs on one's campus. The important concept here is that we wish to make the superb "new" PC-based information products as available as we can to interested scientists.

A critical part of the strategy for delivery of information to the end-user is that one can anticipate marked increased usage of the more traditional, hard-copy based resources of the centralized library. The tools described here are frequently complementary to the pivotal library-based information center. What one can anticipate, however, is a much more focused use of hard-copy based information

## REFERENCES

American Conference of Governmental Industrial Hygienists (ACGIH). (1986). *Documentation of the Threshold Limit Values for Substances in Workroom Air*, 5th ed. ACGIH, Cincinnati.

American Industrial Hygiene Association (AIHA). (1980). *Hygienic Guide Series*, Vols. I and II. AIHA, Akron.

Ash, M. and Ash, I. (1994). *Cosmetic and Personal Care Additives*. Electronic Handbook. Gower, Brookfield, VT.

Ash, M. and Ash, I. (1995). *Food Additives*. Electronic Handbook. Gower, Brookfield, VT.

Barnhart, E.R. (1999). *Physician's Desk Reference*. Medical Economics Company, Oradell, NJ.

Budavari, S. (1989). *The Merck Index*, 11th ed. Merck and Company, Rahway, NJ.

Bingham, E., Cohrssen, B. and Powell, C.H. (Eds.). 2001. *Patty's Toxicology*, 5th rev. ed. Vols. 1–7. Wiley, New York.

Cronin, E. (1980). *Contact Dermatitis*. Churchill Livingston, Edinburgh.

Ellenhorn, M.J. (1997). *Medical Toxicology*, 2nd ed. Elsevier, New York.

Finkel, A.J. (1983). *Hamilton and Hardy's Industrial Toxicology*, 4th ed. John Wright PSG Inc., Boston.

Gad, S.C. and Chengelis, C.P. (1998). *Acute Toxicology*, 2nd ed. Academic Press, San Diego, CA.

Gosselin, R.E., Smith, R.P. and Hodge, H.C. (1984). *Clinical Toxicology of Commercial Products*, 5th ed. Williams & Wilkins, Baltimore.

Grant, W.M. (1993). *Toxicology of the Eye*, 4th ed. Charles C. Thomas, Springfield, IL.

Institute for Scientific Information (ISI). (1986). *Current Contents—Life Sciences*. ISI, Philadelphia.

Klassen, C.D. (2001). *Casarett and Doull's Toxicology*, 6th ed. McGraw-Hill, New York.

Lewis, R.J. (1991). *Carcinogenically Active Chemicals*. Van Nostrand Reinhold, New York.

Mackison, F., National Institute for Occupational Health and Safety/Occupational Safety and Health Administration (1981). *Occupational Health Guidelines for Chemical Hazards*. Department of Health and Human Services (NIOSH)/Department of Labor (OSHA) DHHS no. 81–123, Government Printing Office, Washington, D.C.

National Institute for Occupational Safety and Health. *NIOSH Criteria for a Recommended Standard for Occupational Exposure to* XXX. Department of Health, Education and Welfare, Cincinnati, OH.

National Institute for Occupational Safety and Health. (19XX). *NIOSH Current Intelligence Bulletins*. Department of Health, Education and Welfare, Cincinnati, OH.

National Institute for Occupational Safety and Health. (1984). *Registry of Toxic Effects of Chemical Substances*, 11th ed., Vols. 1–3. Department of Health and Human Services DHHS No. 83–107, 1983 and RTECS Supplement DHHS 84–101, Washington, D.C.

National Toxicology Program. (2000). *Nineteenth Annual Report on Carcinogens*. Department of Health and Human Services, PB 85-134633. Washington, D.C.

National Toxicology Program. (1999). *Annual Plan for Fiscal Year 1999*. Department of Health and Human Services, NTP-85-0055. Government Printing Office, Washington, D.C.

National Toxicology Program. (1999). *Review of Current DHHS, DOE, and EPA Research Related to Toxicology*. Department of Health and Human Services, NTP-85-056. Government Printing Office, Washington, D.C.

Parker, C.M. (1988). Available toxicology information sources and their use. *Product Safety Evaluation Handbook* (Gad, S.C., Ed.). Marcel Dekker, New York, pp. 23–41.

Proctor, N.H. and Hughes, J.P. (1978). *Chemical Hazards of the Workplace*. J.B. Lippincott, Philadelphia.

Sax, N.I. (2000). *Dangerous Properties of Industrial Materials*, 10th ed. Van Nostrand Reinhold, New York.

Schardein, J.L. (1999). *Chemically Induced Birth Defects*, 3rd ed. Marcel Dekker, New York.

Shepard, T.H. (1998). *Catalog of Teratogenic Agents*, 9th ed. Johns Hopkins University Press, Baltimore.

Sidhu, K.S., Stewart, T.M. and Netton, E.W. (1989). Information sources and support networks in toxicology. *J. Amer. Coll. Toxicol.* 8: 1011–1026.

Sittig, M. (1985). *Handbook of Toxic and Hazardous Chemicals*, 2nd ed. Noyes Publications, Park Ridge, NJ.

Society of Toxicology. (XXXX). *Toxicologist* (Abstracts of the Xth annual meeting). Society of Toxicology, Reston, VA.

Turco, S. and Davis, N.M. (1973). Clinical significance of particular matter: A review of the literature. *Hosp. Pharm.* 8: 137–140.

Wexler, P. (2000). *Information Resources in Toxicology*, 3rd ed. Elsevier, New York.

Wexler, P. (1998). *Encyclopedia of Toxicology*, Academic Press, San Diego, CA.

Wolff, M.E. (1997). *Burger's Medicinal Chemistry*, 5th ed. Wiley, New York.

# 4

# SCREENS IN SAFETY AND HAZARD ASSESSMENT

## 4.1. INTRODUCTION

In biological research, screens are tests designed and performed to identify agents or organisms having a certain set of characteristics that will either exclude them from further consideration or cause them to be selected for closer attention. In pharmaceutical safety assessment, our use of screens is usually negative (i.e., no activity is found); agents or objects possessing certain biochemical activities are considered to present enough of a hazard that they are not studied further or developed as potential therapeutic agents without compelling reasons (in cases of extreme benefit such as life-saving qualities).

In the broadest terms what is done in preclinical (and, indeed, in phase I, clinical) studies can be considered a form of screening (Zbinden et al., 1984). What varies is the degree of effectiveness of (or our confidence in) each of the tests used. As a general rule, though we think of the expensive and labor intensive "pivotal" studies required to support regulatory requirements (four-week to one-year toxicity studies, carcinogenicity, and segment I–III studies, etc.) as definitive, in fact, they are highly effective (or at least we generally so believe) but not necessarily efficient screens.

Though toxicologists in the pharmaceutical industry are familiar with the broad concepts of screening, they generally do not recognize the applicability of screens. The principles underlying screening are also not generally well recognized or understood. The objective behind the entire safety assessment process in the pharmaceutical industry is to identify those compounds for which the risk of harming humans does not exceed the potential benefit to them. In most cases this means that if a test or screen identifies a level of risk that we have confidence in (our "activity criterion"), then the compound that was tested is no longer considered a viable candidate for development. In this approach, what may change from test to test is the activity criterion (i.e., our basis for and degree of confidence in the outcome). We are interested in minimizing the number of false negatives in safety assessment. Anderson and Hauck (1983) should be consulted for statistical methods to minimize false-negative results.

Figure 4.1 illustrates how current decisions are more likely to be made on a multidimensional basis, which creates a need for balance between (1) degree of benefit, (2) confidence that there *is* a benefit (efficacy is being evaluated in "models" or screens at the same time safety is), (3) type of risk (with, e.g., muscle irritation, mutagenicity, acute lethality, and carcinogenicity having various degrees of concern attached to them), and (4) confidence in, and degree of, risk. This necessity for balance is commonly missed by many who voice opposition to screens because

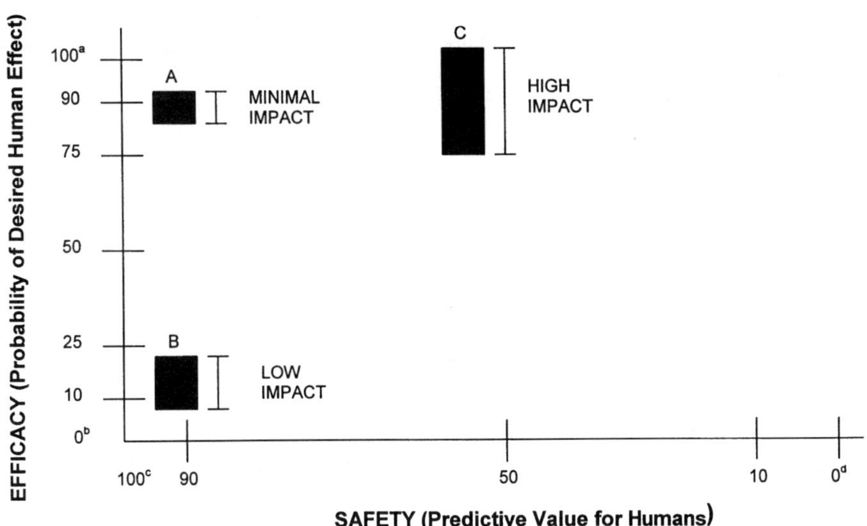


**FIGURE 4.1.** Decision-making for pharmaceutical candidates based on outcome of screening tests. (a) A 100% probability of efficacy means that every compound that has the observed performance in the model(s) used has the desired activity in humans. (b) A 0% probability of efficacy means that every compound that has the observed performance in the model(s) used does not have the desired activity in humans. (c) A 100% probability of a safety finding means that such a compound would definitely cause this toxicity in humans. (d) A 0% probability means this will never cause such a problem in humans. *Note.* These four cases (a, b, c, and d) are almost never found.

The height of the "impact" column refers to the relative importance ("human risk") of a safety finding. Compound 'A' as a high probability of efficacy but also a high probability of having some adverse effect in humans. But if that adverse effect is of low impact, say, transitory muscle irritation for a life-saving antibiotic, 'A' should go forward. Likewise, 'B,' which has low probability of efficacy and high probability of having an adverse effect with moderate impact, should not be pursued. Compound 'C' is at a place where the high end of the impact scale should be considered. Thought there is only a 50% probability of this finding (say, neurotoxicity or carcinogenicity) being predictive in humans, the adverse effect is not an acceptable one. Here a more definitive test is called for or the compound should be dropped.

"they may cause us to throw out a promising compound based on a finding in which we have only (for example) 80% confidence." Screens, particularly those performed early in the research and development process, should be viewed as the biological equivalent of exploratory data analysis. They should be very sensitive, which by definition means that they will have a lot of "noise" associated with them. Screens generally do not establish that an agent is (or is not) a "bad actor" for a certain endpoint. Rather, they confirm that if interest in a compound is sufficient, a more definitive test (a confirmatory test) is required, which frequently will provide a basis for selecting between multiple candidate compounds.

## 4.2. CHARACTERISTICS OF SCREENS

The terminology involved in screen design and evaluation and the characteristics of a screen should be clearly stated and understood. The characteristics of screen performance are defined as

- Sensitivity: the ratio of true positives to total actives;
- Specificity: the ratio of true negatives to total inactives;
- Positive accuracy: the ratio of true to observed positives;
- Negative accuracy: the ratio of true to observed negatives;
- Capacity: the number of compounds that can be evaluated;
- Reproducibility: the probability that a screen will produce the same results at another time (and, perhaps, in some other lab).

These characteristics may be optimized for a particular use, if we also consider the mathematics underlying them and "errors."

A brief review of the basic relationships between error types and power starts with considering each of five interacting factors (Gad, 1982a, 1999) that serve to determine power and define competing error rates.

$\alpha$, the probability of our committing a type I error (a false positive);

$\beta$, the probability of our committing a type II error (a false negative);

$\Delta$, the desired sensitivity in a screen (such as being able to detect an increase of 10% in mutations in a population);

$\sigma$, the variability of the biological system and the effects of chance errors;

$n$, the necessary sample size needed to achieve the desired levels of each of these factors.

We can, by our actions, generally change only this portion of the equation, since $n$ is proportional to

$$\frac{\sigma}{\alpha,\ \beta,\ \text{and}\ \Delta}$$

The implications of this are, therefore, that (1) the greater $\sigma$ is, the larger $n$ must be to achieve the desired levels of $\alpha$, $\beta$, and/or $\Delta$; and (2) the smaller the desired levels of $\alpha$, $\beta$, and/or $\Delta$, if $n$ is constant, the larger $\sigma$ must be.

What are the background response level and the variability in our technique? As any good toxicologist will acknowledge, matched concurrent control (or standardization) groups are essential to minimize within group variability as an "error" contributor. Unfortunately, in *in vivo* toxicology test systems, large sample sizes are not readily attainable, and there are other complications to this problem that we shall consider later.

In an early screen, a relatively large number of compounds will be tested. It is unlikely that one will stand out so much as to have greater statistical significance than all the other compounds (Bergman and Gittins, 1985). A more or less continuous range of activities will be found instead. Compounds showing the highest (beneficial) or lowest (adverse) activity will proceed to the next assay or tier of tests in the series, and may be used as lead compounds in a new cycle of testing and evaluation.

The balance between how well a screen discovers activities of interest versus other effects (specificity) is thus critical. Table 4.1 presents a graphic illustration of the dynamic relationship between discovery and discrimination.

Both discovery and discrimination in screens hinge on the decision criterion that is used to determine if activity has or has not been detected. How sharply such a criterion is defined and how well it reflects the working of a screening system are two of the critical factors driving screen design.

An advantage of testing many compounds is that it gives the opportunity to average activity evidence over structural classes or to study quantitative structure-activity relationships (QSARs). Quantitative structure-activity relationships can be used to predict the activity of new compounds and thus reduce the chance of *in vivo* testing on negative compounds. The use of QSARs can increase the proportion of truly active compounds passing through the system.

It should be remembered that maximization of the performance of a series of screening assays required close collaboration among the toxicologist, chemist, and

**TABLE 4.1. Discovery and Discrimination of Toxicants**

| Screen outcome | Actual activity of agent tested | |
| --- | --- | --- |
| | Positive | Negative |
| Positive | $a$ | $b$ |
| Negative | $c$ | $d$ |

Discovery (sensitivity) $= a/(a + c)$, where $a =$ all toxicants found positive, $a + c =$ all toxicants tested.

Discrimination (specificity) $= d/(b + d)$, where $d =$ all nontoxicants found negative, $b + d =$ all nontoxicants tested.

statistician. Screening, however, forms only part of a much larger research and development context. Screens thus may be considered the biological equivalent of exploratory data analysis (EDA). Exploratory data analysis methods, in fact, provide a number of useful possibilities for less rigid and yet utilitarian approaches to the statistical analysis of the data from screens, and are one of the alternative approaches presented and evaluated here (Tukey, 1977; Redman, 1981; Hoaglin et al., 1983, 1985). Over the years, the author has published and consulted on a large number of screening studies and projects. These have usually been directed at detecting or identifying potential behavioral toxicants or neurotoxicants, but some have been directed at pharmacological, immunotoxic, and genotoxic agents (Gad, 1988, 1989a).

The general principles or considerations for screening in safety assessments are as follows:

1. Screens almost always focus on detecting a single point of effect (such as mutagenicity, lethality, neurotoxicity, or developmental toxicity) and have a particular set of operating characteristics in common.

2. A large number of compounds are evaluated, so ease and speed of performance (which may also be considered efficiency) are very desirable characteristics.

3. The screen must be very sensitive in its detection of potential effective agents. An absolute minimum of active agents should escape detection; that is, there should be very few false negatives (in other words, the type II error rate or beta level should be low). Stated yet another way, the signal gain should be way up.

4. It is desirable that the number of false positives be small (i.e., there should be a low type I error rate or alpha level).

5. Items (2)–(4), which are all to some degree contradictory, require the involved researchers to agree on a set of compromises, starting with the acceptance of a relatively high alpha level (0.10 or more), that is, a higher noise level.

6. In an effort to better serve item (1), safety assessment screens frequently are performed in batteries so that multiple endpoints are measured in the same operation. Additionally, such measurements may be repeated over a period of time in each model as a means of supporting item (2).

7. The screen should use small amounts of compound to make item (1) possible and should allow evaluation of materials that have limited availability (such as novel compounds) early on in development.

8. Any screening system should be validated initially using a set of blind (positive and negative) controls. These blind controls should also be evaluated in the screening system on a regular basis to ensure continuing proper operation of the screen. As such, the analysis techniques used here can then be used to ensure the quality or modify performance of a screening system.

9. The more that is known about the activity of interest, the more specific the form of screen that can be employed. As specificity increases, so should sensitivity. However, generally the size of what constitutes a meaningful change (that is, the $\Delta$) must be estimated and is rarely truly known.

10. Sample (group) sizes are generally small.

11. The data tend to be imprecisely gathered (often because researchers are unsure what they are looking for), and therefore possess extreme within-group variability or modify test performance.

12. Proper dose selection is essential for effective and efficient screen design and conduct. If insufficient data are available, a suitably broad range of doses must be evaluated (however, this technique is undesirable on multiple grounds, as has already been pointed out).

Much of the mathematics involved in calculating screen characteristics came from World War II military-based operations analysis and research, where it was important for design of radar, antiair and antisubmarine warfare systems and operations (Garrett and London, 1970).

## 4.3. USES OF SCREENS

The use of screens that first occurs to most pharmaceutical scientists is in pharmacology (Martin et al., 1988). Early experiences with the biological effects of a new molecule are almost always in some form of efficacy or pharmacology screen. The earliest of these tend to be with narrowly focused models, not infrequently performed *in vitro*. The later pharmacology screens, performed *in vivo* to increase confidence in the therapeutic potential of a new agent or to characterize its other activities (cardiovascular, CNS, etc), can frequently provide some information of use in safety assessment also (even if only to narrow the limits of doses to be evaluated), and the results of these screens should be considered in early planning. In the new millennium, requirements for specific safety pharmacology screens have been promulgated. Additionally, since the late 1990s two new areas of screening have become very important in pharmaceutical safety assessment. The first is the use of screens for detecting compounds with the potential to cause fatal cardiac arrhythmias. These are almost always preceded by the early induction of a prolongation of the Q-T interval. While this should be detected in the EKGs performed in repeat dose canine studies, several early screens (such as the HERG) are more rapid and efficient (though not conclusive) for selecting candidate compounds for further development.

The other area is the use of microassays in toxicogenomic screening, early detection of the potential for compounds to alter gene expressions with adverse consequences (Pennie, 2000; Nuwaysir et al., 1999).

Safety assessment screens are performed in three major settings—discovery support, development (what is generally considered the "real job" of safety assessment), and occupational health/environmental assessment testing. Discovery support is the most natural area of employment of screens and is the place where effective and efficient screen design and conduct can pay the greatest long-range benefits. If compounds with unacceptable safety profiles can be identified before substantial resources are invested in them and structures can be modified to maintain efficacy while avoiding early safety concerns, then long-term success of the entire research and development effort is enhanced. In the discovery support phase, one has the greatest flexibility in the design and use of screens. Here screens truly are used to select from among a number of compounds.

Examples of the use of screens in the development stage are presented in some detail in the next section.

The use of screens in environmental assessment and occupational health is fairly straightforward. On the occupational side, the concerns (as addressed in Chapter 11 of this volume) address the potential hazards to those involved in making the bulk drug. The need to address potential environmental concerns covers both true environmental items (aquatic toxicity, etc.) and potential health concerns for environmental exposures of individuals. The resulting work tends to be either regulatorily defined tests (for aquatic toxicity) or defined endpoints such as dermal irritation and sensitization, which have been (in a sense) screened for already in other nonspecific tests.

The most readily recognized examples of screens in toxicology are those that focus on a single endpoint. The traditional members of this group include genotoxicity tests, lethality tests (particularly recognizable as a screen when in the form of limit tests), and tests for corrosion, irritation (both eye and skin), and skin sensitization. Others that fit this same pattern, as will be shown, include the carcinogenicity bioassay (especially the transgenic mouse models) and developmental toxicity studies.

The "chronic" rodent carcinogenicity bioassay is thought of as the "gold standard" or definitive study for carcinogenicity, but, in fact, it was originally designed as (and functions as) a screen for strong carcinogens (Page, 1977). It uses high doses to increase its sensitivity in detecting an effect in a small sample of animals. The model system (be it rats or mice) has significant background problems of interpretation. As with most screens, the design has been optimized (by using inbred animals, high doses, etc.) to detect one type of toxicant: strong carcinogens. Indeed, a negative finding does not mean that a material is not a carcinogen but rather than it is unlikely to be a potent one.

Many of the studies done in safety assessment are multiple endpoint screens. Such study types as a 90-day toxicity study or immunotox or neurotox screens are designed to measure multiple endpoints with the desire of increasing both sensitivity and reliability (by correspondence–correlation checks between multiple data sets).

## 4.4. TYPES OF SCREENS

There are three major types of screen designs: the single stage, sequential, and tiered. Both the sequential and tiered are multistage approaches, and each of these types also varies in terms of how many parameters are measured. But these three major types can be considered as having the following characteristics.

### 4.4.1. Single Stage

A single test will be used to determine acceptance or rejection of a test material. Once an activity criterion (such as an $X$ score in a righting reflex test) is established, compounds are evaluated based on being less than $X$ (i.e., negative) or equal to or greater than $X$ (i.e., positive). As more data are accumulated, the criterion should be reassessed.

### 4.4.2. Sequential

Two or more repetitions of the same test are performed, one after the other, with the severity of the criterion for activity being increased in each sequential stage. This procedure permits classification of compounds in to a set of various ranges of potencies. As a general rule, it appears that a two-stage procedure, by optimizing decision rules and rescreening compounds before declaring compounds "interesting," increases both sensitivity and positive accuracy; however, efficiency is decreased (or the screen's through-put rate).

### 4.4.3. Tier (or Multistage)

In this procedure, materials found active in a screen are re-evaluated in one or more additional screens or tests that have greater discrimination. Each subsequent screen or test is both more definitive and more expensive.

For purposes of our discussion here, we will primarily focus on the single-stage system, which is the simplest. The approaches presented here are appropriate for use in any of these screening systems, although establishment of activity criteria becomes more complicated in successive screens. Clearly, the use of multistage screens presents an opportunity to obtain increased benefits from the use of earlier (lower-order) screening data to modify subsequent screen performance and the activity criterion.

## 4.5. CRITERION: DEVELOPMENT AND USE

In any early screen, a relatively large number of compounds will be evaluated with the expectation that a minority will be active. It is unlikely that any one will stand out so much as to have greater statistical significance than all the other compounds based on a formal statistical test. A more or less continuous range of activities will be found. Compounds displaying a certain degree of activity will be identified as "active" and handled as such. For safety screens, those which are "inactive" go on to the next test in a series and may be used as lead compounds in a new cycle of testing and evaluation. The single most critical part of the use of screens is how to make the decision that activity has been found.

Each test or assay has an associated activity criterion. If the result for a particular test compound meets this criterion, the compound is "active" and handled accordingly. Such a criterion could have a statistical basis (e.g., all compounds with observed activities significantly greater than the control at the 5% level could be tagged). However, for early screens, a statistical criterion may be too strict, given the power of the assay, resulting in a few compounds being identified as "active." In fact, a criterion should be established (and perhaps modified over time) to provide a desired degree of confidence in the predictive value of the screen.

A useful indicator of the efficiency of an assay series is the frequency of discovery of truly active compounds. This is related to the probability of discovery and to the degree of risk (hazard to health) associated with an active compound passing a screen undetected. These two factors, in turn, depend on the distribution of activities in the series of compounds being tested, and the chances of rejecting and accepting compounds with given activities at each stage.

Statistical modeling of the assay system may lead to the improvement of the design of the system by reducing the interval between discoveries of active compounds. The objectives behind a screen and considerations of (1), costs for producing compounds and testing and (2), the degree of uncertainty about test performance, will determine desired performance characteristics of specific cases. In the most common case of early toxicity screens performed to remove possible problem compounds, preliminary results suggest that it may be beneficial to increase the number of compounds tested, decrease the numbers of animals (or other test models) per assay, and increase the range and number of doses. The result will be less information on more structures, but there will be an overall increase in the frequency of discovery of active compounds (assuming that truly active compounds are entering the system at a random and steady rate).

The methods described here are well suited to analyzing screening data when the interest is truly in detecting the absence of an effect with little chance of false negatives. There are many forms of graphical analysis methods available, including some newer forms that are particularly well suited to multivariate data (the type that are common in more complicated screening test designs). It is intended that these aspects of analysis will be focused on in a later publication.

The design of each assay and the choice of the activity criterion should, therefore, be adjusted, bearing in mind the relative costs of retaining false positives and rejecting false negative (Bickis, 1990). Decreasing the group sizes in the early assays reduced the chance of obtaining significance at any particular level (such as 5%), so that the activity criterion must be relaxed, in a statistical sense, to allow more compounds through. At some stage, however, it becomes too expensive to continue screening many false positives, and the criteria must be tightened accordingly. Where the criteria are set depends on what acceptable noise levels are in a screening system.

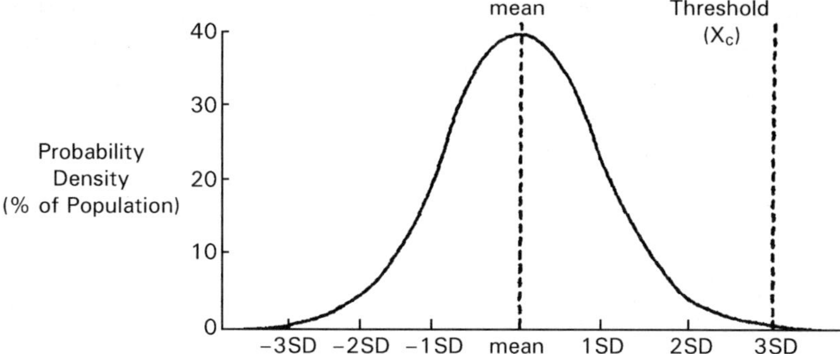


**FIGURE 4.2.** Setting thresholds using historical control data. The figure shows a Gaussian ("normal") distribution of screen parameters; 99.7% of the observations in the population are within three standard deviations (SD) of the historic mean. Here the threshold (i.e., the point at which a datum is outside of "normal") was set at $X_c = \text{mean} + 3$ SD. Note that such a screen is one-sided.

Criteria can be as simple (lethality) or as complex (a number of clinical chemical and hematologic parameters) as required. The first step in establishing them should be an evaluation of the performance of test systems that have not been treated (i.e., negative controls). There will be some innate variability in the population, and understanding this variability is essential to selling some "threshold" for "activity" that has an acceptably low level of occurrence in a control population. Figure 4.2 illustrates this approach.

What endpoints are measured as inputs to an activity criterion are intrinsic in the screen system, but may be either direct (i.e., having some established mechanistic relationship to the endpoint that is being predicted in humans, such as gene mutations as predictive of carcinogenicity in humans) or correlative. Correlated variables (such as many of those measured in *in vitro* systems) are "black box" predictors; compounds causing certain changes in these variables have a high probability of having a certain effect in humans, though the mechanisms (or commonality of mechanism) is not established. There is also, it should be noted, a group of effects seen in animals the relevance of which in humans is not known. This illustrates an important point to consider in the design of a screen: one should have an understanding (in advance) of the actions to be taken given each of the possible outcomes of a screen.

## 4.6. ANALYSIS OF SCREENING DATA

Screening data presents a special case that, due to its inherent characteristics, is not well served by traditional approaches (Gad, 1982b, 1988, 1989a, b, c).

Why? First consider which factors influence the power of a statistical test. Gad (1988) established the basic factors that influence the statistical performance of any bioassay in terms of its sensitivity and error rates. Recently, Healy (1987) presented a review of the factors that influence the power of a study (the ability to detect a dose-related effect when it actually exists). In brief, the power of a study depends on seven aspects of study design.

- Sample size.
- Background variability (error variance).
- Size of true effect to be detected (i.e., objective of the study).
- Type of significance test.
- Significance level.
- Decision rule (the number of false positives one will accept).

There are several ways to increase power, each with a consequence.

| *Action* | *Consequence* |
| --- | --- |
| Increase the sample size | Greater resources required |
| Design test to detect larger differences | Less useful conclusions |
| Use a more powerful significance test | Stronger assumptions required |
| Increase the significance level | Higher statistical false-positive rate |
| Use one-tailed decision rule | Blind to effects in the opposite direction |

Timely and constant incorporation of knowledge of test system characteristics and performance will reduce background variability and allow sharper focus on the actual variable of interest. There are, however, a variety of nontraditional approaches to the analysis of screening data.

### 4.6.1. Univariate Data

***Control Charts.*** The control chart approach (Montgomery, 1985), commonly used in manufacturing quality control in another form of screening (for defective product units), offers some desirable characteristics.

By keeping records of cumulative results during the development of screen methodology, an initial estimate of the variability (such as standard deviation) of each assay will be available when full-scale use of the screen starts. The initial estimates can then be revised as more data are generated (i.e., as we become more familiar with the screen).

The following example shows the usefulness of control charts for control measurements in a screening procedure. Our example test for screening potential muscle strength suppressive agents measures reduction of grip strength by test compounds compared with a control treatment. A control chart was established to monitor the performance of the control agent (1) to establish the mean and variability of the control, and (2) to ensure that the results of the control for a given experiment are within reasonable limits (a validation of the assay procedure).

As in control charts for quality control, the mean and average range of the assay were determined from previous experiments. In this example, the screen had been run 20 times previous to collecting the data shown. These initial data showed a mean grip strength $X$ of 400 g and a mean range $R$ of 90 g. These values were used for the control chart (Figure 4.3). The subgroups are of size five. The action limits for the mean and range charts were calculated as follows:

$$X \pm 0.58\,R = 400 \pm 0.58 \times 90 = 348 - 452 \quad \text{(from the } X \text{ chart)}$$

Then, using the upper limit $(du)$ for an $n$ of 5,

$$2.11\,R = 2.11 \times 90 = 190 \quad \text{(the upper limit for the range)}$$

Note that the range limit, which actually established a limit for the variability of our data, is, in fact, a "detector" for the presence of outliers (extreme values).

Such charts may also be constructed and used for proportion or count types of data. By constructing such charts for the range of control data, we may then use them as rapid and efficient tools for detecting effects in groups being assessed for that same activity end point.

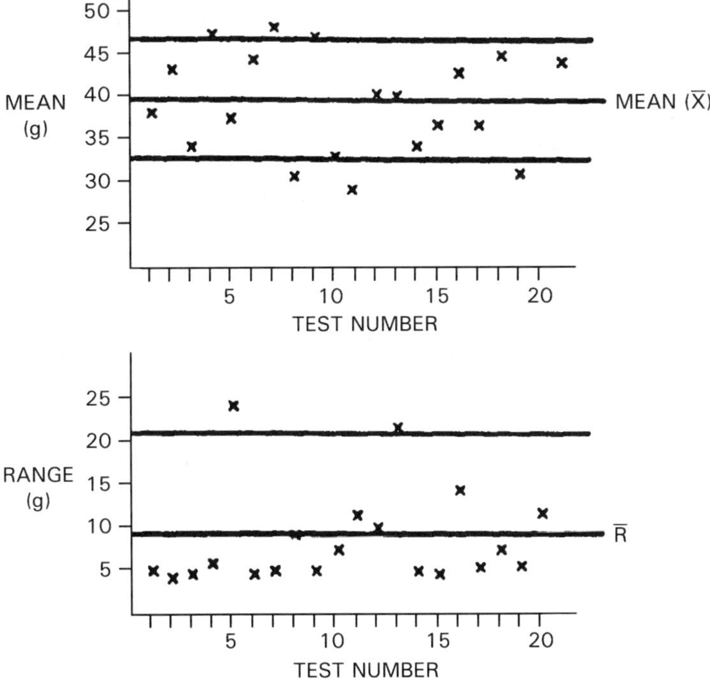


**FIGURE 4.3.** Example of a control chart used to "prescreen" data (actually, explore and identify influential variables), from a portion of a functional observational battery. See text discussion for explanation.

***Central Tendency Plots.***  The objective behind our analysis of screen data is to have a means of efficiently, rapidly, and objectively identifying those agents that have a reasonable probability of being active. Any materials that we so identify may be further investigated in a more rigorous manner, which will generate data that can be analyzed by traditional means. In other words, we want a method that makes out-of-the-ordinary results stand out. To do this we must first set the limits on "ordinary" (summarize the control case data) and then overlay a scheme that causes those things that are not ordinary to become readily detected ("exposed," in exploratory data analysis (EDA) terms (Velleman and Hoaglin, 1981; Tufte, 1983). One can then perform "confirmatory" tests and statistical analysis (using traditional hypothesis testing techniques), if so desired.

If we collect a set of control data on a variable (say scores on our observations of the righting reflex) from some number of "ordinary" animals, we can plot it as a set of two histograms (one for individual animals and the second for the highest total score in each randomly assigned group of five animals), such as those shown in Figure 4.4 (the data for which came from 200 actual control animals).

Such a plot identifies the nature of our data, visually classifying them into those that will not influence our analysis (in the set shown, clearly scores of 0 fit into this category) and those that will critically influence the outcome of an analysis. In so doing, the position of control ("normal") observations is readily revealed as a "central tendency" in the data (hence the name for this technique).

We can (and should) develop such plots for each of our variables. Simple inspection makes clear that answers having no discriminatory power (0 values in Figure 4.4) do not interest us or influence our identifying of an outlier in a group and should simply be put aside or ignored before continuing on with analysis. This first stage, summarizing the control data, thus gives us a device for identifying data with

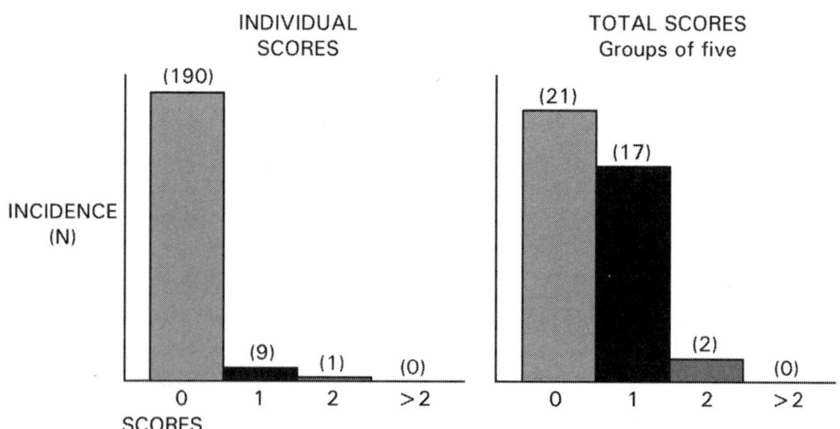



**Figure 4.4.** Plotting central tendency. Possible individual scores for righting reflexes may range from 0 to 8 (Gad, 1982a). Group total scores would thus range from 0 to 40. (Shown are the number of groups that contain individual scores in the individual categories.)

discriminatory power (extreme values), thus allowing us to set aside the data without discriminatory power.

Focusing our efforts on the remainder, it becomes clear that although the incidence of a single, low, nonzero observation in a group means nothing, total group scores of 2 or more occurred only 5% of the time by chance. So we can simply perform an extreme value screen on our "collapsed" data sets, looking for total group values or individual values that are beyond our acceptance criteria.

The next step in this method is to develop a histogram for each ranked or quantal variable, by both individual and group. "Useless" data (those that will not influence the outcome of the analysis) are then identified and dropped from analysis. Group scores may then be simply evaluated against the baseline histograms to identify those groups with scores divergent enough from control to be either true positives or acceptably low-incidence false positives. Additional control data can continue to be incorporated in such a system over time, both increasing the power of the analysis and providing a check on screen performance.

### 4.6.2. Multivariate Data

The traditional acute, subchronic, and chronic toxicity studies performed in rodents and other species also can be considered to constitute multiple endpoint screens. Although the numerically measured continuous variables (body weight, food consumption, hematology values) generally can be statistically evaluated individually by traditional means, the same concerns of loss of information present in the interrelationship of such variables apply. Generally, traditional multivariate methods are not available, efficient, sensitive, or practical (Young, 1985).

***The Analog Plot.*** The human eye is extremely good at comparing the size, shape and color of pictorial symbols (Anderson, 1960; Andrews, 1972; Davison, 1983; Schmid, 1983; Cleveland and McGill, 1985). Furthermore, it can simultaneously appreciate both the minute detail and the broad pattern.

The simple way of transforming a table of numbers to a sheet of pictures is by using analog plots. Numbers are converted to symbols according to their magnitude. The greater the number, the larger the symbol. Multiple variables can be portrayed as separate columns or as differently shaped or colored symbols (Wilk and Gnanadesikan, 1968).

The conversion requires a conversion chart from the magnitude of the number to the symbol size. The conversion function should be monotonic (e.g., dose, and the measured responses should each change in one direction according to a linear, logarithmic, or probit function). Log conversion will give more emphasis to differences at the lower end of the scale, whereas a probit will stabilize the central range of response (16–84%) of a percentage variable. For example, for numbers $x$, symbol radium $r$, and plotting scaling factor $k$, a log mapping will give

$$x = 1 \qquad r = k$$
$$x = 10 \qquad r = 2k$$
$$x = 100 \qquad r = 3k$$

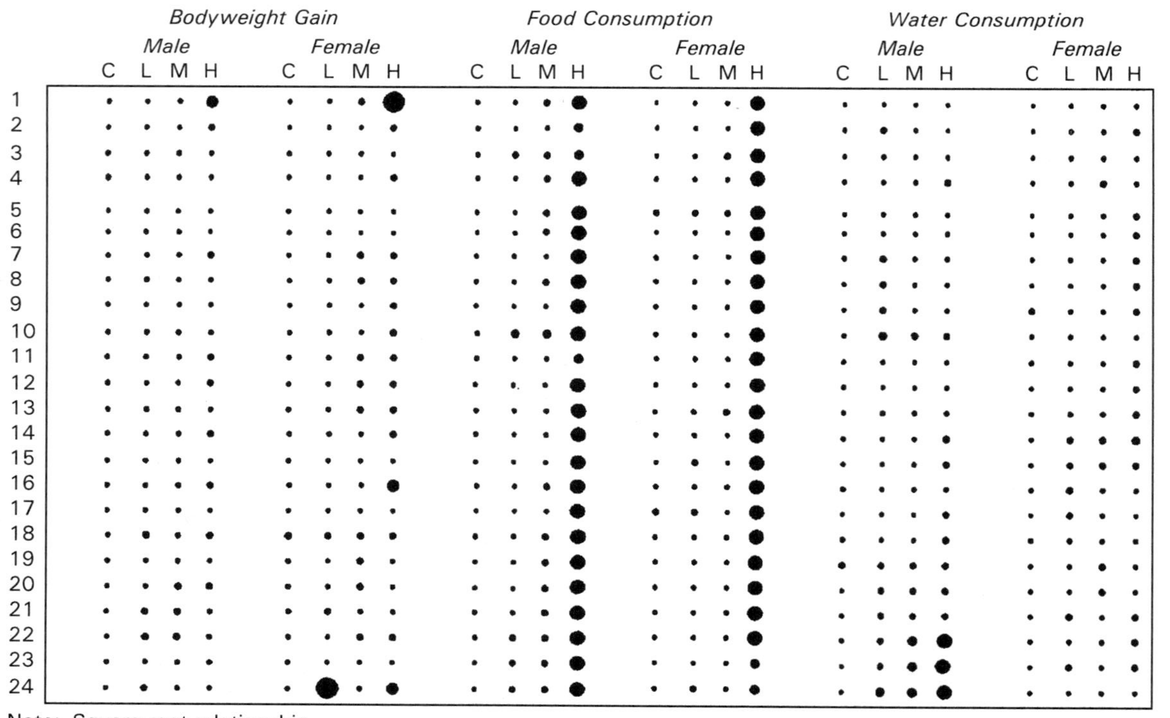



**FIGURE 4.5.**  Analog plot for dose-response contrasts. One of many possible approaches to graphically presenting multidimensional data. In this case, various effects—day of dosing, dose response, and magnitude of response—are simultaneously portrayed, with the size of each circle being proportional to the magnitude of the measured value.

To compare different variables on the same sheet requires some form of standardization to put them on the same scale. Also, a choice must be made between displaying the magnitude of the numbers or their significance (Kruskal, 1964; Kass, 1980). Two possibilities are

1. Express each mean as a percentage change from a control level or overall mean (*a means plot*).
2. Calculate effects for meaningful contrasts (*a contrasts plot*).

The analog plot chart in Figure 4.5 shows relationships for five measures on a time versus dose basis, allowing ready evaluation of interrelationships and patterns.

A study using 50 rats of each sex in each of five groups (two controls and three increasing doses) measured body weight and food and liquid consumption every week or month for two years. This resulted in 3 variables $\times$ 2 sexes $\times$ 5 groups $\times$ 53 times $\times$ 50 animals. Means alone constituted some 1600 four-digit numbers.

Body weight gains from the period immediately preceding each consumption measurement were used, since these were less correlated. For each variable and at each time, the sums of squares for group differences were divided into four meaningful contrasts:

Control A versus control B.

Control A + B versus low.

Control A + B + low versus medium.

Control A + B + low + medium versus high.

To make the variables comparable, the sums of squares were standardized by the within-group standard deviations. Contrast involving doses can be compared with the contrast for the difference between the controls, which should be random. The clearest feature is the high-dose effect for food consumption. However, this seems not to be closely correlated with changes in body weight gains. Certain changes can be seen at the later measurement times, probably because of dying animals.

There are numerous approaches to the problem of capturing all the information in a set of multi endpoint data. When the data are continuous in nature, approaches such as the analog plot can be used (Chernoff, 1973; Chambers et al., 1983; Schmid, 1983). A form of control chart also can be derived for such uses when detecting effect rather than exploring relationships between variables is the goal. When the data are discontinuous, other forms of analysis must be used. Just as the control chart can be adapted to analyzing attribute data, an analog plot can be adapted. Other methods are also available.

## REFERENCES

Anderson, E. (1960). A semigraphical method for the analysis of complex problems. *Technometrics* 2: 387–391.

Anderson, S. and Hauck, W. (1983). A new procedure for testing equivalence in comparative bioavailability and other clinical trials. *Commun. Stat. Thero. Meth.* 12: 2663–2692.

Andrews, D.F. (1972). Plots of high dimensional data. *Biometrics* 28: 125–136.

Bergman, S.W. and Gittins, J.C. (1985). Screening procedures for discovering active compounds. In: *Statistical Methods for Pharmaceutical Research Planning.* (Peace, K. Ed.). Marcel Dekker, New York.

Bickis, M.G. (1990). Experimental design. In: *Handbook of In Vivo Toxicity Testing* Arnold, D.L., Grice, H.C. and Krewski, D.R., Eds.). Academic Press, San Diego, pp. 128–134.

Chambers, J.M., Cleveland, W.S., Kliner, B. and Tukey, P.A. (1983). *Graphical Methods for Data Analysis.* Duxbury Press, Boston.

Chernoff, H. (1973). The use of faces to represent points in $K$-dimensional space graphically. *J. Am. Stat. Assoc.* 68: 361–368.

Cleveland, W.S. and McGill, R. (1985). Graphical perception and graphical methods for analyzing scientific data. *Science* 229: 828–833.

Davison, M.L. (1983). *Multidimensional Scaling.* Wiley, New York.

Gad, S.C. (1982a). A neuromuscular screen for use in industrial toxicology *J. Toxicol. Environ. Health* 9: 691–704.

Gad, S.C. (1982b). Statistical analysis of behavioral toxicology data and studies. *Arch. Toxicol.* (Suppl.) 5: 256–266.

Gad, S.C. (1988). An approach to the design and analysis of screening studies in toxicology. *J. Am. Coll. Toxicol.* 8: 127–138.

Gad, S.C. (1989a). Principles of screening in toxicology with special emphasis on applications to neurotoxicology. *J. Am. Coll. Toxicol.* 8: 21–27.

Gad, S.C. (1989b). Screens in neurotoxicity: Objectives, design and analysis, with the observational battery as a case example. *J. Am. Coll. Toxicol.* 8: 1–18.

Gad, S.C. (1989c). Statistical analysis of screening studies in toxicology with special emphasis on neurotoxicology. *J. Amer. Coll. Toxicol.* 8: 171–183.

Gad, S.C. (1999). *Statistics and Experimental Design for Toxicologists*, 3rd ed. CRC Press, Boca Raton, FL.

Garrett, R.A. and London, J.P. (1970). *Fundamentals of Naval Operations Analysis.* U.S. Naval Institute, Annapolis, Maryland.

Healy, G.F. (1987). Power calculations in toxicology. *A.T.L.A.* 15: 132–139.

Hoaglin, D.C., Mosteller, F.D. and Tukey, J.W. (1983). *Understanding Robust and Exploratory Data Analysis.* Wiley, New York.

Hoaglin, D.C., Mosteller, F.D. and Tukey, J.W. (1985). *Exploring Data Tables, Trends, and Shapes.* Wiley, New York.

Kass, G.V. (1980). An exploratory technique for investigating large quantities of categorical data. *Appl. Stat.* 29: 119–127.

Kruskal, J.B. (1964). Multidimensional scaling by optimizing goodness of fit to a nonmetric hypothesis. *Psychometrika* 29: 1–27.

Martin, Y.C., Kutter, E. and Austel, V. (1988). In: *Modern Drug Research.* Marcel Dekker, New York, pp. 31–34, 155, 265–269, 314–318.

Montgomery, D.C. (1985). *Introduction to Statistical Quality Control.* Wiley, New York.

Nuwaysir, E.F., Bittner, M., Trent, J., Barrett, J.C. and Afshari, C.A. (1999). Microassays and toxicology: the advent of toxicogenomics. *Mol. Carcinog.* 24: 153–159.

Page, N.P. (1977). Concepts of a bioassay program in environmental carcinogenesis. In: *Environmental Cancer* (Kraybill, H.F. and Mehlman, M.A., Eds.). Hemisphere Publishing, New York, pp. 87–171.

Pennie, W.D. (2000). Use of cDNA microassays to probe and understand the toxicological consequences of altered gene expression. *Toxicol. Lett.* 112–113: 473–477.

Redman, C. (1981). Screening compounds for clinically active drugs. In: *Statistics in the Pharmaceutical Industry* (Buncher, C.R. and Tsya, J., Eds.). Marcel Dekker, New York, pp. 19–42.

Schmid, C.F. (1983). *Statistical Graphics*. Wiley, New York.

Tufte, E.R. (1983). *The Visual Display of Quantitative Information*. Graphic Press, Cheshire, CT.

Tukey, J.W. (1977). *Exploratory Data Analysis*. Addison-Wesley, Reading, MA.

Velleman, P.F. and Hoaglin, D.C. (1981). *Applications, Basics and Computing of Exploratory Data Analysis*. Duxbury Press, Boston.

Wilk, M.B. and Gnanadesikan, R. (1986). Probability plotting methods for the analysis of data. *Biometrics* 55: 1–17.

Young, F.W. (1985). Multidimensional scaling. In: *Encyclopedia of Statistical Sciences*, Vol. 5 (Katz, S. and Johnson, N.L., Eds.). Wiley, New York, pp. 649–659.

Zbinden, G., Elsner, J. and Boelsterli, U.A. (1984). Toxicological screening. *Regul. Toxicol. Pharmacol.* 4: 275–286.

# 5

# ACUTE TOXICITY TESTING IN DRUG SAFETY EVALUATION

## 5.1. INTRODUCTION

What is acute toxicity testing and why does it warrant a separate chapter in this book? Of what value is it in ensuring the safety of pharmaceutical agents? Acute toxicity testing is the defining and evaluation of the toxic syndrome (if any) produced by a single dosage (or, in the case of continuously infused intravenous formulation, in a 24-hour course of treatment) of a drug. Historically, the main focus of these tests has been lethality determinations and the identification of overt signs and symptoms of overdosage. For a complete historical perspective, see Gad and Chengelis (1999), Auletta (1998) or Piegorsh (1989). A more enlightened and modern view holds that, especially for pharmaceutical agents, lethality in animals is a relatively poor predictor of hazard in humans (Gad and Chengelis, 1999). The current trend is toward gaining increasing amounts of more sophisticated data from these tests. The various types of acute study designs, their utility in pharmaceutical product testing, and the resultant sample data are discussed in this chapter.

In the pharmaceutical industry, acute toxicity testing has uses other than for product safety determinations. First, as in other industries, acute toxicity determinations are part of industrial hygiene or occupational health environmental impact assessments (Deichmann and Gerarde, 1969). These requirements demand testing not only for finished products but frequently of intermediates as well. These issues and requirements, however, are discussed in Chapter 2 and are not directly addressed here.

Another use, now almost abandoned except for in natural product-derived drugs, is in quality control testing or batch release testing. The latter was once a mandated part of the standardization process for antibiotics, digoxin and insulin in the U.S.

Pharmacopoeia. While, perhaps, this type of testing is part of a broad safety picture, it is not typically part of a "preclinical" safety package used to make decisions on whether to market a new chemical entity, or on what the allowable clinical dosage shall be. These uses also are therefore not discussed here. The emphasis here is on tests used to elucidate the toxicity of new chemical entities, not the safety of finished drug preparations. These tests fall into three general categories: (1) range-finding studies, used primarily to set dosages for initial subchronic or acute testing; (2) complete "heavy" acute toxicity tests, used to thoroughly describe the single-dose toxicity of a chemical; and (3) screening tests, used to select candidates for development.

## 5.2. RANGE-FINDING STUDIES

Range finders are not normally done completely under the auspices of the Good Laboratory Practices Act. They are not used to generate data to support decisions on human safety; rather, they are used to generate information that allows dosages in definitive studies to be rationally set. These dosage-level determinations can be for use in acute studies, *in vivo* genotoxicity or subchronic studies. As discussed by Gad and Chengelis (1999), however, there can be a great deal of difference between the acute toxic dosage and subchronic daily dosage of a drug. Therefore, acute range-finding studies will often include a component (or second phase) whereby animals will receive a short-term treatment (less than seven days) with the drug in question. Accordingly, the definition of "acute" in this chapter is stretched to include "subacute" dosing regimens of very short duration.

### 5.2.1. Lethality Testing

Often, in range-finding tests, the endpoint is simply to determine what is the maximum dosage that can be given without killing an animal. There are numerous designs available for obtaining this information that minimize the expenditure of animals and other resources.

***Classical $LD_{50}$.*** The $LD_{50}$ test has a rich and controversial history (it is one of a number of tests that raises the ire of the animal welfare movement (see Rowan, 1981 and Muller and Kley, 1982). The classical method was originated by Trevan (1927) and required the use of 80 or more animals. In pharmaceutical development, however, there is rarely a need or requirement for an $LD_{50}$ (Office of Science Coordination, 1984; Osterberg, 1983, McClain, 1983, Pendergast, 1984 and LeBeau, 1983). In general, a complete, precisely calculated $LD_{50}$ consumes more resources than is generally required for range-finding purposes. The reader is referred to Chapter 7 of Gad and Chengelis (1999) for a complete discussion of this test.

***Dose Probes.*** Dose probe protocols (see Figure 5.1) are of value when one needs the information supplied by a traditional protocol but has no preliminary data from

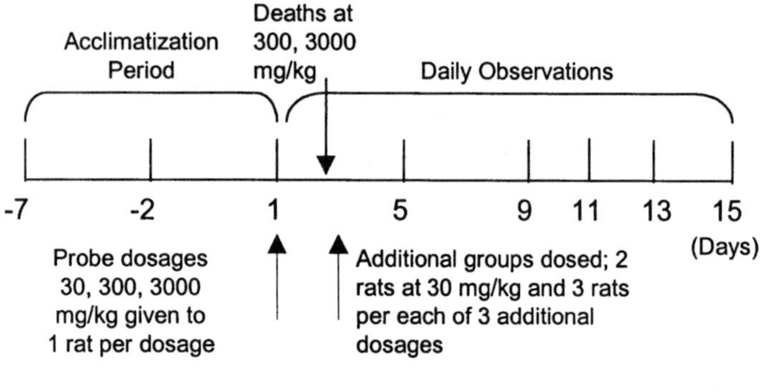

**FIGURE 5.1.**  Example of typical dosage probe protocol.

which to choose dosages. In this acute protocol, one animal is dosed at each of three widely spaced dosages, where the top dosage is generally the maximum deliverable. The method works best if the dosages are separated by constant multiples (e.g., 3000, 300, and 30 mg kg$^{-1}$ a logarithmic progression). Subsequent dosages are selected on the basis of the results from these probe animals. If none of these animals dies, the protocol defaults to a limit test (described below), and two more animals are dosed at the top dosage to confirm the limit.

A dose probe can develop into a more thorough lethality determination. If one or two animals die, then two additional dosages between the lethal and nonlethal dosages are chosen and three animals treated per dosage for defining acute lethality. Selection of these dosages is often a matter of personal judgement. If, for example, one wishes to apply the moving average method of calculation, these subsequent dosages can be either even fractions of the top dosage or even multiples of the low dosage. In either case, two to three animals are dosed at the initial dose and three to four animals are dosed at each of the two to three new dosages. The results should be three to four groups of three to four animals each, which should probably provide sufficient data for calculating the $LD_{50}$ and the slope of the curve. Probing can also be used to define the dosages for subchronic tests. Instead of selecting additional doses for an acute study, one can use the results from the probe to select two dosages for a short (e.g., five days) daily dosing regimen (see later section entitled "Rolling" Acute Tests).

In a few instances, all the animals may die following the first day of dosing. In that case, the probe activity continues on Day 2 with two more animals dosed at two widely spaced lower dosages (i.e., 3 and 0.3 g kg$^{-1}$). This regimen could continue daily until a nonlethal dosage is identified. Unless one has grossly misestimated the toxicity of the test substance, it is unlikely that the probing process would take more than three days. Carrying our example into three days of dosing would have resulted in probing the 3 µg kg$^{-1}$ to the 3 g kg$^{-1}$ range, and it is a rare chemical that is lethal at less than 3 µg kg$^{-1}$. Once a nonlethal dosage is identified, additional animals and/or dosages can be added, as discussed above.

There are two disadvantages to dose probe studies. First, delayed deaths pose difficulties. Hence, all animals should be observed for at least seven days after dosing (though most deaths occur within three days). Second, if the follow-up dosages are not lethal, the next decision point is ill defined. Should more animals be dosed at some different dosage? The resulting data sets may be cumbersome and difficult to analyze by traditional statistical methods. Alternatively (and this is true regardless of protocol design), if no "partial response" (mortality greater than 0 but less than 100%) dosage is identified, one can simply conclude that the LD$_{50}$ is between two dosages, but the data do not permit the calculation of the LD$_{50}$ or the slope of the curve. This can happen if the dosage response is fairly steep.

Lörke (1983) has developed a similar protocol design. His probe (or dose range) experiment consists of three animals per dosage at 10, 100, and 1000 mg kg$^{-1}$. The results of the experiment dictate the dosages for the second round of dosing, as shown in Table 5.1. Animals were observed for 14 days after dosing. Lörke (1983) compared the results obtained when one to five animals were used per dosage group for the second test. He concluded that using only one animal per group gave unreliable results in only 7% of chemicals tested. Hence, the Lörke design can

**TABLE 5.1. Dosage Selection for the Two-Step Dose-Probing Protocol Design**

| Mortality by Dose (mg kg$^{-1}$)[a] | | | Dosages (mg kg$^{-1}$) for the Definitive Experiment as Determined by the Results of the Probe | | | |
|---|---|---|---|---|---|---|
| (10) | (100) | (1000) | | | | |
| 0/3 | 0/3 | 0/3 | | 1600 | 2900 | 5000 |
| 0/3 | 0/3 | 1/3 | 600 | 1000[b] | 1600 | 2900 |
| 0/3 | 0/3 | 2/3 | 200 | 400 | 800 | 1600 |
| 0/3 | 0/3 | 3/3 | 140 | 225 | 370 | 600 |
| 0/3 | 1/3 | 3/3 | 50 | 100[b] | 200 | 400 |
| 0/3 | 2/3 | 3/3 | 20 | 40 | 80 | 160 |
| 0/3 | 3/3 | 3/3 | 15 | 25 | 40 | 60 |
| 1/3 | 3/3 | 3/3 | 5 | 10[b] | 20 | 40 |
| 2/3 | 3/3 | 3/3 | 2 | 4 | 8 | 16 |
| 3/3 | 3/3 | 3/3 | 1 | 2 | 4 | 8 |

[a] Number of animals that died/number of animals used.
[b] The results from the probe are inserted for these doses.
*Source*: Lörke, 1983.

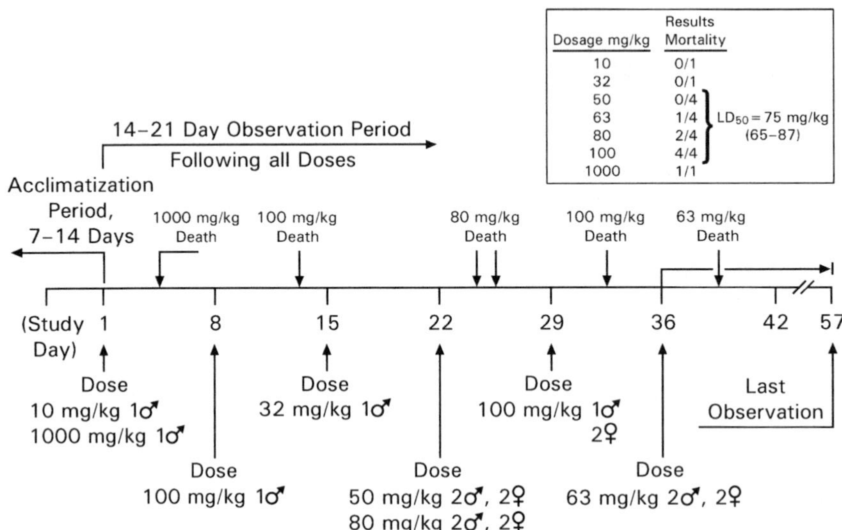



**FIGURE 5.2.** Example of dose probe method with delayed deaths. *Source:* Schultz and Fuchs, 1982.

produce reasonable estimates of lethal dosages using 14 or fewer animals. Schutz and Fuchs (1982) have proposed a dose probe protocol that adequately deals with delayed deaths (Figure 5.2). All animals are observed for seven days before subsequent dosages are given. Dosing is initiated at two widely delivered dosages using one rate for each dosage. A third probe dosage is determined pending the outcome of the first two probes. A fourth may also be used. After that, groups of three to four animals are used at subsequent dosages either as part of a "para-acute" dosing regimen to select or confirm dosages for a subchronic study or to continue with the definition of an acute lethality curve.

***Up/Down Method.*** Using classical or traditional acute lethality protocols, 15 to 30 animals per curve may be required to calculate a singe $LD_{50}$. This is because the method relies on the analysis of group responses. The up/down method can provide lethality information by analyzing the responses on an individual animal basis using appropriate statistical maximum likelihood methods (Bruce, 1985). Deichmann and LeBlanc (1943) published an early method that provided an estimate of lethality using no more than six animals. All animals were dosed at the same time. The dosage range was defined as $1.5 \times$ a multiplication factor (e.g., 1.0, 1.5, 2.2, 3.4, 5.1 ml $kg^{-1}$). The approximate lethal dose (ALD), as they defined it, was the highest dose that did not kill the recipient animal. The resultant ALD differed from the $LD_{50}$ (as calculated by the probit method from more complete data sets) by −22 to +33%.

The Deichmann method proved to be too imprecise. Later, Dixon and Wood (1948), followed by Brownlee et al. (1953), developed the method in which one

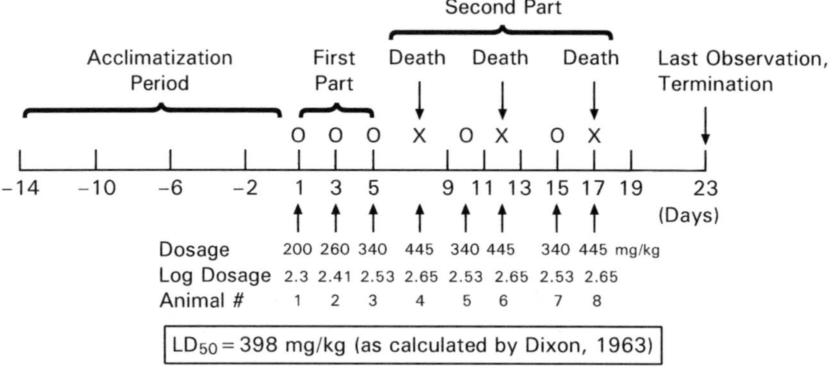


**FIGURE 5.3.** Example of typical up–down acute lethality protocol.

animal was exposed per dosage, but subsequent dosages were adjusted up or down by some constant factor depending on the outcome of the previous dosage. In this method (Figure 5.3), which has been developed more extensively by Bruce (1985), individual animals are dosed at different dosages on successive days. If an animal dies, the dosage for the next animal is decreased by a factor of 1.3. Conversely, if an animal lives, the next dosage is increased by a factor of 1.3. The process is continued until five animals have been dosed after a reversal of the first observation. Alternatively, one can use the tables developed by Dixon (1965). This design can be used not only for range-finding purposes but also to define an $LD_{50}$ if this value is needed. In general, only six to nine animals are required, unless the initial dosages are grossly high or low. When compared to the $LD_{50}$ obtained by other more classical protocols, excellent agreement is obtained with the up/down method (Bruce, 1985). As with classical protocols, sexes should be tested separately. However a further reduction in the numbers of animals used can be accomplished if one is willing to accept that females are of the same or increased sensitivity as males, as is the case approximately 85%–90% of the time (Gad and Chengelis, 1999).

There are three main disadvantages to using the up/down method. The first is regulatory, the second procedural, and the third scientific. First, many regulatory guidelines simply have a requirement for the use of traditional protocols. Some also specify the method of calculation. Second, the sequential dosing design is inappropriate for substances that cause delayed deaths. As reported by various authors (Gad et al., 1984; Bruce, 1985), delayed deaths (beyond two days after dosing) are rare but not unknown. They are most prevalent when animals are dosed by the intraperitoneal route with a chemical that causes peritonitis. Death secondary to severe liver or gastrointestinal damage may also take over two days to occur. To guard against possible spurious results, all animals should be maintained and observed for at least seven days after dosing. If delayed deaths occur, the original data set must be corrected and the $LD_{50}$ recalculated. A substantial number of delayed deaths could result in a data set from which an $LD_{50}$ cannot be calculated, in which case the test should be rerun.

***"Pyramiding" Studies.*** Using this type of design (Figure 5.4), one can obtain information about lethality with the minimum expenditure of animals. A minimum of two animals are dosed throughout the study, usually on alternate days (e.g., Monday, Wednesday, and Friday), but the dosage at session may be 1, 3, 10, 30, 100, 300, 1000, and 3000 mg kg$^{-1}$, or 10, 20, 40, 80, 160, 320, 640, and 1280 mg kg$^{-1}$. One is literally stepping up, or pyramiding, the lethality-dosage curve. Dosing continues in this fashion until one or both animals die or until some practical upward limit is reached. For drugs, there is no longer a need to go higher than 1000 mg kg$^{-1}$ for rodents or nonrodents. An alternative, but similar, design is the "leapfrog" study (Figure 5.5). This consists of two groups of two animals each. They are dosed on alternating days, but the dosages are increased each day. Extending the example of the pyramiding regiment, group 1 would receive 10, 60, and 120 mg kg$^{-1}$, while group 2 would be given 30, 100, and 120 mg kg$^{-1}$. This design is of value when one has to complete the range-finding activity in a short period of time. Because these designs utilize few animals, they are commonly used for assessing lethality in nonrodent species. An exploratory study typically uses an animal of each sex.

There are three conclusions that can be reached on the basis of data from a pyramiding dosage study. First, if none of the animals dies, then both the threshold or minimum lethal dosage (MLD) and the $LD_{50}$ are greater than the top or limit dosage. Second, if all animals die at the same dosage, then both the MLD and the $LD_{50}$ are reported as being between the last two dosages given. This not uncommon finding is an indication that the lethality curve has a steep slope. Third, one animal may die at one dosage and remaining deaths occur at a subsequent dosage. In this case, the MLD is between the lowest nonlethal dosage and the dosage at which the first death occurred, while the $LD_{50}$ is reported as being between this latter dosage

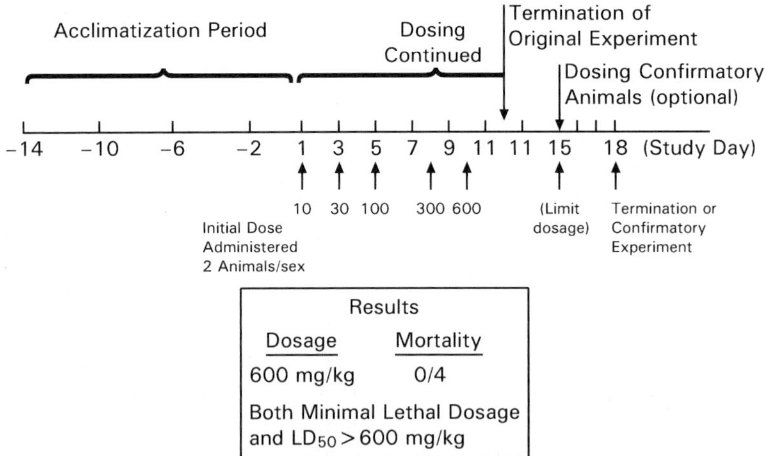


**FIGURE 5.4.** Example of typical pyramiding dose protocol.

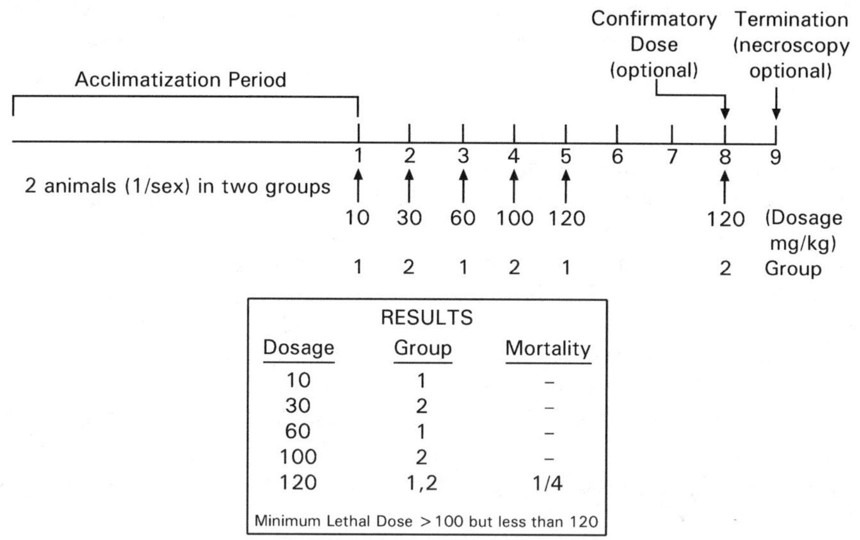

FIGURE 5.5. Example of typical "leapfrog" dosing protocol.

and the dosage at which the last animal dies. A frequently employed variation with nonrodents is, if lethality is not observed, the animals are dosed for five or seven consecutive days at the highest observed tolerated dose. This "phase B" study portion serves to provide more confidence in selecting the top dose in subsequent repeat dose studies.

There are some disadvantages to the pyramiding dose protocol. First, it cannot produce a lethality curve or provide for the calculation of an $LD_{50}$. Second, this method cannot identify delayed deaths. If an animal, for example, dies 1 hour after the second dosage, one has no way of determining whether it was actually the second dosage or a delayed effect of the first. For this reason it is of little value to observe the animals for any more than a few days after the last dosage. Third, if the test article has an unusually long half-life, bioaccumulation can lead to an underestimation of the acute lethal dosage. By contract, the pharmacological accommodation can lead to a spuriously high estimate of lethality. Depending on the importance of the finding, one may wish to confirm that the results obtained at the highest dosage administered were dosing two naïve animals at the same dosage. Fortunately, the minimum 48-hour period between dosing sessions will minimize such effects. Because of this design feature, it may take as long as three weeks to complete the dosing sequence. However, as there is generally no need for a 1- to 2-week post-dosing observation or holding period, the actual study may not take significantly more time than a test of more traditional design.

Keep in mind that the objective of such studies is to gain information about lethality and gross tolerance. For nonrodents (especially monkeys), if none of the animals dies or demonstrates obvious signs of toxicity, little would be gained by euthanizing and necropsying such animals. They can be saved and used again, following a reasonable "washout" period, to assess the lethality, toxicity, or safety pharmacology of a different chemical. In the hands of a skilled toxicologist, such adaptive reuse of animals is a cost-effective way to minimize overall usage.

***Limit Tests.*** There are many relatively innocuous drugs that are simply not potently lethal. The limit test (Figure 5.6) provides the simplest protocol for determining the lethality of such substances. The limit test is designed to obtain clearance at a specific dosage based on the assumption that what may occur at a higher dosage is not of practical relevance. Thus, one dosage only is studied. This limit "dosage" can be set on the basis of the chemical or physical properties of the test article (or vehicle), or on the basis of an upward safety margin. If the preparation is highly acidic (pH < 3), large intravenous dose would be expected to cause systemic acidosis as well as local irritation, but will yield little relevant toxicology information, as such a preparation would never be approved for clinical use. Alternately, if the anticipated human dosage of a drug is 0.3 mg kg$^{-1}$, there is probably little reason to test dosages in excess of 300 mg kg$^{-1}$, (1000 times) the expected human dosage). In general, there is never any reason to use dosages of 5 g kg$^{-1}$ or greater, and rarely any reason to exceed 3 g kg$^{-1}$.

There are three possible outcomes to a limit test. If none of the animals dies, then the conclusion is that the MLD is greater than the limit dosage. If fewer than 50% of the animals die, then the conclusion is that the LD$_{50}$ is greater than the limit dosage. If more than 50% of the animals die, then one has a problem. Depending on the reasons for performing the test, one could reset the limit and repeat the study, or one could assess lethality by a different protocol. Alternatively, the change in the limit could reflect a change in the chemical or biological properties of the test substance that should be evaluated further.

***Fixed Dose Procedure.*** The fixed dose design (Figure 5.7) was proposed by the British Toxicology Society (1984). It is designed to supply the data needed for classification or labeling purposes. It is essentially a three-step limit test.

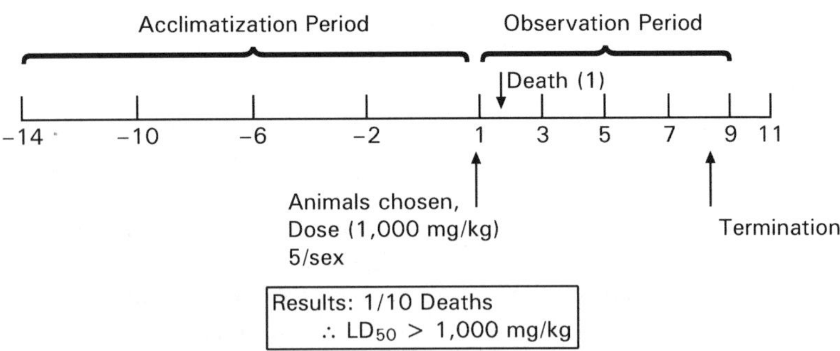


**FIGURE 5.6.** Example of typical limit test protocol.

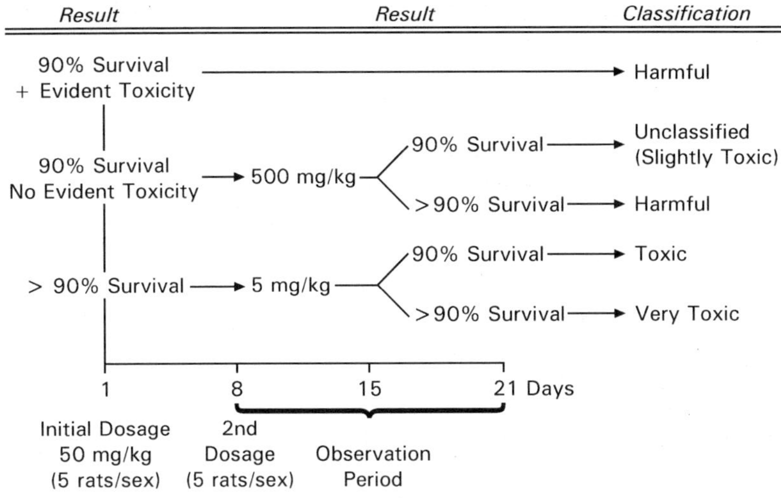


**FIGURE 5.7.** British Toxicology Society fixed dose procedure.

Five rats per sex are given 50 mg kg$^{-1}$. If survival is less than 90%, a second group of animals is given 5 mg kg$^{-1}$. If survival is again less than 90%, the substance is classified as "very toxic;" otherwise, it is classified as "toxic."

If, after the 50 mg kg$^{-1}$ dose, survival is 90% but there is evident toxicity, no further dosages are given and the substance is classified as "harmful." If, on the other hand, there is no evident toxicity at 50 mg kg$^{-1}$, another group of rats is given 500 mg kg$^{-1}$. If there is again 90% survival and no evident toxicity, the substance is given "unclassified" or "slightly toxic" status.

The fixed dose procedure is relatively new and apparently results in a large decrease in animal usage. It is also noteworthy in that it utilizes not only lethality but also "evident toxicity," which, in all likelihood, refers to obvious signs of CNS effect, such as seizures or prostration. Whether or not this protocol design becomes widely accepted by various regulatory agencies remains to be established.

The potential utility of the fixed-dose procedure was demonstrated in an international validation study in which the acute oral toxicity of 20 different chemicals was evaluated using both the fixed dose and classical LD$_{50}$ procedures. Thirty-three laboratories in 11 different countries were involved in the validation project, and the results have been published (van den Heuvel et al., 1990). The results demonstrated that the fixed dose procedure produced consistent evaluations of acute toxicity that were not subject to significant interlaboratory variation, and provided sufficient information for hazard identification and risk assessment based on signs of toxicity (clinical signs, time-to-onset, duration, outcome, etc.). The fixed dose procedure used fewer animals than the classical LD$_{50}$ tests and generally required less time to complete. Because of the emphasis on toxicity (rather than mortality) and the use of fewer animals, the fixed dose procedure could be considered a more "humane" or animal-sparing design than the classical LD$_{50}$

**TABLE 5.2. Comparison of Toxicity Classification Based on LD$_{50}$ versus Fixed Dose Procedure**

| Test Chemical | Toxicity Classification Based on LD$_{50}$ | Fixed-dose: Number of Laboratories Classifying Chemical | | | |
|---|---|---|---|---|---|
| | | Very Toxic | Toxic | Harmful | Unclassified |
| Nicotine | Toxic | — | 23 | 3 | — |
| Sodium pentachlorophenate | Harmful | — | 1 | 25 | — |
| Ferrocene | Harmful/unclassified | — | — | 3 | |
| 2-Chloroethyl alcohol | Toxic | — | 19 | 7 | — |
| Sodium arsenite | Toxic | — | 25 | 1 | — |
| Phenyl mercury acetate | Toxic | 2 | 24 | — | — |
| p-Dichlorobenzene | Unclassified | — | — | — | 26 |
| Fentin hydroxide | Toxic | — | 8 | 17 | 1 |
| Acetanilide | Harmful | — | — | 4 | 22 |
| Quercetin dihydrate | Unclassified | — | — | — | 26 |
| Tetrachlorvinphos | Unclassified | — | — | 1 | 25 |
| Piperidine | Harmful | — | 2 | 24 | — |
| Mercuric chloride | Toxic | — | 25 | 1 | — |
| 1-Phenyl-2-thiourea | Toxic/harmful | 12 | 12 | 2 | — |
| 4-Aminophenol | harmful | — | — | 17 | 9 |
| Naphthalene | Unclassified | — | — | — | 26 |
| Acetonitrile | Harmful | — | — | 4 | 22 |
| Aldicarb (10%) | Very toxic | 22 | — | — | — |
| Resorcinol | Harmful | — | — | 25 | 1 |
| Dimethyl formamide | Unclassified | — | — | — | 26 |

*Source*: van der Heuvel *et al.*, 1990.

test. When the results of the fixed dose and LD$_{50}$ tests were compared for hazard ranking purposes (Table 5.2), comparable results were obtained. Thus, it would appear that the fixed dose procedure has utility. It was recommended late in 2000 for broad regulatory adaptation by ICVAM.

***"Rolling" Acute Test.*** The rolling acute test is a combination protocol that is designed to find a tolerated dose to use for a subchronic toxicity test. The first segment can be either a dose probe or an up/down or pyramiding type of study to define the MLD. In the second segment, three to five animals are dosed for as short period of time, five to seven days. The objective of this design is to compensate for the fact that cumulative toxicity can occur at substantial differences in acute and subchronic toxic dosages. One can be easily misled by selecting subchronic dosages based entirely on acute lethality data. An example is a drug tested where it was found that 360 mg kg$^{-1}$ was acutely nonlethal and the MLD was 970 mg kg$^{-1}$. The dosages selected for the four-week subchronic study were 50,

100, 200 and 400 mg kg$^{-1}$ day$^{-1}$. The top-dose animals all died within a week. Substantial mortality occurred at 200 mg kg$^{-1}$ and evident toxicity was present at 50 mg kg$^{-1}$. A no-effect dosage was not identified, so the entire test had to be repeated with a different dosage structure. The rolling acute structure is a quick and relatively simple "sanity" check that permits one to avoid making such mistakes.

### 5.2.2. Using Range-Finding Lethality Data in Drug Development: The Minimum Lethal Dosage

Range-finding data are often used early in drug development to make preliminary safety estimates. The LD$_{50}$ is simply a calculated point on a curve. The shape or slope of this curve is also an important characteristic of the test substance. However, unless one does a great deal of acute toxicity testing, the difference between a slope of 1.5 and a slope of 4 has very little meaning. Further, for safety considerations, the dosage that kills 50% of the animals is not as important as the dosage at which lethality first becomes apparent (i.e., the threshold dosage or MLD). For example, if the oral LD$_{50}$s of two different drugs (A and B) were 0.6 and 2.0 g kg$^{-1}$, respectively, what would we conclude about the relative safety of these compounds? Further, let us assume that the estimated human dosage of drug A is 0.5 mg kg$^{-1}$ and of drug B is 5 mg kg$^{-1}$. Do our conclusions concerning the relative safety of these two drugs change? In fact, the LD$_{50}$s of both drugs are so high that both are considered only slightly toxic (0.5 to 5.0 g kg$^{-1}$). One can also compute the lethality safety margin or index (LSI, equal to LD$_{50}$/EHD, where EHD is the estimated human dose) for these two drugs; both indices are so large (1200 for A and 400 for B) that there is still no toxicologically relevant difference between the two drugs. Let us now assume that the lethality curve for substance A is very steep, such that 0.4 g kg$^{-1}$ causes death in a very small percentage of animals; it is, in fact, the lowest dose administered that causes death. This is the MLD or estimated MLD (EMLD). Let us now assume that the lethality curve for B is very shallow, such that its MLD is also 0.4 g kg$^{-1}$. Does this change our safety considerations of these two drugs? One can calculate a new more conservative safety index (MLD/EHD) of 800 for A and 80 for B. As a very general rule of thumb, an index for lethality of less than 100 is cause for mild concern, one less than 10 is cause for caution, and one less than 1 should be cause for extreme caution. In the case of our two hypothetical drugs, the development of drug B should be approached with more caution than that of drug A, despite the fact that B has a higher LD$_{50}$. This is demonstrated in Figure 5.8. There are drugs sold over the counter, however, that have lethality safety indices of less than 10. For example, the MLD of indomethacin in rats is 3.7 mg kg$^{-1}$ (from data reported by Schiantarelli and Cadel, 1981), while the maximum recommended human dose is 200 mg (2.9 mg kg$^{-1}$ for a 70-kg person); hence, indomethacin has an LSI of 1.3. Such a finding is only cause for some caution, but does not in and of itself justify restricting the use or sale of a drug. Hence, because it results in a more conservative safety factor and also takes into consideration the slope of the lethality curve, the use of the MLD rather than the LD$_{50}$ is recommended in calculating acute safety indices.

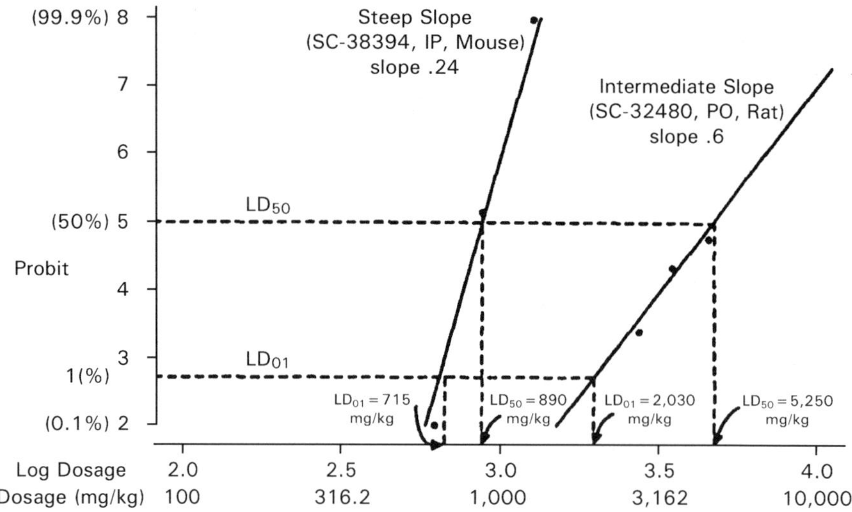


**FIGURE 5.8.** Examples of probit-log dosage response curves illustrating differences in slope curves and the relationship between the slope, $LD_{50}$, and $LD_{01}$.

A number of different safety factors and therapeutic indices have been proposed in the literature. Despite their similarity, some distinction should be made between these two. A therapeutic index applies only to drugs and is the ratio between a toxic dosage (TD or LD: the toxic endpoint does not always have to be death) and the pharmacologically effective dosage (ED) *in the same species*. A safety index can be calculated for all xenobiotics, not just drugs. A safety index is the ratio of likely human exposure (or dosage) and the dosage that causes death or other forms of toxicity in the most sensitive experimental animal species. The most conservative (lethality) safety index (LSI) is obtained by dividing the maximum estimated human dosage or exposure by either the minimum lethal dosage or the maximum nonlethal dosage.

***Minimum Lethal Dosage Protocols.*** Stating that the MLD is preferable to the $LD_{50}$ for safety considerations is one thing; trying to determine what a specific MLD may be or could be is another. There are no commonly used experimental designs that have the MLD as an endpoint. Assuming a log dose response, the MLD may become a function of group size. Theoretically, if enough animals are dosed, at least one animal could die at any reasonable dosage. There are, however, practical considerations that can and should be applied to determining an MLD. As a practical rule of thumb, we recommend that the estimated $LD_{01}$—the dose that would be expected to kill 1% of the experimental animals exposed—be used as an estimate of the MLD. If one already has sufficient data to describe a lethality curve, an $LD_{01}$ can be calculated as easily as the $LD_{50}$. This is often the case with acute toxicity data obtained to support regulatory submission.

How is the MLD calculated without a complete lethality curve? A modified pyramiding dosage design may be the most appropriate approach. With this design, groups of animals are treated with stepwise increases in dosage until death occurs or a limit dosage is attained. If one has no idea as to what the initial dosage should be or how to graduate the dosages, a dose-probing experiment can be conducted. If the dose-probing experiment produces no deaths, two to three more animals can be dosed at the limit dose to confirm the results; the lethality determination is now complete. If the probe experiment does produce death, then the additional dosages can be graduated between the lowest lethal and the highest nonlethal dosages. A typical progression may proceed as follows (Figure 5.9): On Day 1 of the study, three probe animals are dosed at 10, 100, and 1000 mg kg$^{-1}$. The animal at 100 mg kg$^{-1}$ dies within a few hours of dosing. The two remaining animals are dosed at 300 mg kg$^{-1}$ on Day 3. Neither dies. They are then dosed at 500 mg kg$^{-1}$ on Day 5. One dies. Three additional animals should be dosed on Day 7 or 8 at a dosage in between (i.e., 400 mg kg$^{-1}$ is a good estimate of the maximum nonlethal dosage, or MNLD). While different by definition, there is usually not a great deal of distance between the MLD and the MNLD, as this example illustrates. In fact, even for a well-characterized lethality curve; the confidence limits for the LD$_{01}$ will be quite broad and encompass both the MLD and MNLD.

Malmfors and Teiling (1983) have proposed a similar method for determining what they also termed the MNLD (maximum nonlethal dose). Rather than initiating the study with probe animals, their design calls for three consecutive pyramiding-type studies with the steps becoming increasingly smaller. For example, two animals will be sequentially dosed at 2, 200, and 2000 mg kg$^{-1}$. If death occurs at 2000 mg kg$^{-1}$, a new pair of animals is initiated at 200 mg kg$^{-1}$, and sequential dosages are increased by a factor of 1.8 until death occurs. Then another pair of animals is initiated at the highest nonlethal dosage, and successive dosages are increased by a factor of 1.15. The result of this exercise will be two dosages, one apparently nonlethal and the other lethal. Six animals are dosed at each dosage. If none dies at the lower dosage and one dies at the higher dose, then the lower dose is considered to be the MNLD. At least 24 hours between dosing rounds are recommended. While this method may have some utility, there are some disadvantages. First, the

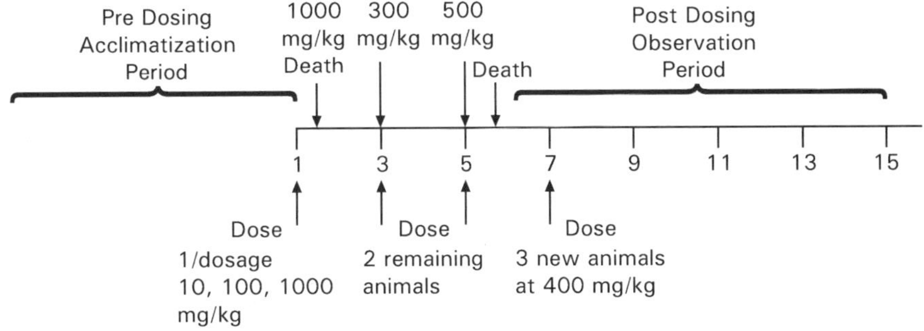


**FIGURE 5.9.** Example of minimum lethal dosage (MLD) pyramiding dose design.

recommended limiting dosage of $6.5\,g\,kg^{-1}$ is too high. Second, 24 hours between doses may be too short a period to allow for recovery. Third, even with only 24 hours between doses, this is a time-consuming procedure; it may take up to two weeks to complete the dosing. Finally, it does not decrease the number of animals needed, since it may use 18 to 20 animals.

Dose probing is not generally used for nonrodents, and the initiating dosage is normally in the range of 1 to 5 times the projected human clinical dosage. The limit is generally in the area of $1\,g\,kg^{-1}$ or 100–200 times the human dosage, whichever is less. The normal study will include two animals of each sex treated with the test article. For simple lethality, there is seldom any need to include control animals. If the projected human dosage is $4\,mg\,kg^{-1}$, for example, the initial dosage in an MLD range finder in dogs will be $20\,mg\,kg^{-1}$ and succeeding dosages will increase stepwise at half-log intervals; thus, 20, 60, 200, and $600\,mg\,kg^{-1}$ doses are separated by at least 48 hours. The MLD is simply reported as being between the highest observable nonlethal and the lowest lethal dosages, or at greater than the limit dosage, in this case, $600\,mg\,kg^{-1}$. Studies should not be done with nonrodents solely for determining lethality, because this would not be an appropriate use of time and animals. Generally, these studies should also include some combination of extensive physical examinations, such as ECGs and rectal temperatures, careful observations of behavior and activity, and extensive clinical laboratory workups after each dose.

The pyramiding dose study is not without disadvantages. The small number of animals used can cause simple random variation resulting in misestimation of lethality. It is a well-accepted statistical maxim that the smaller the sample size, the greater the impact of any random variation (error or outlier) on the population characteristic. This may be especially true for a nonrodent species where experimental animals are drawn from an outbred population. Second, the pyramiding dose regimen can permit the development of tolerance. For example, pyramiding dosage studies were conducted to range-find dosages for a two-week study on a 1,4-benzodiazepine. Lethality in dogs was observed at $600\,mg\,kg^{-1}$ in the pyramiding study. For the subsequent subchronic study, the top dose was set at $300\,mg\,kg^{-1}$; both dogs died of CNS depression on the first day of dosing.

## 5.3. ACUTE SYSTEMIC TOXICITY CHARACTERIZATION

Acute systemic toxicity studies are performed to more completely define the acute toxicity of a drug. They are more extensive and time-consuming than range-finding tests or screens, and are normally the type of study done to satisfy regulatory requirements or to provide a more thorough early characterization or prediction of toxicity. In pharmaceutical development, an acute test would rarely be sufficient to support registration, but it may be required as part of an overall package. These protocols may resemble range-finding tests, but they call for collection of more data. A list of the types of data that can be obtained in well-conducted acute toxicity tests is given in Table 5.3. Given that these studies usually include control groups, the

**TABLE 5.3. Information, Including Lethality, that can be Gained in Acute Toxicity Testing**

Lethality/Mortality
   $LD_{50}$ with confidence limits
   Shape and slope of lethality curves
   Estimation of maximum nonlethal dose or minimum lethal dose ($LD_{01}$)
   Time to dose estimates
Clinical signs
   Times of onset and recovery
   Thresholds
   Agonal vs. nonagonal (i.e., do signs occur only in animals that die?)
   Specific vs. general responses
   Separation of dose-response curves from lethality curves
Body weight changes
   Actual loss vs. decreased gain
   Recovery
   Accompanied by changes in feed consumption
   Changes in animals that die vs. those that survive
Target organ identification
   Gross examinations
   Histological examinations
   Clinical chemical changes
   Hematological changes
Specialized function tests
   Immunocompetency
   Neuromuscular screening
   Behavioral screening
Pharmacokinetic considerations
   Different routes of administration yielding differences in toxicity
   Plasma levels of test article
   Areas under the curves, volume of distribution, half-life
   Metablic pattern of test article
   Distribution to key organs
   Relationship between plasma levels and occurrence of clinical signs

classical or traditional design is the most common because it allows for the most straightforward statistical analyses. In addition, while the use of staggered dosing days for different groups is still a fairly common practice, data analyses may be more sensitive if all animals are dosed on the same day, requiring that one have preliminary range-finder data that permits selection of appropriate dosages. Studies of more than one species and/or more than one route should be limited to those instances where they are required by statute.

In general, traditionally designed acute toxicity tests can be divided into three types that can be called the minimal acute toxicity test, the complete acute toxicity test, and the supplemented acute toxicity test. Of these, the minimal protocol is by far the most common and is discussed first. The other two represent increasing orders of complexity as additional parameters of measurement are added to the basic minimal study.

### 5.3.1.  Minimal Acute Toxicity Test

An example of a typical minimal acute toxicity test protocol is shown in Figure 5.10. This study resembles a traditional lethality test in terms of the number of groups and the number of animals per group. Standard protocols consist of three or four groups of treated animals and one group of control animals, each group consisting of five animals per sex per dosage. Traditionally, the emphasis in these types of studies was on determining the $LD_{50}$, time to death, slope of the lethality curve, and the prominent clinical signs, as illustrated by the data reported by Jenner et al. (1964). More recent designs specify, in addition to lethality and clinical observations, that body weights be recorded during the study and gross necropsies performed at the end of the postdosing observation period. For an excellent example of a well-performed acute toxicity evaluation the reader is referred to the paper by Peterson et al. (1987) of the acute toxicity of the alkaloids of *Lupinus angustifolius*, in which the $LD_{50}$s, time to death, clinical signs, body weight effect, and gross necropsy findings were all discussed. For pharmaceuticals, where acute toxicity data for more than one species are often required, these studies will be done as batteries on both rats and mice. In addition, because many drugs will be given by more than one route to human patients, these batteries will include groups treated by two different routes. Thus, an acute study on a pharmaceutical agent will often result in eight "curves," one per route per species per sex. For tests on nonrodent species, as required for pharmaceuticals, a different design is used (discussed later).

The animals should be acclimated to laboratory conditions for 7 to 14 days prior to dosing. For acute toxicity tests, this pretreatment period should be more than just a holding period. Animals should be checked daily for signs of ill health and/or abnormal behavior. Body weights may also be determined. These data should be used to exclude abnormal animals from the test. Such data also provide an additional basis for interpreting the data gathered during the postdosing period. Finally, these

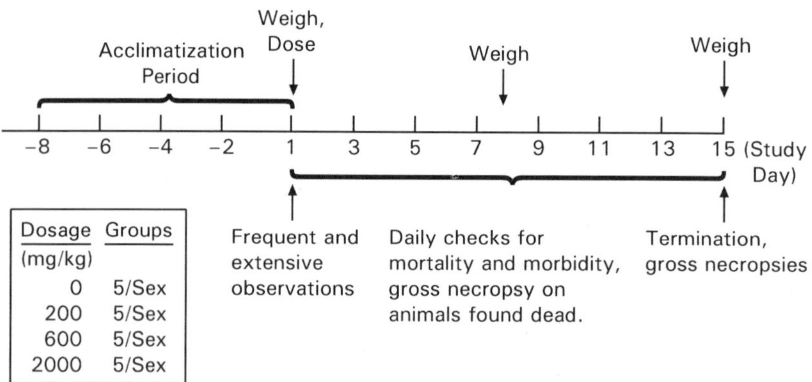


**FIGURE 5.10.** Example of minimal acute toxicity protocol.

activities acclimate the animals to the frequent handling that is a necessary part of an acute toxicity test.

In selecting dosages for an acute systemic toxicity study, the same general guidelines apply as with lethality testing:

1. There is little to be gained from testing dosages that are so high that the physical rather than biological properties become prominent. Generally, little additional information is gained by pushing dosages past $3\,\mathrm{g\,kg}^{-1}$.
2. The highest dosage should be no larger than 100–300 times the anticipated human dosage.
3. Widely spaced dosages are better than narrowly spaced dosages.

This latter point is particularly true in an acute toxicity test on a drug, because pharmacologically based clinical signs may occur at dosages considerably lower than those that cause death. Also, as discussed by Sperling (1976) and Gad (1982), the effects at high dosages may mask the effects that would be observed at low dosages. As human beings are more likely to be exposed to lower dosages than experimental animals, these low-dosage effects may be important parameters to define.

Historically, it has been stated in various regulatory communications that a well-conducted acute toxicity test should contain sufficient data to calculate an $LD_{50}$. This is no longer necessarily the case. Simpler, less resource-intensive range-finding protocols should be used for defining lethality. Because it is rare that an extensive acute protocol would be attempted without preliminary lethality data, the lethality objectives of acute systemic testing are not always critical. Ideally, the highest dosage should elicit marked toxicity (such as lethality), but it does not need to kill all of the animals to satisfy one's need to show due diligence in stressing the test system. If one already has sufficient preliminary data to suspect that the top dosage will be nonlethal or otherwise innocuous, the test can be conducted as a limit test, consisting of one treated group and one control group.

***Clinical Signs.*** The nonlethal parameters of acute toxicity testing have been extensively reviewed by Sperling (1976) and Balazs (1970, 1976). Clinical observations or signs of toxicity are perhaps the most important aspect of a minimal acute toxicity test because they are the first indicators of drug- or chemical-related toxicity or morbidity, and they are necessary in the interpretation of other data collected. For example, body weight loss (or a reduction in body weight gain) would be expected if an animal had profound CNS depression lasting several hours.

With regard to clinical signs and observations, there are some basic definitions that should be kept in mind. Symptomatology is the overall manifestation of toxicity. Signs are overt and observable events (Brown, 1983). Symptoms are the subjective impressions of a human patient (e.g., headache) and cannot be described or reported by speechless animals (Balazs, 1970). Clinical signs can be reversible or irreversible. Reversible signs are those that dissipate as the chemical is cleared from the body or tolerance develops (Chan et al., 1982) and are generally not accompanied by permanent organ damage. Irreversible signs are those that do not dissipate and are generally accompanied by organic damage. Signs can also represent a normal biological or pharmacological response (Chan et al., 1982). For example, an antidepressant would be expected to cause decreased activity and some ataxia. These symptoms are generally reversible and can lead to secondary, nonspecific signs: nonspecific in that any number of agents or stimuli can evoke the same response, and secondary in that they are probably not due (at least, one has no evidence to determine otherwise) to the direct action of the test article. Responses can also be abnormal, in that they are not due to a homeostatic process. The increases in serum urea and creatinine due to kidney damage, for example, are abnormal responses. These are often irreversible, but this is not always the case, depending on the repair capacity or functional reserves of the target organ. These abnormal responses may also be called primary effects because they reflect the direct action of a test article. Agonal signs are those occurring immediately prior to, or concomitantly with, death. They are obviously irreversible, but not necessarily reflective of a specific effect of a test article. For example, regardless of the cause, labored breathing will occur in a moribund animal. It is, therefore, important to distinguish between signs that occur in animals that die and those that do not. It should also be kept in mind that agonal signs may mask (make it difficult or impossible) to observe other signs, including those clearly seen at lower doses.

In their simplest form, clinical observations are those done on an animal in its cage, or, preferably, in an open plane, such as on the top of a counter or laboratory cart. These are considered passive observations. One can gain even more information by active examination of the animal, such as the animal's response to stimulation. Fowler and Rutty (1983) divide their clinical evaluation of toxicity into those signs scored by simple observations (e.g., ataxia), those scored by provocation (e.g., righting reflex), those scored in the hand (e.g., mydriasis) and those scored by monitoring (e.g., rectal temperature). Cage pans should always be examined for unusually large or small amounts of excreta, or excreta of abnormal color or consistency. A list of typical observations is summarized in Table 5.4. A more extensive table has been prepared by Chan et al. (1982). Given the fact that the number of different signs displayed is not infinite and that some signs are simply easier to discern than others, most clinical signs are referable to the CNS (e.g., lack of activity), the GI tract (e.g., diarrhea) or the general autonomic nervous system (e.g., increased salivation or lacrimation). This is illustrated by an actual example set of data from acute toxicity studies summarized in Table 5.5.

Other signs can be detected by a well-trained observer, but are, nonetheless, less common than those described above. Respiratory distress can be diagnosed by examining the animal's breathing motions and listening for breathing noises. Cardiovascular signs are generally limited to pallor, cyanosis, and/or hypothermia. Changes in cardiac function can be difficult to detect in small animals, and generally consist of "weak" or "slow" breathing. Arrhythmias can be difficult to detect because the normal heart rate in a rodent is quite rapid. EKGs are difficult to record from rodents on a routine basis. Therefore, the assessment of potential acute cardiovascular effect of a drug or chemical is usually restricted to a nonrodent species, usually the dog.

**TABLE 5.4. Clinical Observation in Acute Toxicity Tests**

| Organ system | Observation and examination | Common signs of toxicity |
| --- | --- | --- |
| CNS and somatomotor | Behavior | Unusual aggressiveness, unusual vocalization, restlessness, sedation |
|  | Movements | Twitch, tremor, ataxia, catatonia, paralysis, convulsion |
|  | Reactivity to various stimuli | Irritability, passivity, anesthesia, hyperesthesia |
|  | Cerebral and spinal reflexes | Sluggishness, absence of reflex |
|  | Muscle Tone | Rigidity, flaccidity |
| Autonomic nervous system | Pupil size | Miosis, mydriasis |
| Respiratory | Nostrils | Discharge (color vs. uncolored) |
|  | Character and rate | Bradypnea, dyspnea, Cheyne–Stokes breathing, Kussmaul breathing |
| Cardiovascular | Palpation of cardiac region | Thrill, bradycardia, arrhythmia, stronger or weaker beat |
| Gastrointestinal | Events | Diarrhea, constipation |
|  | Abdominal shape | Flatulence, contraction |
|  | Feces consistency and color | Unformed, black or clay colored |
| Genitourinary | Vulva, mammary glands | Swelling |
|  | Penis | Prolapse |
|  | Perineal region | Soiled |
| Skin and fur | Color, turgor, integrity | Reddening, flaccid skinfold, eruptions, piloerection |
| Mucous membranes | Conjunctiva, mouth | Discharge, congestion, hemorrhage, cyanosis, jaundice |
| Eye | Eyelids | Ptosis |
|  | Eyeball | Exophthalmos, nystagmus |
|  | Transparency | Opacities |
| Others | Rectal or paw skin temperature | Subnormal, increased |
|  | Injection site | Swelling |
|  | General condition | Abnormal posture, emaciation |

*Source*: Balazs, 1970.

Given the subjective nature of recognizing clinical signs, careful steps must be taken to ensure uniformity (is the animal depressed or prostrated?) of observation so that the data can be analyzed in a meaningful fashion. There are three ways of achieving this. First, signs should be restricted to a predefined list of simple descriptive terms, such as those listed in Table 5.4 or in Appendix B. Second, if a computerized data acquisition system is unavailable, the use of standardized forms will add uniformity to the observation and recording processes. An example of such

**TABLE 5.5. Summary of Clinical Observations from Actual Acute Toxicity Tests**

| Drug (route) | Indication | Acute Clinical Signs[a] |
|---|---|---|
| SC-37407 (PO) | Analgesic (opiate) | Reduced motor activity, mydriasis, reduced fecal output, hunched posture, convulsions (tonic), ataxia |
| SC-35135 (PO) | Arrhythmias | Reduced motor activity, lost righting reflex, tremors, dyspnea, ataxia, mydriasis |
| SC-32840 (PO) | Intravascular thrombosis | Reduced motor activity, ataxia, lost righting reflex, closed eyes, red/clear tears |
| SC-31828 (PO) | Arrhythmias | Reduced activity, dyspnea, ataxia, lost righting reflex, red/clear tears |
| SC-25469 (PO) | Analgesic (nonopiate) | Reduced motor activity, ataxia, lost righting reflex, dyspnea, convulsions (clonic) |

[a] The five or six most frequent signs in descending order of occurrence.

a form is shown in Figure 5.11. Third, technicians should be trained in studies (not intended for regulatory submission) using material of known toxicity, so that all personnel involved in such evaluations are using the same terminology to describe the same signs.

Animals should be observed continuously for several hours following dosing. Times of observation should be recorded as well as the actual observations. After the first day of the study, observations generally need only to consist of brief checks for sign remission and the development of new signs of morbidity. Data should be collected in such a way that the following could be concluded for each sign: (1) estimated times of onset and recovery, (2) the range of threshold dosages, and (3) whether signs are directly related (primary) to the test article. An example of clinical signs provoked by a specific drug is given in Table 5.6. Incidences are broken down by dosage group and sex. These data illustrate the fact that mortality can censor (preclude) the occurrence of clinical signs. Note that reduced fecal output was a more frequent observation at the intermediate dosages because most of the animals died at the higher dosages.

Therapeutic ratios are traditionally calculated using the $LD_{50}$. A more sensitive therapeutic ratio could be calculated using the $ED_{50}$ (effective dose) for the most prominent clinical sign. However, while it may be possible to describe a dosage-response curve (which may, in fact, have a different slope than the lethality curve) for a clinical sign, and calculate the $ED_{50}$, in practice this is rarely done. It is more common for the approximate threshold dosages or no observable effect levels (NOELs) to be reported. A typical minimal acute toxicity study can be summarized as shown in Table 5.7.

# ACUTE OBSERVATION RECORD

(Days, other than Study Day 1, on which no signs are observed are recorded on the Log of Animal Observations)

Species    Sex    Route    Dose Level    Animals Coded*    Date Dosed

| | | | | | | | | | | | | |
|---|---|---|---|---|---|---|---|---|---|---|---|---|
| Study Day | | | | | | | | | | | | |
| OBSERVATIONS: Time | | | | | | | | | | | | |
| Date | | | | | | | | | | | | |
| No Signs Observed | | | | | | | | | | | | |
| Reduced Motor Activity | | | | | | | | | | | | |
| Ataxia | | | | | | | | | | | | |
| Lost Righting Reflex | | | | | | | | | | | | |
| Convulsions ( ) | | | | | | | | | | | | |
| Mydriasis | | | | | | | | | | | | |
| | | | | | | | | | | | | |
| | | | | | | | | | | | | |
| | | | | | | | | | | | | |
| | | | | | | | | | | | | |
| | | | | | | | | | | | | |
| | | | | | | | | | | | | |
| | | | | | | | | | | | | |
| DEATH | | | | | | | | | | | | |
| Observer | | | | | | | | | | | | |

Page of NOTES:

*An Code    An. ID

*Animal Code for Recording Observations

Read and Understood

_____________________ Date

**FIGURE 5.11.** Example of a form for recording clinical observations in acute systemic toxicity studies.

**TABLE 5.6.  Example of Clinical Observations Broken Down by Dosage Group and Sex in an Acute Toxicity Study of the Drug SC-37407[a]**

| | Dose Levels ($mg\ kg^{-1}$) by sex | | | | | | | | | |
| | 0 | | 50 | | 160 | | 500 | | 1600 | |
| Signs Observed | M | F | M | F | M | F | M | F | M | F |
|---|---|---|---|---|---|---|---|---|---|---|
| Reduced motor activity | — | — | — | — | — | — | 5/5 | 5/5 | 4/5 | 4/5 |
| Mydriasis | — | — | — | — | 3/5 | 4/5 | 4/5 | 5/5 | 5/5 | 5/5 |
| Reduced fecal output | — | — | 5/5 | 5/5 | 3/5 | 5/5 | — | 1/5 | — | — |
| Hunched posture | — | — | — | — | — | 1/5 | 3/5 | 3/5 | — | — |
| Convulsions (tonic) | — | — | — | — | — | — | 5/5 | 1/5 | 5/5 | 3/5 |
| Ataxia | — | — | — | — | — | — | 5/5 | 4/5 | 2/5 | 1/5 |
| Tremors | — | — | — | — | — | — | 1/5 | 2/5 | 1/5 | — |
| Death | 0/5 | 0/5 | 0/5 | 0/5 | 0/5 | 0/5 | 5/5 | 4/5 | 5/5 | 5/5 |

[a] Signs observed in rats treated orally (number exhibiting sign within 14 days after treatment/no. treated). A dash indicates that the sign was not observed at that dose level.

**TABLE 5.7.  Minimal Acute Toxicity Study Summary of the Drug SC-34871**

| Species (route) | Dose ($mg\ kg^{-1}$) | Dead/ Dosed | $LD_{50}$ ($mg\ kg^{-1}$) | Signs Observed | Treatment to Death Intervals |
|---|---|---|---|---|---|
| Rat (PO) | 2400 | 0/10 | > 2400[a] | None | None |
| Rat (IV) | 16 | 0/10 | Approxi- | Reduced motor | 0–2 hours |
| | 50 | 2/10 | mately | activity at 50 mg $kg^{-1}$; | |
| | 100 | 10/10 | 67 | convulsions, dyspnea, lost righiting reflex at 160 mg $kg^{-1}$. | |
| Mouse (PO) | 500 | 0/10 | > 2,400 | None | None |
| | 1600 | 0/10 | | | |
| | 2400 | 0/10 | | | |
| Mouse (IV) | 50 | 1/10 | 120 (75–200)[b] | Reduced motor activity, ataxia at 160 mg $kg^{-1}$; temors, convulsions, dyspnea at 500 mg $kg^{-1}$ | 0–2 hours |
| | 160 | 6/10 | | | |
| | 500 | 10/10 | | | |

[a] Limit dosage.

[b] Fiducial limits.

### 5.3.2. Complete Acute Toxicity Testing

An example of the next-level test, the complete acute toxicity test, is given in Figure 5.12. As stated by Dayan (1983), the value of doing more than the minimal test will depend on the nature of subsequent testing. The complete protocol is designed to provide for a more in-depth search for target organs than the minimal protocol. This type of study, which has been well described by Gad and coworkers (1984), is similar in design to a minimal acute toxicity study, but includes feed consumption data, more frequent body weight determinations, and more detailed and frequent clinical sign assessment. Groups should consist of at least ten animals per group; five per sex per dosage should then be sacrificed 24 to 48 hours for more immediate examination of any pathological changes induced by the test article. Remaining animals will be sacrificed at the end of the two-week period and examined for pathological changes. Blood will be collected at both sacrifices for clinical chemistry and/or hematology determinations.

***Body Weight Considerations.*** Body weight and feed consumption are frequently determined parameters in toxicity testing. To an extent, the ability of an animal to gain or maintain weight may be considered a sensitive, but nonspecific, indicator of health. While this is true in subchronic or chronic studies, its relevance in acute studies must be carefully considered. In most protocols, body weights are determined on Day 1 (prior to dosing), Day 7, and Day 14, which are the days mandated by most regulatory guidelines. Despite being common, the design is not well founded: if an animal has not died within seven days postdosing, it has probably recovered and its body weight may not be noticeably different from controls by Day 14. A complete protocol addresses this problem by specifying more frequent body weight determinations (daily for the first three to five days of the observation period) so that not only can initial decreases (if they occur) be detected, but recovery can also be charted. Feed consumption measurements should be made at the same times,

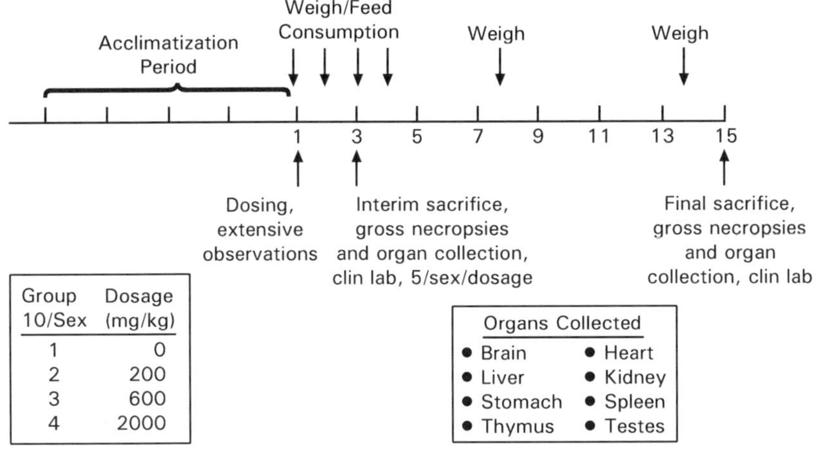


**FIGURE 5.12.** Example of complete acute toxicity protocol.

because it is difficult to determine the causes behind body weight changes in the absence of feed consumption data. Body weight loss accompanied by normal feed consumption implies something very different from body weight loss (or lack of gain) accompanied by lack of feed consumption. In the absence of feed consumption data, however, changes in body weight should still be considered indicative of a change in an animal's health status.

Yet another reason why body weight determinations are of questionable value in acute studies has to do with the statistical analysis of the data. Deaths may substantially alter group size and complicate analysis. The death of two of five animals causes a 40% decrease in group size and a substantial diminution of the power of any statistical test. In addition, the resulting data sets are censored: comparisons will often be between the control group, a dosage group where all the animals survive, and a high-dosage group where less than 50% of the animals survive to the end of the observation period. One has to question the utility of body weight changes if they occur at dosages that are acutely lethal. The data in Table 5.8 illustrate this point. Body weight changes tended to occur only at dosages that were acutely lethal. Additionally, one would suspect that the censoring of body weights in groups where death occurs is not random; that is, the animals that die are most likely those that are most sensitive, while those that survive are the most resistant or robust. This problem can be addressed by building exclusionary criteria into a protocol. For example, one could statistically analyze body weight data in groups that had less than 50% mortality.

Minimal rather than complete protocols tend to be more common in the acute testing of pharmaceutical agents. Drugs will almost always be subjected to at least one subchronic study. Body weight and feed consumption determinations are a standard feature of such studies. Additionally, changes in body weight and feed consumption are more likely in a subchronic than an acute study because the animals are dosed continuously between body weight determinations.

***Pathology Considerations.*** One of the objectives of any well-conducted toxicity study is to identify target organs. There is some question, however, concerning the utility of extensive pathological assessments as part of an acute study. Gross necropsies are generally the minimum assessments requested by most regulatory bodies. Hence, minimal protocols will include necropsies on all animals found dead and those sacrificed following the postdosing observation period. An example of necropsy findings is given in Table 5.9. This table illustrates that gross necropsy observations on acute studies rarely predict the toxicity that will be seen when the chemical is given for longer periods of time. This is not surprising, because most drug-related histological lesions are the result of chronicity; that is, discernible lesions tend to result from the cumulative effect of dosages that are acutely well tolerated.

The data in Table 5.9 also demonstrate that substantial gross macroscopic findings are rare in minimal acute studies and seldom suggestive of a specific effect. There are several reasons for the lack of specificity. The first is the rather limited nature of gross observations, in that they are limited to broad descriptive

**TABLE 5.8. Examples of Body Weight Changes in Rats from Minimal Acute Toxicity Studies**

| Drug (route) | Dosage (mg kg$^{-1}$) | BWT Change (g)[a] | Mortality |
|---|---|---|---|
| SC-32561 | | | |
| (PO) | 0 | $45 \pm 4$ | 0/10 |
| | 5000 | $39 \pm 10$ | 0/10 |
| (IP) | 0 | $43 \pm 4$ | 0/10 |
| | 500 | $43 \pm 9$ | 0/10 |
| | 890 | $44 \pm 11$ | 0/10 |
| | 1600 | $6 \pm 14$[d] | 2/10 |
| | 2800 | $24 \pm 20$[d] | 3/10 |
| SC-36250 | | | |
| (PO) | 0 | $38 \pm 10$ | 0/10 |
| | 5000 | $34 \pm 10$ | 0/10 |
| (IP) | 0 | $34 \pm 6$ | 0/10 |
| | 670 | $50 \pm 8$[d] | 2/10 |
| | 890 | $46 \pm 8$[d] | 3/10 |
| | 1200 | $45 \pm 4$ | 4/10 |
| | 1400 | $35$[b] | 9/10 |
| SC-36602 | | | |
| (IV) | 0 | $38 \pm 9$ | 0/10 |
| | 58 | $38 \pm 3$ | 0/10 |
| | 67 | $36 \pm 7$ | 2/10 |
| | 77 | $49 \pm 5$[d] | 3/10 |
| | 89 | $41 \pm 7$ | 7/10 |
| (PO) | 0 | $38 \pm 5$ | 0/10 |
| | 2100 | $41 \pm 5$ | 3/10 |
| | 2800 | $38 \pm 5$ | 7/10 |
| | 3700 | $26 \pm 6$ | 7/10 |

[a] Mean $\pm$ standard deviation. Body weight (BWT) changes in grams for each group during the first week of the postdosing observation period.

[b] Only one animal survived, so there is no standard deviation.

[d] Statistically different from control (0 dosage group), $P < 0.05$.

terms (size, shape, color, etc.). Second, for animals found dead, it is difficult to separate the chemically associated effects from agonal and/or autolytic changes. Finally, it is difficult to come to a conclusion about the nature of a gross lesion without histological assessment.

If there are any identifiable gross lesions, they often differ between animals that die, and those that survive to the end of the observation period. The reason for these differences is very simple. An animal that dies less than 24 hours after chemical exposure probably has not had sufficient time to develop a well-defined lesion. As mentioned earlier, most deaths occur within 24 hours. Animals that survive for the two-week observation period have probably totally recovered and rarely have apparent lesions. Hence, the animals that provide the best chance to identify test-article-specific lesions are those that die in the region of 24 to 96 hours postdosing.

**TABLE 5.9. Examples of Gross Necropsy Findings from Acute Toxicity Studies**

| Drug | Acute gross pathology | Subchronic Target Organs[a] |
|---|---|---|
| SC-36602 | Distended stomach and intestine, bloody fluid in intestine, congested lung, pale liver | None |
| SC-38394 | None | Liver, testes, bone marrow, thymus, kidney |
| SC-32840 | None | Heart, stomach, kidney, bladder |
| SC-25469 | Peritonitis (IP route only) | None |
| SC-36250 | Peritonitis (IP route only) | Adrenal, liver, thyroid |
| SC-27166 | None | Liver |

[a] Organs that showed any evidence of test-article-related changes in repeated-dose studies of two weeks or longer duration.

This is, in fact, one of the problems with acute pathology data, that is, comparing animals found dead with those sacrificed at a different time, and comparing both to controls. As mentioned, a complete protocol, where groups of animals are sacrificed 24 to 96 hours after dosing, at least partially solves this problem.

Many guidelines suggest microscopic confirmation of gross lesions "when necessary;" however, these are seldom done because of the autolytic nature of many of the tissues collected from animals found dead. Additionally, the practice of collecting and examining only gross lesions is difficult to justify because it does not permit in-depth comparisons. Pathological findings are most easily interpreted when the same organs are collected and examined from all animals on a test regardless of the circumstances of death. Elsberry (1986) recommends that the GI tract, kidney, heart, brain, liver and spleen be specifically examined routinely in acute studies. Given the timing issues discussed in the previous paragraph, the amount of effort may not be worth the result. In an attempt to address these problems, Gad and coworkers (1984) have developed a complete protocol that includes groups of satellite animals that are sacrificed 48 hours after exposure, necropsied, and a standardized organ list collected, weighed, and prepared for histological assessment. This list routinely includes the "first-line" organs: brain, thyroid, liver, kidneys, heart, and adrenals. The same organs are collected from all other animals, that is, those that die as a result of the toxicity as well as control animals. Additional tests can be included if one has a specific concern. For example, the structure of a test article may suggest that it has anticholinesterase potential. Therefore, one could include serum pseudocholinesterase determinations in the clinical laboratory package, as is frequently done for organophosphate and carbamate structures.

### 5.3.3. Supplemented Acute Studies

An example of the third-level acute toxicity test, a supplemented study, is given in Figure 5.13. Such tests are rarely performed but are of use when one wishes to obtain data other than descriptive toxicity data. For example, the addition of satellite groups

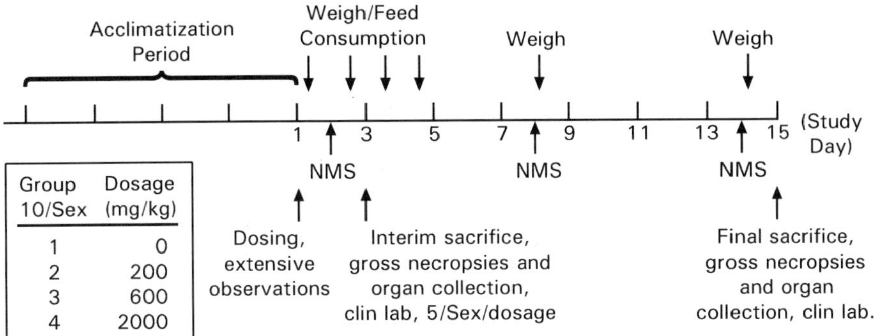


**FIGURE 5.13.** The design and conduct of a supplemented (or "heavy") acute systemic toxicity study. The figure illustrates the approach to such a study when it is to serve as the definitive systemic toxicity study for some period of time.

of animals to be dosed with a radiolabeled compound to gain pharmacokinetic information will turn a "complete" study into a "supplemented" one. Another common practice is the addition of other examinations or measurements to gain more information about a potential target organ. An example of this would be recording EKGs in rats, which is too complicated and time consuming to do on a routine basis, but should be considered if the heart is a potential target organ. One way of describing such a study is that it is a complete toxicity study carrying a specific screen "piggyback."

An excellent example of a supplemented protocol is that described by Gad and colleagues (1984). A neuromuscular screen was developed (Gad, 1982) and incorporated into their routine acute toxicity protocol for testing nonpharmaceuticals. Doing so allowed for a more systematic and quantifiable examination of effects on the CNS than reliance on simple clinical observations. The neuromuscular screen consists of a battery incorporating standard clinical observations plus some behavioral assessment techniques already described in the literature. These are summarized in Table 5.10. This screen has been further developed to become the now regulatorily required FOB (functional observational battery). An advantage of this screen is that is uses noninvasive techniques and, therefore, will require the use of no additional animals. If an animal is displaying signs of severe CNS depression two hours post dosing, little useful data will be gathered by examining behavior. In testing a pharmaceutical it is probably better practice to apply the neuromuscular screen on Days 2, 7, and 14 postdosing in an attempt to identify more subtle or lingering effects, and to chart recovery from these effects. For drugs that produce no observable CNS effect following dosing, the neuromuscular screen can be done a few hours postdosing. The more extensive and detailed nature of the data generated by the neuromuscular screen permits more confidence in the conclusion that the test article had no effect on the CNS. Any suspect target organ can be investigated in a

**TABLE 5.10. Neuromuscular Screen Observations**

| Observation | Nature of Data Generated[a] | Correlates to Which Neutral Component[b] |
|---|---|---|
| Locomotor activity | S/N | M/C |
| Righting reflex | S | C/M |
| Grip strength (forelimb) | N | M |
| Body temperature | N | C |
| Salivation | Q | P |
| Startle response | Q | S/C |
| Respiration | S | M/P/C |
| Urination | S | P/M |
| Mouth breathing | Q | S |
| Convulsions | S | C |
| Pineal response | Q | Reflex |
| Piloerection | Q | P/C |
| Diarrhea | S | GI tract/P/M |
| Pupil size | S | P/C |
| Pupil response | Q | P/C |
| Lacrimation | Q | S/P |
| Impaired gait | S | M/C |
| Stereotypy | Q | C |
| Toe pinch | S | S (Surface pain; spinal reflex) |
| Tail pinch | S | S (deep pain) |
| Wire maneuver | S | C/M |
| Hind-leg splay | N | P/M |
| Positional passivity | S | S/C |
| Tremors | S | M/C |
| Extensor thrust | S | C/M |
| Positive geotropism | Q | C |
| Limb rotation | S | M/C |

[a] Data quantal (Q), scalar (S), or interval (N). Quantal data are characterized by being of an either/or variety, such as dead/alive or present/absent. Scalar data allow one to rank something as less than, equal to, or greater than other values, but one cannot exactly quantitate the difference between such rankings. Interval data is continuous data where one can assign (theoretically) an extremely accurate value to a characteristic that can be precisely related to other values in a quantitative fashion.

[b] Peripheral (P), sensory (S), muscular (M), or central (C).

similar fashion. Depending on the invasiveness of the supplementary techniques, satellite groups may or may not need to be added to the study. Care must be taken in this regard to prevent the study from becoming too cumbersome and too complicated to conduct. It may be better to address some questions as separate studies. For this reason, one should not attempt to address more than one supplemental question in any one study.

### 5.3.4. Acute Toxicity Testing with Nonrodent Species

The designs described thus far for acute toxicity testing generally assume that the test species being used is a rodent. Nonrodent species are also used for acute toxicity testing. Many regulatory bodies require acute testing in at least one nonrodent species. The animals most often used are the dog, pig, or monkey. Veterinary products will also be tested in the target species. For example, a flea collar intended for cats must be tested in cats. While the rabbit is not technically a rodent, it is the species of choice for a variety of tests for assessing acute oral or intravenous toxicity, and is considered a rodent for regulatory purposes. This section is written with the dog and monkey in mind. Clearly, there are some profound differences between these species and rodents with regard to handling, husbandry, and dosing. Here we focus on the design differences in toxicity testing in large species.

For financial, procurement, and ethical reasons, acute systemic toxicity tests on nonrodents are not performed using traditionally designed animal-intensive protocols. The minimal acute study requires thirty to fifty animals. Complete and supplemented studies will usually require even more. At a cost of $475.00 per beagle dog, $650.00 for minipig, or $3500.00 per monkey, the animal costs alone are enough to make such studies with these species prohibitively expensive. Vivarium space and husbandry costs are also much higher with nonrodent species than with rodents. Nonrodents also require a much longer prestudy quarantine period than rodents: at least 6–8 weeks for dogs and pigs and 18–24 weeks for monkeys. Treatment during the quarantine period is more extensive than that given rodents. The animals should be given frequent physical examinations including complete clinical laboratory panels and appropriate tests for common illnesses and parasites. Special care must be taken with monkeys not only because they can be vectors of human disease, but also because they can contract human diseases, and a sick animal can compromise study outcome. All these factors dictate that these animals be sparing used. Hence, it is most common to study acute systemic toxicity in nonrodent animals using a pyramiding dosage design. The typical study will consist of two treated animals per sex and two control animals per sex for a total of eight animals. A typical protocol is shown in Figure 5.14.

The use of fewer but larger animals permits more extensive observations of each individual. Following each dose, animals can be given complete physical examinations that include palpations, behavioral checks, spinal reflex checks, pupillary light reflexes, respiration rate, ECG recording, and rectal temperature measurement. Blood samples can also be collected following each dose to determine standard clinical chemistry and hematology profiles. Hence, while fewer animals are used with the pyramiding dosage protocol, more information per animal is collected.

The small number of animals used in a pyramiding dosage study makes it difficult to do standard statistical comparisons. This difficulty can be overcome to a certain extent by taking advantage of two design aspects of the pyramiding protocol. First, pretreatment data can and should be obtained on all animals for all parameters examined or determined. In-study comparisons should be made both to pretreatment data and to concurrent control animals. Such comparisons can be made not only on

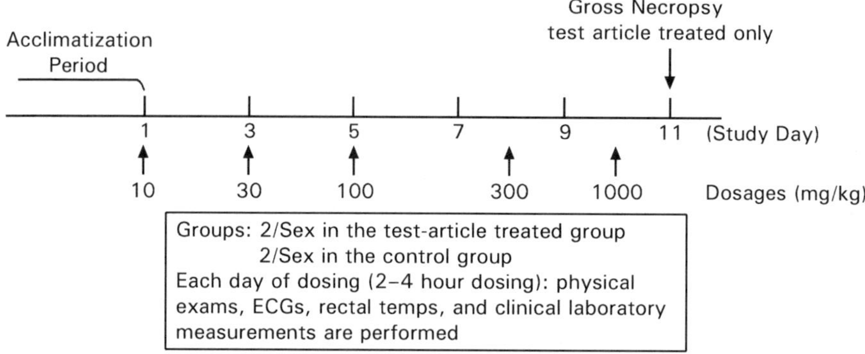


**FIGURE 5.14.** Example of pyramiding dose study for acute toxicity testing in a nonrodent species.

the basis of absolute numbers but also on the magnitude of any changes from pretreatment values. Second, all animals should be measured repeatedly throughout the study. Hence, to reflect a true drug-related effect, the magnitude of change should increase following each dose (though one must be aware of the potential for the development of tolerance as induction of metabolism). This is, in fact, the only way one can make any dosage-response or threshold conclusions using the pyramiding protocol.

Drugs are seldom tested in nonrodent animals via routes other than the intended or likely routes of human exposure. Hence, the most common routes in these types of protocols are oral, intravenous, and respiratory. Rarely is a test article given to nonrodent species by the intraperitoneal route. Routes are discussed elsewhere in detail (Gad and Chengelis, 1999), but some discussion is appropriate here because of design considerations. Test articles are normally given orally by capsule to dogs and pigs, and by gavage to monkeys. Nonrodents have to be restrained if dosed by gavage, making the process very labor intensive. This is minimized by the small number of animals specified by the pyramiding protocol. In contrast, because of the differences in size, it is much easier to deliver a test article intravenously to nonrodents than to rodents. For topical studies, the rabbit is the nonrodent choice because it is easier to prevent a rabbit from grooming the delivery site, and considerably less material is required to deliver a comparable dose to a rabbit than a dog or pig. Acute dermal studies are not, however, usually done with a pyramiding study design, but rather as a limit dose study.

The biggest problem with the pyramiding protocol is the development of tolerance. If no toxicity is observed, the chemical could be innocuous or animals could have developed tolerance during the study. The escalating dosage feature of the pyramiding protocol is an excellent vehicle for fostering the development of tolerance. One can check this by dosing additional naïve animals at the limit dosage to confirm, as it were, a negative result. Another problem, which is most peculiar to the dog, is emesis. Oral administration of a large amount of almost any material will cause a dog to vomit. This is always somewhat of a surprise to toxicologists whose prior experience is primarily with rodents, which cannot vomit. One should pay close attention to dogs the first hour after capsule delivery. If the dog vomits up most of the dose, the actual dosage absorbed could be grossly overestimated. This can be a particular problem if one is using the results of a pyramiding dosage study to set the dosages for a repeated-dose study. Dogs can develop tolerance to the emetic effect of a set dosage. When this occurs, absorption and resulting blood concentrations of a test article can increase dramatically, resulting in more florid toxicity than expected on the basis of the pyramiding study. Another problem is that emesis can result in secondary electrolyte changes, especially decreases in chloride, that may be mistaken for a direct effect of the test article. If emesis is a severe problem, one can study toxicity in a different nonrodent species or divide larger dosages into two or three divided dosages on the day of dosing.

As with traditionally designed rodent studies, the pathology component of pyramiding studies usually consists of gross necropsies followed by (when appropriate and necessary) histological assessment of gross lesions. Unfortunately, this study design does not permit the establishment of a dose-response relationship with regard to gross necropsy findings. In addition, the small number of animals makes definitive conclusions difficult. Usually, gross lesions are defined in absolute terms with few comparisons to control animals. Suspected target organs should be further investigated in subsequent subchronic studies, or in rigorous and specific mechanistic studies. Because of the limited value of the pathology data generated by the pyramiding protocol, control animals should not be terminated, but rather should be saved for reuse.

### 5.3.5. Factors That Can Affect Acute Tests

Many investigations into the sources of variability in acute toxicity testing have been conducted, and these have been reviewed by Elsberry (1986). The factors causing the greatest interstudy variation included lack of specifications for sex, strain, age and weight range. When clearly defined, detailed protocols were used, interlaboratory variation was found to be minimal. Hence, it is equally important that the details of the protocol be well described and followed. It is not appropriate to draw dosage-response conclusions by comparing groups that differ substantially in age or that have been fed, fasted, or otherwise manipulated differently. Guidelines for standardization of acute toxicity testing were proposed by the interagency regulatory liaison group (IRLG, 1981; Elsberry, 1986). These do not differ markedly from those mandated by the Toxic Substance Control Act of 1986 (Gad and Chengelis, 1999).

***Number, Size, and Sex of Dosage Groups.*** The precision with which lethality and signs of toxicity are described will depend on the number of groups (hence, dosages) and the number of animals in each group. Between 1940 and 1980, the standard was to use from four to six dosages with ten animals per dosage. The current emphasis is on limiting the number of animals used for acute testing, particularly with recognition of the limited value of "precise" lethality data (Gad and Chengelis, 1999). Retrospective analyses by DePass (1989) and Olson et al. (1990) have demonstrated that decreasing group size to two to three animals generally has little impact on overall study results. Hence, the number and size of dosage groups will depend, to an extent, on the methods of statistical analysis. The classic statistical methods for analyzing lethality data (or, indeed, any quantal dosage-response data) were published between 1930 and 1960 and have been extensively reviewed by Armitage and Allen (1959) and Morrison et al. (1968). These methods are mentioned here with regard to the demand they make on protocol design, specifi- cally, the number of dosage groups, the spacing of the dosages, and the number of animals per dosage group. The probit and moving average methods are the most commonly used today. In general, all methods of calculation and computation are more precise if the designs are symmetrical (i.e., the dosages are evenly spaced and the group sized are equal). The probit method, first developed by Bliss (1935, 1957) and later refined by Finney (1971, 1985), is considered to be the most precise, but it requires at least two groups of partial responses (i.e., mortality greater than 0, but less than 100%). This may require dosing more than three groups until this criterion is met. It also deals ineffectively with groups that had either 0 or 100% mortality. (The most common correction for these groups is to substitute 0.1% for 0 and 99.7% for 100%.) The moving average method, first described by Thompson and Weil (1952), does not require partial responses, deals effectively with complete responses, and, therefore, can produce an acceptable estimate of an $LD_{50}$ with as few as three groups of three to five animals each. The moving average method can also be used to design the experiment. Groups can be dosed in a sequential fashion as in a pyramiding study, with each step dictated by the moving average method. Once evidence of toxicity is observed, further dosing is discontinued. This method requires that the dosages be separated by a constant geometric factor (e.g., 2, 4, and 8 mg kg$^{-1}$) and that groups be of equal size. Weil (1952), and later Gad (1999, 2001) have published tables that allow for the easy calculation of $LD_{50}$ using $K = 3$ (where $K$ is the number of dosage groups minus one).

The $LD_{50}$ for $K < 3$ can be easily calculated without the aid of tables. In addition, methods for estimating the confidence limits of this calculated $LD_{50}$ have also been published (Gad, 1999). Traditionally, the moving average method has not been extensively used because, while it yielded an estimate of the $LD_{50}$, it did not give the slope of the (probit transformed) lethality curve. However, Weil (1983) has published a method for calculating a slope form the same data. Hence, an estimate of the $LD_{50}$ and slope can be obtained from as few as three groups of three to five animals per group, provided that at least one group shows a response less than 50% and another shows a response greater than 50%.

The Litchfield and Wilcoxon (1949) plotting method was once commonly used. It is certainly a valid method, and it poses no more restrictions on study design than those imposed by the probit method. The Litchfield–Wilcoxon method has become a victim of technology as modern, handheld calculators and the ready availability of simple computer programs have made other methods more convenient to run.

However, at least one software company has adopted the Litchfield–Wilcoxon method for its acute toxicity protocol package.

The normit-chi square, developed by Berkson (1955), is also sometimes used. Like the probit method, the normit-chi square does not absolutely require equally spaced dosages or equal group sizes, but it does require at least one partial response. Hence, fewer dosage groups may be needed with the normit-chi square method than with the probit method. According to Waud (1972), the correction for including complete responses is better than that used for probit analysis but is still "tainted." His method supposedly deals adequately with complete responses, but it is extremely complex and, probably for this reason, is rarely used.

In an early paper, Karber (1931) published a simple method (often described but rarely cited) for calculating an $LD_{50}$. It does not require that dosages be equally spaced, but widely divergent dosages will lead to a biased result. The method was originally described for groups of equal size, but groups of slightly varying sizes can be used, provided they do not differ by more than a few animals each. In this case, mean group size can be inserted into Karber's formula with little change in accuracy. The formula is very simple, and one can calculate an acceptable estimate of the $LD_{50}$ quickly with only a few arithmetic computations. This method, unlike those mentioned above, does not allow for calculating the confidence limit or slope of the probit response curve. Hence, if these calculated parameters are not sought, the Karber method allows one a bit more freedom in picking dosages.

While much has been written about the influence of gender on acute lethality, most authors now agree that there are seldom any substantial differences in the $LD_{50}$ due to sex (DePass et al., 1984; Gad and Chengelis, 1999). In those instances where there is a sex-related difference, females tend to be more sensitive than males (approximately 85% of the time). If one is willing to accept this amount of uncertainty, only one sex needs to be tested. Alternatively, as few as two to three animals per sex per dosage can be used. Schutz and Fuchs (1982) have demonstrated that, by pooling sexes, there are seldom any substantial differences in the $LD_{50}$ calculations between groups consisting of five per sex versus three per sex. If there are no substantial differences between sexes (i.e., 70% mortality for males and 80% for females at a dosage), the results from pooling the sexes can provide a pooled $LD_{50}$. For most safety considerations, an $LD_{50}$ derived on this basis will be acceptable, and will result in the use of fewer animals.

### 5.3.6. Selection of Dosages

In setting dosages for acute studies a few common sense rules have to be applied. First, the intrinsic biological and chemical activity of the test article must be considered. Zbinden and Flury-Roversi (1981) have documented several cases where lethality was of no biological relevance. The oral lethality of tartaric acid, for example, is due to the caustic action of a high concentration of acid in the GI tract. In these instances, limit tests are more appropriate tests. Additionally, it is uncommon that a completely unknown chemical will be tested. Factors such as known pharmacological profile, chemical or physical characteristics including molecular weight, particient coefficient, and the like, and the toxicity of related chemicals should be considered. For example, it is likely that a polymeric, poorly soluble molecule will not be bioavailable at an initial dosage of 100 mg kg$^{-1}$. A full understanding of all available data will permit one to pick dosages with more confidence, and, thereby, save both time and resources.

Second, no protocol will yield high-quality data if all dosages given cause 100% lethality. Therefore, one is best advised to pick widely spaced, rather than closely spaced, dosages. In general, the best dosage regimen includes a dose that will definitely produce a high incidence of severe toxicity, another that will produce marginal toxicity, and one in between. If this pattern is obtained, adding more groups does not generally change the results. This point is illustrated by the data in Table 5.11. For two drugs, an LD$_{50}$ of 300 mg kg$^{-1}$ was obtained using six groups of ten mice each. Essentially the same result was obtained if the second, fourth, and sixth groups were eliminated and not used in the calculations. Behrens (1929) noted this phenomenon almost 60 years ago.

Widely spaced dosages also decrease the likelihood of nonnormotonic data, where mortality does not necessarily increase with dosage (see Table 5.12). This can occur when the test chemical has a shallow dose-response curve and the group size is small (three to four animals). While it is possible to calculate an LD$_{50}$ from such data, the slope and confidence limits will be inaccurate. Nonmonotonic data can also occur if the lethality is indeed biphasic. If one suspects that this is occurring, additional dosages should be examined. For safety considerations, only the first part of the curve, the lowest LD$_{50}$, is of importance.


***Timing.*** The greatest precision in any lethality curve is obtained when the number of experimental variables is kept to a minimum. Hence, it is best if all the animals used for determining a specific curve are dosed on the same day and, if possible, at

**TABLE 5.11. Sample Data Sets: LD$_{50}$ Calculations Using Fewer Dosages[a]**

| SC-27166 | | Theophylline | |
|---|---|---|---|
| Dosage (mg kg$^{-1}$) | Mortality | Dosage (mg kg$^{-1}$) | Mortality |
| 100 | 0/10 | 280 | 0/10 |
| 180 | 0/10 | 320 | 3/10 |
| 240 | 4/10 | 370 | 5/10 |
| 320 | 7/10 | 430 | 9/10 |
| 560 | 9/10 | 500 | 10/10 |
| 1000 | 10/10 | 670 | 10/10 |
| LD$_{50}$ = 300 | | LD$_{50}$ = 300 | |
| Using every other dosage | | | |
| 100 | 0/10 | 280 | 0/10 |
| 240 | 4/10 | 370 | 5/10 |
| 560 | 9/10 | 500 | 10/10 |
| LD$_{50}$ = 290 | | LD$_{50}$ = 290 | |

[a] Adult male mice; drugs given by gavage.

**TABLE 5.12. Sample Data Sets: Homogeneous versus Heterogeneous Data**

| Homogeneous[a] (normotonic) | | Hetereogeneous[b] (nonnormotonic) | |
|---|---|---|---|
| Dosage (mg kg$^{-1}$) | Mortality | Dosage (mg kg$^{-1}$) | Mortality |
| 300 | 0/20 | 620 | 0/10 |
| 600 | 1/20 | 1600 | 2/10 |
| 800 | 10/20 | 2100 | 8/10 |
| 1000 | 17/20 | 2800 | 5/10 |
| | | 3700 | 8/10 |
| | | 5000 | 8/10 |

[a] Data from study of SC-31828, using adult rats of both sexes.
[b] Data from study of SC-3894, using adult male rats.

the same time of day, which limits age-related and diurnal effects. If a total of only 15 animals are being dosed, this is not a difficult task for a single well-trained technician. However, if the test substance is of unknown lethality, it is imprudent to deliver all doses on the same day. It is common practice for a single dosage group to be treated on the first day of an experiment, and the dosages for the second and third groups to be adjusted pending the results of the first group. Generally, most acute deaths will occur within 24 hours of dosing. Delayed deaths (those occurring more than 24 hours after dosing) are relatively rare and generally restricted to the 72-hour period following dosing (Gad et al., 1984; Bruce, 1985). Hence, waiting for 24 hours between doses will generally yield sufficient data to allow the choice of the next dosage. For example, if all but one of the animals dosed in the first groups dies, there is no doubt that the next dosage should be adjusted downward considerably, whether or not the final animal eventually dies. All the dosing for a single curve can be completed in three days. If a test article is being tested in traditional protocols (with two species, two routes, separate sexes), the two initial groups by a route can be treated on the first day of the dosing period, and the second route initiated on the next day. Subsequent dosages can be adjusted on alternate days. Little real impact on the results will occur if there are two to three days between dosing sets. After that, however, the increasing age of the animals may result in a change in sensitivity. As reviewed by Balazs (1976), for example, the ratios of the $LD_{50}$s obtained in adult animals to the $LD_{50}$s obtained in neonates can vary from 0.002 to 160. One can use longer observation periods between dosing days if separate animals orders are timed for delivery to ensure that all animals dosed are closer in age. As a rule of thumb, the animals should not differ in age by more than 15%; hence, the younger the animals, the smaller the age window.

## 5.4. SCREENS

Screens are generally not safety studies in the regulatory sense. These are the studies done, as the name implies, to examine several chemicals in order either to select those with the most desirable properties for development or to eliminate those that have undesirable properties. There is nothing novel about screening; the process has been an integral part of pharmaceutical research for decades (Irwin, 1962). In a pioneering paper, Smyth and Carpenter (1944) described a screening process for gathering preliminary toxicity data for a new chemical. In their discussion they clearly state the underlying rationale for toxicity screening:

> Opinions upon the toxicity, hazards of manufacture, and fields for safe use must be expressed regarding many chemicals which will never be produced in quantity. Large expenditures of time and money upon securing these basic conclusions is not justified. Later, when a few of the new compounds are obviously going to be made commercially, more detailed studies can be undertaken—Smyth and Carpenter (1944).

Screens are designed for speed, simplicity, and minimal resource expenditure. They are designed to answer positive, single-sided questions. For example, the lack of an effect in an initial screen does not mean that toxicity will not be manifested with a different formulation or in a different species. It is for this reason that screens should, as stated by Zbinden (1984), not be seen as replacements for thorough safety testing. An acute toxicity screen can be the first leg in a decision tree or tier testing process for selecting a chemical or drug candidate for development. An example of this process is given in Figure 5.15.

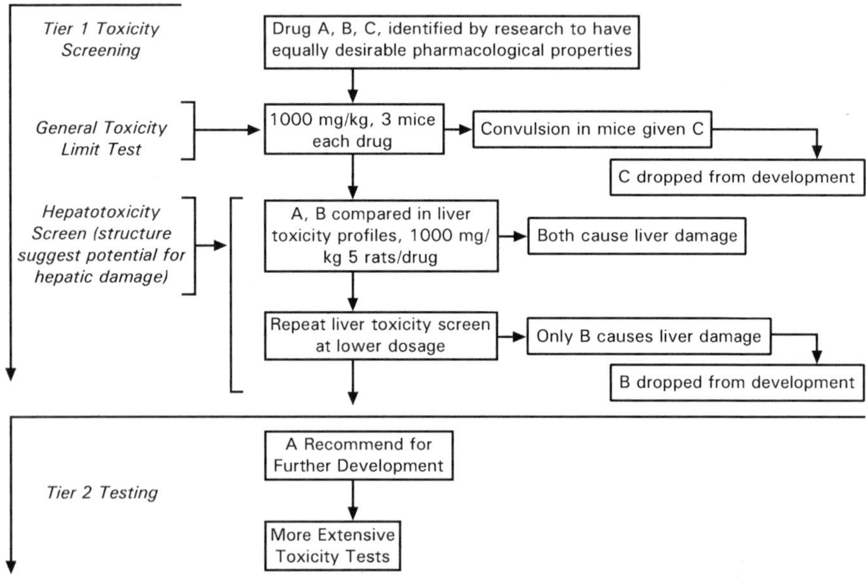


**FIGURE 5.15.** Example of use of screens in selecting drug candidates for development.

### 5.4.1. General Toxicity Screens

There are two types of acute toxicity screens. In the general toxicity screen, animals (often, for economic reasons, mice) are exposed to two or three predefined dosages of chemicals. No more than three mice per dosage are necessary and no control group is required. An example of this type of protocol is shown in Figure 5.16. The animals are carefully observed for mortality and obvious signs of toxicity, such as convulsions, but no attempt should be made to quantify the severity of a response. There is seldom any need to have an observation period of more than four to five days. Because of the quantal nature of the data, interpretation is straightforward. There are four possible outcomes: (1) no death or signs of toxicity seen at dosages up to $X$ mg kg$^{-1}$; (2) no deaths, but evident signs of toxicity seen at $X$ mg kg$^{-1}$; (3) evident signs of toxicity at $X$ mg kg$^{-1}$; (4) deaths and evident signs of toxicity both occurred at $X$ mg kg$^{-1}$. General toxicity screens may also provide the preliminary information for picking the dosages for more definitive acute studies.

There are two ways to apply the data from toxicity screens to the development of a drug or chemical. On a relative basis, the drugs under consideration can be ranked according to screen results and the one that appears to be the least toxic can be chosen for future development. Alternatively, decisions can be made on an absolute basis. All candidates that are positive below a certain dosage are dropped, and all those that are negative at or above that dosage will continue to the next tier of testing. If absolute criteria are used, the screen need be done only at the critical dosage. If only one dosage is examined, the test is a limit test. A limit test of this kind is the simplest form of toxicity screen and, depending on the nature of subsequent testing, it is highly recommended.

Fowler and his colleagues (1979) have described a rat toxicity screen (illustrated in Figure 5.17) that is more extensive and detailed than the one shown in Figure 5.16. It includes two rounds of dosing. In the first round, up to 12 rats are (singly)

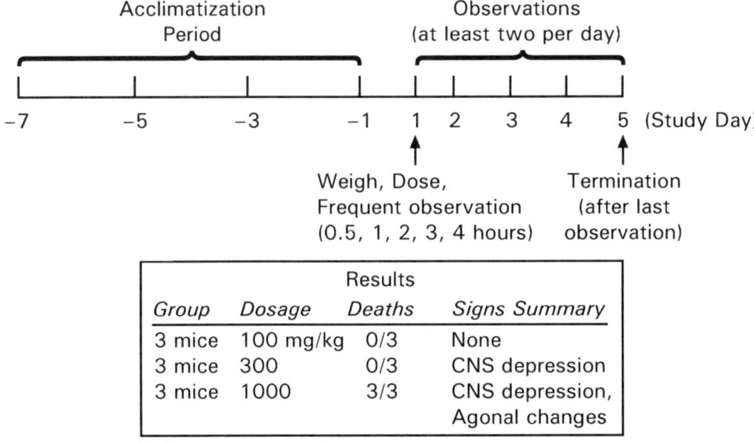



| | | Results | |
| --- | --- | --- | --- |
| *Group* | *Dosage* | *Deaths* | *Signs Summary* |
| 3 mice | 100 mg/kg | 0/3 | None |
| 3 mice | 300 | 0/3 | CNS depression |
| 3 mice | 1000 | 3/3 | CNS depression, Agonal changes |

**FIGURE 5.16.** Example of general toxicity screen.

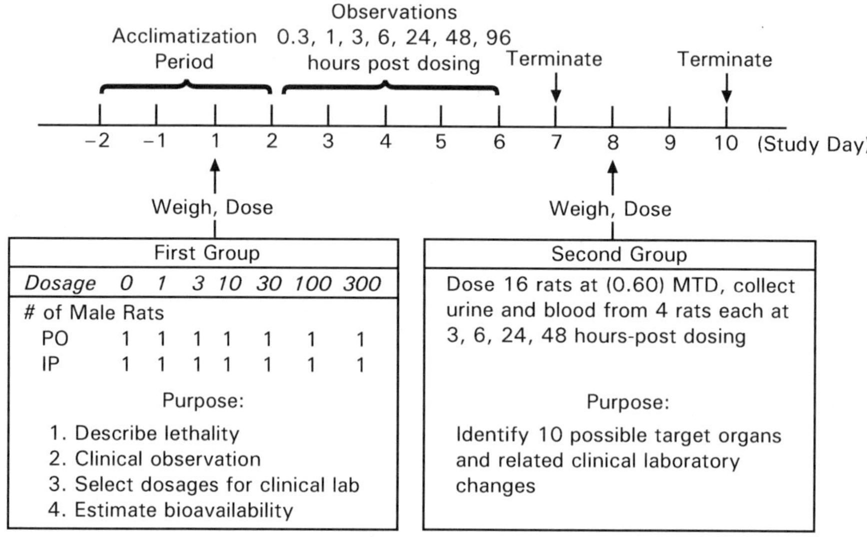


**FIGURE 5.17.** Example of rat toxicity screen for drugs.

exposed to six different dosages by two different routes for the purpose of defining the maximally tolerated dose (MTD). In the second round of dosing, 16 rats are dosed at two-thirds (0.66) of the MTD and sacrificed on a serially timed basis for blood sample collections to determine test-article concentrations and for clinical laboratory tests. These features make this design too complicated, time-consuming, and expensive to run as an initial screen. This design is better suited as a second-tier screen to provide a more extensive follow-up study for a more limited screen. Fowler et al. contend that their screen disclosed most toxicity uncovered by more conventional studies. This screen was most successful in defining acute CNS, liver, or kidney toxicity (Fowler et al., 1979). Lesions that require long-term exposure, such as those generally involving the eyes, may not be detected in this type of screen.

Up–down or pyramiding designs can be used for general toxicity screens, but this is not a common approach because of the time involved. In addition, if several chemicals are being compared, an up–down study where death occurs at different dosages can be complicated to run. It is much easier to test several chemicals at the same time using a limited test design. Because only individual animals are dosed, these designs can be used when there is a very limited amount of test article available and/or there are few prior data on which to base an expected toxic dosage.

Hazelette and colleagues (1987) have described a rather novel pyramiding dosage screen that they term the "rising dose tolerance" (RDT) study (illustrated in Figure 5.18). The study, which uses a subacute rather than an acute dosing regimen, can also be used as a range-finding study design. The rats are exposed for four days to the initial dosage followed by three days of recovery before the next four-day dosing period at the next highest dosage. This process is repeated for the three dosing cycles. Plasma and urine samples are collected for clinical chemistry and urinalysis,

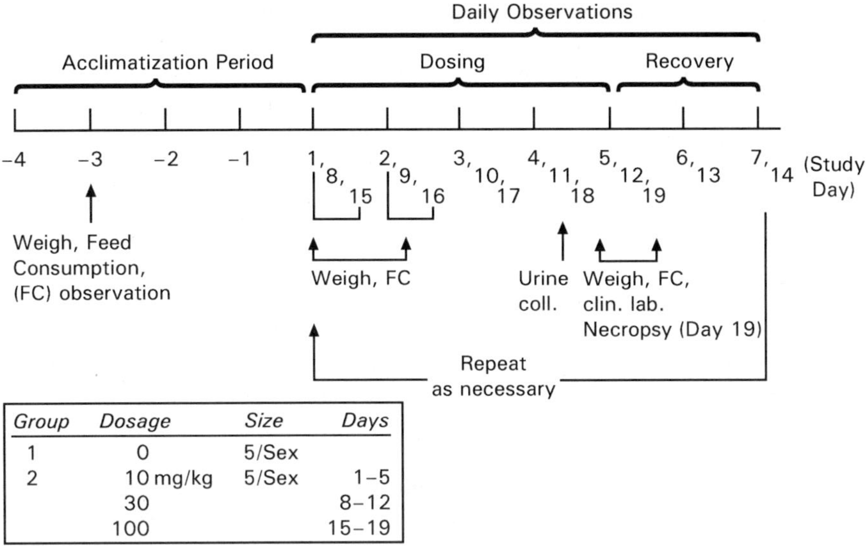



| Group | Dosage | Size | Days |
|---|---|---|---|
| 1 | 0 | 5/Sex | |
| 2 | 10 mg/kg | 5/Sex | 1–5 |
| | 30 | | 8–12 |
| | 100 | | 15–19 |

**FIGURE 5.18.** Example of rising dose tolerance test [no pharmacokinetic (PK) groups].

as well as test-article determinations. Necropsies and microscopic examinations are performed. While this study design is novel, it appears to provide considerable acute data. It is also possible that this design could generate sufficient data to plan a pivotal subchronic study and, therefore, replace a traditional two-week study, resulting in considerable savings of time and animals. This is not a simple study and, therefore, inappropriate as an initial screen, but it would appear to be appropriate for a second-tier test.

### 5.4.2. Specific Toxicity Screening

The second type of acute toxicity screen is the specific toxicity test. This type of test is done when one has a specific toxicological concern, for example, when prior structure-activity data suggest that a family of chemicals can be hepatotoxic. A screen to select the chemical with the least hepatotoxic potential is then in order. These tests are also done, as described by Zbinden (1984), to look for a specific toxicological effect that may be easily overlooked in a route safety study. Zbinden gives, as an example, screens that are designed to detect specific lesions to the hemostatic process. As pointed out by Irwin (1962) over three decades ago, such tests have their greatest power if more than one measure of specific target organ toxicity is used. Dayan (1983) refers to this technique as a matrix of measurements. In a liver toxicity screen, for example, liver weights (both absolute and relative), gross necropsy examinations, and a battery of serum enzyme assays should all be part of the protocol. As a general rule, because of the time and expense involved, screens should be designed to minimize the use of histopathological techniques. The dosages can be standardized or set on the basis of the results of a generalized toxicity screen. Specific toxicity screens can be the next-level test in the decision tree process for selecting a candidate for development (as illustrated in Figure 5.15).

The number of animals and the number of dosages are highly dependent on the type of data gathered. A few rules of thumb should be followed: (1) keep it lean: each additional group, animal, or test article added to a protocol makes the study exponentially more difficult to conduct—simplicity is one of the most important features of a screen; (2) the more parameters examined, the fewer the number of animals required; (3) if normal limits of a test parameter are relatively broad (e.g., serum glucose), more animals will be required than if the parameter is normally tightly controlled (e.g., prothrombin time). In general, three is the minimum and ten is the maximum number of animals required per group. Further, if a single chemical is examined per study, no more than three groups will be required. If more than one chemical is included in the study, then a single dosage (limit) group per chemical is the best design.

Strictly speaking, an acute toxicity study is conducted to examine the effect of a single dose of a single compound. In designing specific toxicity screens, however, deviation from this principle is permissible if it increases screen sensitivity. For example, the sensitivity of mice to many indirect hepatotoxins will be enhanced by prior treatment with phenobarbital. Hence, the sensitivity of a hepatotoxicity screen will be enhanced if the mice are pretreated for three days with phenobarbital.

The screen should be validated for consistency of response with both positive and negative control articles. A positive control article is one that is known to reliably produce the toxic syndrome the screen is designed to detect. Concurrent control groups are not required with each replicate. Rather, control groups should be evaluated on some regular basis to ensure that screen performance is stable. Because a screen relies on a biological system, it is not a bad idea to test the control benchmarks, particularly the positive ones, on a routine period basis. Not only does that give one increased confidence in the screen, but it also provides a historical base against which to compare the results of new test articles. Zbinden and colleagues refer to the positive control as the reference compound, and they have discussed some of the general criteria be applied in the selection of these compounds (Zbinden et al., 1984). Any changes to the design should trigger revalidation. Any analytical methods should be subjected to P.A.S.S. (precision, accuracy, sensitivity, and selectivity) validation.

Interpretation of specific toxicity screen data is not as straightforward as that of a general toxicity screen. This is because the data will often be continuous, following a Gaussian, or normal, distribution. This has two ramifications. First, for results around the threshold, it may be very difficult to differentiate between positive and negative responses. Second, for any one parameter, there is a real chance of false statistical significance (type I errors), especially if small numbers of animals are used. This occurrence is one of the reasons why specific toxicity screens should include the determination of more than one variable, since it is unlikely for multiple false positives to occur in the same group of animals. An undetected false positive could lead to the dropping of a promising candidate in error. False negatives, by contrast, may not be as critical (other than the time lost and the resources spent), because extensive subsequent tests should lead to the more complete description of the test article's toxic properties.

The problems described in the preceding paragraph assume that the screen will include a traditional ("negative," or vehicle) control group, and that the data from the treated groups will be compared to those of the control group by standard methods. These problems will be minimized if no control group and, therefore, no traditional statistical comparisons are included. In addition, a decrease in the number of animals used simplifies the study. Data can be interpreted by comparison to a historical control data base as described by Zbinden et al. (1984). The threshold, or test criterion $X_c$, is calculated according to the following formula:

$$X_c = m + (z)s,$$

where $m$ is the population mean, $s$ is the standard deviation, and $z$ is an arbitrary constant. This formula is essentially a method of converting continuous data to quantal data: it is used to determine if individual animals are over the test threshold, not if the group mean is over the threshold. Analysis of screening data by comparison to experience (i.e., historical control data) and an activity criterion are discussed in greater detail in Chapter 4 and by Gad (2001). The higher the $z$ value, the lower the probability of a false positive, but the lower the sensitivity of the screen. Again, including multiple parameters in the screen helps alleviate this problem. Zbinden has proposed a ranking procedure in which various levels of suspicion (LOS) or a level of certainty (LOC) is assigned to the result of a toxicity screen. This is simply a formalized fashion of stating that the more animals that respond, and the greater the severity of the response, the more certainty one has in drawing a conclusion. If relative comparisons are being made, this system provides a framework for ranking test articles and selecting those to continue to the next tier of testing.

With regard to specific toxicity screening, behavioral toxicity screening is an area currently generating a great deal of interest. As reviewed by Hopper (1986), there are several reasons for this interest. First, the Toxic Substance Control Act of 1976 legislatively recognized behavioral measures as essential to examining chemicals for neurotoxic potential. Second, the structure and function of the CNS are not amenable to traditional methods of examination, in that profound behavioral changes can be induced in the absence of any detectable morphological lesions. This large and somewhat controversial subject is outside the scope of this chapter. Specific screening strategies are presented and critically discussed by Hopper (1986). Other recommended references to consult for different perspectives on acute toxicity testing are Rhodes (2000), Brown (1980), and Arnold et al. (1990).

## REFERENCES

Armitage, P. and Allen, J. (1959). Methods of estimating the $LD_{50}$ in quantal response data. *J. Hygiene* 48: 298–322.

Arnold, D.L., Grice, H.C. and Krewski, D.R. (1990). *Handbook of In Vivo Toxicity Testing.* Academic Press, San Diego, CA.

Auletta, C. (1998). Acute systemic toxicity testing. In: *Handbook of Product Safety Assessment*, 2nd ed. (Gad, S., Ed.). Marcel Dekker, New York.

Balazs, R. (1970). Measurement of acute toxicity. In: *Methods of Toxicology* (Paget, G., Ed.). F. A. Davis Co., Philadelphia, pp. 49–81.

Balazs, R. (1976). Assessment of the value of systemic toxicity studies in experimental animals. In: *Advances in Modern Toxicity*, Vol. 1 Part 1: New Concepts in Safety Evaluation (Mahlman, M., Shapiro, R. and Blumenthal, H., Eds.). Hemisphere Publishing, Washington, D.C., pp. 141–153.

Behrens, B. (1929). Evaluation of *Digitalis* leaves in frog experiments *Arch. Exp. Pathol. Pharmacol.* 140: 236–256 (in German).

Berkson, J. (1955). Estimate of the integrated normal curve by minimum normit chi-square with particular reference to bioassay. *J. Am Stat. Assoc.* 50: 529–549.

Bliss, C. (1935). The calculation of the dosage mortality curve. *Anal. Appl. Biol.* 22: 134–167.

Bliss, C. (1957). Some principles of bioassay. *Am. Scientist* 45: 449–466.

British Toxicology Society (1984). A new approach to the classification of substances and preparations on the basis of their acute toxicity. A report by the British Toxicology Society Working Party on Toxicology. *Human Toxicol.* 3: 85–92.

Brown, V.K. (1980). *Acute Toxicity*, Wiley, New York.

Brown, V.K. (1983). Acute toxicity testing. In: *Animals and Alternatives in Toxicity Testing* (Bals, M., Riddell, R. and Worden, A., Eds.). Academic Press, New York, pp. 1–13.

Brownlee, K., Hodges, J. and Rosenblatt, M. (1953). The up-and-down method with small samples. *J. Am. Stat. Assoc.* 48: 262–277.

Bruce, R. (1985). An up-and-down procedure for acute toxicity testing. *Fund. Appl. Tox.* 5: 151, 157.

Chan, P., O'Hara, G. and Hayes, A. (1982). Principles and methods for acute and subchronic toxicity. In: *Principles and Methods of Toxicology* (Hayes, A., Ed.). Raven Press, New York, pp. 1–51.

Dayan, A. (1983). Complete program for acute toxicity testing—not only $LD_{50}$ determination. *Acta Pharmacol. Toxicol.* 52 (Suppl 2): 31–51.

Deichmann, W. and Gerarde, H. (1969). *Toxicology of Drugs and Chemicals.* Academic Press, New York.

Deichmann, W. and LeBlanc, T. (1943). Determination of the approximate lethal dose with about six animals. *J. Ind. Hyg. Toxicol.* 25: 415–417.

DePass, L. (1989). Alternative approaches in median lethality ($LD_{50}$) and acute toxicity testing. *Tox. Lett.* 49: 159–170.

DePass, L., Myers, R., Weaver, E. and Weil, C. (1984). An assessment of the importance of number of dosage levels, number of animals per dosage level, sex, and method of $LD_{50}$ and slope calculations in acute toxicity studies. In: *Acute Toxicity Testing: Alternative Approaches*, Vol 2 (Goldberg, A., ed.). Mary Ann Liebert, Inc. New York, pp. 139–153.

Dixon, W. (1965). The up-and-down method for small samples. *J. Am. Stat. Assoc.* 60: 967–978.

Dixon, W.J. and Wood, A.M. (1948). A method for obtaining and analyzing sensitivity data. *J. Am. Stat. Assoc.* 43: 109–126.

Elsberry, D. (1986). Screening approaches for acute and subacute toxicity studies. In: *Safety Evaluation of Drugs and Chemicals* (Lloyd, W., Ed.). Hemisphere Publishing, Washington, D.C., pp. 145–151.

Finney, D.J. (1971). *Probit Analysis*, 3rd ed. Cambridge University Press, New York.

Finney, D. (1985). The median lethal dose and its estimation. *Arch. Toxicol.* 56: 215–218.

Fowler, J. and Rutty, D. (1983). Methodological aspects of acute toxicity testing particularly $LD_{50}$ determinations: Present use in development of new drugs. *Acta Pharmacol. Toxicol.* 52 (Suppl. 2): 20–30.

Fowler, J., Brown, J. and Bell, H. (1979). The rat toxicity screen. *Pharmacol. Therapy* 5: 461–466.

Gad, S. (1982). A neuromuscular screen for use in industrial toxicology. *J. Toxicol. Envir. Health* 9: 691–704.

Gad, S. (1999). Statistics and Experimental Design for Toxicologists, CRC Press, Boca Raton, FL.

Gad, S. and Chengelis, C.P. (1999). *Acute Toxicology Testing*, 2nd ed. Academic Press, San Diego, CA.

Gad, S. (2001). Statistics for toxicologists. In: *Principles and Methods in Toxicology*, 4th ed. (Hayes, A., Ed.). Taylor & Francis, Philadelphia.

Gad, S., Smith, A., Cramp, A., Gavigan, F. and Derelanko, M. (1984). Innovative designs and practices for acute systemic toxicity studies. *Drug Chem. Toxicol.* 7: 423–434.

Hazelette, J., Thompson, T., Mertz, B., Vuolo-Schuessler, L., Gree, J., Tripp, S., Robertson, P. and Triana, V. (1987). Rising dose tolerance (RDT) study: A novel scenario for obtaining preclinical toxicology/drug metabolism data. *Toxicologist* 7, Abstract #846.

van den Heuvel, M., Clark, D., Fielder, R., Koundakijian, P., Oliver, G., Pelling, D., Tomlinson, C. and Walker, A. (1990). The international validation of a fixed-dose procedure as an alternative to the classical $LD_{50}$ test, *Fd. Chem. Toxicol.* 28: 469–482.

Hopper, D. (1986). Behavioral measures in toxicology screening. In: *Safety Evaluation of Drugs and Chemicals* (Lloyd W., Ed.). Hemisphere Publishing, New York, pp. 305–321.

Interagency Regulatory Liaison Group (IRLG), Office of Consumer Affairs. (1981). *Testing Standards and Guidelines Work Group* (HFE-88), Washington, D.C.

Irwin, S. (1962). Drug screening and evaluative procedures. *Science* 136: 123–128.

Jenner, P., Hagan, E., Taylor, J., Cook, E. and Fitzhugh, O. (1964). Food flavorings and compounds of related structure. I. Acute oral toxicity. *Food. Cosmet. Toxicol.* 2: 327–343.

Karber, G. (1931). Contribution to the collective treatment of pharmacological serial experiments. *Arch. Exp. Path. Pharmacol.* 162: 480–483.

LeBeau, J. (1983). The role of the $LD_{50}$ determination in drug safety evaluation. *Reg. Tox. Pharmacol.* 3: 71–74.

Litchfield, J. and Wilcoxon, F. (1949). A simplified method of evaluating dose-effect experiments. *J. Pharmacol. Exp. Therap.* 96: 99–113.

Lörke, D. (1983). A new approach to practical acute toxicity testing. *Arch. Toxicol.* 54: 275–287.

Malmfors, T. and Teiling, A. (1983). $LD_{50}$—its value for the pharmaceutical industry in safety evaluation of drugs. *Acta Pharmacol. Toxicol.* 52 (Suppl. 2): 229–246.

McClain, R. (1983). Generating, interpreting and reporting information in toxicity studies. *Drug Info. J.* 17: 245–255.

Morrison, J., Quinton, R. and Reinert, H. (1968). The purpose and value of $LD_{50}$ determinations. In: *Modern Trends in Toxicology*, Vol. I (Boyland, E. and Goulding, R., Eds.). Appleton-Century-Crofts, London, pp. 1–17.

Muller, H. and Kley, H. (1982). Retrospective study on the reliability of an "approximate $LD_{50}$" determined with a small number of animals. *Arch. Toxicol.* 51: 189–196.

Office of Science Coordination, FDA. (1984). *Final Report on Acute Studies Workshop Sponsored by the U.S. Food ,and Drug Administration.* U.S. Government Printshop, Washington, D.C.

Olson, H., Fabian, R., Greener, Y., Pack, F., Zelinger, D. and Dean, J. (1990). Reduction in animals used for acute toxicity testing based on retrospective analysis. *Toxicologist* 141 (abstract).

Osterberg, R. (1983). Today's requirements in food, drug, and chemical control. *Acta Pharmacol. Toxicol.* 52 (Suppl. 2): 201–228.

Pendergast, W. (1984). Biological drug regulation. In: *The Seventy-fifth Anniversary Commemorative Volume of Food and Drug Law.* Edited and Published by the Food and Drug Law Institute, Washington, D.C., pp. 293–305.

Peterson, D., Ellis, Z., Harris, D. and Spadek, Z. (1987). Acute toxicity of the major alkaloids of cultivated *Lupinus angustifolius* seeds to rats. *J. Appl. Toxicol.* 7: 51–53.

Piegorsh, W. (1989). Quantification of toxic response and the development of the median effective dose ($ED_{50}$)—a historical perspective. *Toxicol. Indust. Health.* 5: 55–62.

Rhodes, C. (2000). Principles of Tseting for Acute Toxic Effects. In: *General and Applied Toxicology* (Ballantyne, B., Marrs, T. and Szversen, T., Eds.) Macmillan References, Ltd., London, pp. 33–54.

Rowan, A. (1981). The $LD_{50}$ Test: A critique and suggestions for alternatives. *Pharmaceutical Technology*, April pp. 65–92.

Schiantarelli, P. and Cadel, S. (1981). Piroxicam pharmacological activity and gastrointestinal damage by oral and rectal route: Comparison with oral indomethacin and phenylbutazone. *Arzneim.-Forsch./Drug Res.* 31: 87–92.

Schutz, E. and Fuchs, H. (1982). A new approach to minimizing the number of animals in acute toxicity testing and optimizing the information of the test results. *Arch. Toxicol.* 51: 197–220.

Smyth, H. and Carpenter, C. (1944). The place of the range-finding test in the industrial toxicology laboratory. *J. Indus. Hyg. Tox.* 26: 269–273.

Sperling, F. (1976). Nonlethal parameters as indices of acute toxicity: Inadequacies of the acute $LD_{50}$. In: *Advances in Modern Toxicology*, Vol. 1, Part 1: *New Concepts in Safety Evaluation* (Mehlman, M., Shapiro, R. and Blumenthal, H., Eds.). Hemisphere Publishing, Washington, D.C., pp. 177–191.

Thompson, W. and Weil, C. (1952). On the construction of a table for moving average interpolation. *Biometrics* 8: 51–54.

Trevan, J. (1927). The error of determination of toxicity. *Proc. Roy. Soc., B101*, pp. 483–514.

Waud, D. (1972). Biological assays involving quantal responses. *J. Pharmacol. Exp. Therap.* 183: 577–607.

Weil, C. (1952). Table for convenient calculation of median effective dose ($LD_{50}$ or $ED_{50}$) and instructions in their use. *Biometrics* 8: 249–263.

Weil, C. (1983). Economical $LD_{50}$ and slope determination. *Drug and Chem. Tox.* 6: 595–603.

Zbinden, G. (1984). Acute toxicity testing, purpose. In: *Acute Toxicity Testing: Alternative Approaches* (Goldberg, A., Ed.). Mary Ann Liebert, New York, pp. 5–22.

Zbinden, G. and Flury-Roversi, M. (1981). Significance of the $LD_{50}$ Test for the toxicological evaluation of chemical substances. *Arch. Toxicol.* 47: 77–99.

Zbinden, G., Elsner, J. and Boelsterli, U. (1984). Toxicological screening. *Regul. Toxicol. Pharmacol.* 4: 275–286.

# 6

# GENOTOXICITY

## 6.1. INTRODUCTION

Genotoxicity encompasses all the potential means by which the genetic material of higher organisms may be damaged, with resulting serious consequences. Most forms of genotoxicity are expressions of mutagenicity: the induction of DNA damage and other genetic alterations, with changes in one or a few of DNA bare pairs (gene mutations). Others are clastogenicity, with gross changes in chromosomal structure (i.e., chromosomal aberrations) or in chromosome numbers. Clearly, the potential of any pharmaceutical to cause such damage is a concern.

It has been known for several hundred years that exposure to particular chemicals or complex mixtures can lead to cancer in later life (Doll, 1977), and it has been postulated more recently that chemicals can also induce heritable changes in humans, leading to diseases in the next generation (ICEMC, 1983). There has been accumulating evidence that such changes can arise following damage to DNA and resulting mutations (see, e.g., Bridges, 1976). Therefore, it has become necessary to determine whether widely used drugs or potentially useful new drugs possess the ability to damage DNA. In pharmaceutical development, such information may be used to discard a new candidate drug from further work, to control or eliminate human exposure for a mutagenic industrial compound or, for a drug, to proceed with development if benefits clearly outweigh risks. Data concerning the genotoxicity of a new drug have become part of the safety package, though the timing of the performance of the tests may vary. They are needed for decision-making and to reduce risks that might otherwise be unforeseen.

### 6.1.1. Iso Testing Requirements and ICH Test Profile

ISO 10993-3 (1993) sets forth clear guidance on testing requirements as summarized in Table 6.1. ICH (International Conference on Harmonization) guidance, shown in Table 6.2, has different but also clear requirements. They want to see an *in vivo* test conducted. While FDA has no clear guidelines, it expects that an appropriate adaptation of one of these two be performed.

## 6.2. DNA STRUCTURE

With the exception of certain viruses, the blueprint for all organisms is contained in code by deoxyribonucleic acid (DNA), a giant macro-molecule whose structure allows a vast amount of information to be stored accurately. We have all arisen from a single cell, the fertilized ovum containing two sets of DNA (packaged with protein to form chromatin), one set from our mother, resident in the nucleus of the unfertilized ovum, the second set from our father via the successful sperm. Every cell in the adult has arisen from this one cell and (with the exception of the germ cell and specialized liver cells) contains one copy of these original chromosome sets.

The genetic code is composed of four "letters"—two pyrimidine nitrogenous bases, thymine and cytosine, and two purine bases, guanine and adenine—which can be regarded functionally as arranged in codons (or triplets). Each codon consists of a combination of three letters; therefore, $4^3$ (64) different codons are possible. Sixty-one codons code for specific amino acids (three produce stop signals), and as only 20 different amino acids are used to make proteins, one amino acid can be specified by more than one codon.

The bases on one strand are connected together by a sugar (deoxyribose) phosphate backbone. DNA can exist in a single-stranded or double-stranded form. In the latter state, the two strands are held together by hydrogen bonds between the bases. Hydrogen bonds are weak electrostatic forces involving oxygen and nitrogen atoms. As a strict rule, one fundamental to mutagenesis, the adenine bases on one strand always hydrogen bond to the thymine bases on the sister strand. Similarly, guanine bases pair with cytosine bases. Adenine and thymine form two hydrogen bonds, and guanine and cytosine form three.

Double-stranded DNA has a unique property in that it is able to make identical copies of itself when supplied with precursors, relevant enzymes, and cofactors. In simplified terms, two strands begin to unwind and separate as the hydrogen bonds are broken. This produces single-stranded regions. Complementary deoxyribonu-cleotide triphosphates then pair with the exposed bases under the control of a DNA polymerase enzyme.

A structural gene is a linear sequence of codons which codes for a functional polypeptide, that is, a linear sequence of amino acids. Individual polypeptides may have a structural, enzymatic or regulatory role in the cell. Although the primary structure of DNA is the same in prokaryotes and eukaryotes, there are differences between the genes of these two types of organism, in internal structure, numbers and

**TABLE 6.1. ISO Genotoxicity Guidance[a]**

| Genotoxic Effect to be Assessed for Conformance with ISO 10993-3 | Significance of Test | Tests Meeting Requirements |
|---|---|---|
| DNA effects | Damage to DNA (Deoxyribonucleic acid) by a chemical or material may result in genotoxic effects such as mutations, which in turn may lead to carcinogenicity. Damage to DNA causes the cell to manufacture new DNA to compensate for the loss or damage. This can be assessed by evaluating the formation of newly synthesized DNA. | Unscheduled DNA Synthesis |
| Gene mutations | Gene mutations (changes in the sequences of DNA that code for critical proteins or functions) have been correlated to carcinogenicity and tumorigenicity. | Ames Assay (4 *Salmonella Typhimurium* bacterial strains and *Escherichia Coli*) is a reverse mutation assay. A bacterial mutation event causes the bacteria to become Histidine (a vital amino acid) independent. Normal bacteria will not survive in the absence of Histidine. Hypoxanthine Guanine Phosphoribosyl Transferase (HGPRT) is a forward mutation assay. Mammalian cells that have been exposed to a mutagen will survive in the presence of a toxic substance (6-Thioguanine). |
| Chromosomal aberrations | Physical damage to chromosomes (large ordered stretches of DNA in the nuclei of cells) or clastogenicity can lead to DNA damage, in turn leading to abnormal and/or carcinogenic growth of cells. | Chromosomal aberration assay assesses the potential for physical damage to the chromosomes of mammalian cells by a biomaterial. |

[a]ISO 10993-3 (1993) Biological Evaluation of Medical Devices—Part 3: Tests for Genotoxicity, Carcinogenicity, and Reproductive Toxicity states that at least three *in vitro* tests, two of which use mammalian cells, should be used to test for three levels of genotoxic effects: DNA effects, gene mutations, and chromosomal aberrations. ANSI/AAMI/ISO 10993-3 (1993) Biological Evaluation of Medical Devices—Part 3: Tests for Genotoxicity, Carcinogenicity, and Reproductive Toxicity states that "Suitable cell transformation systems may be used for carcinogenicity prescreening".

**TABLE 6.2. Genotoxicity Tests Recommended by ICH**

| Genotoxicity Test—ICH | Mutation | Cell Type | Method |
| --- | --- | --- | --- |
| A test for gene mutation in bacteria | Gene | Bacterial | *In vitro* |
| *In vitro* cytogenetic assay using mouse lymphomas tk cells | Chromosome | Mammalian | *In vitro* |
| *In vivo* test for chromosomal damage using rodent hematopoietic cells | Gene | Mammalian | *In vivo* |

(ICH, 1996, 1997).

mechanism of replication. In bacteria, there is a single chromosome, normally a closed circle, which is not complexed with protein, and replication does not require specialized cellular structures. In plant and animal cells, there are many chromosomes, each present as two copies, as mentioned earlier, and the DNA is complexed with protein. Replication and cell division require the proteinaceous spindle apparatus. The DNA of eukaryotic cells contains repeated sequences of some genes. Also, eukaryotic genes, unlike prokaryotic genes, have noncoding DNA regions called introns between coding regions called exons. This property means that eukaryotic cells have to use an additional processing step at transcription.

### 6.2.1. Transcription

The relationship between the DNA in the nucleus and proteins in the cytoplasm is not direct. The information in the DNA molecule is transmitted to the protein-synthesizing machinery of the cell via another informational nucleic acid, called messenger RNA (mRNA), which is synthesized by an enzyme called RNA polymerase. Although similar to DNA, mRNAs are single-stranded, and possess the base uracil instead of thymine and the sugar ribose rather than deoxyribose. These molecules act as short-lived copies of the genes being expressed.

In eukaryotic cells, the initial mRNA copy contains homologues of both the intron and exon regions. The intron regions are then removed by enzymes located in the nucleus of the cell. Further enzymes splice the exon regions together to form the active mRNA molecules. In both groups of organisms, mature mRNA molecules then pass out of the nucleus into the cytoplasm.

### 6.2.2. Translation

The next process is similar in both eukaryotes and prokaryotes, and involves the translation of mRNA molecules into polypeptides. This procedure involves many enzymes and two further types of RNA: transfer RNA (tRNA) and ribosomal RNA (rRNA). There is a specific tRNA for each of the amino acids. These molecules are involved in the transportation and coupling of amino acids into the resulting polypeptide. Each tRNA molecule has two binding sites, one for the specific amino acid, the other containing a triplet of bases (the "anticodon") which is complementary to the appropriate codon on the mRNA.

rRNA is complexed with protein to form a subcellular globular organelle called a ribosome. Ribosomes can be regarded as the "reading head" which allows the linear array of mRNA codons each to base-pair with an anticodon of an appropriate incoming tRNA/amino acid complex. The polypeptide chain forms as each tRNA/amino acid comes into register with their RNA codon and with specific sites on the ribosome. A peptide bond is formed between each amino acid as it passes through the reading head of the ribosome (Venitt and Parry, 1984).

### 6.2.3. Gene Regulation

Structural genes are regulated by a special set of codons, in particular "promoter" sequences. The promoter sequence is the initial binding site for RNA polymerase before transcription begins. Different promoter sequences have different affinities for RNA polymerase. Some sets of structural genes with linked functions have a single promoter and their coordinate expression is controlled by another regulatory gene called an operator. A group of such genes is called an operon. The activity of the operator is further controlled by a protein called a repressor, since it stops the expression of the whole operon by binding to the operator sequence, preventing RNA polymerase from binding to the promoter. Repressors can be removed by relevant chemical signals or in a time-related fashion.

In the ways described above, only the genes required at a given moment are expressed. This not only helps to conserve the energy of the cell, but also is critical for correct cellular differentiation, tissue pattern formation and formation of the body plan.

### 6.2.4. DNA Repair

All living cells appear to possess several different major DNA repair processes (reviews: Walker, 1984; Rossman and Klein, 1988). Such processes are needed to protect cells from the lethal and mutating effects of heat-induced DNA hydrolysis; ultraviolet light; ionizing radiation; DNA reactive chemicals; free radicals, and so on. In single-celled eukaryotes such as the yeast *Saccharomyces cerevisiae*, the number of genes known to be involved in DNA repair approaches 100 (Friedberg, 1988). The number in mammalian cells is expected to be at least equal to this and emphasizes the importance of correction of DNA damage.

*Excision Repair.* Some groups of enzymes (light-independent) are apparently organized to act cooperatively to recognize DNA lesions, remove them, and correctly replace the damaged sections of DNA. The most comprehensively studied of these is the excision repair pathway.

Briefly, the pathway can be described as follows

1. *Preincision Reactions*. UvrA protein dimers are formed which bind to the DNA location distant from the damaged site. The UvrB protein then binds to the DNA-UvrA complex to produce an energy-requiring topological unwinding of the DNA via DNA gyrase. This area of unwinding is then translocated, again using ATP as an energy source, to the site of the damaged DNA.

2. *Incision Reactions*. The UvrC protein binds to the DNA-UvrA, B complex and incises the DNA at two sites: seven bases to the 5′ end and three bases to the 3′ end of the damage.

3. *Excision Reactions*. UvrD protein and DNA polymerase 1 excise the damaged bases and then resynthesize the strand, using the sister strand as a template. The Uvr complex then breaks down, leaving a restored, but nicked, strand.

4. *Ligation Reaction*. The nick in the phosphate backbone is repaired by DNA ligase. A similar excision repair mechanism exists in mammalian cells (see, e.g., Cleaver, 1983).

In both cases, the process is regarded as error-free and does not lead to the generation of mutations. However, this pathway can become saturated with excessive numbers of damaged DNA sites, forcing the cell to fall back on other repair mechanisms.

***Error-Prone Repair.*** Exposure of *E. coli* to agents or conditions that either damage DNA or interfere with DNA replication results in the increased expression of the so-called "SOS" regulatory network (Walker, 1984). Included in this network is a group of at least 17 unlinked DNA damage-inducible (*din*) genes. The *din* gene functions are repressed in undamaged cells by the product of the *lexA* gene (Little and Mount, 1982) and are induced when the LexA protein is cleaved by a process that requires modified RecA protein (RecA*), which then acts as a selective protease (Little, 1984). The *din* genes code for a variety of functions, including filamentation, cessation of respiration, and so on. Included are the *umuDC* gene products, which are required for so-called error-prone or mutagenic DNA repair (Kato and Shinoura, 1977). The precise biochemical mechanism by which this repair is achieved is still not fully understood. Bacterial polymerase molecules have complex activities, including the ability to "proof-read" DNA, that is, to ensure that the base-pairing rules of double-stranded DNA are met. It is hypothesized that Umu proteins may suppress this proof-reading activity, so that base mismatches are tolerated (Villani et al., 1978). Recent evidence suggests that DNA lesions are bypassed, and this bypass step requires UmuDC proteins and RecA* proteins (Bridges et al., 1987). The net result is that random base insertion occurs opposite the lesion, which may result in mutation.

Analogues of the *umuDC* genes can be found in locations other than the bacterial chromosome, for example, plasmid pKM101 (Walker and Dobson, 1979), a derivative of the drug resistance plasmid R46 (Mortelmans and Stocker, 1979), which carried *mucAB* genes (Shanabruch and Walker, 1980) (see pp. 879–880).

Mutagenic repair, as controlled by *umuDC*, is not universal even among entero-bacteria (Sedgwick and Goodwin, 1985). For instance, *Salmonella typhimurium* LT2 does not appear to express mutagenic repair (Walker, 1984). Thus, the usefulness of strains of this species is greatly enhanced by using derivatives containing plasmids with genes coding for error-prone repair (MacPhee, 1973; McCann et al., 1975).

***Mismatch Repair.*** Mispairs that break the normal base-pairing rules can arise spontaneously due to DNA biosynthetic errors, events associated with genetic recombination and the deamination of methylated cytosine (Modrich, 1987). With the latter, when cytosine deaminates to uracil, an endonuclease enzyme, *N*-uracil-DNA glycosylase (Lindahl, 1979), excises the uracil residue before it can pair with adenine at the next replication. However, 5-methyl cytosine deaminates to form thymine and will not be excised by a glycosylase. As a result, thymine exits on one strand paired with guanine on the sister strand, that is, a mismatch. This will result in a spontaneous point mutation if left unrepaired. For this reason, methylated cytosines form spontaneous mutation "hot-spots" (Miller, 1985). The cell is able to repair mismatches by being able to distinguish between the DNA strand that exists before replication and a newly synthesized strand.

The mechanism of strand-directed mismatch correction has been demonstrated in *E. coli* (see, e.g., Wagner and Meselson, 1976). In this organism, adenine methylation of d(G-A-T-C) sequences determines the strand on which repair occurs. Thus, parental DNA is fully methylated, while newly synthesized DNA is undermethylated, for a period sufficient for mismatch correction. By this means the organism preserves the presumed correct sequence, i.e., that present on the original DNA strand, and removes the aberrant base on the newly synthesized strand. Adenine methylation is achieved in *E. coli* by the *dam* methylase, which is dependent on *S*-adenosylmethionine. Mutants (*dam*) lacking this methylase are hypermutable, as would be expected by this model (Marinus and Morris, 1974).

***The Adaptive Repair Pathway.*** The mutagenic and carcinogenic effects of alkylat-ing agents such as ethyl methane sulphonate are due to the generation of $O^6$-alkylguanine residues in DNA, which result in point mutations. Bacterial and mammalian cells can repair a limited number of such lesions before DNA replica-tion, thus preventing mutagenic and potentially lethal events from taking place.

If *E. coli* are exposed to low concentrations of a simple alkylating agents, a repair mechanism is induced that causes increased resistance to subsequent challenge with a high dose. This adaptation response was first described by Samson and Cairns (1977) and has recently been reviewed by Lindahl et al. (1988). The repair pathway is particularly well understood.

***Plasmids and DNA Repair.*** Plasmids are extrachromosomal genetic elements that are composed of circular double-stranded DNA. In bacteria some can mediate their own transfer from cell to cell by conjugation; they contain a set of *tra* genes coding for tube-like structures, such as pili, through which a copy of plasmid DNA can pass during transfer. Plasmids range in size from 1.5 to 200 million daltons. The number of copies per cell differs from plasmid to plasmid. Copy number relates to control of replication and this correlates with size; that is, small plasmids tend to have large copy numbers per cell. This may relate to a lack of replication control genes (Mortelmans and Dousman, 1986).

Many plasmids are known to possess three properties: (1) increased resistance to the bactericidal effects of UV and chemical mutagens, (2) increased spontaneous mutagenesis, and (3) increased susceptibility to UV and chemically induced mutagenesis. Some plasmids possess all three properties; others may possess just one, for example, increased susceptibility to mutagenesis (review: Mortelmans and Dousman, 1986). Often the profile of activity depends on the DNA repair status of the host cell (Pinney, 1980). Plasmid pKM101 carries DNA repair genes and has been widely used in strains used in bacterial mutagenicity tests.


### 6.2.5.  Nature of Point Mutations

The word "mutation" can be applied to point-mutations which are qualitative changes involving one or a few bases in base sequences within genes, as described below, as well as to larger changes involving whole chromosomes (and thus many thousands of genes), and even to changes in whole chromosome sets (described later under "Cytogenetics").

Point mutations can occur when one base is substituted for another (base substitution). Substitution of another purine for a purine base or of another pyrimidine for pyrimidine is called a transition, while substitutions of purine for pyrimidine or pyrimidine for purine are called transversions. Both types of base substitution have been identified within mutated genes. These changes lead to a codon change which can cause the "wrong" amino acid to be inserted into the relevant polypeptide and are known as mis-sense mutations. Such polypeptides may have dramatically altered properties if the new amino acid is close to the active center of an enzyme or affects the three-dimensional makeup of an enzyme or a structural protein. These changes, in turn, can lead to change or reduction in function, which can be detected as a change in phenotype of the affected cells.

A base substitution can also result in the formation of a new inappropriate terminator (or non-sense) codon, and are thus known as non-sense mutations. The polypeptide formed from such mutated genes will be shorter than normal and is most likely to be inactive. Owing to the redundancy of the genetic code, about a quarter of all possible base substitutions will not result in an amino acid replacement and will be silent mutations.

Bases can be deleted or added to a gene. As each gene is of a precisely defined length, these changes, if they involve a number of bases that are not a multiple of 3, result in a change in the "reading frame" of the DNA sequence and are thus known as frameshift mutations. Such mutations tend to have a dramatic effect on the polypeptide of the affected gene, as most amino acids will differ from the point of the insertion or deletion of bases onwards. Very often a new terminator codon is produced, so, again, short inactive polypeptides will result.

Both types of mutation result in an altered polypeptide, which, in turn, can have a marked effect on the phenotype of the affected cell. Much use of phenotypic changes is made in mutagenicity tests.

Base substitutions and frameshift changes occur spontaneously and can be induced by radiation and chemical mutagens. It is apparent that the molecular mechanisms resulting in these changes are different in each case, but the potential hazards associated with mutagens capable of inducing the different types of mutation are equivalent.

### 6.2.6. Suppressor Mutations

In some instances a mutation within one gene can be corrected by a second mutational event at a separate site on the chromosome. As a result, the first defect is suppressed and the second mutation is known as a suppressor mutation. Most suppressor mutations have been found to affect genes encoding for transfer RNAs. Usually the mutation causes a change in the sequence of the anticodon of the tRNA. Thus, if a new terminator or non-sense codon is formed as the first mutation, this can be suppressed by a second mutation forming a tRNA species that now has an anticodon complementary to a termination codon. Thus, the new tRNA species will supply an amino acid at the terminator site on the mRNA and allow translation to proceed. Surprisingly, most suppressors of this type do not adversely affect cell growth, which implies that the cell can tolerate translation proceeding through termination signals, producing abnormal polypeptides. An alternative explanation is that the particular DNA sequences surrounding normal terminator codons result in a reduced efficiency of suppressor tRNAs (Bossi, 1985).

Frameshift suppression is also possible. This can be achieved by a second mutation in a tRNA gene such that the anticodon of a tRNA molecule consists of 4 bases rather than 3, for example, an extra C residue in the CCC anticodon sequence of a glycine tRNA gene. This change will allow correction of a $+1$ frameshift involving the GGG codon for glycine (Bossi, 1985).

### 6.2.7. Adduct Formation

The earlier discussion of adaptive repair made reference to the fact that some unrepaired alkylated bases are lethal, owing to interference with DNA replication, while others, such as $O^6$-methylguanine lead to mutation if unrepaired. These differences indicate that not all DNA adducts (i.e., DNA bases with additional chemical groups, not associated with normal DNA physiology) are equivalent. In fact, some adducts appear not to interfere with normal DNA functions or are rapidly repaired, others are mutagenic and yet others are lethal. Chemicals that form electrophilic species readily form DNA adducts. These pieces of information are hard-won, and the reader is recommended to read reviews of the pioneering work of Brook and Lawley (review: Lawley, 1989) summarizing work identifying the importance of DNA adduct formation with polycyclic hydrocarbons and the importance of "minor" products of base alkylation such as $O^6$-methylguanine, and, in addition, the work of the Millers in linking attack of nucleophilic sites in DNA by electrophiles to mutagenesis and carcinogenesis (Miller and Miller, 1971).

If a DNA adduct involves the nitrogen or oxygen atoms involved in base-pairing, and the adducted DNA is not repaired, base substitution can result. Adducts can be small, such as the simple addition of methyl or ethyl groups, or they can be very bulky, owing to reaction with multiringed structures. The most vulnerable base is guanine, which can form adducts at several of its atoms (e.g., $N^7$, $C^8$, $O^6$ and exocyclic $N^2$) (Venitt and Parry, 1984). Adducts can form links between adjacent bases on the same strand (intrastrand cross-links) and can form interstrand cross-links between each strand of double-stranded DNA.

The induction of frameshift mutation does not necessarily require covalent adduct formation. Some compounds that have a flat, planar structure, such as particular polycyclic hydrocarbons, can intercalate between the DNA strands of the DNA duplex. The intercalated molecules interfere with DNA repair enzymes or replication and cause additions and deletions of base-pairs. The precise mechanism is still unclear, although several mechanisms have been proposed. Hotspots for frameshift mutation often involve sections of DNA where there is a run of the same base, for example, the addition of a guanine to a run of 6 guanine residues. Such information leads to a "slipped mispairing" model for frameshift mutation (Streisinger et al., 1966; Roth, 1974). In this scheme single strand breaks allow one strand to slip and loop out one or more base-pairs, the configuration being stabilized by complementary base-pairing at the end of the single-stranded region. Subsequent resynthesis results ultimately in additions or deletions of base-pairs (Miller, 1985).

### 6.2.8. Mutations Due to Insertion Sequences

The subject of mutations due to insertion sequences is reviewed in Cullum (1985). Studies of spontaneous mutation in *E. coli* detected a special class of mutations that were strongly polar, reducing the expression of downstream genes (Jordan et al., 1967). These genes mapped as point mutations and reverted like typical point-mutations. However, unlike point-mutations, mutagens did not increase their reversion frequency. Further studies showed that these mutations were due to extra pieces of DNA that can be inserted into various places in the genome. They are not just random pieces of DNA but are "insertion sequences" 0.7–1.5 kilobases long that can "jump" into other DNA sequences. They are related to transposons, which are insertion sequences carrying easily detected markers such as antibiotic resistance genes, and Mu phages (bacterial viruses).

### 6.2.9. The Link between Mutation and Cancer

The change in cells undergoing normal, controlled cell division and differentiation to cells that are transformed, dividing without check, and are undifferentiated or abnormally differentiated, does not appear to occur as a single step; that is, transformation is multistage. Evidence for this comes from *in vitro* studies, animal models and clinical observations, in particular, the long latent period between exposure to a carcinogen and the appearance of a tumor in the target tissue. There is much evidence for the sequence of events shown in Figure 6.1 (tumor initiation, promotion, malignant conversion, and progression). Such a scheme provides a useful working model but clearly does not apply to all "carcinogens" in all circumstances (Kuroki and Matsushima, 1987).

Study of Figure 6.1 shows that there are several points where genetic change appears to play a role. Such change may occur spontaneously, due to rare errors at cell division such as misreplication of DNA or spindle malfunction, or may be induced by exposure to viruses (e.g., acute transforming retroviruses), ionizing and nonionizing radiations absorbed by DNA (e.g., X-rays; UVC) or particular chemical species capable of covalently interacting with DNA (as discussed earlier) or with vital proteins, such as tubulin, that polymerize to form the cell division spindle apparatus.

### 6.2.10. Genotoxic versus Nongenotoxic Mechanisms of Carcinogenesis

The previous discussions of oncogene activation and human DNA repair deficiencies provide strong evidence for carcinogenesis via genotoxic mechanisms. However, it has been recognized for many years that cancers can arise without biologically significant direct or indirect interaction between a chemical and cellular DNA (see, e.g., Gatehouse et al., 1988). The distinction between nongenotoxic and genotoxic carcinogens has recently been brought into a sharper focus following the identification of a comparatively large number of "nongenotoxic" carcinogens by the United States National Toxicology Program (Tennant et al., 1987). These include a wide range of chemicals acting via a variety of mechanisms, including augmentation of high "spontaneous" tumor yields; disruption of normal hormonal homeostasis in hormone-responsive tissues; peroxisome proliferation; proliferation of urothelial cells following damage via induced kidney stones; etc. (Clayson, 1989). This author points out that a major effort is under way to determine whether many of these compounds can elicit similar effects in humans.

Ashby and Tennant (1988) and Ashby et al. (1989) stress the significance of their observations that 16 tissues are apparently sensitive to genotoxic carcinogens, while a further 13 tissues are sensitive to both genotoxic and nongenotoxic carcinogens (Table 6.3). Also, genotoxic carcinogens tend to induce tumors in several tissues of both males and females in both rats and mice. This contrasts with nongenotoxic carcinogens, which may induce tumors at high doses, in one tissue, of one sex, of one species. Although it is most unlikely that all nongenotoxic carcinogens will prove to be irrelevant in terms of human risk, it appears from the analysis above that a proportion of carcinogens identified by the use of near-toxic levels in rodent bioassays are of dubious relevance to the induction of human cancer. For further discussion, see Butterworth and Slaga (1987).

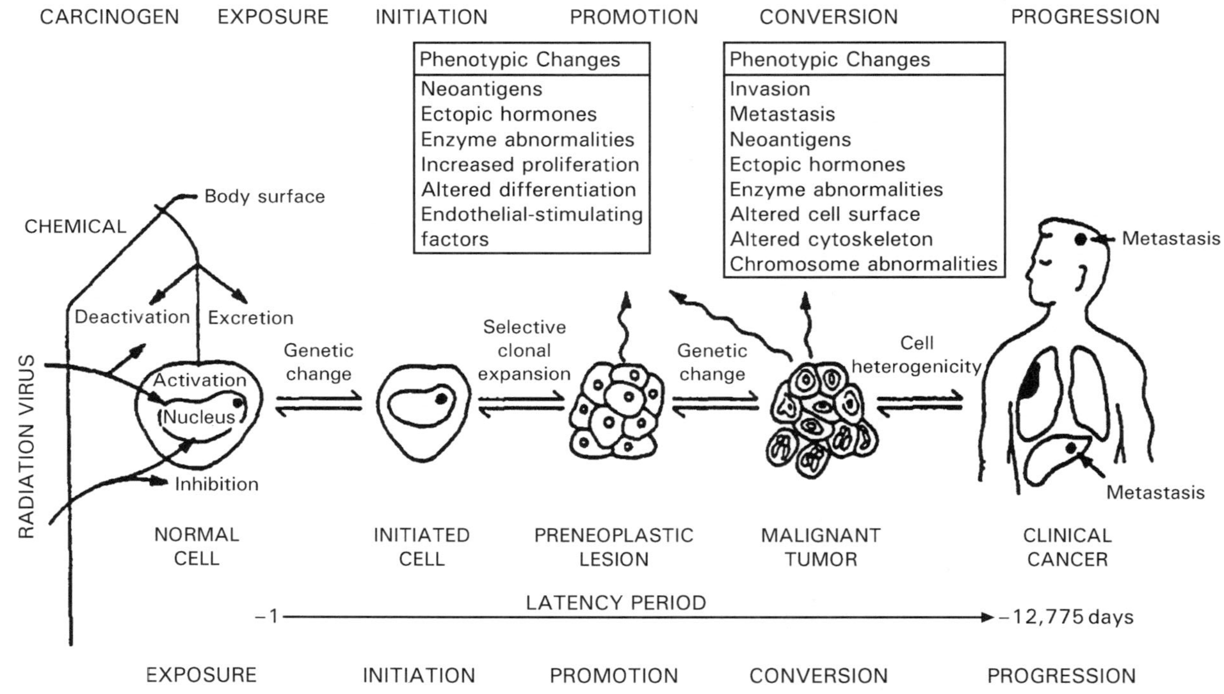


**FIGURE 6.1.**  Schematic representation of events leading to neoplasia. *Source*: Adapted from Harris, et al. (1987).

**TABLE 6.3. Tissues Sensitive to Genotoxic and/or Nongenotoxic Carcinogens**

| Tissues Sensitive Primarily to Genotoxins | Tissues Sensitive to Both Genotoxins and Nongenotoxins |
| --- | --- |
| Stomach | Nose |
| Zymbal gland | Mammary gland |
| Lung | Pituitary gland |
| Subcutaneous tissue | Integumentary system |
| Circulatory system | Kidney |
| Clitoral gland | Urinary bladder |
| Skin | Liver |
| Intestine/colon | Thyroid gland |
| Uterus | Hematopoietic system |
| Spleen | Adrenal gland |
| Tunica vaginalis | Pancreas |
| Bile duct | Seminal vesicle |
| Ovary | Urinary tract |
| Haderian gland | Lymphatic system |
| Preputial gland | |
| [Multiple organ sites] | |

### 6.2.11. Genetic Damage and Heritable Defects

Concern about the effects of radiations and chemicals on the human gene pool, and the resulting heritable malformations and syndromes, has steadily risen during this century. The recognition that changes in morphology would result from changes in the hereditary material due to mutations (from the Latin word *mutare*, to change), was adopted by de Vries following observations on the evening primrose, *Oenothera* (de Vries, 1901). Muller went on to demonstrate that X-rays could induce mutations in the germ cells of the fruit fly *Drosophila melanogaster* (Muller, 1927).

The human gene pool is known to carry many deleterious genes acquired from preceding generations that result in numerous genetic diseases. It is clear that these arise as a result of DNA changes affecting particular chromosomes or genes. They can be grouped as follows

1. Chromosome abnormalities, small changes in either number or structure.
2. Autosomal dominant gene mutations, in which a change in only one copy of the pair of genes is sufficient for the condition to be expressed.
3. Autosomal recessive gene mutations in which both copies of a gene must be mutated for the trait to become manifest.
4. Sex-linked conditions, which may also be recessive or dominant, where the mutant gene is on an X chromosome and will be expressed at high frequency

in males (XY) and at a much lower frequency in females (XX), if the gene acts in a recessive manner.

5. Polygenic mutations, in which the condition results from the interaction of several genes and may include an environmental component.

### 6.2.12. Reproductive Effects

If a potent genotoxin is able to cross the placental barrier, it is very likely to interfere with differentiation of the developing embryo and thus possess teratogenic potential. Indeed, many of the better studied teratogens are also mutagenic (Kalter, 1977). However, mutagens form only one class of teratogens and a large proportion of teratogens are not mutagenic. Alternative mechanisms of teratogenesis include cell death, mitotic delay, retarded differentiation, vascular insufficiency, inhibited cell migration, and so on (Beckman and Brent, 1986).

It is known that more fetal wastage than generally believed and many spontaneous abortions arise as a result of the presence of dominant lethal mutations in the developing embryo, many of which appear to be due to major chromosomal damage. In addition, impairment of male fertility may also be a consequence of exposure to mutagens.

### 6.3. CYTOGENETICS

There are various types of cytogenetic change which can be detected in chromosomes. These are structural chromosome aberrations (Cas), numerical changes which could result in aneuploidy, and sister chromatid exchanges (SCEs). Chromosome aberration assays are used to detect the induction of chromosome breakage (clastogenesis) in somatic or germinal cells by direct observation of chromosome damage during metaphase analysis, or by indirect observation of micronuclei. Chromosome damage detected in these assays is mostly lethal to the cell during the cell cycle following the induction of the damage. Its presence, however, indicates a potential to induce more subtle chromosome damage which survives cell division to produce heritable cytogenetic changes. Cytogenetic damage is usually accompanied by other genotoxic damage such as gene mutation.

### 6.3.1. Cytogenetic Damage and Its Consequences

Structural and numerical chromosomal aberrations in somatic cells may be involved in the etiology of neoplasia and in germ cells can lead to perinatal mortality, dominant lethality or congenital malformations in the offspring (Chandley, 1981), and some tumors (Anderson, 1990).

Chromosome defects arise at the level of the individual chromosome or at the level of the chromosomal set, so affecting chromosomal number in subsequent cell replications.

### 6.3.2. Individual Chromosome Damage

Damage to individual chromosomes consists of breakage of chromatids, which must result from a discontinuity of both strands of the DNA in a chromatid Heddle and Bodycote, 1970). How mutagens produce chromosome breakage is not totally understood, but DNA lesions which are not in themselves discontinuities will produce breakage of a chromosome as a consequence of their interference with the normal process of DNA replication. In haploid microorganisms and prokaryotes chromosome breaks are usually lethal, but not in diploid eukaryotes. According to Bender et al., (1974), in these organisms chromosome breaks may reconstitute in the same order, probably as a result of an enzyme repair process, resulting in no apparent cytogenetic damage; they may remain unjoined as fragments, which could result in cell death at the next or following mitoses, if, for example, unrejoined fragments are introduced into the zygote via treated germ cells, the embryo may die at a very early stage from a dominant lethal mutation; or they may rejoin in a different order from the original one, producing chromosomal rearrangements. There are various types of chromosomal rearrangements.

***Reciprocal Translocations.*** These can result from the exchange of chromosomal segments between two chromosomes and, depending on the position of the centromeres in the rearranged chromosomes, different configurations will result.

1. Asymmetrical exchanges arise when one of the rearranged chromosomes carries both centromeres and is known as dicentric while the other carries none and is acentric. The cell or zygote carrying this anomaly usually dies, death being caused by segregation difficulties of the dicentric or the loss of the acentric fragment at cell division. Such a translocation contributes to dominant lethality.

2. Symmetrical exchanges occur when each rearranged chromosome carries just one centromere. This allows the zygote to develop normally, but when such heterozygoes form germ cells at meiosis, about half of their gametes will be genetically unbalanced, since they have deficiencies and duplications of chromosomal material. The unbalanced gametes which survive produce unbalanced zygotes, which results in death shortly before or after birth, or congenital malformations.

***Centric Fusions.*** These involve the joining together of two chromosomes, each of which has a centromere at or near one end, to produce a single metacentric or submetacentric chromosome. When such translocations are produced in a germ cell and result from breakage and rejoining in the short arms of the two chromosomes, as a consequence of loss of the derived acentric fragments, a genetic deficiency can result. Some Robertsonian translocations are able to survive but others pose a risk. In heterozygotes the two arms of the translocation chromosome may pair with the two separate homologous chromosomes at meiosis but segregate in a disorderly manner. Some of the resultant germ cells lack copies (nullisomy) or carry two copies (disomy) of one or other of the two chromosomes involved, which results in monosomic or trisomic embryos. Monosomics die early but trisomic embryos, which carry three copies of a chromosome, can survive to birth or beyond. If chromosome 21 is involved in the translocation, it can form a translocation trisomy and produce inherited Down's syndrome (this differs from nondisjunctional Down's syndrome trisomy).

***Deletions and Deficiencies.*** When two breaks arise close together in the same chromosome, the two ends of the chromosome join when the fragment between the breaks becomes detached. At the next cell division the unattached piece of chromosome is likely to be lost. Large deletions may contribute to dominant lethality. Small deletions are difficult to distinguish from point mutations. Deletions may uncover preexisting recessive genes. If one gene that is essential for survival is uncovered, it can act as a lethal in a homozygote and as a partial dominant in a heterozygote.

***Inversions.*** When two breaks occur in the same chromosome, the portion between them is detached and becomes reinserted in the opposite way to its original position, that is, the gene order is reversed. This need not cause a genetic problem, but imbalanced gametes could result in congenital malformation or fetal death.


### 6.3.3. Chromosome Set Damage

Accuracy of chromosome replication and segregation of chromosomes to daughter cells requires accurate maintenance of the chromosome complement of a eukaryotic cell. Chromosome segregation in meiosis and mitosis is dependent upon the synthesis and functioning of the proteins of the spindle apparatus and upon the attachment and movement of chromosomes on the spindle. The kinetochores attach the chromosomes to the spindle and the centrioles are responsible for the polar orientation of the division apparatus. Sometimes such segregation events proceed incorrectly and homologous chromosomes separate, with deviations from the normal number (aneuploidy) into daughter cells or as a multiple of the complete karyotype (polyploidy). When both copies of a particular chromosome move into a daughter cell and the other cell receives none, the event is known as nondisjunction.

Aneuploidy in live births and abortions arises from aneuploid gametes during germ cell meiosis. Trisomy or monosomy of large chromosomes leads to early embryonic death. Trisomy of the smaller chromosomes allows survival but is detrimental to the health of an affected person, for example, Down's syndrome (trisomy 21), Patau syndrome (trisomy 13) and Edward's syndrome (trisomy 18). Sex chromosome trisomies (Klinefelter's and XXX syndromes) and the sex chromosome monosomy (XO), known as Turner's syndrome, are also compatible with survival.

Aneuploidy in somatic cells is involved in the formation of human tumors. Up to ten percent of tumors are monosomic and trisomic for a specific chromosome as the single observable cytogenetic change. Most common among such tumors are trisomy 8, 9, 12, and 21 and monosomy for chromosomes 7, 22, and Y.

**TABLE 6.4. Fifteen Common Assays Described by OECD**

|  | *In vitro* | *In vivo* |
|---|:---:|:---:|
| ***Assays for Gene Mutations*** |  |  |
| *Salmonella Typhimurium* reverse mutation assay (Ames test, bacteria) [OECD 471] | ✓ |  |
| *Escherichia coli* reverse mutation assay (bacteria) [OECD472] | ✓ |  |
| Gene mutation in mammalian cells in culture [OECD 476] | ✓ |  |
| *Drosophila* sex-linked recessive lethal assay (fruit fly) [OECD 477] |  | ✓ |
| Gene mutation in *Saccaromyces cerevisiae* (yeast) [OECD 480] | ✓ |  |
| Mouse Spot test [OECD 484] |  | ✓ |
| ***Assays for Chromosomal and Genomic Mutations*** |  |  |
| *In vitro* cytogenetic assay [OECD 473] | ✓ |  |
| *In vivo* cytogenetic assay [OICD 475] |  | ✓ |
| Micronucleus test [OECD 474] |  | ✓ |
| Dominant lethal assay [OECD 478] |  | ✓ |
| Heritable translocation assay [OECD 485] |  | ✓ |
| Mammalian germ cell cytogenetic assay [OECD 483] |  | ✓ |
| ***Assays for DNA Effects*** |  |  |
| DNA damage and repair: unscheduled DNA synthesis *in vitro* [OECD 482] | ✓ |  |
| Mitotic recombination in *Saccharomyces cerevisiae* (yeast) [OECD 481] | ✓ |  |
| *In vitro* sister chromatid exchange assay [OECD 479] | ✓ |  |

### 6.3.4. Test Systems

*In vivo* and *in vitro* techniques are available to test mutagenic properties to demonstrate presence or lack of ability of the test material to cause mutation or chromosomal damage or cause cancer, as summarized in Table 6.4. The material intended for intimate contact and long exposure should not have any genotoxic properties. The presence of unpolymerized materials and traces of monomers, oligomers, additives or biodegration products can cause mutations. Mutation can be a point mutation or chromosomal rearrangement caused by DNA damage. Therefore, the material's ability to cause point mutation, chromosomal change, or evidence of DNA damage are tested. As we have seen, correlations exist between mutagenic and carcinogenic properties. Most carcinogens are mutagens, but not all mutagens are human carcinogens.

The Ames salmonella–microsome test is a principal sensitive mutagen screening test. Compounds are tested on the mutants of *Salmonella typhimurium* for reversion from a histidine requirement back to prototrophy. A positive result is seen by the growth of revertant bacteria (which do not require an external histidine source). A microsomal activation system should be included in this assay. The use of five different bacterial test strains are generally required.

Two mammalian mutagenicity tests are generally required to support the lack of mutagenic or carcinogenic potential. Some well known tests are

- The L5178Y mouse lymphoma assay (MLA) for mutants at the TK locus.
- The induction of recessive lethals in *Drosophilia melanogaster.*
- Metaphase analysis of cultured mammalian cells and of treated animals.
- Sister Chromatid Exchange Assay (SCE).
- Unscheduled DNA Synthesis Assay (UDS).
- Cell Transformation Assay.
- SOS Repair System Assay.
- Gene mutation in cultured mammalian cells such as Chinese Hamster V79 cell/HGPRT mutation system.

ICH guidelines specifically require three genotoxicity assays for all devices (see Table 6.2). The assays should preferably evaluate DNA effects, gene mutations and chromosomal aberrations, and two of the assays should preferably use mammalian cells. Guidance for providing tests for selection to meet these needs are the OECD guidelines, which include 8 *in vitro* and 7 *in vivo* assays.

### 6.3.5. *In Vitro* Test Systems

The principal tests can be broadly categorized into microbial and mammalian cell assays. In both cases the tests are carried out in the presence and absence of *in vitro* metabolic activation enzymes, usually derived from rodent liver.

***In Vitro* Metabolic Activation.** The target cells for *in vitro* mutagenicity tests often possess a limited (often overlooked) capacity for endogenous metabolism of xenobiotics. However, to simulate the complexity of metabolic events that occur in the whole animal, there is a critical need to supplement this activity.

***Choice of Species.*** A bewildering variety of exogenous systems have been used for one purpose or another in mutagenicity tests. The choice begins with plant or animal preparations. The attraction of plant systems has stemmed from a desire to avoid the use of animals, where possible, in toxicity testing. In addition, plant systems have particular relevance when certain chemicals are being tested, for example, herbicides.

If animal systems are chosen, preparations derived from fish (see, e.g., Kada, 1981) and birds (Parry et al., 1985) have been used. However, by far the most widely used and validated are those derived from rodents, in particular, the rat. Hamsters may be preferred as a source of metabolizing enzymes when particular chemical classes are being screened, for example, aromatic amines, heterocyclic amines, *N*-nitrosamines and azo dyes (Prival and Mitchell, 1982; Haworth et al., 1983).

***Choice of Tissue.*** The next choice is that of source tissue. Preparations derived from liver are the most useful, as this tissue is a rich source of mixed-function oxygenases capable of converting procarcinogens to genetically active electrophiles. However, many extrahepatic tissues (e.g. kidney, lung, etc.) are also known to possess important metabolic capacity which may be relevant to the production of mutagenic metabolites in the whole animal.

***Cell-Free versus Cell-Based Systems.***  Most use has been made of cell-free systems, in particular, crude homogenates such as 9000 g supernatant (S9 fraction) from rat liver. This fraction is composed of free endoplasmic reticulum, microsomes (membrane-bound packets of "membrane-associated" enzymes), soluble enzymes and some cofactors. Hepatic S9 fractions do not necessarily completely reflect the metabolism of the whole organ, in that they mainly possess phase I metabolism (e.g., oxygenases) and are deficient in phase II systems (e.g., conjugation enzymes). The latter are often capable of efficient detoxification, while the former are regarded as "activating." This can be a strength in that S9 fractions are used in screening tests as a surrogate for all tissues in animals, some of which may be exposed to reactive metabolites in the absence of efficient detoxification. Many carcinogens are organ-specific in extrahepatic tissues, yet liver S9 fraction will reveal their mutagenicity. The deficiency of S9 fractions for detoxification can also be a weakness, in that detoxification may predominate in the whole animal, such that the potential carcinogenicity revealed *in vitro* is not realized *in vivo*.

Cell-free systems, when supplemented with relevant cofactors, are remarkably proficient, despite their crudity in generating reactive electrophiles from most procarcinogens. However, they provide at best a broad approximation of *in vivo* metabolism and can fail to produce sufficient quantity of a particular reactive metabolite to be detectable by the indicator cells or they can produce inappropriate metabolites that do not play a role *in vivo* (see Gatehouse and Tweats, 1987, for discussion).

Some of these problems can be overcome by the use of cell-based systems, in particular, primary hepatocytes. Hepatocytes closely simulate the metabolic systems found in the intact liver and do not require additional cofactors for optimal enzyme activity. However, apart from greater technical difficulties in obtaining hepatocytes as opposed to S9 fraction, hepatocytes can effectively detoxify particular carcinogens and prevent their detection as mutagens. Despite these difficulties, hepatocytes have a role to play in mutagenicity screening, in both bacterial and mammalian-based systems (Tweats and Gatehouse, 1988).

***Inducing Agents.***  The final choice considered here is whether to use "uninduced" liver preparations or those derived from animals pretreated with an enzyme inducer to promote high levels of metabolic activity. If induced preparations are preferred, which inducer should be used?

It appears that uninduced preparations are of limited use in screening assays, because they are deficient in particular important activities such as cytochrome P-$450_{IA1}$ cytochrome oxygenases. In addition, species and organ differences are most divergent with uninduced enzyme preparations (Brusick, 1987).

The above differences disappear when induced microsomal preparations are used. A number of enzyme inducers have been used, the most popular being Aroclor 1254, which is a mixture of polychlorinated bipheynyls (as described by Ames et al., 1975). However, concern about the toxicity, carcinogenicity and persistence of these compounds in the environment has led to the use of alternatives, such as a combination of phenobarbitone (phenobarbital) and $\beta$-naphthoflavone (5, 6-benzoflavone). This combination results in the induction of a range of mono-oxygenases similar to that induced by Aroclor 1254 (see, e.g., Ong et al., 1980). More selective inducers such as phenobarbitone (cytochrome P-450$_{IIA1}$, P-450$_{IIB1}$) or 3-methylcholanthrene (cytochrome P-450$_{IA1}$) have also been used.

In summary, genetic toxicity tests with both bacterial and mammalian cells are normally carried out with rat liver cell-free systems (S9 fraction) from animals pretreated with enzyme inducers. However, investigations should not slavishly follow this regimen: there may be sound scientifically based reasons for using preparations from different species or different organs, or for using whole cells such as hepatocytes.

***Standard Method of S9 Fraction Preparation.*** The following describes the production of hepatic S9 mix from rats induced with a combination of phenobarbitone and $\beta$-naphthoflavone, and is an adaptation of the method described by Gatehouse and Delow (1979).

Male albino rats within the weight range 150–250 g are treated with phenobarbitone sodium 16 mg ml$^{-1}$, 2.5 ml kg$^{-1}$ in sterile saline, and $\beta$-naphthoflavone 20 mg ml$^{-1}$ in corn oil. A fine suspension of the latter is achieved by sonicating for 1 h. These solutions are dosed by intraperitoneal injection on days 1, 2, and 3.

Phenobarbitone sodium is normally administered between 0.5 and 2 h prior to $\beta$-naphthoflavone.

The animals are killed on day 4 by cervical dislocation and the livers removed as quickly as possible and placed on ice-cold KCI buffer (0.01 M Na$_2$ HPO$_4$ + KCl 1.15%). The liver is cleaned, weighed, minced and homogenized (in an Ultra Turrx homogenizer) in the above buffer to give a 25% (w/v) liver homogenate. The homogenate is stored at 4°C until it can be centrifuged at 9000 g for 15 min. The supernatant is decanted, mixed and divided into 2 ml volumes in cryotubes. These are then snap-frozen in liquid nitrogen. Storage at $-196$°C for up to three months results in no appreciable loss of most P-450 isoenzymes (Ashwood-Smith, 1980).

Quality control of S9 batches is usually monitored by the ability to activate compounds known to require metabolism to generate mutagenic metabolites. This is a rather crude approach; more accurate data can be obtained by measuring biochemical paramets, for example, protein, cytochrome P-450 total activity (from crude S9) and related enzyme activities (from purified microsomes) such as 7-ethoxyresorufin-0-deethylase and 7-methoxycoumarin-0-demethylase to give an indication of S9 batch-to-batch variation and to set standards for rejecting suboptimal batches (Hubbard et al., 1985). For further details on critical features affecting the use and limitations of S9 fraction, see Gatehouse and Tweats (1987).

***S9 Mix.*** The S9 fraction prepared as described above is used as a component in "S9 mix" along with buffers and various enzyme cofactors. The amount of S9 fraction in the S9 mix can be varied, but a "standard" level of 0.1 ml ml$^{-1}$ of S9 mix (or ten per cent S9) is often recommended for general screening.

No single concentration of S9 fraction in the S9 mix will detect all classes of genotoxic carcinogen with equal efficiency (Gatehouse et al., 1990). Some mutagens, including many polycyclic aromatic hydrocarbons, are activated to mutagens by higher than normal levels of S9 fraction in the S9 mix (see, e.g., Carver et al., 1985).

The mixed-function oxidases in the S9 fraction require NADPH, normally generated from the action of glucose-6-phosphate dehydrogenase acting on glucose-6-phosphate and reducing NADP, both of which are normally supplied as cofactors. As an alternative, isocitrate can be substituted for glucose-6-phosphate (to be used as a substrate by isocitrate dehydrogenase) (Linblad and Jackim, 1982). Additional cofactors may be added (e.g., flavin mononucleotide), when particular classes of compounds such as azo dyes are being tested (Prival et al., 1984), or acetyl coenzyme A when aromatic animes such as benzidine are being tested (Kennelly et al., 1984).

The composition of a "standard" S9 mix is given in Table 6.5.

### 6.3.6. Bacterial Mutation Tests

The study of mutation in bacteria (and bacterial viruses) has had a fundamental role in the science of genetics in the twentieth century. In particular, the unraveling of biochemical anabolic and catabolic pathways, the identification of DNA as the hereditary material, knowledge of the fine structure of the gene, and the nature of gene regulation, and so on, have all been aided by bacterial mutants.

As an offshoot of studies of genes concerned with the biosynthesis of amino acids, a range of *E. coli* (see, e.g., Yanofsky, 1971) and *Salmonella typhimurium* strains (see, e.g., Ames, 1971) with relatively well-defined mutations in known genes

**TABLE 6.5. Composition of Standard S9 Mix**[a]

| Constituent | Final Conc. in Mix (mM) |
| --- | --- |
| Glucose-6-phosphate | 5 |
| Nicotinamide adenine dinucleotide phosphate | 4 |
| MgCl$_2$6H$_2$O  Salt solution | 8 |
| KCl | 33 |
| Phosphate buffer 90.2 M | 100 |
| Distilled water to make up to the required volume | |
| S9 fraction added at 0.1 ml per ml of S9 mix | |

[a] *Note:* For assays using cultured mammalian cells, phosphate buffer and distilled water are replaced by tissue culture medium, as high concentrations of Na and K salts are toxic to such cells. The concentration of S9 fraction in the S9 mix varies, depending on the relevant assay (see individual sections). Once prepared, S9 mix should be used as soon as possible and should be stored on ice until required. S9 fraction, once thawed, should not be refrozen for future use.

became available. Thus, bacteria already mutant at an easily detectable locus are treated with a range of doses of the test material to determine whether the compound can induce a second mutation that directly reverses or suppresses the original mutations. Thus, for amino acid auxotrophs, the original mutation has resulted in loss of ability to grow in the absence of the required amino acid. The second mutation restores prototrophy; that is, the affected cell is now able to grow in the absence of the relevant amino acid, if provided with inorganic salts and a carbon source. This simple concept, in fact, underlines the great strength of these assays, for it provides enormous selective power, which can identify a small number of the chosen mutants from a population of millions of unmutated cells and cells mutated in other genes. The genetic target, that is, the mutated DNA bases in the gene in question (or bases in the relevant tRNA genes; see the discussion of suppressor mutations) can thus be very small, just one or a few bases in length.

An alternative approach is to use bacteria to detect "forward mutations." Genetic systems which detect forward mutations have an apparent advantage, in that a wide variety of genetic changes may lead to a forward mutation, for example, point mutation, deletions, insertions, and so on. In addition, forward mutations in a number of different genes may lead to the same change in phenotype; thus, the genetic target is much larger than that seen in most reverse mutation assays. However, if a particular mutagen causes rare specific changes, these changes may be lost against the background of more common events (Gatehouse et al., 1990). Spontaneous mutation rates tend to be relatively high in forward mutation systems. Acquisition of resistance to a toxic chemical (e.g., an amino acid analogue or antibiotic) is a frequently used genetic marker in these systems. For instance, the use of resistance to the antibiotic streptomycin preceded the reversion assays in common use today.

***Reversion Tests: Background.*** There are several excellent references describing the background and use of bacteria for reversion tests (Brusick, 1987; Gatehouse et al., 1990). Three different protocols have been widely used: plate incorporation assays, treat and plate tests, and fluctuation tests. These methods are described in detail in the following sections. Fundamental to the operation of these tests is the genetic compositions of the tester strains selected for use.

***Genetic Make up of Tester Strains.*** The most widely used strains are those developed by Bruce Ames and colleagues which are mutant derivatives of the organism *Salmonella typhimurium*. Each strain carries one of a number of mutations in the operon coding for histidine biosynthesis. In each case the mutation can be reverted either by base-change or by frameshift mutations. The genotype of the commonly used strains is shown in Table 6.6.

***The Use of the Plasmid pKM101.*** *Salmonella typhimurium* LT2 strains do not appear to possess classical "error-prone" repair as found in *E. coli* strains and some other members of the Enterobacteria (Walker, 1984; Sedgwick and Goodwin, 1985). This is due to a deficiency in *umu D* activity in these *Salmonella* strains (Herrera et

**TABLE 6.6. Genotype of Commonly Used Strains of *Salmonella typhimurium* LT2 and their Reversion Events**

| Strain | Genotype[a] | Reversion Events |
| --- | --- | --- |
| TA1535 | $hisG_{46}$ rfa *f* gal chlD bio uvrB | Subset of base-pair substitution events |
| TA100 | $hisG_{46}$ *f*rfa gal chlD bio uvrB (pKM101) | Subset of base-pair substitution events |
| TA1537 | $hisC_{3076}$ *f*rfa gal chlD bio uvrB | Frameshifts |
| TA1538 | $hisD_{3052}$ *f*rfa gal chlD bio uvrB | Frameshifts |
| TA98 | $hisD_{3052}$ *f*rfa gal chlD bio uvrB (pKM101) | Frameshifts |
| TA97 | $hisD_{6610}$ $hisO_{1242}$ rfa *f* gal $chl^{D}$ bio uvrB (pKM101) | Frameshifts |
| TA102 | his *f* $(G)_{8476}$ rfa galE (pAQ1) (pKM101) | All possible transitions and transversions; small deletions |

al., 1988; Thomas and Sedgewick, 1989). One way to overcome this deficiency and to increase sensitivity to mutagens is to use strains containing a plasmid carrying analogues to the *umu DC* genes, such as are present in the pKM101 pasmid.

***Ames* Salmonella/*Plate Incorporation Method.*** The following procedure is based on that described by Ames and colleagues (Maron and Ames, 1983), with additional modifications.

1. Each selected test strain is grown for 10 h at 37°C in nutrient broth (Oxoid No. 2) or supplemented minimal media (Vogel-Bonner) on an orbital shaker. A timing device can be used to ensure that cultures are ready at the beginning of the working day.

2. 2.0 ml aliquots of soft agar overlay medium are melted just prior to use and cooled to 50°C, and relevant supplements added: L-histidine, final concentration 9.55 µg ml$^{-1}$, and D-biotin, 12 µg ml$^{-1}$. (Note.: If *E. coli* WP2 tester strains are used, the only supplement required is tryptophan 3.6 µg ml$^{-1}$.) The medium is kept semimolten by holding the tubes containing the medium in a hot aluminum dry block, held at 45°C. It is best to avoid water baths as microbial contamination can cause problems.

3. The following additions are made to each tube of top agar: the test article (or solvent control) in solution (10–200 µl), the test strain (100 µl) and, where necessary, S9 mix (500 µl). The test is carried out in the presence and absence of S9 mix. The exact volume of test article or solvent may depend on toxicity or solubility, as described in the preceding section.

4. There should be at least three replicate plates per treatment with at least five test doses plus untreated controls. Duplicate plates are sufficient for the positive and sterility control treatments. The use of twice as many negative control plates as used

in each treatment group will lead to more powerful tests from a statistical standpoint (Mahon et al., 1989).

5. Each tube of top agar is mixed and quickly poured onto dried prelabeled Vogel-Bonner basal agar plates.

6. The soft agar is allowed to set at room temperature and the plates are inverted and incubated (within 1 h of pouring) at 37°C in the dark. Incubation is continued for 2–3 days.

7. Before scoring the plates for revertant colonies, the presence of a light background lawn of growth (due to limited growth of nonrevertant colonies before the trace of histidine or tryptophan is exhausted) should be confirmed for each concentration of test article by examination of the plate under low power of a light microscope. At concentrations that are toxic to the test strains, such a lawn will be deplated and colonies may appear that are not true revertants but surviving, nonprototrophic cells. If necessary, the phenotype of any questionable colonies (pseudorevertants) should be checked by plating on histidine or tryptophan-free medium.

8. Revertant colonies can be counted by hand or with an automatic colony counter. Such machines are relatively accurate in the range of colonies normally observed (although regular calibration against manual counts is a wise precaution). Where accurate quantitative counts of plates with large numbers of colonies are required, only manual counts will give accurate results.


### 6.3.7. Controls

***Positive Controls.*** Where possible, positive controls should be chosen that are structurally related to the test article. This increases confidence in the results. In the absence of structurally related mutagens, the set of positive controls given in Table 6.7 can be used. The use of such controls validates each test run and helps to confirm the nature of each strain. Pagano and Zeiger (1985) have shown that it is possible to store stock solutions of most routinely used positive controls (sodium azide, 2-aminoanthracene, benzo[*a*]phyene, 4-nitroquinoline oxide) at −20°C to −80°C for several months, without loss of activity. This measure can help reduce potential exposure of laboratory personnel.


***Untreated and Vehicle Controls.*** Untreated controls omit the test article, but are made up to volume with buffer. The vehicle control is made up to volume with the solvent used to dissolve the test substance. It is preferable to ensure that each of the treated plates contain the same volume of vehicle throughout.

As detailed by Gatehouse and Tweats (1987), the nature and concentration of solvent may have a marked effect on the test result. Dimethysolphoxide is often used as the solvent of choice for hydrophibic compounds. However, there may be unforeseen effects, such as an increase in mutagenicity of some compounds, for example, *p*-phenylenediamne (Burnett et al., 1982) or a decrease in mutagenicity of others, such as simple aliphatic nitrosamines (Yahagi et al., 1977). It is essential to

**TABLE 6.7. Positive Controls for Use in Plate Incorporation Assays**

| Species | Strain | Mutagen | Conc. (µg plate$^{-1}$)[a] |
|---|---|---|---|
| *In the absence of S9 mix* | | | |
| *S. typhimurium* | TA1535 | Sodium azide | 1–5 |
| | TA100 | | |
| | TA1538 | Hycanthone methane sulphonate | 5–20 |
| | TA98 | | |
| | TA1537 | ICR 191 | 1 |
| *E. coli* | WP2 uvrA | Nifuroxime | 5–15 |
| *In the presence of S9 mix* | | | |
| *E. coli* | WP2 uvraA (pKM101) | | |
| *S. typhimurium* | TA1538 | 2-Aminoanthracene | 1–10 |
| | TA1535 | | |
| | TA100 | | |
| | TA90 | | |
| | TA1537 | Neutral red | 10–20 |

[a] *Note:* The concentration given above will give relatively small increases in revertant count above the spontaneous level. There is little point in using large concentrations of reference mutagens, which invariably give huge increases in revertant counts. This would give little information on the day-to-day performance of the assay.

use fresh batches of the highest purity grade available and to prevent decomposition/oxidation on during storage. The products after oxidation, and so forth are toxic and can induce base-pair substitutions in both bacterial and mammalian assays. Finally, DMSO and other organic solvents can inhibit the oxidation of different premutagens by microsomal mono-oxygenases (Wolff, 1977a,b). To reduce the risk of artifactual results, it is essential to use the minimum amount of organic solvent (e.g., less than 2 percent w/w) compatible with adequate testing of the test chemical.

It is important to keep a careful check of the number of mutant colonies present on untreated or vehicle control plates. These numbers depend on the following factors.

1. *The repair status of the cell,* that is, excision repair-deficient strains tend to have more "spontaneous mutants" than repair-proficient cells.

2. *The presence of mutator plasmids.* Excision-deficient strains containing pKM101 have a higher spontaneous mutation rate at both base substitution and frameshift loci than excision-proficient strains.

3. *The total number of cell divisions that take place in the supplemented top agar.* This is controlled by the supply of nutrients, in particular, histidine. Rat liver extracts may also supply trace amounts of limiting nutrients, resulting in a slight increase in the spontaneous yield of mutants in the presence of S9 mix.

4. *The size of the initial inoculum.* During growth of the starting culture, mutants will arise. Thus, if a larger starting inoculum is used, more of these "pre-existing" mutants will be present per plate. In fact, the "plate mutants" arising as described in point (3) predominate.

5. *The intrinsic mutability of the mutation in question.* In practice the control mutation values tend to fall within a relatively precise range for each strain. Each laboratory should determine the normal range of revertant colonies per plate for each strain.

Deviations in background reversion counts from the normal range should be investigated. It is possible that cross-contamination, variations in media quality, and so on, have occurred that may invalidate particular experiments.

Frequent checks should also be made on the sterility of S9 preparations, media and test articles. These simple precautions can prevent loss of valuable time and resources.

***Evaluation of Results.*** At least two independent assays are carried out for each test article. The criterion for positive response is a reproducible and statistically significant result at any concentration for any strain. When positive results are obtained, the test is repeated, using the strain(s) and concentration range with which the initial positive results were observed. This range may be quite narrow for toxic agents.

Several statistical approaches have been applied to the results of plate incorporation assays (Wahrendorf et al., 1985 and Mahon et al., 1989). These authors make a number of important suggestions to maximize the power of statistical analyses; those that relate to the method of analysis are reproduced below.

1. Unless it is obvious that the test agent has had no effect, the data should be plotted, to give a visual impression of the form of any dose response and the pattern of variability.

2. Three methods of analysis—linear regression (Gad, 1999; Steel and Torrie, 1960); a multiple comparison analysis, Dunnett's method (Dunnett, 1955); and a nonparametric analysis, such as Kruskal–Wallis (Gad, 1999)—can all be recommended. Each has its strengths and weaknesses, and other methods are not excluded.

3. Linear regression assumes that variance across doses is constant and that the dose response is linear. If the variance is not approximately constant, then a transformation may be applied or a weighted analysis may be carried out. If the dose scale tends to a plateau, then the dose scale may be transformed. If counts decline markedly at high doses, then linear regression is inappropriate.

4. Dunnett's method, perhaps with a transformation, is recommended when counts decline markedly at one or two high doses. However, when the dose response shows no such decline, other methods may be more powerful.

5. Kruskal–Wallis's nonparametric method avoids the complications of transformations of weighting and is about as powerful as any other method. However, it is inappropriate when the response declines markedly at high dose.

***Preincubation Tests.*** Some mutagens are poorly detected in the standard plate incorporation assay, particularly those that are metabolized to short-lived reactive electrophiles, for example, short-chain aliphatic *N*-nitroso compounds (Bartsch et al., 1976). It is also possible that some metabolites may bind to components within the agar. Such compounds can be detected by using a preincubation method first described by Yahagi et al. (1975) in which the bacteria, test compound and S9 mix are incubated together in a small volume at 37°C for a short period (30–60 min) before the soft agar was added and poured as for the standard assay. In this variation of the test, during the preincubation step, the test compound, S9 mix and bacteria are incubated in liquid at higher concentrations than in the standard test, and this may account for the increased sensitivity with relevant mutagens. In the standard method the soluble enzymes in the S9 mix, cofactors and the test agent may diffuse into the bottom agar. This can interfere with the detection of some mutagens, a problem that is overcome in the preincubation method (Forster et al., 1980; Gatehouse and Wedd, 1984).

The test is carried out as follows:

1. The strains are cultured overnight, and the inocula and S9 mix are prepared as in the standard Ames test.

2. The soft agar overlays are prepared and maintained at 45°C prior to use.

3. To each of 3–5 tubes maintained at 37°C in a Driblock are added 0.5 ml of S9 mix, 0.1 ml of the tester strain (10–18 h culture) and a suitable volume of the test compound, to yield the desired range of concentrations. The S9 mix is kept on ice prior to use.

4. The reaction mixtures are incubated for up to 1 h at 37°C.

5. 2.0 ml of soft agar is added to each tube. After mixing, the agar and reaction mixture are poured onto previously labeled, dried Vogel-Bonner plates.

6. Once the agar has set, the plates are incubated for 2–3 days before revertant colonies are scored.

The use of controls is as described for the plate incorporation assay. It is crucial to use the minimum amount of organic solvent in this assay, as the total volume of the incubation mixture is small relative to the solvent component.

This procedure can be modified to provide optimum conditions for particular chemical classes. For instance, preincubation times greater than 60 min plus aeration have been found necessary in the detection of allyl compounds (Neudecker and Henschler, 1985).

***E. coli* Tester Strains.** Ames and colleagues have made an impressive contribution to mutagenicity testing by the development of the *Salmonella* microsome test and, in particular, its application in the study of environmental mutagens. In genetic terms, *Salmonella* strains are, in some ways, not the best choice (see, e.g., Venitt and Croften-Sleigh, 1981). Unlike the *Salmonella* strains, *E. coli* B strains such as the WP2 series developed by Bridges, Green and colleagues (Bridges, 1972; Green and Muriel, 1976) inherently possess the *umuDC*$^+$ genes involved in generating mutations; they are also part-rough and thus allow many large molecules to enter the cell.

In addition to being effective general strains for mutagen detection, studies by Wilcox et al. (1990) have shown that a combination of *E. coli* WP2 *trp E* (pKM101), which has a functioning excision repair system for the detection of cross-linking agents, and *E. coli* WP2 *trp E uvrA* (pKM101) can be used as alternatives to *Salmonella* TA102 for the detection of oxidative mutagens. The *E. coli* strains have the advantage of lower spontaneous mutation rate and are somewhat less difficult to use and maintain. The *Salmonella* strains are, however, more commonly employed.

***Storage and Checking of Tester Strains.*** Detailed instructions for maintenance and confirmation of the phenotypes of the various tester strains are given in Maron and Ames (1983) and Gatehouse et al. (1990). Permanent master cultures of tester strains should be stored in liquid nitrogen or on dry ice. Such cultures are prepared from fresh nutrient broth cultures, to which DMSO is added as a cryopreservative. These cultures are checked for the various characteristics before storage as described below. Cultures for use in individual experiments should be set up by inoculation from the master culture or from a plate made directly from the master culture, not by passage from a previously used culture. Passage in this way will inevitably increase the number of pre-existing mutants, leading to unacceptably high spontaneous mutation rates (Gatehouse et al., 1990).

The following characteristics of the tester strains should be confirmed at monthly intervals or if the internal controls of a particular experiment fail to meet the required limits:

- Amino acid requirement;
- Sensitivity to the lethal effects of the high-molecular-weight dye crystal violet for those strains carrying the *rfaE* mutation;
- Increased sensitivity to UV irradiation for those strains carrying the *uvrA* or *uvrB* mutations;
- Resistance to ampicillin for strains carrying pKM101 and resistance to tetracycline for strains carrying pAQ1;
- Sensitivity to diagnostic mutagens. This can be measured very satisfactorily be testing pairs of strains, one giving a strongly positive response, the partner a weak response.

The importance of these checks together with careful experiment-to-experiment controls of spontaneous mutation rates, response to reference mutation rates and response to reference mutagens cannot be overstressed; failure to apply them can result in much wasted effort.

### 6.3.8. Plate Incorporation Assay

***Protocol for Dose Ranging and Selection.*** Before carrying out the main tests, it is necessary to carry out a preliminary toxicity dose ranging test. This should be carried out following the same basic protocol as the mutation test, except that instead of scoring the number of mutants on, for example minimal media plates with limiting amounts of a required amino acid, the number of survivors is scored on fully supplemented minimal media. A typical protocol is outlined below.

1. Prepare a stock solution of the test compound at a concentration of 50 mg ml$^{-1}$ in an appropriate solvent. It may be necessary to prepare a lower concentration of stock solution, depending on the solubility of the test compound.

2. Make dilutions of the stock solution.

3. To 2.0 ml aliquots of soft agar overlay medium (0.6% and 0.5% sodium chloride in distilled water) containing a trace of histidine and excess biotin and maintained at 45°C in a dry block, add 100 µl at a solution of the test article. Use only one plate per dilution.

4. Mix and pour onto dried Vogel and Bonner minimal medium plates as in an Ames test, including an untreated control and a solvent control, if necessary. The final concentrations of test compound will be 5000, 1500, 500, 150 and 50 µg plate$^{-1}$.

5. Repeat step (3), using 0.5 ml of 8 percent S9 mix per 2.0 ml aliquot of soft agar in addition to the test compound and tester strain. The S9 mix is kept on ice during the experiment.

6. Incubate the plates for 2 days at 37°C and examine the background lawn of growth with a microscope ($\times 8$ eyepiece lens, $\times 10$ objective lens). The lowest concentration giving a depleted background lawn is regarded as a toxic dose.

This test will also demonstrate excess growth, which may indicate the presence of histidine or tryptophan or their precursors in the test material, which could make testing for mutagenicity impracticable by this method.

When setting the maximum test concentration, it is important to test into the mg plate$^{-1}$ range where possible (Gatehouse et al., 1990), as some mutagens are only detectable when tested at high concentrations. However, for nontoxic, soluble mutagens an upper limit of 5 mg plate$^{-1}$ is recommended (DeSerres and Shelby, 1979). For less soluble compounds at least one dose exhibiting precipitation should be included.

***Forward Mutation Tests.*** Forward mutation is an endpoint that may arise from various events, including base substitutions, frameshifts, DNA deletions, and so on, as mentioned earlier.

### 6.3.9. Eukaryotic Mutation Tests

Prokaryotic systems, as described, have proved to be quick, versatile, and in many cases surprisingly accurate in identifying potential genetic hazards to humans. However, there are intrinsic differences between eukaryotic and prokaryotic cells in the organization of the genome and the processing of the genetic information. Thus, there is a place for test systems based on mammalian cells for fundamental studies to understand the mutation process in higher cells and for the use of such tests for screening for genotoxic effects.

The early work of Muller showed the usefulness of the fruit fly *Drosophila melanogaster* as a higher system for measuring germ line mutations in a whole animal. The *Drosophila* sex-linked recessive lethal test has yielded much useful information and in the 1970s was a popular system for screening chemicals for mutation, but this test failed to perform well in international collaborative trials to study the utility of such tests to detect carcinogens and its popularity waned. Another *Drosophila* test devised in the 1980s, the SMART assay (Somatic Mutation and Recombination Test) shows much promise and has revived the popularity of *Drosophila* for screening for genotoxic agent.

There are a number of test systems that use cultured mammalian cells, from both established and primary lines, that now have a large database of tested chemicals in the literature, are relatively rapid, and are feasible to use for genetic toxicity screening. These are discussed in the next section.

### 6.3.10. In Vitro Tests for the Detection of Mammalian Mutation

There have been a variety of *in vitro* mutation systems described in the literature, but only a small number have been defined adequately for quantitative studies (Kakunaga, Yamasaki, 1984; Cole et al., 1990). These are based on the detection of forward mutations in a similar manner to the systems described earlier for bacteria. A defined large number of cells are treated with the test agent and then, after a set interval, exposed to a selective toxic agent, so that only cells that have mutated can survive. As cultured mammalian cells are diploid (or near-diploid), normally, there are two copies of each gene. Recessive mutations can be missed if a normal copy is present on the homologous chromosome. As mutation frequencies for individual genes are normally very low, an impossibly large population of cells would need to be screened to detect cells in which both copies are inactivated by mutation. This problem is overcome by measuring mutation in genes on the X chromosome in male cells where only one copy of the gene will be present, or using heterozygous genes where two copies of a gene may be present but one copy is already inactive through mutation or deletion.

Many genes are essential for the survival of the cell in culture, and thus mutations in such genes would be difficult to detect. However, use has been made of genes that are not essential for cell survival but allow the cell to salvage nucleotides from the surrounding medium. This saves the cell energy, as it does not have to make these compounds from simpler precursors by energy-expensive catabolism. These enzymes are located at the cell membrane. If the cell is supplied with toxic nucleotides, the "normal" unmutated cells will transport these into the cell and kill the cell. However, if the cells have lost the enzyme as a result of mutation (or chromosomal deletion, rearrangement, etc.), they will not be able to "salvage" the exogenous toxic nucleotides and will survive. The surviving mutant cells can be detected by the formation of colonies on tissue culture plates or, in some cases, in the wells of microtitre plates.

One factor to take into account with these tests is that of expression time. Although a gene may be inactivated by mutation, the mRNA existing before the mutational event may decay only slowly, so that active enzyme may be present for some time after exposure to the mutagen. Thus, the cells have to be left for a period before being challenged with the toxic nucleotide; this is the expression time, and differs between systems.

***Chinese Hamster Lines.***  Chinese hamster cell lines have given much valuable data over the past 15 years but their use for screening is limited by lack of sensitivity, because only a relatively small target cell population can be used, owing to metabolic co-operation (see Cole et al., 1990); however, they are still in use, so a brief description follows.

Chinese hamster CHO and V79 lines have high plating efficiencies and short generation times (less than 24 h). These properties make the lines useful for mutagenicity experiments. Both cell lines have grossly rearranged chromosomal complements, which has an unknown effect on their responsiveness to mutagens (Tweats and Gatehouse, 1988). There is some evidence that Chinese hamster lines are undergoing genetic drift in different culture collections (Kirkland, 1992).

***V79 System.***  The Chinese hamster V79 line was established in 1958 (Ford and Yerganian, 1958). Publication of the use of the line for mutation studies (by measuring resistance to purine analogues due to mutation of the *Hgprt* locus) occurred 10 years later (Chu and Malling, 1968). The V79 line was derived from a male Chinese hamster; hence, V79 cells possess only a single X chromosome.

V79 cells grow as a cell sheet or monolayer on glass or plastic surfaces. If large numbers of cells are treated with a mutagen, when plated out, cells in close contact can link via intracellular bridges. These allow the transfer of cellular components between cells such as messenger RNA. Thus, if a cell carries a mutation in the *Hgprt* gene resulting in the inactivation of the relevant mRNA, it can receive viable mRNA or intact enzyme from adjacent nonmutated cells. Therefore, when the mutated cell is challenged with a toxic purine, it is lost, owing to the presence of active enzyme derived from the imported mRNA. This phenomenon is termed "metabolic co-operation" and severely limits the sensitivity of lines such as V79 for mutagen detection. This drawback can be overcome to an extent by carrying out the detection of mutant clones in semisolid agar (see, e.g., Oberly et al., 1987) or by using the "respreading technique" (Fox, 1981).

The preferred expression time for *Hgprt* mutants is 6–8 days, although care needs to be taken when testing chemicals well into the toxic range, where the "expression time" needs to be extended to allow recovery.

***Preliminary Cytotoxicity Testing.***  An essential first step is to carry out a preliminary study to evaluate the toxicity of the test material to the indicator cells, under the conditions of the main mutagenicity test. When selecting dose levels, the solubility of the test compound, the resulting pH of the media, and the osmolality of the test solutions all need to be considered. The latter two parameters have been known to induce false positive effects in *in vitro* mammalian tests (Brusick, 1986). The experimental procedure is carried out as follows.

1. Seek T75 plastic tissue culture flasks with a minimum of $2.5 \times 10^6$ cells in 120 ml of Eagle's medium containing 20 mM L-glutamine: $0.88\,g\,l^{-1}$ sodium bicarbonate; 20 mM HEPES; $50\,\mu g\,ml^{-1}$ streptomycin sulphate; $50\,IU\,ml^{-1}$ benzylpenicillin; and 7.5% fetal bovine serum. The flasks are incubated for 18–24 h at $37°C$ in a $CO_2$ incubator to establish monolayer cultures.

2. Prepare treatment medium containing various concentrations of test compound: 19.7 ml of Eagle's medium (without serum) plus $300\,\mu l$ of stock concentration of compound in a preferred solvent (e.g., water, ethanol, DMSO, etc.). The final concentration of solvent other than water should not exceed 1% v/v. Normally a range of $0$–$5000\,\mu g\,ml^{-1}$ (final concentration) is covered. For a sparingly soluble compound, the highest concentration will be the lowest at which visible precipitation occurs. Similarly, if a compound has a marked effect on osmolality, concentrations should not be used that exceed 500 milliosmoles (mosm) per kg. In addition, a pH range of 6.5–7.5 should be maintained.

3. Each cell monolayer is rinsed with a minimum of 20 ml phosphate buffered saline (PBS) and then 20 ml of treatment medium is carefully added. The flasks are incubated for 3 h at $37°C$ in a $CO_2$ incubator.

4. After treatment, carefully discard the medium from each flask and wash each monolayer twice with PBS. Care needs to be taken to dispose of contaminated solutions safely.

5. Add 10 ml of trypsin solution (0.025% trypsin in PBS) to each flask. Once the cells have rounded up, the trypsin is neutralized by the addition of 10 ml of complete medium. A cell suspension is obtained by vigorous pipetting to break up cell clumps.

6. The trypsinized cell suspension is counted and diluted in complete media before assessing for survival. For each treatment set up five Petri dishes containing 200 cells per dish.

7. Incubate at $37°C$ in a $CO_2$ incubator for 7–10 days.

8. The medium is removed and the colonies are fixed and stained, using 5% Giemsa in buffered formalin. Once the colonies are stained, the Giemsa is removed and the colonies are counted.

The method can be repeated including 20% v/v S9 mix.

To calculate percentage survival, the following formula is used:

$$\frac{\text{cell titre in treated culture}}{\text{cell titre in control culture}} \times \frac{\text{mean number of colonies on treated plates}}{\text{mean number of colonies on control plates}} \times 100$$

The cloning efficiency (CE) of the control culture is calculated as follows:

$$\text{CE} = \frac{\text{mean number of colonies per plate}}{\text{number of cells per plate (i.e., 200)}} \times 100$$

In the absence of precipitation or effects on pH or osmolality, the maximum concentration of the main mutagenicity study is a concentration that reduces survival to approximately 20% of the control value.

***Procedure for the Chinese Hamster V79/Hgprt Assay.*** The assay usually comprises three test concentrations, each in duplicate, and four vehicle control replicates. Suitable positive controls are ethylmethane sulphonate ($-$S9) and dimethyl benzanthracene ($+$S9). V79 cells with a low nominal passage number should be used from frozen stocks to help minimize genetic drift. The procedure described includes a reseeding step for mutation expression.

Steps 1–5 are the same as the cytotoxicity assay. As before, tests can be carried out in the presence and in the absence of S9 mix.

6. The trypsinized cultures are counted and a sample is assessed for survival as for the cytotoxicity assay. In addition, an appropriate number of cells are reseeded for estimation of mutation frequency at the day 8 expression time. The cells are transferred to roller bottles (usually $490\,\text{cm}^2$) for this stage. The bottles are gassed with pure $CO_2$, the tops are tightened and the bottles are incubated at $37°C$ on a roller machine (approximate speed 0.5–1.0 rev $\text{min}^{-1}$). Usually $10^6$ viable cells are reseeded in 50 ml of Eagle's medium containing serum, but more cells are required at the toxic dose levels.

7. The bottles are subcultured as necessary throughout the expression period to maintain subconfluency. This involves retrypsinization and determining the cell titre for each treatment. For each culture a fresh roller bottle is reseeded with a minimum of $10^6$ cells.

8. On day 8, each culture is again trypsinized, counted and diluted so that a sample cell population can be assessed for cloning efficiency and a second sample can be assessed for the induction of 6TG-resistant cells.

9. The cell suspension is diluted in complete medium and $2 \times 10^5$ cells added per petri dish (10 petri dishes per treatment). 6-Thioguanine is added to the medium at a final concentration of $10\,\mu\text{g}\,\text{ml}^{-1}$.

10. The petri dishes are incubated for 7–10 days and the medium is then removed. The colonies are fixed and stained as previously. The colonies (more than 50 cells per clone) are then counted.

Mutation frequency in each culture is calculated as

$$\frac{\text{mean number colonies on thioguanine plates}}{1000 \times \text{mean number colonies on survival plates}}$$

***Data Analysis. (Arlett et al., 1989).***  A weighted analysis of variance is performed on the mutation frequencies, as the variation in the number of mutations per plate usually increases as the mean increases. Each dose of test compound is compared with the corresponding vehicle control by means of a one-sided Dunnett's test and, in addition, the mutation frequencies are examined to see whether there is a linear relationship with dose.

The criterion employed for a positive response in this assay is a reproducible statistically significant increase in mutation frequency (weighted mean for duplicate treated cultures) over the concurrent vehicle control value (weighted mean for four independent control cultures). Ideally, the response should show evidence of a dose-response relationship. When a small isolated significant increase in mutation frequency is observed in only one of the two duplicate experiments, then a third test should be carried out. If the third test shows no significant effects, the initial increase is likely to be a chance result. In cases where an apparent treatment-related increase is thought to be a result of unusually low variability or a low control frequency, comparison with the laboratory historical control frequency may be justified.

***Chinese Hamster CHO/Hgprt System.***  Chinese hamster ovary (CHO) cells have 21 or 22 chromosomes with one intact X chromosome and a large acrocentric marker chromosome (Natarajan and Obe, 1982). The use of these cells in mammalian mutation experiments was first reported by Hsie et al. (1975), and was refined into a quantitative assay for mutagenicity testing by O'Neill. The performance of this system has been reviewed by the USA EPA Gene-Tox Program. The experimental procedure for this assay is similar to the V79/Hgprt system already described, and for more detailed descriptions the reader is referred to Li et al. (1987).

***Mouse Lymphoma L5178Y TK$^{+/-}$ Assay.***  Whereas the Chinese hamster cell systems are regarded as relatively insensitive, the mouse lymphoma L5178Y TK$^{+/-}$ test is undoubtedly more sensitive. Unfortunately, there are persistent doubts regarding its specificity, the ability to distinguish between carcinogens and noncarcinogens (see, e.g., Tennant et al., 1987). However, a great advantage is the ability of these cells to grow in suspension culture in which intracellular bridges do not occur. Thus, the problems of metabolic co-operation are avoided, which allows a large number of cells to be treated for optimum statistical analysis of results.

A candid historical overview of the development of the mouse lymphoma $TK^{+/-}$ mutagenicity assay is given by its originator, Clive (1987). Initially methodologies were developed for producing the three TK genotypes ($TK^{+/+}$ and $TK^{-/-}$ homozygotes and the $TK^{+/-}$ heterozygotes (Clive et al., 1972). This first heterozygote was lost; however, it was recognized that subsequent heterozygotes produced distinctly bimodal distributions of mutant-colony sizes, owing to differences in growth rate. These were interpreted in terms of single-gene (large-colony mutants) and viable chromosomal mutations (small-colony mutants). A period of diversification of the mouse lymphoma assay was followed by controversy over the significance of small-colony mutants (Amacher et al., 1980).

Following this, a series of cytogenetic studies confirmed the cytogenetic interpretation for small-colony mutants (see, e.g., Hozier et al., 1982). Molecular studies showed that most mutations resulting in small-colony mutants involve large-scale deletions (Evans et al., 1986). A current theory states that, for many cómpounds, deletion mutants are induced by binding of the compound to complexes between topoisomerase II and DNA (Clive, 1989). Topoisomerases are enzymes that control supercoiling via breakage and reunion of DNA strands; it is the latter strep that is disrupted, which leads to chromosome damage and deletions. Further molecular studies (Applegate et al., 1990) have shown that a wide variety of genetic events can result in the formation of $TK^{+/-}$ genotype from the heterozygote, including recombinations and mitotic nondisjunction.

The $TK^{+/-}$ line was originally isolated as a spontaneously arising revertant clone from a UV-induced $TK^{-/-}$ clone. The parental $TK^{+/+}$ cell and the heterozygote were then the only TK-competent mouse lymphoma cells that could be maintained in THMG medium ($3\,\mu g\ ml^{-1}$ thymidine, $5\,\mu g\ ml^{-1}$ hypoxanthine, $0.1\,\mu g\ ml^{-1}$ methotrexate and $7.5\,\mu g\ ml^{-1}$ glycine) (Clive, 1987). Thus, like most established lines, these cells are remote from wild-type cells. The karyotype of the $TK^{+/-}$ $-3.7.2C$ line has a modal chromosome number of 40 like wild-type, but has a variety of chromosomal rearrangements and centromeric heteromorphisms (Blazak et al., 1986).

Two main protocols have been devised for carrying out mutation assays with mouse lymphoma L5178Y cells, plating the cells in soft agar or a fluctuation test approach. The latter is described in the following section, based on Cole et al. (1986). The reader is referred to Clive et al. (1987) for a full description of the soft-agar method.

*Preliminary Cytotoxicity Assay.* The cells are maintained in RPMI 1640 medium containing 2.0 mM glutamine, 20 mM HEPES, $200\,\mu g\ ml^{-1}$ sodium pyruvate, 50 IU $ml^{-1}$ benzylpenicillin, $50\,\mu g\ ml^{-1}$ streptomycin sulphate and 10% donor horse serum (heat-inactivated for 30 min at 56°C). This medium is designated CM10. Conditioned medium is CM10 in which cells have grown exponentially for at least one day. Treatment medium contains 3% horse serum and 30% conditioned media (CM3). Medium without serum is known as incomplete medium (ICM). If treatment time exceeds 3 h, treatment is carried out in CM10.

The method is as follows.

1. The cell titer of an exponentially growing culture of cells in CM10 is determined with a Coulter counter. The cell suspension is centrifuged at 70 g for 5 min and the supernatant is reduced such that 3 ml contains approximately $5 \times 10^6$ cells (3-h treatment) or $2 \times 10^6$ (treatment more than 3 h).

2a. For tests in the absence of S9 mix, treatment groups are prepared by mixing 3 ml of solution of test compound and 6.9 ml of ICM (3-h treatment) or 6.9 ml of CM10 (treatment more than 3 h).

2b. Tests in the presence of S9 mix are carried out in the same way, except the treatment medium contains 10% v/v S9 mix at the expense of ICM: 3 ml cell suspension, 5.9 ml ICM, 1 ml S9 mix, and 0.1 ml test compound solution/vehicle. The composition of the S9 mix is as described earlier. It is prepared immediately before required and kept on ice until it is added to the test system. For the vehicle controls, if an organic solvent is used, it should not exceed 1% v/v.

3. After the treatment period, cells are spun down at 70 g for 5 min and the supernatant is transferred for assessment of pH and osmolality. The cell pellet is washed twice in PBS and then resuspended in 10 ml CM10. (All contaminated material and waste should be disposed of safely.)

4. The cell titer of each culture is counted and a sample diluted in CM10 for assessment of posttreatment survival. For this, two 96-well microtiter plates are charged with 200 μl of a diluted cell suspension, using a multichannel pipette such that each well contains on average one cell.

5. Plates are incubated for 7–8 days at 37°C and 5% $CO_2$ in $95 \pm 3\%$ relative humidity.

6. The plates are removed from the incubator and 20 μl of MTT [3-(4,5-dimethylthiazol-2-yl)-2,5-diphenyltetrazolium bromide] at 5 mg ml$^{-1}$ (in PBS) is added to each well with a multichannel pipette. The plates are left to stand for 1–4 h and are then scored for the presence of colonies with a Titertek mirror-box, which allows direct viewing of the bottom surface of the plates.

7. Cytotoxicity can also be determined post-treatment as follows: T25 flasks are set up after treatment containing $0.75 \times 10^5$ cells per ml in 5 ml CM10. Flasks are incubated with loose lids at 37°C with 5 percent $CO_2$ in $95 \pm 3$ percent relative humidity. Two days later the cell titre of each culture is determined with a Coulter counter.

8. Following this procedure, various calculations are carried out to aid selection of dose levels for the main mutation assay.

    (a) *Cloning efficiency.* In microtiter assays, calculations are based on the Poisson distribution:

$$P_{(o)} = \frac{\text{number of wells without a colony}}{\text{total number of cells}}$$

(b) *Relative survival.* Relative survival ($S$) is calculated as follows:

$$S = \frac{\text{CE of treated group}}{\text{CE of control group}}$$

(c) *Growth.* Growth in suspension ($SG$) is calculated as follows:

$$SG = \frac{\text{cell count after 3 days}}{0.75 \times 10^5}$$

Relative suspension growth ($RSG$) is calculated as follows:

$$RSG = \frac{SG \text{ of treated group}}{SG \text{ of control group}} \times 100 \text{ percent}$$

***Selection of Dose Levels.*** The highest test concentration is selected from one of the following options, whichever is lowest:

- A concentration which reduces survival to about 10–20% of the control value.
- A concentration which reduces RSG to 10–20% of the control value.
- The lowest concentration at which visible precipitation occurs.
- The highest concentration which does not increase the osmolality of the medium to greater than $400 \text{ mmol kg}^{-1}$ or 100 mmol above the value for the solvent control.
- The highest concentration that does not alter the pH of the treatment medium beyond the range 6.8–7.5.
- If none of these conditions are met, $5 \text{ mg ml}^{-1}$ should be used.

Lower test concentrations are selected as fractions of the highest concentration, usually including one dose that causes 20–70% survival and one dose that causes more than 70% survival.

***Main Mutation Assay.*** The assay normally comprises three test concentrations, a positive control and vehicle control. All treatment groups are set up in duplicate. The expression time is two days, unless there are indications that the test agent inhibits cell proliferation, where an additional or possibly alternative expression time should be employed.

Stock cultures are established from frozen ampoules of cells that have been treated with thymidine, hypoxanthine, methotrexate and glycine for 24 h, which purges the culture of pre-existing $TK^{-/-}$ mutants. This cell stock is used for a maximum of two months.

Treatment is normally carried out in 50 ml centrifuge tubes on a roller machine. During the expression time the cells are grown in T75 plastic tissue culture flasks.

For estimation of cloning efficiency and mutant induction, cells are plated out in 96-well microtiter plates. Flasks and microtitre plates are incubated at 37°C in a $CO_2$ incubator as in the cytotoxicity assays.

Cell titres are determined by diluting of the cell suspension in Isoton and counting an appropriate volume (usually 0.5 ml) with a Coulter counter. Two counts are made per suspension.

The experimental procedure is carried out as follows:

1. On the day of treatment stock solutions for the positive control and the various concentrations of test compound (selected as per the previous selection) are prepared.

2. Treatment is carried out in 30% conditioned media. The serum concentration is 3% (3-h treatment) or 10% (treated more than 3 h).

3. Cell suspensions of exponentially growing cells are prepared as in the cytotoxicity assay, except that 6 ml of media required for each treatment culture contains $10^7$ cells (3-h treatment) or $3 \times 10^6$ cells (more than 3 h treatment). The number of cells per treatment may be increased if marked cytotoxicity is expected, to allow enough cells to survive (e.g., if 20% survival or less is expected, $2 \times 10^7$ cells may be treated).

4. For tests in the absence of S9 mix, 6 ml of cell suspension, 0.2 ml test compound/vehicle and 13.8 ml ICM (3-h treatment) or 13.8 ml CM10 (treatment more than 7 h) are mixed in the presence of S9 mix and 0.2 ml of test compound or vehicle are prepared.

5. After treatment the cells are centrifuged at 70 g for 5 min, and supernatant is discarded and the cell pellet is resuspended in PBS (pH 7). This washing procedure is repeated twice, and finally the cell pellet is resuspended in CM10.

6. Each culture is counted so that a sample of cells can be assessed for posttreatment survival, and the remaining cell population assessed for estimation of mutation frequency.

7. For survival estimation, cells are placed into 96-well microtitre trays at a cell density of 1 cell per well as per the cytotoxicity assay.

8. For mutation estimation, the cells are diluted to a cell density of $2 \times 10^5$ cells per ml with CM10 in tissue culture flasks and the culture is incubated at 37°C in a $CO_2$ incubator. On day 1 each culture is counted and diluted with fresh medium to a cell density of $2 \times 10^5$ cells per ml in a maximum of 100 ml of medium.

9. On day 2 each culture is counted again and an aliquot of cells taken so that. (i) a sample of the cell population can be assessed for cloning efficiency. Plates are incubated at 37°C in a $CO_2$ incubator for 7 days (ii) a sample of the cell population can be assessed for the induction of TFT-resistant cells (mutants). For this $2 \times 10^3$ cells are plated per well in 200 µl CM10 containing 4 µg ml$^{-1}$ TFT. TFT and TFT-containing cultures must not be exposed to bright light, as the material is light-sensitive. The plates are incubated for 10–12 days at 37°C in a $CO_2$ incubator.

10. At the end of incubation 20 µl MTT is added to each well. The plates are left to develop for 1–4 h at 37°C and then scored for colony-bearing wells. Colonies are scored by eye and are classified as small or large.

The calculation for cloning efficiency is made as for the cytotoxicity assay.

Relative total growth ($RTG$) is a cytotoxicity parameter which considers growth in suspension during the expression time and the cloning efficiency of the end of the expression time as follows:

$$\text{Suspension growth } (SG) = \frac{24\,\text{h cell count}}{2 \times 10^4} \times \frac{48\,\text{h cell count}}{2 \times 10^5}$$

$$RTG = \frac{SG \text{ treated culture}}{SG \text{ control culture}} \times \frac{CE \text{ of treated culture}}{CE \text{ of control culture}}$$

Mutation frequency ($MF$) is calculated as follows:

$$MF = \frac{\text{InP}_o \text{ for mutation plates}}{\text{Number of cells per well} \times CE/100}$$

***Data Analysis.*** Data from the fluctuation test described above are analyzed by an appropriate statistical method as described in Robinson et al. (1989). Data from plate assays are analyzed as described in Arlett et al. (1989) for treat and plate tests.

***Status of Mammalian Mutation Tests.*** At present the only practical assays for screening new chemical entities for mammalian mutation are the mammalian cell assays described above. The protocols are well defined, and mutant selection and counting procedures are simple and easily quantified. In general, the genetic endpoints are understood and relevant to deleterious genetic events in humans. For these reasons the assays are still regarded as valuable in safety evaluation (Li et al., 1991). It is, however, recognized that there are still unknown factors and molecular events that influence test results. This can be illustrated by the conclusions of the third UKEMS collaborative trial, which focused on tests with cultured mammalian cells. The following points were made:

- The number of cells to be cultured during expression imposes a severe limitation in the use of surface attached cells.
- The importance of a careful determination of toxicity.
- That S9 levels may need to be varied.
- That the aromatic amine benzidine is mutagenic only at the TK locus in L5178Y TK$^{+/-}$ cells. The most disturbing finding was that benzidine (detectable without metabolism by S9 mix) did not produce detectable DNA adducts (as shown by [32]P-post-labeling) in L5178Y cells. Thus, the mechanism

for mutagenesis in L5178Y cells benzidine remains to be elucidated (Arlett and Cole, 1990).

### 6.3.11. *In Vivo* **Mammalian Mutation Tests**

Mammalian mutation studies of chemicals in the whole animal have provided fundamental information on mutation parameters in germ cells such as dose response, dose fractionation, sensitivity of various stages in gametogenesis, and so on, just as is known for ionizing radiation (Russell, 1984, 1989). This has led to estimations of the possible impact chemical mutagens may have on heritable malformation, inborn errors of metabolism, and so on. Today germ cell studies are still required when estimating the heritable damage a mutagen may inflict on exposed human populations.

The existing tests tend to be cumbersome and are not used for routine genetic toxicology screening, and thus only brief descriptions will follow. Reviews of existing data, particularly by Holden (Holden, 1982; Adler and Ashby, 1989), have indicated that most if not all germ cell mutagens also induce DNA damage in somatic cells, as detected by well-established assays such as the rodent micronucleus test. The converse is not true; some mutagens and clastogens can induce somatic cell damage but do not induce germ cell changes, which probably reflects the special protection afforded to the germ cells, such as that provided by the blood-testes barrier. In other words, it appears that germ cell mutagens are a subset of somatic cell mutagens.

*In vivo* mammalian mutation tests are not restricted to germ cell tests. The mouse spot test described below is, again, a test used first for studying radiation-induced mutation but has also been used for screening chemicals for *in vivo* mutagenic potential. This test has had several proponents but compared with *in vivo* chromosomal assays is not widely used.

***The Mouse Specific Locus Test.*** The mouse somatic spot test is a type of specific locus test. The classical specific locus test was developed independently by Russell at Oak Ridge in the late 1940s (Russell, 1951, 1989) and Carter in Edinburgh (Carter et al., 1956). The test consists of treatment of parental mice homozygous for a wild-type set of marker loci. The targets for mutation are the germ cells in the gonads of the treated mice. These are mated with a tester stock that is homozygous recessive at the marker loci. The $F_1$ offspring that result are normally heterozygous at the marker loci and thus express the wild-type phenotype. In the event of a mutation from the wild-type allele at any of these loci, the $F_1$ offspring express the recessive phenotype.

The test marker strain (T) developed by Russell uses seven recessive loci: *a* (nonagouti), *b* (brown), $c^{ch}$ (chinchilla), *d* (dilute), *p* (pink-eyed dilution), *s* (piebald) and *se* (short-ear). As for the mouse spot test, these genes control coat pigmentation, intensity or pattern, and, for the *se* gene, the size of the external ear.

Because the occurrence of mutation is rare even after mutagen treatment, the specific locus test is the ultimate study of mutation, requiring many thousands of offspring to be scored, plus significant resources of time, space, and animal husbandry. Because of these constraints it is often difficult to define a negative result, as insufficient animals are scored or all stages of spermatogenesis are not covered. Of the 25 compounds tested in the assay, as reviewed by Ehling et al. (1986), 17 were regarded as "inconclusive" and 8 positive. The scale studies can reach is illustrated by the test of ethylene oxide described by Russell (1984), where exposures of 101,000 and 150,000 ppm were used for 16–23 weeks. A total of 71,387 offspring were examined. The spermatogonial stem-cell mutation rate in the treated animals did not differ significantly from the historical control frequency!

With regard to the design of the test, mice are mated when 7–8 weeks old. By this age all germ cell stages are present. The test compound is normally administered by the IP route to maximize the likelihood of germ cell exposure. The preferred dose is just below the toxic level so long as fertility is not compromised. One lower dose should also be included.

In males spermatogonia are most at risk but it is desirable that later stages also be exposed. Thus, the mice are mated immediately after treatment to 2–4 females. This is continued each week for 7 weeks. Then the first group has completed its rearing of the first set of offspring and is remated. This cycle can be continued for the lifetime of the males. Tests can also be carried out by dosing females, when treatment is carried out for 3 weeks to cover all stages of ogenesis (Brook and Chandley, 1985).

The offspring are examined immediately after birth for identification of malformations (dominant visibles) and then at weaning for the specific locus mutations. Presumptive mutant mice are checked by further crosses to confirm their status (Searle, 1984).

Comparison of mutation frequencies is made with the historical database. For definition of a positive result the same principles are recommended as for the mouse spot test (Selby and Olson, 1981). A minimum size of 18,000 offspring per group is recommended by those authors for definition of a negative result.


## 6.4. *IN VITRO* CYTOGENETIC ASSAYS

The *in vitro* cytogenetic assay is a short-term mutagenicity test for detecting chromosomal damage in cultured mammalian cells.

Cultured cells have a limited ability metabolically to activate some potential clastogens. This can be overcome by adding an exogenous metabolic activation system such as S9 mix to the cells (Ames et al., 1975; Natarajan et al., 1976; Maron and Ames, 1983; Madle and Obe, 1980).

Observations are made in metaphase cells arrested with a spindle inhibitor such as colchicine or colcemid to accumulate cells in a metaphase-like stage of mitosis (c-metaphase) before hypotonic treatment to enlarge cells and fixation with alcohol–acetic acid solution. Cells are then dispersed on to microscope slides and stained and slides are randomized, coded and analyzed for chromosome aberrations with high-power light microscopy. Details of the procedure are given in Dean and Danford (1984) and Preston et al. (1981, 1987). The UKEMS guidelines (Scott et al., 1990) recommend that all tests be repeated regardless of the outcome of the first test and that, if a negative or equivocal result is obtained in the first test, the repeat should include an additional sampling time. In the earlier version of the guidelines (Scott et al., 1983) a single sampling at approximately 1.5 normal cycle times ($-24$ h for a 1.5 cell cycle) from the beginning of treatment was recommended, provided that a range of concentrations was used which induced marginal to substantial reductions in mitotic index, usually an indicator of mitotic delay. However, Ishidate (1988a) reported a number of chemicals which gave negative responses with a fixation time of 24 h but which were positive at 48 h. This was when a Chinese hamster fibroblast line (CHO) with a doubling time of 15 h was used. It would appear, therefore, that there are chemicals which can induce extensive mitotic delay at clastogenic doses and may be clastogenic only when cells have passed through more than one cell cycle since treatment (Thust et al., 1980). A repeat test should include an additional sample at approximately 24 h later but it may only be necessary to score cells from the highest dose at this later fixation time. When the first test gives a clearly positive result, the repeat test need only utilize the same fixation time. The use of other sampling times is in agreement with other guidelines: (European Community EEC Directive (OECD, 1983); American Society for Testing and Materials (Preston et al., 1987); Japanese Guidelines (JMHW, 1984); Joint Directives, 1987; Ishidate, 1988b).

### 6.4.1. Cell Types

Established cell lines, cell strains or primary cell cultures may be used. The most often used are Chinese hamster cell lines and human peripheral blood lymphocytes. The merits of these two cell lines have been reported (Ishidate and Harnois, 1987; Kirkland and Garner, 1987). The cell system must be validated and consistently sensitive to known clastogens.

### 6.4.2. Chinese Hamster Cell Lines

Chinese hamster ovary cells in which there has been an extensive rearrangement of chromosome material and the chromosome number may not be constant from cell to cell, are frequently used. Polyploidy, endoreduplication and high spontaneous chromosome aberration frequencies can sometimes be found in these established cell lines, but careful cell culture techniques should minimize such effects. Cells should be treated in exponential growth when cells are in all stages of the cell cycle.

### 6.4.3. Human Peripheral Blood Lymphocytes

Blood should be taken from healthy donors not known to be suffering from viral infections or receiving medication. Staff handling blood should be immunized against hepatitis B and regular donors should be shown to be hepatitis B antigen negative. Donors and staff should be aware of AIDS implications, and blood and cultures should be handled at containment level 2 (Advisory Committee on Dangerous Pathogens, 1984).

Peripheral blood cultures are stimulated to divide by the addition of a T cell mitogen such as phytohaemagglutinin (PHA) to the culture medium. Mitotic activity is at a maximum at about 3 days but begins at about 40 h after PHA stimulation and the chromosome constitution remains diploid during short-term culture (Evans and O'Riordan, 1975). Treatments should commence at about 44 h after culture initiation. This is when cells are actively proliferating and cells are in all stages of the cell cycle. They should be sampled about 20 h later. In a repeat study the second sample time should be about 92 h after culture initiation. Morimoto et al. (1983) report that the cycle time for lymphocytes averages about 12–14 h except for the first cycle.

Female donors can give higher yields of chromosome damage (Anderson et al., 1989).

### 6.4.4. Positive and Negative Controls

When the solvent is not the culture medium or water, the solvent, liver enzyme activation mixture and solvent and untreated controls are used as negative controls.

Since cultured cells are normally treated in their usual growth medium, the solubility of the test material in the medium should be ascertained before testing. As pointed out earlier, extremes of pH can be clastogenic (Cifone et al., 1987), so the effect of the test material on pH should also be determined, but buffers can be utilized.

Various organic solvents are used, such as dimethyl sulfoxide (DMSO), dimethylformamide, ethanol and acetone. The volume added must not be toxic to cells. Greater than 10% water v/v can be toxic because of nutrient dilution and osmolality changes.

A known clastogen should always be included as a positive control. When metabolic activation is used, a positive control chemical known to require metabolic activation should also be used to ensure that the system is functioning properly. Without metabolic activation, a direct-acting positive control chemical should be used. A structurally related positive control can also be used. Appropriate safety precautions must be taken in handling clastogens (IARC, 1979; MRC, 1981).

Positive control chemicals should be used to produce relatively low frequencies of aberrations so that the sensitivity of the assay for detecting weak clastogens can be established (Preston et al., 1987).

Aberration yields in negative and positive controls should be used to provide a historical database.

### 6.4.5. Treatment of Cells

When an exogenous activation system is employed, short treatments (about 2 h) are usually necessary because S9 mix is often cytotoxic when used for extended lengths of time. However, cells may be treated with chemicals either continuously up to harvest time or for a short time followed by washing and addition of fresh medium to allow cell cycle progression. Continuous treatment avoids centrifugation steps required with washing of cells and optimizes the endogenous metabolic capacity of the lymphocytes.

When metabolic activation is used, S9 mix should not exceed 1–10 percent of the culture medium by volume. It has been shown that the S9 mix is clastogenic in CHO cells and mouse lymphoma cells (Cifone et al., 1987; Kirkland et al., 1989) but not in human lymphocytes, where blood components can inactivate active oxygen species which could cause chromosome damage. When S9 mix from animals treated with other enzyme-inducing agents such as phenobarbitone/beta-naphtho-flavone, is used, clastogenesis may be minimized (Kirkland et al., 1989).

Prior to testing, it is necessary to determine the cytotoxicity of the test material, in order to select a suitable dose range for the chromosome assay both with and without metabolic activation. The range most commonly used determines the effect of the agent on the mitotic index (MI), that is, the percentage of cells in mitoses at the time of cell harvest. The highest dose should inhibit mitotic activity by approximately 50% (EEC Annex V), 75% (UKEMS: Scott et al., 1990) or exhibit some other indication of cytotoxicity. If the reduction in MI is too great, insufficient cells can be found for chromosome analysis. Cytotoxicity can also be assessed by making cell counts in the chromosome aberration test when using cell lines. In the lymphocyte assay total white cell counts can be used in addition to MI. A dose which induces 50–75 percent toxicity in these assays should be accompanied by a suitable reduction in mitotic index.

If the test material is not toxic, it is recommended that it be tested up to $5\,mg\,ml^{-1}$. It is recommended that chemicals be tested up to their maximum solubility in the treatment medium and not just their maximum solubility in stock solutions.

For highly soluble nontoxic agents, concentrations above 10 mM may produce substantial increases in the osmolality of the culture medium which could be clastogenic by causing ionic imbalance within the cells (Ishidate et al., 1984; Brusick, 1987). At concentrations exceeding 10 mM the osmolality of the treatment media should be measured and if the increase exceeds $50\,mmol\,kg^{-1}$, clastogenicity resulting from high osmolality should be suspected and, according to the UKEMS, is unlikely to be of relevance to human risk. The UKEMS also does not recommend the testing of chemicals at concentrations exceeding their solubility limits as suspensions or precipitate.

A minimum of three doses of the test material should be used, the highest chosen as described above, the lowest on the borderline of toxicity, and an intermediate one. Up to six doses can be managed satisfactorily, and this ensures the detection of any dose response and that a toxic range is covered. MIs are as required for the preliminary study (at lease 1000 cells per culture). It is also useful to score endoreduplication and polyploidy for historical data. Cells from only three doses need to be analyzed.

The range of doses used at the repeat fixation time can be those which induce a suitable degree of mitotic inhibition at the earlier fixation time, but if the highest dose reduces the MI to an unacceptably low level at the second sampling time, the next highest dose should be chosen for screening.

A complete assay requires the test material to be investigated at a minimum of three doses together with a positive (untreated) and solvent-only control can be omitted if tissue culture medium is used as a solvent. When two fixation times are used in repeat tests, the positive control is necessary at only one time but the negative or solvent control is necessary at both times.

Duplicates of each test group and quadruplicates of solvent or negative controls should be set up. The sensitivity of the assay is improved with larger numbers scored in the negative controls (Richardson et al., 1989).

### 6.4.6. Scoring Procedures

Prior to scoring, slides should be coded, randomized and then scored "blind." Metaphase analysis should only be carried out by an experienced observer. Metaphase cells should be sought under low-power magnification and those with well-spread, that is, nonoverlapping, clearly defined non fuzzy chromosomes examined under high power with oil immersion. It is acceptable to analyze cells with total chromosome numbers or that have lost one or two chromosomes during processing. In human lymphocytes ($2n - 46$) 44 or more centromeres and in CHO cells ($2n = 22$; range 21–24) 20 or more centromeres can be scored. Chromosome numbers can be recorded for each cell, to give an indication of aneuploidy. Only cells with increases in numbers (above 46 in human lymphocytes and 24 in CHO cells) should be considered in this category, since decreases can occur through processing.

Recording microscope co-ordinates of cells is necessary and allows verification of abnormal cells. A photographic record is also useful of cells with aberrations. Two hundred cells (100 from each of two replicates) should be scored per treatment group. When ambiguous results are obtained, there may be further "blind" reading of these samples.

### 6.4.7. Data Recording

The classification and nomenclature of the International System for Human Cytogenetic Nomenclature (ISCN, 1985) as applied to acquired chromosome aberrations is recommended. Score sheets giving the slide code, microscope scorer's name, date, cell number, number of chromosomes and aberration types should be used. These should include chromatid and chromosome gaps, deletions, exchanges and others. A space for the vernier reading for comments and a diagram of the aberration should be available.

From the score sheets, the frequencies of various aberrations should be calculated and each aberration should be counted only once. To consider a break as one event and an exchange as two events is not acceptable, since unfounded assumptions are made about mechanisms involved (Revell, 1974).

### 6.4.8. Presentation of Results

The test material, test cells, used, method of treatment, harvesting of cells, cytotoxicity assay, and so on, should be clearly stated as well as the statistical methods used. Richardson et al. (1989) recommend that comparison be made between the frequencies in control cells and at each dose level using Fisher's Exact Test.

In cytogenetic assays the absence of a clear positive dose-response relationship at a particular time frequently arises. This is because a single common sampling time may be used for all doses of a test compound. Chromosome aberration yields can vary markedly with post-treatment sampling time of an asynchronous population, and increasing doses of clastogens can induce increasing degrees of mitotic delay (Scott et al., 1990). Additional fixation times should clarify the relationship between dose and aberration yield.

Gaps are by tradition excluded from quantification of chromosome aberration yields. Some gaps have been shown to be real discontinuities in DNA (e.g., Heddle and Bodycote, 1970). Where chromosome aberration yields are on the borderline of statistical significance above control values, the inclusion of gaps could be useful. Further details on this approach may be found in the UKEMS guidelines (Scott et al., 1990).

Since chromosome exchanges are relatively rare events, greater biological significance should be attached to their presence than to gaps and breaks.

Chemicals which are clastogenic *in vitro* at low doses are more likely to be clastogenic *in vivo* than those where clastogenicity is detected only at high concentrations (Ishidate et al., 1988). Negative results in well-conducted *in vitro* tests are a good indication of a lack of potential for *in vivo* clastogenesis, since almost all *in vivo* clastogens have given positive results *in vitro* when adequately tested (Thompson, 1986; Ishidate 1988a, b).

## 6.5. *IN VIVO* CYTOGENETICS ASSAYS

Damage induced in whole animals can be detected in *in vivo* chromosome assays in either somatic or germinal cells by examination of metaphases or the formation of micronuclei. The micronucleus test can also detect whole chromosome loss or aneuploidy in the absence of clastogenic activity and is considered comparable in sensitivity to chromosome analysis (Tsuchimoto and Matter, 1979).

Rats and mice are generally used for *in vivo* studies, with the mouse being employed for bone marrow micronucleus analysis and the rat for metaphase analysis, but both can be used for either. Mice are cheaper and easier to handle than rats, and only a qualitative difference in response has been found between the species (Albanese et al., 1987). Chinese hamsters are also widely used for metaphase analysis because of their low diploid chromosome number of 22. However, there are few other historical toxicological data for this species.

### 6.5.1. Somatic Cell Assays

***Metaphase Analysis.*** Metaphase analysis can be performed in any tissue with actively dividing cells, but bone marrow is the tissue most often examined. Cells are treated with a test compound and are arrested in metaphase by the administration of colcemid or colchicine at various sampling times after treatment. Preparations are examined for structural chromosome damage. Because the bone marrow has a good blood supply, the cells should be exposed to the test compound or its metabolites in the peripheral blood supply. Additionally, these cells are sensitive to S-dependent and S-independent mutagens (Topham et al., 1983).

Peripheral blood cells can be stimulated to divide even though the target cell is relatively insensitive (Newton and Lilly, 1986). It is necessary to stimulate them with a mitogen since the number of lymphocytes which are dividing at any one time is very low. Cells are in $G_0$ when exposure is taking place, so they may not be sensitive to cell cycle stage specific mutagens and any damage might be repaired before sampling.

### 6.5.2. Micronuclei

The assessment of micronuclei is considered simpler than the assessment of metaphase analysis. This assay is most often carried out in bone marrow cells, where polychromatic erythrocytes are examined. Damage is induced in the immature erythroblast and results in a micronucleus outside the main nucleus, which is easily detected after staining as a chromatid-containing body. When the erythroblast matures, the micronucleus, whose formation results from chromosome loss during cell division or from chromosome breakage forming centric and acentric fragments, is not extruded with the nucleus. Micronuclei can also be detected in peripheral blood cells (MacGregor et al., 1980). In addition, they can be detected in liver (Tates et al., 1980; Collaborative Study Group for the Micronucleus Test, 1986 & 1988; Braithwaite and Ashby, 1988) after partial hepatectomy or stimulation with 4-acetylaminofluorene, or they can be detected in any proliferating cells.

### 6.5.3. Germ Cell Assays

The study of chromosome damage is highly relevant to the assessment of heritable cytogenetic damage. Many compounds which cause somatic cell damage have not produced germ cell damage (Holden, 1982) and, so far, all germ mutagens have also produced somatic damage.

Germ cell data, however, are needed for genetic risk estimation, and testing can be performed in male or female germ cells. The former are most often used, owing to the systemic effects in females. Testing in the male is performed in mitotically proliferating premeiotic spermatogonia, but chromosomal errors in such cells can result in cell death or prevent the cell from passing through meiosis. Damage produced in postmeiotic cells, the spermatids or sperm are more likely to be transmitted to the $F_1$ progeny (Albanese, 1987). In females it is during early fetal development of the ovary that öocyte stage is the most commonly tested stage in the adult female. To test other stages during the first or second meiotic divisions demands the use of öocytes undergoing ovulation which occur naturally or are hormone-stimulated. It is thus more difficult technically to test female germ cells.

### 6.5.4. Heritable Chromosome Assays

Damage may be analyzed in the heritable translocation test, which involves the examination in male $F_1$ animals if diakinesis metaphase 1 spermatocytes for multivalent association fall within the acceptable range for the laboratory for a substance to be considered positive or negative under the conditions of the study.

### 6.5.5. Germ Cell Cytogenetic Assays

Either mouse or rat can be used but the mouse is generally the preferred species. Normally such assays are not conducted for routine screening purposes.

Spermatogonial metaphases can be prepared by the air-drying technique of Evans et al. (1964) for the first and second meiotic metaphase (MI and MII) in the male mouse. This method is not so suitable for rat and hamster. The numbers of spermatogonial metaphases can be boosted if, prior to hypotonic treatment, the testicular tubules are dispersed in trypsin solution (0.25%). At least one month between treatment and sample should be allowed to pass in the mouse to allow treated cells to reach meiosis. Brook and Chandley (1986) established that 11 days and 4 h was the time required for spermatogonial cells to reach preleptotene and 8 days and 10 h to reach zygotene. It takes 4 h for cells to move from MI to MII but test compounds can alter this rate. A search for multivalent formation can be made at MI for the structural rearrangements induced in spermatogonia. Cawood and Breckon (1983) examined the synaptonemal complex at pachytene, using electron microscopy. Errors of segregation should be searched for at the first meiotic division in the male mouse, MII cells showing 19 (hypoploid) and 21 (hyperploid) chromo-somes (Brook and Chandley, 1986). Hansmann and El-Nahass (1979), Brook (1982) and Brook and Chandley (1985) describe assays in the female mouse and procedures used for inducing ovulation by hormones and treatment of specific stages of meiosis.

## 6.6. SISTER CHROMATID EXCHANGE ASSAYS

SCEs are reciprocal exchanges between sister chromatids. They result in a change in morphology of the chromosome but breakage and reunion are involved although the exact mechanism is unclear. They are thought to occur at homologous loci.

In 1958 Taylor demonstrated SCEs, using autoradiographic techniques to detect the disposition or labeled DNA following incorporation of [3H]-thymidine. 5-Bromo-2′-deoxyuridine (drdU) has now replaced [3H]-thymidine and various stain-ing methods have been used to show the differential incorporation of BrdU between sister chromatids: fluorescent: Hoechst 33258 (Latt, 1973); combined fluorescent and Giemsa (Perry and Wolff, 1974); and Giemsa (Korenberg and Freedlander, 1974). The fluorescent plus Giemsa procedure is recommended in view of the fact that stained slides can be stored and microscope analysis is simpler.

So that SCEs can be seen at metaphase, cells must pass through S phase (Kato, 1973, 1974; Wolff and Perry, 1974). SCEs appear to occur at the replication point, since SCE induction is maximal at the beginning of DNA synthesis but drops to zero at the end of S phase (Latt and Loveday, 1978).

For SCE analysis *in vitro*, any cell type that is replicating or can be stimulated to divide is suitable. The incorporation of BrdU into cells *in vivo* allows the examination of a variety of tissues (Latt et al., 1980). Edwards et al. (1993) suggest that is necessary to standardize protocols measuring SCE since different responses can be obtained depending on the extent of simultaneous exposure of test compound and BrdU.

### 6.6.1. Relevance of SCE in Terms of Genotoxicity

SCEs do not appear to be related to other cytogenetic events, since potent clastogens such as bleomycin and ionizing radiation induce low levels of SCE (Perry and Evans, 1975). The mechanisms involved in chromosome aberrations and SCE formation are dissimilar (e.g., Galloway and Wolff, 1979). There is no evidence that SCEs are in themselves lethal events, since there is little relationship to cytotoxicity (e.g., Bowden et al., 1979). It was suggested by Wolff (1977a, b) that they relate more to mutational events due to a compatibility with cell survival. However, there are examples of agents that induce significant SCE increases in the absence of mutation (Bradley et al., 1979) as well as they converse (Connell, 1979; Connell and Medcalf, 1982).

The SCE assay is particularly sensitive for alkylating agents and base analogues, agents causing single-strand breaks in DNA and compounds acting through DNA binding (Latt et al., 1981). The most potent SCE inducers are S-phase-dependent. Painter (1980) reports that agents such as X-irradiation, which inhibits replicon initiation, are poor SCE inducers, whereas mitomycin C, which inhibits replication fork progression, is a potent SCE inducer.

### 6.6.2. Experimental Design

Established cell lines, primary cell cultures of rodents, may be used. Detailed information on *in vitro* and *in vivo* assays may be obtained in reviews of SCE methods by Latt et al. (1977, 1981), Perry and Thompson (1984) and Perry et al. (1984). The *in vitro* methods will be briefly explored here.

Either monolayer or suspension cultures can be employed, or human lymphocytes. Human fibroblasts are less suitable because of their long cell cycle duration.

The concentration of organic solvents for the test compound should not exceed 0.8% v/v, as higher concentrations could lead to slight elevations in the SCE level (Perry et al., 1984).

For monolayer cultures, the cultures are set up the day before BrdU treatment so that the cells will be in exponential growth before the addition of BrdU or the test compound. After BrdU addition the cells are allowed to undergo the equivalent of two cell cycles before cell harvest. A spindle inhibitor such as colchicine or colcemid is introduced for the final 1–2 h of culture to arrest cells in metaphase, after which the cells are harvested and chromosome preparations are made by routine cytogenetic techniques.

In the absence of metabolic activation, BrdU and the test agent can be added simultaneously and left for the duration of BrdU labeling. Shorter treatments should be used in the presence of metabolic activation or to avoid synergistic effects with BrdU, when cells can be pulse treated for, for example, 1 h before BrdU addition (see Edwards et al. (1993).

Peripheral blood cultures are established in medium containing BrdU and PHA. Cocemid is added 1–2 h before harvest and the cells are harvested between 60 and 70 h post-PHA stimulation. Cell harvest and slide preparations are conducted according to routine cytogenetic methods.

Heparinized blood samples may be stored at 4°C for up to 48 h without affecting the SCE response (Lambert et al., 1982). If the test agent is known to react with serum or red blood cells, the mononuclear lymphocytes may be isolated by use of a Ficoll/Hypaque gradient (Boyum, 1968).

If metabolic activation is not required, treatment is best conducted over the whole of the final 24 h of culture, or if metabolic activation is required, a pulse exposure may be employed to treat cultures at the first S phase at around 24–30 h, or at 48 h for an asynchronous population.

Exposure of cells to fluorescent light during the culture period, leads to photolysis of BrdU-containing DNA and a concomitant increase in SCE frequency (Wolff and Perry, 1974). Consequently, SCE cultures should be kept in the dark and manipulated under subdued light conditions such as yellow safe light. Furthermore, media used in SCE assays should be stored in the dark, since certain media components produce reactive SCE-inducing intermediates on exposure to fluorescent light (Monticone and Schneider, 1979).

Coded and randomized slides should be read. All experiments should be repeated at least once (Perry et al., 1984) with higher and lower concentrations of S9 mix if a negative response is achieved. Even for an apparently unambiguous positive response with a greater than twofold increase in SCEs over the background level at the highest dose, and with at least two consecutive dose levels with an increased SCE response, a repeat study is necessary to show a consistent response.

The quality of differential staining will determine the ease and accuracy of SCE scoring, and, to eliminate variation, results from different observers should occasionally be compared. Furthermore, to avoid observer bias, scorers should have slides from different treatment groups equally distributed among them, as with all cytogenetic studies.

## REFERENCES


Adler, I.D. and Ashby, J. (1989). The present lack of evidence for unique rodent germ-cell mutagens. *Mutation Res.* 212: 55–66.

Advisory Committee on Dangerous Pathogens (1984), *Hazards and Precaution for Handling of Blood Borne Pathogens*, HHG, Washington, D.C.

Albanese, R. (1987). Mammalian male germ cell cytogenetics. *Mutagenesis* 2: 79–85.

Amacher, D.E., Paillet, S.C., Turner, G.N., Ray, V.A. and Salsburg, D.S. (1980). Point mutations at the thymidine kinase locus in L5178Y mouse lymphoma cells. 2. Test validation and interpretation. *Mutation Res.* 72: 447–474.

Ames, B.N. (1971). The detection of chemical mutagens with enteric bacteria. In: *Chemical Mutagens, Principles and Methods for Their Detection*, (Hollaender, A., Ed.) Vol. 1. Plenum Press, New York, pp. 267–282.

Ames, B.N., McCann, J. and Yamasaki, E. (1975). Methods for detecting carcinogens and mutagens with the Salmonella/mammalian-microsome mutagenicity test. *Mutation Res.* 31: 237–364.

Anderson, D. (1990). Male mediated $F_1$ abnormalities. *Mutation Res.* 229: 103–246.

Applegate, M.L., Moore, M.M., Broder, C.B. et al. (1990). Molecular dissection of mutations at the heterozygous thymidine canise locus in mouse lymphoma cells. *Proc. Nat. Acad. Sci. U.S.A.* 87: 51–55.

Arlett, C.F. and Cole, J. (1990). The third United Kingdom Environmental Mutagen Society collaborative trial: overview, a summary and assessment. *Mutagenesis* 5 (Suppl.) 85–88.

Arlett, C.F., Smith, D.M., Clark, G.M., Green, J.H.L., Cole, J., McGregor, D.B. and Asquith, J.C. (1989). Mammalian cell assays based upon colony formation. In: *UKEMS Subcommittee on Guidelines for Mutagenicity Testing. Report Part III: Statistical Evaluation of Mutagenicity Test Data*, (Kirkland, D.J., Ed.). Cambridge University Press, pp. 66–101.

Ashby, J. and Tennant, R.W. (1988). Chemical structure, *Salmonella* mutagenicity and extent of carcinogenicity as indices of genotoxic carcinogens among 222 chemicals tested in rodents by the US NCI/NTP. *Mutation Res.* 204: 17–115.

Ashby, J., Tennant, R.W., Zeiger, E. and Stasiewiczs, S. (1989). Classification according to chemical structure, mutagenicity to *Salmonella* and level of carcinogenicity of a further 42 chemicals tested for carcinogenicity by the U.S. National Toxicology Program. *Mutation Res.* 223: 73–104.

Ashwood-Smith, M.J. (1980). Stability of frozen microsome preparations for use in the Ames Salmonella mutagenicity assay. *Mutation Res.* 69: 199–200.

Bartsch, H., Camus, A.-M. and Malaveille, C. (1976). Comparative mutagenicity of *N*-nitrosamines in a semi-solid and in a liquid incubation system in the presence of rat or human tissue fractions. *Mutation Res.* 37: 149–162.

Beckman, D.A. and Brent, R.L. (1986). Mechanism of known environmental teratogens: drugs and chemicals. *Clin. Perinatol.* 13: 649–687.

Bender, M.A., Griggs, H.G. and Bedford, J.S. (1974). Mechanisms of chromosomal aberration production. III. Chemicals and ionizing radiation. *Mutation Res.* 23: 197–212.

Blazak, W.F., Steward, B.E., Galperin, I., Allen, K.L., Rudd, C.J., Mitchell, A.D. and Caspary, W.J. (1986). Chromosome analysis of triflourothymidine-resistant L5178Y mouse lymphoma cells colonies. *Environ. Mutagen.* 8: 229–240.

Bossi, L. (1985). Information suppression. In: *Genetics of Bacteria*, (Scaife, J., Leach, D. and Galizzi, A., Eds.), Academic Press, New York, pp. 49–64.

Bowden, G.T., Hsu, I.C., and Harris, C.C. (1979). The effect of caffeine on cytotoxicity, mutagenesis and sister chromatid exchanges in Chinese hamster cells treated with dihydrodiol epoxide derivatives of benzo(a)pyrene. *Mutation Res.* 63: 361–370.

Boyum, A. (1968). Separation of lymphocytes and erythrocytes by centrifugation. *Scand. J. Clin. Invest.* 21: 77–85.

Bradley, M.O., Hsu, I.C. and Harris, C.C. (1979). Relationships between sister chromatid exchange and mutagenicity, toxicity and DNA damage. *Nature* 282: 318–320.

Braithwaite, I. and Ashby, J. (1988). A non-invasive micronucleus assay in rat liver. *Mutation Res.* 203: 23–32.

Bridges, B.A. (1972). Simple bacterial systems for detecting mutagenic agents. *Lab. Pract.* 21: 413–419.

Bridges, B.A. (1976). Short-term screening tests for carcinogens. *Nature* 261: 195–200.

Bridges, B.A., Woodgate, R., Ruiz-Rubio, M., Sharif, F., Sedgwick, S.G. and Hubschere, U. (1987). Current understanding of UV-induced base pair substitution mutation in *E. coli* with particular reference to the DNA polymerase III complex. *Mutation Res.* 181: 219–226.

Brook, J.D. (1982). The effect of 4CMB on germ cells of the mouse. *Mutation Res.* 100: 305–308.

Brook, J.D. and Chandley, A.C. (1985). Testing of 3 chemical compounds for aneuploidy induction in the female mouse. *Mutation Res.* 157: 215–220.

Brook, J.D. and Chandley, A.C. (1986). Testing for the chemical induction of aneuploidy in the male mouse. *Mutation Res.* 164: 117–125.

Brusick, D. (1986). Genotoxic effects in cultures mammalian cells produced by low pH treatment conditions and increased ion concentrations. *Environ. Mutagen.* 8: 879–886.

Brusick, D. (1987). Genotoxicity produced in cultures mammalian cell assays by treatment conditions. Special issue. *Mutation Res.* 189: 1–80.

Brusick, D. (1987). *Principles of Genetic Toxicology*, 2nd ed. Plenum Press, New York.

Burnett, C., Fuchs, C., Corbett, J. and Menkart, J. (1982). The effect of dimethylsulphoxide on the mutagenicity of the hair-dye, *p*-phenylenediamine. *Mutation Res.* 103: 1–4.

Butterworth, B.E. and Slaga, T.J. (1987). *Nongenotoxic Mechanisms in Carcinogenesis*. Banbury Report No. 25. Cold Spring Harbor Laboratory, NY.

Carter, T.C., Lyon, M.F. and Philips, R.J.S. (1956). Induction of mutations in mice by chronic gamma irradiation; interim report. *Br. J. Radiol.* 29: 106–108.

Carver, J.H., Machado, M.L. and MacGregor, J.A. (1985). Petroleum distillates suppress *in vitro* metabolic activation: Higher (S9) required in the *Salmonella*/microsome mutagenicity assay. *Environ. Mutagen.* 7: 369–380.

Cawood, A.D. and Breckon, G. (1983). Synaptonemal complexes as indicators of induced structural change in chromosomes after irradiation of spermatogonia. *Mutation Res.* 122: 149–154.

Chandley, A.C. (1981). The origin of chromosomal aberrations in man and their potential for survival and reproduction in the adult human population. *Ann. Genet.* 24: 5–11.

Chu, E.H.Y. and Malling, H.U. (1968). Mammalian cell genetics. II. Chemical induction of specific lucus mutations in Chinese hamster cells *in vitro*. *Proc. Nat. Acad. Sci. U.S.A.* 61: 1306–1312.

Cifone, M.A., Myhr, B., Eiche, A. and Bolisfodi, G. (1987). Effect of pH shifts on the mutant frequency at the thymidine kinase locus in mouse lymphoma L5178Y TK+/− cells. *Mutation Res.* 189: 39–46.

Clayson, D.B. (1989). ICPEMC publication No. 17: Can a mechanistic rationale be provided for non-genotoxic carcinogens identified in rodent bioassays? *Mutation Res.* 221: 53–67.

Cleaver, J.E. (1983). Xeroderma pigmentosum. In: *The Metabolic Basis of Inherited Disease*, (Stanbury, J.B., Wyngaarden, J.B., Fredrickson, D.S., Goldstein, J.C. and Brown, M.S. Eds.). McGraw-Hill, New York, pp. 1227–1248.

Clive, D. (1989). Mammalian cell genotoxicity: A major role for non-DNA targets? *Mutation Res.* 223: 327–328.

Clive, D. (1987). Historical overview of the mouse lymphoma $TK^{+/-}$ mutagenicity assay. In: *Mammalian Cell Mutagenesis*, (Moore, M.M., Demarini, D.M., De Serres, F.J. and Tindall, K.R., Eds.). Banbury Report 28. Cold Spring Harbor Laboratory, NY, pp. 25–36.

Clive, D., Caspary, W., Kirkby, P.E., Krehl, R., Moore, M., Mayo, J. and Oberly, T.J. (1987). Guide for performing the mouse lymphoma assay for mammalian cell mutagenicity. *Mutation Res.* 189: 145–146.

Clive, D., Flamm, W.G. and Patterson, J.B. (1972). A mutational assay system using the thymidine kinase locus in mouse lymphoma cells. *Mutation Res.* 16: 77–87.

Collaborative Study Group for the Micronucleus Test (1986). Sex Differences in the micronucleus test. *Mutation Res.* 172: 151–163.

Collaborative Study Group for the Micronucleus Test (1988). Strain differences in the micronucleus test. *Mutation Res.* 204: 307–316.

Cole, J., Fox, M., Garner, R.C., McGregor, D.B. and Thacker, J. (1990). Gene mutation assays in cultured mammalian cells. In: *UKEMS Subcommittee on Guidelines for Mutagenicity Testing. Report Part I rev.* (Kirkland, D.J., Ed.). Cambridge University Press, pp. 87–114.

Cole, J., Muriel, W.J. and Bridges, B.A. (1986). The mutagenicity of sodium flouride to L5178Y (wildtype and $TK^{+/-}$ 3.7.2c) mouse lymphoma cells. *Mutagenesis* 1: 157–167.

Connell, J.R. (1979). The relationship between sister chromatid exchange, chromosome aberration and gene mutation induction by several reactive polycyclic hydrocarbon metabolites in cultured mammalian cells. *Int. J. Cancer* 24: 485–489.

Connell, J.R. and Medcalf, A.S. (1982). The induction of SCE and chromosomal aberrations with relation to specific base methylation of DNA in Chinese hamster cells by N-methyl-*n*-nitrosourea and dimethyl sulphate. *Carcinogenesis* 3: 385–390.

Cullum, J. (1985) Insertion sequences. In: (Scaife, J., Leach, D. and Galizzi, A., Eds.). *Genetics of Bacteria*, Academic Press, New York, pp. 89–96.

Dean, B.J. and Danford, N. (1984). Assays for the detection of chemically induced chromosome damage in cultures mammalian cells. In: *Mutagenicity Testing. A Practical Approach*, (Venitt, S. and Parry, J.M., Eds.). IRL Press, Oxford, pp. 187–232.

DeSerres, F.J. and Shelby, M.D. (1979). Recommendations on datas production and analysis using the *Salmonella*/microsome mutagenicity assay. *Mutation Res.* 64: 159–165.

deVries, J.H. (1901). *The Mutation Theory*, Verlag von Veit, Leipzig.

Doll, R. (1977). Strategy for detection of cancer hazards to man. *Nature* 265: 589–596.

Dunnett, C.W. (1955). A multiple comparison procedure for comparing several treatments with a control. *J. Am. Stat. Assoc.* 50: 1096–1121.

Edwards, A.J., Moon, E.Y., Anderson, D. and McGregor, D.B. (1993). The effect of simultaneous exposure to bromodeoxyuridine and methyl methansulphonate on sister chromatid exchange frequency in culture human lymphocytes and its mutation research. *Mutation Res.* 247: 117–125.

Ehling, U.H., Chu, E.H.Y., DeCarli, L., Evans, H.J., Hayashi, M., Lambert, B., Neubert, D., Thilly, W.G. and Vainio, H. (1986). Report 8. Assays for germ-cell mutations in mammals. In: *Long-term and Short-term Assays for Carcinogens.* (Montesano, R., Bartsch, H., Vainio, H., Wilbourn, J. and Yamasaki, H., Eds.). *A Critical Appraisal.* IARC Scientific Publications, No. 83, Lyon, pp. 245–265.

Evans, E.P., Breckon, G. and Ford, C.E. (1964). An air-drying method for meiotic preparations from mammalian testes. *Cytogenet. Cell Genet.* 3: 289–294.

Evans, H.H., Mencl, J., Horng, M.F., Ricanti, M., Sanchez, D. and Hozier, J. (1986). Lucus specificity in the mutability of L5178Y mouse lymphoma cells: the role of multilocus lesions. *Proc. Nat. Acad. Sci. U.S.A.* 83: 4379–4385.

Evans, H.J. and O'Riordan, M.L. (1975). Human peripheral blood lymphocytes for the analysis of chromosome aberrations in mutagen tests. *Mutation Res.* 31: 135–148.

Ford, D.K. and Yerganian, G. (1958). Observations on the chromosomes of Chinese hamster cells in tissue culture. *J. Nat. Cancer Inst.* 21: 393–425.

Forster, R., Green, M.H.L. and Priestley, A. (1980). Optimal Levels of S9 fraction in Ames and fluctuation tests: apparent importance of diffusion of metabolites from top agar. *Carcinogenesis* 2: 1081–1085.

Fox, M. (1981). Some quantitative aspects of the response of mammalian *in vitro* to induced mutagenesis. In: *Cancer Biology Reviews* (Marchelonis, J.J. and Hanna, M.G., Eds.). Vol. 3, Marcel Dekker, New York, pp. 23–62.

Friedberg, E.C. (1988). DNA repair in the yeast *Saccharomyces cerevisiae. Microb. Rev.* 52: 70–102.

Gad, S.C. (1999). *Statistics and Experimental Design for Toxicologists*, 3rd ed. CRC Press, Boca Raton, FL.

Galloway, S.M. and Wolff, S. (1979). The relation between chemically induced SCEs and chromatid breakage. *Mutation Res.* 61: 297–307.

Gatehouse, D.G. and Delow, G.F. (1979). The development of a "Microtitre[®]" fluctuation test for the detection of indirect mutagens and its use in the evaluation of mixed enzyme induction of the liver. *Mutation Res.* 60: 239–252.

Gatehouse, D.G. and Tweats, D.J. (1987). Letter to the Editor. *Mutagenesis* 1: 307–308.

Gatehouse, D. and Wedd, D.J. (1984). The differential mutagenicity of isoniazid in fluctuation assays and *Salmonella* plate tests. *Carcinogenesis* 5: 391–397.

Gatehouse, D.G., Wedd, D.J., Paes, D., Delow, G., Burlinson, B., Pascoe, S., Brice, A., Stemp, G. and Tweats, D.J. (1988). Investigations into the genotoxic potential of Ioxtidine, a long-acting $H_2$-receptor antagonist. *Mutagenesis* 3: 57–68.

Gatehouse, D.G., Wilcox, P., Forster, R., Rowland, I.R., and Callander, R.D. (1990). Bacterial mutation assays. In: *Basic Mutagenicity Tests: UKEMS Recommended Procedures* (Kirkland, D.J., Ed.). Cambridge University Press, pp. 13–61.

Green, M.H.L. and Muriel, W.J. (1976). Mutagen testing using $TRP^+$ reversion in *E. coli. Mutation Res.* 38: 3–32.

Hansmann, I. and El-Nahass, E. (1979). Incidence of non-disjunction in mouse öocytes. *Cytogenet. Cell Genet.* 24: 115–121.

Haworth, S., Lawlor, T., Mortelmanns, K., Speck, W. and Zeiger, E. (1983). Salmonella mutagenicity results for 250 chemicals *Environ. Mutagen. Suppl.* 1: 3–142.

Heddle, J.A. and Bodycote, D.J. (1970). On the formation of chromosomal aberrations. *Mutation Res.* 9: 117–126.

Herrera, G., Urios, A., Alexandre, V., and Blanco, M., (1988). UV light induced mutability in *Salmonella* strains containing the *umu DC* or the *muc AB* operon: evidence for a *umu C* function. *Mutation Res.* 198: 9–13.

Holden, H.E. (1982). Comparison of somatic and germ cell models for cytogenetic screening. *J. Appl. Toxicol.* 2: 196–200.

Hozier, J., Sawger, D., Clieve, D. and Moore, M. (1982). Cytogenetic distinction between the $TK^+$ and $TK^-$ chromosomes in $L5178Y/TK^{+/-}$-3.7.2.C mouse lymphoma cell line. *Mutation Res.* 105: 451–456.

Hsie, A.W., Brimer, P.A., Mitchell, T.J. and Gosslee, D.G. (1975). The dos-response relationship for ethyl methane sulfonate-induced mutation at the hypoxanthine-guanine phosphoribosyl transferase locus in Chinese hamster ovary cells. *Somatic Cell Genet.* 1: 247–261.

Hubbard, S.A., Brooks, T.M., Gonzalez, L.P. and Bridges, J.W. (1985). Preparation and characterization of S9-fractions. In: *Comparative Genetic Toxicology.* (Parry, J.M. and Arlett, C. F., Eds.). Macmillan, London, pp. 413–438.

IARC (1979). *Handling Chemical Carcinogens in the Laboratory; Problems of Safety,* Scientific Publications No. 33. International Agency for Research on Cancer, Lyons, France.

ICEMC (1983). Committee & Final Report: screening strategy for chemicals that are potential germ-cell mutagens in mammals. *Mutation Res.* 114: 117–177.

ICH (1996). Technical Requirements for Registration of Pharmaceuticals for Human Use. Guidance on Specific Aspects of Regulatory Genotoxicity Tests for Pharmaceuticals. S2A document recommended for adoption at step 4 of the ICH process on July 19, 1995. Federal Register 61: 18198–18202, April 24, 1996.

ICH (1997). Technical Requirements for Registration of Pharmaceuticals for Human Use. Genotoxicity: A Standard Battery for Genotoxicity Testing of Pharmaceuticals. S2B document recommended for adoption at step 4 of the ICH process on July 16, 1997. Federal Register 62: 16026–16030, November 21, 1997.

ISCN (1985). *An International System for Human Cytogenetic Nomenclature.* In: Report of the Standing Committee on Human Cytogenetic Nomenclature (Harnden, D.G. and Klinger H.P., Eds.). Karger, Basel, Switzerland.

Ishidate, M., Jr. (1988a). *Data Book of Chromosomal Aberration Tests in vitro,* Elsevier, Amsterdam.

Ishidate, M., Jr. (1988b). A proposed battery of tests for the initial evaluation of the mutagenic potential of medicinal and industrial chemicals. *Mutation Res.* 205: 397–407.

Ishidate, M., Jr. and Harnois, M.C. (1987). The clastogenicity of chemicals in mammalian cells. Letter to the editor. *Mutagenesis* 2: 240–243.

Ishidate, M., Jr., Sofuni, T., Yoshikawa, K., et al. (1984). Primary mutagenicity screening of food additives currently used in Japan *Food Chem. Toxicol.* 22: 623–636.

ISO (1993). *Biological Evaluation of Medical Devices. Part 3: Tests for Genotoxicity, Carcinogenicity, and Reproductive Toxicity.* ISO 10993–3.

JMHW (1984). *Guidelines for Testing of Drugs for Toxicity.* Pharmaceutical Affairs Bureau, Notice No. 118. Ministry of Health and Welfare, Japan.

Joint Directives of the Japanese Environmental Protection Agency, Japanese Ministry of Health and Welfare and Japanese Ministry of International Trade and Industry, 31 March 1987.

Jordan, E., Saedler, H., and Starlinger, P. (1967). Strong polar mutations in the transferase gene of the galactose operon in *E. coli. Molec. Gen. Genet.* 100: 296–306.

Kada, T. (1981). The DNA damaging activity of 42 coded compounds in the Rec-assay. In: *Evaluation of Short-term Tests for Carcinogens. Report of the International Collaborative Program* (de Serres F. and Ashby J., Eds.). Elsevier/North Holland, Amsterdam, pp. 175–182.

Kalter, K. (1977). Correlation between teratogenic and mutagenic effects of chemicals in mammals. In: *Chemical Mutagens: Principles and Methods for Their Detection* (Hollanender, A., Ed.). Vol. 6, Plenum Press, New York, pp. 57–82.

Kato, H. (1973). Induction of sister chromatid exchanges by UV light and its inhibition by caffeine, *Exp. Cell Res.*, 82: 383–390.

Kato, H. (1974). Induction of sister chromatid exchanges by chemical mutagens and its possible relevance to DNA repair. *Exp. Cell Res.* 85: 239–247.

Kato, T. and Shinoura, Y. (1977). Isolation and characterization of mutants of *Escherichia coli* deficient in induction of mutation by ultraviolet light. *Mol. Gen. Genet.* 156: 121–132.

Kennelly, J.C., Stanton, C. and Martin, C.N. (1984). The effect of acetyl-CoA supplementation on the mutagenicity of benzidines in the Ames assay. *Mutation Res.* 137: 39–45.

Kirkland, D.J. and Garner, R.C. (1987). Testing for genotoxicity-chromosomal aberrations *in vitro*. CHO cells or human lymphocytes? *Mutation Res.* 189: 186–187.

Kirkland D.J., Marshall R.R., McEnaney, S., Bidgwood, J., Rutter, A. and Mulliheux, S. (1989). Aroclor-1254 induced rat liver S-9 causes chromosome aberrations in CHO cells but not in human lymphocytes, a role for active oxygen? *Mutat. Res.* 214: 115–122.

Korenberg, J.R. and Freedlender, E.F. (1974). Giesma technique for the detection of sister chromatid exchanges. *Chromasoma* 48: 355–360.

Kuroki, T. and Matsushima, T. (1987). Performance of short-term tests for detection of human carcinogens. *Mutagenesis* 2: 33–37.

Lambert, B., Lindblad, A., Holmberg, K. and Francesconi, D. (1982). The use of sister chromatid exchange to monitor human populations for exposure to toxicologically harmful agents. In: *Sister Chromatid Exchange* (Wolff, S., Ed.). Wiley, New York, pp. 149–182.

Latt, S.A. (1973). Microfluorometric detection of deoxyribonucleic acid replication in human metaphase chromosomes. *Proc. Nat. Acad. Sci. U.S.A.* 770: 3395–3399.

Latt, S., Allen, J.W., Bloom, S.E., Carr A., Falke, E., Schneider, E., Schreck, R., Jice, R., Whitfield, B. K, and Wolff, S. (1981). Sister chromatid exchanges: a report of the gene-tox program. *Mutation Res.* 87: 17–62.

Latt, S.A., Allen, J.W., Rogers, W.E., and Jurgens, L.A. (1977). *In vitro* and *in vivo* analysis of sister chromatid exchange formation. In: *Handbook of Mutagenicity Test Procedures* (Kilbey, B.J., Legator, M., Nichols, W. and Ramel, C., Eds.). Elsevier, Amsterdam, pp. 275–291.

Latt, S.A. and Loveday, K.S. (1978). Characterization of sister chromatid exchange induction by 8-methoxypsoralen plus UV light. *Cytogenet. Cell Genet.* 21: 184–200.

Latt, S.A., Schreck, R.R., Loveday, K.S., Dougherty, C.P. and Shuler, C.F. (1980). Sister chromatid exchanges. *Adv. Human Genet.* 31: 291–298.

Lawley, P. (1989). Mutagens as carcinogens: development of current concepts. *Mutation Res.* 213: 3–26.

Li, A.P., Aaron, C.S., Aueltta, A.E., Dearfield, K.L., Riddle, J.C., Slesinski, R.S. and Stankowski, L.F., Jr. (1991). An evaluation of the roles of mammalian cell mutation assays in the testing of chemical genotoxicity. *Regulatory Toxicol. Pharmacol.* 14: 24–40.

Li, A.P., Carver, J.H., Choy, W.N., Bupta, R.S., Loveday, K.S., O'Neill, J.P., Riddle, J.C., Stankowski, L.F. and Yang, L.C. (1987). A guide for the performance of the Chinese Hamster ovary cell/hypoxanthine guanine phosphoribosyl transferase gene mutation assay. *Mutation Res.* 189: 135–141.

Linblad, W.J. and Jackim, E. (1982). Mechanism for the differential induction of mutation by kS9 activated benzo(*a*)pyrene employing either a glucose-6-phosphate dependent NADPH-regenerating system or an isocitrate dependent system. *Mutation Res.* 96: 109–118.

Lindahl, T. (1979). DNA glycoslylases, endonucleases for apurinic/apyrimidinic sites and base excision repair. *Proc. Nuc. Acid Res. Mol. Biol.* 22: 109–118.

Lindahl, T., Sedwick, B., Sekiguchi, M. and Nakabeppu, Y. (1988). Regulation and expression of the adaptive response to alkylating agents, *Ann. Rev. Biochem.* 57: 133–157.

Little, J.W. (1984). Autodigestion of *lex A* and phage T repressors. *Proc. Nat. Acad. Sci. U.S.A.* 81: 1375–1379.

Little, J.W. and Mount, D.W. (1982). The SOS regulatory system of *Escherichia coli. Cell.* 29: 11–22.

McCann, J., Spingarn, N.-E., Kobori, J. and Ames, B.N. (1975b). Detection of carcinogens as mutagens: Bacterial tester strains with R factor plasmids. *Proc. Natl. Acad. Sci. USA* 72: 979–983.

MacGregor, J.T., Wehr, C.M. and Gould, D.H. (1980). Clastogen-induced micronuclei in peripheral blood erythrocytes: the basis of an improved micronucleus test. *Environ. Mutagen.* 2: 509–514.

MacPhee, D.G. (1973). *Salmonella typhimurium* hisG46 (R-Utrecht): possible use in screening mutagens and carcinogens. *Appl. Microbiol.* 26: 1004–1005.

Madle, S. and Obe, G. (1980). Methods for the analysis of the mutagenicity of indirect mutagens/carcinogens in eukaryotic cells. *Human Genet.* 56: 7–20.

Mahon, G.A.T., Green, M.H.L., Middleton, B., Mitchell, I.DeG., Robinson, W.D. and Tweats, D.J. (1989). Analysis of data from microbial colon assays. In: *Statistical Evaluation of Mutagenicity Test Data* (Kirkland, D.J., Ed.). Cambridge University Press, pp. 26–65.

Marinus, M.G. and Morris, R.N. (1974). Biological function for the 6-methyladenine residues in the DNA of *Escherichia coli* K12. *J. Mol. Biol.* 85: 309–322.

Maron, D.M. and Ames, B.N. (1983). Revised methods for the *Salmonella* mutagenicity test. *Mutation Res.* 113: 173–215.

Miller, E.C. and Miller, J.A. (1971). The mutagenicity of chemical carcinogens: correlations, problems and interpretations. In: *Chemical Mutagens, Principles and Methods for Their Detection* (Hollaender, A., Ed.), Vol. 1. Plenum Press, New York, pp. 83–120.

Miller, J.H. (1985). Pathways of mutagenesis revealed by analysis of mutational specificity. In: *Genetics of Bacteria*, (Scaife, J., Leach, D. and Galizzi, A., Eds.). Academic Press, New York, pp. 25–40.

Modrich, P. (1987). DNA mismatch correction. *Ann. Rev. Biochem.* 56: 435–466.

Monticone, R.E. and Schneider, E.L. (1979). Induction of SCEs in human cells by fluorescent light. *Mutation Res.* 59: 215–221.

Morimoto, K., Sato, M. and Koizumi, A. (1983). Proliferative kinetics of human lymphocytes in culture measure by autoradiography and sister chromatid differential staining. *Epithel. Cell Res.*, 145: 249–356.

Mortelmanns, K.E. and Dousman, L. (1986). Mutagenesis and plasmids. In: *Chemical Mutagens, Principles and Methods for Their Detection*, (de Serres, F.J., Ed.). Vol. 10, Plenum Press, New York, pp. 469–508.

Mortelmanns, K.E. and Strocker, B.A.D. (1979). Segregation of the mutator property of plasmid R46 from its ultraviolet-protecting property. *Mol. Gen. Genet.* 167: 317–328.

MRC (1981). *Guidelines for Work with Chemical Carcinogens in Medical Research Council Establishments*, Medical Research Council, London.

Muller, H.J. (1927). Artificial transmutation of the gene. *Science* 66: 84–87.

Natajaran, A.T., Tates, A.D., van Buul, P.P.W., Meijers, M. and de Vogel, N. (1976). Cytogenetic effects of mutagens/carcinogens after activation in a microsomal system *in vitro. Mutat. Res.* 37: 83–90.

Natarajan, A.T. and Obe, G. (1982). Mutagenicity testing with cultured mammalian cells: cytogenetic assays. In: *Mutagenicity, New Horizons in Genetic Toxicology*, (Heddle, J.A., Ed.). Academic Press, New York, pp. 172–213.

Neudecker, T. and Henschler, D. (1985). Allyl isothiocyanate is mutagenic in *Salmonella typhimurium. Mutation Res.* 30: 143–148.

Newton, M.F. and Lilly, L.J. (1986). Tissue specific clastogenic effects of chromium and selenium salts *in vivo. Mutation Res.* 169: 61–69.

Oberly, T.J., Bewsey, B.J. and Probst, G.S. (1987). A procedure for the CHO/HGPRT mutation assay involving treatment of cells in suspension culture and selection of mutants in soft agar. *Mutation Res.* 182: 99–111.

OECD (1983). *OECD Guidelines for the Testing of Chemicals*. No. 475. Genetic toxicology: *in vivo* mammalian bone marrow cytogenetic test: chromosomal analysis. Adopted 4 April 1984.

Ong. T., Mukhtar, M., Wolf, C.R. and Zeiger, E. (1980). Differential effects of cytochrome P450-inducers on promutagen activation capabilities and enzymatic activities of S-9 from rat liver. *J. Environ. Pathol. Toxicol.* 4: 55–65.

Pagano, D.A. and Zeiger, E. (1985). The stability of mutagenic chemicals tested in solution. *Environ. Mutagen.* 7: 293–302.

Painter, R.B. (1980). A replication model of sister-chromatid exchange. *Mutation Res.* 70: 337–341.

Parry, J.M., Arlett, C.F. and Ashby, J. (1985). An overview of the results of the *in vivo* and *in vitro* test systems used to assay the genotoxicity of BZD, DAT, DAB and CDA in the second UKEMS study. In: *Comparative Genetic Toxicology: The Second UKEMS Collaborative Study*, (Parry, J.M. and Arlett, C.F., Eds.). Macmillan, London, pp. 597–616.

Perry, P.E. and Evans, H.J. (1975). Cytoitological detection of mutagen/carcinogen exposure by sister chromatid exchange. *Nature* 258: 121–125.

Perry, P., Henderson, L. and Kirkland, D. (1984). Sister chromatid exchange in cultured cells. In: *UKEMS Subcommittee on Guidelines for Mutagenicity Testing. Report Part IIA*, pp. 89–121.

Perry, P.E. and Thomson, E.J. (1984). Sister chromatid exchange methodology. In: *Handbook of Mutagenicity Test Procedures*, (Kilbey, B.J., Legator, M., Nichols, W. and Ramel, C., Eds.). Elsevier, Amsterdam, pp. 495–529.

Perry, P.E. and Wolff, S. (1974). New Giemsa method for the differential staining of sister chromatids. *Nature* 251: 156–158.

Pinney, R.J. (1980). Distribution among incompatibility groups of plasmids that confer UV mutability and UV resistance. *Mutation Res.* 72: 155–159.

Preston. R.J., Au, W., Bender, M., Brewen J.G., Carrano A.C., Heddle, J.A., McFee, A.F., Wolff, G. and Wassom, J. (1981). Mammalian *in vivo* and *in vitro* cytogenetic assays. *Mutation Res.* 87: 143–188.

Preston, R.J., San Sebastian, J.R. and McFee, A.F. (1987). The *in vitro* human lymphocyte assay for assessing the clastogenicity of chemical agents. *Mutation Res.* 189: 175–183.

Prival, M.J., Bell, S.J., Mitchell, V.D., Peiperi, M.D. and Vaughn, V.L. (1984). Mutagenicity of benzidine and benzidine-congener dyes and selected monoazo dyes in a modified *Salmonella* assay. *Mutation Res.* 136: 33–47.

Prival, M.J. and Mitchell, V.D. (1982). Analysis of a method for testing azo-dyes for mutagenic activity in *S. typhimurium* in the presence of FMN in hamster liver S9. *Mutation Res.* 97: 103–116.

Revell, S.H. (1974). The breakage-and-reunion theory and the exchange theory for chromosome aberrations induced by ionizing radiations: A short history. In: *Advances in Radiation Biology* (Lett, J.T. and Zelle, M., Eds.). Vol. 4, Academic Press, New York, pp. 367–415.

Richardson, C., Williams, D.A., Allen, J.A., Amphlett, G., Changer, D.O. and Phillips, B. (1989). Analysis of data from *in vitro* cytogenetic assays. In: *UKEMS Sub-committee on Guidelines for Mutagenicity Testing. Report. Part III. Statistical Evaluation of Mutagenicity Test Data.* (Kirkland, D.J., Ed.). Cambridge University Press, pp. 141–154.

Robinson, W.D., Green, M.H.L., Cole, J., Healy, M.J.R., Garner, R.C. and Gatehouse, D. (1989). Statistical Evaluation of bacterial mammalian fluctuation tests. In: *Statistical Evaluation of Mutagenicity Test Data* (Kirkland, D.J., Ed.). Cambridge University Press, pp. 102–140.

Rossman, T.G. and Klein, C.B. (1988). From DNA damage to mutation in mammalian cells: A review. *Environ. Molec. Mutagen.* 11: 119–133.

Roth, J.R. (1974). Frameshift mutations. *Ann. Rev. Genet.* 8: 319–346.

Russell, L.B. (1984). Procedures and evaluation of results of the mouse spot test. In: *Handbook of Mutagenicity Test Procedures* (Kilbey, B.J., Legator, M., Nichols, W. and Ramel, C., Eds.). Elsevier, Amsterdam, pp. 393–403.

Russell, W.L. (1951). X-ray induced mutations in mice. *Cold Spring Harbor Symp. Quantum Biol.*, 16: 327–336.

Russell, W.L. (1989). Reminiscences of a mouse specific-locus addict. *Environ. Mol. Mutagen.*, 14 (Suppl. 16): 16–22.

Samson, L. and Cairns, J. (1977). A new pathway for DNA repair in *E. coli. Nature* 267: 281–282.

Scott, D., Danford, N., Dean, B., Kirkland, D. and Richardson, C. (1983). *In vitro* chromosome aberration assays. In: *UKEMS Subcommittee on Guidelines for Mutagenicity Testing, Report Part I, Basic Test Battery* (Dean, B.J., Ed.). UKEMS, Swansea, U.K., pp. 63–86.

Scott, D., Dean, B.J., Danford, N.D. and Kirkland, D.J. (1990). Metaphase chromosome aberration assays *in vitro*. In: *UKEMS Subcommittee on Guidelines for Mutagenicity Testing, Report. Part I: Revised Basic Mutagenicity Tests, UKEMS Recommended Procedures* (Kirkland, D.J., Ed.). Cambridge University Press, pp. 63–86.

Searle, A.G. (1984). The specific locus test in the mouse. In: *Handbook of Mutagenicity Test Procedures* (Kilbey, B.J., Legator, M., Nichols, W. and Ramel, C., Eds.). Elsevier, Amsterdam, pp. 373–391.

Sedgwick, S.G. and Goodwin, P.A. (1985). Differences in mutagenic and recombinational DNA repair in enterobacteria. *Proc. Nat. Acad. Sci. U.S.A.* 82: 4172–4176.

Selby, P.B. and Olson, W.H. (1981). Methods and criteria for deciding whether specific-locus mutation-rate data in mice indicates a positive, negative or inconclusive result. *Mutation Res.* 83: 403–418.

Shanabruch, W.G. and Walker, G.C. (1980). Localization of the plasmid (pKM101) gene(s) involved in $recA^+lexA^+$-dependent mutagenesis. *Mol. Gen. Genet.* 129: 289–297.

Steel, R.G.D. and Torrie, J.H. (1960). *Principles and Procedures of Statistics*, McGraw-Hill, New York.

Streisinger, G., Okada, T., Emrich, J., Newton J., Tougita, A., Terzaghi, E. and Inouye, M. (1966). Frameshift mutations and the genetic code. *Cold Spring Harbor Symp. Quantum Biol.* 31: 77–84.

Tates, A.D., Neuteboom, I., Hofker, M. and den Engelese, L. (1980). A micronucleus technique for detecting clastogenic effects of mutagens/carcinogens (DEN, DMN) in hepatocytes of rat liver *in vivo. Mutation Res.* 74: 11–20.

Taylor, J.H. (1958). Sister chromatid exchanges in tritium labeled chromosomes. *Genetics* 43: 515–529.

Tennant, R.W., Margolin, B.H., Shelby, M.D., Zeiger, E., Haseman, J.K., Spalding, J., Caspary, W., Resnick, M., Stasiewicz, S., Anderson, B. and Minor, R. (1987). Prediction of chemical carcinogenicity in rodents from *in vitro* genetic toxicity assays. *Science* 236: 933–941.

Thomas, S.M. and Sedgwick, S.G. (1989). Cloning of *Salmonella typimurium* DNA encoding mutagenic DNA repair. *J. Bacteriol.* 171: 5776–5782.

Thompson, E.D. (1986). Comparison of *in vivo* and *in vitro* cytogenetic assay results. *Environ. Mutagen.* 8: 753–767.

Thust, R., Mendel, J., Schwarz, H. and Warzoki, R. (1980). Nitrosated urea pesticide metabolites and other nitrosamides. Activity in clastogenicity and SCE assays, and aberration kinetics in Chinese hamster V79-E cells. *Mutation Res.* 79: 239–248.

Topham, J., Albanese, R., Bootman, J., Scott, D. and Tweats, D. (1983). *In vivo* cytogenetic assays. In: *Report of UKEMS Sub-committee on Guidelines for Mutagenicity Testing. Part I* (Dea, B., Ed.). pp. 119–141.

*Transformation Assays of Established Cell Lines: Mechanisms and Application.* (Kakunaga, T. and Yamasaki, H., Eds). Proceedings of a Workshop Organized by IARC in Collaboration with the U.S. National Cancer Institute and the U.S. Environmental Protection Agency, Lyon 15–17 Feb. 1984. IARC Scientific Publication No. 67.

Tsuchimoto, T. and Matter, B.E. (1979). *In vivo* cytogenetic screening methods for mutagens with special reference to the micronucleus test. *Arch. Toxicol.* 42: 239–248.

Tweats, D.J. and Gatehouse, D.G. (1988). Discussion forum: Further debate of testing strategies. *Mutagenesis* 3: 95–102.

Venitt, S. and Crofton-Sleigh, C. (1981). Mutagenicity of 42 coded compounds in a bacterial assay using *Escherichia coli* and *Salmonella typhimurium*. In: *Evaluation of Short-term Tests for Carcinogens. Report of the International Collaborative Program. Progress in Mutational Research* (de Serres, F.J. and Ashby J., Eds.). Vol 1. Elsevier, New York, pp. 351–360.

Venitt, S. and Parry, J.M. (1984). Background to mutagenicity testing. In: *Mutagenicity Testing, a Practical Approach* (Venitt, S. and Parry, J.M., Eds.). IRL Press, Oxford, pp. 1–24.

Villani, G., Boiteux, S. and Radman, M. (1978). Mechanisms of ultraviolet-induced mutagenesis: extent and fidelity of *in vitro* DNA synthesis on irradiated template. *Proc. Nat. Acad. Sci. USA* 75: 3037–3041.

Wagner, R. and Meselson, M. (1976). Repair tracts in mismatched DNA heteroduplexes. *Proc. Natl. Acad. Sci. USA.* 73: 4135–4139.

Wahrendorf, J., Mahon, G.A.T. and Schumacher, M. (1985). A non-parametric approach to the statistical analysis of mutagenicity data. *Mutation Res.* 147: 5–13.

Walker, G.C. (1984). Mutagenesis and inducible responses to deoxyribonucleic acid damage in *Escherichia coli. Microbiol. Rev.* 48: 60–93.

Walker, G.C. and Dobson, P.P. (1979). Mutagenesis and repair deficiencies of *Escherichia coli umu C* mutants are suppressed by the plasmid pKM101. *Proc. Gen. Genet.* 172: 17–24.

Wilcox, P., Naidoo, A., Wedd, D.J. and Gatehouse, D.G. (1990). Comparison of *Salmonella Typhimurium* TA102 with *Escherichia coli* WP2 tester strains. *Mutagenesis* 5: 285–291.

Wolff, S. (1977a). Lesions that lead to SCEs are different from those that lead to chromosome aberrations. *Mutation Res.* 46: 164.

Wolff, S. (1977b). *In vitro* inhibition of mono-oxygenase dependent reactions by organic solvents. *International Conference on Industrial and Environmental Xenobiotics*, Prague, Czechoslovakia.

Wolff, S. and Perry, P. (1974). Differential staining of sister chromatids and the study of sister chromatid exchange with out autoradiography. *Chromosomes* 48: 341–353.

Yahagi, T., Degawa, M., Seino, Y., Matsushima, T. and Okada, M. (1975). Mutagenicity of carcinogen azo dyes and their derivatives. *Cancer Lett.* 1: 91–96.

Yahagi, T., Nagao, M., Seino, Y., Matsushima, T., Sugimura, T. and Okada, M. (1977). Mutagenicities of *N*-nitrosamines in *Salmonella. Mutation Res.* 48: 120–130.

Yanofsky, C. (1971). Mutagenesis studies with *Escherichia coli* mutants with known amino acid and base-pair) changes. In: *Chemical Mutagens, Principles and Methods for Their Detection* (Hollaender A., Ed.). Vol. 1, Plenum Press, New York, pp. 283–287.

7

# SUBCHRONIC AND CHRONIC TOXICITY STUDIES

## 7.1. INTRODUCTION

In the broadest sense, subchronic and chronic studies for pharmaceutical products can incorporate any of the routes used to administer a therapeutic agent, use any of a number of animal models, and conform to a broad range of experimental designs. They can be two weeks long (what used to be called "subacute" studies because they were conducted at dose levels below those employed for single-dose or acute studies) or last up to a year. Another name for these studies is repeat-dose studies (Ballantyne, 2000), that is, those studies whereby animals have a therapeutic agent administered to them on a regular and repeated basis by one or more routes over a period of one year or less. There is great flexibility and variability in the design of such studies.

This chapter seeks to provide a firm grasp of the objectives for repeat-dose studies, the regulatory requirements governing them, the key factors in their design and conduct, and the interpretation of their results. There are a number of review chapters which deal with the general case of such studies (Wilson et al., 2001 being the most recent) that provide useful background.

## 7.2. OBJECTIVES

As with any scientific study or experiment (but especially for those in safety assessment), the essential first step is to define and understand the reason(s) for the conduct of the study, its objectives. There are three major (scientific) reasons for conducting subchronic and chronic studies, but a basic characteristic of all but a few

237

subchronic studies needs to be understood. The subchronic study is (as are most other studies in whole animal toxicology) a broad screen. It is not focused on a specific endpoint; rather, it is a broad exploration of the cumulative biological effects of the administered agent over a range of doses. So broad an exploration, in fact, that it can be called a "shotgun" study.

The objectives of the typical subchronic study fall into three categories. The first is to broadly define the toxicity (and, if one is wise, the pharmacology and hyperpharmacology) of repeated doses of a potential therapeutic agent in an animal model (Traina, 1983). This definition is both qualitative (what are the target organs and the nature of the effects seen?) and quantitative (at what dose levels, or, more important, at what plasma and tissue levels, are effects definitely seen and not seen?).

The second objective (and the one that in the pharmaceutical industry lab usually compels both timing and compromising of design and execution) is to provide support for the initiation of and/or continued conduct of clinical trials in humans (O'Grady and Linet, 1990; Smith, 1992). As such, subchronic studies should provide not only adequate clearance (therapeutic margin) of initial dose levels and duration of dosing, but also guidance for any special measures to be made or precautions to be taken in initial clinical trials. Setting inadequate dose levels (either too low or too high) may lead to the failure of a study. A successful study must both define a safe, or "clean," dose level (one that is as high as possible, to allow as much flexibility as possible in the conduct of clinical studies), and demonstrate and/or characterize signs of toxicity at some higher dose. The duration of dosing issue is driven by a compromise between meeting regulatorily established guidelines (as set out in Table 7.1) and the economic pressure to initiate clinical trials as soon as possible.

The third objective is one of looking forward to later studies. The subchronic study must provide sufficient information to allow a prudent setting of doses for later, longer studies (including, ultimately, carcinogenicity studies). At the same time, the subchronic study must also provide guidance for the other (than dose) design features of longer-term studies (such as what parameters to measure and when to measure them, how many animals to use and how long to conduct the study).

**TABLE 7.1. Duration of Treatment Supported by Preclinical Studies**

| Animal Study Length | Generally Allowed Human Dosing |
| --- | --- |
| 2 weeks | Up to 3 doses |
| 1 month | 10 days |
| 3 months | 1 month |
| 1 year (rodent) | Unlimited |
| 9 months (dog) (U.S.) | |
| 6 months (dog) (EEC & Japan) | |

These objectives are addressed by the usual subchronic study. Some subchronic studies, however, are unusual in being conceived, designed, and executed to address specific questions raised (or left unanswered) by previous preclinical or early clinical studies. Such a special purpose is addressed separately.

Chronic studies (those that last six or nine months or a year) may also be conducted for the above purposes but are primarily done to fulfill registration requirements for drugs that are intended for continuous long-term (lifetime) use or frequent intermittent use.

## 7.3. REGULATORY CONSIDERATIONS

Much of what is done (and how it is done) in repeat-dose studies is a response to a number of regulations. Three of these have very broad impact. These are the Good Laboratory Practices requirements, Animal Welfare Act requirements, and regulatory requirements that actually govern study design.

### 7.3.1. Good Laboratory Practices (GLPs)

Since 1978, the design and conduct of preclinical safety assessment studies for pharmaceuticals in the United States (and, indeed, internationally) have been governed and significantly influenced by GLPs. Strictly speaking, these regulations cover qualifications of staff and facilities, training, record-keeping, documentation, and actions required to insure compliance with and the effectiveness of these steps. Though the initial regulations were from the U.S. Food and Drug Administration (FDA, 1983), they have always extended to cover studies performed overseas (FDA, 1988a). Most other countries have adopted similar regulations. A discussion of these regulations is beyond the scope of the current chapter, but several aspects are central to this effort. Each technique or methodology to be employed in a study (such as animal identification, weighing and examination, blood collection, data recording, and so on) must be adequately described in a standard operating procedure (SOP) before the study begins. Those who are to perform such procedures must be trained in them beforehand. The actual design of the study, including start date and how it is to be ended and analyzed, plus the principal scientists involved (particularly the study director), must be specified in a protocol that is signed before the study commences. Any changes to these features must be documented in amendments once the study has begun. It is a good practice for the pathologist who is to later perform or oversee histopathology to be designated before the start of the study, and that the design be a team effort involving the best efforts of the toxicologist, pathologist, and (usually, for subchronic studies) the drug metabolism scientist.

### 7.3.2. Animal Welfare Act

Gone are the days when the pharmaceutical scientist could conduct whatever procedures or studies that were desired using experimental animals. The Animal

Welfare Act (APHIS, 1989) (and its analogues in other countries) rightfully requires careful consideration of animal usage to ensure that research and testing uses as few animals as possible in as humane a manner as possible. As a start, all protocols must be reviewed by an Institutional Animal Care and Use Committee. Such review takes time, but should not serve to hinder good science. When designing a study or developing a new procedure or technique, the following points should be kept in mind.

1. Will the number of animals used be sufficient to provide the required data yet not constitute excessive use? (It ultimately does not reduce animal use to utilize too few animals to begin with and then have to repeat the study.)
2. Are the procedures employed the least invasive and traumatic available? This practice is not only required by regulations, but is also sound scientific practice, since any induced stress will produce a range of responses in test animals that can mask or confound the chemically induced effects.

### 7.3.3. Regulatory Requirements for Study Design

The first consideration in the construction of a study is a clear statement of its objectives, which are almost always headed by meeting regulatory requirements to support drug development and registration. Accordingly, the relevant regulatory requirements must be analyzed, which is complicated by the fact that new drugs are no longer developed for registration and sale in a single-market country. The expense is too great, and the potential for broad international sales too appealing. While each major country has its own requirements as to study designs and studies required (with most of the smaller countries adhering to the regulations of one of the major players), harmonization has done much to smooth these differences (Adler and Zbinden, 1988). Meeting these regulatory requirements is particularly challenging for several reasons. First, the only official delineation of general requirements in the Untied States is outdated (FDA, 1971), because recently special cases have arisen (anti-HIV agents, biotechnologically derived agents, therapeutic agents for neonates and the very elderly, etc.) that try the utility of these requirements. These needs have led to a stream of points-to-consider which seek to update requirements. Second, the term "guidelines" means different things in different countries (in the United States it means "requirements," and in Japan, "suggestions").

Agents intended to treat or arrest the progress of rapidly spreading life-threatening diseases (such as AIDS) are subject to less stringent safety assessment requirements prior to initial clinical evaluations than are other drugs. However, even though approval (if clinical efficacy is established) for marketing can be granted with preclinical testing still under way, all applicable safety assessments (as with any other class of drugs) must still be completed (FDA, 1988b).

Drugs intended for use in either the elderly or the very young have special additional requirements for safety evaluation, in recognition of the special characteristics and potential sensitivities of these populations. For the elderly, these requirements call for special consideration of renal and hepatic effects [Center for Drug Evaluation and Research (CDER), 1989]. Likewise, drugs intended for the young require special studies to be performed in neonates and juvenile animals (usually of two or four weeks' duration in rats).

In the last five to six years, a number of potentially important drugs have been produced by recombinant DNA technology. These biomacromolecules, which are primarily endogenously occurring proteins, present a variety of special considerations and concerns, including the following:

- Because they are endogenously occurring molecules, assessing their pharmacokinetics and metabolism presents special problems.

- Is the externally commercially produced molecule biologically equivalent to the naturally occurring one?

- As proteins, are they immunogenic or do they provoke neutralizing antibodies that will limit their usefulness?

- Because they are available only in very small quantities, the use of traditional protocols (such as those that use ever-increasing doses until an adverse effect is achieved) is impractical.

- Agents with such specific activity in humans may not be appropriately evaluated in rodents or other model species.

Each of these points must be addressed in any safety testing plan (Weissinger, 1989). The requirements set out in this chapter are designed to do this (for repeat-dose testing).

## 7.4. STUDY DESIGN AND CONDUCT

### 7.4.1. Animals

In all but a few rare cases, for pharmaceutical safety assessment, separate studies in at least two species are required. Regulations require that both species be mammalian, and one of these must be a nonrodent; practice and economics dictate that the other species will be a rodent. With extremely rare exceptions, the rodent species employed is the rat (though the mouse also sees significant use). There is considerably more variability in the nonrodent species, with a range of factors determining whether the dog (most common choice), a primate species (typically the rhesus or cynomolgus, though some others are used in particular cases), the pig (particularly in Europe), or some other animal (the ferret, for example) is selected. The factors that should and do govern species selection are presented in detail in Gad and Chengelis (1992). The use of multiple species is a regulatory requirement arising from experience and the belief (going back to 1944, at least) that such use will provide a better chance of detecting the full range of biological responses (adverse and otherwise) to the new molecular entity being evaluated. This belief has

**TABLE 7.2. Numbers of Animals for Chronic and Subchronic Study per Test Group**

| Study Length | Rats per Sex | Dogs per Sex | Primates per Sex |
| --- | --- | --- | --- |
| Two–four weeks | 5–10 | 3–4 | 3 |
| Three months[a] | 20 | 6 | 5 |
| Six months | 30 | 8 | 5 |
| One year | 50 | 10 | 10 |

[a]Starting with 13-week studies, one should consider adding animals (particularly to the high-dose group) to allow evaluation of reversal (or progression) of effects.

come under fire in recent years (Zbinden, 1993), but is unlikely to be changed soon. Along the same lines, unless an agent is to be used by only one sex or the other of humans, equal numbers of both sexes of an animal species are utilized in the studies, with the sexes being treated as unrelated for purposes of statistical analysis. Also except in rare cases, the animals used are young, healthy adults in the logarithmic phase of their growth curve. (The FDA specifies that rodents be less than six weeks of age at the initiation of dosing; FDA, 1993.)

The number of animals to be used in each dose group of a study are presented in Table 7.2. Though the usual practice is to use three different dose groups and at least one equal-sized control group, this number is not fixed and should be viewed as a minimum (see the section on study design later in this chapter). Use of more groups allows for a reduction in the risk of not clearly defining effects and establishing the highest possible safe dose at a modest increase in cost. There must be as many control animals as are in the largest-size test group to optimize statistical power.

Animals are assigned to groups (test and control) by one or another form of statistical randomization. Prior to assignment, animals are evaluated for some period of time after being received in house (usually at least one week for rodents and two for nonrodents) to ensure that they are healthy and have no discernible abnormalities. The randomization is never pure; it is always "blocked" in some form or another (by initial body weight, at least) so that each group is not (statistically) significantly different from the others in terms of the "blocked" parameters.

Proper facilities and care for test animals is not only a matter of regulatory compliance (and a legal requirement), but also essential for a scientifically sound and valid study. Husbandry requires clean cages of sufficient size and continuous availability of clean water and food (unless the protocol requires some restriction on their availability). Environmental conditions (temperature, humidity, and light–dark cycle) must be kept within specified limits. All of these must, in turn, be detailed in the protocols of studies. The limits for these conditions are set forth in relevant NIH and USDA publications.

### 7.4.2. Routes and Setting Doses

Route (how an agent is administered to a test animal) and dose (how much of and how frequently an agent is administered) are inseparable in safety assessment studies, and really cannot be defined independently. The selection of both begins with an understanding of the intended use of the drug in humans. The ideal case is to have the test material administered by the same route, at the same frequency (once a day, three times a day, etc.), and for the same intervals (continuously, if the drug is an intravenously infused agent, for example) as the drug's eventual use in people. Practical considerations such as the limitations of animal models (i.e., there are some things you can't get a rat to do), limitations on technical support,* and the like, and regulatory requirements (discussed below as part of dose setting) frequently act or interact to preclude this straightforward approach.

Almost 30 routes exist for administration of drugs to patients, but only a handful of these are commonly used in preclinical safety studies (Gad, 1994). The most common deviation from what is to be done in clinical trials is the use of parenteral (injected) routes such as IV (intravenous) and SC (subcutaneous) deliveries. Such injections are loosely characterized as bolus (all at once or over a very short period, such as five minutes) and infusion (over a protracted period of hours, days, or even months). The term *continuous infusion* implies a steady rate over a protracted period, requiring some form of setup such as an implanted venous catheter or infusion port.

It is rare that the raw drug (drug substance) itself is suitable (in terms of stability, local tissue tolerance, and optimum systemic absorption and distribution) for direct use as a dosage form. Either it must be taken into a solution or suspension in a suitable carrier, or a more complex formulation (a prototype of the commercial form) must be developed. Gad and Chengelis (1999) should be consulted for a more complete discussion of dose formulation for animals or humans. One formulation or more must be developed (preferably the same one for both animals and humans) based on the specific requirements of preclinical dosage formulation. For many therapeutic agents, limitations on volumes that can be administered and concentrations of active ingredients that can be achieved impact heavily on dose setting.

Setting of doses for longer-term toxicity studies is one of the most difficult tasks in study design. The doses administered must include one that is devoid of any adverse effect (preferably of *any* effect) and yet still high enough to "clear" the projected clinical dose by the traditional or regulatory safety factors ($10\times$ for rodents, $5\times$ for nonrodents). At the same time, if feasible, at least one of the doses should characterize the toxicity profile associated with the agent (for some biotechnologically derived agents, particularly those derived from endogenous human molecules, it may only be possible to demonstrate biological effects in appropriate disease models, and impossible to demonstrate toxicity). Because of limitations on availability of proto-drugs, it is generally undesirable to go too high to achieve this second (toxicity) objective.

Traditionally, studies include three or more dose groups to fulfill these two objectives. Based on earlier results (generally, single-dose or two-week studies),

---

*Many antiviral agents, particularly some anti-HIV agents, have rather short plasma half-lives, which require frequent oral administration of the agent. Thirteen-week studies have been conducted with t.i.d. dosing of rats and monkeys, requiring around-the-clock shift work for technical staff of the laboratory.

doses are selected. It is, by the way, generally an excellent idea to observe the "decade rule" in extrapolation of results from shorter to longer studies; that is, do not try to project doses for more than an order-of-magnitude-longer study (thus the traditional progression from single-dose to fourteen-day to ninety-day studies). Also, one should not allow the traditional use of three dose groups plus a control to limit designs. If there is a great deal of uncertainty, it is much cheaper in every way to use four or five dose groups in a single study than to have to repeat the entire study. Finally, remember that different doses may be appropriate for the different sexes.

It should also be kept in mind that formulating materials may have effects of their own, and a "vehicle" control group may be required in addition to a negative control group.

### 7.4.3. Parameters to Measure

As was stated earlier, subchronic studies are "shotgun" in nature; that is, they are designed to look at a very broad range of endpoints with the intention of screening as broadly as indications of toxicity. Meaningful findings are rarely limited to a single endpoint; rather, what typically emerges is a pattern of findings. This broad search for components of toxicity profile is not just a response to regulatory guidelines intended to identify potentially unsafe drugs. An understanding of all the indicators of biological effect can also frequently help one to understand the relevance of findings, to establish some as unrepresentative of a risk to humans, and even to identify new therapeutic uses of an agent.

Parameters of interest in the repeat-dose study can be considered as sets of measures, each with its own history, rationale, and requirements. It is critical to remember, however, that the strength of the study design as a scientific evaluation lies in the relationships and patterns of effects that are seen not in simply looking at each of these measures (or groups) as independent findings, but rather as integrated profiles of biological effects.

***Body Weight.*** Body weight (and the associated calculated parameter of body weight gain) is a nonspecific, broad screen for adverse systemic toxicity. Animals are initially assigned to groups based on a randomization scheme that includes having each group vary insignificantly from one another in terms of body weight. Weights are measured prior to the initial dose, then typically one, three, five, seven, eleven, and fourteen days thereafter. The frequency of measurement of weights goes down as the study proceeds. After two weeks, weighing is typically weekly through six weeks, then every other week through three months, and monthly thereafter. Because the animals used in these studies are young adults in the early log phase of their growth, decreases in the rate of gain relative to control animals is a very sensitive (albeit nonspecific) indicator of systemic toxicity.

***Food Consumption.*** Food consumption is typically measured with one or two uses in mind. First, it may be explanatory in the interpretation of reductions (either absolute or relative) in body weight. In cases where administration of the test compound is via diet, it is essential to be able to adjust dietary content so as to accurately maintain dose levels. Additionally, the actual parameter itself is a broad and nonspecific indicator of systemic toxicity. Food consumption is usually measured over a period of several days, first weekly and then on a once-a-month basis. Water consumption, which is also sometimes measured, is similar in interpretation and use. Giving measured quantities of food (as opposed to the traditional *ad libitum* feeding) is recommended for studies of more than 90 days, as it precludes excessive body weight gain and the complications thereof (Allaben and Hart, 1998).

***Clinical Signs.*** Clinical signs are generally vastly underrated in value, probably because insufficient attention is paid to care in their collection. Two separate levels of data collection are actually involved here. The first is the morbidity and mortality observation, which is made twice a day. This generally consists of a simple cage-side visual assessment of each animal to determine if it is still alive, and, if so, whether it appears in good (or at least stable) health. Historically, this regulatory required observation was intended to ensure that tissues from intoxicated animals were not lost for meaningful histopathologic evaluation due to autolysis (Arnold et al., 1990).

The second level of clinical observation is the detailed hands-on examination analogous to the human physical examination. It is usually performed against a checklist (see Gad and Chengelis, 1999, for an example), and evaluation is of the incidence of observations of a particular type in a group of treated animals compared to controls. Observations range from being indicative of nonspecific systemic toxicity to fairly specific indicators of target organ toxicity. These more detailed observations are typically taken after the first week of a study and on a monthly basis thereafter.

Ophthalmologic examinations are typically made immediately prior to initiation of a study (and thus serve to screen out animals with preexisting conditions) and toward the end of a study.

Particularly when the agent under investigation either targets or acts via a mechanism likely to have a primary effect on a certain organ for which functional measures are available, an extra set of measurements of functional performance should be considered. The organs or organ systems that are usually of particular concern are the kidneys, liver, cardiovascular, nervous, and immune. Special measures (such as creatinine clearance as a measure of renal function) are combined with other data already collected (organ weights, histopathology, clinical pathology, etc.) to provide a focused "special" investigation or evaluation of adverse effects on the target organ system of concern. In larger animals (dogs and primates) some of these measures (such as ECGs) are made as a matter of course in all studies.

***Clinical Pathology.*** Clinical pathology covers a number of biochemical and morphological evaluations based on invasive and noninvasive sampling of fluids from animals that are made periodically during the course of a subchronic study. These evaluations are sometimes labeled as clinical (as opposed to anatomical) pathology determinations. Table 7.3 presents a summary of the parameters measured under the headings of clinical chemistry, hematology, and urinalysis, using samples

**TABLE 7.3. Clinical Pathology Measures**

| Clinical Chemistry | Hematology | Urinalysis |
| --- | --- | --- |
| Albumin | Erythrocyte count (RBC) | Chloride |
| Alkaline phosphatase (ALP) | Hemoglobin (HGB) | Bilirubin |
| Blood urea nitrogen (BUN) | Hematocrit (HCT) | Glucose |
| Calcium | Mean corpuscular hemoglobin | Occult blood |
| Chloride |   (MCH) | pH |
| Creatine | Mean corpuscular volume | Phosphorus |
| Creatine phosphokinase (CPK) |   (MCV) | Potassium |
| Direct bilirubin | Platelet count | Protein |
| Gamma glumly transferees | Prothrombin time | Sodium |
|   (GGT) | Reticulocyte count | Specific gravity |
| Globulin | White cell count (WBC) | Volume |
| Glucose | White cell differential count | |
| Lactic dehydrogenase (LDH) | | |
| Phosphorus | | |
| Potassium | | |
| Serum glutamic-oxaloacetic | | |
|   transaminase (SGOT) | | |
| Serum glutamic-pyruvic | | |
|   transaminase (SGPT) | | |
| Sodium | | |
| Total bilirubin | | |
| Total cholesterol | | |
| Total protein | | |
| Triglycerides | | |

of blood and urine collected at predetermined intervals during the study. Conventionally, these intervals are typically evenly spaced at three points over the course of the study, with the first being one month after study initiation and the last being immediately prior to termination of the test animals. For a three-month study, this means that samples of blood and urine would be collected at one, two, and three months after study initiation (i.e., after the first day of dosing of the animals). There are some implications of these sampling plans that should be considered when the data are being interpreted. Many of the clinical chemistry (and some of the hematologic) markers are really the result of organ system damage that may be transient in nature (see Table 7.4 for a summary of interpretations of clinical chemistry findings and Table 7.5 for a similar summary for hematologic findings). The samples on which analysis is performed are from fixed points in time, which may miss transient changes (typically, increases) in some enzyme levels.

***Pharmacokinetics and Metabolism.*** Pharmaceutical subchronic toxicity studies are always accompanied by a parallel determination of the pharmacokinetics of the material of interest administered by the same route as that used in the safety study.

**TABLE 7.4. Association of Changes in Biochemical Parameters with Actions at Particular Target Organs**

| Parameter | Organ System | | | | | | | | Notes |
|---|---|---|---|---|---|---|---|---|---|
| | Blood | Heart | Lung | Kidney | Liver | Bone | Intestine | Pancreas | |
| Albumin | | | | ↓ | ↓ | | | | Produced by the liver. Very significant reductions indicate extensive liver damage. |
| ALP (alkaline phosphatase | | | | | ↑ | ↑ | ↑ | | Elevations usually associated with cholestasis. Bone alkaline phosphatase tends to be higher in young animals. |
| Bilirubin (total) | ↑ | | | | ↑ | | | | Usually elevated due to cholestasis either due to obstruction or hepatopathy. |
| BUN (blood urea nitrogen) | | | | ↑ | ↓ | | | | Estimates blood-filtering capacity of the kidneys. Doesn't become significantly elevated until kidney function is reduced 60–75%. |
| Calcium | | | | ↑ | | | | | Can be life threatening and result in acute death. |
| Cholinesterase | | | | ↑ | ↓ | | | | Found in plasma, brain, and RBC. |

*(continued)*

**TABLE 7.4. Association of Changes in Biochemical Parameters with Actions at Particular Target Organs**

| Parameter | Organ System | | | | | | | | Notes |
| --- | --- | --- | --- | --- | --- | --- | --- | --- | --- |
| | Blood | Heart | Lung | Kidney | Liver | Bone | Intestine | Pancreas | |
| CPK (creatinine phosphokinase) | | ↑ | | | | | | | Most often elevated due to skeletal muscle damage but can also be produced by cardiac muscle damage. Can be more sensitive than histopathology. |
| Creatine | | | | ↑ | | | | | Also estimates blood-filtering capacity of kidney as BUN does. More specific than BUN. |
| Glucose | | | | | | | | ↑ | Alterations other than those associated with stress are uncommon and reflect an effect on the pancreatic islets or anorexia. |
| GGT (gamma glutamyl transferase) | | | | | ↑ | | | | Elevated in cholestasis. This is microsomal enzyme and levels often increase in response to microsomal enzyme induction. |
| HBDH (hydroxybutyric dehydrogenase) | | ↑ | | | ↑ | | | | Most prominent in cardiac muscle tissue. |

| Test | | | | | | Comments |
|---|---|---|---|---|---|---|
| LDH (lactic dehydrogenase) | ↑ | ↑ | ↑ | ↑ | | Increase usually due to skeletal muscle, cardiac muscle, and liver damage. Not very specific unless isozymes are evaluated. |
| Protein (total) | | | ↑ | ↑ | | Absolute alterations are usually associated with decreased production (liver) or increased loss (kidney). |
| SGOT (serum glutamic oxaloacetic transaminase); also called AST (asparate amino transferase) | ↑ | | ↑ | ↑ | ↑ | Present in skeletal muscle and heart and most commonly associated with damage to these. |
| SGPT (serum glutamic-pyruvic transaminase); also called ALT (alanide amino transferase) | | | | ↑ | | Evaluations usually associated with hepatic damage or disease. |
| SDH (sorbitol dehydrogenase) | | | | ↑ or ↓ | | Liver enzyme which can be quite sensitive but is fairly unstable. Samples should be processed as soon as possible. |

**TABLE 7.5. Some Probable Conditions Affecting Hematological Changes**

| Parameter | Elevation | Depression |
| --- | --- | --- |
| Red blood cells | Vascular shock | Anemias |
| | Excessive diuresis | Blood loss |
| | Chronic hypoxia | Hemolysis |
| | Hyperadrenocorticism | Low RBC production |
| Hematocrit | Increased RBC | Anemias |
| | Stress | Pregnancy |
| | Shock | Excessive hydrdation |
| | (a) Trauma | |
| | (b) Surgery | |
| | Polycythemia | |
| Hemoglobin | Polycythemia (increase in production of RBC) | Anemias |
| | | Lead poisonings |
| Mean cell volume | Anemias | Iron deficiency |
| | B-12 deficiency | |
| Mean corpuscular hemoglobin | Reticulocytosis | Iron deficiency |
| White blood cells | Bacterial infections | Bone marrow depression |
| | Bone marrow stimulation | Cancer chemotherapy |
| | | Chemical intoxication |
| | | Splenic disorders |
| Platelets | | Bone marrow depression |
| | | Immune disorder |
| Neutrophilis | Acute bacterial infections | Viral infections |
| | Tissue necrosis | |
| | Strenuous exercise | |
| | Convulsions | |
| | Tachycardia | |
| | Acute hemorrhage | |
| Lymphocytes | Leukemia | |
| | Malnutrition | |
| | Viral infections | |
| Monocytes | Protozoal infections | |
| Eosinophils | Allergy | |
| | Irradiation | |
| | Pernicious anemia | |
| | Parasitism | |
| Basophils | Lead poisoning | |

This parallel determination consists of measuring plasma levels of the administered agent and its major metabolites either in animals that are part of the main study or in a separate set of animals (in parallel with the main study) that are dosed and evaluated to determine just these endpoints. The purpose of these determinations is both to allow a better interpretation of the findings of the study and to encourage the most accurate possible extrapolation to humans. The first data of interest are the absorption, distribution, and elimination of the test material, but a number of other types of information can also be collected (Yacobi et al., 1989; Tse and Jaffe, 1991). For nonparenteral routes it is essential to demonstrate that systemic absorption and distribution of the test material did occur; otherwise, it is open to question whether the potential safety of the agent in man has been adequately addressed (not to mention the implication for potential human therapeutic efficacy).

### 7.4.4. Other In-Life Endpoints for Evaluation

***Ophthalmology.*** Ophthalmological examination of all animals in study (particularly nonrodents) should be performed both before study initiation and at the completion of the period at which the drug is administered. This should be performed by an experienced veterinary ophthalmologist.

***Cardiovascular Function.*** Particularly in light of recent concerns with drug-induced arrhythmias, careful consideration must be given to incorporating adequate evaluation of drug induced alterations on cardiovascular function. This is usually achieved by measuring blood pressure, heart rate, and by an EKG pre-study and periodically during the course of the study (usually at at least one intermediate period and at the end of the study) in the nonrodent species being employed. The Q to T interval should specifically be evaluated.

***Neurotoxicology.*** Table 7.6 presents the FDA's current draft criteria (FDA, 1993, 2000) for endpoints to be incorporated in studies as a screen for neurotoxicity. IN practice, a functional observation battery is employed at several endpoints (usually one and three months in to the study) to fill these requirements.

***Immunotoxicology.*** In response to concerns about potential effects of drugs on the immune system, FDA (2000) has proposed that a basic set of criteria (Table 7.7) be evaluated and considered in standard subchronic and chronic studies. Most of these endpoints are, it should be noted, already collected in traditional subchronic designs.

***Pharmacokinetics.*** All subchronic and chronic toxicity studies now incorporate (either in the study itself or in a parallel study) evaluation of the basic pharmacokinetics of a compound. This is discussed in detail in Chapter 18.

### 7.4.5. Histopathology

Histopathology is generally considered the single most significant portion of data to come out of a repeat-dose toxicity study. It actually consists of three related sets of data (gross pathology observations, organ weights, and microscopic pathology) that are collected during the termination of the study animals. At the end of the study, a number of tissues are collected during termination of all surviving animals (test and

**TABLE 7.6. FDA Draft Criteria for a Neurotoxicity Screen as a Component of Short-Term and Subchronic Studies**

Histopathological examination of tissues representative of the nervous system, including the brain, spinal cord, and peripheral nervous system

Quantitative observations and manipulative test to detect neurological, behavioral, and physiological dysfuntions. These may include:

    general appearance
    body posture
    incidence and severity of seizure
    incidence and severity of tremor, paralysis, and other dysfunction
    level of motor activity and arousal
    level of reactivity to stimuli
    motor coordination
    strength
    gait
    sensorimotor response to primary sensory stimuli
    excessive lacrimation or salivation
    pilorection
    diarrhea
    ptosis
    other signs of neurotoxicity deemed appropriate

**TABLE 7.7.  FDA Draft Recommendation for Type I Immunotoxicity Test That Can Be Included in Repeated Dose Toxicity Studies**

Hematology:
    white blood cell counts
    differential white blood cell counts
    lymphocytosis
    lymphopenia
    eosinophilia
Histopathology:
    lymphoid tissues
    spleen
        lymph nodes
        thymus
        Peyer's patches in gut
        bone marrow
    cytology (if needed)[a]
        prevalence of activated macrophages
        tissue prevalence and location of lymphocytes
        evidence of B-cell germinal centers
        evidence of T-cell germinal centers
    necrotic or proliferative changes in lymphoid tissues

Clinical chemistry:
    total serum production
    albumin
    albumin-to-globulin ratio
    serum transaminases

[a]More comprehensive cytological evaluation of the tissues would not be done unless there is evidence of potential immunotoxicity from the preceding evaluations.

control). Organ weight and terminal body weights are recorded at study termination, so that absolute and relative (to body weight) values can be statistically evaluated.

These tissues, along with the organs for which weights are determined, are listed in Table 7.5. All tissues collected are typically processed for microscopic observation, but only those from the high-dose and control groups are necessarily evaluated microscopically. If a target organ is discovered in the high-dose group, then successively lower-dose groups are examined until a "clean" (devoid of effect) level is discovered (Haschek and Rousseaup, 1991).

In theory, all microscopic evaluations should be performed blind (without the pathologist knowing from which dose group a particular animal came), but this is difficult to do in practice and such an approach frequently degrades the quality of the evaluation. Like all the other portions of data in the study, proper evaluation benefits from having access to all data that addresses the relevance, severity, timing, and potential mechanisms of a specific toxicity. Blind examination is best applied in peer review or consultations on specific findings.

In addition to the "standard" set of tissues specified in Table 7.8, observations during the course of the study or in other previous studies may dictate that additional tissues be collected or special examinations (e.g., special stains, polarized light or electron microscopy, immunocytochemistry, or quantitative morphometry) be undertaken to evaluate the relevance of, or understand the mechanisms underlying, certain observations.

Histopathology testing is a terminal procedure, and, therefore, sampling of any single animal is a one-time event (except in the case of a tissue collected by biopsy). Because it is a regulatory requirement that the tissues from a basic number of

**TABLE 7.8. Tissues for Histopathology**

| | |
|---|---|
| Adrenals[a] | Mainstream bronchi |
| Body and cervix | Major salivary gland |
| Brain, all three levels[a] | Mesenteric lymph nodes |
| Cervical lymph nodes | Ovaries and tubes |
| Cervical spinal cord | Pancreas |
| Duodenum | Pituitary |
| Esophagogastric junction | Prostate |
| Esophagus | Skeletal muscle from proximal hind limb |
| Eyes with optic nerves | Spleen[a] |
| Femur with marrow | Sternebrae with marrow |
| Heart | Stomach |
| Ileum | Testes with epididymides[a] |
| Kidneys[a] | Thymus and mediastinal contents[a] |
| Large bowel | Thyroid with parathyroid[a] |
| Larynx with thyroid and parathyroid | Trachea |
| Liver[a] | Urinary bladder |
| Lungs[a] | Uterus including horns |

[a]Organs to be weighed.

animals be examined at the stated end of the study, an assessment of effects at any other time course (most commonly, to investigate recovery from an effect found at study termination) requires that satellite groups of animals be incorporated into the study at start-up. Such animals are randomly assigned at the beginning of the study, and otherwise treated exactly the same as the equivalent treatment (or control) animals.

### 7.4.6. Study Designs

The traditional design for a repeat-dose toxicity study is very straightforward. The appropriate number of animals of each sex are assigned to each of the designated dose and control groups. Unfortunately, this basic design is taken by many to be dogma, even when it does not suit the purposes of the investigator. There are many possible variations to study design, but four basic factors should be considered: controls, the use of interval and satellite groups, balanced and unbalanced designs, and staggered starts.

Classically, a single control group of the same size as each of the dose groups is incorporated into each study. Some studies incorporate two control groups (each the same size as the experimental groups) to guard against having a statistically significant effect due to one control group being abnormal for one or more parameters (a much more likely event when laboratory animals were less genetically homogeneous than they are now). The belief is that a "significant" finding that differs from one (but not both) of the concurrent control groups, and does not differ from historical control data, can be considered as not biologically significant. This is, however, an indefensible approach. Historical controls have value, but it is the concurrent control group(s) in a study that is of concern.

Interval or satellite groups have been discussed at two earlier points in this chapter. They allow measurement of termination parameters at intervals other than at termination of the study. They are also useful when the manipulation involved in making a measurement (such as the collection of an extensive blood sample), while not terminal, may compromise (relative to other animals) the subject animals. Another common use of such groups is to evaluate recovery from some observed effect at study termination.

Usually, each of the groups in a study is the same size, with each of the sexes being equally represented. The result is called a balanced design, with statistical power for detection of effects optimized for each of the treatment groups. If one knows little about the dose-toxicity profile, this is an entirely sound and rational approach. However, there are situations when one may wish to utilize an unbalanced design, that is, to have one or more dose groups larger than the others. This is usually the case when either greater sensitivity is desired (typically in a low-dose group), or an unusual degree of attrition of test animals is expected (usually due to mortality in a high-dose group), or as a guard against a single animal's idiopathic response being sufficient to cause "statistical significance."

As it is the normal practice to have a balanced design, it is also traditional to initiate treatment of all animals at the same time. This may lead to problems at study termination, however. It is a very uncommon toxicology laboratory that can "bring a study down" on a single day. In fact, there are no labs that can collect blood and perform necropsies in a single day on even the 48 to 80 dogs involved in a study, much less the 160 to 400+ rats in the rodent version. Starting all animals on study the same day presents a number of less than desirable options. The first is to terminate as many animals as can be done each day, continuing to dose (and therefore, further affect) the remaining test animals. Assuming that the animals are being terminated in a random, balanced manner, this means that the last animals terminated will have received from three to ten additional days of treatment. At the least, this is likely to cause some variance inflation (and therefore both decrease the power of the study design and possibly confound interpretation). If the difference in the length of treatment of test animals is greater than 3% of the intended length of the study, one should consider alternative designs.

An alternative approach to study design that addresses this problem employs one of several forms of staggered starts. In these, distinct groups of animals have their dosing initiated at different times. The most meaningful form recognizes that the two sexes are in effect separate studies anyway (they are never compared statistically, with the treatment groups being compared only against the same-sex control group). Thus if the termination procedure for one sex takes three to five days, then one sex should be initiated on dosing one week and the other on the following week. This maximizes the benefits of common logistical support (such as dose formulation) and reduces the impact of differential length of dosing on study outcome.

A variation on this is to stagger the start-up either of different dose groups, or of the satellite and main study portions of dose groups. The former is to be avoided (it will completely confound study outcome), while the latter makes sense in some cases (pharmacokinetics and special measures) but not others (recovery and interval sacrifice).

## 7.5. STUDY INTERPRETATION AND REPORTING

For a successful repeat-dose study, the bottom line is the clear demonstration of a no-effect level, characterization of a toxicity profile (providing guidance for any clinical studies), enough information on pharmacokinetics and metabolism to scale dosages to human applications, and at least a basic understanding of the mechanisms involved in any identified pathogenesis. The report that is produced as a result of the study should clearly communicate these points—along with the study design and experimental procedures, summarized data and their statistical analysis—and it should be GLP compliant, suitable for FDA submission format.

Interpretation of the results of a study should be truly scientific and integrative. It is elementary to have the report state only each statistically and biologically significant finding in an orderly manner. The meaning and significance of each in relation to other findings, as well as the relevance to potential human effects, must be evaluated and addressed.

The author of the report should insure that it is accurate and complete, but also that it clearly tells a story and concludes with the relevant (to clinical development) findings.

## REFERENCES


Adler, S. and Zbinden, G. (1988). *National and International Drug Safety Guidelines*. M.T.C. Verlag, Zollikon, Switzerland.

Allaben, W.T. and Hart, R.W. (1998). Nutrition and toxicity modulation: the impact of animal body weight on study outcome. *Int. J. Toxicol.* 17, Suppl 2: 1–3.

Animal and Plant Health Inspection Service (APHIS). (1989). United States Department of Agriculture. (August 31, 1989) *Federal Register* 54 (168), 36112–36163.

Arnold, D.L., Grice, H.C. and Krawksi, D.R. (1990). *Handbook of in Vivo Toxicity Testing*. Academic Press, San Diego.

Ballantyne, B. (2000). Repeated Exposure Toxicity. In: *General and Applied Toxicology* Ballantyne, B., Marrs, T., and Syversen, T., Eds.). MacMillan, London, pp. 55–66.

CDER (Center for Drug Evaluation and Research) (1989). *Guideline for the Study of Drugs Likely to Be Used in the Elderly*. FDA, November, 1989.

Ellaben, W.T. and Hart, R.W. (1998). Nutrition and toxicity modulation: the impact of animal body weight on study outcome. *Int. J. Toxicol.* 17, Suppl. 2: 1–3.

FDA (Food and Drug Administration). (1971). *FDA Introduction to Total Drug Quality*. U.S. Government Printing Office, Washington, D.C.

FDA (Food and Drug Administration). (1983). Good Laboratory Practices for Nonclinical Laboratory Studies, *CFR* 21 Part 58, March, 1983.

FDA (Food and Drug Administration). (1988a). Good Laboratory Practices, *CFR* 21 Part 58, April, 1988.

FDA (Food and Drug Administration). (1988b). Investigational new drug, antibiotic, and biological drug product regulations, procedures for drugs intended to treat life-threatening and severely debilitating illness. *Federal Register* 53 (204): 41516–41524.

FDA (1993). *Toxicological Principles for the Safety Assessment of Direct Food Additives and Color Additives Used in Food*, "Redbook II," p. 86. Center for Food Safety and Applied Nutrition, FDA, Washington, D.C.

FDA (2000). *Toxicological Principles for the Safety of Food Ingredients, Redbook 2000*, Center for Food Safety and Applied Nutrition, FDA, Washington, D.C.

Gad, S.C. (1994). Routes in Safety Assessment Studies. *J. Amer. Coll. Toxicol.* 13: 1–17.

Gad, S.C. and Chengelis, C.P. (1999). *Acute Toxicology*, 2nd ed. Academic Press, San Diego.

Gad, S.C. and Chengelis, C.P. (1992). *Animal Models in Toxicology*. Marcel Dekker, New York.

Haschek, W.M. and Rousseaup, C.G. (1991). *Handbook of Toxicology Pathology*. Academic Press, San Diego.

O'Grady, J. and Linet, O.I. (1990). *Early Phase Drug Evaluation in Man*. CRC Press, Boca Raton, FL.

Smith, C.G. (1992). *The Process of New Drug Discovery and Development*. CRC Press, Boca Raton, FL.

Traina, v. M. (1983). The role of toxicology in drug research and development. *Med. Res. Rev.* 3: 45–72.

Tse, F.L.S. and Jaffe, J.M. (1991). *Preclinical Drug Disposition.* Marcel Dekker, New York.

Weissinger, J. (1989). Nonclinical pharmacologic and toxicologic considerations for evaluating biologic products. *Regul. Toxicol. Pharmacol.* 10: 255–263.

Wilson, N.H., Hardisty, J.F. and Hayes, J.R. (2001). Short-term, Subchronic and Chronic Toxicity Studies. In: *Principles and Methods of Toxicicology,* 4th ed. (Hayes, A.W., Ed.). Taylor & Francis, Philadelphia, PA, pp. 917–958.

Yacobi, A., Skelly, J.P. and Batra, V.K. (1989). *Toxicokinetics and New Drug Development.* Pergamon Press, New York.

Zbinden, G. (1993). The concept of multispecies testing in industrial toxicology. *Regul. Toxicol. Pharmacol.* 17: 84–94.

# 8

# DEVELOPMENTAL AND REPRODUCTIVE TOXICITY TESTING

## 8.1. INTRODUCTION

The goal of testing the developmental and reproductive toxicity of drug candidates in laboratory animals is to predict which agents would adversely affect the ability to achieve and maintain pregnancy and normal development of offspring in humans. This testing involves an extensive battery of studies based historically on guidelines promulgated by the Food and Drug Administration of the United States (FDA) in 1966 (see Food and Drug Administration, 1966, 1982, 1984 and D'Aguanno, 1973). These guidelines established three basic types of studies, Segments I, II, and III, which are based on dosing during sequential phases of the reproductive cycle. These guidelines represented a dramatic increase in the extent and sophistication of testing expected of new drug candidates. The impetus for this intensified interest was the tragic epidemic of phocomelia and other congenital malformations caused in the early 1960s by the exposure of pregnant women to the sedative thalidomide (for an excellent discussion of the history of the thalidomide tragedy, see pp. 228–249 in Schardein, 1993). Table 8.1 presents the most recent guidelines.

The types of developmental and reproductive toxicity studies performed prior to 1993 and the methods used have been extensively documented (see Palmer, 1981; Christian, 1983; Heinrichs, 1985; Heywood and James, 1985; Persaud, 1985; Schardein, 1988; Tyl, 1988; Christian and Hoberman, 1989; Khera et al., 1984; and Manson and Kang, 1989). Since June 20, 1979, the FDA has required that these studies be conducted according to Good Laboratory Practice (GLP) regulations (see FDA, 1978, 1987). The conduct of these studies had been complicated by the need to satisfy worldwide regulatory guidelines that varied from country to country. As a result, studies were conducted for regulatory purposes that, from a scientific

**258**

**TABLE 8.1. Current Regulatory Guidelines: ICH, FDA**

| Medical Agents | |
| --- | --- |
| ICH | Detection of Toxicity to Reproduction for Medicinal Products (Proposed Rule endorsed by the ICH Steering Committee at Step 4 of the ICH Process, 1994). |
| ICH | Detection of Toxicity to Reproduction for Medicinal Products. (Proposed Rule endorsed by the ICH Steering Committee at Step 4 of the ICH Process, 1995). |
| FDA | International Conference on Harmonization: Guideline on detection of toxicity to reproduction for medicinal products. Federal Register, September 22, 1994, Vol. 59, No. 183. |
| FDA | International Conference on Harmonization: Guideline on detection of toxicity to reproduction for medicinal products; Addendum on toxicity to male fertility. Federal Register, April 5, 1996, Vol. 61, No. 67. |

viewpoint, were redundant, superfluous, and/or unnecessarily complex. This situation was changed in 1993 when the International Conference on Harmonization of Technical Requirements for the Registration of Pharmaceuticals for Human Use (ICH) standardized worldwide requirements in the guideline "Detection of Toxicity to Reproduction for Medicinal Products."

This chapter briefly describes the current standard study designs and then focuses on current issues in developmental and reproductive toxicity testing.

## 8.2. ICH STUDY DESIGNS

The ICH guideline allows for various combinations of studies. The studies conducted must include evaluation of the following components

1. Male and female fertility and early embryonic development to implantation.
2. Embryo-fetal development.
3. Pre-and postnatal development including maternal function.

Table 8.2 presents a comparison of ICH, FDA, European, and Japanese guidelines.

These components would normally be evaluated in a rodent species (preferably rats) and, in addition, embryo-fetal development would be evaluated in a second species, typically the rabbit. The "most probable option" in the ICH guideline is the case where three rodent studies would be conducted that separately addressed each of the components listed above. These study designs are described below. The day of insemination or detection of evidence of mating is considered Day 0 of gestation and the day of birth is considered postpartum and postnatal Day 0. Figure 8.1 presents line charts for the ICH Stage-Study Designs.

**TABLE 8.2. Comparison of ICH Stages and Study Types with Similar Regulatory Protocols**

| ICH Stage | FDA Guidelines | Great Britain and EEC Guidelines | Japanese Guidelines | EPA OPPTS, OECD and FDA Redbook Guidelines |
|---|---|---|---|---|
| **A. Premating to conception:** Reproductive functions in adult animals, including development and maturation of gametes, mating behavior, and fertilization | Segment I | Segment I | Segment I | Multigeneration One-generation |
| **B. Conception to implantation:** Reproductive functions in the adult female, preimplantation and implantation stages of the conceptus. | Segment I | Segment I | Segment I | Multigeneration One-generation developmental toxicity |
| **C. Implantation to closure of the hard palate:** Adult female reproductive functions and development of the embryo through major organ formation. | Segment I Segment II | Segment I Segment II | Segment II | Multigeneration One-generation developmental toxicity Developmental neurotoxicity |
| **D. Closure of the hard palate to the end of pregnancy:** Adult female reproductive function, fetal development, and growth and organ development and growth. | | | | |

| | | | | |
|---|---|---|---|---|
| Segment I<br>Segment II<br>Segment III | Segment I<br>Segment II | Segment II | Multigeneration<br>One-generation developmental<br>  toxicity<br>Developmental neurotoxicity | |
| **E.  Birth to weaning:**<br>Adult female reproduction function, adaptation of the neonate to extrauterine life, including preweaning development and growth (postnatal age optimally based ;on postcoital age). | Segment I<br>Segment III<br>Pediatric | Segment I<br>Segment II<br>Segment III | Segment II<br>Segment III | Multigeneration<br>One-generation developmental<br>  toxicity<br>Developmental neurotoxicity |
| **F.  Weaning to sexual maturaity:**<br>(pediatric evaluation when treated) postweaning development and growth, adaptation to independent life and attainment of full sexual development. | Pediatric | Segment I | Segment II<br>Segment III | Multigeneration<br>Developmental neurotoxicity<br>Developmental immunotoxicity |

[a]Bolded information in stub column indicates treatment interval.

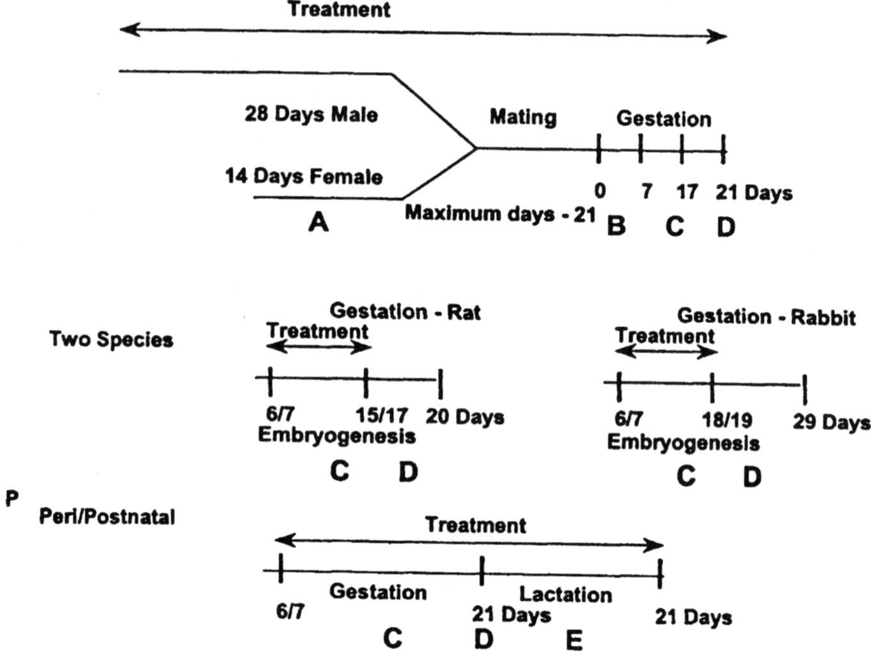


**FIGURE 8.1.** Line Charts for ICH Stage-Study Designs.

### 8.2.1. Male and Female Fertility and Early Embryonic Development to Implantation

The purpose of this component is to assess the effects that result from treatment during maturation of gametes, during cohabitation, and, in females, during gestation up through the time of embryo implantation (typically last dose on Day 6 of gestation). Assuming that the findings from a toxicity study of at least one month in duration do not contraindicate, the treatment period begins in males four weeks before male/female cohabitation and, in females, two weeks prior to cohabitation. A group size of 16 to 24 litters would generally be considered acceptable.

Minimal in-life observations include

1. Clinical signs and mortality daily.
2. Body weight twice weekly.
3. Food consumption weekly.
4. Vaginal cytology daily during cohabitation.
5. Valuable target effects seen in previous toxicity studies.

Females are sacrificed after the middle of the gestation period. Males are sacrificed at any time after the end of the cohabitation period, but it is generally advisable to retain the males until after the outcome of the first mating is known, to ensure that a repeat cohabitation with untreated females will not be needed to determine if an observed effect on mating performance is a male effect. Males are treated until termination. Terminal examination of adults includes

1. Necropsy.
2. Preservation of organs with gross changes and sufficient control organs for comparison.
3. Preservation of testes, epididymides, ovaries, and uteri.
4. Sperm count and sperm viability.
5. Count of corpora lutea and implantation sites.
6. Count of live and dead conceptuses.

Among the study designs conducted before the ICH guidelines, the Segment I fertility study conducted according to Japanese guidelines is most similar to this ICH study design. The major differences are the shortening of the treatment period of males prior to cohabitation from the duration of spermatogenesis (60 to 80 days) to four weeks and the addition of sperm evaluation. The justifications given for shortening the treatment period of males are

1. Careful organ weight and histopathological evaluation of testes in general toxicity studies will detect most testicular toxins.
2. Fertility is an insensitive measure of testicular effects.
3. Compounds known to affect spermatogenesis generally exert their effects during the first four weeks of treatment.

Sperm counts can be performed with sperm from either the testis or the epididymis. Sperm motility is commonly being treated as a measure of sperm viability. The addition of sperm evaluation greatly increases the sensitivity of the study to detect effects on sperm maturation and the current study design will likely detect more male effects than previous designs even though the treatment period has been shortened.

### 8.2.2. Embryo-Fetal Development

The purpose of this component is to detect anatomical effects on the developing conceptus by treating during the period of organogenesis from implantation to closure of the secondary palate. The study design is very similar to the historical Segment II developmental toxicity study. A group size of 16 to 24 litters would generally be considered acceptable. The following is recommended:

|  | Rat | Rabbit | Mouse |
|---|---|---|---|
| Treatment period (gestational days) | 6–17 | 6–18 | 6–15 |
| Group size (mated or inseminated) | 25 | 20 | 25 |

Minimal in-life observations include

1. Clinical signs and mortality daily.
2. Body weight twice weekly.
3. Food consumption weekly.
4. Valuable target effects seen in previous toxicity studies.

Females are sacrificed at the end of the gestation period, about one day prior to parturition (Day 20 or 21 for rats, Day 28 or 29 for rabbits, and Day 17 or 18 for mice). Terminal examinations include

1. Necropsy.
2. Preservation of organs with gross changes and sufficient control organs for comparison.
3. Count of corporea lutea and live and dead implantations.
4. Fetal body weight.
5. External, visceral, and skeletal examination of fetuses.
6. Gross evaluation of placenta.

A minimum of 50% of fetuses are to be examined for visceral alterations and a minimum of 50% for skeletal abnormalities. When a fresh tissue microdissection technique is being used for the visceral examination of rabbit fetuses, all fetuses should be examined for both visceral and skeletal abnormalities.

Interpretation of results requires understanding and utilizing the following definitions.

*Malformation.* Structural change that is likely to be permanent and detrimental to the survival or well-being of the fetus, in the species/strain of animal being tested.

*Alteration.* Change that is, in isolation, unlikely to be detrimental to the survival or well-being of the fetus, in the species/strain of animal being tested.

*Variant.* Observation occurring frequently in a particular strain of animal.

### 8.2.3. Adverse Effects

The following definitions should be referred to when considering whether an observed effect of treatment is adverse or not:

1. Treatment related trend in incidence of specific or related malformations.
2. Treatment related increase in alterations, the cumulative effect of which is considered to be detrimental to the wellbeing of the fetus.
3. Treatment related increase in alterations, which are related in nature or derivation to treatment related malformations evident on the study.

4. Treatment related marked change in the incidence of a group of alterations, which although their form is normal for a previous or future stage of development, that is, their occurrence suggests precocious or delayed development, their presence in a marked degree suggests some permanent change in the rate of development of the fetus and could be detrimental to its future development.

5. Marked treatment related increase in the occurrence of a specific alteration, in which the form is not predictive of the normal chronological order of development (e.g., bent scapula).

### 8.2.4. Pre- and Postnatal Development

The purpose of this component is to detect effects of treatment from implantation through lactation on the pregnant and lactating female and on the development of the conceptus and offspring though sexual maturity. The study design is similar to the previous Segment III study design except that dosing begins on Day 6 of gestation instead of Day 15. A group size of 16 to 24 litters would generally be considered acceptable (with 25 mated females being recommended).

Minimal in-life observations for parental (F0 generation) females include

1. Clinical signs and mortality daily.
2. Body weight twice weekly.
3. Food consumption weekly.
4. Valuable target effects seen in previous toxicity studies.
5. Length of gestation.
6. Parturition.

Parental females are sacrificed after weaning of the F1 generation. The age of sacrifice of the F1 generation animals is not specified in the ICH guideline and varies among laboratories. Typically, they are sacrificed intermittently with some laboratories reducing litter size on postnatal Day 0, 3, or 4, on postnatal Day 21 or at weaning, at male/female cohabitation to produce an F2 generation, and the terminal sacrifice, after production of the F2 generation. Terminal examinations for maternal animals and offspring include

1. Necropsy of all parental and F1 adults.
2. Preservation of organs with gross changes and sufficient control organs for comparison.
3. Count of implantations.

Additional observations of the F1 generation include

1. Abnormalities.
2. Live and dead offspring at birth.

3. Body weight at birth.

4. Pre- and postnatal survival, growth, maturation, and fertility.

5. Physical development including vaginal opening and preputial separation.

6. Sensory function, reflexes, motor activity, learning, and memory.

### 8.2.5. Single-Study and Two-Study Designs for Rodents

Except for the embryo and fetal development component in rabbits, the components described above can be combined into fewer, larger studies instead of conducting each component separately. Acceptable alternatives include the "single-study design" and "two-study design." The choice may be made based on when study results are needed (how soon are females to be incorporated in clinical studies) and compound availability.

In the "single-study design," all of the above components are combined into one study. The dosing period, extending from before mating through lactation, is a combination of that for the fertility study together with that for the pre- and postnatal development study. Subgroups of animals are terminated at the end of gestation for fetal examination.

There are a variety of possible "two-study designs." One is to conduct the single study described above except that, instead of having subgroups for fetal examination, a separate embryo-fetal development study in rodents is conducted. Another two-study design consists of combining the embryo-fetal development study with the pre- and postnatal development study such that the two studies to be conducted would be (1) the fertility study and (2) the pre- and postnatal development study with subgroups terminated at the end of gestation for fetal examination. A third possible two-study design is to combine the fertility study with the embryo-fetal development study. In the first study, treatment would extend through the end of organogenesis and then, at termination at the end of gestation, there would be a complete fetal examination. The second study would be the pre- and postnatal development study.

For all the options described above, effects on male and female fertility can be evaluated separately by conducting separate studies in which only one sex is treated. The treatment periods are the same, but the treated animals are cohabited with untreated animals of the opposite sex. In the male fertility study, the untreated females are terminated after the middle of gestation and terminal observations include embryo survival and possibly external examination of fetuses (if terminated at the end of gestation) (Tanimura, 1990). The advantage of conducting separate male and female studies is that, if there are effects, is it clear which sex was affected by treatment. Often when effects are seen in a combined male and female study, additional work is required to resolve which sex was affected. Either a second cohabitation of the treated males with untreated females is added or studies with only one sex treated must then be conducted.

With the possible exception of combining the female fertility component with the embryo-fetal development component, the combined-study approach is used often. The female fertility and embryo-fetal development components are needed to support clinical trials in women of childbearing potential in most countries and thus will be conducted early in the development of a drug. However, since the pre- and postnatal development component is not routinely required for clinical studies of women of childbearing potential and represents a large commitment of resources, it will not generally be conducted until late in the drug development process.

### 8.2.6. Preliminary Studies

According to the ICH guideline, "some minimal toxicity is to be expected to be induced in the high dose dams" in the reproductive toxicity studies. In some cases, particularly for the fertility and early embryonic development study, available information from general toxicity studies in the selected rodent species may be sufficient to allow the selection of dosage levels for a reproductive toxicity study with the goal of achieving minimal toxicity in high-dose dams. However, pregnant females sometimes respond differently to toxins than nonpregnant females, the duration of dosing for reproductive toxicity studies is different than for general toxicity studies, and toxicity may not have been achieved in the subacute toxicity studies. Thus, it is often necessary to conduct a range-finding study in pregnant rodents prior to the embryo-fetal development study. A range-finding study in rabbits is almost always required since only rarely are results available from other toxicity studies.

The range-finding study in pregnant animals (rodents or rabbits) is similar to the embryo-fetal development study discussed above except that there may be more dosage groups, group size is smaller (six to ten inseminated or mated females per group), and there is no need to examine fetuses for visceral or skeletal abnormalities. Evaluating litters from range-finding studies for resorption, fetal weight, and external abnormalities is valuable for providing an early indication of marked developmental toxicity. This is particularly important if conceptus survival at a particular dosage level would be inadequate to evaluate effects on development in the subsequent embryo-fetal development study. Once it has been determined during a range-finding study that a particular dosage level causes toxicity exceeding the minimal toxicity desired for the embryo-fetal development study, it is best to terminate that dosage group since continued treatment and evaluation unnecessarily expose animals to toxicity, any subsequent data collected are not useful for risk assessment (since it is known that excessive maternal toxicity itself causes developmental toxicity), and investment of resources is therefore unwarranted.

### 8.2.7. Toxicokinetics

The ICH guidelines do not require that toxicokinetic studies be conducted except that "at the time of study evaluation further information on kinetics in pregnant or lactating animals may be required according to the results obtained." In addition, the guidelines state that "it is preferable to have some information on kinetics before initiating reproduction studies."

The major toxicokinetic issue for reproductive toxicity studies is whether systemic exposure in the selected species and route is adequate relative to the systemic exposure with the clinical regimen. Often, this information is available for the selected rodent species from studies conducted independently from the reproductive toxicity studies. For rabbits, though, there is rarely toxicokinetic information available from other studies. Accordingly, it is advisable to conduct at least a crude evaluation of systemic exposure in the rabbit. It is best if these data are available prior to the embryo-fetal development study so that, if the rabbit is found to have inadequate systemic exposure, an alternative species may be selected before the investment of resources in a large rabbit study. The collection of blood samples for toxicokinetic evaluations may be incorporated into the range-finding study in pregnant rabbits. However, rabbits stressed by multiple bleedings should not be retained for evaluation of developmental toxicity and satellite groups of toxicokinetic animals for bleeding only may be needed.

It would be ideal to have data from five to eight time points following the first and last doses to examine accumulation and other changes in kinetic parameters during pregnancy and, since physiology changes rapidly during gestation, to have data periodically during gestation as well. However, from a practical point of view, the question being asked (what is the approximate systemic exposure?) does not justify a comprehensive kinetic evaluation. When circumstances dictate that a toxicokinetic evaluation be performed, determining maternal plasma levels at a few postdosing intervals during a single 24-hour period of gestation, preferably during the period when serious adverse effects are most likely to be induced (Days 9 through 12 of gestation), will generally provide adequate information.

Only in special circumstances will the determination of embryo levels of drug add meaningfully to the assessment of human risk from a drug. In such studies, even if it is found that the embryo is not exposed, the lack of exposure of the embryo would not necessarily indicate an invalid study or increased human risk since there may also be no exposure in human embryos. When embryo level studies are conducted, the selection of day(s) of gestation to harvest embryos is severely restricted by the sensitivity of the assay. Often, the earliest day that allows the collection of sufficient tissue for assay is gestational Day 10 or 11.

### 8.2.8.  Timing of Studies

The definition of which studies need to be performed in advance of clinical trials has not been addressed yet by the ICH process and is currently monitored by the regulatory agencies of individual countries and institutional review boards (IRBs). Embryo-fetal development studies in two species are almost universal prerequisites for clinical studies in women of childbearing potential. Some regulatory agencies also request that a fertility study in female rodents be conducted before clinical trials in women of childbearing potential. A fertility study in male rodents is required before clinical trials in men in Japan. Some pharmaceutical companies have internal guidelines that specify compliance with all the guidelines listed above, regardless of the location of the clinical trials.

The most conspicuous exception to the policy described above is the position of the U.S Food and Drug Administration (FDA, 1993). The FDA withdrew the restriction on the participation of women of childbearing potential in early clinical trials, citing "(1) exclusion of women from early trials is not medically necessary because the risk of fetal exposure can be minimized by patient behavior and laboratory testing, and (2) initial determinations about whether that risk is adequately addressed are properly left to patients, physicians, local IRBs and sponsors with appropriate review and guidance by FDA, as are all other aspects of the safety of proposed investigations." The policy of excluding women has been replaced by one that specifies that "the patients included in clinical trials should, in general, reflect the population that will receive the drug when it is marketed." In fact, inclusion of women at the earliest possible stages is frequently mandated.

To comply with FDA policy, at least for the conduct of clinical trials in the United States, pharmaceutical companies have a few choices. They can conduct the standard battery of reproductive studies prior to enrolling women of childbearing potential in early clinical trials. The possible negative impact would be a delay in the initiation of clinical trials. Alternatively, pharmaceutical companies can enroll women of child-bearing potential in early clinical trials without having conducted any reproductive toxicity studies and accept the additional risk resulting from exposure to untested drugs during inadvertent or undetected pregnancy. In either case, the incidence of pregnancy during clinical trials can be decreased by pregnancy testing and/or assurances of contraception.


## 8.3. METHODOLOGICAL ISSUES

### 8.3.1. Control of Bias

An important element to consider when designing developmental and reproductive toxicity studies is the control of bias. For example, animals should be assigned to groups randomly and preferably blocked by body weight. This can be accomplished by first ranking the animals in order of body weight and then, starting with the lightest or heaviest, assigning by rank to groups based on a list of sets of random permutations of numbers (e.g., 1, 2, 3, and 4 if there are four groups, where 1 represents the control group, 2 represents the low-dose group, etc.). Housing of treatment groups should also be unbiased. This can be done by "Latin square" design where each block of four cages (if there are four groups) includes an animal from each group. It is often an acceptable compromise to have animals from different groups in alternating vertical columns with all the animals in a column from the same group. This provides equal vertical balancing for all groups. Historically, it has proven unwise to have groups segregated on separate racks.

The order of sacrifice on the day of cesarean sectioning should be balanced by group (again using random permutations) since fetuses continue to grow during the day and an unbalanced time of sacrifice would bias fetal weights, particularly for rodents. Alternatively, all animals can be killed at about the same time in the morning and the fetuses stored for examination later the same day. Fetal examinations should be conducted blind, that is, without knowledge of treatment group.

### 8.3.2. Diet

It is known that rodents require a diet relatively rich in protein and fats for successful reproduction (Zeman, 1967; Chow and Rider, 1973; Turner, 1973; Mulay et al., 1982). Consequently, rodents are fed high-protein, high-fat diets *ad lib* for reproductive toxicity studies and also generally as a maintenance diet for all toxicity studies. Female rats fed in this manner begin to show decreases in fertility, litter size, and the incidence of normal estrus cycling at the age of six months (Matt et al., 1986, 1987). The disadvantage of this feeding practice is that the animals more quickly acquire age-related diseases and sexual dysfunction and die sooner than if they are fed a restricted amount of calories (for review, see Weindruch and Walford, 1988). In relatively short-term studies (such as standard ICH studies), this rapid aging does not present a problem. However, for male breeding colonies or multigeneration studies with multiple litters per generation, it could be advantageous to restrict caloric intake, at least when the animals are not being bred. Restriction of food intake to achieve a 30% decrease in body weight gain compared to *ad lib*-fed controls has no adverse effect on male rat reproduction (Chapin et al., 1991), although it does affect reproduction in mice (Gulati et al., 1991) and female rats (Chapin et al., 1991).

Dietary restriction is even more important for rabbits. Rabbits fed *ad lib* fare very poorly. Some laboratories restrict New Zealand white rabbits to 150 to 180 g per day of a high- (at least 13.5%) fiber diet. However, even this regimen results in some rabbits going off feed late in gestation. It has been observed that by restricting New Zealand white rabbits to only 125 g of food per day nearly all control animals retain appetite throughout gestation and fewer of these animals abort (Clark et al., 1991). More uniform food consumption late in gestation is associated with greater uniformity in maternal body weight change and fetal weight. This decreased variability makes these measures more sensitive indicators of maternal and developmental toxicity. Thus, 125 g is the preferred daily ration for New Zealand white rabbits.

### 8.3.3. Clinical Pathology

Regulatory guidelines require that there be maternal toxicity at the highest dosage level in embryo-fetal developmental toxicity studies. It is important to avoid excessive toxicity in these studies since it is known that marked maternal toxicity can cause secondary developmental toxicity (see discussion in Section 8.4.3, "Association between Developmental and Maternal Toxicity"). This secondary developmental toxicity is irrelevant to the assessment of the developmental hazard of the test agent and thus simply confounds the interpretation of the data.

The traditional indicators of maternal toxicity in range-finding studies in pregnant animals (mortality, body weight, food consumption, and clinical signs) do not always provide a sensitive measure of toxicity. This insensitivity is a particular problem for rabbit studies since typically no other toxicity studies are conducted in rabbits and body weight change in rabbits is very variable (typically $-100$ to $+400\,\mathrm{g}$ during gestation), making it a particularly insensitive indicator of toxicity.

Thus, it is desirable to improve the assessment of toxicity in range-finding studies in pregnant animals. Complete histopathologic examination is not practical. However, it is often feasible to perform hematologic and serum biochemical analyses that can significantly increase the changes of detecting significant toxicity and provide important information for selecting an appropriate highest dosage level for the embryo-fetal developmental toxicity study.

Based on more than twenty years of experience, body weight effects most often provided the basis for the selection of dosage levels in the Segment II study. However, there have been cases where clinical pathology was or would have been useful to justify dosage selection. For example, nonsteroidal anti-inflammatory drug diflunisal caused a decrease in erythrocyte count from 6.0 (million/mm$^3$) to 2.9 at a dosage level ($40\,\mathrm{mg\,kg^{-1}\,day^{-1}}$) that caused only a 1% decrease in body weight in pregnant rabbits. The severe hemolytic anemia caused by this excessively high dosage level in turn caused secondary axial skeletal malformations in the fetuses (Clark et al., 1984). Also, the angiotensin-converting enzyme (ACE) inhibitor enalapril caused an increase in serum urea nitrogen from $16\,\mathrm{mg\,dl^{-1}}$ to $46\,\mathrm{mg\,dl^{-1}}$ (highest value $= 117$) at a dosage level ($10\,\mathrm{mg\,kg^{-1}\,day^{-1}}$) that had no apparent effect on body weight but caused a significant ($p < 0.05$) increase in resorptions (Minsker et al., 1990). Serum urea nitrogen concentration was used to select dosage levels for a subsequent ACE inhibitor, lisinopril. Likewise, the routine use of clinical pathology in range-finding studies had previously been proposed (Wise et al., 1988). The animals can be bled on the day after the last dose or sooner to detect transient effects or to allow an evaluation of the data prior to cesarean section.

### 8.3.4. Gravid Uterine Weights

Effects of treatment on maternal body weight gain are commonly evaluated as indicators of maternal toxicity. However, maternal body weight gain is influenced by fetal parameters such as live fetuses per litter and fetal body weight. Thus, effects indicative of developmental toxicity could contribute to decreased maternal body weight gain and confound the interpretation of maternal toxicity. In addition, other maternal but pregnancy-related parameters, such as volume of intrauterine fluid, could be affected by treatment and contribute to effects on overall body weight gain.

In an attempt to correct this complication, some laboratories weigh the gravid uterus at cesarean section and then subtract the weight of the gravid uterus from the body weight gain to obtain an adjusted weight gain that is more purely maternal. This adjustment is imprecise, but not inappropriate for rats for which gravid uterine weight is correlated with and generally substantially less than maternal body weight change during gestation (e.g., see Figure 8.2 for which the correlation coefficient $r$ was 0.63 and $p < 0.001$). However, the subtraction of gravid uterine weight from maternal weight gain is an over-adjustment for rabbits. The maternal body weight

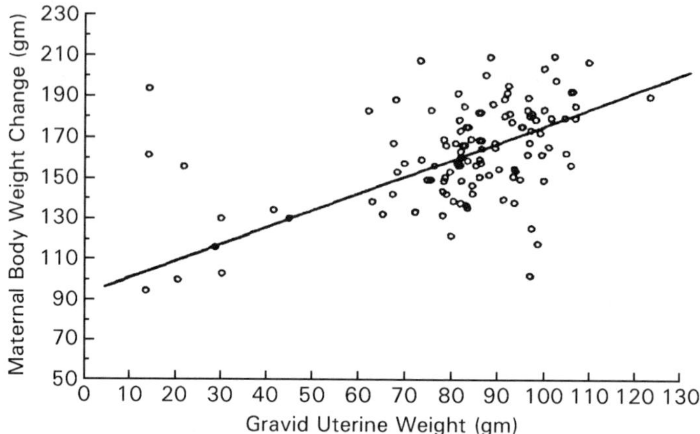

**FIGURE 8.2.** The relationship between gravid uterine weight and maternal body weight change in control rats between Days 0 and 20 of gestation. One hundred and twenty pregnant Sprague-Dawley (Crl: CD(SD)BR) rats were dosed orally with 0.5% aqueous methylcellulose on Days 6 through 17 of gestation and cesarean sectioned on Day 20 of gestation. The gravid uterus from each animal was removed and weighed.

gain of rabbits during gestation is generally less than the weight of the gravid uterus (see Figure 8.3). Moreover, gravid uterine weight is correlated with maternal body weight change in some but not all studies. For example, in the 53 untreated rabbits from the study shown in Figure 8.3, $r = 0.54$ and $p < 0.001$. However, in a study of 32 rabbits treated with a methylcellulose vehicle, $r = 0.21$ and $p = 0.25$. Thus,

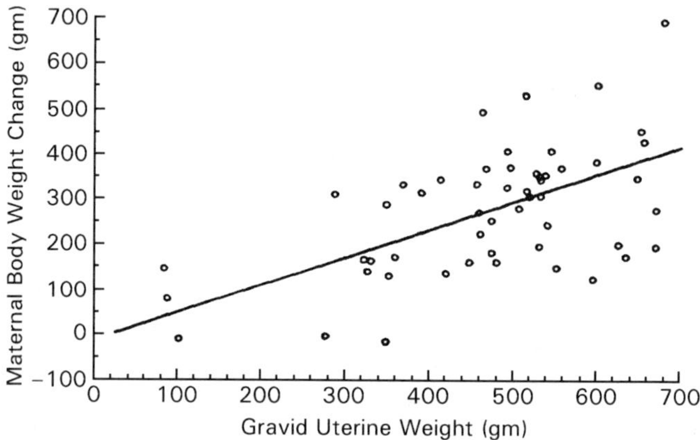

**FIGURE 8.3.** The relationship between gravid uterine weights and maternal body weight change in untreated rabbits between Days 0 and 28 of gestation. Fifty-three pregnant New Zealand white rabbits that had not been treated with control article or test agent were cesarean sectioned on Day 28 of gestation. The gravid uterus from each animal was removed and weighed.

subtracting the gravid uterine weight from the maternal weight gain is not always appropriate. A preferred method for adjusting maternal body weight gain for possible developmental effects is to test and, if appropriate, use gravid uterine weight as a covariate (J. Antonello, personal communication, 1990). This method can be used for both rats and rabbits and for body weight change intervals in addition to those ending at study termination.

Alternatively, to avoid weighing the uterus (or if the analysis is being performed retrospectively and uterine weights are unavailable) or if a more purely fetal adjustment is desired, one can use the sum of the live fetal weights within the litter (total live fetal weight) as the covariate instead of gravid uterine weight. As expected, total live fetal weight is very highly correlated with gravid uterine weight in control animals ($r = 0.99$ in control rats and 0.95 in control rabbits; J. Antonello, personal communication, 1990). Thus, in general, using either gravid uterine weight or total live fetal weight as the covariate will yield similar results. However, if treatment was to have an effect on gravid uterine weight that was not reflected in total live fetal weight (e.g., if the volume of amniotic, extracoelomic, or intrauterine fluid was affected), then total live fetal weight may not be highly correlated with gravid uterine weight and, hence, not interchangeable as a covariate. In that case, only weighing the gravid uterus would allow the detection of these effects not revealed by total live fetal weight.

### 8.3.5. Implant Counts and Determination of Pregnancy

Two observations suggest that the remnants of embryos that die soon after implantation are not apparent at gross examination of the uterus near term. First, embryos that were observed to be resorbing at laparotomy early in gestation left no readily visible trace near term (Staples, 1971). Second, occult implantation sites can be revealed near term by staining the uterus with ammonium sulfide or sodium hydroxide (Salewski, 1964; Yamada et al., 1988). It is not known if the uterine staining techniques reveal all implantation sites. It is clear, though, that when uterine staining techniques are not used, very early resorptions may not be included in what is termed the "resorption rate" but instead may contribute to the apparent "preimplantation loss" or, if no implantation sites were detected, the rate of "nonpregnant" animals.

In normal circumstances, probably very few implantation sites are not detected without staining. However, cases have occurred in which probable treatment effects were detected only as a result of uterine staining. For example, in one rabbit study with drug treatment starting on Day 6 of the gestation, a drug-treated group had four litters that had implantation sites that were seen only after staining with ammonium sulfide, indicating very early drug-induced resorption. For critical studies in rabbits designed to determine early effects on resorption and abortion rates, it would be advantageous to measure plasma levels of progesterone on Day 6 of gestation since low levels indicate nonpregnant animals (Adams et al., 1989, 1990).

### 8.3.6. Fetal Examinations

Many fetal anomalies, such as cleft palate, exencephaly, ectrodactyly, and missing vertebrae, are discrete and distinct and therefore easy to recognize objectively. Some anatomical structures, though, occur along a continuous gradation of size and shape and are only considered anomalous if the deviation from the typical exceeds a somewhat arbitrarily selected threshold. These anomalies are observed in all examination types and include, for example, micrognathia, reduced gallbladder, enlarged heart, distended ureter, wavy rib, and incomplete ossification at many sites. In many cases, it cannot be said with certainty whether a specific degree of variation from normal would have resulted in an adverse consequence to the animal and should therefore be considered abnormal. In the absence of certainty about outcome, the best approach is to uniformly apply a single criterion within a study (and preferably among studies) so that all treatment groups are examined consistently. The subjectivity (and hence fetus-to-fetus variability) of the examination can be minimized by having the criteria be as clear and objective as possible. For example, when examining for incompletely ossified thoracic centra or supraoccipitals, it can be required that the ossification pattern be absent (unossified), unilateral, or bipartite (which are objective observations) before recording as an observation. Subjective criteria such as being dumbbell- or butterfly-shaped would not be applied.

***Examination of External Genitalia.*** One aspect of external anatomy that is largely overlooked in the examination of offspring exposed *in utero* to test agents is the external genitalia, even though major malformations can occur in those structures. For example, hypospadias is a malformation in the male in which the urethra opens on the underside of the penis or in the perineum. Hypospadias can occur in the male rat following *in utero* exposure to antiandrogens (e.g., Neumann et al., 1970), testosterone synthesis inhibitors (e.g., Bloch et al., 1971), or finasteride, a 5$\alpha$-reductase inhibitor (Clark et al., 1990b). However, it is impractical to detect hypospadias in fetuses or young pups. Although the genital tubercle of the normal male rat fetus is grossly distinguishable from that or the normal female as early as Day 21 of gestation (the female has a groove on the ventral side), the difference is very subtle and partial feminization of the male genital tubercle would be very difficult to ascertain. Routine histological examination is obviously too labor intensive to be considered. Hypospadias can readily be determined, though, by expressing and examining the penis of the adult. Thus, it is recommended that adult $F_1$ males be examined for hypospadias. If the timing of the separation of the balano-preputial membrane is being included in the pre- and postnatal development study as a developmental sign (see Korenbrot et al., 1977), the examination of the penis for hypospadias can be conducted at the same time.

The critical period for the induction of hypospadias by finasteride in rats is Days 16 to 17 of gestation (Clark et al., 1990a). It is unlikely that other agents would have a much earlier critical period since testosterone synthesis, which is required for the development of the penile urethra, begins in the rat on Day 15 of gestation (Habert and Picon, 1984). Thus, if treatment in the embryo-fetal development study terminates on Day 15 of gestation (as is done in some laboratories), it is doubtful that hypospadias could be induced. However, hypospadias could be induced in the pre- and postnatal development study. Since the formation of the penile urethra in the rat is not completed until Day 21 of gestation (Anderson and Clark, 1990), it could be argued that "major organogenesis" continues until that time.

One parameter that is readily and commonly measured as an indicator of effects on differentiation of the external genitalia in rodent fetuses is the sexually dimorphic distance between the anus and the genital tubercle (anogenital distance). However, it should not be assumed that anogenital distance is synonymous with hypospadias, since effects on anogenital distance are not necessarily predictive of hypospadias. Finasteride caused both hypospadias and decreased anogenital distance in male offspring but with very different dose-response relationships and only a slight tendency for animals with hypospadias to have a shorter anogenital distance (Clark et al., 1990b). Also, the effects on anogenital distance were largely reversible, whereas hypospadias was not. Another agent, triamcinolone acetonide, caused dramatic (reversible) decreases in anogenital distance in male rat fetuses on Day 20 of gestation but did not affect the development of the genital tubercle and did not cause hypospadias (Wise et al., 1990b). Thus, decreased anogenital distance per se does not necessarily indicate a serious congenital anomaly.

When evaluating effects of treatment on fetal anogenital distance, it is obviously important to correct for effects on fetal weight. One approach is to calculate "relative" anogenital distance, the ratio between anogenital distance and another linear measure, for example, biparietal diameter (head width). The cube rood of fetal weight simulates a linear measure (Wise et al., 1990b) and can also be used to normalize anogenital distance. Another approach is to compare the anogenital distance in a weight-reduced treatment group to that in a weight-matched control group at a younger age.

***Visceral Fetal Examinations.*** The examination of the abdominal and thoracic viscera of fetuses is performed either fresh without fixation ("Staples technique") or after Bouin's fixation by making freehand razor blade sections ("Wilson's technique"; Wilson, 1965). Both techniques have advantages. The fresh examination technique, which may require less training for thorough proficiency, provides a more easily interpreted view of heart anomalies. The examination must be performed on the day the dam is terminated, however, so having a large number of litters to examine in one day requires that a large team of workers be committed to the task.

With both techniques, the heads of one-half of the fetuses can be fixed in Bouin's fixative for subsequent freehand sectioning and examination. A common artifact induced by fixation in rabbit fetal heads is retinal folding.

Whether or not the kidneys are sliced transversely to examine the renal pelvis varies among laboratories. Hydronephrosis, delayed papillary development, and distended renal pelvis are most readily detected in this manner. However, it is not necessary to slice the kidneys to detect the urinary retention that can lead to distended renal pelvis and hydronephrosis. This point was demonstrated in a study in which 200,000 IU kg$^{-1}$ day$^{-1}$ of vitamin A administered orally on Days 8 to 10 of gestation induced hydronephrosis and/or distended renal pelvis in 29 fetuses (R. Clark, personal communication). In all of these 29 fetuses (and two others), distended ureter also occurred. Thus, a distended ureter may be a more sensitive indicator of urinary retention than a distended renal pelvis.

***Skeletal Fetal Examination.*** There is variability in the development of the fetal skeleton, including numbers of vertebrae and ribs, patterns of sternebral ossification, alignment of ribs with sternebrae, and alignment of ilia with lumbar and sacral vertebrae. There is also extensive plasticity in the development of the skeleton beyond the fetal stage. For example, it is known that markedly wavy ribs in fetuses can resolve so that the ribs in the adult are normal (Saegusa et al., 1980; Nishimura et al., 1982) and supernumerary ribs can be resorbed (Wickramaratne, 1988). This variability and plasticity complicates the classification of anomalies as true malformations as opposed to variations of normal. There is no unanimity on terminology, but, in general, a variation tends to be an alteration that occurs at relatively high spontaneous incidence (> 1%), is often reversible, and has little or not adverse consequence for the animal.

When tabulating and interpreting fetal skeleton data, a distinction is made between alterations in the pattern of development and simple delays in development that are considered to be less serious. A delay in skeletal development is usually apparent as a delay in ossification, as evidenced by an increased incidence of specific, incompletely ossified sites or decreases in counts of ossified bones in specific regions (e.g., sacrocaudal vertebrae). These delays are normally associated with decreases in fetal weight and commonly occur at dosage levels of the test agent that also cause decreased maternal body weight gain.

When determining the criteria for recording skeletal alterations, particularly sites of incomplete ossification, it is legitimate to consider the resulting incidences. For example, including an unossified fifth sternebra in the criteria for recording incomplete sternebral ossification may increase the control incidence to a very high proportion (over 95%) of fetuses affected, which would then reduce the sensitivity for detecting treatment effects. The additional effort expended in recording the extra observations due to sternebra 5 would be wasted. In addition, recording high incidences of incomplete ossification at many sites is not worth the effort involved. The ossification at various sites is highly correlated, so recording at multiple sites is redundant. In some cases, the incidences can be reduced to reasonable levels (1 to 20% of control fetuses) and the criteria simultaneously being made more objective by requiring that the bone be entirely unossified before recording.

### 8.3.7. Developmental Signs

The postnatal evaluation of $F_1$ pups includes the observation of developmental signs in two or more pups per sex per litter. In general, the acquisition of these developmental landmarks, including anatomical changes (e.g., ear pinna detachment, incisor eruption, hair growth, and eye opening) and reflexes (negative geotaxis, surface righting, and free-fall righting), are highly correlated with body weight but as indicators of developmental toxicity they are not as sensitive as body weight (Lochry et al., 1984; Lochry, 1987) and thus have minimal value. Possible exceptions to this generality are the ontogeny of the auditory startle reflex and the markers of sexual maturation (vaginal patency, testes descent, and balano-preputial separation in males).

The examinations for developmental signs should be performed daily starting before and continuing until criterion is achieved. The separation of the balano-preputial membrane of the penis (occurring at postnatal week 6 to 7; Korenbrot et al., 1977) is becoming the preferred landmark of sexual maturation in males. The timing of the testes descent is more variable and very dependent on the achievement criteria used. Another advantage of determining the time of the balano-preputial separation is that anomalies of the penis may be observed at the same time (as noted above).

### 8.3.8. Behavioral Tests

The trend within reproductive toxicology is to move from simple determinations of developmental landmarks and reflexes to more sophisticated and sensitive behavioral tests. This process was accelerated by the Environmental Protection Agency (EPA) of the United States, which issued guidelines requiring a "developmental neuro-toxicity" study of compounds that meet any of several broad criteria (EPA, 1991). The behavioral tests to be performed in this study are extensive and rigidly defined. As laboratories become equipped and trained to meet these guidelines, they are adding such tests to their evaluations of pharmaceuticals. The suggestions for routine testing made below are considered reasonable for pre- and postnatal development studies intended as routine screens. It is suggested that testing be conducted on one or two adults per sex per litter, keeping the range of actual ages as tight as possible.

Measurement of motor activity is commonly performed in the dark in cages or plastic boxes (open field) or residential mazes in which movement is quantitated by infrared detectors or by recording the interruption of light beams as the test subject moves through a horizontal grid of light beams. Possible parameters to evaluate include horizontal activity (light beams interrupted), number of movements, and time spent in the middle of the cage. The test period is selected to be long enough (normally 30 to 50 min) to allow the activity of the animals to decrease to an approximately constant level (asymptote). Testing of young pups (e.g., 13 days of age) is not recommended as their activity level is fairly constant during the test period and young unweaned pups should not be separated from their mothers for extended periods of time.

Another test paradigm for detecting treatment effects on brain functioning in $F_1$ offspring measures auditory startle habituation. In this test, the animal is placed in a chamber with a floor that detects movement. The animal is exposed to a sequence of 50 to 60 auditory stimuli, each at 110 to 120 decibels for 20 to 50 sec and separated by 5 to 20 sec. The gradual diminution of the animal's movement response is indicative of normal habituation.

There is not a consensus about the procedures to use to test for effects on learning and memory. The two most commonly used techniques are the water-filled maze, which is preferred for measuring learning, and passive avoidance, which is preferred for measuring memory (see Buelke-Sam et al., 1985). Retention is tested in a repeat test conducted approximately 1 week later.

### 8.3.9. Detecting Effects on Male Reproduction

Male fertility studies with typical group sizes (15 to 30 males per group) are very insensitive for detecting effects on male fertility. If the control fertility rate is 80%, even a group size of 30 will only detect (at the 5% significance level) a 38% decrease in fertility 80% of the time and a 50% decrease 95% of the time (J. Antonello, personal communication, 1990). To detect slight effects on male fertility would require enormous group sizes. Mating each male with more than one female provides a more precise estimate of the reproductive capacity of each male, but does not greatly increase statistical power. If multiple matings are to be done, it is recommended that the cohabitations with multiple females be sequential rather than concurrent.

Not only is it difficult to detect effects on male fertility because of group-size considerations, effects on male fertility mediated by decreased sperm production are also difficult to detect because of the normally huge excess of sperm included in a rat ejaculate. Sperm production can be decreased by up to 90% without effect on fertility (either pregnancy rate or litter size) in the rat. This is not the case for men, so the sperm excess in the rat represents a serious flaw in the rat model (see Working, 1988). To address this deficiency and improve the sensitivity of the model, it is advisable to determine the effects of the test agent on testes weights, testicular spermatid counts, and histopathology of the testes (preferably plastic sections) in the male fertility study and/or the 14-week toxicity study. In some cases, these parameters may be more predictive of possible effects on male fertility in humans than the fertility rate in rats.

### 8.4. DATA INTERPRETATION

### 8.4.1. Use of Statistical Analyses

Statistical analysis is a very useful tool for evaluating the effects of treatment on many developmental and reproductive toxicity parameters. For some parameters, such as maternal body weight changes, fetal weight, and horizontal activity in an open field, the comparison to the concurrent control is the primary consideration and, assuming adequate group size, the investigator relies heavily on the results of appropriate statistical analyses to interpret differences from control.

For other parameters, though, statistical analysis is just one of several considerations that include historical control data and other relevant information about the test agent and related test agents. For example, statistical analysis of a low incidence of an uncommon fetal malformation will usually not be significant ($p = 0.05$) even if treatment related, due to the low power for detecting such effects with typical group sizes. In such cases, examination of the historical control data becomes paramount. If two fetuses with a particular malformation occur in separate litters only in a high-dose group, the finding is of much more concern if it is a very rare malformation than if recent historical control groups have had a few fetuses with that malformation.

Other known effects of the test agent or related agents also sometimes contribute to data interpretation. For example, a low incidence of a malformation may be considered treatment related if it is at the low end of a typical dose-response curve or if it is in a high-dose group and that malformation is an expected effect of the test agent. In general, though, a single occurrence of a fetal malformation in a treatment group (with none in control) is not cause for alarm, since this occurs in almost every study (together with occurrences of some malformations only in the control group).

Statistical methods exist to appropriately analyze most developmental and reproductive toxicity parameters. Exceptions to this are the $r/m$ litter parameters in which, for each litter, there is a number affected divided by the number in the litter. These parameters include preimplantation loss ($r =$ corpora lutea $-$ implants, $m =$ corpora lutea), resorption rate ($r =$ resorptions, $m =$ implants), and the family of alteration rates ($r =$ affected fetuses, $m =$ fetuses). There are two factors complicating the statistical analysis of these data that have heretofore been inadequately handled (Clark et al., 1989). One is that almost all of these parameters have a strong dependence on $m$. For example, both preimplantation loss (Figure 8.4)

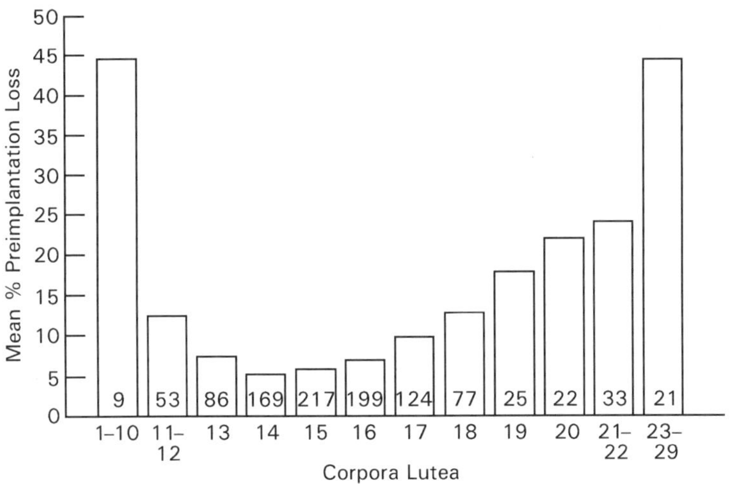


**FIGURE 8.4.** Effect of litter size on mean percentage preimplantation loss in 1035 control rat litters. Between 1970 and 1988, 1035 control rats were cesarean sectioned on Day 20 of gestation and the numbers of resorptions and implants were counted. Numbers within the bars indicate number of litters.

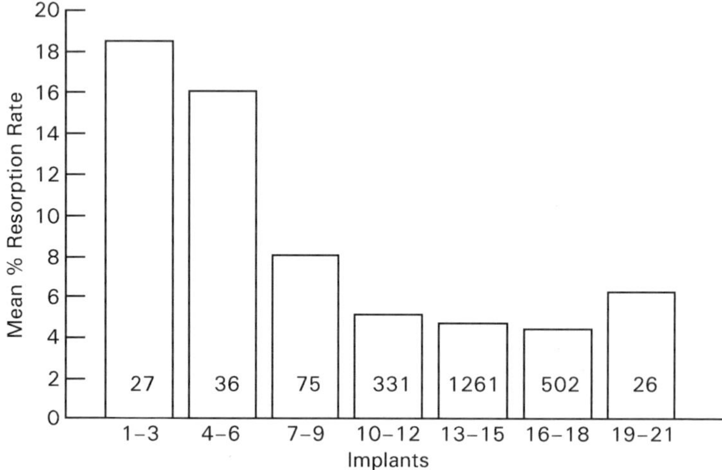

**FIGURE 8.5.** Effect of litter size on mean percentage resorption rate in 2258 control rat litters. Between 1970 and 1988, 2258 control rats were cesarean sectioned on Day 20 of gestation and the numbers of resorptions and implants were counted. Numbers within the bars indicate number of litters.

and resorption rate (Figure 8.5) are normally higher at both the low and high extremes of $m$. In contrast, supernumerary rib tends to occur at higher incidences in average-size litters (Figure 8.6). The second factor that complicates the statistical analysis of $r/m$ data is that affected implants tend to occur in clusters within litters ("litter effects"); that is, the intralitter correlation is greater than the interlitter correlation. For example, the total number of litters affected with anasarca, missing vertebra, and supernumerary rib is much less than would be expected by change based on the number of affected fetuses (Table 8.3 and Figure 8.7).

These problems have been resolved for analysis of resorption rate (and preimplantation loss) in Sprague-Dawley rats using a three-step process (Soper and Clark, 1990). First, based on an analysis of data from 1379 control rat litters examined since 1978, a likelihood score was derived for each $(r, m)$ couplet based on the incidence of that couplet given the value of $m$. These scores were approximately equal to $r$. Second, an analysis of 136 litters from groups with slight effects on resorption rate revealed that, at low-effect doses of embryocidal test agents, the increases in resorptions tended to occur as increased numbers of resorptions within affected litters rather than as an increased proportion of affected litters. To maximize the difference in scores between control and affected litters, the scores for control-like litters ($r = 1$, 2, or 3) were downgraded from $r$ (1, 2, and 3) to 0.4, 1, and 2.4, respectively. Third, to arrive at the final score for each litter, the modified $r$ score for each litter was divided by the expected control value for that value of $m$. This last step makes the litter score immune to spontaneous or treatment-related effects on $m$. The final "robust" scores have more power for detecting effects than various other

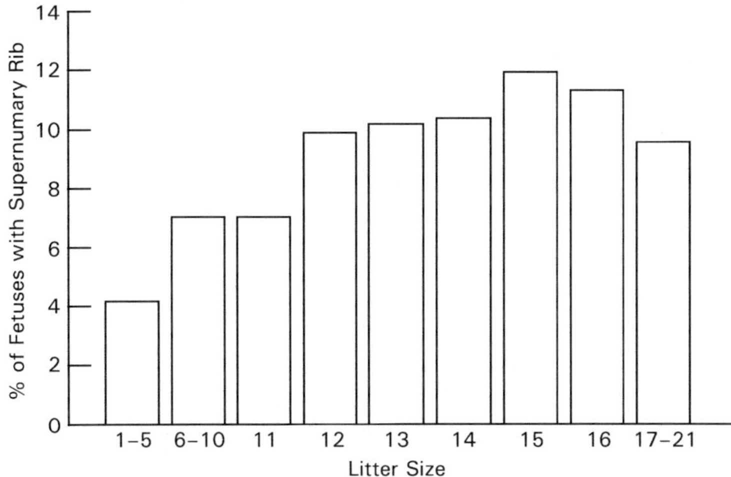


**FIGURE 8.6.** Effect of litter size (live fetuses per litter) on incidence of supernumerary rib in 1379 control rat litters. Between 1978 and 1988, fetal skeletons from 1379 litters of control rats were stained with alizarin red and examined for supernumerary rib.

measures (raw $r/m$, affected litters/litters, $r$, $\Sigma r/\Sigma n$, and the likelihood score) and has a lower false positive rate with fluctuations in $m$.

Covariance analysis (Snedecor and Cochran, 1980) can be used to reduce variability in a parameter and thereby increase sensitivity. For example, much of the variability in fetal weight data is due to variable litter size and, for rats, litters being sacrificed at different times during the workday. The variability due to these sources can be reduced by using litter size and time of sacrifice as potential covariates. Similarly, litter size and length of gestation can be used as covariates for neonatal pup weights and body weight at the beginning of treatment can be used as a covariate for maternal body weight changes during the treatment period of an embryo-fetal development study.

### 8.4.2. Potential Hazard Categories of Developmental Toxins

It is generally agreed that an agent that causes developmental toxicity in laboratory animals at dosage levels that cause no maternal toxicity (i.e., "selective" develop-

**TABLE 8.3.  Examples of Litter Effects in Control Litters**

| Effect | Affected Fetuses | Affected Litters | Litters Examined |
| --- | --- | --- | --- |
| Anasarca | 22 | 12 | 2203 |
| Missing vertebra | 53 | 13 | 1951 |
| Supernumerary rib | 1817 | 621 | 1379 |

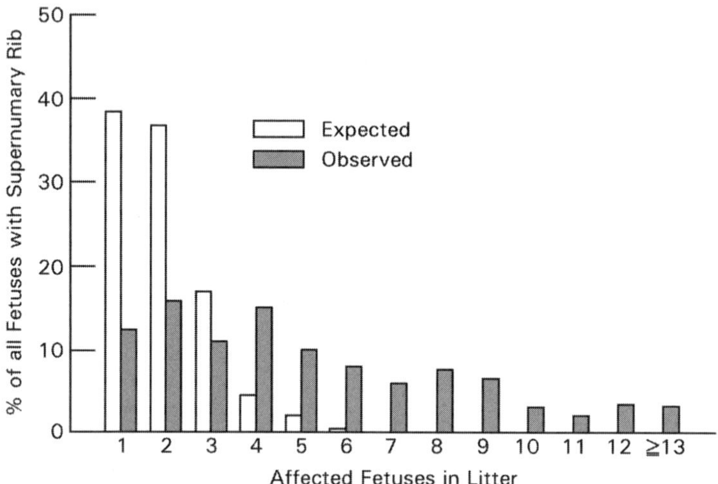


**FIGURE 8.7.** Litter effect with supernumerary rib in 1379 control litters. Between 1978 and 1988, fetal skeletons from 1379 litters of control rats were stained with alizarin red and examined for supernumerary rib in addition to other anomalies. The calculation of the expected number of fetuses with supernumerary rib in each litter was based on the assumption that each fetus had an equally likely chance of having supernumerary rib independent of the incidence among littermates (K. Soper, personal communication, 1990).

mental toxins) are potentially more hazardous to humans than agents that cause developmental toxicity only at maternotoxic dosages ("nonselective" developmental toxins; e.g., see Johnson, 1981; Schwetz, 1981; Fabro et al., 1982; Johnson, 1984; Johnson and Christian, 1984). This position is based on the supposition that pregnant women will avoid being exposed to toxic dosages of pharmaceuticals (which is usually but not always true). Developmental toxins can also be categorized as acting directly on the embryo or indirectly via an effect on the mother. All selective developmental toxins are presumably direct-acting. Nonselective developmental toxins can either act directly or indirectly.

Direct-acting developmental toxins may be potentially more hazardous to humans than indirectly acting ones even if the direct developmental toxicity occurred only at maternotoxic dosages in the species of laboratory animals tested. When the developmental toxicity of an agent is secondary to maternal toxicity in all species tested, the dose-response curves for developmental and maternal toxicity in various species may be invariably linked and developmental toxicity would never occur at nonmaternotoxic dosages. However, when an agent acts directly on the embryo to cause developmental toxicity, the dose-response curves may not be linked and, although they may be superimposed in the species of laboratory animals tested, they may not be superimposed in other species including humans. Thus, a direct-acting developmental toxin that is nonselective in one species may be selective in another species.

The ranking of potential developmental hazard in terms of selective, direct/nonselective, and indirect is more meaningful than the use of the terminology of specific/nonspecific and malformation/variation. However, when it cannot be determined if observed developmental toxicity is a direct or indirect effect, the alternative terminology becomes useful. A nonspecific effect (including in some cases decreased fetal weight, supernumerary rib, cleft palate in mice, and abortion in rabbits) is one that occurs commonly in response to high toxic dosages of a test agent. What makes a nonspecific effect generally less important than a specific effect is that nonspecific effects commonly occur only at maternally toxic dosages ("coeffective") and may be secondary to maternal toxicity, that is, indirect. However, when an apparently nonspecific adverse developmental effect is selective (direct), that is, it occurs at nonmaternotoxic dosages, it may nevertheless be indicative of a potential developmental hazard.

In general, an agent that induces a malformation (i.e., a teratogen) is considered to be more of a potential hazard than one that induces only a minor variation. Also, there has traditionally been more of a stigma associated with an agent that induces malformations than one that causes resorptions, even though embryo death is obviously a seriously adverse outcome. The point that makes the distinction among malformations, variations, or resorptions less important is that an agent that perturbs development to cause one effect in one species may cause a different effect in another species. Thus, any developmental toxic effect at nonmaternotoxic dosages should be considered carefully.

### 8.4.3. Associations between Developmental and Maternal Toxicity

The developmental toxicity of many pharmaceuticals occurs only at maternally toxic dosages (Khera, 1984, 1985; Schardein, 1987). Also, there are several compounds for which there is evidence that their developmental toxicity is secondary to their maternal toxicity. The decreased uterine blood flow associated with hydroxyurea treatment of pregnant rabbits may account for the embryotoxicity observed (Millicovsky et al., 1981). The teratogenicity of diphenylhydantion in mice may be secondary to decreased maternal heart rate (Watkinson and Millicovsky, 1983) as supported by the amelioration of the teratogenicity by hyperoxia (Millicovsky and Johnston, 1981) and the dependence on maternal genotype in genetic crosses between sensitive and resistant strains (Johnston et al., 1979; Hansen and Hodes, 1983). The hemolytic anemia caused in pregnant rabbits by diflunisal was severe enough to explain the concomitant axial skeletal malformations (Clark et al., 1984). Acetazolamide-induced fetal malformations in mice are apparently related to maternal hypercapnia (Weaver and Scott, 1984a, b) and hypokalemia (Ellison and Maren, 1972). The increased resorption rate induced in rabbits by the antibiotic norfloxacin depends on exposure of the maternal gastrointestinal tract (Clark et al., 1984).

In addition, various treatments that simulate effects that can result from pharmaceutical treatment have been shown to cause developmental toxicity. Food deprivation can cause embryo-fetal toxicity and teratogenicity in mice (Szabo and

Brent, 1975; Hemm et al., 1977) and rats (Ellington, 1980) and fetal death, decreased fetal weight, and abortions in rabbits (Matsuzawa et al., 1981; Clark et al., 1986). Treatments that result in maternal hypoxia, such as hypobaric exposure (Degenhardt and Kladetzky, 1955) and blood loss (Grote, 1969), have been shown to be teratogenic. Also, the results from testing with numerous agents suggest that supernumerary rib in mice is caused by maternal stress (Kavlock et al., 1985; Beyer and Chernoff, 1986).

Thus, in any case where developmental toxicity occurs at dosage levels with only moderate to severe maternal toxicity, the possibility of the developmental toxicity being secondary to the maternal toxicity can be considered. That is not to say, however, that it can be concluded that the developmental toxicity is secondary any time there is coincident maternal toxicity. To the contrary, it is usually very difficult to establish a causal relationship. Superficially similar types of maternal toxicity do not always cause the same pattern of developmental toxicity (Chernoff et al., 1990). This may be because the developmental toxicity is secondary to maternotoxicity, but, since typical developmental toxicity studies include only a very cursory evaluation of maternal toxicity, the developmental toxicity may be secondary to an aspect of maternotoxicity that is not even being measured.

To demonstrate that a developmental effect is secondary to a particular parameter of maternal toxicity, it is necessary but not sufficient to show that all mothers with developmental toxicity also had maternal toxicity and that the severity of the developmental effect was correlated with the maternal effect. An example of such a correlation is shown in Figure 8.8, in which a drug-induced effect on maternal

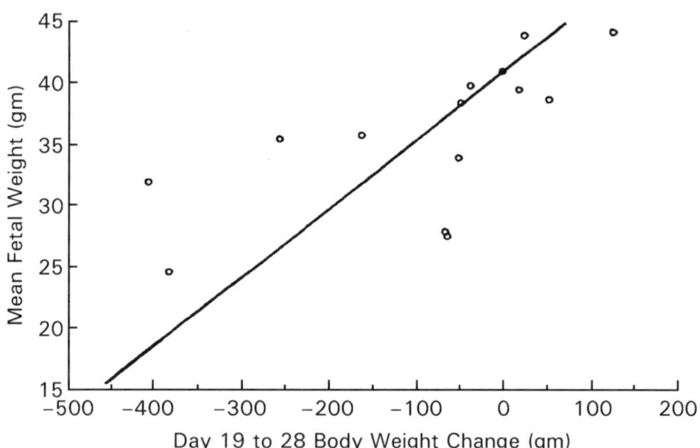

**FIGURE 8.8.** Correlation between drug-induced effects on maternal body weight change and fetal weight in rabbits. The data were collected from the high-dosage group of a developmental toxicity study of a prospective drug candidate. The rabbits were dosed orally with the test agent from Days 6 through 18 of gestation. On Day 28 of gestation, the rabbits were cesarean sectioned and the live fetuses weighed.

body weight change in rabbits is correlated ($r = 0.45$, $p < 0.05$) with a drug-induced decrease in fetal weight. Other examples where this approach has been used to evaluate the relationship between maternal and developmental toxicity include: (1) the negative correlation between resorption rate and maternal body weight change in norfloxacin-treated rabbits (Clark et al., 1984), supporting the contention that the developmental toxicity was secondary; and (2) the lack of correlation between embryotoxicity and maternal body weight change in pregnant mice treated with caffeine and L-phenylisopropyladenosine (Clark et al., 1987), suggesting no causal relationship between developmental and maternal toxicity may be required.

### 8.4.4. Assessment of Human Risk

Most test agents can be demonstrated to be developmentally toxic if tested under extreme conditions. This fact has been popularized as Karnofsky's Law: "Any drug administered at the proper dosage, at the proper stage of development, to embryos of the proper species...will be effective in causing disturbances in embryonic development" (Karnofsky, 1965, p. 185). In practice, about 37% of 3301 chemicals tested have been found to be teratogenic according to one tabulation (Schardein, 1993, p viii; see also Shepard, 1998). Contributing to this high rate is the practice of testing maternotoxic doses (to satisfy regulatory guidelines) that in some cases result in developmental toxicity secondary to maternal toxicity. Despite the high rate of positives in animal tests, very few xenobiotics are known to cause developmental toxicity in humans as commonly used. Thus, simply the induction of developmental toxicity by a test agent in animals does not necessarily indicate that that test agent will be a developmental hazard to human conceptuses under normal exposure conditions.

When a prospective drug under development for use in women of childbearing potential is determined to cause developmental toxicity in laboratory animals, the first question to be considered is whether that agent would cause developmental toxicity in humans at the anticipated therapeutic dosage level. This assessment and the related decision of whether to continue development of the drug candidate are currently based on the following

1. The ratio between the estimated systemic exposure at the lowest effect level (or highest no-observed-effect-level: NOEL) and the estimated systemic exposure at the anticipated therapeutic dosage level (the "safety factor").
2. Whether the effect is selective, direct, and/or specific.
3. The potential benefit to the patient population (compared to other available therapies).

The most common finding is that minor, nonselective, nonspecific developmental toxicity (e.g., decreased fetal weight) is observed at dosages at least tenfold above the anticipated therapeutic dosage level. In this situation, development of the agent would normally proceed even if the "safety factor" were only 3 to 5. This is the case since (1) many pharmaceuticals cause maternal toxicity in laboratory animals at low multiple (e.g., 10) of the clinical exposure, (2) nonspecific developmental toxicity commonly accompanies maternal toxicity, and (3) pharmaceuticals fitting this pattern do not usually cause developmental effects as used clinically (which often includes the practice of not prescribing for women known to be pregnant).

In contrast, a drug candidate that selectively causes major malformations at a dosage threefold higher than the clinical dosage would likely not be developed to treat a non-life-threatening disease. However, it might be developed if the disease to be treated was particularly debilitating, no other effective therapy was available, and it was felt that the exposure of pregnant women could be largely avoided.

Once a new pharmaceutical is approved by the FDA, it is placed in one of five pregnancy categories (A, B, C, D, or X) based on the results of animal developmental toxicity studies and, when available (usually not), information from human usage experience (see Table 8.4 and Frankos, 1985). Note that the categorization does not depend on the safety factor for a developmental effect or whether the effect is major, selective, direct, or specific (although these factors may be considered when determining if a drug is to be approved). Most often, there are positive findings in animals, no experience in pregnant women, and the drug is placed in Pregnancy Category C, indicating that it is to be used in pregnancy only if the potential benefit justifies the risk to the conceptus. Thus, it is left to the prescribing physician to regulate the exposure of pregnant women to the drug. If animal studies were negative and there is no information on effects on pregnant women, the agent is placed in Pregnancy Category B, indicating that the agent is to be used in pregnancy only if clearly needed. If developmental toxicity has been established in women (or, in some cases, is only strongly suspected), the agent is placed in category D or X. With category D, women may be prescribed the drug if the benefit outweighs the risk and the patient is informed of the potential hazard to the conceptus. Category X drugs are contraindicated in women who are or may become pregnant. Table 8.5

**TABLE 8.4. Pregnancy Categories (Use-in-pregnancy ratings, FDA, 1979)**

A: Adequately tested in humans, no risk (0.7% of approved drugs)
B/C/D: (Increasing levels of concern) (92.3% of approved drugs—66% in C)
X: Contraindicated for use in pregnancy (7.0% of approved drugs)

A: Animal studies and well-controlled studies in pregnant women failed to demonstrate a risk to the fetus.
B: Animal studies have failed to demonstrate risk to fetus; no adequate and well-controlled studies in pregnant women.
C: Animal studies showed adverse effect on fetus; no well-controlled human studies.
D: Positive evidence of human fetal risk based upon human data, but potential drug benefit outweighs risk.
X: Studies show fetal abnormalities in animals and humans; drug is contraindicated in pregnant women.

**TABLE 8.5. Pregnancy Categories**[a]

|  | Outcome of Animal Studies | | |
| --- | --- | --- | --- |
| Outcome of Human Studies | + | − | Not Available |
| + | X or D | X or D | X or D |
| − | B | A | A or B |
| Not available | $C_1$ | B | $C_2$ |

[a]A, B, $C_2$: Use during pregnancy only if clearly needed.
$C_1$: Use during pregnancy only if the potential benefit justifies the potential risk to the fetus.
D: If used during pregnancy, the patient should be apprised of the potential hazard to the fetus.
X: Contraindicated in women who are or may become pregnant.

summarizes these categories and the proportions of drugs in each in 2000 (according to the PDR).

Using the highest no-observed-effect level (NOEL) for determining a safety factor has the following flaws:

1. The determination of a true no-effect level (should one actually exist, which is debatable in some cases) is impossible given the statistical power associated with the group sizes typically used; thus, the reported NOEL is very dependent on the selected group size.

2. The NOEL depends greatly on the selection of dosage levels; unless the selected dosage is just below the threshold for detectable effects, the reported NOEL is an underestimate; thus, tightly spaced dosage levels favor the determination of a higher NOEL.

Accordingly, FDA has developed a sequential method of evaluating and dealing with reproductive and developmental analysis. This is called Wedge Analysis and is demonstrated in Figures 8.9 through 8.11.

## 8.5. *IN VITRO* TESTS FOR DEVELOPMENTAL TOXICITY

Many *in vitro* systems have been proposed as tests for developmental toxicity (for review, see Brown and Freeman, 1984; Lin, 1987; *In Vitro* Teratology Task force, 1987; and Gad, 2000). Various uses have been suggested for these *in vitro* tests including the following:

1. A general prescreen to select likely developmental toxins for subsequent whole-animal studies.

2. A prescreen to select among possible backups to a lead drug candidate that had been found to be developmentally toxic.

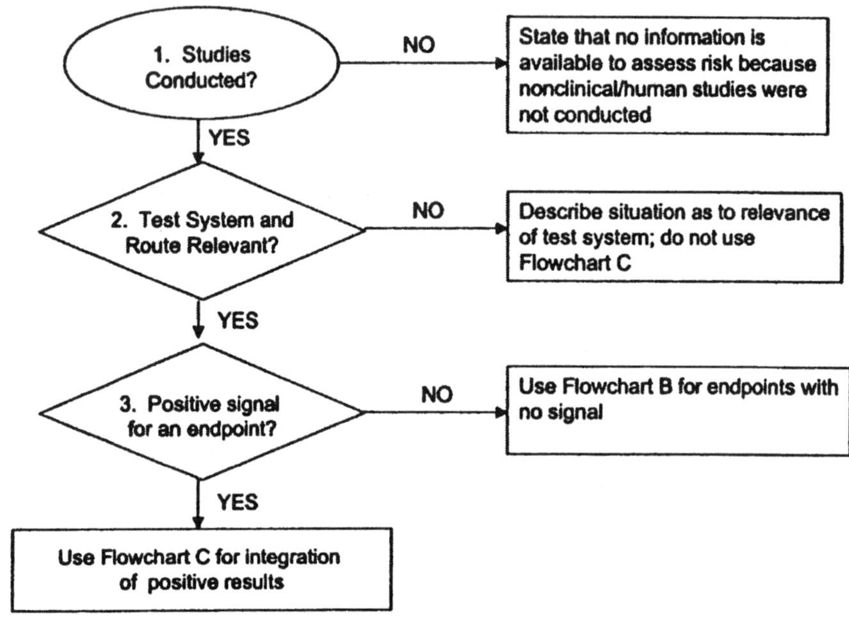


**FIGURE 8.9.** Flowchart A. Overall decision tree for evaluation on repro/developmental toxicity risk from Wedge Document, 1999, distributed through www.FDA.gov (June, 1999).

3. To study mechanisms of developmental toxicity.
4. To provide supplementary information about developmental toxicity in addition to that provided by whole-animal studies.
5. To replace whole animals for evaluating developmental toxicity.

Uses (1) and (5) above are very unlikely to be applicable to the pharmaceutical industry. One problem with *in vitro* systems for these purposes is that the percentages of the agents that are positive are very high, for example, 69% of agents tested in the mouse ovarian tumor cell attachment (MOT) test and 72% of agents tested in the mouse limb bud (MLB) assay. High correlations between *in vivo* and *in vitro* results have been reported based on the limited number of validation work completed. But these correlations have compared an *in vitro* end-point to teratogenicity in laboratory animals without regard to maternotoxicity. Thus, the question that these screen seem to be answering is: Can this agent be teratogenic or developmentally toxic in laboratory animals at any dosage level? However, as discussed above, it is not important for the purpose of safety assessment if an agent can be developmentally toxic in laboratory animals at high, maternotoxic dosages. The important question for prospective screens to answer is this: Is the agent a selective or direct developmental toxin? For these reasons, a promising drug candidate would not be dropped from development due to a positive result in a

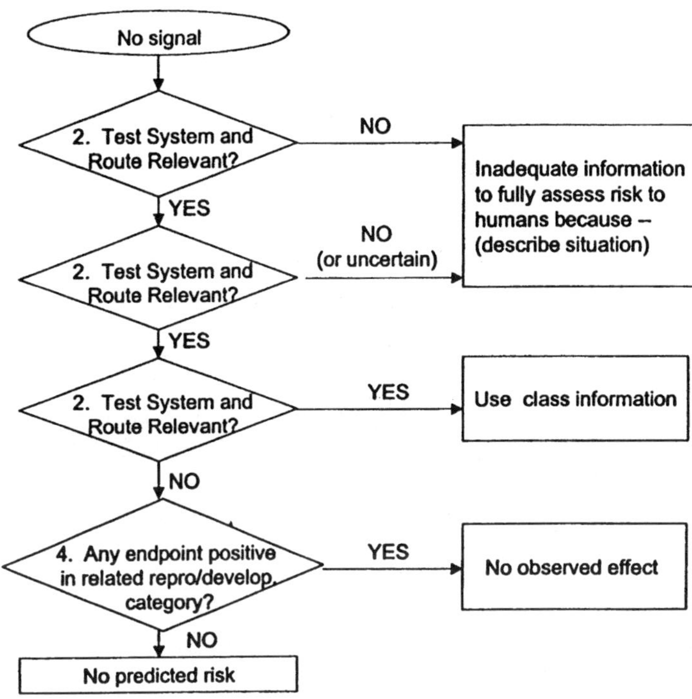


**FIGURE 8.10.** Flowchart B. Decision tree for endpoints with no signal from Wedge Document, 1999, distributed through www.FDA.gov (June, 1999).

current *in vitro* test and a negative result would not preclude the need for whole animal studies.

To relate a positive finding in an *in vitro* test to the *in vivo* situation, one must either compare the concentration that caused the positive developmental effect *in vitro* to the exposure level of the embryo *in vivo* or compare the *in vitro* concentration for a developmental effect to the maternotoxicity that would be associated with exposure at that concentration *in vivo*. To do the necessary pharmacokinetic studies *in vivo* would defeat the purpose of using an *in vitro* test. It would be very desirable and may be possible, though, to have an endpoint in an *in vitro* test that would correlate with maternal toxicity.

Currently, only the *Hydra* system incorporates a measurement of "toxicity" to the adult to provide a comparison of the sensitivity of the "embryo" with that of the adult (Johnson et al., 1988). However, the *Hydra* screen has not been fully validated as being predictive of results in mammals, and has fallen from favor. Thus, a major goal of research directed toward developing an *in vitro* teratogen screen should be to find a simple yet appropriate measure of toxicity unrelated to development. This would allow the comparison of the dose for a 50% effect ($ED_{50}$) on "developmental toxicity" as measured *in vitro* to an $ED_{50}$ for "adult" toxicity *in vitro*. The validation

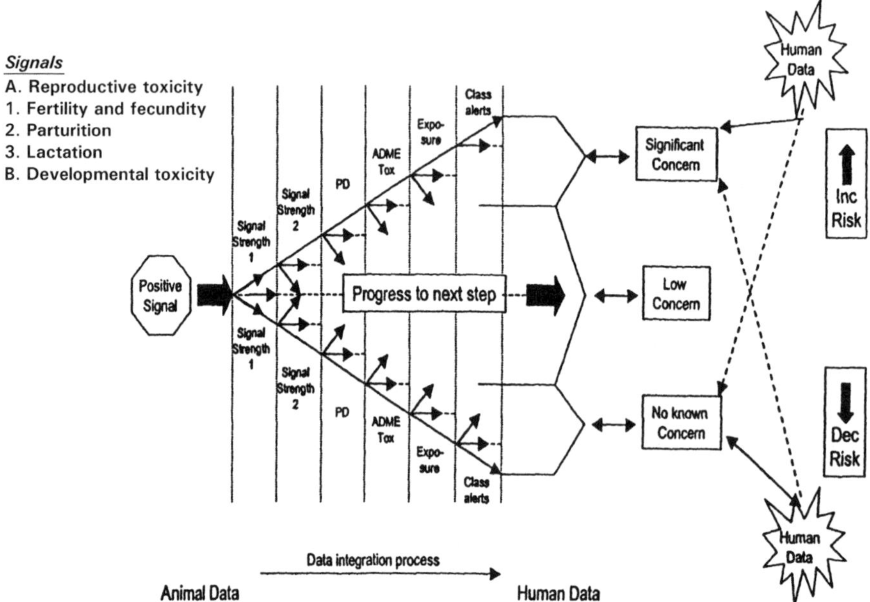


**FIGURE 8.11.** Flowchart C. Integration of positive repro/ancillary study results from Wedge Document, 1999, distributed through www.FDA.gov (June, 1999).

of such a dual *in vitro* system would involve comparing the developmental selectivity *in vitro* to that *in vivo* for a large number of compounds. In a preliminary effort in this regard, effects on cell division in the rat limb bud micromass assay were considered as a possible correlate of maternal toxicity (Wise et al., 1990a).

Another possible use of *in vitro* developmental toxicity tests would be to select the least developmentally toxic backup from among a group of structurally related compounds with similar pharmacological activity [use (2) in the list above], for example, when a lead compound causes malformations *in vivo* and is also positive in a screen that is related to the type of malformation induced. However, even for this limited role for a developmental toxicity screen, it would probably also be desirable to have a measure of the comparative maternotoxicity of the various agents and/or information on the pharmacokinetics and distribution of the agents *in vivo*.

*In vitro* developmental toxicity systems have clearly been useful for studies of mechanisms of developmental effects (e.g., Datson et al., 1989); — use (3) in the list above. It is unclear, though, whether *in vitro* developmental toxicity tests will provide useful information about developmental toxicity that is not derived from whole animal studies [use (4) from the list]. As is true for a possible use as a prescreen, the interpretation of a positive finding in an *in vitro* test will depend on knowing the exposure level *in vivo*. When this is known, the *in vitro* information could be helpful. The results of *in vivo* studies, though, would still likely be considered definitive for that species.

## 8.6. APPRAISAL OF CURRENT APPROACHES FOR DETERMINING DEVELOPMENTAL AND REPRODUCTIVE HAZARDS

The current system for testing new pharmaceuticals for developmental and reproductive toxicity has been largely intact since 1966. In that time, no thalidomide-like disasters have occurred. It cannot be proven, but there is a good chance that these two statements are linked: that is, that the testing system has prevented potent, selective, human teratogens from being marketed. Indeed, the development of many compounds has been terminated because of positive findings in standard developmental toxicity studies. We do not know for certain if any of these agents would have been developmental hazards in humans, but it seems very likely. Due to the limited information on developmental toxicity of chemical agents in humans and the obvious inability to conduct controlled human studies, the correlation between animal studies and human findings is uncertain and it is difficult to extrapolate precisely from animals to humans (see Frankos, 1985). However, the worst hazards—the few dozen selective developmental toxins that are known to be teratogens in humans—are generally also selective teratogens in animals. Thus, although the current battery of animal studies is not perfect, it appears to have been adequate and effective in performing the important task of preventing the widespread exposure of pregnant women to dangerous developmental toxins. In the few cases where new pharmaceuticals have been shown to cause malformations in humans, animal studies had been positive and provided an early warning to the potential problem.

## REFERENCES


Adams, M.J., Hicks, P.G. and York, M.J. (1989). Detection of pregnancy in the rabbit by assay of plasma progesterone. *Teratology* 40: 275.

Adams, M.J., Hicks, P.G. and York, M.J. (1990). Detection of pregnancy in the rabbit by assay of progesterone: An update. *Teratology* 42: 25A–26A.

Anderson, C. and Clark, R.L. (1990). External genitalia of the rat: Normal development and the histogenesis of 5$\alpha$-reductase inhibitor-induced abnormalities. *Teratology* 42: 483–496.

Beyer, P.E. and Chernoff, N. (1986). The induction of supernumerary ribs in rodents: The role of maternal stress. *Teratog. Carcinog. Mutag.* 6: 149–429.

Bloch, E., Lew, M. and Klein, M. (1971). Studies on the inhibition of fetal androgen formation. Inhibition of testosterone synthesis in rat and rabbit fetal testes with observations on reproductive tract development. *Endocrinology* 89: 16–31.

Brown, N.A. and Freeman, S.J. (1984). Alternative tests for teratogenicity, *ATLA* 12: 7–23.

Buelke-Sam, J., Kimmel, C.A. and Adams, J. (1985). Design considerations in screening for behavioral teratogens: Results of the collaborative behavioral teratology study. *Neurobehav. Toxicol. Teratol.* 7: 537–789.

Chapin, R.E., Gulati, D.R. and Barnes, L.H. (1991). The effects of dietary restriction on reproductive endpoints in Sprague-Dawley rats. *Toxicologist* 11: 112.

Chernoff, N., Setzer, R.W., Miller, D.B., Rosen, M.B. and Rogers, J.M. (1990). Effects of chemically induced maternal toxicity on prenatal development in the rat. *Teratology* 42: 651–658.

Chow, B.F. and Rider, A.A. (1973). Implications of the effects of maternal diets in the various species. *J. Anim. Sci.* 36: 167–173.

Christian, M.S. (1983). Assessment of reproductive toxicity: State of the art. In: *Assessment of Reproductive and Teratogenic Hazards* (Christian, M.S., Galbraith, M., Voytek, P. and Mehlman, M.A., Eds.). Princeton Scientific Publishers, Princeton, pp. 65–76.

Christian, M.S. and Hoberman, A.M. (1989). Current *in vivo* reproductive toxicity and developmental toxicity (teratology) test methods. In: *A Guide to General Toxicology*, 2nd ed. (Marquis, J.A. and Hayes, A.W., Eds.). S. Karger, Basel, Switzerland, pp. 91–100.

Clark, R.L., Robertson, R.T., Minsker, D.H., Cohen, S.M., Tocco, D.J., Allen, H.L., James, M.L. and Bokelman, D.L. (1984). Association between adverse maternal and embryo-fetal effects in norfloxacin-treated and food-deprived rabbits. *Fund. Appl. Toxicol.* 7: 272–286.

Clark, R.L., Robertson, R.T., Peter, C.P., Bland, J.A., Nolan, T.E., Oppenheimer, L. and Bokelman, D.L. (1986). Association between adverse maternal and embryo-fetal effects in norfloxacin-treated and food-deprived rabbits. *Fund. Appl. Toxicol.* 7: 272–286.

Clark, R.L., Eschbach, K., Cusick, W.A. and Heyse, J.F. (1987). Interactions between caffeine and adenosine agonists in producing embryo resorptions and malformations in mice. *Toxicol. Appl. Pharmacol.* 91: 371–385.

Clark, R.L., Antonello, J.M., Soper, K.A., Bradstreet, T.C., Heyse, J.F. and Ciminera, J.L. (1989). Statistical analysis of developmental toxicity data. *Teratology* 39: 445–446.

Clark, R.L., Anderson, C.A., Prahalada, S., Leonard, Y.M., Stevens, J.L. and Hoberman, A.M. (1990a). 5α-reductase inhibitor-induced congenital abnormalities in male rat external genitalia. *Teratology* 41: 544.

Clark, R.L., Antonello, J.M., Grossman, J.T., Wise, L.D., Anderson, C., Bagdon, W.J., Prahalada, S., MacDonald, J.S. and Robertson, R.T. (1990b). External genitalia abnormalities in male rats exposed *in utero* to finasteride, a 5α-reductase inhibitor. *Teratology* 42: 91–100.

Clark, R.L., Antonello, J.M., Wenger, J.D., Deyerle-Brooks, K. and Duchai, D.M. (1991). Selection of food allotment for New Zealand white rabbits in developmental toxicity studies. *Fund. Appl. Toxicol.* 17: 584–592.

D'Aguanno, W. (1973). Guidelines of reproduction studies for safety evaluation of drugs for human use. In: *FDA Introduction to Total Drug Quality*, DHEW Publ. (FDA) 74-3006, DHEW/PHS/FDA.

Datson, G.P., Yonker, J.E., Powers, J.F. and Heitmeyer, S.A. (1989). Difference in teratogenic potency of ethylenethiourea in rats and mice: Relative contribution of embryonic and maternal factors. *Teratology* 40: 555–556.

Degenhardt, K. and Kladetzky, J. (1955). Spinal deformation and chordal attachment. *Z. Menschl. Vererb. Konstitutionsl.* 33: 151–192.

Ellington, S. (1980). *In vivo* and *in vitro* studies on the effects of maternal fasting during embryonic organogenesis in the rat. *J. Reprod. Fertil.* 60: 383–388.

Ellison, A.C. and Maren, T.H. (1972). The effect of potassium metabolism on acetazolamide-induced teratogenesis. *Johns Hopkins Med. J.* 130: 105–115.

Environmental Protection Agency (1991). *Pesticide Assessment Guidelines: Subdivision F, Hazard Evaluation: Human and Domestic Animals.* Addendum 10, Neurotoxicity Series

81, 82, and 83. Publication No. PB-91-154617. National Technical Information Service, Washington, D.C.

Fabro, S., Shull, G. and Brown, N.A. (1982). The relative teratogenic index and teratogenic potency: Proposed components of developmental toxicity risk assessment. *Teratog. Carcinog. Mutag.* 2: 61–76.

Food and Drug Administration (1966). *Guidelines for Reproduction Studies for Safety Evaluation of Drugs for Human Use.* Drug Review Branch, Division of Toxicological Evaluation, Bureau of Science, Food and Drug Administration, Washington, D.C.

Food and Drug Administration (1978). Good Laboratory Practice Regulations. *Federal Register,* Friday, December 22, 1978. Title 21, Part II, Part 58.

Food and Drug Administration, Bureau of Foods (1982). *Toxicological Principles for Safety Assessment of Direct Food Additives and Color Additives and Color Used in Food.* No. PB83-170696, pp. 80–117. National Technical Information Service, Washington, D.C. [Also cited as (Red Book). *Guidelines for a Three-Generation Reproduction Toxicity Study with Optional* Teratology Phase. Guidelines for Reproduction Testing with a Teratology Phase.]

Food and Drug Administration (1984). *Final Report of Task Force on Reproductive and Developmental Toxicity. Review of Current Recommendations and Requirements for Reproductive and Developmental Toxicity Studies,* Department of Health and Human Services, Washington, D.C., 24 pp.

Food and Drug Administration (1987). Good Laboratory Practice Regulations: Final Rule. *Federal Register,* Friday, September 4, 1987. Part IV, Vol. 52, No. 172.

Food and Drug Administration (1993). *Guideline for the Study and Evaluation of Gender Differences in the Clinical Evaluation of Drugs. Federal Register,* Thursday, July 22, 1993. Vol. 58, No. 139, pp. 39405–39416.

Frankos, V. (1985). FDA perspectives on the use of teratology data for human risk assessment. *Fund. Appl. Toxicol.* 5: 615–625.

Gad, S.C. (2000). *In Vitro Toxicology,* 2nd ed. Taylor & Francis, Philadelphia, PA.

Grote, W. (1969). Trunk skeletal malformations following blood loss in gravid rabbits. *Z. Anat. Entwicklungsgesch.* 128: 66–74.

Gulati, K., Hope, E. and Chapin, R.E. (1991). The effects of dietary restriction on reproductive endpoints in Swiss mice. *Toxicologist.* 11: 112.

Habert, R. and Picon, R. (1984). Testosterone, dihytrostestosterone and estradiol-17$\beta$ levels in maternal and fetal plasma and in fetal testes in the rat. *J. Steroid Biochem.* 21: 183–198.

Hansen, D.K. and Hodes, M.E. (1983). Comparative teratogenicity of phenytoin among several inbred strains of mice. *Teratology* 28: 175–179.

Heinrichs, W.L. (1985). Current laboratory approaches for assessing female reproductive toxicity. In: *Reproductive Toxicology* (Dixon, R.L., Ed.). Raven Press, New York, pp. 95–108.

Hemm, R., Arslanoglou, L. and Pollock, J. (1977). Cleft palate following prenatal food restriction in mice: Association with elevated maternal corticosteroids. *Teratology* 15: 243–248.

Heywood, R. and James, R.W. (1985). Current laboratory approaches for assessing male reproductive toxicity: Testicular toxicity in laboratory animals. In: *Reproductive Toxicology* (Dixon, R.L., Ed.). Raven Press, New York, pp. 147–160.

ICH (1994). Detection of toxicity to reproduction for medicinal products, *Federal Register* 59 (183): 48746–48752.

*In vitro* Teratology Task Force (1987). Report. *Environ. Health Perspect.* F72: 201–249.

Johnson, E.M. (1981). Screening for teratogenic hazards: Nature of the problems. *Ann. Rev. Pharmacol. Toxicol.* 21: 417–429.

Johnson, E.M. (1984). A prioritization and biological decision tree for developmental toxicity safety evaluations. *J. Am. Coll. Toxicol.* 3: 141–147.

Johnson, E.M. and Christian, M.S. (1984). When is a teratology study not an evaluation of teratogenicity? *J. Am. Coll. Toxicol.* 3: 431–434.

Johnson, E.M., Newman, L.M., Gabel, B.E.G., Boerner, T.F. and Dansky, L.A. (1988). An analysis of the Hydra assay's applicability and reliability as a developmental toxicity prescreen. *J. Am. Coll. Toxicol.* 7: 111–126.

Johnston, M.C., Sulik, K.K. and Dudley, K.H. (1979). Genetic and metabolic studies of the differential sensitivity of A/J and C57BL/6J mice to phenytoin ("Dilantin")-induced cleft lip. *Teratology* 19: 33 A.

Karnofsky, D. (1965). Mechanisms of action of certain growth-inhibiting drugs. In: *Teratology: Principles and Techniques* (Wilson, J. and Warkany, J., Eds.). University of Chicago Press, pp. 185–213.

Kavlock, R.J., Chernoff, N. and Rogers, E.H. (1985). The effect of acute maternal toxicity on fetal development in the mouse. *Teratog. Carcinog. Mutag.* 5: 3–13.

Khera, K.S. (1984). Maternal toxicity-A possible factor in fetal malformations in mice. *Teratology* 29: 411–416.

Khera, K.S. (1985). Maternal toxicity: A possible etiological factor in embryo-fetal deaths and fetal malformations of rodent–rabbit species.

Korenbrot, C.C., Huhtaniemi, I.T. and Weiner, R.I. (1977). Preputial separation as an external sign of pubertal development in the male rat. *Biol. Reprod.* 17: 298–303.

Lin, G.H.Y. (1987). Prediction of teratogenic potential and a proposed scheme for teratogenicity screening of industrial research and development materials. *In Vitro Toxicology* 1: 203–217.

Lochry, E.A. (1987). Concurrent use of behavioral/functional testing in existing reproductive and developmental toxicity screens: Practical consideration. *J. Am. Coll. Toxicol.* 6: 433–439.

Lochry, E.A., Hoberman, A.M. and Christian, M.S. (1984). Positive correlation of pup body weight with other commonly used developmental landmarks. *Teratology* 29: 44A.

Manson, J.M. and Kang, Y.J. (1989). Test methods for assessing female reproductive and developmental toxicology. In: *Principles and Methods of Toxicology*, 2nd ed. (Hayes, A.W., Ed.). Raven Press, New York, pp. 311–359.

Matt, D.W., Lee, J., Sarver, P.L., Judd, H.L. and Lu, J.K.H. (1986). Chronological changes in fertility, fecundity, and steroid hormone secretion during consecutive pregnancies in aging rats. *Biol. Reprod.* 34: 478–487.

Matt, D.M., Sarver, P.L. and Lu, J.K.H. (1987). Relation of parity and estrous cyclicity to the biology of pregnancy in aging female rats. *Biol. Reprod.* 37: 421–430.

Matsuzawa, T., Nakata, M., Goto, I. and Tsushima, M. (1981). Dietary deprivation induces fetal loss and abortions in rabbits. *Toxicology* 22: 255–259.

Millicovsky, G. and Johnston, M.C. (1981). Maternal hyperoxia greatly reduces the incidence of phenytoin-induced cleft lip and palate in A/J mice. *Science* 212: 671–672.

Millicovsky, G., DeSesso, J.M., Kleinman, L.I. and Clark, K.E. (1981). Effects of hydroxyurea on hemodynamics of pregnant rabbits: A maternally mediated mechanism of embryotoxicity. *Am. J. Obstet. Gynecol.* 140: 747–752.

Minsker, D., Bagdon, W., MacDonald, J., Robertson, R. and Bokelman, D. (1990). Maternotoxicity and fetotoxicity of an angiotensin-converting enzyme inhibitor, enalapril, in rabbits. *Fund. Appl. Toxicol.* 14: 461–479.

Mulay, S., Varma, D.R. and Solomon, S. (1982). Influence of protein deficiency in rats on hormonal status and cytoplasmic glucocorticoid receptors in maternal and fetal tissues. *J. Endocrinol.* 95: 49–58.

Neumann, F., von Berswordt-Wallrabe, R., Elger, W., Steinbeck, H., Hahn, J.D. and Kramer, M. (1970). Aspects of androgen-dependent events as studied by antiandrogens. *Recent Prog. Horm. Res.* 26: 337–410.

Nishimura, M., Iizuka, M., Iwaki, S. and Kast, A. (1982). Repairability of drug-induced "wavy ribs" in rat offspring. *Arzneim.-Forsch./Drug Res.* 32: 1518–1522.

Palmer, A.K. (1981). Regulatory requirements for reproducing toxicology: Theory and practice. In: *Developmental Toxicology* (Kimmel, C.A., and Buelke-Sam, J., Eds.). Raven Press, New York, pp. 259–287.

Persaud, T.V.N. (1985). Teratogenicity testing. In: *Basic Concepts in Teratology* (Persaud, T.V.N., Chudley, A.E., and Skalko, R.G., Eds.). Alan R. Liss, New York, pp. 155–181.

Saegusa, T., Kaneko, Y., Sato, T., Nrama, I. and Segima, Y. (1980). BD40A-induced wavy ribs in rats. *Teratology* 22: 14A.

Salewski, V.E. (1964). Färbemethode zum makroskopischen Nachweis von Implantationsstellen am Uterus der Ratte. Nauyn-Schmiedebergs. *Arch. Exp. Path. U. Pharmak.* 247: 367.

Schardein, J. (1987). Approaches to defining the relationship of maternal and developmental toxicity. *Teratog. Carcinog. Mutag.* 7: 255–271.

Schardein, J. (1988). Teratologic testing: Status and issues after two decades of evolution. *Rev. Environ. Contam. Toxicol.* 102: 1–78.

Schardein, J. (1993). *Chemically Induced Birth Defects*, 2nd ed. Marcel Dekker, New York.

Schwetz, B.A. (1981). Monitoring problems in teratology. In: *Scientific Considerations in Monitoring and Evaluating Toxicological Research* (Gralla, E.J., Ed.). Hemisphere, Washington, D.C., pp. 179–192.

Shepard, T. (1998). *Catalog of Teratogenic Agents*, 9th ed. Johns Hopkins University Press, Baltimore.

Snedecor, G.W. and Cochran, W.G. (1980). *Statistical Methods*, 7th ed., Chapter 10. Iowa State University Press, Ames.

Soper, K.A. and Clark, R.L. (1990). Exact permutation trend tests for fetal survival data. *Proc. Biopharm. Section Am. Stat. Assoc.*, pp. 263–268.

Staples, R.E. (1971). Blastocyst transplantation in the rabbit. In: *Methods in Mammalian Embryology* (Daniel, J.C., Jr., Ed.). W.H. Freeman, San Francisco, pp. 290–304.

Szabo, K. and Brent, R. (1975). Reduction of drug-induced cleft palate in mice. *Lancet* (June), 1296–1297.

Tanimura, T. (1990). The Japanese perspectives on the reproductive and developmental toxicity evaluation of pharmaceuticals. *J. Am. Coll. Toxicol.* 9: 27–38.

Turner, M.R. (1973). Perinatal mortality, growth, and survival to weaning in offspring of rats reared on diets moderately deficient in protein. *Br. J. Nutr.* 29: 139–147.

Tyl, R.W. (1988). Developmental toxicity in toxicological research and testing. In: *Perspectives in Basic and Applied Toxicology* (Ballantyne, B., Ed.). Butterworth, Woburn, MA, pp. 206–241.

Watkinson, W.P. and Millicovsky, G. (1983). Effect of phenytoin on maternal heart rate in A/J mice: Possible role in teratogenesis. *Teratology* 28: 1–8.

Weaver, T.E. and Scott, W.J. (1984a). Acetazolamide teratogenesis: Association of maternal respiratory acidosis and ectrodactyly in C57Bl/6J mice. *Teratology* 30: 187–193.

Weaver, T.E. and Scott, W.J. (1984b). Acetazolamide teratogenesis: Interaction of maternal metabolic and respiratory acidosis in the induction of ectrodactyly in C57Bl/6J mice. *Teratology* 30: 195–202.

Weindruch, R. and Walford, R.L. (1988). *The Retardation of Aging and Disease by Dietary Restriction*. Charles C. Thomas, Springfield, IL.

Wickramaratne, G.A. de S. (1988). The post-natal fate of supernumerary ribs in rat teratogenicity studies. *J. Appl. Toxicol.* 8: 91–94.

Wilson, J. (1965). Methods for administering agents and detecting malformations in experimental animals. In: *Teratology, Principles and Techniques* (Wilson, J.G. and Warkany, J., Eds.). University of Chicago Press, pp. 262–277.

Wise, L.D., Clark, R.L., Minsker, D.H. and Robertson, R.T. (1988). Use of hematology and serum biochemistry data in developmental toxicity studies. *Teratology* 37: 502–503.

Wise, L.D., Clark, R.L., Rundell, J.O. and Robertson, R.T. (1990a). Examination of a rodent limb bud micromass assay as a prescreen for developmental toxicity. *Teratology* 41: 341–351.

Wise, L.D., Vetter, C.M., Anderson, C., Antonello, J.M. and Clark, R.L. (1990b). Reversible effects on external genitalia in rats exposed *in vitro* to triamcinolone acetonide. *Teratology* 41: 600.

Working, P.K. (1988). Male reproductive toxicology: Comparison of the human to animal models. *Environ. Health. Perspec.* 77: 37–44.

Yamada, T., Ohsawa, K. and Ohno, H. (1988). The usefulness of alkaline solutions for clearing the uterus and staining implantation sites in rats. *Exp. Anim.* (Tokyo) 37: 325–332.

Zeman, F.J. (1967). Effect on the young rat of maternal protein restriction. *J. Nutr.* 93: 167–173.

# 9

# CARCINOGENICITY STUDIES

## 9.1. INTRODUCTION

In the experimental evaluation of substances for carcinogenesis based on experimental results of studies in a nonhuman species at some relatively high dose or exposure level, an attempt is made to predict the occurrence and level of tumorogenesis in humans at much lower levels. In this chapter we will examine the assumptions involved in this undertaking and review the aspects of design and interpretation of traditional long-term (lifetime) animal carcinogenicity studies as well as some alternative short-term models.

At least in a general way, we now understand what appears to be most of the mechanisms underlying chemical and radiation induced carcinogenesis. The most recent regulatory summary on identified carcinogens (NIH, 2000) lists 44 agents classified as "Known to be Human Carcinogens." Several hundred other compounds are also described as having lesser degrees of proof. A review of these mechanisms is not germane to this chapter (readers are referred to Miller and Miller, 1981, for a good short review), but it is now clear that cancer as seen in humans is the result of a multifocal set of causes.

The mechanisms and theories of chemical carcinogenesis are as follows (Powell and Berry, 2000; Williams and Iatropoulos, 2001):

1. Genetic (all due to some mutagenic event).
2. Epigenetic (No mutagenic event).
3. Oncogene activation.
4. Two-Step (induction/promotion).
5. Multistep (combination of above).

Looked at another way, the four major carcinogenic mechanisms are DNA damage, cell toxicity, cell proliferation and oncogene activation. Any effective program to identify those drugs which have the potential to cause or increase the incidence of neoplasia in humans must effectively screen for these mechanisms (Kitchin, 1999).

The single most important statistical consideration in the design of bioassays in the past was based on the point of view that what was being observed and evaluated was a simple quantal response (cancer occurred or it didn't), and that a sufficient number of animals needed to be used to have reasonable expectations of detecting such an effect. Though the single fact of whether or not the simple incidence of neoplastic tumors is increased due to an agent of concern is of interest, a much more complex model must now be considered. The time-to-tumor, patterns of tumor incidence, effects on survival rate, and age of first tumor all must now be captured in a bioassay and included in an evaluation of the relevant risk to humans.

The task of interpreting the results of any of the animal-based bioassays must be considered from three different potential perspectives as to organ responsiveness.

I.   Those organs with high animal and low human neoplasia rates.
II.  Those organs with high neoplasia rates in both animals and humans.
III. Those organs with low animal but high human neoplasia rates.

Note that not considered is the potential other case, where the neoplasia rates are low for both animals and humans. This is a very rare case and one for which our current bioassay designs probably lack sufficient power to be effective.

In group I, the use of animal cancer data obtained in the liver, kidney, forestomach, and thyroid gland are perceived by some as being hyperresponsive, too sensitive, and of limited value and utility in the animal cancer data obtained in group I organs. The liver is such a responsive and important organ in the interpretation of cancinogenesis data that the discussion of this subject area has been broken up into three chapters for human, rat, and mouse data. Peroxisome proliferation in the liver, particularly in mice, is an area of interpretive battle, as in many cases the metabolism and mechanisms involved are not relevant to man.

Group II organs (mammary gland, hematopoietic, urinary bladder, oral cavity, and skin) are less of an interpretive battleground than group I organs. For group II organs, all four major mechanisms of carcinogenesis (electrophile generation, oxidation of DNA, receptor-protein interactions, and cell proliferation) are known to be important. The high cancer rates for group B organs in both experimental animals and humans may at first give us a false sense of security about how well the experimental animal models are working. As we are better able to understand the probable carcinogenic mechanism(s) in the same organ in the three species, we may find that the important differences between the three species are more numerous than we suspect. This is particularly true for receptor-based and for cell-proliferation-based carcinogenic mechanisms.

Animal cancer data of group III organs are the opposite of group I organs. Group III organs have low animal cancer rates and high human cancer rates. In contrast to the continuing clamor and interpretive battleground associated with group A organs, there is little debate over group III organs. Few voices have questioned the adequacy of the present-day animal bioassay to protect the public health from possible cancer risks in these group III organs. Improved efforts must be made toward the development of cancer-predictive systems or short-term tests for cancer of the prostate gland, pancreas, colon and rectum, cervix and uterus.

Carcinogenicity bioassays are the longest and most expensive of the extensive battery of toxicology studies required for the registration of pharmaceutical products in the United States and in other major countries. In addition, they are often the most controversial with respect to interpretation of their results. These studies are important because, as noted by the International Agency for Research on Cancer (1987), " . . . in the absence of adequate data on humans, it is biologically plausible and prudent to regard agents for which there is sufficient evidence of carcinogenicity in experimental animals as if they presented a carcinogenic risk to humans."

In this chapter, we consider the major factors involved in the design, conduct, analysis, and interpretation of carcinogenicity studies as they are performed in the pharmaceutical industry.

## 9.2. REGULATORY REQUIREMENTS AND TIMING

The prior FDA guidance on the need for carcinogenicity testing of pharmaceuticals presented a dual criteria: that such studies were required to support registration of a drug that was to be administered for a period of three months or more (in Japan and Europe this was stated to be six months or more), and such testing had to be completed before filing for registration in such cases. ICH guidelines (ICH, 1996) now fix this triggering human exposure period at six months, excluding agents given infrequently through a lifetime or for shorter periods of exposure unless there is reason for concern (such as positive findings in genotoxicity studies, structure-activity relationships suggesting such risk, evidence of preneoplastic lesions in repeat dose studies or previous demonstration of carcinogenic potential in the product class that is considered relevant to humans). Such studies are still only required to be completed before filing for registration. Most developers conduct carcinogenicity studies in parallel with phase III clinical studies.

Endogenous peptides, protein substances and their analogs are generally not required to be evaluated for carcinogenicity. There are three conditions which call the need into question:

- Products where there are significant differences in biological effects to the natural counterparts.
- Products where modifications lead to significant changes in structure compared to the natural substance.

- Products resulting in humans having a significant increase over the existing local or systemic concentration.

ICH has also given guidance on design, dose selection, statistical analysis and interpretation for such studies (1995, 1996, 1997). FDA has also offered guidance, the most recent form (FDA, 2001) in a 44-page document available on line.

There has been extensive debate and consideration on the relevance and value of the traditional long-term rodent bioassays. The FDA looked at rat and mouse studies for 282 human pharmaceuticals, resulting in the conclusion that "sufficient evidence is now available for some alternative *in vivo* carcinogenicity models to support their application as complimentary studies *in combination with a single two-year carcinogenicity study* [emphasis added] to identify trans-species tumorigens (Contrera et al., 1997).

The Europeans, meanwhile, have focused on the need for better care in study design, conduct and interpretation (Spindler et. al., 2000), aiming to incorporate these in the revision of the CPMP (Center for Proprietary Medicinal Products) carcinogenicity guidelines.

## 9.3. SPECIES AND STRAIN

Two rodent species are routinely used for carcinogenicity testing in the pharmaceutical industry, the mouse and the rat. Sprague–Dawley derived rats are most commonly used in American pharmaceutical toxicology laboratories. However, the Wistar and Fischer 344 strains are favored by some companies, while the Long Evans and CFE (Carworth) strains are rarely used [Pharmaceutical Manufacturers Association (PMA), 1988].

With respect to mice, the CD-1 is by far the most commonly used strain in the pharmaceutical industry. Other strains used less frequently are the B6C3F1, CF-1, NMRI, C57B1, Balb/c, and Swiss (PMA, 1988; Rao et al., 1988). "Swiss" is the generic term since most currently used inbred and outbred strains were originally derived from the "Swiss" mouse.

If either the mouse or the rat is considered to be an inappropriate species for a carcinogenicity study, the hamster is usually chosen as the second species.

The use of two species in carcinogenicity studies is based on the traditional wisdom that no single species can be considered an adequate predictor of carcinogenic effects in humans. Absence of carcinogenic activity in two different species is thought to provide a greater level of confidence that a compound is "safe" for humans than data derived from a single species.

One may question this reasoning on the basis that data from two "poor predictors" may not be significantly better than data from a single species. It is also reasonable to expect that the ability of one rodent species to predict a carcinogenic effect in a second rodent species should be at least equal to, if not better than, its ability to predict carcinogenicity in humans. The concordance between mouse and rat carcinogenicity data has been investigated and a summary of the results is presented in the next paragraph.

A review of data from 250 chemicals found an 82% concordance between results of carcinogenicity testing in the mouse and the rat (Purchase, 1980). Haseman et al. (1984a) reported a concordance of 73% for 60 compounds studies in both species. However, 30 to 40% of 186 National Cancer Institute (NCI) chemicals were found to be positive in one species and negative in the other (Gold et al., 1984). It is reasonable to conclude that neither rodent species will always predict the results in the other rodent species or in humans, and that the use of two species will continue until we have a much better understanding of the mechanisms of carcinogenesis.

The choice of species and strain to be used in a carcinogenicity study is based on various criteria including susceptibility to tumor induction, incidence of spontaneous tumors, survival, existence of an adequate historical data base, and availability.

Susceptibility to tumor induction is an important criterion. There would be little justification for doing carcinogenicity studies in an animal model that did not respond when treated with a "true" carcinogen. Ideally, the perfect species/strain would have the same susceptibility to tumor induction as the human. Unfortunately, this information is usually unavailable, and the tendency has been to choose animal models that are highly sensitive to tumor induction to minimize the probability of false negatives.

The incidence of spontaneous tumors is also an important issue. Rodent species and strains differ greatly in the incidence of various types of spontaneous tumors. The Sprague–Dawley stock, although preferred by most pharmaceutical companies, has a very high incidence of mammary tumors in aging females, which results in substantial morbidity during the second year of a carcinogenicity study. If one chooses the Fischer 344 (F344) strain, the female mammary tumor incidence will be lower, but the incidence of testicular tumors will be higher (close to 100%) than that in Sprague–Dawley rats.

A high spontaneous tumor incidence can compromise the results of a carcinogenicity study in two ways. If a compound induces tumors at a site that already has a high spontaneous tumor incidence, it may be impossible to detect an increase above the high background "noise." Conversely, if a significant increase above control levels is demonstrated, one may question the relevance of this finding to humans on the basis that the species is "highly susceptible" to tumors of this type.

The ability of a species/strain to survive for an adequate period is essential for a valid assessment of carcinogenicity. Poor survival has caused regulatory problems for pharmaceutical companies and is, therefore, an important issue (PMA, 1988). The underlying concept is that animals should be exposed to the drug for the greater part of their normal life span to make a valid assessment of carcinogenicity. If animals on study die from causes other than drug-induced tumors, they may not have been at risk long enough for tumors to have developed. The sensitivity of the bioassay would be reduced and the probability of a false negative result would be increased.

The availability of an adequate historical data base is often cited as an important criterion for species/strain selection. Historical control data can sometimes be useful in evaluating the results of a study. Although such data are not considered equal in value to concurrent control data, they can be helpful if there is reason to believe that the concurrent control data are "atypical" for the species/strain.

Although outbred stocks (e.g., Sprague–Dawley rats and CD-1 mice) are generally favored in the pharmaceutical industry, inbred strains are also used (e.g., Fischer 344 rats and B6C3F1 mice). Inbred strains may offer greater uniformity of response, more predictable tumor incidence, and better reproducibility than outbred strains. However, their genetic homogeneity may also result in a narrower range of sensitivity to potential carcinogens than exists in random-bred animals. In addition, extrapolation of animal data to humans is the ultimate goal of carcinogenicity studies, and the human population is anything but genetically homogenous.

The ideal species for carcinogenicity bioassays should absorb, metabolize, and excrete the compound under study exactly as humans do. Unfortunately, because of the small number of species that meet the other criteria for selection, there is limited practical utility to this important scientific concept, as applied to carcinogenicity studies.

Before concluding this discussion of species/strain selection, it may be worthwhile to take a closer look at the animals preferred by pharmaceutical companies to determine to what extent they meet the conditions described above. Advantages of the CD-1 mouse are (1) a good historical data base including various routes of exposure, (2) demonstrated susceptibility to induction of tumors, and (3) relatively low spontaneous incidence of certain tumors to which other strains are highly susceptible, especially mammary and hepatic tumors. Disadvantages are (1) lack of homogeneity, (2) relatively low survival, (3) moderate to high incidence of spontaneous pulmonary tumors and leukemias, and (4) high incidence of amyloidosis in important organs, including the liver, kidney, spleen, thyroid, and adrenals (Sher et al., 1982).

There has recently been a reduction in survival of Sprague–Dawley rats and rats of other strains [Food and Drug Administration (FDA), 1993]. This reduction may be the result of *ad libitum* feeding, as preliminary results suggest that caloric restriction may improve survival. Leukemia appears to be the major cause of decreasing survival in the F344 rat. The problem of reduced survival may necessitate a reevaluation of the survival requirements for carcinogenicity studies by regulatory agencies.

## 9.4. ANIMAL HUSBANDRY

Because of the long duration and expense of carcinogenicity studies, the care of animals used in these studies is of paramount importance. Various physical and biological factors can affect the outcome of these studies. Some important physical factors include light, temperature, relative humidity, ventilation, atmospheric conditions, noise, diet, housing, and bedding (Rao and Huff, 1990). Biological factors include bacteria and viruses that may cause infections and diseases.

The duration, intensity, and quality of light can influence many physiological responses, including tumor incidence (Greenman et al., 1984; Wiskemann et al., 1986). High light intensity may cause eye lesions, including retinal atrophy and opacities (Bellhorn, 1980; Greenman et al., 1982). Rats housed in the top row and the side columns of a rack may be the most severely affected.

The influence of light on the health of animals may be managed in several ways. The animals may be randomly assigned to their cages on a rack such that each column contains animals of a single dose group. The location of the columns on the rack may also be randomized so that the effect of light is approximately equal for all dose groups. In addition, the cages of each column of the rack may be rotated from top to bottom when the racks are changed.

Room temperature has been shown to influence the incidence of skin tumors in mice (Weisbrode and Weiss, 1981). Changes in relative humidity may alter food and water intake (Fox, 1977). Low humidity may cause "ringtail," especially if animals are housed in wire mesh cages (Flynn, 1960).

Diets for rodents in carcinogenesis studies should ideally be nutritionally adequate while avoiding excesses of nutrients that may have adverse effects.

Types of caging and bedding have been shown to affect the incidence and latency of skin tumors in mice. In a study by DePass et al. (1986), benzo-(a)pyrene-treated mice were housed either in stainless steel cages or polycarbonate shoebox cages with hardwood bedding. The mice housed in shoebox cages developed tumors earlier and with higher frequency than those housed in steel cages.

Housing of rats in stainless steel cages with wire mesh floors may result in decubitous ulcers on the plantar surfaces. This condition may be a significant clinical problem associated with high morbidity, and may affect survival of the animals if euthanasia is performed for humane reasons. Ulcers are particularly frequent and severe in older male Sprague–Dawley rats, perhaps because of their large size and weight compared with females and rats of other strains.

Common viral infections may affect the outcome of carcinogenicity studies by altering survival or tumor incidence. Nevertheless, viral infections did not cause consistent adverse effects on survival or tumor prevalence in control F344 rats from 28 NCI-NTP studies, though body weights were reduced by Sendai and pneumonia viruses of mice (Rao et al., 1989). The probability of such infections can be minimized by using viral-antibody-free animals, which are readily available.

## 9.5. DOSE SELECTION

### 9.5.1. Number of Dose Levels

In the pharmaceutical industry, most carcinogenicity studies have employed at least three dose levels in addition to the controls, but four levels have occasionally been used (PMA, 1988). The use of three or four dose levels satisfies regulatory requirements (Speid et al., 1990) as well as scientific and practical considerations. If a carcinogenic response is observed, information on the nature of the dose-response relationship will be available. If excessive mortality occurs at the highest dose level, a valid assessment of carcinogenicity is still possible when there is adequate survival at the lower dose levels. These lead to the first two great sins of toxicology (testing at too high a dose and not testing at a high enough dose), and regulatory guidance for dose selection is broad (ICH, 1995).

### 9.5.2. Number of Control Groups

Pharmaceutical companies have most frequently favored the use of two control groups of equal size (PMA, 1988). A single control group of the same size as the treated groups is also used and, less frequently, one double-sized control group may be used. The diversity of study designs reflects the breadth of opinion among toxicologists and statisticians on this issue.

Use of two control groups has the advantage of providing an estimate of the variation in tumor incidence between two groups of animals in the absence of a drug effect. If there are no significant differences between the control groups, the data can be pooled, and the analysis is identical to that using a single, double-sized group. When significant differences occur between the control groups, one must compare the data from the drug-treated groups separately with each control group.

There will be situations in which the incidence of a tumor in one or more drug-treated groups is significantly higher than that of one control group but similar to that of the other control group. In such a situation, it is often helpful to compare the tumor incidences in the control groups to appropriate historical control data. One may often conclude that, for this tumor, one of the control groups is more "typical" than the other, and should, therefore, be given more weight in interpreting the differences in tumor incidence.

In spite of its current popularity in the pharmaceutical industry, the use of two control groups is opposed by some statisticians on the grounds that a significant difference between the two groups may indicate that the study was compromised by excessive, uncontrolled variation. Haseman et al. (1986), however, analyzed tumor incidence data from 18 color additives tested in rats and mice and found that the frequency of significant pairwise differences between the two concurrent control groups did not exceed that which would be expected by chance alone.

The use of one double-sized group is sometimes preferred because it may provide a better estimate of the true control tumor incidence than that provided by a smaller group. Nevertheless, more statistical power would be obtained by assigning the additional animals equally to all dose groups rather than to the control group only, if power is a primary consideration (Weaver and Brunden, 1998).

### 9.5.3. Criteria for Dose Selection

Dose selection is one of the most important activities in the design of a toxicology study. It is especially critical in carcinogenicity studies because of their long duration. Whereas faulty dose selection in an acute or subchronic toxicity study can easily be corrected by repeating the study, this situation is much less desirable in a carcinogenicity study, especially since such problems may not become evident until the last stages of the study.

The information used for dose selection usually comes from subchronic toxicity studies, but other information about the pharmacological effects of a drug and its metabolism and pharmacokinetics may also be considered. The maximum recommended human dose (MRHD) of the drug may be an additional criterion, if this is known when the carcinogenicity studies are being designed.

For most pharmaceutical companies, the doses selected are as follows. The highest dose is selected to be the estimated maximum tolerated dose (MTD). The lowest dose is usually a small multiple (1 to 5 times) of the MRHD, and the mid-dose approximates the geometric mean of the other two doses (PMA, 1988; McGregor, 2000).

The MTD is commonly estimated to be the maximum dose that can be administered for the duration of the study that will not compromise the survival of the animals by causes other than carcinogenicity. It should be defined separately for males and females. ICH (1995) states that the MTD is "that dose which is predicted to produce a minimum toxic effect over the course of the carcinogenicity study, usually predicted from the results of a 90-day study." Factors used to define minimum toxicity include no more than a 10% decrease in body weight gain relative to controls, target organ toxicity, and/or significant alterations in clinical pathology parameters. If the MTD has been chosen appropriately, there should be no adverse effect on survival, only a modest decrement in body weight gain and minimal overt signs of toxicity. The procedures for dose selection described above are generally consistent with major regulatory guidelines for carcinogenicity studies (Speid et al., 1990; Food and Drug Administration, 1993*). There are, however, exceptions to the general approach described above. For example, for nontoxic drugs, the difference between the high and the low doses may be many orders of magnitude, if the high dose is set at the estimated MTD and the low dose is a small multiple of the clinical dose. Some guidelines request that the low dose be no less than 10% of the high dose (Speid et al., 1990). In this situation, it may be acceptable to set the high dose at 100 times the MRHD, even if the MTD is not achieved (Speid et al., 1990). Similarly, when a drug is administered in the diet, the highest concentration should not exceed 5% of the total diet, whether or not the MTD is achieved (Japanese Ministry of Health and Welfare, 1989).

Metabolism and/or pharmacokinetic data, when available, should also be considered in the dose selection process. It is desirable that a drug not be administered at such a high dose that it is excreted in a different manner than at lower doses, such as the MRHD. Similarly, the high dose should not lead to the formation of metabolites other than those formed at lower (clinical) doses. If data show that a given dosage produces maximum plasma levels, administration of higher

---

* Note that the *FDA Redbook* applies, strictly speaking, only to food additives. It is cited here because it is a well-known toxicology guideline routinely applied to animal pharmaceuticals to which humans may be exposed. The *Redbook* has recently been updated by the FDA (Food and Drug Administration, 1993).

doses should be unnecessary. These considerations may be very useful when interpreting the results of the study or attempting to extrapolate the results to humans.

## 9.6. GROUP SIZE

The minimum number of animals assigned to each dose group in pharmaceutical carcinogenicity studies is 50 of each sex (PMA, 1988). Most companies, however, use more than the minimum number, and some use up to 80 animals per sex per group. The most important factor in determining group size is the need to have an adequate number of animals for a valid assessment of carcinogenic activity at the end of the study. For this reason, larger group sizes are used when the drug is administered by daily gavage because this procedure may result in accidental deaths by perforation of the esophagus or aspiration into the lungs. Larger group sizes are also used when the carcinogenicity study is combined with a chronic toxicity study in the rat. In this case, serial sacrifices are performed at 6 and 12 months to evaluate potential toxic effects of the drug.

In the final analysis, the sensitivity of the bioassay for detecting carcinogens is directly related to the sample size. Use of the MTD has often been justified based on the small number of animals at risk compared to the potential human population, in spite of the difficulties inherent in extrapolating effects at high doses to those expected at much lower clinical doses. A reasonable compromise may be the use of doses lower than the MTD combined with a larger group size than the 50 per sex minimum accepted by regulatory agencies.

## 9.7. ROUTE OF ADMINISTRATION

In the pharmaceutical industry, the two most common routes of administration are via diet and gavage (PMA, 1988). Some compounds are given by drinking water, topical (dermal) application, or injection, depending on the expected clinical exposure route, which is the primary criterion for determining the route of administration in carcinogenicity studies. When more than one clinical route is anticipated for a drug, the dietary route is often chosen for practical reasons.

Dietary administration is often preferred over gavage because it is far less labor intensive. Another advantage is the MTD has rarely been overestimated in dietary studies, whereas it has often been overestimated in gavage studies, according to data from the NTP (Haseman, 1985). The dietary route is unsuitable for drugs that are unstable in rodent chow or unpalatable. The dietary route is also disadvantaged by the fact that dosage can only be estimated based on body weight and food intake data, in contrast with gavage by which an exact dose can be given. Disadvantages of gavage testing are the likelihood of gavage-related trauma, such as puncture of the trachea or esophagus, and possible vehicle (e.g., corn oil) effects.

When doing studies by the dietary route, the drug may be administered as a constant concentration at each dose level, or the concentration may be increased as body weight increases to maintain a constant dose on a milligram per kilogram basis. The later method allows greater control of the administered dose and avoids age- and sex-related variations in the dose received, which occur with the former method. Both methods are acceptable to regulatory agencies.

## 9.8. STUDY DURATION

The duration of carcinogenicity studies for both rats and mice is two years in most pharmaceutical laboratories (PMA, 1988). Occasionally, rat studies are extended to 30 months, while some companies terminate mouse studies at 18 months. The difference in duration between mouse and rat studies is based on the belief that rats have a longer natural life span than mice. Recent data indicate, however, that this is not the case. The most commonly used strains, the Sprague–Dawley rat and the CD-1 mouse, have approximately equal survival at two years, based on industry data (PMA, 1988). The same is true for the most popular inbred strains, the Fischer 344 rat and the B6C3F1 mouse (PMA, 1988). Data from NCI studies confirm that the two-year survival of the B6C3F1 mouse is at least equal to, if not greater than, that of the Fischer 344 rat (Cameron et al., 1985).

## 9.9. SURVIVAL

As stated earlier, adequate survival is of primary importance in carcinogenicity studies because animals must be exposed to a drug for the greater part of their life span to increase the probability that late-occurring tumors can be detected. Early mortality, resulting from causes other than tumors, can jeopardize the validity of a study because dead animals cannot get tumors.

In general, the sensitivity of a carcinogenicity bioassay is increased when animals survive to the end of their natural life span, because weak carcinogens may induce late-occurring tumors. The potency of a carcinogen is often inversely related to the time to tumor development. By analogy, as the dose of a carcinogen is reduced, the time to tumor occurrence is increased (Littlefield et al., 1979; DePass et al., 1986).

Why do we not allow all animals on a carcinogenicity study to live until they die a natural death if by so doing we could identify more drugs as carcinogens? In fact, the sensitivity of a bioassay may not be improved by allowing the animals to live out their natural life span because the incidence of spontaneous tumors tends to increase with age. Thus, depending on the tumor type, the ability of the bioassay to detect a drug-related increase in tumor incidence may actually decrease, rather than increase, with time. Therefore, the optimum duration of a carcinogenicity study is that which allows late-occurring tumors to be detected but does not allow the incidence of spontaneous tumors to become excessive.

Reduced survival in a carcinogenicity study may or may not be drug related. Sometimes, the MTD is exceeded and increased mortality occurs at the highest dose level and occasionally, at the mid-dose level as well. This situation may not necessarily invalidate a study; in fact, the protocol may be amended to minimize the impact of the drug-induced mortality. For example, cessation of drug treatment may enhance the survival of the animals in the affected groups, and allow previously initiated tumors to develop. As shown by Littlefield et al. (1979) in the CNTR ED01 study, liver tumors induced by 2-acetylaminofluorene, which appeared very late in the study, were shown to have been induced much earlier and not to require the continuous presence of the carcinogen to develop. By contrast, bladder tumors that occurred in the same study were dependent on the continued presence of the carcinogen.

Whether drug treatment is terminated or not, drug-related toxicity may also be managed by performing complete histopathology on animals in the lower-dose groups rather than on high-dose and control animals only. If there is no increase in tumor incidence at a lower-dose level that is not compromised by reduced survival, the study may still be considered valid as an assessment of carcinogenicity.

When reduced survival is related to factors other than excessive toxicity, the number of animals at risk for tumor development may be inadequate, and the validity of the study may be compromised even in the absence of a drug effect on survival. Obviously, the adjustments described above for excessive, drug-related toxicity are not relevant to this situation.

There is no unanimity of opinion among regulatory agencies as to the minimum survival required to produce a valid carcinogenicity study or as to the best approach for dealing with survival problems. Even within a single agency such as the FDA, different opinions exist on these issues. For example, the recently issued *FDA Redbook II Draft Guideline* requires that rats, mice, or hamsters be treated for 24 months. Early termination due to decreased survival is not recommended. The EEC guidelines differ in that they suggest termination of the study when survival in the control group reaches 20%, while Japanese guidelines suggest termination at 25% survival in the control or low-dose groups (Speid et al., 1990). These provisions make good sense in that they do not request termination of the study when drug-related mortality may be present only at the highest dose.

## 9.10. ENDPOINTS MEASURED

A carcinogenicity study is more focused than a chronic toxicity study; fewer endpoints are evaluated, and as such it is a simpler study. The key endpoints are actually few.

Pathology (limited to neoplastic and preneoplastic tissue transformations);
Body weight (to ensure that toxicity is not so great as to invalidate the assays and also that it is just sufficient to validate the assay);

Survival (key to determining when to terminate the study);

Clinical pathology (limited to evaluating the morphology of white blood cells, and usually this is actually deferred until there are indications that such data is needed);

Food consumption (actually measured to ensure that dietary administration doses are accurate).

Only pathology will be considered in detail.

The primary information for carcinogenicity evaluation is generated by pathologists. Table 9.1 lists the tissues normally collected, processed and evaluated. These professionals, like any other group of professionals, vary in their training and experience, and these are characteristics which may influence the evaluation in a number of ways. Some of these are listed here.

1. Differences in terminology may be important when considering controversial lesions.

2. Lack of consistency throughout a study is likely when a pathologist has only recently become involved with rodent carcinogenicity. Training is often in a clinical situation (especially in Europe), where each animal or person is unique and there is in a rodent carcinogenicity study consisting of 500 inbred animals.

3. Unfamiliarity with the observed lesion in a particular species may cause problems in interpretation.

**TABLE 9.1. Standard Tissue List**

| | | |
|---|---|---|
| Kidney | Urinary bladder | Aorta |
| Heart | Trachea | Lungs |
| Liver | Gall bladder | Pancreas |
| Fat | Salivary gland | Spleen |
| Cervical lymph node | Mesenteric lymph node | Thymus |
| Tongue | Esophagus | Stomach |
| Duodenum | Jejunum | Ileum |
| Cecum | Colon | Mammary gland |
| Skin | Skeletal muscle | Sciatic nerve |
| Parathyroid | Thyroid | Adrenal |
| Pituitary | Prostate | Seminal vesicles |
| Testes | Epididymides | Ovaries |
| Oviducts | Uterine horns | Uterine body |
| Cervix | Vagina | Brain |
| Spinal cord | Sternum | Rib/bone |
| Eyes | Harderian glands | BM smear |
| Nares | Clitoral/preputial gland | Zymbal's gland |
| Gross lesions | | |

Possible bias introduced by knowledge of treatment can be corrected in several ways, but the use of a two-stage process would seem to be most efficient.

1. An initial evaluation is performed with full knowledge of the animal's history, including treatment.
2. A second evaluation of specific lesions is then carried out. This should be done blind, either by the same pathologist or, preferably, by the same and a second pathologist.

Differences in evaluation between pathologists should always be discussed by them to resolve the differences; they may be due to subtle differences in diagnosis and do not indicate incompetence in one of the pathologists. It is unacceptable for a study sponsor to shop around until he finds a pathologists who gives, for whatever reason, the result he is looking for without giving an opportunity for interaction with all of the other evaluators. Sometimes these diagnoses are given years apart, during which time understanding of the pathogenesis of lesions may change, and even the first pathologist may not arrive at the same conclusion as he did some years ago.

Evaluation of the data is not purely a statistical exercise. A number of important factors should be considered: (1) dose-effect relationship; (2) a shift towards more anaplastic tumors in organs where tumors are common; (3) earlier appearance of tumors, and (4) presence of preneoplastic lesions.

The language used to describe the carcinogenic response has masked its complexity and presents a stumbling block to its understanding among nonhisto-pathologists. Benign or malignant neoplasms do not arise without some precursor change within normal tissue. An important concept in carcinogenicity evaluation is that of neoplastic progression, which was derived from studies on skin tumors (Berenblum and Shubik, 1947) and expanded to a number of other tissues (Foulds, 1969, 1975). There is, on many occasions, a far from clear distinction between hyperplastic and "benign" neoplasia and between benign and malignant neoplasia.

Hyperplasia and benign and malignant neoplasia are convenient medical terms with prognostic significance. Hyperplasia can occur either as a regenerative response to injury, with no neoplastic connotations, or as a sustained response to a carcinogenic agent. It is an increase in the number of normal cells retaining normal intercellular relationships within a tissue. This normally may break down, resulting in altered growth patterns and altered cellular differentiation, a condition which may be described as atypical hyperplasia or presumptively as preneoplastic lesions. Possible sequelae to hyperplasia are: (1) persistence without qualitative change in either structure or behavior, (2) permanent regression, (3) regression, with later reappearance, and (4) progression to develop new characteristics indicating increased probability of malignancy. The last of these is the least likely to occur in experimental multistage models, such as in mouse skin or rat liver, where large numbers of hyperplastic lesions may occur, but notably fewer carcinomas develop from them.

Benign neoplasms in most rodent tissues apparently arise in hyperplastic foci, for example, squamous-cell papillomas of the skin and forestomach. Furthermore, these papillomas seldom demonstrate autonomous growth and even fewer progress to squamous-cell carcinomas (Burns et al., 1976; Colburn, 1980). This decisive progression to carcinoma, when it occurs, provides powerful evidence for the multistage theory of carcinogenesis: the new, malignant cells arising as a focus within the papilloma or even in an area of hyperplasia, since the papilloma is not a necessary intermediate stage. In other organs, benign neoplasia is usually characterized by well-differentiated cell morphology, a fairly uniform growth pattern, clear demarcation from surrounding tissues and no evidence of invasion. The progression towards malignancy involves anaplasia (loss of differentiation) and pleomorphism (variety of phenotypic characteristics within the neoplasm). These changes may be focal in an otherwise benign neoplasm and may vary in degree and extent. Evidence of invasion of the surrounding tissues or of metastasis are not essential characteristics of malignancy, although their presence strengthens the diagnosis.

The grouping together of certain tumor types can aid statistical analysis, but it must be done carefully, with full appreciation of the biology and whatever is known of the pathogenesis of the lesions. Grouping for analysis of all animals showing neoplasia, irrespective of the tumor type, is inappropriate because the incidence in most treatment control groups can be very high and, in U.S. National Toxicology Program studies, approaches 100% in rats and 50–70% in mice (Table 9.2).

There may be similar incidences of tumors in aging people, but the real prevalence of tumors in human populations is uncertain. In the United States, where autopsies are uncommon, over one-third reveal previously undiagnosed cancers when they are conducted (Silverberg, 1984). A single type of neoplasm, renal adenoma, is present in 15–20% of all adult kidneys (Holm–Nielson and Olsen,

**TABLE 9.2. Tumor-bearing Animals in Control Groups from Rodent Studies**

| Control animals for two-year NTP bioassay | No. of Animals | % with Tumors | | |
|---|---|---|---|---|
| | | Malignant | Benign | Total |
| B6C3F1 mice | | | | |
|   Male | 1692 | 42 | 35 | 64 |
|   Female | 1689 | 45 | 33 | 64 |
| F344 rats | | | | |
|   Male | 1596 | 55 | 95 | 98 |
|   Female | 1643 | 38 | 76 | 88 |
| Osborne–Mendel rats | | | | |
|   Male | 50 | 26 | 68 | 78 |
|   Female | 50 | 12 | 80 | 88 |
| Sprague–Dawley rats | | | | |
|   Male | 56 | 9 | 36 | 39 |
|   Female | 56 | 30 | 68 | 79 |

*Source*: Haseman, unpublished summary of US NTP data

1988), although it is unclear whether these 2–6 mm foci of proliferating tubular and papillary epithelium represent small carcinomas or benign precursors of renal-cell carcinomas. Irrespective of the significance of these lesions in human pathology, the presence of similar foci in a rodent carcinogenicity experiment would trigger the recording of renal tumor-bearing animals and, hence, their consideration in the statistical and pathological evaluation processes. Evaluation is further complicated by the increased background incidences of tumors as animals get older.

The independent analysis of every different diagnosis in rodent studies would also mask significant effects in many cases, while enhancing them in others. Benign and malignant neoplasms of a particular histogenesis are often grouped because the one is seen as a progression from the other. However, this grouping may result in a nonsignificant difference from the controls because there has been an acceleration of progression towards malignancy, the incidence of benign neoplasms decreasing while the malignant neoplasms increase. Guidelines are available for "lumping" or "splitting" tumor types, but in using them, the basis for the classification of neoplastic lesions should be clarified, especially when data generated over several or many years are coupled, since diagnostic criteria and ideas regarding tumor histogenesis may have changed. Reliance on tabulated results alone can lead to serious misinterpretation by those not closely connected with a particular study. For this very important reason, the pathology and toxicology narrative should be full and clear. If it is not, then there will always be doubts about future interpretations, even if these doubts are not, in reality, justified.


## 9.11. STATISTICAL ANALYSIS

Irrespective of the specific protocols used, all carcinogenicity studies end with a statistical comparison of tumor proportions between treated and control groups. This analysis is necessary because the control incidence of most tumor types is rarely zero. In the unlikely case that a type of tumor is found in treated animals but not in concurrent or appropriate historical controls, it is reasonable to conclude that the tumor is drug-related without statistical analysis.

Most pharmaceutical companies analyze tumor data using mortality-adjusted methods (PMA, 1988). Peto/International Agency for Research on Cancer (IRC) methodology is most commonly used, perhaps because this method is currently favored by the FDA (Peto et al., 1980). The use of life-table methods is most appropriate for "lethal" tumors, that is, those that cause the death of the animals. Various statistical methods are available for analyzing the incidence of lethal and nonlethal tumors (e.g., Gart et al., 1979, 1986; Dinse and Lagakos, 1983; McKnight, 1988; Portier and Bailer, 1989). These methods are especially useful when there are drug-related differences in mortality rates. When there is no drug effect on survival, unadjusted methods will generally give the same results.

As a general approach, most pharmaceutical statisticians begin by testing for the presence of a dose-related trend in tumor proportions. If the trend test is significant, that is, the $p$ value is less than or equal to 0.05, pairwise comparisons are performed between the treated and control groups. Trend and pairwise analyses may be adjusted for mortality as stated earlier, or performed without mortality adjustment using such simple methods as chi-square or Fisher's exact tests.

Although in most cases the use of trend tests is appropriate since most biological responses are dose related, there are exceptions to this rule. Certain drugs, especially those with hormonal activity, may not produce classical dose responses and may even induce inverse dose-response phenomena. In these cases, a pairwise comparison may be appropriate in the absence of a significant positive trend.

Most (70%) pharmaceutical companies use one-tailed comparisons, and a substantial number use two-tailed methods (PMA, 1988). Since regulatory agencies are primarily interested in identifying carcinogenic drugs, as opposed to those that inhibit carcinogenesis, the use of one-tailed tests is generally considered more appropriate. Some companies prefer two tailed comparisons because, in the absence of a true carcinogenic effect, there is an equal probability of seeing significant decreases as well as significant increases by chance alone.

One of the most important statistical issues in the analysis of carcinogenicity data is the frequency of "false positives," or type I errors. Because of the multiplicity of tumor sites examined and the number of tests employed, there is concern that noncarcinogenic drugs may be erroneously declared carcinogens. If an $p < 0.05$ increase in tumor incidence is automatically regarded as a biologically meaningful result, then the false positive rate may be as high as 47–50% (Haseman et al., 1986).

Several statistical procedures designed to correct for the multiplicity of significance tests have been published (and reviewed by Haseman, 1990). One approach to the problem of multiple tumor site/type testing is a procedure attributed to Tukey by Mantel (1980). This method is used to adjust a calculated $p$ value based on the number of tumor types/sites for which there are minimum number of tumors in the particular study. The reasoning here is that, for tumor sites, the number of tumors found is so small that it is impossible to obtain a significant result for that tumor site no matter how the tumors might have been distributed among the dose groups. Only those sites for which a minimum number of tumors is present can contribute to the false positive rate for a particular study.

A method proposed by Schweder and Spjotvoll (1982) is based on a plot of the cumulative distribution of observed $p$ values. Farrar and Crump (1988) have published a statistical procedure designed not only to control the probability of false positive findings, but also to combine the probabilities of a carcinogenic effect across tumor sites, sexes, and species.

Another approach to controlling the false positive rate in carcinogenicity studies was proposed by Haseman (1983). Under this "rule," a compound would be declared a carcinogen if it produced an increase significant at the 1% level in a common tumor or an increase significant at the 5% level in a rear tumor. A rare neoplasm was defined as a neoplasm that occurred with a frequency of less than 1% in control animals. The overall false positive rate associated with this decision rule was found to be not more that 7–8%, based on control tumor incidences from NTP studies in rats and mice. This false positive rate compares favorably with the expected rate of 5%, which is the probability at which one would erroneously conclude that a compound was a carcinogen. The method is notable for its simplicity and deserves serious consideration by pharmaceutical statisticians and toxicologists. Without resorting to sophisticated mathematics, this method recognizes the fact that tumors differ in their spontaneous frequencies and, therefore, in their contribution to the overall false positive rates in the carcinogenicity studies. False positive results are much less likely to occur at tissue sites with low spontaneous tumor incidences than at those with high frequencies.

As a final point that has special relevance to pharmaceutical carcinogenicity studies, one may question whether the corrections for multiple comparisons and their effect on the overall false positive rate are appropriate for all tumor types. For example, if a compound is known to bind to receptors and produce pharmacological effects in a certain organ, is it justified to arbitrarily correct the calculated $p$ value for the incidence of tumors in that organ, using the methods described above? It is difficult to justify such a correction considering that the basis for correcting the calculated $p$ value is that the true probability of observing an increased incidence of tumors at any site by chance alone may be much higher than the nominal alpha level (usually 0.05). It is reasonable to expect that, when a drug has known pharmacological effects on a given organ, the probability of observing an increased tumor incidence in that organ by chance alone is unlikely to be higher than the nominal 5% alpha level.

Although most pharmaceutical statisticians and toxicologists agree on the need to control the probability of false positive results, there is no consensus as to which method is most appropriate or most acceptable to regulatory agencies, The FDA and other such agencies will accept a variety of statistical procedures but will often reanalyze the data and draw their own conclusions based on their analyses.

## 9.12. TRANSGENIC MOUSE MODELS

Since the early 1970s, the standard for adequate evaluation of the carcinogenic potential of a candidate pharmaceutical has been the conduct of lifetime, high dose assays in two species, almost always the rat and the mouse.

The relevance (and return on investment) for the bioassays preformed in mice have been questioned for some time. In 1997, ICH opened the possibility for the substitution of some form of short- or medium-term mouse test as an alternative for the traditional lifetime mouse bioassay. FDA has subsequently stated that it would accept "validated" forms of a set of medium-term mouse studies based on transgenic models, and significant effort has since gone into such validation.

The huge advances made in molecular biology since the late 1980s have provided the possibility of approaches to evaluating chemicals and potential drugs for carcinogenic potential in approaches which are different, less expensive and which take a shorter period of time than traditional long-term bioassays. This work has also been stimulated by dissatisfaction with the performance of traditional test systems.

The traditional long-term bioassays use highly inbred animals, developed with the goal of reducing the variability in background tumor incidences as a means of increasing the statistical sensitivity of the bioassays. This inbreeding has led to narrowing of the allelic pool in the strains of animals that are currently used for testing, as opposed to the wild-type populations (of humans) that the tests are intended to protect (Festing, 1979). Transgenic models should serve to improve the identification of carcinogens by providing the gene-specific mechanistic data, minimizing the influence of spontaneous tumors and strain-specific effects, and reducing time required, cost and animal usage (Eastin et al., 1998).

As it has become possible to transfer new or engineered genes to the germ lines of mammals, the results have been transgenic mice that can be used in shorter term *in vivo* assays for carcinogenicity and which are also useful for research into the characterization of genotoxic events and mechanisms in carcinogenesis. By coupling reporter phenotypes (such as papilomas in the $Tg \cdot AC$ mouse, the task of "reading" results in test animals is made much less complex.

There are four transgenic mouse models that have been broadly evaluated: the $TSPp53^{+/-}$, the Tg.AC, the Hras2 and the $XPA^{-/-}$. Each of these has its own characteristics. Each of these merits some consideration. They are each made by either zygote injection or specific gene targeting in embryonic cells (McAnulty, 2000; French et al., 1999).

### 9.12.1. The $Tg \cdot AC$ Mouse Model

This was the earliest of the models to be developed, and its use in mouse skin carcinogenicity studies was first reported in 1990. The mice have four copies of the v-H-ras oncogene in tandem on chromosome 11, and the transgene is fused with a fetal $\zeta$-globin gene which acts as a promoter. The transgene codes for a switch protein which is permanently "on" and this results in the mice having genetically initiated skin. The application of tumor promoters to the surface of the skin causes the rapid induction of predunculate papillomas that arise from the follicular epithelium. This is despite the fact that the transgene is not expressed in the skin, although it is present in the papillomas that form, and also in the focal follicular hyperplastic areas that are the precursors to the papillomas. In about 40% of the mice, the papillomas become malignant skin tumors, mainly squamous cell carcinomas and sarcomas.

The first assessments of this model as an alternative to traditional carcinogenicity studies were performed by the U.S. NIEHS and NTP, and the results with over 40 chemicals have been published. The majority of studies were performed by skin painting, regardless of whether the product was a dermal or systemic carcinogen. However, a good correlation was found with the known carcinogenicity of the test compounds, and both mutagenic and nonmutagenic were identified. It was found that great care had to be taken with the skin, because damage could also induce papillomas, which means that these animals cannot be identified using transponder chips. This sensitivity may also explain some of the false-positive results that have occurred with resorcinol and rotenone. Of more concern is that there have been false-negatives with known carcinogens, namely ethyl acrylate and *N*-methyl-*o*-acrylamide. The model was designed for use in the context of the two-stage model of carcinogenesis with the underlying mechanistic pathway involving specific transcription factors, hypomethylation and cell-specific expression of the results, along with the p53, this model has seen the widest use and evaluation (in terms of number of agents evaluated) so far. The carrier mouse strain employed, the FVB/N, is not commonly employed in toxicology and is prone to sound-induced seizures. It may be that the dermal route is not suitable for all systemic carcinogens, and this is the reason that in the ILSI program, both the dermal and systemic routes are being investigated in this model.

Another problem with this model was the occurrence of a nonresponder genotype to positive control agents. This was found to be attributable to a rearrangement of the $\zeta$-globin promoter region, but it is claimed that this problem has been resolved. However, this has considerably delayed the ILSI studies with this model, but the data was available in time for the November 2001 meeting (Cohen et al., 2001). It is already clear that the model gives a robust response to the positive control agent, 12-*o*-tetradecanoylphorbol 13-acetate (TPA).

### 9.12.2. The Tg · rasH2 Mouse Model

This model was developed at CIEA in Japan, and the first information about the mouse was published in 1990. The mice have five or six copies of the human H-ras proto-oncogene inserted in tandem into their genome surrounded by their own promoter and enhancer regions. This transgene has been very stabile, with no loss of responsiveness since the model was developed. The transgene codes for a molecular switch protein in the same way as the previous model, but the transgene is expressed in all organs and tissues. Thus the response endpoint is not primarily dermal.

The initial studies with this model revealed a rapid appearance of forestomach papillomas with *N*-methyl-*N*-nitrosourea (MNU), and this compound has already been used as the positive control agent in subsequent studies with this strain. A study duration of six months is sufficient to obtain a positive response, and longer periods should be avoided because the mice start to develop various spontaneous tumors, such as splenic haemangiosarcomas, forestomach and skin papillomas, lung and Harderian gland adenocarcinomas, and lymphomas. It has a high level of constitutive expression and some spontaneous tumors even when the animals are younger. It is, however, very responsive to carcinogens; one gets a rapid onset after exposure and a higher response incidence than with the other models. The underlying mechanism is still not certain.

A large number of studies have been run in this strain in Japan in advance of the ILSI program. The model is sensitive to both mutagenic and nonmutagenic carcinogens, although cyclophosphamide and furfural have given equivocal results in each category, respectively. The majority of noncarcinogens have also been identified correctly, although again, there are a small number of compounds that have given equivocal results. In the ILSI program, 24 of the 25 studies were completed in time for the November 2000 meeting, and the final study competed was is 2001.

### 9.12.3. The P53$^{+/-}$ Mouse Model

The TSP p53$^{+/-}$ (hereafter referred to as the p53), the designation of the tumor suppressor gene involved) is a heterozygous knockout with (up to seven or so months of age), a low spontaneous tumor incidence. It is responsive to the genotoxic carcinogens by a mechanism based on the fact that many (but not all) tumors show a loss of the wild-type allele. The p53 has been extensively worked on by Tennant's group at NIEHS (Tennant et al., 1995 and 1999). This model was developed in the United States and carries a hemizygous knockout of the p53 gene which was developed by integrating a mutated copy of the gene into the genome of mice. The p53 gene is known as a tumor-suppressor gene, and it is the most commonly mutated gene in human malignancies. It searches for a protein transcription factor which activates multiple genes when damage to DNA strands occurs, and this in turn leads to either the arrest of the cell cycle while DNA repair occurs, or to apoptosis (programmed cell death) which removes the damaged cell. The heterozygote is used because homozygotes show a very high incidence of spontaneous tumors within a few months of birth. The heterozygotes have a low background incidence of tumors up to 12 months, but during this time there is a high chance of a second mutagenic event occurring, following exposure to a carcinogen, for example, and this would result in a loss of suppressor function, or an increase in transforming activity.

The initial studies with this model as an alternative in traditional carcinogenicity testing were performed at the United States NIEHS, and these suggested that it was sensitive to mutagenic carcinogens such as benzene and *p*-cresidine within six months. Nonmutagenic carcinogens were negative in the assay, as were mutagenic noncarcinogens. However, subsequent studies and some parts of the ILSI program have shown clear indications that a six-month duration may be insufficient. In particular, benzene has given negative or equivocal results within six months, although positive results have been obtained by extending the study to nine months. It will be very important to assess the results of the ILSI program when deciding the best study duration for this model. This is the most popular model in the United States.

### 9.12.4. The XPA$^{-/-}$ Mouse Model

This was the last of the models to be developed, and was created using a knockout technique after the XPA gene had been cloned. The first data were published by RIVM in the Netherlands in 1995 (Tennant, et al., 1999). Both alleles of the XPA gene have been inactivated by a homologous recombination in ES cells, resulting in a homozygous deletion of the gene spanning exons three and four. The protein coded by this gene is essential for the detection and repair of DNA damage, using the nucleotide excision repair (NER) pathway. This model only has between 2% and 5% of residual NER-activity.

The initial studies at RIVM demonstrated that exposure of these mice to IV-B radiation or 7,12-dimethylbenz[*a*]anthracene resulted in the rapid induction of skin tumors. It was also shown that various internal tumors could be induced following oral administration of mutagenic carcinogens such as benzo[*a*]pyrene (B[*a*]P) and 2-acetylaminofluorine (2-AAF). The early studies suggested that this response could occur within six months, but further experience has indicated that a nine-moth treatment period is essential in order to obtain a response with positive control agents such as B[*a*]P,2-AAF and *p*-cresidine.

All of the 13 studies that have been undertaken with this model were available for review at the November 2000 meeting. The model is sensitive to both UV and genotoxic carcinogens, and also to some nonmutagenic carcinogens, such as diethylstilboestrol (DES), Wy-14,643 and cyclosporin A. There have been no false-positives with noncarcinogens. Some laboratories have also investigated a double transgenic XPA$^{-/-}$ p53$^{+/-}$ model, and this seems to increase the sensitivity of the assay. For example, in a DES study, seven animals with metastasizing osteosarcomas were found in the double transgenic group, compared with one in the XPA group and none among the wild type animals. There remains concern (as with any new model) that these models may be overly sensitive, or (put another way), that the relevance of positive findings to risk in humans may not be clear. The results of the ILSI/HESI workshop seem to minimize these concerns.

It is generally proposed that while such models can improve the identification of carcinogens in three ways (providing gene-specific mechanistic data, minimizing the influence of spontaneous tumors and strain specific effects, and reducing the time, cost and animal usage involved), they have two potential uses in pharmaceutical development. These are either in lieu of the mouse two-year cancer bioassay or in subchronic toxicity assessments prior to making a decision to commit to a pair of two-year carcinogenicity bioassays.

As performance data has become available on these strains, ICH (1997) has incorporated their use into pharmaceutical testing guidelines in lieu of the second rodent species tests (that is, to replace the long-term mouse bioassay when the traditional rat study has been performed). FDA has stated that they would accept such studies when "performed in a validated model." In fact, CBER has accepted such studies as a sole carcinogenicity bioassay in some cases where there was negative traditional genotoxicity data and strong evidence of a lack of a mechanistic basis for concern.

A joint ILSI and HESI validation program has been completed, looking at the results of the four prime candidate models in identifying carcinogens as compared to the results of traditional long-term rodent bioassays. This validation program involved 51 different laboratories, and imposed protocol standards to allow comparison of results. Three dose levels were studied per chemical, with 15 males and 15 females being used for each dose group. A vehicle and high dose control in wild-type animals was also included, with information from NTP bioassays and 4-week range-finding assays being used to help set doses. Animals were dosed for 26 weeks. The issues in and coming out of these validation programs bear consideration (Tennant, et al., 1999).

- Is the proper comparator data for evaluating performance human or rodent bioassay data? It should be kept in mind that there are sets of rodent bioassay data (particularly those involving liver tumors in mice) that are widely accepted as irrelevant in the prediction of human risk.

- How will the data from these assays be incorporated into any weight-of-evidence approach to assessing human health risk?
- What additional mechanistic research needs to be undertaken to improve our understanding of the proper incorporation and best use of the data from these assays?
- How can the results of current validation efforts be best utilized in the timely evaluation of the next generation of assays?
- Given that, at least under some conditions, assays using these models tend to "blow up" (have high spontaneous tumor rates) once the animals are more than eight or nine months of age, how critical are age and other not currently apprehended factors to optimizing both sensitivity and specificity?
- How wide and unconditional will FDA (and other regulatory bodies) acceptance be of these models in lieu of the traditional two-year mouse bioassay?

## 9.13. INTERPRETATION OF RESULTS

### 9.13.1. Criteria for a Positive Result

There are three generally accepted criteria for a positive result in a carcinogenicity study. The first two are derived directly from the results of the statistical analysis: (1) a statistically significant increase in the incidence of a common tumor and (2) a statistically significant reduction in the time-to-tumor development. The third criterion is the occurrence of very rare tumors, that is, those not normally seen in control animals, even if the incidence is not statistically significant.

## 9.14. STATISTICAL ANALYSIS

The actual statistical techniques used to evaluate the results of carcinogenicity bioassays basically utilize four sets of techniques, three of which have been presented earlier in this book:

- Exact tests;
- Trend tests;
- Life tables (such as log rank techniques);
- Peto analysis.

These are then integrated into the decision-making schemes discussed earlier in this chapter. The methods themselves and alternatives are discussed elsewhere in detail (Gart et al., 1979, Gad, 1998; Chow and Lin, 1998).

### 9.14.1. Exact Tests

The basic forms of these (the Fisher exact test and chi-square) have previously been presented, and the reader should review these. Carcinogenicity assays are, of course, conducted at doses that are at least near those that will compromise mortality. As a consequence, one generally encounters competing toxicity producing differential mortality during such a study. Also, often, particularly with certain agricultural chemicals, latency of spontaneous tumors in rodents may shorten as a confounded effect of treatment with toxicity. Because of such happenings, simple tests on proportions, such as $\chi^2$ and Fisher–Irwin exact tests on contingency tables, may not produce optimal evaluation of the incidence data. In many cases, however, statisticians still use some of these tests as methods of preliminary evaluation. These are unadjusted methods without regard for the mortality patterns in a study. Failure to take into account mortality patterns in a study sometimes causes serious flaws in interpretation of the results. The numbers at risk are generally the numbers of animals histopathologically examined for specific tissues.

Some gross adjustments on the numbers at risk can be made by eliminating early deaths or sacrifices by justifying that those animals were not at risk to have developed the particular tumor in question. Unless there is dramatic change in tumor prevalence distribution over time, the gross adjusted method provides fairly reliable evidence of treatment effect, at least for nonpalpable tissue masses.

### 9.14.2. Trend Tests

Basic forms of the trend tests (such as that of Tarone) have previously been presented in this text. These are a natural development from earlier methods of regression testing (Dinse and Lagakes, 1983), but are much more powerful. (Gaylor and Kodell, 2001).

Group comparison tests for proportions notoriously lack power. Trend tests, because of their use of prior information (dose levels) are much more powerful. Also, it is generally believed that the nature of true carcinogenicity (or toxicity for that matter), manifests itself as dose-response. Because of the above facts, evaluation of trend takes precedence over group comparisons. In order to achieve optimal test statistics, many people use ordinal dose levels (0,1,2..., etc.) instead of the true arithmetic dose levels to test for trend. However, such a decision should be made *a priori*. The following example demonstrates the weakness of homogeneity tests.

**Example:  Trend versus Heterogeneity**

| Number at Risk | Number with Tumor | Dose Level |
| --- | --- | --- |
| 50 | 2 | 0 |
| 50 | 4 | 1 |
| 50 | 6 | 2 |
| 50 | 7 | 3 |

*Cochran–Armitage Test for Trend*

|  | Calculated chi$^2$ subgroup | DF | Alpha | 2-tail $p$ |
|---|---|---|---|---|
| Trend | 3.3446 | 1 | 0.0500 | 0.0674 |
| Departure | 0.0694 | 2 | 0.0500 | 0.9659 |
| Homogeneity | 3.4141 | 3 | 0.0500 | 0.3321 |

*One-Tail Tests for Trend*

| Type | Probability |
|---|---|
| Uncorrected | 0.0337[a] |
| Continuity corrected | 0.0426[a] |
| Exact | 0.0423[a] |

*Multiple Pairwise Group Comparisons by Fisher–Irwin Exact Test*

| Groups compared | Alpha | One-tail probability |
|---|---|---|
| 1 vs 2 | 0.0500 | 0.33887 |
| 2 vs 3 | 0.0500 | 0.13433 |
| 1 vs 4 | 0.0500 | 0.07975 |

[a]Direction $= +$

As is evident from this example, often group comparison tests will fail to identify significant treatment but trend tests will. Same arguments apply to survival adjusted tests on proportions as well. In an experiment with more than one dose group ($K > 1$), the most convincing evidence for carcinogenicity is given by tumor incidence rates that increase with increasing dose. A test designed specifically to detect such dose-related trends is Tarone's (1975) trend test.

Letting $\mathbf{d} = (O, d_1, d_2 \cdots d_k)^T$ be the vetor of dose levels in *all $K + 1$* groups and letting

$$(\mathbf{O} - \mathbf{E}) = (O_o - E_0, \cdots O_k - E_k)^T \text{ and } V = \begin{pmatrix} V_{00} & \cdots & V_{0K} \\ \vdots & \vdots & \vdots \\ V_{K0} & \cdots & V_{KK} \end{pmatrix}$$

contain elements as described in the previous section but for *all $K + 1$ groups*, the trend statistic is given by

$$X\frac{2}{T} = \frac{[d^T(Q - E)]^2}{d^T V d}.$$

The statistic $X^{2/T}$ will be large when there is evidence of a dose-related increase or decrease in the tumor incidence rates, and small when there is little difference in the tumor incidence between groups or when group differences are not dose related. Under the null hypothesis of no differences between groups, $X^{2/T}$ has approximately a chi-squared distribution with one degree of freedom.

Tarone's trend test is most powerful at detecting dose-related trends when tumor onset hazard functions are proportional to each other. For more power against other dose related group differences, weighted versions of the statistic are also available; see Breslow (1984) or Crowley and Breslow (1984) for details.

These tests are based on the generalized logistic function (Cox, 1972). Specifically one can use the Cocrhan–Armitage test (or its parallel, Mantel–Haenszel verson) for monotonic trend as heterogeneity test.

### 9.14.3. Life Table and Survival Analysis

These methods are essential when there is any significant degree of mortality in a bioassay. They seek to adjust for the differences in periods of risk individual animals undergo. Life table techniques can be used for those data where there are observable or palpable tumors. Specifically, one should use Kaplan–Meier product limit estimates from censored data graphically, Cox–Tarone binary regression (log-rank test), and Gehan–Breslow modification of Kruskal–Wallis tests (Thomas et al., 1977; Portier and Bailer, 1989) on censored data.

The Kaplan–Meier estimates produce a step function for each group and are plotted over the lifetime of the animals. Planned, accidentally killed, and lost animals are censored. Moribund deaths are considered to be treatment related. A graphical representation of Kaplan–Meier estimates provide excellent interpretation of survival adjusted data except in the cases where the curves cross between two or more groups. When the curves cross and change direction, no meaningful interpretation of the data can be made by any statistical method because proportional odds' characteristic is totally lost over time. This would be a rare case where treatment initially produces more tumor or death and then, due to repair or other mechanisms, becomes beneficial.

Cox–Tarone Binary Regression (Tarone, 1975; Thomas, Breslow, and Gart, 1977): Censored survival and tumor incidence data are expressed in a logistic model in dose over time. The log-rank test (Peto, 1974), tests based on the Weibull distribution, and Mantel–Haenszel (Mantel and Haenszel, 1952) test are very similar to this test when there are no covariates or stratifying variables in the design. The logistic regression based Cox–Tarone test is preferable because one can easily incorporate covariates and stratifying variables, which one cannot do in the IARC methods.

Gehan–Breslow Modification of Kruskal–Wallis Test is a nonparametric test on censored observations. It assigns more weight to early incidences compared to Cox–Tarone test.

Survival Adjusted Tests on Proportions: As mentioned earlier, in the case of survival adjusted analyses, instead of having a single $2 \times k$ table, one has a series of such $2 \times k$ tables across the entire lifetime of the study. The numbers at risk for such analyses will depend on the type of tumor one is dealing with.

1. Palpable or lethal tumors: Number at risk at time $t$ = number of animals surviving at the end of time $t - 1$.
2. Incidental tumors: The number at risk at time $t$ = number of animals that either died or were sacrificed whose particular tissue was examined histopathologically.

The methods of analyzing the incidences, once the appropriate numbers at risk are assigned for these tumors are rather similar, either binary regression-based or by evidence pooled from individual tables (Gart et al., 1986).

### 9.14.4. Peto Analysis

The Peto method of analysis of bioassay tumor data is based on careful classification of tumors into five different categories, as defined by IARC.

1. Definitely incidental;
2. Probably incidental.

*Comment*: Combine (1) and (2)

3. Probably lethal;
4. Definitely lethal.

*Comment*: These categories may be combined into one (otherwise it requires a careful cause of death determination).

5. Mortality Independent (such as mammary, skin, and other observable or superficial tumors).

### 9.14.5. Interval Selection for Occult (Internal Organ) Tumors

1. FDA : 0–50, 51–80, 81–104 weeks, interim sacrifice, terminal sacrifice
2. NTP: 0–52, 53–78, 79–92, 93–104 weeks, interim sacrifice, terminal sacrifice.
3. IARC: *ad hoc* selection method (Peto et al., 1980).

*Comment*: Any of the above may be used. Problems with IARC selection method include two sexes, two or more strains will have different intervals for the same compound. Different interval selection methods will produce different statistical significance levels. This may produce bias and requires an isotonic tumor prevalence for ready analysis.

### 9.14.6. Logistic Regression Method for Occult (Internal Organ) Tumors (Dinse, 1985)

Tumor prevalence is modeled as logistic function of dose and polynomial in age.

*Comment*: Logistic tumor prevalence method is unbiased. Requires maximum likelihood estimation. Allows for covariates and stratifying variables. It may be time-consuming and have convergence problem with sparse tables (low tumor incidences) and clustering of tumors.

### 9.14.7. Methods To Be Avoided

The following methods and practices should be avoided in evaluation of carcinogenicity.

1. Use of only the animals surviving after one year in the study.
2. Use of a two-strata approach: separate analyses for animals killed during the first year of the study and the ones thereafter.
3. Exclusion of all animals in the study that died on test and analyze only the animals that are sacrificed at the end of the study.
4. Exclusion of interim sacrifice animals from statistical analyses.
5. Evaluation of number of tumors of all sites as opposed to the number of animals with tumors for specific sites of specific organs.

Another issue is subjectivity in slide reading by most pathologists, who do not want to read them in a coded fashion whereby they will not know the dose group an animal is coming from. This is not under statisticians, control but they should be aware of this tendency in any case.

Often a chemical being tested is both toxic as well as potentially carcinogenic. When competing toxicity causes extreme differences in mortality or there is clustering effect in tumor prevalence in a very short interval of time, none of the adjusted methods works. One then must use biological intuition to evaluate the tumor data.

Use of historical control incidence data for statistical evaluation is controversial. There are too many sources of variation in these data. For example, different pathologists use different criteria for categorizing tumors (in fact, the same pathologist may change opinion over time); there is laboratory-to-laboratory variation; there may be genetic drift over time; location of suppliers may make a difference; and finally, these data are not part of the randomized concurrent control. Regulatory agencies and pathologists generally use these data for qualitative evaluation. My personal view is that that is where the data belong.

### 9.14.8. Use of Historical Controls

When the study is over, the data analyzed, and the $p$ values corrected, as appropriate, one may find that one or more tumor types increased in drug-treated groups relative to concurrent controls. Although the FDA and other regulatory agencies play down the importance of historical control data, it is common practice in the pharmaceutical industry to use historical data in the interpretation of tumor findings. The first and most appropriate comparison of a treated group is with concurrent control group(s), but it is of interest to see how tumor incidences in the treated groups compare with the historical incidence and that such a comparison is an accepted practice in toxicology and biostatistics (Gart et al., 1979; Hajian, 1983; Haseman et al., 1984b). A treated group may have a tumor incidence significantly higher than that of the concurrent control groups(s), but comparable to or lower than the historical incidence. Occasionally, a small number of tumors may be found in a treated group and the incidence may be significant because of the absence of this tumor in the concurrent controls. Review of appropriate historical control data may reveal that the low tumor incidence in the treated group is within the "expected" range for this tumor.

The role of historical control data in interpreting carcinogenicity findings depends on the "quality" of the historical data. Ideally, the data should be derived from animals of the same age, sex, strain, and supplier, housed in the same facility, and the pathology examinations should have been performed by the same pathologist or using the same pathological criteria for diagnosis. Since genetic drift occurs even in animals of a given strain and supplier, recent data are more useful than older data. The value of historical control data is directly proportional to the extent to which these conditions are fulfilled.

Although methods are available for including historical control data in the formal statistical analysis (Tarone, 1982; Dempster et al., 1983; Haseman, 1990), this is usually not done and for good reason. The heterogeneity of historical data requires that they be used qualitatively and selectively to aid in the final interpretation of the data, after completion of the formal statistical analysis. Table 9.3 presents a summary of background tumor incidences for the most commonly employed rodent strains.

### 9.14.9. Relevance to Humans

After statistical analyses have been performed and historical data consulted, the final interpretation may be that a drug appears to cause tumors at one or more tissue sites in the mouse or the rat. But what does this mean for the species to which the drug will be administered, namely, the human? Extrapolation of rodent carcinogenicity data to humans remains one of the greatest challenges of modern toxicology. There is no simple formula, and each case must be evaluated on its own merits. Very generally speaking, the FDA and other major regulatory agencies consider compounds that are tumorigenic in one or more animal species to be "suspect" tumorigens in humans. The actual impact of this conclusion on the approval of a drug depends on the target population and the indication. For example, even a

**TABLE 9.3. Comparative Percent Incidence of Pertinent Neoplasia in Different Strains of Rats and Mice (104 weeks old)**

| Types of neoplasia | F344 rats | | S-D rats | | Wistar rats | | B6C3F$_1$ mice | | CD-1 mice | |
|---|---|---|---|---|---|---|---|---|---|---|
| | Males | Females | Males | Females | Males | Females | Males | Females | Males | Females |
| Hepatocellular adenoma | 4 | < 1 | 5 | < 1 | 1 | 2 | 29 | 30 | 26 | 5 |
| Hepatocellular carcinoma | 2 | 0 | 2 | 0 | < 1 | < 1 | 26 | 16 | 10 | 1 |
| Pancreas islet adenoma | 12 | 2 | 8 | 9 | 4 | 2 | 2 | 0 | < 1 | < 1 |
| Pancreas islet carcinoma | 3 | 0 | < 1 | 5 | < 1 | < 1 | 0 | 0 | 0 | 0 |
| Pancreas acinar adenoma | 6 | 0 | 1 | 0 | 13 | < 1 | 2 | 0 | < 1 | 0 |
| Pheochromocytoma | 21 | 4 | 23 | 5 | 10 | 2 | 0 | 2 | < 1 | < 1 |
| Adrenocortical adenoma | 0 | 2 | 3 | 0 | 8 | 9 | < 1 | 0 | 1 | < 1 |
| Pituitary adenoma | 49 | 42 | 62 | 85 | 34 | 55 | 2 | 8 | 0 | 5 |
| Thyroid C-cell adenoma | 17 | 8 | 7 | 6 | 6 | 8 | 0 | 0 | 0 | 0 |
| Thyroid follicular adenoma | 0 | 0 | 4 | 2 | 2 | 1 | 2 | 6 | 1 | < 1 |
| Mammary-gland fibroadenoma | 4 | 57 | 2 | 54 | 3 | 36 | 0 | 0 | < 1 | 1 |
| Mammary-gland carcinoma | 0 | 4 | < 1 | 26 | 1 | 13 | 0 | 0 | 0 | 6 |
| Skin fibroma | 10 | 2 | 2 | < 1 | 5 | 1 | 1 | 2 | < 1 | < 1 |
| Skin papilloma | 6 | 0 | 2 | 0 | 2 | < 1 | 0 | 0 | < 1 | 0 |
| Pulmonary adenoma | 4 | 4 | < 1 | < 1 | < 1 | 0 | 22 | 6 | 15 | 15 |
| Preputial-gland neoplasia | 10 | NA | > 1 | NA | < 1 | NA | < 1 | NA | < 1 | NA |
| Leydig-cell neoplasia | 89 | NA | 7 | NA | 11 | NA | 0 | NA | 1 | NA |
| Clitoral-gland neoplasia | NA | 14 | NA | < 1 | NA | < 1 | NA | < 1 | NA | 0 |
| Uterine polyps | NA | 14 | NA | 6 | NA | 16 | NA | 1 | NA | < 1 |
| Ovarian neoplasia | NA | 6 | NA | 1 | NA | 8 | NA | 6 | NA | 1 |
| Mononuclear-cell leukemia | 62 | 42 | 0 | 0 | < 1 | < 1 | 0 | 0 | 2 | 2 |
| Lymphoma | 0 | 0 | 2 | 1 | 3 | 5 | 14 | 24 | 8 | 22 |
| Forestomach papilloma | 0 | 2 | < 1 | < 1 | 0 | < 1 | 4 | 2 | < 1 | < 1 |
| Scrotal mesothelioma | 5 | NA | 1 | NA | 2 | NA | 0 | NA | 0 | NA |

*Note:* F344, Fischer 244 rats; S-D, Sprague–Dawley rats; B6C3F$_1$, mice (C57BL/6N + C3H/HeN)F$_1$; CD-1, 1CRCr: CD-1 mice; NA, non-applicable; the average number used by species/strain/gender was in excess of 750 animals.

suspicion of carcinogenic activity may be fatal for a potential contraceptive drug intended for use in a very large population of healthy people. By contrast, clear evidence of carcinogenic activity may be overlooked in a drug being considered for use in a restricted population with a life-threatening disease.

Regardless of the target population and indication, the FDA and other agencies have, in recent years, attempted to consider the mechanism of tumor induction in rodents and its relevance for humans. If a drug is known to cause tumors in a rodent via a mechanism that does not exist in humans, the importance of the tumor findings may be markedly reduced. For example, drugs that cause tumors by a secondary hormonal mechanism shown to be inapplicable to humans may be given special consideration. It is the sponsor's responsibility to provide pertinent data on the mechanism of tumor induction and its relevance, or irrelevance, for humans. If the sponsor can show that an apparently drug-related tumor is species specific, the importance of the tumor in the overall evaluation of the drug will be greatly minimized. Table 9.4 presents a list of neoplastic or tumorigenic responses seen in rodents which have limited relevance to human safety. Part of the consideration must also be a recognition of the main characteristics of nongenotoxic carcinogins. These are recognized to be dose dependent responses with operative thresholds. The major characteristics are (Spindler, et al., 2000)

- Specificity (of species, sex and organ).
- A threshold is operative, and must be exceeded for cell proliferation and tumor development to occur.
- There is a step-wise dose response curve/relationship between exposure, cell proliferation and tumor development.
- The response is reversible with a cessation of dosing unless a point of no return has been passed.

One must then consider all of the available relevant information in a weight-of-evidence approach, such as that presented in Table 9.5.

## 9.15. CONCLUSIONS

The design, conduct, and interpretation of carcinogenicity studies is one of the major challenges for the pharmaceutical toxicologist, pathologist, biostatistician, and regulator. This is a rapidly changing field generating more questions than answers. The largest question continues to be the extrapolation of rodent data to humans, especially when data on mechanisms of tumor induction are unavailable or controversial. Much has been written on the difficulties inherent in extrapolating results from rodents treated with MTDs of a compound to humans who will be exposed to much lower doses and often for shorter periods. A discussion of these and other aspects of carcinogenic risk assessment is beyond the scope of this chapter.

**TABLE 9.4. Examples of Neoplastic Effects in Rodents with Limited Significance for Human Safety**

| Neoplastic effect | Pathogenesis (agents) |
|---|---|
| Renal tubular neoplasia in male rats | $\alpha_{2\mu}$-globulin nephropathy/hydrocarbons ($d$-limonene, $p$-dichlorpbenzene) |
| Hepatocellular neoplasia in rats and mice | Peroxisome proliferation (clofibrate, phthalate esters, phenoxy agents) Phenobarbital-like promotion |
| Urinary-bladder neoplasia in rats | Crystalluria, carbonic anhydrase inhibition, urine pH extremes, melamine, saccharine, carbonic anhydrase inhibitors, dietary phosphates |
| Hepatocellular neoplasia in mice | Enzymatic-metabolic activation (in part unknown)/phenobarbital-like promotion |
| Thyroid follicular-cell neoplasia in rats | Hepatic enzyme induction, thyroid enzyme inhibition/axazepam, amobarbital, sulphonamides, thioureas |
| Gastric neuroendocrine-cell neoplasia mainly in rats | Gastric secretory suppression, gastric atrophy induction (climetidine, omeprazole, butachlor |
| Adenohypophysis neoplasia in rats | Feedback interference/neuroleptics (dopamine inhibitors) |
| Mammary-gland neoplasia in female rats | Feedback interference/neuroleptics, antiemetics, antihypertensives (calcium channel blockers), serotonin agonists, anticholinergics, exogenous estrogens |
| Pancreatic islet-cell neoplasia in rats | Feedback interference/neuroleptics |
| Harderian-gland neoplasia in mice | Feedback interference/misoprostol ($PGE_1$), nalidixic acid, aniline dyes |
| Adrenal medullary neoplasia in rats | Feedback interference (lactose, sugar alcohols) |
| Forestomach neoplasia in rats and mice | Stimulation of proliferation/butylated hydroxyanisole, phthalate esters, proprionic acid |
| Lymphomas in mice | Immunosuppression/cyclosporin |
| Mononuclear-cell leukemia in rats (mainly F344) | Immunosuppression (in part unknown)/furan, iodinated glycerol |
| Splenic sarcomas in rats | Methemoglobonemia (in part unknown)/dapsone |
| Osteomas in mice | Feedback interference/lactose, sugar alcohols, $H_2$ antagonists, carbamazepine, vidarabine, isradipine, dopaminergics, finasteride |
| Leydig-cell testicular neoplasia in mice | Feedback interference (proestrogens, finasteride, methoxychlor, cadmium) |
| Endometrial neoplasia in rats | Feedback interference (proestrogens, dopamine agonists) |
| Uterine leiomyoma in mice | Feedback interference ($\beta_1$-antagonists) |
| Mesovarial leiomyoma in rats (occasionally in mice) | Feedback interference ($\beta_2$-agonists) |
| Ovarian tubulostromal neoplasia in mice | Feedback interference (cytotoxic agents, nitrofurantoin) |

**TABLE 9.5. Interpretation of the Analysis of Tumor Incidence and Survival Analysis (Life Table)**

| Outcome Type | Tumor association with treatment[a] | Mortality association with treatment | Interpretation[b] |
|---|---|---|---|
| A | − | + | Unadjusted test may underestimate tumorigenicity of treatment. |
| B | + | + | Unadjusted test gives valid picture of tumorigenicity of treatment. |
| C | + | − | Tumors found in treated groups may reflect longer survival of treated groups. Time adjusted analysis is indicated. |
| D | − | + | Apparent negative findings on tumors may be due to the shorter survival in treated groups. Time adjusted analysis and/or a retest at lower doses is indicated. |
| E | − | 0 | Unadjusted test gives a valid picture of the possible tumor-preventive capacity of the treatment. |
| F | − | − | Unadjusted test may underestimate the possible tumor-preventive capacity of the treatment. |
| G | 0 | + | High mortality in treated groups may lead to unadjusted test missing a possible tumorigen. Adjusted analysis and/or retest at lower doses is indicated |
| H | 0 | 0 | Unadjusted test gives a valid picture of lack of association with treatment. |
| I | 0 | − | Longer survival in treated groups may mask tumor-preventive capacity of treatment. |

[a] + = Yes, − = No and 0 = No bearing on discussion

[b] The unadjusted test referred to here is a contingency table type of analysis of incidence, such as Fisher s Exact test.

Regulatory agencies are very aware of these challenges and deserve credit for attempting to respond to changes in the state of knowledge, while still discharging their responsibility to protect the public health. For example, the latest version of the Japanese guidelines (Speid et al., 1990) acknowledges that the highest does in a carcinogenicity study may be set at 100 times the clinical dose, instead of requiring that the MTD be achieved. It is also noteworthy that the FDA Center for Drug Evaluation has announced the formation of a Carcinogenicity Assessment Committee representing all drug review divisions. This group will advise all the divisions on issues related to carcinogenicity. Creation of such a group reflects the importance that the agency places on carcinogenicity data in evaluating the safety of new drug candidates.

## REFERENCES

Bellhorn, R.W. (1980). Lighting in the animal environment. *Lab Anim. Sci.* 30: 440–450.

Berenblum, I. And Shubik, P. (1947). The role of croton oil applications associated with a single painting of a carcinogen, in tumour induction in the mouse's skin. *Br. J. Cancer* 1, 379–383.

Breslow, N. (1984). Comparison of survival curves. In: *Cancer Clinical Trials: Methods and Practice* (Buyse, M.E., Staquet, M.J. and Sylvester, R.J., Eds.). Oxford University Press, Oxford, pp. 381–406.

Burns, F.J., Vanderlan, M., Snyder, E. and Albert, R.E. (1976). Induction and progression kinetics of mouse skin papillomas. In Slaga, T.J., Sivak, A. And Boutwell, R.K. (Eds). *Carcinogenesis, Vol. 2. Modifiers of Chemical Carcinogenesis*. Raven Press, New York, pp. 91–96.

Cameron, T.P., Hickman, R.L., Kornreich, M.R. and Tarone, R.E. (1985). History, survival, and growth patterns of B6C3F1 mice and F344 rats in the National Cancer Institute Carcinogenesis Testing Program. *Fundam. Appl. Toxicol.* 5: 526–538.

Chu, K., Cueto. C. and Ward, J. (1981). Factors in the evaluation of 20 NCI carcinogenicity bioassays. *J. Toxicol. Environ. Health* 8: 251–280.

Chow, S.C. and Liu, J-P. (1998). *Design and analysis of animal studies in Pharmaceutical Development*. Marcel Dekker, New York.

Cohen, S.M., Robinson, B. and MacDonald, J. (2001) Alternative Models for Carcinogenicity Testing, *Tox. Sci* 64: 14–19.

Colburn, N.H. (1980). Tumour promotion and preneoplastic progression. In Slaga, T.J., Sivak, A. and Boutwell, R.K. (Eds). *Carcinogenesis, Vol. 5. Modifiers of Chemical Carcinogenesis*. Raven Press, New York, pp. 33–56.

Contrera, J.F., Jacobs, A.C. and DeGeorge, J.J. (1997). Carcinogenicity testing and the evaluation of regulatory requirements for pharmaceuticals, *Reg. Tox. Pharmacol.* 25: 130–145.

Cox, D.R. (1972): Regression models and life-tables. *J Royal Stat. Soc.* 34B, 187–220.

Crowley, J. and Breslow, N. (1984). Statistical analysis of survival data. *Ann. Rev. Public Health* 5: 385–411.

Dempster, A.P., Selivyn, M.R. and Weeks, B.J. (1983). Combining historical and randomized controls for assessing trends in proportions. *J. Amer. Stat. Assoc.* 78: 221–227.

DePass, L.R., Weil, C.S., Ballantyne, B., Lewis, S.C., Losco, P.E., Reid, J.B. and Simon, G.S. (1986). Influence of housing conditions for mice on the results of a dermal oncogenicity bioassay. *Fundam. Appl. Toxicol.* 7: 601–608.

Dinse, G.E. (1985). Estimating Tumor Prevalence, Lethality and Mortality, Presented at the Symposium on Long-Term Animal Carcinogenicity Studies: A Statistical Perspective, March 4–6, 1985, Bethesda.

Dinse, G.E. and Lagakos, S.W. (1983). Regression analysis of tumor prevalence data. *Appl. Stat.* 32: 236–248.

Eastin, W.C., Haseman, J.K., Mahler, J.F. and Bucher, J.R. (1998). The National Toxicology Program evaluation of genetically altered mice predictive models for identifying carcinogens. *Toxicol. Pathol.* 26: 461–584

Farrar, D.B. and Crump, K.S. (1988). Exact statistical tests for any carcinogenic effect in animal bioassays. *Fundam. Appl. Toxicol.* 11: 652–663.

Festing, M.W. (1979). Properties of inbreed strains and outbreed stocks, with special reference to toxicity testing, *J Toxicol Environ Health* 5: 53–68.

Flynn, R.J. (1960). Studies on the aetiology of ringtail in rats. *Proc. Anim. Care Panel* 9: 155–160.

Food and Drug Administration (FDA) (2001). Guidance for Industry: Statistical Aspects of the Design, Analysis and Interpretation of Chronic Rodent Carcinogenicity Studies of Pharmaceuticals. USDHEW, Washington, D.C.

Food and Drug Administration (FDA). (1993). Toxicological principles for the safety assessment of direct food additives and color additives used in food. In *Redbook II* (draft). Food and Drug Administration: Washington, D.C., pp. 111–115.

Foulds, L. (1969). *Neoplastic Development*, Vol. 1. Academic Press, New York.

Foulds, L. (1975). *Neoplastic Development*, Vol. 2. Academic Press, New York.

Fox, J.G. (1977). Clinical assessment of laboratory rodents on long term bioassay studies. *J. Environ. Pathol. Toxicol.* 1: 199–226.

French, J.E., Spalding, J.W., Dunnick, J.K., Tice, R.R., Furedi-Marchacck, M. and Tennant, R.W. (1999). The use of transgenic animals in cancer testing. *Inhalation Toxicol*, 11: 541–544.

Gad, S.C. (1998). *Statistics and Experimental Design for Toxicologists*, 3rd ed. CRC Press: Boca Raton, FL.

Gart, J.J., Chu, K.C. and Tarone, R.E. (1979). Statistical issues in interpretation of chronic bioassay tests for carcinogenicity. *J. Nat. Cancer Inst.* 62: 957–974.

Gart, J. J., Krewski, D., Lee, P. N., Tarone, R. E. and Wahrendorf, J. (1986). The design and analysis of long-term animal experiment, in *Statistical Methods in Cancer Research*, Vol. III. IARC Scientific Publication No. 79. International Agency for Research on Cancer: Lyon.

Gaylor, D.W. and Kodell, R.L. (2001). Dose-response trend tests for tumorogenesis adjusted for differences in survival and body weight across doses. *Toxicol. Sci.*, 59: 219–225.

Gold, L.S., Sawyer, C.B., Magaw, R., Blackman, G., deVeciana, M, Levenson, R., Hooper, N.K., Havender, W.R., Bernstein, L., Peto, R., Pike, M.C. and Ames, B.N. (1984). A carcinogenic potency data base of the standardized results of animal bioassays. *Environ. Health Perspect.* 58: 9–319.

Greenman, D.L., Bryant, P., Kodell, R.L. and Sheldon, W. (1982). Influence of cage shelf level on retinal atrophy in mice. *Lab. Anim. Sci.* 32: 353–356.

Greenman, D.L., Kodell, R.L. and Sheldon, W.G. (1984). Association between cage shelf level and spontaneous induced neoplasms in mice. *J. Nat. Cancer Inst.* 73: 107–113.

Hajian, G. (1983). Statistical issues in the design and analysis of carcinogenicity bioassays. *Toxicol. Pathol.* 11: 83–89.

Haseman, J.K. (1983). A reexamination of false-positive rates for carcinogenicity studies. *Fundam. Appl. Toxicol.* 3: 334–339.

Haseman, J.K. (1985). Issues in carcinogenicity testing: Dose selection. *Fundam. Appl. Toxicol.* 5: 66–78.

Haseman, J.K. (1990). Use of statistical decision rules for evaluating laboratory animal carcinogenicity studies. *Fundam. Appl. Toxicol.* 14: 637–648.

Haseman, J.K., Crawford, D.D., Huff, J.E., Boorman, G.A. and McConnell, E.E. (1984a). Results for 86 two-year carcinogenicity studies conducted by the National Toxicology Program. *J. Toxicol. Environ. Health* 14: 621–639.

Haseman, J.K., Huff, J. and Boorman, G.A. (1984b). Use of historical control data in carcinogenicity studies in rodents. *Toxicol. Pathol.* 12: 126–135.

Haseman, J.K., Winbush, J.S. and O Donnell, M.W. (1986). Use of dual control groups to estimate false positive rates in laboratory animal carcinogenicity studies. *Fundam. Appl. Toxicol.* 7: 573–584.

Holm-Nielsen, P. And Olsen, T.S. (1988). Ultrastructure of renal adenoma. *Ultrastruct. Pathol,* 12: 27–39.

ICH. (1996). *The Need for Long-Term Rodent Carcinogenicity Studies of Pharmaceuticals.*

ICH. (1997). *Testing for Carcinogenicity of Pharmaceuticals.*

ICH. (1995). *Dose Selection for Carcinogenicity Studies of Pharmaceuticals.*

International Agency for Research on Cancer (1987). IARC Monographs on the Evaluation of Carcinogenic Risks to Humans: Preamble. *IARC Internal Technical Report* 87/001, IARC: Lyon.

Japanese Ministry of Health and Welfare (MHW). (1989). *Revised Guidelines for Toxicity Studies Required for Application for Approval of Manufacturing/Importing Drugs.* Ministry of Health and Welfare: Tokyo, pp. 37–48.

Kitchin, K.T. (1999). *Carcinogenicity.* Marcel Dekker, New York.

Littlefield, N. A., Farmer, J. H., Gaylor, D. W. and Sheldon, W. G. (1979). Effects of dose and time in a long-term, low-dose carcinogenic study. In: *Innovations in Cancer Risk Assessment (ED01Study)* (Staffa, J.A. and Mehlman, M.A. Eds.). Pathotox Publishers, Chicago, IL, pp. 17–34.

Mantel, N. (1980). Assessing laboratory evidence for neoplastic activity. *Biometrics* 36: 381–399.

Mantel, N. and Haenszel, W. (1952): Statistical aspects of the analysis of data from the retrospective studies of disease, *J. Nat. Cancer Inst.,* 22: 719–748.

McAnulty, P.A. (2000). Transgenic Mouse models in carcinogenicity testing, *European Pharmaceutical Contractor,* July, 2000, pp. 84–90.

McGregor, D. (2000). Carcinogenicity and Genotoxic Carcinogens, in *General and Applied Toxicology*, 2nd ed. (Ballantyne, B., Marrs, T. and Syversen, T. Eds.). MacMillan, London.

McKnight, B. And Crowley, J. (1984). Tests for Differences in Tumor Incidence Based on Animal Carcinogenesis Experiments. *J. Am. Stat. Assoc.* 79: 639–648.

Miller, E.C. and Miller, J.A. (1981). Mechanisms of chemical carcinogenesis. *Cancer*, 47: 1055–1064.

NIH (2000). *Ninth Report on Carcinogens*. U.S. Department of Health and Human Services. Washington, D.C.

Peto, R. (1974): Guidelines on the analysis of tumor rates and death rates in experimental animals. *Br. J. Cancer* 29: 101–105.

Peto, R., Pike, M.C., Day, N.E., Gray, R.G., Lee, P.N., Parish, S., Peto, J., Richards, S. and Wahrendorf, J. (1980). Guidelines for simple, sensitive significance tests for carcinogenic effects in long-term animal experiments, In: *IARC Monographs on the Evaluation of the Carcinogenic Risk of Chemicals to Humans*. International Agency for Research on Cancer: Lyon.

Pharmaceutical Manufacturers Association (PMA). (1988). *Results of a Questionnaire Involving the Design of and Experience with Carcinogenicity Studies*. This document has not been published in the open literature but is widely available within the pharmaceutical industry. It may be obtained by writing to the Pharmaceutical Manufacturers Association, Washington, DC.

Portier, C.J. and Bailer, A.J. (1989). Testing for increased carcinogenicity using a survival-adjusted quantal response test. *Fundam. Appl. Toxicol.* 12: 731–737.

Powell, C.J. and Berry, C.L. (2000). Non-genotoxic or Epigenetic Carcinogenesis. In *General and Applied Toxicology*, 2nd ed. (Ballantyne, B., Marrs, T. and Syversen, T. Eds.). MacMillan, London.

Purchase, I.F.H. (1980). Interspecies comparisons of carcinogenicity. *Br. J. Cancer* 41: 454–468.

Rao, G.N. and Huff, J. (1990). Refinement of long-term toxicity and carcinogenesis studies. *Fundam. Appl. Toxicol.* 15: 33–43.

Rao, G.N., Birnbaum, L.S., Collins, J.J., Tennant, R.W. and Skow, L.C. (1988). Mouse strains for chemical carcinogenicity studies: Overview of a workshop. *Fundam. Appl. Toxicol.* 10: 385–394.

Rao, G.N., Haseman, J.K. and Edmondson, J. (1989). Influence of viral infections on body weight, survival, and tumor prevalence in Fisher 344 rats on two-year studies. *Lab. Anim. Sci.* 39: 389–393.

Schweder, T. and Spjotvoll, E. (1982). Plots of $p$-values to evaluate many tests simultaneously. *Biometrika* 69: 493–502.

Sher, S.P., Jensen, R.D. and Bokelman, D.L. (1982). Spontaneous tumors in control F344 and Charles River CD rats and Charles River CD-1 and B6C3F1 mice. *Toxicol. Lett.* 11: 103–110.

Silverberg, S.G. (1984). The autopsy and cancer. *Arch. Pathol. Lab. Med.*, 108: 476–478.

Speid, L.H., Lumley, C.E. and Walker, S.R. (1990). Harmonization of guidelines for toxicity testing of pharmaceuticals by 1992. *Reg. Toxicol. Pharmacol.* 12: 179–211.

Spindler, P., Loan, J., Ceuppens, P., Harling, R., Eittlin, R. and Lima, B.S. (2000). Carcinogenicity testing of pharmaceuticals in the European Union: a workshop report, *Drug Information J.* 34: 821–828.

Tarone, R.E. (1975). Tests for trend in life table analysis, *Biometrika* 62: 679–682.

Tarone, R.E. (1982). The use of historical control information in testing for a trend in proportions. *Biometrics* 38: 215–220.

Tennant, R.W., French, J.E. and Spalding, J.W. (1995). Identification of chemical carcinogens and assessing potential risks in short-term bioassays using transgenic mouse models. *Environ. Health Perspect.* 103: 942–950.

Tennant, R.W., Stasiewicz, S., Mennear, J., French, J.E. and Spalding, J.W. (1999). Genetically altered mouse models for identifying carcinogens. In *The Use of Short and Medium-Term Tests for Carcinogens and Data on Genetic Effects in Carcinogenic Hazard Evaluation,* (McGregor, D.B., Rice, J.M. and Venith, S., Eds.) IARC Science Publications No. 146, Lyon, France, pp. 23–148.

Thomas, D.G., Breslow, N. and Gart, J.J. (1977). Trend and homogeneity analyses of proportions and life table data. *Comput. Biomed. Res.* 10: 373–381.

Weaver, R.J. and Brunden, M.N. (1998). The design of long-term carcinogenicity studies. In *Design and Analysis of Animal Studies in Pharmaceutical Development* (Chow, S. and Liu, J., Eds.), Marcel Dekker: New York.

Weisbrode, S.E. and Weiss, H.S. (1981). Effect of temperature on benzo(*a*)pyrene induced hyperplastic and neoplastic skin lesions in mice. *J. Nat. Cancer Inst.* 66: 978–981.

Williams, G.M. and Iatropoulos, M.J. (2001). Principles of testing for carcinogenic activity, in *Principles and Methods of Toxicology,* 4th ed. (Hayes, A.W., ed.), Taylor and Francis, Philadelphia, PA.

Wiskemann, A., Sturm, E. and Klehr, N.W. (1986). Fluorescent lighting enhances chemically induced papilloma formation and increases susceptibility to tumor challenge in mice. *J. Cancer Res. Clin. Oncol.* 112: 141–143.

# 10

# SAFETY ASSESSMENT OF INHALANT DRUGS

## 10.1. INTRODUCTION

Drugs and medicinal agents administered by the inhalation route include the gaseous and vaporous anesthetics, coronary vasodilators, the aerosols of bronchodilators, corticosteroids, mucolytics, expectorants, antibiotics, and peptides and proteins where there is significant nasal absorption (Cox et al., 1970; Williams, 1974; Paterson et al., 1979; Hodson et al., 1981; Lourenco and Cotromanes, 1982). Concerns with the environmental affects of chloroflurocarbons has also led to renewed interest in dry powder inhalers, which have additionally shown promise for better tolerance and absorption for some new drugs. Excessive inhalation of a drug into the pulmonary system during therapy or manufacturing may result in adverse local and/or systemic effects. Consequently, safety assessment of inhaled medicinal preparations with respect to pulmonary toxicity and the therapeutic-to-toxicity ratio are essential. The data generated is essential for charting the course of evaluation and development of a potential therapeutic agent.

## 10.2. THE PULMONARY SYSTEM

An average man inhales approximately 7.5, 28.6, and 42.9 liters of air per minute during resting, light work, and heavy work periods, respectively, and the corresponding mean tidal volumes of 750, 1673 and 2030 ml (National Academy of Sciences, 1958). Each breath is distributed between 300–400 million alveoli, where gas exchange takes place. The total alveoli surface area is approximately $75\,m^2$, which is penetrated by approximately 200 km of capillary blood vessels (Hatch and Gross, 1964). The high vascularity and large surface area of the lung ensure rapid gas exchange and entry of an inhaled drug into the bloodstream. A drug is then quickly carried to the heart and brain before reaching the liver, where first-pass metabolism occurs. The pulmonary system is, therefore, a very effective portal through which gases, vapors, and aerosols can enter the body to exert desirable therapeutic effects and undesirable side effects locally and/or systemically.

Anatomically, the pulmonary system is divided into extrathoracic and thoracic regions. The extrathoracic, or head, region includes the nasal and pharyngeal passages. The thoracic region is subdivided into tracheobronchial (TB) and alveolar (AL) regions. The TB region consists of the trachea, primary and secondary bronchi, and primary through-ciliated bronchioles. The alveolar region consists of nonciliated terminal bronchioles, alveolar ducts, and alveoli (Lippmann, 1981). The anatomical structure of the pulmonary system maximizes gas exchange but minimizes the penetration of extraneous particulate matter into the lungs. The formalized anatomy (Davis, 1961; Weibel, 1963; Horsfield and Cumming, 1968; Weibel, 1983; Parent, 1991) of the branchings, the dimensions of the airways, the penetrability by particles of certain sizes, and the distribution of cell types in the respiratory tract and lungs are summarized in Figure 10.1.

## 10.3 PENETRATION AND ABSORPTION OF INHALED GASES AND VAPORS

Pulmonary dynamics, the dimension and geometry of the respiratory tract and the structure of the lungs, together with the solubility and chemical reactivity of the inhalants greatly influence the magnitude of penetration, retention, and absorption of inhaled gases, vapors (Dahl, 1990), and aerosols (Raabe, 1982; Phalen, 1984). The quantity of an inhalant effectively retained in the pulmonary system constitutes the inhaled "dose" that causes pharmacotoxic responses.

Highly reactive and soluble gaseous or vaporous drugs react and dissolve readily in the mucosal membrane of the nasopharynx and the upper respiratory tract (URT), thereby exerting pharmacological effects or causing local irritation and/or adverse effects on the ciliated, goblet, brush border columnar, and squamous cells of the epithelium. The dissolved drug is also absorbed into the bloodstream and transported to the target organ where it exerts systemic effects. Less reactive and less soluble gaseous or vaporous drugs are likely to penetrate beyond the URT and reach the bronchial and alveolar regions, causing local and systemic effects. The unabsorbed gases or vapors are then exhaled. For example, ammonia gas generated from a 10% ammonia water may be inhaled for reflex respiratory stimulation purposes (Budavari, 1989). Ammonia is extremely soluble in water at a concentration of 715 ml of ammonia per milliliter (mL) of water (Phalen, 1984), and is readily solubilized in the mucous lining causing URT irritation. By contrast, oxygen is only sparingly soluble in water (0.031 cc of oxygen per mL of water ) and capable of penetrating deeply into the alveoli where gas exchange takes place. Oxygen that binds reversibly with the hemoglobin of erythrocytes is unloaded at the target tissues, while the unbound

| Regions | | | Generations | Total Cross section (cm²) | Particle size penetration limits (μm) | Distribution | | | |
| --- | --- | --- | --- | --- | --- | --- | --- | --- | --- |
| | | | | | | Cell types | Mucous Glands | Smooth Muscle | p-sym. Innerv. |
| Extrathoracic | Head | Nasopharynx | | | 60 | | | | |
| Intrathoracic | Tracheo-bronchial | Trachea | 0 | 2.54 | | Cilliated | | | |
| | | Primary bronchi | 1 | 2.33 | 20 | Goblet | | | |
| | | Secondary bronchi | 2 | 2.13 | 10 | Brush Border Squamus Columnar | | | |
| | | | 3 | 2.00 | | | | | |
| | | | 4 | 2.48 | | | | | |
| | | | 10 | 13.4 | | | | | |
| | | Bronchioles | 11 | 19.6 | 6 | | | | |
| | | | 15 | 113 | | | | | |
| | Alveolar | Terminal bronchioles | 16 | 180 | 4 | Cuboidal Less ciliated | | | |
| | | Respiratory bronchioles | 17 | 300 | 3 | Less goblet Non cilicated clara | | | |
| | | | 18 | 534 | | | | | |
| | | | 19 | 944 | | | | | |
| | | Alveoli ducts | 10 | 1.60K | <3 | Type I | | | |
| | | | 21 | 3.22K | | | | | |
| | | | 22 | 5.88K | | | | | |
| | | Alveoli | 23 | 11.8K | <3 | Type II | | | |

**FIGURE 10.1.** The distribution of cell types in the respiratory tract and lungs.

oxygen is exhaled. Inhalation of properly humidified oxygen is life supporting, but inhalation of unhumidified oxygen may cause a reduction in the mucociliary clearance of secretions in the trachea of animals (Pavia, 1984) and humans (Lichtiger et al., 1975; Gamsu et al., 1976). Gases or vapors of low lipid solubility are also poorly absorbed in the lungs, with much of the inhaled vapor exhaled. Other pharmacological gases and vapors, such as the anesthetics (nitrous oxide, halothane, enflurane, isoflurane, etc.) and the coronary vasodilators (amyl nitrite), likewise affect the epithelium of the respiratory tract and the lungs. The absorbed drugs exert local effects on various types of epithelial cells of the respiratory tract, and on Type I and II cells and the alveolar macrophages (AM)s in the alveoli. Repeated inhalation of some halogenated hydrocarbon anesthetics will result in accumulation of the vapors and systemic toxicity (Chenoweth et al., 1972). By contrast, vapors such as the fluorocarbons (FC 11 and FC 12), which are used extensively as propellants for bronchodilator and corticosteroid aerosols, are absorbed rapidly but are not accumulated in the body even upon repeated inhalation (Aviado and Micozzi, 1981).

In general, dissolved gases or vapors at a nontoxic concentration are absorbed and metabolized locally by the lungs and systemically by the liver. The unchanged parent drug and its metabolites may be excreted to some extent via exhalation but mainly via the renal system. A dissolved gas or vapor at a toxic concentration, however, is likely to exert local effects such as altering the surface tension of the alveoli linings or disrupting the normal functions of the epithelial cells, the pneumocytes, and the AMs. The disrupted AMs in turn release their intracellular enzymes, causing destruction of the alveolar septa and contributing to histopathologic changes of the respiratory tract and the lungs. Again, the magnitude of the adverse effects is dependent on pulmonary dynamics and the solubilities of the inhalants in the mucous membrane of the URT and in the plasma or lipids of the erythrocytes.

## 10.4. DEPOSITION OF INHALED AEROSOLS

For inhaled aerosols, particle size is the major factor affecting the penetration, deposition, and hence the "dose" and site of pharmacological action (Dautrebande, 1962a, b; Agnew, 1984). Particle size is expressed in terms of *aerodynamic diameter* (AD), defined as the diameter of a spherical particle of unit density ($1g/cm^3$) that has the same terminal settling velocity as the particle in question, regardless of its shape and density (Marple and Rubow, 1980). The unit for AD is micrometers ($\mu m$). A sample of aerosol particles having ADs within a narrow size range is considered to be a monodisperse aerosol, whereas a sample of aerosols with a wide range of ADs is a heterodisperse, or polydisperse, aerosol. The pattern of particle-size distribution is usually bell shaped, with smaller and larger particles on both sides of the mean AD. An aerosol sample with a high proportion of particles of similar size has a narrow particle-size distribution, or small geometric standard deviation (GSD). An aerosol sample with a GSD of less than 2 is considered to be a monodisperse aerosol. Thus, both the AD and GSD of 2 or less is considered to be optimal for pulmonary penetration and distribution in the respiratory tract and the lungs. For example, in nose breathing, aerosol particles with ADs > 15 µm are likely to be trapped in the nasopharynx (extrathoracic, or head, region) by filtration and impaction. Particles deposited in the nasopharynx are considered to be "noninhalable" (Lippmann, 1977; Miller et al., 1979).

In mouth breathing, only 10–15% of 15 µm particles penetrate through the larynx to the intrathoracic TB region. Particles reaching the TB region are considered to be "inhalable" (Lippmann, 1977; Miller et al., 1979).

In natural nose and mouth breathing, only a negligible proportion of aerosol particles of AD > 10 µm reach the lungs (Swift and Proctor, 1982). Aerosol particles of 3 to 4 µm in AD are considered to be optimal sizes for TB deposition. The mechanisms of deposition are by impaction along the trachea and at bronchial branchings where the direction of airflow changes; and by gravity settlement in the fine airways in amounts proportional to the particle-settling velocity and the time available for settlement (Hatch and Gross, 1964; Heyder et al., 1980). Aerosol particles of 1 to 2 µm in AD, however, decrease in TB deposition because the particles are too small for effective impaction and sedimentation (Lippmann, 1977; Chan and Lippmann, 1980; Stahlhofen et al., 1980). Consequently, the majority of the very fine particles are exhaled. However, the deposition of the ultrafine particles of approximately 0.5 µm in AD on the walls of the finest bronchioles and the alveoli increases again due to molecular diffusion processes. Even so, some 90% of the inhaled 0.5 µm particles will still be exhaled during quiet tidal breathing and much more under forced exhalation (Davis et al., 1972; Taulbee et al., 1978). Those fine particles reaching the finest bronchioles and alveoli are considered to be "respirable" (Lippmann, 1970).

In general, particles of AD > 10 µm deposit mainly in the URT, whereas particles of 1 to 5 µm AD, with a GSD of less than 2, are likely to reach the lower respiratory tract, which includes the TB region and the alveoli, with small oropharyngeal loss.

The proportion of an aerosol sample suitable for inhalation can also be determined on the basis of mass median aerodynamic diameter (MMAD), which is defined as the percentage (50%) by weight of an aerosol sample having ADs equal to or less than the stated median AD. For example, a sample with an MMAD of 5 µm means that 50% by weight of that sample has ADs of 5 µm and smaller. The MMAD is, therefore, a good index for determining the proportion of an aerosol sample that is "noninhalable," "inhalable," or "respirable." An aerosol sample with an MMAD of 5 µm and a GSD of less than 2 is considered to be optimal for pulmonary deposition and retention (Task Group on Lung Dynamics, 1966).

In addition to AD and GSD, the pulmonary dynamics of a subject also greatly influence the distribution of aerosol particles in various regions of the respiratory tract (Agnew, 1984). For example, the velocity of airflow in the respiratory tract significantly influences the pattern of TB deposition. An increase in airflow velocity in the airways increases the effectiveness of particle impaction at the bifurcations of the large airways (Dennis, 1961; Hatch and Gross, 1964; Parent, 1991). As a result, spots impacted with a high concentration of particles (hot spots) are frequently present at the carina and the bifurcations of the airways (Lee and Wang, 1977; Bell, 1978; Stahlhofen et al., 1981). Furthermore, the depth of each breath (tidal volume) also influences the distribution of aerosols. A small tidal volume permits greater impaction in the proximal conducting airways and less sedimentation in the distal airways.

In general, slow, deep inhalation followed by a period of breath holding increases the deposition of aerosols in the peripheral parts of the lungs, whereas rapid inhalation increases the deposition in the oropharynx and in the large central airways. Thus, the frequency of respiration (the flow velocity) and the depth of breath (tidal volume) influence the pattern of pulmonary penetration and deposition of inhaled aerosols. Therefore, an aerosol of ideal size will penetrate deeply into the respiratory tract and the lungs only when the aerosols are inhaled in the correct manner (Sackner, 1978 and Sackner et al., 1975).

## 10.5. ABSORPTION AND CLEARANCE OF INHALED AEROSOLS

Soluble aerosols deposited on the epithelial linings of the respiratory tract are absorbed and metabolized in the same way as soluble gases and vapors.

Insoluble medicinal aerosols are few in number. Sodium cromoglycate (SCG) is probably the only insoluble powder to be administered as a prophylactic antiasthmatic (Wanner, 1979). Insoluble particles deposited on the ciliated linings of the URT are removed by a mucociliary clearance mechanism. Particles deposited on a terminal airway devoid of ciliated cells may be endocytosed into the epithelial cells. At a toxic concentration, the cells die and the debris is then phagocytosed and transported into the interstitial space for removal via the lymph or vascular drainages, or re-enters the ciliated zone of the airway. Particles deposited in the alveolar walls are phagocytosed by the AMs and transported from the low surface tension surfactant in the alveolar lining to the high surface tension bronchial fluid of the ciliate airways for elimination by the mucociliary clearance mechanism (Laurweryns and Baert, 1977). The particle sizes optimal for phagocytosis are 2–3 µm, while particles smaller than 0.26 µm are less effective in activating the macrophages (Holma, 1967). In any case, AMs can phagocytose only a small fraction of a large number of deposited particles. The nonphagocytosed particles are translocated to the lymphatic system for elimination (Ferin, 1977).

Like the inhaled gases or vapors, soluble and insoluble aerosol particles can directly exert desirable and undesirable local effects at the site of deposition and/or systemic effects after solubilization, absorption, and metabolization.

## 10.6. PHARMACOTOXICITY OF INHALED AEROSOLS

The inhalation route for administering drugs into the pulmonary system for treatment of respiratory diseases eliminates many bioavailability problems such as plasma binding and "first-pass" metabolism, which are encountered in parenteral or oral administration. Consequently, a small inhalation dose is adequate for achieving the desirable therapeutic response without inducing many undesirable side effects. Furthermore, the direct contact of the drug with the target site ensures rapid action. Nevertheless, the effects from inhaled drug aerosols also depend on the pharmacological properties of the aerosols and the location of their deposition in the respiratory system. For example, the classic experiments on bronchodilation drugs (Dautrebande, 1962a, b; Paterson, 1977) showed that fine aerosol particles of isoproterenol penetrate deeply in to the lower respiratory airways (LRA). In this way, a high concentration of the drug aerosol can reach the beta-adrenergic receptors of the bronchial smooth muscles. Stimulation of the receptors causes relaxation of the smooth muscle fibers and results in brochodilation (Weiner, 1984; McFadden, 1986). Such rapid bronchial responses can be produced in healthy and asthmatic subjects without inducing any cardiac effects. By contrast, the same dose of isoproterenol of large particle sizes deposits mainly along the URT, with a minimal amount reaching the smooth muscles of the LRA. The drug is quickly absorbed into the tracheal and bronchial veins and delivered immediately to the left ventricle of the heart. A high plasma concentration of the drug in the heart causes prominent cardiovascular effects such as tachycardia and hypertension. Other aerosols of beta-adrenergic drugs, such as epinephrine, isoprenaline, terbutaline, and salbutamol, induce bronchodilation effects in animals and humans (Pavia, 1984) via inhalation and stimulate ciliary beat frequency and mucus production at the site of deposition in the trachea (Wanner, 1981). Thus the tracheobronchial mucociliary clearance mechanism is also stimulated. By contrast, anticholinergic bronchodilators, such as atropine and ipratropium bromide, cause mucus retention in the lungs (Pavia et al., 1983a, b). Therefore, in pharmacological or safety assessments of inhalant beta-adrenergic bronchial dilatation drugs, aerosols should be of small particle sizes suitable for deposition in the peripheral airways to minimize side effects. However, anticholinergic agents should be of larger particle sizes suitable for deposition in the large airways (Ingram et al., 1977; Hensley et al., 1978).

Other therapeutic aerosols, such as beclomethasone dipropionate, betamethasone valerate, and budesonide corticosteroid (Williams, 1974); the carbenicillin and gentamicin antibiotics (Hodson et al., 1981); the 2-mercaptoethane-sulfonate (Pavia et al., 1983b) and n-acetylcysteine (Hollinger, 1985) mucolytics; and even vaccines for the prevention of influenza and tuberculosis (Lourenco and Cotromanes, 1982), are active by inhalation and/or oral administration. When these drugs are administered as aerosols, certain particle sizes may be targeted to a specific region or to multiple regions of the pulmonary system depending on the therapeutic target site(s). In any case, when aerosols are delivered as fine particles, the rate of absorption is increased because of an increase in the distribution area per unit mass of the drug. Thus, an effective aerosol dose of corticosteroid for treatment of asthma and bronchitis is merely a fraction of an oral dose (Williams, 1974). An aerosol of SCG dry powder, a prophylactic for preventing the onset of bronchoconstriction in asthmatic attacks (Cox, 1970), is effective mainly by local inhibition of the release of chemical mediators from mast cells in bronchial smooth muscle. Therefore, SCG particle sizes should be approximately 2 $\mu$m in AD for the most effective penetration into the bronchial regions (Godfrey et al., 1974; Curry et al., 1975). Likewise, therapeutic aerosols of local anesthetics and surfactants may require appropriate particle sizes to be targeted to a specific region of the pulmonary system.

Other than undesirable pharmacological effects, toxic concentrations of soluble or insoluble aerosol particles may lead to adverse physiological and/or histophathologic responses. For example, irritating aerosols cause dose-related reflex depression of the respiratory rate (Alarie, 1966, 1981a), while phagocytosed particles cause chemotaxis of AMs and neutrophils to the site of deposition (Brain, 1971). The maximum response usually occurs at 24 h and returns to normal in approximately 3 days postexposure (Kavet et al., 1978). Furthermore, a toxic quantity of phagocytosed particles may interact with the lysosomal membrane within a macrophage, releasing cytotoxic lysosomal enzymes, proteases, and free radicals that in turn damage the adjacent lung tissue (Hocking and Golde, 1979).

In general, a specific category of drug delivered to a specific site of the pulmonary system will exert a specific pharmacological or toxicological action locally or systemically. Therefore, in safety assessments of inhalants, a drug should be delivered to the target sites of the pulmonary system according to the toxicological information required.

Finally, there are many drugs in the categories of amphetamines, anorectics, antihistamines, antipsychotics, tricyclic antidepressants, analgesics and narcotics, and beta-adrenergic blocking agents that are known to accumulate in the lung (Wilson, 1982; Hollinger, 1985) even though these drugs are not administered via the inhalation route. Therefore, in safety assessments of these drugs, their pulmonary toxicity should also be evaluated.

## 10.7. METHODS FOR SAFETY ASSESSMENT OF INHALED THERAPEUTICS

Methods for evaluation of inhalation toxicity should be selected according to the pharmacological and/or the toxicological questions asked, and the design of experiments should specify the delivery route of a drug to the target sites in the pulmonary system. For example, if an immunologic response of the lungs to a drug is in question, then the lymphoid tissues of the lungs should be the major target of evaluation. The following are some of the physiological, biochemical, and pharmacological tests that are applicable for safety assessment of inhaled medicinal gases, vapors, or aerosols.

Upper respiratory tract irritation can occur from inhalation of a medicinal gas, vapor, or aerosol. For assessing the potential of an inhalant to cause URT irritation, the mouse body plethysmographic technique (Alarie, 1966, 1981a, b) has proven to be extremely useful. This technique operates on the principle that respiratory irritants stimulate the sensory nerve endings located at the surface of the respiratory tract from the nose to the alveolar region. The nerve endings in turn stimulate a variety of reflex responses (Alarie, 1973; Widdicombe, 1974) that result in characteristic changes in inspiratory and expiratory patterns and, most prominently, depression of respiratory rate. Both the potency of irritation and the concentration of the irritant are positively related to the magnitude of respiratory rate depression. The concentration response can be quantitatively expressed in terms of "$RD_{50}$," defined as the concentration (in logarithmic scale) of the drug in the air that causes a 50% decrease in respiratory rate. The criteria for positive URT irritation in intact mice exposed to the drug atmosphere are depression in breathing frequency and a qualitative alteration of the expiratory patterns. Numerous experimental results have shown that the responses of mice correlated almost perfectly with those of humans (Alarie et al., 1980; Alarie and Luo, 1986). Thus, this technique is useful for predicting the irritancy of airborne medicinal compounds in humans. From the drug-formulating point of view, an inhalant drug with URT-irritating properties indicates the need for an alternate route of administration. From the industrial hygiene point of view, the recognition of the irritant properties is very important. If a chemical gas, vapor, or aerosol irritates, it has a "warning property." With an adequate warning property a worker will avoid inhaling damaging amounts of the airborne toxicant; without a warning property a worker may unknowingly inhale an injurious amount of the toxicant.

Inhalation of a cardiovascular drug, such as an aerosol of propranolol (a beta-adrenergic receptor agonist), may affect the respiratory cycle of a subject. For evaluating the cardiopulmonary effects of an inhalant, the plethysmograph technique using a mouse or a guinea pig model is useful. The criteria for a positive response in intact mice or guinea pigs are changes in the duration of inspiration and expiration, and the interval between breaths (Schaper et al., 1989).

Pulmonary sensitization may occur from inhalation of drug vapors such as enflurane (Schwettmann and Casterline, 1976), and antibiotics such as spiramycin (Davies and Pepys, 1975) and tetracycline (Menon and Das, 1977). To detect pulmonary sensitization from inhalation of drug and chemical aerosols, the body plethysmographic technique using a guinea pig model has been shown to be useful (Patterson and Kelly, 1974; Karol, 1988; Karol and Thorne, 1988; Karol et al., 1989; Thorne and Karol, 1989). The criteria for positive pulmonary sensitization in intact guinea pigs are changes in breathing frequency and their extent, and the time of onset of an airway constrictive response after induction, and after a challenge dose of the test drug (Karol et al., 1989).

The mucociliary transport system of the airways can be impaired by respiratory irritants, local analgenesics and anesthetics, and parasympathetic stimultants (Pavia, 1984). Any one of the above agents will retard the beating frequency of the cilia and the secretion of the serous fluid of the mucous membranes. As a result, the propulsion of the inhaled particles, bacteria, or endogenous debris toward the oral pharynx for expectoration or swallowing will be retarded. Conversely, inhalation of adrenergic agonists increases the activity of the mucociliary transport system and facilitates the elimination of noxious material from the pulmonary system. Laboratory evaluation of the adverse drug effects on mucociliary transport in animal models can be achieved by measuring the velocity of the linear flow of mucus in the trachea of surgically prepared animals (Rylander, 1966). Clinically, the transportation of markers placed on the tracheal epithelium of normal human subjects can also be observed using a fiber-optic bronchoscopic technique (Pavia et al., 1980; Mussatto et al., 1988). The criteria of a positive response are changes in the transport time over a given distance of markers placed on the mucus, or changes in the rate of mucus secretion (Davis et al., 1976; Johnson et al., 1983, 1987; Webber and Widdicombe, 1987). More comprehensive discussion on mucociliary clearance can be found in several reviews (Newhouse et al., 1976; Last, 1982; Pavia, 1984). The fluid also contains a unique set of surfactants (Oyarzun and Clements, 1977, 1978) which can also be degraded by surfactants.

Cytological studies on the bronchial alveolar lavage fluid (BALF) permit the evaluation of the effects of an inhaled drug on the epithelial lining of the respiratory tract. This fluid can be obtained from intact animals or from excised lungs (Henderson, 1984, 1988, 1989). Quantitative analyses of fluid constituents such as neutrophils, antibody-forming lymphocytes, and antigen-specific IgG provide information on the cellular and biochemical responses of the lungs to the inhaled agent (Henderson 1984; Henderson et al., 1985, 1987). For example, BALF parameters were found to be unperturbed by the inhalation of halothane (Henderson and Lowrey, 1983). The criteria of a positive response are increases in protein content, increase in number of neutrophils and macrophages for inflammation; increase in number of lymphocytes and alteration of lymphocytes profiles for immune response; increase in cytoplasmic enzymes (lactate dehydrogenease) for cell lysis (Henderson, 1989); and the presence of antigen-specific antibodies for specific immune responses (Bice, 1985).

Morphological examination of the cellular structure of the pulmonary system is the foundation of most inhalation toxicity studies. Inhalation of airborne drug vapors or aerosols at harmful concentrations results mainly in local histopathologic changes in the epithelial cells of the airways, of which there are two types: nonciliated and ciliated cells. The nonciliated cells are the Clara cells, which contain secretory granules and smooth endoplasmic reticulum (SER); the cilliated cells have secretory granules but lack SER; and the brush cells, which have stubby microvilli and numerous cytoplasmic fibers on their free surfaces. If the concentration gradient of the drug in the lung is high enough to reach the alveoli, the Type I alveoli cells will also be affected (Davis et al., 1976; Evans, 1982). Drugs that affect the lungs via the bloodstream, such as bleomycin (Aso et al., 1976), cause changes to the endothelial cells of the vascular system that result in diffuse damage to the alveoli. The criteria of cellular damage are loss of cilia, swelling, and necrosis and sloughing of cell debris into the airway lumina. Tissues recovering from injuries are characterized by increases in the number of dividing progenitor cells followed by increases in intermediate cells that eventually differentiate into normal surface epithelium.

Pulmonary drug disposition studies are essential in research and development of new inhalant drugs. Inhaled drugs are usually absorbed and metabolized to some extent in the lungs because the lungs, like the liver, contain active enzyme systems. A drug may be metabolized to an inactive compound for excretion or to a highly reactive toxic metabolite(s) that causes pulmonary damage. In most pulmonary disposition studies, a gas or vapor is delivered via whole-body exposure (Paustenbach et al. 1983) or head-only exposure (Hafner et al., 1975). For aerosols, over 90% of a dose administered by mouth breathing is deposited in the oropharynx and swallowed. Consequently, the disposition pattern reflects that of ingestion in combination with a small contribution from pulmonary metabolism. For determining the disposition of inhaled drugs by the pulmonary system alone, a dosimetric endotracheal nebulization technique Leong et al., 1988) is useful. In this technique, microliter quantities of a radiolabeled drug solution can be nebulized within the trachea using a miniature air-liquid nebulizing nozzle. Alternatively, a small volume of liquid can be dispersed endotrachially using a microsyringe. In either technique, an accurate dose of a labeled drug solution is delivered entirely into the respiratory tract and lungs. Subsequent radioassay of the excreta thus reflects only the pulmonary disposition of the drug without complication from aerosols deposited in the oropharyngeal regions if the drug had been delivered by mouth inhalation. For example, in a study of the antiasthmatic drug lodoximide tromethamine, the urinary metabolites produced by beagle dogs after receiving a dose of the radiolabeled drug via endotracheal nebulization showed a high percentage of the intact drug. However, metabolites produced after oral administration were mainly nonactive conjugates. The differences were due to the drug's escape from first-pass metabolism in the liver when it was administered through the pulmonary system. The results thus indicated that the drug had to be administered by inhalation to be effective. This crucial information was extremely important in the selection of the most effective route of administration and formulation of this antiasthmatic drug (Leong et al., 1988).

Cardiotoxicity of inhalant drugs should also be evaluated. For example, adverse cardiac effects may be induced by inhaling vapors of fluorocarbons, which are used extensively as propellants in drug aerosols. Inhalation of vapors of anesthetics also has been shown to cause depression of the heart rate and alteration of the rhythm and blood pressure (Merin, 1981; Leong and Rop, 1989). More important, inhalation of antiasthmatic aerosols of beta-receptor agonists delivered in a fluorocarbon propellant has been shown to cause marked tachycardia, electrocardiogram (ECG) changes, and sensitization of the heart to arrhythmia (Aviado, 1981; Balazs, 1981). Chronic inhalation of drug aerosols can also result in cardiomyopathy (Balazs, 1981). For detection of cardiotoxicity, standard methods of monitoring arterial pressures, heart rate, and ECGs of animals during inhalation of a drug, or at frequent intervals during a prolonged treatment period, should be useful in safety assessments of inhalant drugs.

Since the inhalation route is just a method for administering drugs, other nonpulmonary effects, such as behavioral effects (Ts'o et al., 1975) and renal and liver toxicity, should also be evaluated. In addition, attention should also be given to drugs that are not administered via the inhalation route, but that accumulate in the lungs where they cause pulmonary damage (Wilson, 1982; Hollinger, 1985).

## 10.8. PARAMETERS OF TOXICITY EVALUATION

Paracelsus stated over 400 years ago that "All substances are poison. The right dose differentiates a poison and a remedy." Thus, in safety assessments of inhaled drugs, the "dose," or magnitude of inhalation exposure, in relation to the physiological, biochemical, cytological, or morphological response(s) must be determined. Toxicity information is essential to establishing guidelines to prevent the health hazards of acute or chronic overdosage during therapy, or of unintentional exposure to the bulk drugs and their formulated products during manufacturing and industrial handling.

### 10.8.1. The Inhaled "Dose"

Most drugs are designed for oral or parenteral administration in which the dose is calculated in terms of drug weight in milligrams (mg) divided by the body weight in kilograms (kg):

$$\text{dose} = \frac{\text{drug weight (mg)}}{\text{body weight (kg)}} = \text{mg/kg}$$

For inhalant drugs, the inhaled "dose" has been expressed in many mathematical models (Dahl, 1990). However, the practical approach is based on exposure concentration and duration rather than on theoretic concepts. Thus, an inhaled "dose" is expressed in terms of the exposure concentration ($C$) in milligrams per liter (mg/liter) or milligrams per cubic meter (mg/m$^3$) or parts per million (ppm) of air, the duration of exposure ($t$) in minutes, the ventilatory parameters including the respiratory rate ($R$) in number of breaths per minute and the tidal volume ($Tv$) in liters per breath, and a retention factor $\alpha$ (alpha), which is related to the reactivity and the solubility of the drug. The product of these parameters divided by the body weight in kilograms gives the dose:

$$\text{dose} = \frac{C \cdot t \cdot R \cdot Tv \cdot \alpha}{\text{body weight}} = \text{mg/kg}$$

In critical evaluation of the effect of a gas, vapor, or aerosol inhaled in to the respiratory tract of an animal, the dosimetric method has been recommended (Oberst, 1961). However, due to the complexity of measuring the various parameters simultaneously, only a few studies on gaseous drugs or chemicals have employed the dosimetric method (Weston and Karel, 1946; Adams et al., 1952; Leong and MacFarland, 1965; Landy et al., 1983; Stott and McKenna, 1984; Dallas et al., 1986, 1989). For studies on liquid or powdery aerosols, modified techniques such as intratracheal instillation (Brain et al., 1976) or endotracheal nebulization (Leong et al., 1988) were used to deliver an exact dose of the test material into the lower respiratory tract (LRT) while bypassing the URT and ignoring the ventilatory parameters.

In routine inhalation studies, it is generally accepted that the respiratory parameters are relatively constant when the animals are similar in age, sex, and body weight. This leaves only $C$ and $t$ to be the major variables for dose consideration.

$$\text{"Dose"} = C \cdot t = \text{mg} \cdot \text{min/liter}$$

The product $Ct$ is not a true dose because its unit is mg · min/liter rather than mg/kg. Nevertheless, $Ct$ can be manipulated as though it were a dose, an approximated dose (MacFarland, 1976).

The respiratory parameters of an animal will dictate the volume of air inhaled and hence the quantity of test material entering the respiratory system. Commonly used parameters for a number of experimental species and humans are given in Table 10.1 to illustrate this point and include the alveolar surface area because this represents the target tissue for most inhaled materials. It can be seen that by taking the ratios of these parameters and comparing the two extremes, that is, the mouse and man, that (1) a mouse inhales approximately 30 times its lung volume in one minute whereas a man at rest inhales approximately the same volume as that of his lung. This can increase with heavy work up to the same ratio as the mouse, but is not sustained for long periods. This means that the dose per unit lung volume is up to 30 times higher in the mouse than man at the same inhaled atmospheric concentration. (2) The minute volume of the mouse is in contact with five times less alveolar surface area than man, hence the dose per unit area is up to five times greater in the mouse. (3) The lung volume in comparison with the alveolar surface area in experimental animals is less than in humans, meaning that the extent of contact of inhaled gases with the alveolar surface is greater in experimental animals.

While it is possible, and common, to refer to standard respiratory parameters for different species in order to calculate inhaled dose and deposited dose with time, it is usually the case that inhaled materials influence the breathing patterns of test animals. The most common examples of this are irritant vapors, which can reduce the respiratory rate by up to 80%. This phenomenon results from a reflexive pause during the breathing cycle due to stimulation by the inhaled material of the trigeminal nerve endings situated in the nasal passages. The duration of the pause and hence the reduction in the respiratory rate are concentration related, permitting concentration-response relationships to be plotted. This has been investigated extensively by Alarie (1981a) and forms the basis of a test screen for comparing quantitatively the irritancy of different materials, and has found application in

**TABLE 10.1. Respiratory Parameters for Common Experimental Species and Humans**

| Species | Body Weight (kg) | Lung Volume (ml) | Minute Volume (ml min$^{-1}$) | Alveolar Surface Area (m$^2$) | Lung Volume % Surface Area | Minute Volume % Lung Volume | Minute Volume % Surface area |
|---|---|---|---|---|---|---|---|
| Mouse | 0.023 | 0.74 | 24 | 0.068 | 10.9 | 32.4 | 353 |
| Rat | 0.14 | 6.3 | 84 | 0.39 | 16.2 | 13.3 | 215 |
| Monkey | 3.7 | 184 | 694 | 13 | 14.2 | 3.77 | 53 |
| Dog | 22.8 | 1501 | 2923 | 90 | 16.7 | 1.95 | 33 |
| Human | 75 | 7000 | 6000 | 82 | 85.4 | 0.86 | 73 |

*Source*: Altman and Ditmar, 1974.

assessing appropriate exposure limits for human exposure when respiratory irritancy is the predominant cause for concern.

While irritancy resulting from the above reflex reaction is one cause of altered respiratory parameters during exposure, there are many others. These include other types of reflex response, such as bronchoconstriction, the narcotic effects of many solvents, the development of toxic signs as exposure progresses, or simply a voluntary reduction in respiratory rate by the test animal due to the unpleasant nature of the inhaled atmosphere. The extent to which these affect breathing patterns and hence inhaled dose can only be assessed by actual measurement.

By simultaneous monitoring of tidal volume and respiratory rate, or minute volume, and the concentration of an inhaled vapor in the bloodstream and the vapor in the exposure atmosphere, pharmacokinetic studies on the $C \cdot t$ relationship have shown that the effective dose was nearly proportional to the exposure concentration for vapors such as 1,1,1-trichloroethane (Dallas et al., 1986), which has a saturable metabolism, found that the steady-state plasma concentrations were disproportionally greater at higher exposure concentrations.

Acknowledging the possible existence of deviations, this simplified approach of using $C$ and $t$ for dose determination provides that basis for dose-response assessments in practically all inhalation toxicological studies.

### 10.8.2. The Dose-Response Relationship

The first principle of dose-response determination in inhalation toxicology is based on Haber's rule, which states that responses to an inhaled toxicant will be the same under conditions where $C$ varies in complementary manner to $t$ (Haber, 1924). For example, if $C \cdot t$ elicits a specific magnitude of the same response; that is, $Ct = K$, where $K$ is a constant for the stated magnitude of response (as shown in Figure 10.2).

This rule holds reasonably well when $C$ or $t$ varies within a narrow range for acute exposure to a gaseous compound (Rinehart and Hatch, 1964) and for chronic exposure to an inert particle (Henderson et al., 1991). Excursion of $C$ or $t$ beyond these limits will cause the assumption $Ct = K$ to be incorrect (Adams et al., 1950, 1952; Sidorenko and Pinigin, 1976; Andersen et al., 1979; Uemitsu et al., 1985). For example, an animal may be exposed to 1000 ppm of diethyl ether for 420 min or 1400 ppm for 300 min without incurring any anesthesia. However, exposure to 420,000 ppm for 1 min will surely cause anesthesia or even death of the animal. Furthermore, toxicokinetic study of liver enzymes affected by inhalation of carbon tetrachloride (Uemitsu et al., 1985), which has a saturable metabolism in rats, showed that $Ct = K$ does not correctly reflect the "toxicity value" of this compound. Therefore, the limitations of Haber's rule must be recognized when it is used in interpolation or extrapolation of inhalation toxicity data.

### 10.8.3. Exposure Concentration versus Response

In certain medical situations (e.g., a patient's variable exposure duration to a surgical concentration of an inhalant anesthetic, or the repeated exposures of surgeons and

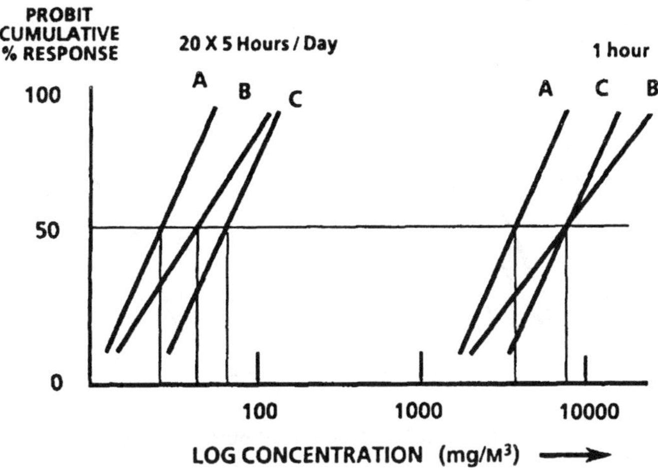



**FIGURE 10.2.** Dose-response is plotted in terms of the probit of cumulative percentage response to logarithm of the exposure concentrations.

nurses to subanesthetic concentrations of an anesthetic in the operating theater) it is necessary to know the duration of safe exposure to a drug. Duration safety can be assessed by determining a drug's median effective time ($Et_{50}$) or median lethal time ($Lt_{50}$). These statistically derived quantities represent the duration of exposure required to affect or kill 50% of a group of animals exposed to a specified concentration of an airborne drug or chemical in the atmosphere.

The graph in Figure 10.3 is the probit plot of cumulative percentage response to logarithm of exposure duration. It shows the 1000 mg/m$^3$ for 10 h or to 10 mg/m$^3$ for 1000 h, each with a $Ct$ (an approximated dose) of $\sim 10,000$ h mg/m$^3$. Similar to concentration-response graphs, the slopes indicate the differences in the mechanism of action and the margins of safe exposure of the three drugs. The ratio of the $ET_{50}$ or $LT_{50}$ of two drugs indicates their relative toxicity, and the ratio of $ET_{50}$ over $LT_{50}$ of the same drug is the therapeutic ratio.

### 10.8.4. Product of Concentration and Duration ($Ct$) versus Responses

To evaluate inhalation toxicity in situations where workers are exposed to various concentrations and durations of a drug vapor, aerosol, or powder in the work environment during manufacturing or packaging, a more comprehensive determination of $E(Ct)_{50}$ or $L(Ct)_{50}$ values are used. The $E(Ct)_{50}$ or $L(Ct)_{50}$ values are statistically derived values that represent the magnitude of exposure, expressed as a function of the product of $C$ and $t$, that is expected to affect or kill less than 50% and more than 50% of the animals. The other curve represents exposures that kill 50% or more than 50% of each group of animals (Irish and Adams, 1940).

The graph in Figure 10.4 illustrates inhalation exposures to a drug using various combinations of $C$ and $t$ that kill 50% of the animals. For example, a 50% mortality

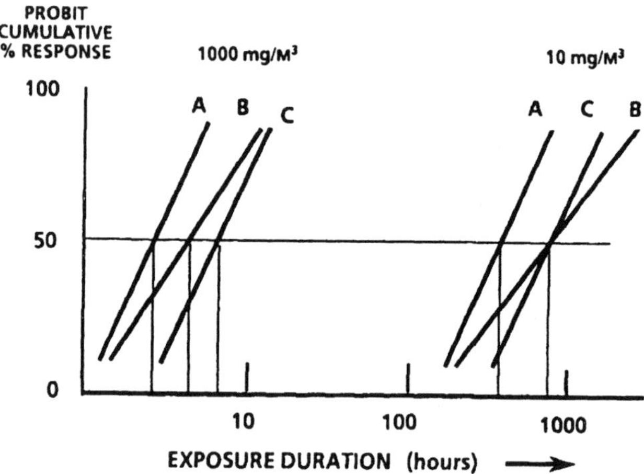



**FIGURE 10.3.** Dose-response plotted in terms of the probit plot of cumulative percentage response to logarithm of exposure duration.

occurs when a group of animals is exposed to drug A at a concentration of $1000\,\text{mg/m}^3$ for a duration of approximately 2 h, or at a concentration of $100\,\text{mg/m}^3$ for a duration of approximately 20 h. Furthermore, the graph also illustrates that the inhalation toxicity of drug A is more than one order of magnitude higher than that of drug B. For example, an exposure to drug A at the concentration of $100\,\text{mg/m}^3$ for 100 h kills 100% of the animals whereas an exposure to drug B at the concentration of $1000\,\text{mg/m}^3$ for 100 h does not kill any animals.

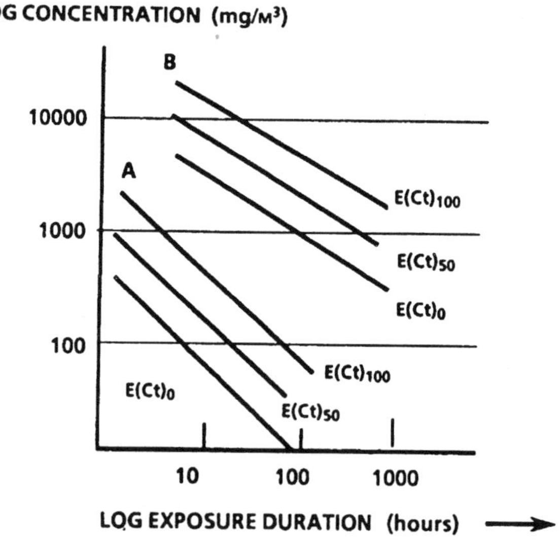



**FIGURE 10.4.** Dose-response plotted in terms of logarithms of exposure concentration and durations.

### 10.8.5. Units for Exposure Concentration

For gases and vapors, exposure concentrations are traditionally expressed in parts per million (ppm). The calculation for the ppm of a gas or vapor in an air sample is based on Avogadro's Law, which states that "Equal volumes contain equal numbers of molecules under the same temperature and pressure." In other words, under standard temperature and pressure (STP), one gram-molecular weight (mole) of any gas under a pressure of one atmosphere (equivalent to the height of 760 mm mercury) and a temperature of 273 K has the same number of molecules and occupies the same volume of 22.4 liters. However, under ambient conditions, the volume of 22.4 liters has to be corrected to a larger volume based on Charles' Law, which states that at constant pressure the volume of gas varies directly with the absolute temperature. Thus, at a room temperature of 25°C, one mole of a gas occupies a volume of 24.5 liters.

$$22.4 \text{ liters} \times \frac{298 \text{ K}}{273 \text{ K}} = 24.5 \text{ liters}$$

Further correction of volume for an atmospheric pressure deviation from one atmosphere may be done by applying Boyle's Law, which states that the volume of a gas without change of temperature varies inversely with the pressure applied to it.

$$24.5 \text{ liters} \times \frac{758 \text{ mm Hg}}{760 \text{ mm Hg}} = 24.4 \text{ liters}$$

In practice, atmospheric pressure in most animal experimental environments usually varies only a few mm Hg, so little or no correction is required.

Using the aforementioned principles, the volume of a vapor generated from a given weight of a liquid can be calculated. For example, 1 mole of water weighs 18 g, while 1 mole of ethanol weighs 46 g. When 1 mole of each liquid is totally vaporized, each will occupy the same volume of 24.5 liters at room temperature (25°C) and pressure (760 mm Hg). In an inhalation experiment, if the volume of test liquid and the rate of airflow being mixed in the animal exposure chamber are known, the vapor concentration in the chamber atmosphere can be calculated in parts per million or milligrams per liter. A conversion table published by the U. S. Bureau of Mines enables quick conversion between parts per million and milligrams per liter for compounds with molecular weights up to 300 g (Fieldner et al., 1921; Patty, 1958).

For aerosols of nonvolatile liquid and powdery compounds, the concentration of the mist or dust atmosphere must be expressed in terms of milligrams per liter or milligrams per cubic meter ($mg/m^3$) of air. With advances in biotechnology, many pharmacological testing techniques are based on specific receptor bindings, in which the ratio of the number of molecules to those of the receptors are considered, in which case the exposure concentration may be more appropriately expressed in micromoles per unit volume of air ($\mu mol/m^3$).

## 10.9. INHALATION EXPOSURE TECHNIQUES

Many inhalation exposure techniques, such as the whole-body, nose-only, mouth-only, or head-only technique (Drew and Laskin, 1973; MacFarland, 1976; Leong et al., 1981; Phalen, 1984; Nelson, 1980), the intranasal exposure technique (Elliott and DeYoung, 1970; Smith et al., 1981), the endotracheal nebulization technique (Leong et al., 1985, 1988; Schreck et al., 1986), and the body plethysmographic techniques (Alarie, 1966; Thorne and Karol, 1989), have been developed for inhalation toxicity studies. Table 10.2 provides a summary of the advantages and disadvantages of each of the major inhalation exposure methodologies.

The main criteria for the design and operation of any dynamic (as opposed to static) inhalation exposure system are the following

1. The concentration of the test atmosphere must be reasonably uniform throughout the chamber and should increase and decrease at a rate close to theoretical at the start or end of the exposure. Silver (1946) showed that the time taken for a chamber to reach a point of equilibrium was proportional to the flow rate of atmosphere passing through the chamber and the chamber volume. From this, the concentration-time relationship during the "run-up" and "run-down" phase could be expressed by the equation

$$t_x = k\frac{V}{F}$$

   where $t_x$ = time required to reach $x\%$ of the equilibrium concentration, $k$ = a constant of value determined by the value of $x$, $V$ = chamber volume and $F$ = chamber flow rate. The $t_{99}$ value is frequently quoted for exposure chambers, representing the time required to reach 99% of the equilibrium concentration and providing an estimate of chamber efficiency. Thus, at maximum efficiency, the theoretical value of $k$ at $t_{99}$ is 4.605, and the closer to this that the results of evaluation of actual chamber performance fall, the greater is the efficiency and the better the design of the chamber.

2. Flow rates must be controlled in such a way that they are not excessive, which might cause streaming effects within the chamber, but must be adequate to maintain normal oxygen levels, temperature and humidity in relation to the number of animals being exposed. A minimum of 10 air changes per hour is frequently advocated and is appropriate in most cases. However, the chamber design and housing density also need to be taken into account and some designs, such as that of Doe and Tinston (1981), function effectively at lower air change rates.

3. The chamber or exposure manifold materials should not affect the chemical or physical nature of the test atmosphere.

The whole-body exposure technique is useful for acute and chronic toxicity studies of gases and vapors. For acute whole-body exposure, a few animals are exposed for 1 to 4 h to a gas, vapor, or aerosol of a drug or chemical in a simple glass jar. The gaseous drug is metered with a precision flow meter into the stream of filtered room air being drawn through the glass jar or chamber. For vapor generation from a volatile liquid, a stream of clean air is bubbled at a constant rate onto the walls of a temperature-regulated flask, which vaporizes the liquid droplets rapidly and continuously. In either method, the vapor emerging from the vaporizer is directed into the filtered airstream being drawn through the glass jar or chamber. For the generation of drug aerosols from liquids or powders, various types of atomizers or nebulizers and dust generators are available (Drew and Laskin, 1973; Drew and Lippmann, 1978; Leong et al., 1981; Phalen, 1984). For more critical and precision studies, an adequate number of animals per group is calculated by an appropriate statistical method (Gad, 1999) and the exposure is carried out in an elaborate dynamic airflow chamber with precision control of the chamber airflow, temperature, and humidity.

Regardless of the exposure apparatus used, the most important aspect of an exposure study is the generation of a constant concentration of the airborne drug vapor or aerosol in the chamber atmosphere. This has to be sampled (Drew and Lippmann, 1978) and analyzed using an appropriate analytical instrument, such as an infrared spectrophotometer for halogenated propellants, or a gas chromatograph for other gases and vapors. The concentration of the drug as detected by the analyzer is the "analytical concentration." For characterizing the aerosol atmosphere, particle sizing, in additional to concentration analyses, is essential. Because the breathing patterns of the experimental animals cannot be regulated, it is extremely important to generate aerosols of the appropriate size for bioavailability.

For critical laboratory studies on inhaled drugs, a monodisperse aerosol of a specified range of MMAD should be used to increase the probability that the aerosol reaches the specified target area of the lungs. The Dautrebande aerosol generators (Dautrebande, 1962c) and the DeVilbiss nebulizer (Drew and Lippmann, 1978) are the classic single-reservoir generators for short-duration inhalation studies. For long-duration inhalation studies, the multiple-reservoir nebulizer (Miller et al., 1981) or the continuous syringe metering and elutriating atomizer (Leong et al., 1981) are frequently used. The nebulizers generate a polydisperse droplet aerosol either by the shearing force of a jet of air over a fine stream of liquid or by ultrasonic disintegration of the surface liquid in a reservoir (Drew and Lippmann, 1978). The aerosols emerging from a jet nebulizer generally have MMADs ranging between 1.2 and 6.9 μm with GSDs of 1.7 to 2.2, and aerosols from an ultrasonic nebulizer have MMADs ranging between 3.7 and 10.5 μm with GSDs of 1.4 to 2.0 (Mercer, 1981).

For testing therapeutic formulations, the liquid aerosols are usually generated by the pressurized metered-dose inhaler (Newman, 1984; Newton, 2000; Gad and Chengelis, 1998). The pressurized metered-dose inhaler (MDI) generates a bolus of aerosols by atomizing a well-defined quantity of a drug that is solubilized in a fluorocarbon propellant. The aerosols, thus, consist of the drug particles with a coating of the propellant. As the aerosols emerge from the orifice, the mean particle

**TABLE 10.2. Advantages, Disadvantages, and Considerations Associated with Patterns of Inhalation Exposure**

| Mode of Exposure | Advantages | Disadvantages | Design Considerations |
| --- | --- | --- | --- |
| Whole body | Variety and number of animals<br>Chronic studies possible<br>Minimum restraint<br>Large historical database<br>Controllable environment<br>Minimum stress<br>Minimum labor | Messy<br>Multiple routes of exposure: skin, eyes, oral<br>Variability of "dose"<br>Cannot pulse exposure easily<br>Poor contact between animals and investigators<br>Capital intensive<br>Inefficient compound usage<br>Difficult to monitor animals during exposure | Cleaning effluent air<br>Inert materials<br>Losses of test material<br>Even distribution in space<br>Sampling<br>Animal care<br>Observation<br>Noise, vibration, humidity<br>Air temperature<br>Safe exhaust<br>Loading<br>Reliability |
| Head only | Good for repeated exposure<br>Limited routes of entry into animal<br>More efficient dose delivery | Stress to animal<br>Losses can be large<br>Seal around neck<br>Labor in loading/unloading | Even distribution<br>Pressure fluctuations<br>Sampling and losses<br>Air temperature, humidity<br>Animal comfort<br>Animal restraint |
| Nose/mouth only | Exposure limited to mouth and respiratory tract<br>Uses less material (efficient)<br>Containment of material<br>Can pulse the exposure | Stress to animal<br>Seal about face<br>Effort to expose large number of animals | Pressure fluctuations<br>Body temperature<br>Sampling<br>Airlocking<br>Animals' comfort<br>Losses in plumbing/masks |

| Lung only (Tracheal administration) | Precision of dose<br>One route of exposure<br>Uses less material (efficient)<br>Can pulse the exposure | Technically difficult<br>Anesthesia or tracheostomy<br>Limited to small numbers<br>Bypasses nose<br>Artifacts in deposition and response<br>Technically more difficult | Air humidity/temperature<br>Stress to the animal<br>Physiologic support |
| Partial lung | Precision of total dose<br>Localization of dose<br>Can achieve very high local doses<br>Unexposed control tissue from same animal | Anesthesia<br>Placement of dose<br>Difficulty in interpretation of results<br>Technically difficult<br>Possible redistribution of material within lung | Stress to animal<br>Physiologic support |

*Source*: Gad and Chengelis, 1998.

size may be as large as 30 µm (Moren, 1981). After traveling through a tubular or cone-shaped spacer, the propellant may evaporate, reducing the MMADs to a range of 2.8 to 5.5 µm with GSDs of 1.5 to 2.2 (Hiller et al., 1978; Sackner et al., 1981; Newman, 1984) and making the aerosols more stable for inhalation studies. In a prolonged animal exposure study, multiple metered-dose inhalers have to be actuated sequentially with an electromechanical gadget (Ulrich et al., 1984) to maintain a slightly pulsatile but relatively consistent chamber concentration.

For generating an aerosol from dry powders, various dust generators, such as the Wright dust feed, air elutriator or fluidized-bed dust generator, and air impact pulverizer, have been developed for acute and chronic animal inhalation studies and described in many articles (Hinds, 1980; Leong et al., 1981; Phalen, 1984; Gad and Chengelis, 1998; Valentine and Kennedy, 2001; Hext, 2000). For generating powdery therapeutic agents, a metered-dose dry powder inhaler, spinhaler, or a rotahaler is used (Newman, 1984). The particle size of the drug powder is micronized to a specific size range during manufacture and the spinhaler or the rotahaler only disperse the powders.

More recently, another approach for administering dry powders to both humans and test animals has arisen. Dry powders, while less frequently used in nasal drug delivery, are becoming more popular. Powders can be administered from several devices, the most common being the insufflator. Many insufflators work with predosed powder in gelatin capsules. To improve patient compliance a multidose powder inhaler has been developed which has been used to deliver budesonide. These devices can also be used for administration to test animals, both in terms of amounts and aerodynamic size of the particles. Early dry powder inhalers such as the Rotohaler® used individual capsules of micronized drug which were difficult to handle. Modern devices use blister packs (e.g., Diskus®) or reservoirs (e.g., Turbuhaler®). The dry powder inhalers rely on inspiration to withdraw the drug from the inhaler to the lung and hence the effect of inhalation flow rate through various devices has been extensively studied. The major problem to be overcome with these devices is to ensure that the finely micronized drug is thoroughly dispersed in the airstream. It has been recommended that patients inhale as rapidly as possible from these devices in order to provide the maximum force to disperse the powder. The quantity of drug and deposition pattern varies enormously depending on the device, for example, the Turbuhaler® produces significantly greater lung delivery of salbutamol than the Diskus®. Vidgren and coworkers (1987) demonstrated by gamma scintigraphy that a typical dry powder formulation of sodium cromoglycate suffers losses of 44% in the mouth and 40% in the actuator nozzle itself.

It must also be emphasized that the major mass of a heterodispersed aerosol may be contained in a few relatively large particles, since the mass of a particle is proportional to the cube of its diameter. Therefore, the particle-size distribution and the concentration of the drug particles in the exposure atmosphere should be sampled using a cascade impactor or membrane filter sampling technique, monitored using an optical or laser particle-size analyzer, and analyzed using optical or electron microscopy techniques.

In summary, many techniques have been developed for generating gas, vapor, and aerosol atmospheres for inhalation toxicology studies. By proper regulation of the operating conditions of the nebulizers and the formulation of metered-dose inhalers, together with the use of spacer or reservoir attachments to MDIs, more particles within the respirable range can be generated for inhalation. An accurately controlled exposure concentration is essential to an accurate determination of the dose-response relationship in a safety assessment of an inhalant drug.

Finally, comparisons of various techniques for animal exposures indicate that the whole-body exposure technique is the most suitable for safety assessment of gases and vapors and permits simultaneous exposure of a large number of animals to the same concentration of a drug; however, this technique is not suitable for aerosol and powder exposures because the exposure condition represents the resultant effects from inhalation, ingestion, and dermal absorption of the drug (Phalen, 1984; Gad and Chengelis, 1998).

## 10.10. THE UTILITY OF TOXICITY DATA

Regardless of the type of test and the parameters to be monitored, the ultimate goal is to interpolate or extrapolate from the dose-response data to find a no-observable-adverse-effect level (NOAEL) or a no-observable-effect level (NOEL). By applying a safety factor of 1 to 10 to the NOAEL, a safe single-exposure dose for a Phase I clinical trial may be obtained. By applying a more stringent safety factor, a multiple-exposure dose for a clinical trial may also be obtained. After the drug candidate has successfully passed all the drug safety evaluations and entered in the production stage, more toxicity tests may be needed for the establishment of a threshold limit value-time-weighted average (TLV-TWA). A TLV-TWA is defined as "the time weighted average concentration for a normal 8-hour workday and a 40-hour workweek, to which nearly all workers may be repeatedly exposed, day after day, without adverse effect" (ACGIH, 1991). Using TLVs as guides, long-term safe occupational exposures during production and industrial handling of a drug may be achieved. Appropriate safety assessments of pharmaceutical chemicals and drugs will ensure the creation and production of a safe drug for the benefit of humans and animals. Further, inhalation toxicity data are needed for compliance with many regulatory requirements of the Food and Drug Administration, the Occupational Health and Safety Administration, and the Environmental Protection Agency (Gad and Chengelis, 1998).

More comprehensive descriptions and discussions on inhalation toxicology and technology may be found in several recent monographs, reviews, and textbooks (Willeke, 1980; Leong et al., 1981; Witschi and Nettesheim, 1982; Clarke and Pavia, 1984; Phalen, 1984; Witschi and Brain, 1985; Barrow, 1986; McFadden, 1986; Menzel and Amdur, 1986; Salem, 1986; Gardner, 1988; Gad and Chengelis, 1998; Valentine and Kennedy, 2001; McClellan, 1989; Hext, 2000).

## REFERENCES

Adams, E.M., Spencer, H.C., Rowe, V.K. and Irish, D.D. (1950). Vapor toxicity of 1,1,1,-trichloroethane (methylchloroform) determined by experiments on laboratory animals. *Arch. Ind. Hyg. Occup. Med.* 1: 225–236.

Adams, E.M., Spencer, H.C., Rowe, V.K., McCollister, D.D. and Irish, D.D. (1952). Vapor toxicity of carbon tetrachloride determined by experiments on laboratory animals. *Arch. Ind. Hyg. Occup. Med.* 6: 50–66.

Agnew, J.E. (1984). Physical properties and mechanisms of deposition of aerosols. In: *Aerosols and the Lung, Clinical Aspects* (Clarke, S.W. and Pavia, D., Eds.). Butterworth, London, pp. 49–68.

Alarie, Y. (1966). Irritating properties of airborne material to the upper respiratory tract. *Arch. Environ. Health* 13: 433–449.

Alarie, Y. (1973). Sensory irritation by airborne chemicals. *CRC Crit. Rev. Toxicol.* 2: 299–363.

Alarie, Y. (1981a). Toxicological evaluation of airborne chemical irritants and allergens using respiratory reflex reactions. In: *Inhalation Toxicology and Technology* (Leong, B.K.J., Ed.). Ann Arbor Science, Ann Arbor, pp. 207–231.

Alarie, Y. (1981b). Bioassay for evaluating the potency of airborne sensory irritants and predicting acceptable levels of exposure in man. *Food Cosmet. Toxicol.* 19: 623–626.

Alarie, Y. and Luo, J.E. (1986). Sensory irritation by airborne chemicals: A basis to establish acceptable levels of exposure. In: *Toxicology of the Nasal Passages* (Barrow, C.S., Ed.). Hemisphere, New York, pp. 91–100.

Alarie, Y., Kane, L. and Barrow, C. (1980). Sensory irritation: The use of an animal model to establish acceptable exposure to airborne chemical irritants. In: *Toxicology: Principles and Practice 1* (Reeves, A.L., Ed.). Wiley, New York.

Altman, P.L. and Dittmer, D.S. (1974). *Biological Data Book*, Vol. III. Federation of American Societies for Experimental Biology, Bethesda, MD.

Andersen, M.E., French. J.E., Gargas, M.L. Jones, R.A. and Jenkins, L.J., Jr. (1979). Saturable metabolism and the acute toxicity of 1,1-dichloroethylene. *Toxicol. Appl. Pharmacol.* 47: 385–393.

Aso, Y., Yoneda, K. and Kikkawa, Y. (1976). Morphologic and biochemical study of pulmonary changes induced by bleomycin in mice. *Lab. Invest.* 35: 558–568.

Aviado, D.M. (1981). Comparative cardiotoxicity of fluorocarbons. In: *Cardiac Toxicology,* Vol. II (Balazs, T., Ed.). CRC Press: Boca Raton, FL, pp. 213–222.

Aviado, D.M. and Micozzi, M.S. (1981). Fluorine-containing organic compounds. In: *Patty's Industrial Hygiene and Toxicology,* vol. 2B (Clayton, G.D. and Clayton, F.E., Eds.). Wiley, New York, pp. 3071–3115.

Balazs, T. (1981). Cardiotoxicity of adrenergic bronchodililator and vasodilating antihypertensive drugs. In: *Cardiac Toxicology,* Vol. II (Balazs, T., Ed.). CRC Press: Boca Raton, FL, pp. 61–73.

Barrow, C.S. (1986). *Toxicology of the Nasal Passages.* Hemisphere: New York.

Bell, K.A. (1978). Local particle deposition in respiratory airway models. In: *Recent Developments in Aerosol Science* (Shaw, D.T., Ed.). Wiley: New York, pp. 97–134.

Bice, D.E. (1985). Methods and approaches to assessing immunotoxicology of the lower respiratory tract. *In Immunotoxicology and Immunopharmacology* (Dean, J.H., Luster, M.I., Munson, A.E. and Amos, H.A., Eds.). Raven Press, New York, pp. 145–157.

Brain, J.D. (1971). The effects of increased particles on the number of aveolar macrophages. In: *Inhaled Particles* III, Proceeding of BOHS Symposium. Unwin Brothers Ltd., London, pp. 200–233.

Brain, J.D., Knudson, D.E., Sorokin, S.P. and Davis, M.A. (1976). Pulmonary distribution of particles given by intratracheal instillation or be aerosol inhalation. *Environ. Res.* 11: 13–33.

Budavari, S. (Ed.) (1989). *Merck Index*, Eleventh ed. Merck & Co., Rahway, NJ., p. 82.

Chan, T.L. and Lippmann, M. (1980). Experimental measurements and empirical modelling of the regional deposition of inhaled particles in humans. *Am. Ind. Hyg. Assoc. J.* 41: 399–409.

Chenoweth, M.B., Leong, B.K.J., Sparschu, G.L. and Torkelson, T.R. (1972). Toxicities of methoxyflurane, halothane and diethyl ether in laboratory animals on repeated inhalation at subanesthetic concentrations. In: *Cellular Biology and Toxicity of Anesthetics* (Fink, B.R., Ed.). Williams & Wilkins, Baltimore, pp. 275–284.

Clarke, S.W. and Pavia, D. (eds.) (1984). *Aerosol and the Lung: Clinical and Experimental Aspects*. Butterworth, London.

Cox, J.S.G., Beach, J.E., Blair, A.M.J.N., Clarke, A.J., King, J., Lee, T.B., Loveday, D.E.E., Moss, G.F., Orr, T.S.C., Ritchie, J.T. and Sheard, P. (1970). Disodium cromoglycate. *Adv. Drug. Res.* 5: 115–196.

Curry, S.H., Taylor, A.J., Evans, S., Godfrey, S. and Zeidifard, E. (1975). Disposition of disodium cromoglycate administered in three particle sizes. *Br. J. Clin. Pharmacol.* 2: 267–270.

Dahl, A.R. (1990). Dose concepts for inhaled vapors and gases. *Toxicol. Appl. Pharmacol.* 103: 185–197.

Dallas, C.E., Bruckner, J.V., Maedgen, J.L. and Weir, F.W. (1986). A method for direct measurement of systemic uptake and elimination of volatile organics in small animals. *J. Pharmacol. Methods* 16: 239–250.

Dallas, C.E., Ramanathan, R., Muralidhara, S., Gallo, J.M. and Bruckner, J.V. (1989). The uptake and elimination of 1,1,1-trichloroethane during and following inhalation exposure in rats. *Toxicol. App. Pharmacol.* 98: 385–397.

Dautrebande, L. (1962a). Importance of particle size for therapeutic aerosol efficiency. In: *Microaerosols*. Academic Press, New York, pp. 37–57.

Dautrebande, L. (1962b). Practical recommendation for administering pharmacological aerosols. In *Microaerosols*. Academic Press, New York, pp. 86–92.

Dautrebande, L. (1962c). Production of liquid and solid micromicellar aerosols. In: *Microaerosols*. Academic Press, New York, pp. 1–22.

Davis, C.N. (1961). A formalized anatomy of the human respiratory tract. In: *Inhaled Particles and Vapours*. (Davis, C.N., Ed.). Pergamon Press, London, pp. 82–91.

Davis, C.N., Heyder, J. and Subba Ramv, M.C. (1972). Breathing of half micron aerosols. I. Experimental. *J. Appl. Physicol.* 32: 591–600.

Davis, B., Marin, M.G., Fischer, S., Graf, P., Widdicombe, J.G. and Nadel, J.A. (1976). New method for study of canine mucus gland secretion *in vivo*: Cholinergic regulation. *Am. Rev. Respir. Dis.* 113: 257 (abstract).

Davies, R.J. and Pepys, J. (1975). Asthma due to inhaled chemical agents—The macrolide antibiotic spiramycin. *Clin. Allergy* 5: 99–107.

Dennis, W.L. (1961). The discussion of a paper by C.N. Davis: a formalized anatomy of the human respiratory tract. In: *Inhaled Particles and Vapours* (Davis, C.N., Ed.). Pergamon Press, London, p. 88.

Doe, J.E. and Tinston, D.J. (1981). Novel chamber for long-term inhalation studies, in *Inhalation Toxicology and Technology*, (Leong, K.J., Ed.). Ann Arbor Science: Ann Arbor, MI.

Drew, R.T. and Laskin, S. (1973). Environmental inhalation chambers. In: *Methods of Animal Experimentation* Vol. IV. Academic Press, New York, pp. 1–41.

Drew, R.T. and Lippmann, M. (1978). Calibration of air sampling instruments. In: *Air Sampling Instruments for Evaluation of Atmospheric Contaminants*, 5th ed. American Conference of Governmental Industrial Hygienists, Cincinnati, Ohio, Section I. pp. 1–32.

Elliot, G.A. and DeYoung, E.N. (1970). Intranasal toxicity testing of antiviral agents. *Am. New York Acad. Sci*, 173: 169–175.

Evans, M.J. (1982). Cell death and cell renewal in small airways and alveoli. In: *Mechanisms in Respiratory Toxicology*, Vol. 1. (Witschi, H. and Nettesheim, P., Eds.). CRC, Boca Raton, FL, pp. 189–218.

Ferin, J. (1977). Effect of particle content of lung on clearance pathways. In: Pulmonary *Macrophage and Epithelial Cells* (Sanders, C.L., Schneider, R.P., Dagle, G.E. and Ragan, H.A., Eds.). Technical Information Center, Energy Research and Development Administration, Springfield, VA, pp. 414–423.

Fieldner, A.C., Kazt, S.H. and Kinney, S.P. (1921). *Gas masks for gases met in fighting fires*. U.S. Bureau of Mines, Technical paper No. 248.

Gad, S. and Chengelis, C.P. (1998). *Acute Toxicology Testing: Perspectives and Horizons*, 2nd ed. Academic Press, San Diego, CA, pp. 404–466.

Gad, S. (1999). *Statistics and Experimental Design for Toxicologists*, 3rd ed. CRC Press, Boca Raton, FL.

Gamsu, G., Singer, M.M., Vincent, H.H., Berry, S. and Nadel, J.A. (1976). Postoperative impairment of mucous transport in the lung. *Am. Rev. Respir. Dis.* 114: 673–679.

Gardner, D.E., Crapo, J.D. and Massaro, E.J. (1988). *Toxicology of the Lung*. Raven Press, New York.

Godfrey, S., Zeidifard, E., Brown, K. and Bell, J.H. (1974). The possible site of action of sodium cromoglycate assessed by exercise challenge. *Clin. Sci. Mol. Med.* 46: 265–272.

Haber, F.R. (1924). Funf Vortage aus den jahren 1920–23, No. 3, *Die Chemie im Kriege*. Julius Springer, Berlin.

Hafner, R.E., Jr., Watanabe, P.G. and Gehring, P.J. (1975). Preliminary studies on the fate of inhaled vinyl chloride monomer in rats. *Am. New York Acad. Sci.* 246: 135–148.

Hatch, T.F. and Gross, P. (1964). *Pulmonary Deposition and Retention of Inhaled Aerosols*. Academic Press, New York, pp. 16–17, 51–52, 147–168.

Henderson, R.F. (1984). Use of bronchoalveolar lavage to detect lung damage. *Environ. Health Persp.* 56: 115–129.

Henderson, R. (1988). Use of bronchoalveolar lavage to detect lung damage. In: *Toxicology of the Lung* (Gardner, D.E., Crapo, J.D. and Massaro, E.J., Eds.). Raven Press, New York, pp. 239–268.

Henderson, R. (1989). Bronchoalveolar lavage: A tool for assessing the health status of the lung. In: *Concepts in Inhalation Toxicology* (McClellan R.O. and Henderson R.F., Eds.). Hemisphere, Washington D.C., pp. 414–442.

Henderson, R.F. and Loery, J.S. (1983). Effect of anesthetic agents on lavage fluid parameters used as indicators of pulmonary injury. *Lab. Anim. Sci.* 33: 60–62.

Henderson, R.F., Benson J.M., Hahn, F.F., Hobbs, C.H., Jones, R.K., Mauderly, J.L., McClellan, R.O. and Pickrell, J.A. (1985). New approaches for the evaluation of pulmonary toxicity: Bronchoalveolar lavage fluid analysis. *Fund. Appl. Toxicol.* 5: 451–458.

Henderson, R.F., Mauderly, J.L., Pickrell, J.A., Hahn, F.F., Muhle, H. and Rebar, A.H. (1987). Comparative study of bronchoalveolar lavage fluid: Effect of species, age, method of lavage. *Exp. Lung Res.* 1: 329–342.

Henderson, R.F., Barr, E.B. and Hotchkiss, J.A. (1991). Effect of exposure rate on response of the lung to inhaled particles. (abstr.) *Toxicologists* 11: 234.

Hensley, M.J., O Cain, C.F., McFadden, E.R., Jr. and Ingram, R.H., Jr. (1978). Distribution of bronchodilatation in normal subjects: Beta agonist versus atropine. *J. Appl. Physicol.* 45: 778–782.

Hext, P.M. (2000). Inhalation Toxicology, in *General and Applied Toxicology*, (Ballantyne, B., Marrs, T. and Syversen, T., Eds.). Macmillan: London, pp. 587–601.

Heyder, J., Gebhart, J. and Stahlhofen, W. (1980). Inhalation of aerosols: Particle deposition and retention. In: *Generation of Aerosols and Facilities for Exposure Experiments* (Willeke, K., Ed.). Ann Arbor Science, Ann Arbor, pp. 80–99.

Hiller, F.C., Mazunder, M.K., Wilson, J.D. and Bone, R.C. (1978). Aerodynamic size distribution of metered dose bronchodilator aerosols. *Am. Rev. Respir. Dis.* 118: 311–317.

Hinds, W.C. (1980). Dry dispersion aerosol generators. In: *Generation of Aerosols and Facilities for Exposure Experiments* (Willeke, K., Ed.). Ann Arbor Science, pp. 171–187.

Hocking, W.G. and Golde, D.W. (1979). The pulmonary alveolar macrophage. *New Eng. J. Med.* 310: 580–587, 639–645.

Hodson, M.E., Penketh, A.R. and Batten, J.C. (1981). Aerosol carbenicillin and gentamicin treatment of *Pseudomonas aeruginosa* infection I patients with cystic fibrosis. *Lancet* 2: 1137–1139.

Hollinger, M.A. (1985). Mucokinetic agents, radionuclides, and anticoagulant-thrombolytic agents. In: Respiratory Pharmacology and Toxicology. W. B. Saunders, Philadelphia, pp. 133–134.

Holma, B. (1967). Lung clearance of mono- and di-disperse aerosols determined by profile scanning and whole body counting: A study on normal and $SO_2$ exposed rabbits. *Acta Med. Scand.* (Suppl.) 473: 1–102.

Horsfield, K. and Cunning, G. (1968). Morphology of the bronchial tree in man. *J. Appl. Physicol.* 24: 373–383.

Ingram, R.H., Wellman, J.J., McFadden, E.R., Jr. and Mead, J. (1977). Relative contributions of large and small airways to flow limitation in normal subjects before and after atropine and isoproterenol. *J. Clin. Invest.* 59: 696–703.

Irish, D.D., Adams, E.M. (1940). Apparatus and methods for testing the toxicity of vapors. *Indust. Med. Surgery* 1: 1–4.

Johnson, H.G., McNee, M.L., Johnson, M.A. and Miller, M.D. (1983). Leukotriene $C_4$ and dimethylphenylpiperazinium-induced responses in canine airway tracheal muscle contraction and fluid secretion. *Int. Arch. Allergy Appl. Immun.* 71: 214–218.

Jonhnson, H.G., McNee, M.L. and Braughler, J.M. (1987). Inhibitors of metal catalyzed lipid peroxidation reactions inhibit mucus secretion and 15 HETE levels in canine trachea. *Prostaglandins Leukotrienes and Med.* 30: 123–132.

Jones, J.G. (1984). Clearance of inhaled particles from alveoli. In: *Aerosols and the Lung: Clinical and Experimental Aspects* (Clarke, S.W. and Pavia, D., Eds.). Butterworth, London, p. 172–196.

Karol, M.H. (1988). Immunologic responses of the lung to inhaled toxicants. In: *Concepts in Inhalation Toxicology* (McClellan, R.O. and Henderson, R., Eds.). Hemisphere Publishing, Washington, D.C., pp. 403–413.

Karol, M.H., Hillebrand, J.A. and Thorne, P.S. (1989). Characteristics of weekly pulmonary hypersensitivity responses elicited in the guinea pig by inhalation of ovalbumin aerosols. *Toxicology of the Lung* (Gardner, D.E., Crapo, J.D. and Massaro, E.J., Eds.). Raven Press, New York, pp. 427–448.

Karol, M.H. and Thorne, P.S. (1988). Hypersensitivity and hyperreactivity. In: *Toxicology of the Lung* (Gardner, D.E., Crapo, J.D. and Massaro, E.J., Eds.). Raven Press, New York, pp. 427–448.

Kavet, R.I., Brain, J.D. and Levens, D.J. (1978). Characteristics of weekly pulmonary macrophages lavaged from hamsters exposed to iron oxide aerosols. *Lab. Invest.* 38: 312–319.

Landy, T.D., Ramsey, J.C. and McKenna, M.J. (1983). Pulmonary physiology and inhalation dosimetry in rats: Development of a method and two examples. *Toxicol. Appl. Pharmacol.* 71: 72–83.

Last, J.A. (1982). Mucus production and ciliary escalator. In: *Mechanisms in Respiratory Toxicology*, Vol. 1. (Witschi, H. and Nettesheim, P., Eds.). CRC Press, Boca Raton, FL, pp. 247–268.

Lauweryns, J.M. and Baert, J.H. (1977). Alveolar clearance and the role of the pulmonary lymphatics. *AM. Rev. Resp. Dis.* 115: 625–683.

Lee, W.-C. and Wang, C.-S. (1977). Particle deposition in systems of repeated bifurcating tubes. In: *Inhaled Particles IV* (Walton, W.H., Ed.). Oxford, Pergamon, pp. 49–60.

Leong, B.K.J. and MacFarland, H.N. (1965). Pulmonary dynamics and retention of toxic gases. *Arch. Environ. Health* 11: 555–563.

Leong, B.K.J. and Rop, D.A. (1989). The combined effects of an inhalation anesthetic and an analgesic on the electrocardiograms of beagle dogs. *Abstract-475. International Congress of Toxicology.* Taylor & Francis, London, p. 159.

Leong, B.K.J., Powell, D.J. and Pochyla, G.L. (1981). A new dust generator for inhalation toxicological studies. In: *Inhalation Toxicology and Technology* (Leong, B.K.J., Ed.). Ann Arbor Science, pp. 157–168.

Leong, B.K.J., Coombs, J.K., Petzold, E.N., Hanchar, A.H. and McNee, M.L. (1985). Endotracheal nebulization of drugs into the lungs of anesthetized animals (abstr.). *Toxicologist* 5: 31.

Leong, B.K.J., Lund, J.E., Groehn, J.A., Coombs, J.K., Sabaitis, C.P., Weaver, R.J. and Griffin, L. (1987). Retinopathy from inhaling 4,4′-methylenedianiline aerosols. *Fund. Appl. Toxicol.* 9: 645–658.

Leong, B.K.J., Coombs, J.K., Petzold, E.N. and Hanchar, A.J. (1988). A dosimetric endotracheal nebulization technique for pulmonary metabolic disposition studies in laboratory animals. *Inhal. Toxicol.* (premier issue): 37–51.

Lichtiger, M., Landa, J.F. and Hirsch, J.A. (1975). Velocity of tracheal mucus in anesthetized women undergoing gynaecologic surgery. *Anesthesiology* 42: 753–756.

Lippmann, M. (1970). "Respirable" dust sampling. *Am. Ind. Hyg. Assoc. J.* 31: 138–159.

Lippmann, M. (1977). Regional deposition of particles in the human respiratory tract. In: *Handbook of Physiology. Section 9: Reactions of Environmental Agents* (Lee, D.H.K., Falk, L.K. and Murphy, S.D., Eds.). American Physiology Society, Bethesda, Maryland, pp. 213–232.

Lippmann, M., Yeates, D.B. and Albert, R.E. (1980). Deposition, retention and clearance of inhaled particles. *Br. J. Ind. Med.* 37: 337–362.

Lourenco, R.V. and Cotromanes, E. (1982). Clinical aerosols. II. Therapeutic aerosols. *Arch. Intern. Med.* 142: 2299–2308.

MacFarland, H.N. (1976). Respiratory toxicology. In: *Essays in Toxicology*, Vol. 7 (Hayes, W.J., Ed.). Academic Press, New York, pp. 121–154.

Marple, V.A. and Rubow, K.L. (1980). Aerosol generation concepts and parameters. In: *Generation of Aerosols and Facilities for Exposure Experiments* (Willeke, K., Ed.). Ann Arbor Science, Ann Arbor, p. 6.

McClellan, R.O. and Henderson, R.F. (1989). *Concepts in Inhalation Toxicology.* Hemisphere, Washington, D.C.

McFadden, E.R., Jr. (1986). *Inhaled Aerosol Bronchodilators.* Williams & Wilkins, Baltimore, pp. 40–41.

Menon, M.P.S. and Das, A.K. (1977). Tetracycline asthma—A case report. *Clin. Allergy* 7: 285–290.

Menzel, D.B. and Amdur, M.O. (1986). Toxic responses of the respiratory system. In: *Casarett and Doull's Toxicology* 3rd ed. (Klaassen, C.D., Amdur, M.O. and Doull, J., Eds.). Macmillan, New York, pp. 330–358.

Mercer, T.T. (1981). Production of therapeutic aerosols; principles and techniques. *Chest* 80 (Suppl. 6): 813–818.

Merin, R.G. (1981). Cardiac toxicity of inhalation anesthetics. In: *Cardiac Toxicology*, Vol. II (Balazs, T., Ed.). CRC Press, Boca Raton, FL, pp. 4–10.

Miller, F.J., Gardner, D.E., Graham, J.A., Lee, R.E., Jr., Wilson, W.E. and Bachmann, J.D. (1979). Size considerations for establishing a standard for inhalable particles. *J. Air Poll. Cont. Assoc.* 29: 610–615.

Miller, J.L., Stuart, B.O., Deford, H.S. and Moss, O.R. (1981). Liquid aerosol generation for inhalation toxicology studies. In: *Inhalation Toxicology and Technology* (Leong, B.K.J., Ed.). Ann Arbor Science, Ann Arbor, pp. 121–207.

Moren, F. (1981). Pressurized aerosols for oral inhalation. *Int. J. Pharm.* 8: 1–10.

Mussatto, D.J., Garrad, C.S. and Lourenco, R.V. (1988). The effect of inhaled histamine on human tracheal mucus velocity and bronchial mucociliary clearance. *Am. Rev. Respir. Dis.* 138: 775–779.

National Academy of Sciences (NAS). (1958). *Handbook of Respiration.* NAS National Research Council. W.B. Saunders, Philadelphia, p. 41.

Nelson, G.O. (1980). *Controlled Test Atmospheres.* Ann Arbor Science, Ann Arbor.

Newhouse, M., Sanchis, J. and Bienenstock, J. (1976). Lung defense mechanisms. *New Eng. J. Med.* 295: 1045–1052.

Newman, S.P. (1984). Therapeutic aerosols. In: *Aerosols and the Lung, Clinical and Experimental Aspects* (Clarke, S.W. and Pavia, D., Eds.). Butterworth, London, pp. 197–224.

Newman, S.P., Pavia, D. and Clarke, S.W. (1981). How should a pressurized beta-adrenergic bronchodilator be inhaled? *Eur. J. Respir. Dis.* 62: 3–21.

Newman, S.P., Moren, F., Pavia, D., Corrado, O. and Clarke, S.W. (1981). The effects of changes in metered volume and propellant vapour pressure on the deposition of pressurized inhalation aerosols. *Int. J. Pharm.* 11: 337–344.

Newton, P.E. (2000). Techniques for Evaluating Hazards of Inhaled Products. In: *Product Safety Evaluation Handbook*, 2nd ed. Marcel Dekker, New York, pp. 243–298.

Oberst, F.W. (1961). Factors affecting inhalation and retention of toxic vapours. In: *Inhaled Particles and Vapours* (Davis, C.N., Ed.). Pergamon Press, New York, pp. 249–266.

Oyarzun, M.J. and Clements, J.A. (1977). Ventilatory and cholinergic control of pulmonary surfactant in rabbit. *J. Appl. Physiol.* 43: 39–45.

Oyarzun, M.J. and Clements, J.A. (1978). Control of lung surfactant by ventilation, adrenergic mediators and prostaglandins in the rabbits. *Am. Rev. Respir. Dis.* 117: 879–891.

Parent, R.A. (1991). *Comparative Biology of the Normal Lung.* CRC Press: Boca Raton, FL.

Paterson, J.W. (1977). Bronchodilators. In: *Asthma* (Clark, T.J.H. and Godfrey, S., Eds.). Chapman and Hall, London, pp. 251–271.

Paterson, J.W., Woocock, A.J. and Shenfield, G.M. (1979). Bronchodilator drugs. *Am. Rev. Respir. Dis.* 120: 1149–1188.

Patterson, R. and Kelly, J.F. (1974). Animal models of the asthmatic state. *Ann. Rev. Med.* 25: 53–68.

Patty, F.A. (1958). *Industrial Hygiene and Toxicology,* 2nd ed. Interscience, New York.

Paustenbach, D.J., Carlson, G.P., Christian, J.E., Born, G.S. and Rausch, J.E. (1983). A dynamic closed-loop recirculating inhalation chamber for conducting pharmacokinetic and short-term toxicity studies. *Fund. Appl. Toxicol.* 3: 528–532.

Pavia, D. (1984). Lung mucociliary clearance. In: *Aerosols and the Lung, Clinical and Experimental Aspects* (Clarke, S.W. and Pavia, D., eds.). Butterworth, London, pp. 127–155.

Pavia, D., Bateman, J.R.M., Sheahan, N.F., Agnew, J.E., Newman, S.P. and Clarke, S.W. (1980). Techniques for measuring lung mucociliary clearance. *Eur. J. Respir. Dis.* 67 (Suppl 110): 157–177.

Pavia, D., Sutton, P.P., Agnew, J.E., Lopez-Vidriero, M.T., Newman,. S.P. and Clarke, S.W. (1983a). Measurement of bronchial mucociliary clearance. *Eur. J. Respir. Dis.* 64 (Suppl 127): 41–56.

Pavia, D., Sutton, P.P., Lopez-Vidriero, M.T., Agnew, J.E. and Clarke, S.W. (1983b). Drug effects on mucociliary function. *Eur. J. Respir. Dis.* 64 (Suppl 128): 304–317.

Phalen, R.F. (1984). *Inhalation Studies: Foundations and Techniques.* CRC Press, Boca Raton, FL, pp. 35–46, 51–57.

Raabe, O.G. (1982a). Deposition and clearance of inhaled aerosols. In: *Mechanisms in Respiratory Toxicology,* Vol. I (Witschi, H. And Nettesheim, P., Eds.). CRC Press, Boca Raton, FL, pp. 35–46, 51–57.

Rinehart, W.E. and Hatch, T. (1964). Concentration–time product ($Ct$) as an expression of dose in sublethal exposures to phosgene. *Am. Ind. Hyg. Assoc. J.* 25: 545–553.

Rylander, R. (1966). Current techniques to measure alterations in the ciliary activity of intact respiratory epithelium. *Am. Rev. Respir. Dis.* 93 (Suppl): 67–85.

Sackner, M.A. (1978). Effect of respiratory drugs on mucociliary clearance. *Chest* 73 (Suppl. 6): 958–966.

Sackner, M.A., Landa, J., Hirsch, J. and Zapata, A. (1975). Pulmonary effects of oxygen breathing. A 6-hour study in normal men. *Ann. Intern. Med.* 82: 40–43.

Sackner, M.A., Brown, L.K. and Kim, C.S. (1981). Basis of an improved metered aerosol delivery system. *Chest* 80 (Suppl. 6): 915–918.

Salem, H. (1986). Principles of inhalation toxicology. In: *Inhalation Toxicology: Research Methods, Applications, and Evaluation.* Marcel Dekker, New York, pp. 1–33.

Schaper, M., Detwiler, K. and Alarie, Y. (1989). Alteration of respiratory cycle timing by propranolol. *Toxicol. Appl. Pharmacol.* 97: 538–547.

Schreck, R.W., Sekuterski, J.J. and Gross, K.B. (1986). Synchronized intratracheal aerosol generation for rodent studies. In: *Aerosols, Formation and Reactivity*, Second International Aerosol Conference, Berlin. Pergamon Press, New York, pp. 37–51.

Schwettmann, R.S. and Casterline, C.L. (1976). Delayed asthmatic response following occupational exposure to enflurane. *Anesthesiology* 44: 166–169.

Sidorenko, G.I. and Pinigin, M.A. (1976). Concentration-time relationship for various regimens of inhalation of organic compounds. *Environ. Health Perspect.* 13: 17–21.

Silver, S.D. (1946). Constant flow gassing chambers: Principles influencing design and operation. *J. Lab. Clin. Med.* 31: 1153–1161.

Smith, D.M., Ortiz, L.W., Archuleta, R.F., Spalding, J.F., Tillery, M.I., Ettinger, H.J. and Thomas, R.G. (1981). A method for chronic nose-only exposure of laboratory animals to inhaled fibrous aerosols. In: *Inhalation Toxicology and Technology* (Leong, B.K.J., Ed.). Ann Arbor Science, Ann Arbor, pp. 89–105.

Stahlhofen, W., Gebhart, J. and Heyder, J. (1980). Experimental determination of the regional deposition of aerosol particles in the human respiratory tract. *Am. Ind. Hyg. Assoc. J.* 41: 385–398.

Stahlhofen, W., Gebhart, J. and Heyder, J. (1981). Biological variability of regional deposition of aerosol particles in the human respiratory tract. *Am. Ind. Hyg. Assoc. J.* 42: 348–352.

Stott, W.T. and McKenna, M.J. (1984). The comparative absorption and excretion of chemical vapors by the upper, lower and intact respiratory tract of rats. *Fund. Appl. Toxicol.* 4: 594–602.

Swift, D.B. and Proctor, D.F. (1982). Human respiratory deposition of particles during oronasal breathing. *Atmos. Environ.* 16: 2279–2282.

Task Group on Lung Dynamics. (1966). Deposition and retention models for internal dosimetry of the human respiratory tract. *Health Phys.* 12: 173–207.

Taulbee, D.B., Yu, C.P. and Heyder, J. (1978). Aerosol transport in the human lung from analysis of single breaths. *J. Appl. Physiol.* 44: 803–812.

Thorne, P.S. and Karol, M.H. (1989). Association of fever with late-onset pulmonary hypersensitivity responses in the guinea pig. *Toxicol. Appl. Pharmacol.* 100: 247–258.

Ts'o, T.O.T., Leong, B.K.J. and Chenoweth, M.B. (1975). Utilities and limitations of behavioral techniques in industrial toxicology. In: *Behavioral Toxicology* (Weiss, B. and Laties, V.G., Eds.). Plenum Press, New York. pp. 265–291.

Uemitsu, N., Minobe, Y. and Nakayoshi, H. (1985). Concentration-time-response relationship under conditions of single inhalation of carbon tetrachloride. *Toxicol. Appl. Pharmacol.* 77: 260–266.

Ulrich, C.E., Klonne, D.R. and Church, S.V. (1984). Automated exposure system for metered-dose aerosol pharmaceuticals. *Toxicologist* 4: 48.

Valentine, R. and Kennedy, G.L., Jr. (2001). Inhalation toxicology. In: *Principles and Methods of Toxicology*, 4th ed. (Hayes, W., Ed.). Raven Press, New York, pp. 1085–1143.

Vidgren, M.T., Karkkainen, A., Paronen, T.P. and Karjalainen, P. (1987). Respiratory tract deposition of $^{99}$Tc-labeled drug particles administered via a dry powder inhaler. *Int J Pharmaceut* 39: 101–105.

Wanner, A. (1979). The role of mucociliary dysfunction in bronchial asthma. *Am. J. Med.* 67: 477–485.

Wanner, A. (1981). Alteration of tracheal mucociliary transport in airway disease. Effect of pharmacologic agents. *Chest* 80 (Suppl. 6): 867–870.

Webber, S.E. and Widdicombe, J.G. (1987). The actions of methacholine, phenylephrine, salbutamol and histamine on mucus secretion from the ferret *in vitro* trachea. *Agents and Actions* 22: 82–85.

Weibel, E.R. (1963). *Morphometry of the Human Lung*. Springer, Heidelberg.

Weibel, E.R. (1983). How does lung structure affect gas exchange? *Chest* 83: 657–665.

Weiner, N. (1984). Norepinephrine, epinephrine, and the sympathomimetic amines. In: *Goodman and Gilman's, The Pharmacological Basis of Therapeutics*, 7th ed. (Gilman, A.G., Goodman, L.S., Rall, T.W. and Murad, F., Eds.). Macmillan, New York, pp. 145–180.

Weston, R. and Karel, L. (1946). An application of the dosimetric method for biologically assaying inhaled substances. *J. Pharmacol. Expt. Ther.* 88: 195–207.

Widdicombe, J.G. (1974). Reflex control of breathing. In: *Respiratory Physiology*, Vol. 2 (Widdicombe, J.G., Ed.). University Park Press, Baltimore, MD.

Willeke, K. (1980). *Generation of Aerosols and Facilities for Exposure Experiments*. Ann Arbor Science, Ann Arbor.

Williams, M.H. (1974). Steroids and antibiotic aerosols. *Am Rev. Respir. Dis.* 110: 122–127.

Wilson, A.G.E. (1982). Toxicokinetics of uptake, accumulation, and metabolism of chemicals by the lung. In: *Mechanisms in Respiratory Toxicology*, Vol. 1. (Witschi, H. and Nettesheim, P., Eds.). CRC Press, Boca Raton, FL, pp. 162–178.

Witschi, H.P. and Nettesheim, P. (1982). *Mechanisms in Respiratory Toxicology*, Vol. 1. CRC Press, Boca Raton, FL.

Witschi, H.P. and Brain, J.D. (1985). *Toxicology of Inhaled Materials*. Springer, New York.

# 11

# IRRITATION AND LOCAL TISSUE TOLERANCE IN PHARMACEUTICAL SAFETY ASSESSMENT

## 11.1. INTRODUCTION

Both irritation and local tolerance studies assess the short-term hazard of pharmaceutical agents in the immediate region of their application or installation. In particular, these studies are done (expected) to assess topically or parenterally administered drugs.

Topical local tolerance effects are almost entirely limited to irritation. Though this usually means dermal irritation, it can also be intracutaneous, mucosal, penile, perivascular, vaginal, rectal, nasal, ocular or to the bladder, depending on the route of drug administration. All but ocular irritation use some version of a common subjective rating scale (see Table 11.1) to evaluate responses. The outcome of all of these tests primarily serves to evaluate the response of the first region of tissue (which is exposed to the highest concentration) to an administered drug substance. In general, any factor which enhances absorption through this tissue is likely to decrease tissue tolerance.

For the skin, this scale is used in the primary dermal irritation test, which is performed for those agents that are to be administered to patients by application to the skin. As with all local tolerance tests, it is essential that the material be evaluated in "condition of use," that is, in the final formulated form, applied to test animals in the same manner that the agent is to be used clinically.

**TABLE 11.1. Evaluation of Local Tissue Reactions in Tissue Irritation Studies**

| Skin Reaction | Value |
| --- | --- |
| Erythema and eschar formation | |
| No erythema | 0 |
| Very slight erythema (barely perceptible) | 1 |
| Well-defined erythema | 2 |
| Moderate to severe erythema | 3 |
| Severe erythema (beet redness) to slight eschar formation (injuries in depth) | 4 |
| Necrosis (death of tissue) | +N |
| Eschar (sloughing or scab formation) | +E |
| Edema formation | |
| No edema | 0 |
| Very slight edema (barely perceptible) | 1 |
| Slight edema (edges of area well-defined by definite raising) | 2 |
| Moderate edema (raised approximately 1 mm) | 3 |
| Severe edema (raised more than 1 mm and extending beyond the area of exposure) | 4 |
| Total possible score for primary irritation | 8 |

## 11.2. PRIMARY DERMAL IRRITATION TEST

### 11.2.1. Rabbit Screening Procedure

1. A group of at least 8–12 New Zealand white rabbits are screened for the study.

2. All rabbits selected for the study must be in good health; any rabbit exhibiting sniffles, hair loss, loose stools, or apparent weight loss is rejected and replaced.

3. One day (at least 18 h) prior to application of the test substance, each rabbit is prepared by clipping the hair from the back and sides using a small animal clipper. A size No. 10 blade is used to remove long hair and then a size No. 40 blade is used to remove the remaining hair.

4. Six animals with skin sites that are free from hyperemia or abrasion (due to shaving) are selected. Skin sites that are in the telogen phase (resting stage of hair growth) are used; those skin sites that are in the anagen phase (stage of active growth, indicated by the presence of a thick undercoat of hair) are not used.

### 11.2.2. Study Procedure

1. As many as four areas of skin, two on each side of the rabbit's back, can be utilized for sites for administration.

2. Separate animals are not required for an untreated control group. Each animal serves as its own control.

3. Besides the test substance, a positive control substance (a known skin irritant, 1% sodium lauryl sulfate in distilled water) and a negative control (untreated patch) are applied to the skin. When a vehicle is used for diluting, suspending, or moistening the test substance, a vehicle control patch is required, especially if the vehicle is known to cause any toxic dermal reactions or if there is insufficient information about the dermal effects of the vehicle.

4. The intact (free of abrasion) sites of administration are assigned a code number. Up to four sites can be used, as follows

   #1. Test substance;

   #2. Negative control;

   #3. Positive control;

   #4. Vehicle control (if required).

5. Application sites should be rotated from one animal to the next to ensure that the test substance and controls are applied to each position at least once.

6. Each test or control substance is held in place with a 1 in. × 1 in. 12-ply surgical gauze patch. The gauze patch is applied to the appropriate skin site and secured with 1 in.-wide strips of surgical tape at the four edges, leaving the center of the gauze patch nonoccluded.

7. If the test substance is a solid or a semisolid, a 0.5-g portion is weighed and placed on the gauze patch. The test substance patch is placed on the appropriate skin site and secured. The patch is subsequently moistened with 0.5 ml of physiological saline.

8. When the test substance is in flake, granule, powder, or other particulate form, the weight of the test substance that has a volume of 0.5 ml (after compacting as much as possible without crushing or altering the individual particles, such as by tapping the measuring container) is used whenever this volume is less than 0.5 g. When applying powders, granules, and the like, the gauze patch designated for the test sample is secured to the appropriate skin site with one of the four strips of the tape at the most ventral position of the animal. With one hand, the appropriate amount of sample measuring 0.5 ml is carefully poured from a glycine weighing paper onto the gauze patch that is held in a horizontal (level) position with the other hand. The patch containing the test sample is then carefully placed into position on the skin and the remaining three edges secured with tape. The patch is subsequently moistened with 0.5 ml of physiological saline.

9. If the test substance is a liquid, a patch is applied and secured to the appropriate skin site. A 1-ml tuberculin syringe is used to measure and apply 0.5 ml of test substance to the patch.

10. The negative control site is covered with an untreated 12-ply surgical gauze patch (1 in. × 1 in.).

11. The positive control substance and vehicle control substance are applied to a gauze patch in the same manner as a liquid test substance.

12. The entire trunk of the animal is covered with an impervious material (such as Saran Wrap) for a 24-h period of exposure. The Saran Wrap is secured by wrapping several long strips of athletic adhesive tape around the trunk of the animal. The impervious material aids in maintaining the position of the patches and retards evaporation of volatile test substances.

13. An Elizabethan collar is fitted and fastened around the neck of each test animal. The collar remains in place for the 24-h exposure period. The collars are utilized to prevent removal of wrappings and patches by the animals, while allowing the animals food and water *ad libitum*.

14. The wrapping is removed at the end of the 24-h exposure period. The test substance skin site is wiped to remove any test substance still remaining. When colored test substances (such as dyes) are used, it may be necessary to wash the test substance from the test site with an appropriate solvent or vehicle (one that is suitable for the substance being tested). This is done to facilitate accurate evaluation for skin irritation.

15. Immediately after removal of the patches, each 1 in. × 1 in. test or control site is outlined with indelible marker by dotting each of the four corners. This procedure delineates the site for identification.

### 11.2.3. Observations

1. Observations are made of the test and control skin sites 1 h after removal of the patches (25 h post-initiation of application). Erythema and edema are evaluated and scored on the basis of designated values presented earlier in Table 11.1.

2. Observations are again performed 48 and 72 h after application and scores are recorded.

3. If necrosis is present or the dermal reaction is unusual, the reaction should be described. Severe erythema should receive the maximum score (4), and +N should be used to designate the presence of necrosis and +E the presence of eschar.

4. When a test substance produces dermal irritation that persists 72 h postapplication, daily observations of test and control sites are continued on all animals until all irritation caused by the test substance resolves or until Day 14 postapplication.

### 11.2.4. Evaluation of Results

1. A Subtotal Irritation Value for erythema or eschar formation is determined for each rabbit by adding the values observed at 25, 48, and 72 h postapplication.

2. A Subtotal Irritation Value for edema formation is determined for each rabbit by adding the values observed at 25, 48, and 72 h postapplication.

3. A Total Irritation Value is calculated for each rabbit by adding the subtotal irritation value for erythema or eschar formation to the subtotal irritation value for edema formation.

4. The Primary Dermal Irritation Index is calculated for the test substance or control substance by dividing the sum of the Total Irritation Scores by the number of observations (three days × six animals = 18 observations).

5. The categories of the Primary Dermal Irritation Index (PDII) are as follows [this categorization of dermal irritation is a modification of the original classification described by Draize et al. (1944)]:

| | |
|---|---|
| PDII = 0.0 | nonirritant |
| > 0.0–0.5 | negligible irritant |
| > 0.5–2.0 | mild irritant |
| > 2.0–5.0 | moderate irritant |
| > 5.0–8.0 | severe irritant |

Other abnormalities, such as atonia or desquamation, should be noted and recorded.

## 11.3. OTHER NONPARENTERAL ROUTE IRRITATION TESTS

The design of vaginal, rectal, and nasal irritation studies is less formalized, but follows the same basic pattern as the primary dermal irritation test. The rabbit is the preferred species for vaginal and rectal irritation studies, but the monkey and dog have also been used for these (Eckstein et al., 1969). Both the rabbit and rat have commonly seen use for nasal irritation evaluations. Defined quantities (typically 1.0 ml) of test solutions or suspensions are instilled into the orifice in question. For the vagina or rectum inert bungs are usually installed immediately thereafter to continue exposure for a defined period of time (usually the same period of hours as future human exposure). The orifice is then flushed clean, and 24 h after exposure it is examined and evaluated (graded) for irritation using the scale in Table 11.1.

## 11.4. FACTORS AFFECTING IRRITATION RESPONSES AND TEST OUTCOME

The results of local tissue irritation tests are subject to considerable variability due to relatively small differences in test design or technique. Weil and Scala (1971) arranged and reported on the best known of several intralaboratory studies to establish this fact clearly. Though the methods presented above have proven to give reproducible results in the hands of the same technicians over a period of years (Gad et al., 1986) and contain some internal controls (the positive and vehicle controls in the PDI) against large variabilities in results or the occurrence of either false positives or negatives, it is still essential to be aware of those factors that may systematically alter test results. These factors are summarized in the following (Gad and Chengdis, 1998).

A.  In general, any factor that increases absorption through the stratum corneum or mucous membrane will also increase the severity of an intrinsic response. Unless this factor mirrors potential exposure conditions, it may, in turn, adversely affect the relevance of test results.

B.  The physical nature of solids must be carefully considered both before testing and in interpreting results. Shape (sharp edges), size (small particles may abrade the skin by being rubbed back and forth under the occlusive wrap), and rigidity (stiff fibers or very hard particles will be physically irritating) of solids may all enhance an irritation response.

C.  Solids frequently give different results when they are tested dry than if wetted for the test. As a general rule, solids are more irritating if moistened (going back to item A, wetting is a factor that tends to enhance absorption). Care should also be taken as to moistening agent; some (few) batches of U.S. Pharmacopeia physiological saline (used to simulate sweat) have proven to be mildly irritating to the skin and mucous membrane on their own. Liquids other than water or saline should not be used.

D.  If the treated region on potential human patients will be a compromised skin surface barrier (e.g., if it is cut or burned) some test animals should likewise have their application sites compromised. This procedure is based on the assumption that abraded skin is uniformly more sensitive to irritation. Experiments, however, have shown that this is not necessarily true; some materials produce more irritation on abraded skin, while others produce less (Guillot et al., 1982; Gad et al., 1986).

E.  The degree of occlusion (in fact, the tightness of the wrap over the test site) also alters percutaneous absorption and therefore irritation. One important quality control issue in the laboratory is achieving a reproducible degree of occlusion in dermal wrappings.

F.  Both the age of the test animal and the application site (saddle of the back versus flank) can markedly alter test outcome. Both of these factors are also operative in humans, of course (Mathias, 1983), but in dermal irritation tests, the objective is to remove all such sources of variability. In general, as an animal ages, sensitivity to irritation decreases. For the dermal test, the skin middle of the back (other than directly over the spine) tends to be thicker (and therefore less sensitive to irritations) than that on the flanks.

G.  The sex of the test animals can also alter study results, because both regional skin thickness and surface blood flow vary between males and females.

H. Finally, the single most important (yet also most frequently overlooked) factor that influences the results and outcome of these (and, in fact most) acute studies is the training of the staff. In determining how test materials are prepared and applied and in how results are "read" against a subjective scale, both accuracy and precision are extremely dependent on the technicians involved. To achieve the desired results, initial training must be careful and all-inclusive. Equally important, some form of regular refresher training must be exercised, particularly in the area of scoring results. Use of a set of color photographic standards as a training and reference tool is strongly recommended; such standards should clearly demonstrate each of the grades in the Draize dermal scale.

I. It should be recognized that the dermal irritancy test is designed with a bias to preclude false negatives and, therefore, tends to exaggerate results in relation to what would happen in humans. Findings of negligible irritancy (or even in the very low mild irritant range) should therefore be of no concern unless the product under test is to have large-scale and prolonged dermal contact.

## 11.5. PROBLEMS IN TESTING (AND THEIR RESOLUTIONS)

Some materials, by either their physicochemical or toxicological natures, generate difficulties in the performance and evaluation of dermal irritation tests. The most commonly encountered of these problems are presented below.

A. *Compound Volatility.* One is sometimes required or requested to evaluate the potential irritancy of a liquid that has a boiling point between room temperature and the body temperature of the test animal. As a result, the liquid portion of the material will evaporate off before the end of the testing period. There is no real way around the problem; one can only make clear in the report on the test that the traditional test requirements were not met, though an evaluation of potential irritant hazard was probably achieved (for the liquid phase would also have evaporated from a human that it was spilled on).

B. *Pigmented Material.* Some materials are strongly colored or discolor the skin at the application site. This makes the traditional scoring process difficult or impossible. One can try to remove the pigmentation with a solvent; if successful, the erythema can then be evaluated. If use of a solvent fails or is unacceptable, one can (wearing thin latex gloves) feel the skin to determine if there is warmth, swelling, and/or rigidity, all secondary indicators of the irritation response.

C. *Systemic Toxicity.* On rare occasions, the dermal irritation study is begun only to have the animals die very rapidly after test material is applied.

## 11.6. OCULAR IRRITATION TESTING

Ocular irritation is significantly different from the other local tissue irritation tests on a number of grounds. For the pharmaceutical industry, eye irritation testing is performed when the material is intended to be put into the eye as a means or route of application for ocular therapy. There are a number of special tests applicable to pharmaceuticals or medical devices that are beyond the scope of this volume, since they are not intended to assess potential acute effects or irritation. In general, however, it is desired that an eye irritation test that is utilized by this group be both sensitive and accurate in predicting the potential to cause irritation in humans. Failing to identify human ocular irritants (lack of sensitivity) is to be avoided, but of equal concern is the occurrence of false positives.

The primary eye irritation test was originally intended to predict the potential for a single splash of chemical into the eye of a human being to cause reversible and/or permanent damage. Since the introduction of the original Draize test 50 years ago (Draize et al., 1944), ocular irritation testing in rabbits has both developed and diverged. Indeed, clearly there is no longer a single test design that is used and different objectives are pursued by different groups using the same test. This lack of standardization has been recognized for some time and attempts have been made to address standardization of at least the methodological aspects of the test, if not the design aspects.

One widely used study design, which begins with a screening procedure as an attempt to avoid testing severe irritants or corrosives in animals, goes as follows.

### 11.6.1. Test Article Screening Procedure

1. Each test substance will be screened in order to eliminate potentially corrosive or severely irritating materials from being studied for eye irritation in the rabbit.

2. If possible, the pH of the test substance will be measured.

3. A primary dermal irritation test will be performed prior to the study.

4. The test substance will not be studied for eye irritation if it is a strong acid (pH of 2.0 or less) or strong alkali (pH of 11.0 or greater), and/or if the test substance is a severe dermal irritant (with a PDII of 5 to 8) or causes corrosion of the skin.

5. If it is predicted that the test substance does not have the potential to be severely irritating or corrosive to the eye, continue to Section 11.4.2, Rabbit Screening Procedure.

### 11.6.2. Rabbit Screening Procedure

1. A group of at least 12 New Zealand white rabbits of either sex are screened for the study. The animals are removed from their cages and placed in rabbit restraints. Care should be taken to prevent mechanical damage to the eye during this procedure.

2. All rabbits selected for the study must be in good health; any rabbit exhibiting sniffles, hair loss, loose stools, or apparent weight loss is rejected and replaced.

3. One hour prior to installation of the test substance, both eyes of each rabbit are examined for signs of irritation and corneal defects with a hand-held slit lamp. All eyes are stained with 2.0% sodium fluorescein and examined to confirm the absence of corneal lesions.

   *Fluorescein Staining.* Cup the lower lid of the eye to be tested and instill one drop of a 2% (in water) sodium fluorescein solution onto the surface of the cornea. After 15 s, thoroughly rinse the eye with physiological saline. Examine the eye, employing a hand-held long-wave ultraviolet illuminator in a darkened room. Corneal lesions, if present, appear as bright yellowish-green fluorescent areas.

4. Only 9 of the 12 animals are selected for the study. The 9 rabbits must not show any signs of eye irritation and must show either a negative or minimum fluorescein reaction (due to normal epithelial desquamation).

### 11.6.3.  Study Procedure

1. At least 1 h after fluorescein staining, the test substance is placed in one eye of each animal by gently pulling the lower lid away from the eyeball to form a cup (conjunctival cul-de-sac) into which the test material is dropped. The upper and lower lids are then gently held together for 1 s to prevent immediate loss of material.

2. The other eye remains untreated and serves as a control.

3. For testing liquids, 0.01 ml of the test substance is used.

4. For solids or pastes, 100 mg of the test substance is used.

5. When the test substance is in flake, granular, powder, or other particulate form, the amount that has a volume of 0.01 ml (after gently compacting the particles by tapping the measuring container in a way that will not alter their individual form) is used whenever this volume weighs less than 10 mg.

6. For aerosol products, the eye should be held open and the substance administered in a single, 1-s burst at a distance of about 4 inches directly in front of the eye. The velocity of the ejected material should not traumatize the eye. The dose should be approximated by weighing the aerosol can before and after each treatment. For other liquids propelled under pressure, such as substances delivered by pump sprays, an aliquot of 0.01 ml should be collected and instilled in the eye as for liquids.

7. The treated eyes of six of the rabbits are not washed following the instillation of the test substance.

8. The treated eyes of the remaining three rabbits are irrigated for 1 min with room temperature tap water, starting 20 s after instillation.

9. To prevent self-inflicted trauma by the animals immediately after instillation of the test substance, the animals are not immediately returned to their cages. After the test and control eyes are examined and graded at 1-h postexposure, the animals are returned carefully to their respective cages.

### 11.6.4. Observations

1. The eyes are observed for any immediate signs of discomfort after instilling the test substance. Blepharospasm and/or excessive tearing are indicative of irritating sensations caused by the test substance, and their duration should be noted. Blepharospasm does not necessarily indicate that the eye will show signs of ocular irritation.

2. Grading and scoring on ocular irritation are performed in accordance with Table 11.2. The eyes are examined and grades of ocular reactions are recorded.

3. If signs or irritation persist at Day 7, readings are continued on Days 10 and 14 after exposure or until all signs of reversible toxicity are resolved.

4. In addition to the required observation of the cornea, iris, and conjunctiva, serious effects (such as pannus, rupture of the globe, or blistering of the conjunctivae) indicative of a corrosive action are reported.

5. Whether or not toxic effects are reversible depends on the nature, extent, and intensity of damage. Most lesions, if reversible, will heal or clear within 21 days. Therefore, if ocular irritation is present at the 14-day reading, a 21-day reading is required to determine whether the ocular damage is reversible or nonreversible.


## 11.7. VAGINAL IRRITATION

Few, if any, products are administered via the vagina that are intended for systemic absorption. Thus, this route has not been as widely studied and characterized as others. On the other hand, large numbers of different products (douches, spermicides, antiyeast agents, etc.) have been developed that require introduction into the vagina in order to assert their localized effects. Increased research into different birth control and antiviral prophylaxis will result in more vaginal products in the future. All these must be assessed for vaginal irritation potential, and this serves as an example of the other tissue tolerance issues.

Considerable research (Eckstein et al., 1969; Auletta, 1994) has indicated that the rabbit is the best species for assessing vaginal irritation. There are those investigators, however, who consider the rabbit too sensitive and recommend the use of ovariectomized rats. Ovariectomy results in a uniformly thin, uncornified epithelium which is more responsive to localized effects. This model is used when the results from a study with rabbits are questionable (Auletta, 1994). The routine progression of studies consists of first doing an acute primary vaginal irritation study, then a 10-day repeated dose study in rats. These protocols are summarized below. Longer-term vaginal studies have been conducted in order to assess systemic toxicity of the active agents, when administered by these routes (while the intended effects may be local, one cannot assume that there will be no systemic exposure).

**TABLE 11.2. Scale of Weighted Scores for Grading the Severity of Ocular Lesions**[a]

| Reaction Criteria | Score |
|---|---|
| I. Cornea | |
| A. Opacity degree of density (area that is most dense is taken for reading) | |
|    1. Scattered or diffuse area, details of iris clearly visible | 1 |
|    2. Easily discernible translucent area, details of iris slightly obscured | 2 |
|    3. Opalescent areas, no details of iris visible, size of pupil barely discernible | 3 |
| B. Area of cornea involved | |
|    1. One-quarter (or less) but not zero | 1 |
|    2. Greater than one-quarter, less than one-half | 2 |
|    3. Greater than one-half, less that whole area | 3 |
|    4. Greater than three-quarters up to whole area | 4 |
| Scoring equals A $\times$ B $\times$ 5; total maximum $= 80$[b] | |
| II. Iris | |
| A. Values | |
|    1. Folds above normal, congestion, swelling, circumcorneal ingestion (any one or all of these or combination of any thereof), iris still reacting to light (sluggish reaction is possible) | 1 |
|    2. No reaction to light, hemorrhage, gross destruction (any one or all of these) | 2 |
| Scoring equals A $\times$ B (where B is the area of the iris involved, graded as "under cornea"); total maximum $= 10$ | |
| III. Conjunctivae | |
| A. Redness (refers to palpebral conjunctivae only) | |
|    1. Vessels definitely injected above normal | 1 |
|    2. More diffuse, deeper crimson red, individual vessels not easily discernible | 2 |
|    3. Diffuse beefy red | 3 |
| B. Chemosis | |
|    1. Any swelling above normal (includes nictitating membrane) | 1 |
|    2. Obvious swelling with partial eversion of the lids | 2 |
|    3. Swelling with lids about half closed | 3 |
|    4. Swelling with lids about half closed to completely closed | 4 |
| C. Discharge | |
|    1. Any amount different from normal (does not include small amount observed in inner canthus of normal animals) | 1 |
|    2. Discharge with moistening of the lids and hair just adjacent to the lids | 2 |
|    3. Discharge with moistening of the lids and considerable area around the eye | 3 |
| Scoring (A + B + C) $\times$ 2; total maximum $= 20$ | |

[a]The maximum total score is the sum of all scores obtained for the cornea, iris and conjunctivae.
[b]All A $\times$ B $= \Sigma$ (1–3) $\times$ $\Sigma$S (1–4) for six animals.

## 11.7.1. Acute Primary Vaginal Irritation Study in the Female Rabbit

1. *Overview of Study Design.* One group of six adult rabbits received a single vaginal exposure and was observed for three days with periodic examination (1, 24, 48, and 72 h postdosing) of the genitalia. Animals are then euthanized and the vagina is examined macroscopically.

2. *Administration*

   Route: The material is generally introduced directly into the vagina using a lubricated 18 French rubber catheter attached to a syringe for quantification and delivery of the test material. Gentle placement of the catheter is important because one needs to ensure complete delivery of the dose without mechanical trauma. For rabbits, the depth of insertion is about 7.5 cm, and the catheter should be marked to about that depth. After delivery is completed, the tube is slowly withdrawn. No attempt is made to close or seal the vaginal orifice. Alternative methods may be used to administer more viscous materials. The most common is to backload a lubricated 1-ml tuberculine syringe, then warm the material to close to body temperature. The syringe is then inserted into the vagina and the dose administered by depressing the syringe plunger.

   Dosage: The test material should be one (concentration, vehicle, etc.) that is intended for human application.

   Frequency: once.

   Duration: 1 day.

   Volume: 1 ml per rabbit.

3. *Test System*

   Species, age, and weight range: Sexually mature New Zealand white rabbits are generally used, weighing between 2 and 5 kg. The weight is not as important as the fact that the animals need to be sexually mature.

   Selection: Animals should be multiparous and nonpregnant. Animals should be healthy and free of external genital lesions.

   Randomization: Because there is only one group of animals, randomization is not a critical issue.

4. *In-Life Observations*

   Daily observations: At least once daily for clinical signs.

   Detailed physical examination: Once during the week prior to dosing.

   Body weight: Day of dosing.

   Vaginal irritation: Scored at 1, 24, 48, and 72 h postdosing. Scoring criteria are shown in Table 11.3.

5. *Postmortem Procedures.* Rabbits are euthanized by lethal dose of a barbiturate soon after the last vaginal irritation scores are collected. The vagina is opened by longitudinal section and examined for evidence of mucosal damage such as erosion, localized hemorrhage, and so on. No other tissues are examined. No tissues are collected. After the macroscopic description of the vagina is recorded, the animal is discarded.


## 11.7.2. Repeated Dose Vaginal Irritation in the Female Rabbit

1. *Overview of Study Design.* Four groups of five adult rabbits each receive a single vaginal exposure daily for 10 days. The genitalia are examined daily. Animals are then euthanized and the vagina is examined macroscopically and microscopically.

**TABLE 11.3. Scoring Criteria for Vaginal Irritation**

Value

*Erythema*

| | |
|---|---|
| 0 | No erythema |
| 1 | Very slight erythema (barely perceptible) |
| 2 | Slight erythema (pale red in color) |
| 3 | Moderate to severe erythema (definite red in color) |
| 4 | Severe erythema (beet or crimson red) |

*Edema*

| | |
|---|---|
| 0 | No edema |
| 1 | Very slight edema (barely perceptible) |
| 2 | Slight edema (edges of area well defined by definite raising |
| 3 | Moderate edema (raised approximately 1 mm) |
| 4 | Severe edema (raised more than 1 mm and extending beyond area of exposure) |

*Discharge*

| | |
|---|---|
| 0 | No discharge |
| 1 | Very slight discharge |
| 2 | Slight discharge |
| 3 | Moderate discharge |
| 4 | Severe discharge (moistening of considerable area around vagina) |

2. *Administration*

   Route: The test materials are introduced directly into the vagina using a lubricated 18 French rubber catheter, using the techniques described previously for acute studies.

   Dosage: The test material should be one (concentration, vehicle, etc.) that is intended for human application. There will also be a sham-negative control (catheter in place but nothing administered), a vehicle control, and a positive control (generally 2% nonoxynol-9).

   Frequency: once daily.

   Duration: 10 days.

   Volume: 1 ml per rabbit for each material.

3. *Test System*

   Species, age and weight range: Sexually mature New Zealand white rabbits are generally used, weighing between 2 and 5 kg. The weight is not as important as the fact that the animals need to be sexually mature.

   Selection: Animals should be nuliparous and nonpregnant. Animals should be healthy and free of external genital lesions.

   Randomization: At least 24 animals should be on pretest. Randomization to treatment groups is best done using a computerized blocking by body weight method or a random number generation method.

4. *In-Life Observations*

   Daily observations: At least once daily for clinical signs.

**TABLE 11.4. Microscopic Scoring Procedure for Vaginal Sections**

|  | Value |
| --- | --- |
| Epithelium | |
|   Intact—normal | 0 |
|   Cell degeneration or flattening of the epithelium | 1 |
|   Metaplasia | 2 |
|   Focal erosion | 3 |
|   Erosion or ulceration, generalized | 4 |
| Leukocytes | |
|   Minimal— < 25 per high-power field | 1 |
|   Mild—25–50 per high-power field | 2 |
|   Moderate—50–100 per high-power field | 3 |
|   Marked— > 100 per high-power field | 4 |
| Injection | |
|   Absent | 0 |
|   Minimal | 1 |
|   Mild | 2 |
|   Moderate | 3 |
|   Marked with disruption of vessels | 4 |
| Edema | |
|   Absent | 0 |
|   Minimal | 1 |
|   Mild | 2 |
|   Moderate | 3 |
|   Marked | 4 |

*Source*: Eckstein et al. (1969).

Detailed physical examination: Once during the week prior to dosing and immediately prior to necropsy.

Body weight: First, fifth, and last day of dosing.

Vaginal irritation: Scored once daily. Scoring criteria shown in Table 11.3.

5. *Postmortem Procedures.* Rabbits are euthanized by lethal dose of a barbiturate soon after the last vaginal irritation scores are collected. The vagina is isolated using standard prosection techniques and then opened by longitudinal section and examined for evidence of mucosal damage such as erosion, localized hemorrhage, and so on. No other tissues are examined. The vagina and cervix are collected and fixed in 10% neutral buffered formalin. Standard hematoxylin/eosin stained, paraffin-embedded histologic glass slides are prepared by routing methods. Three levels of the vagina (low, mid, and upper) are examined and graded using the scoring system shown in Table 11.4. Each level is scored separately and an average is calculated. Irritation is rated as follows:

| Score | Rating |
|---|---|
| 0 | Nonirritating |
| 1–4 | Minimal irritation |
| 5–8 | Mild irritation |
| 9–11 | Moderate irritation |
| 12–16 | Marked irritation |

The score for each rabbit is then averaged and acceptability ratings are given as follows:

| Average Score | Acceptability Ratings |
|---|---|
| 0–8 | Acceptable |
| 9–10 | Marginal |
| 11 or greater | Unacceptable |

### 11.7.3. Repeated Dose Vaginal Irritation in the Ovariectomized Rats

This study is very similar in design to that described previously for rabbits, with the following (sometimes obvious) exceptions. Mature ovariectomized female rats can be obtained from a commercial breeder. A 15% surplus should be obtained. Ten animals per group should be used (40 total for the study). The vaginal catheter is placed to a depth of approximately 2.5 cm and the treatment volume should be 0.2 ml.

### 11.8. PARENTERAL IRRITATION/TOLERANCE

There are a number of special concerns about the safety of materials that are routinely injected (parenterally administered) into the body. By definition, these concerns are all associated with materials that are the products of the pharmaceutical and (in some minor cases) medical device industries. Such parenteral routes include three major ones; IV (intravenous), IM (intramuscular), and SC (subcutaneous); and a number of minor routes (such as intra-arterial) that are not considered here.

These unusual concerns include irritation (vascular, muscular, or subcutaneous), pyrogenicity, blood compatibility, and sterility (Avis, 1985). The background of each of these, along with the underlying mechanisms and factors that influence the level of occurrence of such an effect, are briefly discussed below.

*Irritation.* Tissue irritation upon injection, and the accompanying damage and pain, is a concern that must be addressed for the final formulation, which is to be either tested in humans or marketed, rather than for the active ingredient. This is because most irritation factors are either due to or influenced by aspects of formulation design (see Avis, 1985, for more information or parenteral preparations). These factors are not independent of the route (IV, IM, or SC) that will be used and, in fact (as discussed later), are part of the basis for selecting between the various routes.

Lack of irritation and tissue damage at the injection site is sometimes called *tolerance*. Some of the factors that affect tolerance are not fully under the control of an investigation and are also unrelated to the material being injected. These include body movement, temperature, and animal age. Factors that can be controlled, but that are not inherent to the active ingredient, include solubility, tonicity, and pH. And, finally, the active ingredient and vehicle can have inherent irritative effects and factors such as solubility (in the physiological milieu into which they are being injected), concentration, volume molecular size, and particle size. Gray (1978) and Ballard (1968) discuss these factors and the morphological consequences that may occur if they are not addressed.

*Pyrogenicity.* Pyrogenicity is the induction of a febrile (fever) response induced by the parenteral (usually IV or IM) administration of exogenous material. Pyrogenicity is usually associated with microbiological contamination of a final formulation, but it is now of increasing concern because of the growing interest in biosynthetically produced materials. Generally, ensuring sterility of product and process will guard against pyrogenicity for traditional pharmaceuticals. For biologically produced products, the FDA has promulgated the general guideline that no more than 5.0 units of endotoxin may be present per milligram of drug substance.

*Blood compatibility.* It is important that cellular components of the blood are not disrupted and that serum- or plasma-based responses are not triggered by parenteral administration. Therefore, two mechanisms must be assessed regarding the blood compatibility of component materials. These include the material's effect on cellular components that cause membrane destruction and hemolysis and the activation of the clotting mechanism resulting in the formation of the thromboeboli.

Many of the nonactive, ingredient-related physicochemical factors that influence irritation (tonicity, pH, and particle size, for example) also act to determine blood compatibility. But the chemical features of a drug entity itself, its molecular size and reactivity, can also be of primary importance.

*Sterility.* Sterility is largely a concern to be answered in the process of preparing a final clinical formulation, and it is not addressed in detail in this chapter. However, it should be clear that it is essential that no viable microorganisms are present in any material to be parenterally administered (except for vaccines).

### 11.8.2. Parenteral Routes

There are at least 13 different routes by which to inject material into the body, including the following:

| | |
|---|---|
| 1. Intravenous | 8. Intrathecal |
| 2. Subcutaneous | 9. Intracisternal |
| 3. Intramuscular | 10. Intracardiac |
| 4. Intraarterial | 11. Intraventricular |
| 5. Intradermal | 12. Intraocular |
| 6. Intralesional | 13. Intraperitoneal |
| 7. Epidural | |

Only the first three are discussed in any detail here. Most of these routes of administration place a drug directly or indirectly into systemic circulation. There are a number of these routes, however, by which the drug exerts a local effect, in which case most of the drug does not enter systemic circulation (e.g., intrathecal, intraventricular, intraocular, intraracisternal). Certain routes of administration may exert both local and systemic effects depending on the characteristics of the drug and excipients (e.g., subcutaneous).

The choice of a particular parenteral route will depend on the required time of onset of action, the required site of action, and the characteristics of the fluid to be injected, among other factors.

***Bolus versus Infusion.*** Technically, for all the parenteral routes (but in practice only for the IV route), there are two options for injecting a material into the body. The bolus and infusion methods are differentiated on the single basis of rate of injection, but they actually differ on a wide range of characteristics.

The most commonly exercised option is the bolus, or "push," injection, in which the injection device (syringe or catheter) is appropriately entered into the vein and a defined volume of material is introduced through the device. The device is then removed. In this operation, it is relatively easy to restrain an experimental animal and the stress on the animal is limited. Though the person doing the injection must be skilled, it takes only a short amount of time to become so. The one variable to be controlled in determining dosage is the total volume of material injected (assuming dosing solutions have been properly prepared).

There are limitations and disadvantages to the bolus approach, however. Only a limited volume may be injected, which may prohibit the use of bolus when volumes to be introduced are high (due to, e.g., low active compound solubility or a host of other reasons). Only two devices (syringe and catheter) are available for use in the bolus approach. If a multiple-day course of treatment is desired (say, every day for 15 days), separate injections must be made at discreet entry sites.

The infusion approach involves establishing a fixed entry point into the vein, then slowly passing the desired test material through that point over a period of time (30 minutes is about minimum, while continuous around-the-clock treatment is at least therapeutically possible). There are a number of devices available for establishing their entry point; catheter, vascular port (Garramone, 1986), or osmotic pump (Theeuwes and Yum, 1976). Each of these must, in turn, be coupled with a device to deliver the dosing solution at a desired rate. The osmotic pump, which is implanted, is also its own delivery device. Other options are gravity driven "drips," hand-held syringes (not practical or accurate over any substantial period of time), or syringe pumps. Very large volumes can be introduced by fusion over a protracted period of time, and only a single site need be fitted with an entry device.

However, infusion also has its limitations. Skilled labor is required, and the setup must be monitored over the entire period of infusion. Larger animals must be restrained, while there are special devices that make this requirement unnecessary for smaller animals. Restraint and protracted manipulation are very stressful on animals. Over a period of time, one must regularly demonstrate patency of a device, that is, that entry into the vascular system continues to exist. Finally, one is faced with having to control two variables in controlling the dose: both total volume and rate.

When are the two approaches (bolus and infusion) interchangeable? And why select one over the other? The selection of infusion is usually limited to two reasons: (1) when a larger volume must be introduced than is practical in a bolus injection or (2) tolerance is insufficient if the dose is given all at once (i.e., an infusion will "clear" a higher daily dose than will a bolus injection). For safety studies, when a bolus can be used to clear a human infusion, dosing is a matter of judgement. If the planned clinical infusion will take less than a half an hour, this practicality dictates that the animal studies be accomplished by bolus. In other situations, pharmacokinetics (in particular, the half-life of the drug entity) should be considered in making the decision.

### 11.8.3. Test Systems for Parenteral Irritation

There are no regulatory guidelines or suggested test methods for evaluating agents for muscular or vascular irritation. Since such guidelines are lacking, but the evaluation is necessary, those responsible for these evaluations have tried to develop and employ the most scientifically valid procedures.

Hagan (1959) first suggested a method for assessing IM irritation. His approach, however, did not include a grading system for evaluation of the irritation, and the method used the sacrospinalis muscles, which are somewhat difficult to dissect or repeatedly inject.

Shintani et al. (1967) developed and proposed the methodology that currently seems to be more utilized. It uses the lateral vastus muscle and includes a methodology for evaluation, scoring, and grading of irritation. Additionally, Shintani et al. investigated the effects of several factors such as pH of the solution, drug concentration, volume of injection, the effect of repeated injections, and the time to maximum tissue response. This method also constitutes the USP method (USP, 1985).

### *Acute Intramuscular Irritation in the Male Rabbit*

1. *Overview of Study Design.* Each rabbit is injected as follows:

| Site (m. vastus lateralis) | Treatment (1.0 ml/site) |
| --- | --- |
| Left | (Test article) |
| Right | (Vehicle) |

| Day 1. | Injection of all treatment groups—9 rabbits. |
| --- | --- |
| Day 2. | Sacrifice and evaluation: 24-h posttreatment group—3 rabbits. |
| Day 3. | Sacrifice and evaluation: 48-h posttreatment group—3 rabbits. |
| Day 4. | Sacrifice and evaluation: 72-h posttreatment group—3 rabbits. |

2. Administration
  2.1. Route: The test article is injected into the vastus lateralis of each rabbit.
  2.2. Dose: The dose selected is chosen to evaluate the severity of irritation, and represents a concentration that might be used clinically. This volume has been widely used in irritation testing.
  2.3. Frequency: once only.
  2.4. Duration: 1 day.
  2.5. Volume: 1.0 ml per site.

3. *Test System*
  3.1. Species, age, and weight range: Male New Zealand white rabbits weighing 2 to 5 kg are used. The New Zealand white rabbit has been widely used in muscle irritation research for many years, and is a reasonable sized, even-tempered animal that is well adapted to the laboratory environment.
  3.2. Selection: Animals to be used in the study are selected on the basis of acceptable findings from physical examinations and body weights.
  3.3. Randomization: Animals are ranked by body weight and assigned a number between one and three. The order of number assigned (e.g., 1-3-2) is chosen from a table of random numbers. Animals assigned number 1 are in the 24-h posttreatment group; those assigned number 2 are in the 48-h posttreatment group; and those assigned number 3 are in the 72-h posttreatment group.

4. *In-Life Observations*
  4.1. Daily observations: Once daily following dosing.
  4.2. Physical examinations: Once within the two weeks before the first dosing day.
  4.3. Body weight: Should be determined once before the start of the study.
  4.4. Additional examinations may be done by the study director to elucidate any observed clinical signs.

5. *Postmortem Procedures*
  5.1. Irritation is evaluated as follows: Three rabbits are sacrificed by a lethal dose of barbiturate at approximately 24, 48, or 72-h after dosing. The left and right lateral vastus of each rabbit are excised. The lesions resulting from injection are scored for muscle irritation on a numerical scale of 0 to 5 as follows (Shintani et al., 1967):

| Reaction Criteria | Score |
| --- | --- |
| No discernable gross reaction | 0 |
| Slight hyperemia | 1 |
| Moderate hyperemia and discoloration | 2 |
| Distinct discoloration in comparison with the color of the surrounding area | 3 |
| Brown degeneration with small necrosis | 4 |
| Widespread necrosis with an appearance of "cooked meat" and occasionally an abscess involving the major portions of the muscle | 5 |

The average score for the nine rabbits is then calculated, and a category of irritancy then assigned based on the following table:

| Average score | Grade |
| --- | --- |
| 0.0 to 0.4 | None |
| 0.5 to 1.4 | Slight |
| 1.5 to 2.4 | Mild |
| 2.5 to 3.4 | Moderate |
| 3.5 to 4.4 | Marked |
| 4.5 or greater | Severe |

***Acute Intravenous Irritation in the Male Rabbit.*** The design here is similar to the intramuscular assay, except that injections are made into the veins in specific muscle masses.

1. *Overview of study design.* Rabbits will be injected as follows:

| Group | No. of animals | Treatment site | Evaluation |
| --- | --- | --- | --- |
| 1 | 2 | m. vastus lateralis (left) and cervicodorsal subcutis (left) | 24 h |
| | | m. vastus lateralis (right) and cervicodorsal subcutis (right) | 24 h |
| 2 | 2 | m. vastus lateralis (left) and cervicodorsal subcutis (left) | 72 h |
| | | m. vastus lateralis (right) and cervicodorsal subcutis (right) | 72 h |
| 3 | 2 | Auricular vein (left) Auricular Vein (right) | 24- and 72-h evaluations |

Day 1: Injection of all groups (6 rabbits)

Day 2: Evaluation of Group 3 (2 rabbits). Sacrifice and evaluation of Group 1 (2 rabbits)

Day 4: Evaluation of Group 3 (2 rabbits). Sacrifice and evaluation of Group 2 (2 rabbits)

2. *Administration*

    2.1. Intramuscular: m. vastus lateralis.

    2.2. Subcutaneous: cervicodorsal subcutis.

    2.3. Intravenous: auricular vein.

    2.4. Dose: The doses and concentration selected are chosen to evaluate the severity of irritation. The dose volumes have been widely used in irritation testing.

2.5. Frequency: Once only.

2.6. Duration: 1 day.

2.7. Volume: M. vastus lateralis and cervicodorsal subcutis: 1.0 ml per site; auricular vein: 0.5 ml per site.

3. *Test System*

3.1. Species, age, and weight range: Male New Zealand white rabbits, weighing 2 to 5 kg, are used.

3.2. Selection: Animals to be used in the study are selected on the basis of acceptable findings from physical examinations.

3.3. Randomization: Animals are ranked by body weight and assigned a number between 1 and 3. The order of numbers assigned (e.g., 1-3-2) is chosen from a table of random numbers. Animals assigned number 1 are in Group 1; those assigned number 2 are in Group 2; and those assigned number 3 are in Group 3.

4. *In-Life Observations*

4.1. Daily observations: Once daily following dosing.

4.2. Physical examinations: Once within the two weeks before the first dosing day.

4.3. Body weight: Determined once before the start of the study.

4.4. Additional examinations may be done by the study director to elucidate any observed clinical signs

5. *Postmortem Procedures*

5.1. Intramuscular irritation is evaluated as follows: Rabbits are sacrificed by lethal dose of barbiturate approximately 24 and 72 h after dosing. The left and right lateral vastus muscles of each rabbit are excised. The reaction resulting from injection is scored for muscle irritation using the scale shown here.

5.2. Subcutaneous irritation is evaluated as follows: Rabbits are euthanized by a lethal dose of barbiturate approximately 24 and 72 h after dosing. The subcutaneous injection sites are exposed by dissection, and the reaction is scored for irritation on a scale of 0 to 5 as follows (Shintani et al., 1967; USP, 1995a):

| Reaction criteria | Score |
|---|---|
| No discernible gross reaction | 0 |
| Slight hyperemia and discoloration | 1 |
| Moderate hyperemia and discoloration | 2 |
| Distinct discoloration in comparison with the color of the surrounding area | 3 |
| Small areas of necrosis | 4 |
| Widespread necrosis, possibly involving the underlying muscle | 5 |

| Average score per site | Irritancy grade |
|---|---|
| 0.0 to 0.4 | None |
| 0.5 to 1.4 | Slight |
| 1.5 to 2.4 | Mild |
| 2.5 to 3.4 | Moderate |
| 3.5 to 4.4 | Marked |
| 4.5 or greater | Severe |

5.3. Intravenous irritation is evaluated as follows: Rabbits are sacrificed by a lethal dose of barbiturate following the 72-h irritation evaluation. The injection site and surrounding tissue are grossly evaluated at approximately 24 and 72 h after dosing on a scale of 0 to 3 as follows.

| Reaction Criteria | Score |
|---|---|
| No discernible gross reaction | 0 |
| Slight erythema at injection site | 1 |
| Moderate erythema and swelling with some discoloration of the vein and surrounding tissue | 2 |
| Severe discoloration and swelling of the vein and surrounding tissue with partial or total occlusion of the vein | 3 |

| Average score per site | Irritancy grade |
|---|---|
| 0.0 to 0.4 | None |
| 0.5 to 1.4 | Slight |
| 1.5 to 2.4 | Moderate |
| 2.5 or greater | Severe |

5.4. Additional examinations may be done by the study director to elucidate the nature of any observed tissue change.

### 11.8.3 Alternatives

Intramuscular (IM) and intravenous (IV) injection of parenteral formulations of pharmaceuticals can produce a range of discomfort including pain, irritation, and/or damage to muscular or vascular tissue. These are normally evaluated for prospective formulations before use in humans by histopathologic evaluation of damage in intact animal models, usually the rabbit. Attempts have been made to make this *in vivo* methodology both more objective and quantitative based on measuring the creatinine phosphokinase released in the tissue surrounding the injection site (Sidell et al., 1974). Currently, a protocol utilizing a cultured skeletal muscle cell line (L6) from the rat as a model has been evaluated in an interlaboratory validation program among 11 pharmaceutical laboratories. This methodology (Young et al., 1986) measures creatine kinase levels in media after exposure of the cells to the formulation of interest, and predicts *in vivo* IM damage based on this endpoint. It is reported to give excellent rank-correlated results across a range of antibiotics (Williams et al., 1987). The current multilaboratory evaluation covers a broader structural range of compounds and has shown a good quantitative correlation with *in vivo* results for antibiotics and a fair correlation for a broader range of parenteral drug products. Likewise, Kato et al. (1992) have proposed a model that uses cultured primary skeletal muscle fibers from the rat. Damage is evaluated by the release of creatinine phosphokinase. An evaluation using six parenterally administered antibiotics (ranking their $EC_{50}$ values) showed good relative correlation with *in vivo* results.

Another proposed *in vitro* assay for muscle irritancy for injectable formulations is the red blood cell hemolysis assay (Brown et al., 1989). Water-soluble formulations in a 1 : 2 ratio with freshly collected human blood are gently mixed for 5 min. The percentage of red blood cell survival is then determined by measuring differential absorbance at 540 nm; this value is then compared to values for known irritants and nonirritants. Against a very small group of compounds (four), this assay reportedly accurately predicts muscle irritation.

## 11.9. PHOTOTOXICITY

The potential for sunlight (or selected other light frequencies) to transform a drug or product is both a useful tool for activating some drugs and a cause of significant adverse effects for others (such as the quinolone antibiotics [Horio et al., 1995 and Lambert et al., 1996)].

### 11.9.1 Theory and Mechanisms

The portion of the solar spectrum containing the biologically most active region is from 290 to 700 mm.

The ultraviolet (UV) part of the spectrum includes wavelengths from 200 to 400 nm. Portions of the UV spectrum have distinctive features from both the physical and biological points of view. The accepted designations for the biologically important parts of the UV spectrum are UVA, 400 to 315 nm; UVB, 315 to 280 nm; and UVC, 280 to 220 nm. Wavelengths less than 290 nm (UVC) do not occur at the earth's surface because they are absorbed, predominantly by ozone in the stratosphere. The most thoroughly studied photobiological reactions that occur in skin are induced by UVB. The quinolones, for example, absorb light strongly in the 300- to 400-nm wavelength range. Although UVB wavelengths represent only approximately 1.5% of the solar energy received at the earth's surface, they elicit most of the known chemical phototoxic and photoallergic reactions. The visible portions of the spectrum, representing about 50% of the sun's energy received at sea level, includes wavelengths from 400 to 70 nm. Visible light is necessary for such biological events as photosynthesis, the regulation circadian cycles, vision, and pigment darkening. Furthermore, visible light in conjunction with certain chromophores (e.g., dyes, drugs, and endogenous compounds which absorb light and therefore "give" color) and molecular oxygen induces photodynamic effects.

Understanding the toxic effects of light impinging on the skin requires knowledge of both the nature of sunlight and the skin's optical properties. Skin may be viewed as an optically heterogeneous medium, composed of three layers that have distinct refractive indices, chrmophore distributions, and light-scattering properties. Light entering the outermost layer, the stratum corneum, is in part reflected—4–7% for wavelengths between 250 and 3000 nm (Anderson and Parrish, 1981)—due to the difference in refractive index between air and the stratum corneum. Absorption by urocanic acid (a deamination product of histidine), melanin, and proteins containing the aromatic amino acids tryptophan and tyrosine in the stratum corneum produces further attenuation of light, particularly at shorter UV wavelengths. Approximately 40% of UVB is transmitted through the stratum corneum to the viable epidermis. The light entering the epidermis is attenuated by scattering and, predominantly, absorption. Epidermal chromophores consist of proteins, urocanic acid, nucleic acids, and melanin. Passage through the epidermis results in appreciable attenuation of UVA and UVB radiation. The transmission properties of the dermis are largely due to scattering, with significant absorption of visible light by melanin, $\beta$-carotene, and the blood-borne pigments bilirubin, hemoglobin, and oxyhemoglobin. Light traversing these layers of the skin is extensively attenuated, most drastically for wavelengths less than 400 nm. Longer wavelengths are more penetrating. It has been noted that there is an "optical window," that is, greater transmission, for light at wavelengths of 600–1300 nm, which may have important biological consequences.

Normal variations in the skin's optical properties frequently occur. The degree of pigmentation may produce variations in the attenuation of light, particularly between 300 and 400 nm, by as much as 1.5 times more in blacks than in Caucasians (Pathak, 1967). Alterations in the amount or distribution of other natural chromophores account for further variations in skin optical properties. Urocanic acid, deposited on the skin's surface during perspiration (Anderson and Parrish, 1981), and UV-absorbing lipids, excreted in sebum, may significantly reduce UV transmission through the skin. Epidermal thickness, which varies over regions of the body and increases after exposure to UVB radiation, may significantly modify UV transmission.

Certain disease states also produce alterations in the skin's optical properties. Alterations of the skin's surface, such as by psoriatic plaques, decrease transmitted light. The effect may be lessened by application of oils whose refractive index is similar to that of skin (Anderson and Parrish, 1981). Disorders such as hyperbilirubinemia, porphyrias, and blue skin nevi result in increased absorption of visible light due to accumulation or altered distribution of endogenous chromophoric compounds.

The penetration of light into and through dermal tissues has important consequences. This penetration is demonstrated in Fig. 11.1. Skin, as the primary organ responsible for thermal regulation, is overperfused relative to its metabolic requirements (Anderson and Parrish, 1981).

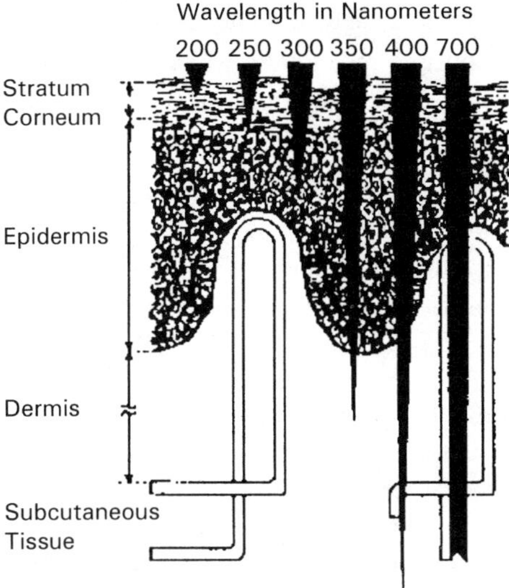


**FIGURE 11.1.** Schematic representation of light of varying wavelengths penetrating the skin.

It is estimated that the average cutaneous blood flow is 20–30 times that necessary to support the skin's metabolic needs. The papillary boundaries between epidermis and dermis allow capillary vessels to lie close to the skin's surface, permitting the blood and important components of the immune system to be exposed to light. The equivalent of the entire blood volume of an adult may pass through the skin, and potentially be irradiated, in 20 min. This corresponds to the time required to receive 1 or 2 MEDs (the MED is defined as the minimal dose of UV irradiation that produces definite, but minimally perceptible, redness 24 hr after exposure). The accessibility of incidence radiation to blood has been exploited in such regimens and phototherapy of hyperbilirubinemia in neonates, where light is used as a therapeutic agent. However, in general, there is a potential for light-induced toxicity due to irradiation of blood-borne drugs and metabolites.

### 11.9.2 Factors Influencing Phototoxicity/Photosensitization

There are a number of factors that can influence an agent acting either as a phototoxin or a photoallergen. In addition to all those factors previously reviewed in Chapter 5, there are also the following.

1. The quantity and location of photoactive material present in or on the skin.
2. The capacity of the photoactive material to penetrate into normal skin by percutaneous absorption as well as into skin altered by trauma, such as maceration, irritation, and sunburn.

3. The pH, enzyme presence, and solubility conditions at the site of exposure.

4. The quantity of activating radiation to which the skin is exposed.

5. The capacity of the spectral range to activate the materials on or within the skin.

6. The ambient temperature and humidity.

7. The thickness of the horny layer.

8. The degree of melanin pigmentation of the skin.

9. The inherent "photoactivity" of the chemical; does it weakly or strongly absorb light?

Basically, any material that has both the potential to absorb ultraviolet light (in the UVA or UVB regions) and the possibility of dermal exposure or distribution into the dermal region should be subject to some degree of suspicion as to potential phototoxicity. As shown in Table 11.5, a large number of agents have been identified as phototoxic or photoallergenic agents. Of these, tetrachlorosalicylanilide (TCSA) is the most commonly used as a positive control in animal studies.

### 11.9.3 Predictive Tests for Phototoxicity

Before we start on our description of the different methods, we will first cover some basics on light dosimetry. The intensity of the irradiation used in phototoxicity testing is determined with a light meter, which provides output as watts per $m^2$. The shelves on which the animals rest during the exposure periods are normally adjustable in order to control the dose of light to the exposure area. The irradiation from fluorescent lights will vary somewhat from day to day, depending on temperature, variations in line current, and so on. The dose the animals receive is generally represented as joules/$cm^2$. A joule is equal to 1 watt/s. Therefore, the dose of light is dependent on the time of exposure. For example, in their review, Lambert et al. (1996) discuss dosages of UVA light of 9 or 10 J/$cm^2$ in the UVA spectral region. If the irradiation from the light is found to be 20 W/$m^2$ at the exposure site, then the time of exposure required to obtain the target dose of light (in J) is calculated as

$$(\text{time of exposure}) = \frac{\text{W s}}{\text{J}} \frac{9 \text{ J}}{\text{cm}^2} \frac{\text{m}^2}{20 \text{ W}} \frac{10^4 \text{ cm}^2}{\text{m}^2} \frac{\text{min}}{60 \text{ s}} = 75 \text{ min}$$

If, with the same set of lights, two weeks later the irradiation is determined to be 19 W/$m^2$, then the exposure period would have to be 79 min.

There are three recommended protocols for assessing topical phototoxicity potential: rabbit, guinea pig, and mouse. The first described here is that for the rabbit. The traditional methodology for a predictive test for phototoxicity has been an intact rabbit test (Marzulli and Maibach, 1970). This test is conducted as follows (and illustrated diagrammatically in Figure 11.2).

**TABLE 11.5. Known Phototoxic Agents**

| In Humans | | In Animals | |
| --- | --- | --- | --- |
| Compounds | Route | Compound | Route |
| Aminobenzoic acid derivatives | Topical | Acradine | Topical |
| | | Amiodarone | Oral |
| Amyldimethylamino benzoate, mixed *ortho* and *para* isomers | Topical | Anthracine | Topical |
| | | Bergapten (5-methoxypsolaren) | Topical |
| Anthracene acridine | Topical | Bithionol | Topical |
| Bergapten (5-methoxypsoralen) | Topical | Chlorodiazepoxide | ip |
| Cadmium sulfide | Tattoo | Chlorprothiazide | ip |
| Chlorothiazides | Oral | Chlorpromazine | Topical |
| Coal tar (multicomponent) | Topical | Demeclocycline | ip |
| Dacarbazine | Infusion | Griseofulvin | ip |
| Disperse blue 35 (anthaquinone-base dye) | Topical | Kynuremic acid | Oral |
| Nalidixic acid | Oral | Nalidixic acid | Oral |
| Padimate A or Escolol 506 (amyl-*p*-dimethylamino benzoate) | Topical | Prochlorperazine | ip |
| | | Quinokine methanol | ip |
| | | Quinolone (antibacterial) | Oral |
| Psoralens | Oral, topical | Tetracyclines | ip, topical |
| Quinolone (antibacterial) | Oral | Xanthotoxin (8-methoxypsoralen) | Oral, ip, im |
| Tetracyclines | Oral | | |
| Xanthotoxin (8-methoxypsoralen) | Topical, oral | | |

393

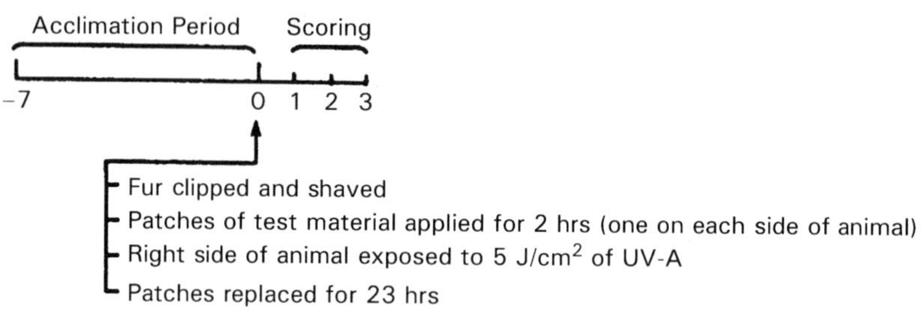


**FIGURE 11.2.** Line chart for the design and conduct of phototoxicity assay using rabbits.

A. Animals and animal husbandry:
   1. Strain/species: Female New Zealand white rabbits.
   2. Number: 6 rabbits per test; 2 rabbits for positive control.
   3. Age: Young adult.
   4. Acclimation period: At least 7 days prior to study.
   5. Food and water: Commercial laboratory feed and water are freely available.
B. Test Article:
   1. A dose of 0.5 ml of liquid or 500 mg of a solid or semisolid will be applied to each test site.
   2. Liquid substances will be used undiluted.
   3. For solids, the test article will be moistened with water (500 mg test article/0.5 ml water or another suitable vehicle) to ensure good contact with the skin.
   4. The positive control material will be a lotion containing 1% 8-methoxypsoralen.
C. Experimental procedures:
   1. Animals will be weighed on the first day of dosing.
   2. On the day prior to dosing, the fur of the test animals will be clipped from the dorsal area of the trunk using a small animal clipper, then shaved clean with a finer bladed clipper.
   3. On the day of dosing, the animals will be placed in restraints.
   4. One pair of patches (approximately 2.5 × 2.5 cm) per test article will be applied to the skin of the back, with one patch on each side of the backbone.

5. A maximum of two pairs of patches may be applied to each animal and the patches must be at least 2 in. apart.

6. The patches will be held in contact with the skin by means of an occusive dressing for the 2-h exposure period.

7. After the 2-h exposure period, the occlusive dressing, as well as the patches on the right side of the animal, will be removed.

8. The left side of the animal will be covered with opaque material (aluminum foil).

9. The animal will then be exposed to approximately 5 J/cm$^2$ of UVA (320–400 nm).

10. After exposure to the UVA light, the patches on the right side of the animal, as well as the occlusive dressing, will be replaced.

11. The dressing will again be removed approximately 23 h after the initial application of the test article. Residual test article will be carefully removed, where applicable, using water (or another suitable vehicle).

12. Animals will be examined for signs of erythema and edema and the responses scored at 24, 48, and 72 h after the initial test article application according to the Draize reaction grading system previously presented in this Chapter.

13. Any unusual observation and mortality will be recorded.

D. Analysis of data: The data from the irradiated and nonirradiated sites are evaluated separately. The scores from erythema and eschar formation, and edema at 24, 48, and 72 hr, are added for each animal (six values). The six values are then divided by 3, yielding six individual scores. The mean of the six individual animal irritation scores represents the mean primary irritation score (maximum score $= 8$, as in the primary dermal irritation study). This method was developed after a human model had been developed.


### 11.9.4. Guinea Pig

Recently, a standardized protocol for using the guinea pig for phototoxicity testing has been proposed (Nilsson et al., 1993), which has been the subject of an international validation exercise. This is detailed below in Figure 11.3.

A. Animals and animal husbandry:

1. Strain/species: Males Hartley guinea pig

2. Number: At least 10 (two groups)
Irradiation control: 4 animals
Test material treated: 6 animals

3. Age: Young adult, 300–500 g

4. Acclimation period: At least 5 days

5. Feed/water: *ad libitum*

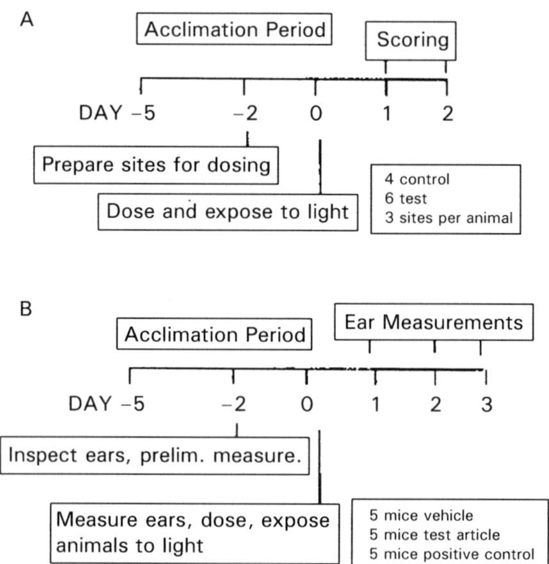


**FIGURE 11.3.** (A) Guinea pig and (B) mouse for phototoxicity testing.

B. Test material:

1. Vehicle: Test assumes that material will be in solution. Use the most volatile, nonirritating organic solvent possible, e.g., ethanol, acetone, dimethylacetamide, or some combination.

2. Treatment: There can be up to four sites per animal, each measuring $1.5 \times 1.5\,cm$ ($2.25\,cm^2$). In general, one side should be for a vehicle control, and another for a positive control [8-methoxypsoralen (8-MOP), 0.005% in ethanol].

3. Dosage: A dose of 0.025–0.050 ml is applied using a micropipetor to each site.

C. Experimental procedure:

1. Animals will be weighed on the first day of dosing.

2. Preparation: Approximately 48 h prior to treatment, removed the hair from a $6 \times 8\,cm$ area on the back with a fine clipper. On the day of dosing, animals are dosed as described previously. Tests are situated to prevent mixing of test solutions after application. No patches or wraps are used.

3. Immediately after the dose application, the animals are placed in a restraint while the test sites are kept uncovered. Prior to irradiation the heads are covered to prevent ocular damage from the light exposure.

4. Thirty minutes after dosing, animals are exposed to a nonerythmogenic dose of light in the UVA band (should have peak intensity between 335 and 365 nm). The dose of light should be 9 or $10\,J/cm^2$ for UVA and $0.1$–$0.3\,J/cm^2$ for UVB.

5. Immediately after light exposure, the animals are wiped clean if necessary and returned to their home cages.

6. Animals are inspected and scored at 24 and 48 h postexposure according to the following:

   —0: No reaction

   —1: Slight erythema

   —2: Moderate erythema

   —3. Severe erythema, with or without edema.

   (The reader should note that this scoring scheme is the same one used for dermal sensitization scoring, whereas the scoring method for the rabbit model discussed previously is that used for dermal irritation studies.)

7. Any unusual clinical signs seen during exposure should be noted. The following descriptive parameters can be calculated from the data.

   Phototoxic irritation Index (PTII) = (number of positive sites $\times 100/$ number of exposure sites)

$$\text{Phototoxicity severity index (PSI)} = \frac{\text{(total of scores)}}{\text{(total of observations)}}$$

Lovell and Sanders (1992) had previously proposed a similar model of assessing topical phototoxicity potential in the guinea pig. Their model differed from the proposed by Nilsson et al. (1993) with regard to the following:

Only one test site per animal was used.

Test sites were smaller (about 1.6 cm$^2$).

Amounts applied were less (about 10 µl).

Light intensity was set at 15 J/cm$^2$.

Their paper made no reference to the use of a restrainer.

Assessments were conducted at 4, 24, 48, and 72 h.

The scoring system was as follows:

0: Normal.

2: Faint/trace erythema.

4: Slight erythema.

6: Definite erythema.

8: Well-developed erythema.

   (Intermediate scores were indicated by odd numbers.)

   They recommended the use of acidine (weak phototoxin) or anthracene (strong phototoxin) for positive controls.

### 11.9.5. Pyrogenicity

The United States Pharmacopeia describes a pyrogen test using rabbits as a model (USP, 1995b). This test, which is the standard for limiting risks of a febrile reaction to an acceptable level, involves measuring the rise in body temperature in a group of three rabbits for 3 h after injection of 10 ml of test solution.

1. *Apparatus and Diluents.* Render the syringes, needles, and glassware free of pyrogens by heating at 250°F for not less than 30 min or by any other suitable method. Treat all diluents and solutions for washing and rinsing of devices or parenteral injection assemblies in a manner that will ensure that they are sterile and pyrogen-free. Periodically perform control pyrogen tests on representative portions of the diluents and solutions that are used for washing or rinsing of the apparatus.

2. *Temperature Recording.* Use an accurate temperature-sensing device, such as a clinical thermometer or thermistor or similar probe, that has been calibrated to ensure an accuracy of $\pm 0.1°$ and has been tested to determine that a maximum reading is reached in less than 5 min. Insert the temperature-sensing probe into the rectum of the test rabbit to a depth of not less than 7.5 cm and, after a period of time not less than that previously determined as sufficient, record the rabbit's temperature.

3. *Test Animals.* Use healthy, mature rabbits. House the rabbits individually in an area of uniform temperature (between 20°C and 23°C) free from disturbances likely to excite them. The temperature should vary no more than $\pm 3°C$ from the selected temperature. Before using rabbit for the first time in a pyrogen test, condition it for not more than seven days before use by a sham test that includes all of the steps as directed under "Procedure," except injection. Do not use a rabbit for pyrogen testing more frequently than once every 48 h, nor prior to two weeks following a maximum rise in its temperature of 0.6° or more while being subjected to the pyrogen test, or following its having been given a test specimen that was adjusted to be pyrogenic.

4. *Procedure.* Perform the test in a separate area designated solely for pyrogen testing and under environmental conditions similar to those under which the animals are housed. Withhold all food from the test rabbits during the period of the test. Access to water is allowed at all times, but may be restricted during the test. If probes measuring rectal temperature remain inserted throughout the testing period, restrain the rabbits with loose-fitting Elizabethan collars that allow the rabbits to assume a natural resting posture. Not more than 30 min prior to the injection of the test dose, determine the "control temperature" of each rabbit; this is the base for the determination of any temperature increase resulting from the injection of a test solution. In any one group of test rabbits, use only those rabbits whose control temperatures do not vary by more than 1°C from each other, and do not use any rabbit having a temperature exceeding 39.8°C.

Unless otherwise specified in the individual protocol, inject 10 ml of the test solution per kilogram of body weight into an ear vein of each of three rabbits, completing each injection within 10 min after the start of administration. The test solution is either the product, constituted if necessary as directed in the labeling, or the material under test. For pyrogen testing of devices or injection assemblies, use washings or rinsings of the surfaces that come in contact with the parenterally administered material or with the injection site or internal tissues of the patient. Ensure that all test solutions are protected from contamination. Perform the injection after warming the test solution to a temperature of $37°C \pm 2°$. Record the temperature at 1, 2, and 3 h subsequent to the injection.

5. *Test Interpretation and Continuation.* Consider any temperature decreases as zero rise. If no rabbit shows an individual rise in temperature of $0.6°$ or more above its respective control temperature, and if the sum of the three individual maximum temperature rises does not exceed $1.4°$, the product meets the requirements for the absence of pyrogens. If any rabbit shows an individual temperature rise of $0.6°$ or more, or if the sum of the three individual maximum temperature rises exceeds $1.4°$, continue the test using five other rabbits. If not more than three of the eight rabbits show individual rises in temperature of $0.6°$ or more, and if the sum of the eight individual maximum temperature rises does not exceed $3.7°$, the material under examination meets the requirements for the absence of pyrogens.

**In Vitro *Pyrogenicity.*** *In vitro* pyrogenicity testing (or bacterial endotoxin testing) is one of the great success stories for *in vitro* testing. Some 15 years ago, the limulus amebocyte lysate (LAL) test was developed, validated, and accepted as an *in vitro* alternative (Cooper, 1975; Weary and Baker, 1977) to the rabbit test. An *in vitro* test for estimating the concentration of bacterial endotoxins that may be present in or on a sample of the article(s) to which the test is applied uses LAL that has been obtained from aqueous extracts of the circulating amebocytes of the horseshoe crab, *Limulus polyphemus*, and that has been prepared and characterized for use as an LAL reagent for gel-clot formation. The test's limitation is that it detects only the pyrogens of gram-negative bacteria. This is generally not significant, since most environmental contaminants that gain entrance to sterile products are gram-negative (Devleeshouwer et al., 1985).

Where the test is conducted as a limit test, the specimen is determined to be positive or negative to the test judged against the endotoxin concentration specified in the individual monograph. Where the test is conducted as an assay of the concentration of endotoxin, with calculation of confidence limits of the result obtained, the specimen is judged to comply with the requirements if the result does not exceed (1) the concentration limit specified in the individual monograph and (2) the specified confidence limits for the assay. In either case the determination of the reaction endpoint is made with parallel dilutions of redefined endotoxin units.

Since LAL reagents have also been formulated to be used for turbidimetric (including kinetic) assays or colorimetric readings, such tests may be used if shown to comply with the requirements for alternative methods. These tests require the establishment of a standard regression curve and the endotoxin content of the test material is determined by interpolation from the curve. The procedure includes incubation for a preselected time of reacting endotoxin and control solutions with LAL reagent and reading the spectrophotometric light absorbance at suitable wavelengths. In the case of the turbidimetric procedure, the reading is made immediately at the end of the incubation period. In the kinetic assays, the absorbance is measured throughout the reaction period and rate values are determined from those readings. In the colorimetric procedure the reaction is arrested at the end of the preselected time by the addition of an appropriate amount of acetic acid solution prior to the readings. A possible advantage in the mathematical treatment of results, if the test is otherwise validated and the assay suitably designed, could be the confidence interval and limits of potency from the internal evidence of each assay itself.

### 11.9.6 Blood Compatibility

The standard test (and its major modifications) currently used for this purpose is technically an *in vitro* one, but it requires a sample of fresh blood from a dog or other large donor animal. The test was originally developed by the National Cancer Institute for use in evaluating cancer chemotherapeutic agents (Prieur et al., 1973) and is rather crude, though definitive.

The variation described here is one commonly utilized. It uses human blood from volunteers, eliminating the need to keep a donor colony of dogs. The test procedure is described in the following.

1. *Test System* Human blood. Collect 30 ml heparinized blood for whole blood and plasma (three tubes) and 30 ml clotted blood for serum (two tubes) from each of six donors.
2. *Precipitation Potential*
    - 2.1. For each donor, set up and label eight tubes 1 through 8.
    - 2.2. Add 1 ml serum to tubes 1 through 4.
    - 2.3. Add 1 ml plasma to tubes 5 through 8.
    - 2.4. Add 1 ml formulation to tubes 1 through 5.
    - 2.5. Add 1 ml vehicle to tubes 2 and 6.
    - 2.6. Add 1 ml physiological saline to tubes 3 and 7 (negative control).
    - 2.7. Add 1 ml 2% nitric acid to tubes 4 and 8 (positive control).
    - 2.8. Observe tubes 1 through 8 for qualitative reactions (e.g., precipitation or clotting) before and after mixing.
    - 2.9. If a reaction is observed in the formulation tubes (tubes 1 and/or 5), dilute the formulation in an equal amount of physiological saline ($\frac{1}{2}$ dilution) and test 1 ml of the dilution with an equal amount of plasma and/or serum. If a reaction still occurs, make serial dilutions of the formulation in saline (i.e., $\frac{1}{4}$, $\frac{1}{8}$, etc.).
    - 2.10. If a reaction occurs in the vehicle tubes (tubes 2 and/or 6), repeat in a manner similar to that in step 2.9.
3. *Hemolytic Potential*
    - 3.1. For each donor, set up and label 8 tubes: 1 through 8.
    - 3.2. Add 1 ml whole blood to each tube.

3.3.  Add 1 ml formulation to tube 1.

3.4.  Add 1 ml vehicle to tube 2.

3.5.  Add 1 ml of $\frac{1}{2}$ dilution of formulation in saline to tube 3.

3.6.  Add 1 ml of $\frac{1}{2}$ dilution of vehicle in saline to tube 4.

3.7.  Add 1 ml of $\frac{1}{4}$ dilution of formulation in saline to tube 6.

3.8.  Add 1 ml of $\frac{1}{4}$ dilution of vehicle in saline to tube 6.

3.9.  Add 1 ml of physiological saline to tube 7 (negative control).

3.10.  Add 1 ml of distilled water to tube 8 (positive control).

3.11.  Mix by gently inverting each tube three times.

3.12.  Incubate tubes for 45 min at 37°C.

3.13.  Centrifuge 5 min at 1000 g.

3.14.  Separate the supernate from the sediment.

3.15.  Determine hemoglobin concentrations to the nearest $0.1\,g\,dl^{-1}$ on the supernate (plasma).

3.16.  If hemoglobin concentrations of the above dilutions are $0.2\,g\,dl^{-1}$ (or more) greater than the saline control, repeat the procedure, adding 1 ml of further serial dilutions (1/8, 1/16, etc.) of formulation or vehicle to 1 ml of blood until the hemoglobin level is within $0.2\,g\,dl^{-1}$ of the saline control.

There are two proposed, true *in vitro* alternatives to this procedure (Mason et al., 1974; Kambric et al., 1976), but neither has been either widely evaluated or accepted.


## REFERENCES


Anderson, R.R. and Parrish, J.A. (1981). The optics of skin. *J. Invest. Dermatol.* 77: 13–19.

Auletta, C. (1994). Vaginal and rectal administration. *J. Am. Col. Toxicol.*13: 48–63.

Avis, K.E. (1985). Parenteral preparations. In: *Remington's Pharmaceutical Sciences* (Gennaro, A. R., Ed.). Mack Publishing Company, Easton, PA, pp. 1518–1541.

Ballard, B.E. (1968). Biopharmaceutical considerations in subcutaneous and intramuscular drug administration. *J. Pharm. Sci* 57: 357–378.

Brown, S., Templeton, D., Prater, D.A. and Potter, C.C. (1989). Use of an *in vitro* hemolysis test to predict tissue irritancy in an intramuscular formation. *J. Parenter. Sci. Technol.* 43: 117–120.

Cooper, J.F. (1975). Principles and applications of the limulus test for pyrogen in parenteral drugs. *Bull. Parenter. Drug Assoc.* 3: 122–130.

Develeeshouwer, M.J., Cornil, M.F. and Dony, J. (1985). Studies on the sensitivity and specificity of the limulus amebocyte lysate test and rabbit pyrogen assays. *Appl. Environ. Microbiol.* 50: 1509–1511.

Draize, J.H., Woodard, G. and Calvery, H.O. (1944). Method for the study of irritation and toxicity of substances applied topically to the skin and mucous membranes. *J. Reprod. Fert.* 20: 85–93.

Eckstein, P., Jackson, M., Millman, N. and Sobero, A. (1969). Comparison of vaginal tolerance test of spermical preparations in rabbits and monkeys. *J. Reprod. Fertil.* 20, 85–93.

Gad, S.C. and Chengelis, C.P. (1998). *Acute Toxicity: Principles and Methods.* 2nd ed., Academic Press, San Diego, CA.

Gad, S.C., Walsh, R.D. and Dunn, B.J. (1986). Correlation of ocular and dermal irritancy of industrial chemicals. *Ocular Dermal Toxicol.* 5(3): 195–213.

Garramone, J.P. (1986). *Vascular Access Port Model SLA. User's Manual.* Norfolk Medical Products, Skokie, IL.

Gray, J.E. (1978). Pathological evaluation of injection injury. In: *Sustained and Controlled Release Drug Delivery Systems* (Robinson, J., Ed.). Marcel Dekker, New York, pp. 351–405.

Hagan, E.C. (1959). *Appraisal of the Safety of Chemicals in Foods, Drugs and Cosmetics.* Association of Food and Drug Officials of the United States, Austin, Texas, p. 19.

Horio, T., Kohachi, K., Ogawa, A., Inoue, T. and Ishirara, M. (1995). Evaluation of photosensitizing ability of quinolones in guinea pigs. *Drugs* 49 (Suppl 2), 283–285.

Kambic, H.E., Kiraly, R.J. and Yukihiko, N. (1976). A simple *in vitro* screening test for blood compatibility of materials. *J. Biomed. Mat. Res. Sympos.* 7: 561–570.

Kato, I., Harihara, A. and Mizushima, Y. (1992). An *in vitro* method for assessing muscle irritation of antibiotics using rat primary cultured skeletal muscle fibers. *Toxicol. Appl. Pharmacol.* 117: 194–199.

Lambert, L., Warmer, W. and Kornhauser, A. (1996). Animal models for phototoxicity tesing. *Toxicol. Methods* 2, 99–114.

Lovell, W.W. and Sanders, D.J. (1992). Phototoxicity testing in guinea pigs, *Fd. Chem. Toxicol.* 30: 155–160.

Mason, R.G., Shermer, R.W., Zucker, W.H., Elston, R.C. and Blackwelder, W.C. (1974). An in vitro test system for estimation of blood compatibility of biomaterials. *J. Biomed. Mat. Res.* 8: 341–356.

Marzulli, F.M. and Maibach, H.K. (1970). Perfume phototoxicity. *J. Soc. Cosmet. Chem.* 21, 685–715.

Mathias, C.G.T. (1983). Clinical and experimental aspects of cutaneous irritation. In: *Dermatotoxicology* (Margulli, F.M. and Maiback, H.T., Eds.). Hemisphere Publishing, New York, pp. 167–183.

Nilsson, R., Maurer, T. and Redmond, N. (1993). A standard protocol for phototoxicity testing: Results from an interlaboratory study. *Contact Dermatitis* 28, 285–290.

Pathak, M.A. (1967). Photobiology of melanogenesis: Biophysical aspects in *Advances in Biology of Skin,* Vol. 8, *The Pigmentary System* (Montagna W. and Uh, F., Eds.), pp. 400–419, Pergamon, New York.

Prieur, D.J., Young, D.M., Davis, R.D., Cooney, D.A., Homan, E.R., Dixon, R.L. and Guarino, A.M. (1973). Procedures for preclinical toxicologic evaluation of cancer chemotherapeutic agents: Protocols of the laboratory of toxicology. *Cancer Chemotherapy Reports,* Part 3, 4: 1–30.

Shintani, S., Yamazaki, M., Nakamura, M. and Nakayama, I. (1967). A new method to determine the irritation of drugs after intramuscular injection in rabbits. *Tox. Appl. Pharm.* 11: 293–301.

Sidell, F.R., Calver, D.L. and Kaminskis, A. (1974). Serum creatine phosphokinase activity after intramuscular injection. *JAMA* 228: 1884–1887.

Theeuwes, F. and Yum, S.I. (1976). Principles of the design and operation of generic osmotic pumps for the delivery of semisolid or liquid drug formulations. *Ann. Biomed. Eng.* 4: 343–353.

USP (1985). Intramuscular irritation test. *United States Pharmacopeia.* USP Convention, Rockville, Maryland, pp. 1180–1183.

USP (1995). Intracutaneous Test, *United States Pharmacopoeia*, USP Convention, Rockville, MD, pp. 1201–1202.

USP (1995). Bacterial endotoxins test. *United States Pharmacopeia.* USP Convention, Rockville, Maryland, pp. 1696–1697.

Wearly, M. and Baker, B. (1977). Utilization of the limulus amebocyte lysage test for pyrogen testing of large-volume parenterals, administration sets and medical devices. *Bull. Parenter. Drug Assoc.* 31: 127–133.

Weil, C.S. and Scala, R.A. (1971). Study of intra- and interlaboratory variability in the results of rabbit eye and skin irritation tests. *Toxicol. Appl. Pharmacol.* 19: 276–360.

Williams, P.D., Masters, B.G., Evans, L.D., Laska, D.A. and Hattendorf, G.H. (1987). An *in vitro* model for assessing muscle irritation due to parenteral antibiotics. *Fundam. Appl. Toxicol.* 9: 10–17.

Young, M.F., Tobretta, L.D. and Sophia, J.V. (1986). Correlative *in vitro* and *in vivo* study of skeletal muscle irritancy. *Toxicologist* 6 (1): 1225.

# 12

# SPECIAL CONCERNS FOR THE PRECLINICAL EVALUATION OF BIOTECHNOLOGY PRODUCTS

## 12.1 INTRODUCTION

Although many assume that biotechnology is a new concept, the application of this science has been understood for many years and utilized in its simplest form in the fermentation of beer, wine, and bread by microbial agents. Modern biotechnology can be divided into three research and development areas: recombinant DNA technology (rDNA), monoclonal antibody technology, and bioprocess technology. The commercialization of these three processes is based on the premise that biotechnology can cost-effectively produce large quantities of a highly purified product.

Biotechnology as a promising source of new and more efficient targeted therapeutics has been with us since the mid-1980s. While (as one should expect) some of the early promises have not quite been met, biotechnology has turned out to be a valuable source of new and valuable therapeutics. Table 12.1, summarizing the first 15 years of biologic approvals, demonstrates this (Malinowski, 1999; Maulik and Patel, 1997).

Protein and other biotechnology derived therapeutics have some fundamental differences from traditional small (synthetic organic) molecules. Table 12.2 presents a comparative summary of these differences.

Among all the other aspects of increasing understanding of what is involved in the evaluation and development of biologically derived therapeutics has been a very real evolution of what is needed to evaluate the safety of these products. In the beginning, there was a stark duality of expectations. On one side, early advocates of

404

**TABLE 12.1. First Biologic Approvals 1980–1994[a]**

| Generic (trade) name | Firm receiving FDA approval for PLA/NDA | FDA Submission date | FDA Approval date | Review phase (mo.) |
|---|---|---|---|---|
| New recombinant entities | | | | |
| Epoetin Alpha (Procrit, Epogen)*o | Amgen | 11/03/87 | 06/01/89 | 18.9 |
| B-CSF (Neupogen)* | Amgen | 01/05/90 | 02/20/91 | 13.5 |
| Interferon Beta 1B (Betaseron)*o,f | Chiron | 07/23/92 | 07/23/93 | 12 |
| Aldesleukin (Proleukin)*o | Chiron | 12/01/88 | 05/05/92 | 12.2 |
| Alteplase (Activase)* | Genetech | 05/01/86 | 11/13/87 | 18.4 |
| Gamma Interferon (Actimmune)*o | Genetech | 12/22/89 | 12/20/90 | 11.9 |
| Dornase Alfa (Pulmozyme)*o,f | Genetech | 04/01/93 | 12/30/93 | 9 |
| Alpha Interferon 2A (Roferon-A)* | Genetech | 10/24/84 | 06/04/86 | 7.3 |
| Sagramostim (Leukine, Prokine)*o,t | Immunex | 02/24/90 | 03/05/91 | 12.2 |
| Alpha Interferon 2B (Intron-A)* | Schering-Plough | 06/15/83 | 06/04/86 | 35.6 |
| New recombinant versions | | | | |
| Somatrem (Protropin)o,[#] | Genetech | 08/31/83 | 10/17/85 | 25.6 |
| Anti Hemophilic Factor (Recombinate)* | Genetics Institute | 05/03/90 | 12/10/92 | 31.3 |
| Imiglucerase (Cerezyme)o,f,[#] | Genzyme | 05/20/93 | 05/23/94 | 12.1 |
| Insulin (Humulin)[#] | Lilly | 05/15/82 | 10/28/82 | 5.5 |
| Somatropin (Humatrope)o,[#] | Lilly | 10/16/86 | 03/08/87 | 4.7 |
| Hepatitis-B Vaccine (Reombivax HB)* | Merck | 12/21/84 | 07/23/86 | 19 |
| Monoclonal antibodies | | | | |
| Centorx 2b/3A 7E3 (Reopro)* | Centocor | 12/15/83 | 12/22/94 | 12.2 |
| Satumomab Pendetide (Oncoscint OC103)*o | Cytogen | 09/28/89 | 12/29/92 | 39 |

*(continued)*

**TABLE 12.1.** (*continued*)

| Generic (trade) name | Firm receiving FDA approval for PLA/NDA | FDA Submission date | FDA Approval date | Review phase (mo.) |
|---|---|---|---|---|
| CD3 Muromonab (Orthoclone)OKT3)* | Ortho | 03/29/84 | 06/19/86 | 26.7 |
| Nonrecombinant proteins | | | | |
| Factor IX (Alphanine)o,* | Alpha Therapeutics | 01/29/88 | 12/21/90 | 35.1 |
| Anti Hemophilic Factor VIII (Monoclate)* | Armour | 12/20/85 | 10/16/87 | 21.8 |
| Calcitonin (Cibacalcin)o,[#] | Ciba-Geigy | 12/08/80 | 10/31/86 | 70.7 |
| PEG-ADA (Adagen)o,[#] | Enzon | 01/13/88 | 03/21/90 | 26.2 |
| PEG-Asparaginase (Oncospar)*o | Enzon | 01/01/91 | 02/01/94 | 37 |
| Alpha Interferon IV (Alferon)* | Interferon-NPDC | 12/15/85 | 10/10/89 | 45.8 |
| Cerebrosidase (Ceredase)o,f,[#] | Genzyme | 04/14/90 | 04/05/91 | 11.7 |
| Alpha Proteinase Inhibitor (Prolastin)o,[#] | Miles | 05/15/86 | 12/02/87 | 18.6 |
| Aprotinin (Trasylolo)o,[#] | Miles | 11/24/92 | 12/29/93 | 13.1 |
| Antistreplase (Eminase)[#] | SmithKline-Beecham | 06/08/88 | 11/27/89 | 17.6 |

[a]Above are the 29 new biologic entities (NBEs) approved during 1980–1994. The review phase (in months) is the time encompassed between the FDA product license application or new drug application submission date and the FDA approval date. Abbreviations are as follows: o = orphan drug, a product intended for the treatment of rare conditions and diseases; t = treatment IND, a "promising investigational drug" and was distributed outside of but concurrent with ongoing clinical trials; f = fast-track review, product was reviewed at the FDA under the SubPart E and/or Accelerated Approval regulations. * indicates the product was reviewed at the Center for Biologics Evaluation and Research at the FDA and [#] indicates the product was reviewed at the Center for Drug Evaluation and Research at the FDA.

**TABLE 12.2 Comparison of Protein Therapeutic Agents with Small Molecule Drugs**

|  | Proteins | Small molecules |
|---|---|---|
| Drug substance | Heterogeneous mixture<br>Broad specifications during development<br>Specifications may change during development | Single entity; high chemical purity<br>Exception: racemic mixtures<br><br>Specifications well defined early in development |
| Drug product | Usually intravenously or subcutaneously | Generally oral; few formulations during development |
| Impurities | Difficult to standardize | Purity standards well established |
| Bridging requirements | Significant for drug substance | Bioequivalence procedures |
| Biological activity | May mimic naturally occurring molecules<br>Primary mechanism of toxicity<br>Predictive based on mechanism | Less predictive |
| Nonspecificity | Variable significance | Usually significant<br>Drug–drug interactions |
| Chronic toxicity | Lack of models because of species-determined biological specificity and antigenicity | Models sometimes relevant |
| Impurities | Toxicity not a major issue<br>May impact immunogenicity | May be significant<br>Purity standards well established |

biotechnology held that there were unlikely to be any safety concerns other than those due to hyperpharmacology overactivity at the target receptors. On the other hand, there were those who cautioned against the possibility of extreme and unforeseeable toxicities. The truth, as is usually the case, has turned out to be in between.

The principle purposes of preclinical safety evaluation in this context remain

To detect harmful (toxic) effects.

To exclude other potentially harmful effects.

To determine their relationship to dose and duration of treatment

If possible, to discover their mechanism or at least pathogenesis.

This information should be used to predict possible adverse actions in the target species, in order for toxicologists to:

- Warn clinicians about unacceptable risks.
- Warn clinicians about risks that should be monitored.

- Remind themselves and others of the possibility of toxic effects not detected because they could not be displayed by the test systems used (e.g., headache in a nonhuman species, or carcinogenicity in a 1-month experiment), or were not sought.

In addition, toxicologists, as general biological scientists, should always be alert to physiological and pharmacological effects manifested in their experiments, because they may illuminate mechanisms of health and disease both of academic and practical importance.

The objectives of the preclinical safety studies on biologically derived therapeutics are to identify the pharmacological and toxicological effects that are likely to be encountered throughout the course of clinical development and beyond (Dorato and Vodicnik, 2001). The selection and design of such studies should be begun by considering what may be known about other products which are structurally and/or pharmacologically similar. The program and study design should then proceed to consider:

1. Intended manner of use, including dose, route of administration and particulars of dosing regimen.
2. Age of intended patient population.
3. Selection of relevant model species.
4. Stability of the formulated drug substance under the conditions of use.
5. Physiologic (disease) state of intended patients.

In the area of bioengineered products, many of which are complex proteins of potent but sparsely studied activities in living systems, the investigative responsibilities of the toxicologist are likely to be very important, because he/she may be the first observer able to study the effects of repeated administration of a range of doses on a living system. It is now possible to frame a classification of the types of biologically derived therapeutic products (Table 12.3).

Each type of product has some specific considerations. The range of materials is enormous. The deciding factors for the toxicologist should be the precision with which the material can be characterized by physico-chemical means, as that should be inversely related to the burden of repeated biological testing necessary to assure safety, and the extent of prior knowledge of its biological properties. The greater our ignorance of the latter, the more searching should be the toxicologist's studies in order to discern the biological ($=$ pharmacological) properties of the substance. Exposure of the individual must also be considered, as different criteria may apply to deliberate administration of a living organism, which could spread in the community.

As in any safety evaluation, the planned work should be related to the intended use and treatment of humans, for example one dose in a few gravely ill patients or multiple doses of the entire healthy community as prophylaxis against a trivial condition. Contrast, say, what might be appropriate for tumor necrosis factor, as in an experimental trial in a few sufferers from late-stage cancer, with the requirements

**TABLE 12.3. Classification of Bioengineered Products on Practical Grounds**

| Type | Bioengineering involvement | Pharmacological properties | Physico-chemical characterization | Example |
|---|---|---|---|---|
| 1 Low molecular weight substance | New production route | Well-known | Rigorous | Amino acid 6-APA |
| 2 High molecular weight substance | New production route | Fairly well-known | Extensive | Human hormones, e.g., hGH, hPTH |
| 3a Endogenous high molecular weight substance. | First ever production | Some knowledge | Moderate | IFN |
| 3b Endogenous high molecular weight substance. | First ever production perhaps gene splicing to make hybrid molecule | Scanty to limited knowledge | Moderate | Other lymphokines, tumor necrosis factor, etc. |
| 4 Engineered antigen | Partly or totally synthetic ag + rDNA production | Probably predictable | Rigorous | Synthetic vaccine for polio myelitis or hepatitis B |
| 5 Monoclonal antibody (or component) | Hybridoma ?human cell line | Probably predictable ?anitgenicity | Moderate | Anti-tumor antibody for imaging anti-idiotype antibody as vaccine |
| 6 Living organism | Removal of pathogenicity by genetic manipulation | uncertain | limited | As vaccine immunogen, e.g., S. typhimurium TY21a, modified herpes or to carry antigen, e.g., vaccinia. |

for a candidate vaccine against dental caries to be widely administered to healthy children.

Because of the rapid development of new biotechnology products, toxicology and safety assessment departments at most chemical or pharmaceutical companies are presently or soon will be confronted with the development of testing protocols for the safety evaluation of rDNA products. Routine toxicology assessment as performed in the past using standard protocols may not apply, and may in fact represent unnecessary or inappropriate studies. Because of the relatively nontoxic nature and species-specificity of many of the new biotechnology products, less evaluation in rodent species may be required than for some of the chemicals of the past. What is needed in dealing with the products of this new technology is the rethinking of traditional toxicology testing approaches.

## 12.2. REGULATION

The regulation of biologically derived therapeutics actually has a long history, and has also continued to evolve (see Table 12.4) (Weissinger, 1989, Korwek, 1997). This history led to the PHS Act providing a somewhat mixed description of the products under its authority, which in turn serves to define biologics for CBER: "[A biologic is] any virus, therapeutic serum, toxin, antitoxin, vaccine, blood, blood

**TABLE 12.4. Historical Perspectives of Biologic Therapeutics Regulation**

| | |
|---|---|
| 1902 | Federal Virus, Serum and Toxin Act/PHS (after tenatnus contaminated diphtheria antitoxin led to deaths of ten children). Intent was to ensure safety, purity, and potency. |
| 1906 | Pure Food and Drugs Act (Upton Sinclair's *The Jungle*) |
| 1937 | Division of Biologics Control/NIH |
| 1938 | FD&C Act (Sulfanilamide Elixir), biologics exempt! |
| 1955 | Division of Biological Standards Established (polio virus) |
| 1962 | FD&C Amendments (thalidomide) |
| 1972 | Bureau of Biologics/FDA |
| 1978 | Good Manufacturing Practices Regulations |
| 1979 | Good Laboratory Practices Regulations |
| 1982 | Bureau of Biologics merged with Bureau of Drugs → National Center for Drugs and Biologics |
| 1983 | Orphan Drug Act |
| 1984 | Drug Price Competition and Patent Term Restoration Act |
| 1992 | User Fees |
| 1997 | ICH Harmonized Guidelines |
| Today | FDA Center for Biologics Evaluation and Research (CBER) regulates *most* biological substances, still located at NIH! |

component or derivative, allergenic product, or analogous product, or arsphenamine or its derivative (or any other trivalent organic arsenic compound), applicable to the prevention, treatment, or cure of disease, or injuries in man . . . " 21 CFR 600.3 states that, "(h) Biological product means any virus, therapeutic serum, toxin, antitoxin, or analogous product applicable to the prevention, treatment or cure of diseases or injuries in man." Confusion of authority and responsibility between the three human health product centers of FDA (CDER, CBER and CDRH) led in 1992 to the promulgation of three intercenter agreements. The agreement between CDER and CBER states that the following biological products require licensure and come under CBER's authority (Mathieu, 1997).

- Vaccines, regardless of the method of manufacture (vaccines were defined as agents administered for the purpose of eliciting an antigen-specific cellular or humoral response).
- *In vivo* diagnostic allergenic products and allergens intended for use as "hyposensitization agents."
- Human blood or human blood-derived products, including placental blood-derived products, animal-derived procoagulant products and animal- or cell culture-derived hemoglobin-based products intended to act as red blood cell substitutes.
- Immunoglobulin products.
- Products composed of, or intended to contain, intact cells or intact micro-organisms.
- Proteins, peptides, or carbohydrate products produced by cell culture, excluding antibiotics, hormones, and products previously derived from human or animal tissue regulated as drugs.
- Protein products made in animal body fluid by genetic alteration of transgenic animals.
- Animal venoms or constituents of venoms.

Other classes of products identified as CBER-regulated products include

- Synthetically produced allergenic products intended to specifically alter the immune response to a specific antigen or allergen.
- Certain drugs used in conjunction with blood banking or transfusion.

As will be seen at the end of this chapter in the section on gene therapy products (where NIH also has some regulatory role), there is still some ambiguity of authority in areas where technology has outrun regulatory foresight. The situation is similar internationally (see CPMP, 1989 and ICH, 1997 for example).

Within the United States, the regulation of therapeutics is split on relatively arbitrary grounds. This is presented in Table 2.5 in Chapter 2. This chapter reflects both current FDA practices and the ICH guidelines.

**TABLE 12.5. Points to Consider in the Preclinical Safety Assessment of Biologics**

---

Rationale
   *In vitro* or *in vivo* studies
    Potency assays
    Receptor characteristics (across species)
    Physiological modeling
    Scientific literature
    Scientific speculation
Indication
    Replacement therapy (long-term)
    Nonpharmacodynamic treatment (prophylactic or diagnostic)
    Pharmacodynamic treatment (short-term or long-term)
Pharmacological activity (pharmacodynamics)
    Primary endpoints
    Secondary endpoints
*In vivo* model selection
    Species-specific effects
    Effects independent of species
    Animal model of disease
Pharmacokinetics and ADME: Correlation with Pharmacodynamics
    Low dose
    High dose
General Toxicity
    Single dose (acute)
    Repeated dose (subacute or subchronic)
Specific Toxicity (may include one or more of the following studies)
    Local irritation (local reactogenicity)
    Antigenicity
    Chronic toxicity
    Reproduction toxicity, including teratogenic potential
    Mutagenicity
    Tumorigenicity
    Carcinogenicity
    Other toxicity concerns (e.g., neurotoxicity, immunotoxicity, etc.)

---

## 12.3. PRECLINICAL SAFETY ASSESSMENT

Because of the complexity and wide diversity of biologic products, their safety is evaluated on a case-by-case basis (in accordance with CBER's promulgated points-to-consider as summarized in Table 12.5) until such time as enough data on either specific products or a class of products are available.

Generally, *in vivo* nonclinical studies should be designed to include a sufficient number of animals per group to permit a valid estimation of a drug's toxicologic and pharmacologic effects in terms of incidence, severity and the dose–response relationships involved (Thomas and Myers, 1998). The latter point requires, as pointed out throughout this text, thoughtful selection of doses. Comparable formulation, routes and regiments of administration, duration of exposure and suitable time to allow expression of expected response are also important proper design features.

The number of species necessary in preclinical testing programs varies. However, there is no specific requirement for the routine use of two species (e.g., one rodent and one nonrodent) in toxicology studies of biological products.

In each stage of product development, it is important to determine exposure by measuring pharmacokinetic (including ADME) or pharmacodynamic endpoints. This includes the following, for example: (1) measurements of the biologic in plasma or target organs; (2) the distribution and persistence of cells for cellular therapies; (3) measurements of viral shedding and recovery of certain values; (4) localization of targeted novel delivery systems; and (5) tissue tropism, including germline tissue, of vectors used in gene therapies.

Such studies provide important information for a better interpretation of the toxicity observed in animals, and aid in the selection of not only the proposed initial human dose but of the dose-escalation scheme and the frequency of dosing in the clinical trial(s). Further, once such exposure data are available in humans, the data can be used to better correlate the human and animal findings. Toxicity studies should be performed in the same species used to assess exposure. Often, exposure and toxicity are measured in the same study, particularly when nonrodents are used.

Toxicity studies should be designed not only to identify a safe dose, but also a toxic dose(s) to anticipate the product's safety and to better define the therapeutic index in humans. Specific product considerations that may complicate the process of defining a toxic dose may include limits based on formulation, lack of significant systemic absorption, or the amount of the product available. The lack of significant toxicity in animals does not necessarily mean that the product is safe. The margin of safety for the initial starting dose, however, will likely be adequate.

Historically, the goal of acute toxicity studies was to define a lethal dose range following a single administration or the administration of a few closely spaced doses. More recently, these studies have been designed to evaluate a high dose that causes significant toxicity but not necessarily lethality. If deaths occur, rarely are such studies expected to provide sufficient information to determine the cause of death.

Studies are often one to two weeks in duration and routinely include body weight determinations, clinical observations, and gross necropsy findings. Additional antemortem studies may be performed as appropriate, especially in large animals (e.g., observation of local reactogenicity, pharmacokinetic evaluations, hematological and/or clinical biochemistry measurements). Histological evaluations may also be performed.

The duration of repeat-dose studies should be at least as long as the proposed clinical study. These studies are designed to establish a dose-response relationship, define target organ(s) of toxicity, and determine whether observed toxicities are reversible. Evaluation parameters should include not only those routinely performed in the acute studies, but those performed in the additional studies as well. Special tests, such as ophthalmoscopic, electrocardiograph, body temperature, and blood pressure monitoring are often included. Depending on the study duration, sampling at multiple time points may be necessary to better characterize the kinetics of response. As mentioned, a group of animals will be examined at term, and some may be reserved for a treatment-free or recovery period to evaluate the reversibility of any findings.

Specific (local tissue tolerance) toxicity studies may be necessary due to special characteristics of the product or the clinical indication. Adjuvanted vaccines are routinely evaluated for local (injection site) reactions, and cellular therapies are routinely screened for tumorigenic potential. Research is also needed to better predict the sensitizing potential of biological products and to determine the relevance of serum antibody levels following repeat dosing in animals and humans.

While carcinogenicity studies have not been performed routinely for biological products, they may be appropriate for products proposed for chronic use. Reproductive toxicology studies will probably become more common, especially as more women of child-bearing potential participate in early clinical trials. In the past, such studies have not been conducted for biologics. Reproductive toxicology studies have been performed with many of the recently approved therapeutics (e.g., interferons, interleukins, cytokines, growth factors, etc.) (Klaff et al., 1978; CBER, 1997 and Fent and Zbinden, 1997). Such studies also have been conducted in the development of AIDS vaccines intended for use in pregnant women. The standard protocol designs were modified to address specific vaccine-related concerns, including dosing in relationship to immunologic effects.

The recent development of biologics to treat various nervous system diseases has involved additional, specific neurotoxicological studies on these products. However, despite the fact that most products regulated as biologics have an immune component or impact directly or indirectly on the immune system, standardized immunotoxicity tests that are potentially useful in screening large numbers of chemicals for their ability to adversely affect the immune system have not proven essential in assessing the safety of biological products.

Throughout the various phases of product development, additional preclinical safety studies may be necessary due to unexpected toxicity, significant changes in the manufacturing process or the final formulation, or changes in the clinical indications. In some cases, the ideal assessment of the safety of novel biological therapies may require alternative approaches, such as *in vitro* or *in vivo* organogenesis model systems, animal models of tolerance, animal models of disease, or transgenic animal models.

## 12.4. RECOMBINANT DNA TECHNOLOGY

The concept of recombinant DNA technology is based on the premise that a gene sentence may be taken from an animal or human gene responsible for the production of a particular protein and inserted into the DNA of *Escherichia coli*, a single-cell bacterium. The bacterial cells then divide very rapidly, making billions of copies of themselves, including a replica of the gene that has been inserted.

There are unique ways to insert human genes into bacteria. In addition to chromosomal DNA, bacteria have numerous copies of extrachromosomal circular DNA called plasmids, which are not attached to the bacterial chromosome. These plasmids can be transferred from one bacteria to another by conjugation (e.g., mating) and can be isolated from bacteria and easily purified. Through use of restriction enzymes (i.e., a family of enzymes that can cut DNA at specific base sequences), the gene sentence to be inserted can be isolated and the plasmid DNA can be opened. While in the open state, the desired piece of animal or human DNA can be inserted. Through the use of ligase enzymes, complementary ends of the plasmid can be connected, thereby producing a recombinant plasmid recombined by joining two heterologous pieces of DNA. This recombinant plasmid can then be put back into the bacteria, and the bacteria will express the new gene function that has been inserted.

A unique characteristic of plasmids is that thousands are produced within each bacterium, to the point that up to 40% of the total DNA of the bacterium may in fact be plasmid DNA. Hence, a single piece of human DNA that heretofore could only be obtained in low concentrations can be recombined with a plasmid, and the DNA sequence multiplied by a million- or a billion-fold (i.e., cloned). Use of cloning techniques may produce many grams of a particular human protein, instead of the few molecules that are produced in normal cells.

Examples of the early application of recombinant DNA technology in medicine are the development of recombinant human growth hormone; human insulin; human interferons, thought to have anticancer activity in addition to antiviral activity; interleukins (regulatory proteins from lymphocytes that are believed to be important in the treatment of immunodeficiency diseases and cancer); tumor necrosis factor; epidermal and bone marrow progenitor cell growth factors; and the production of vaccines (Table 12.1).

Human growth hormone and insulin produced by rDNA technology are already registered with the U.S. Food and Drug Administration for therapeutic use. The applications of rDNA technology agriculture should improve the quality of domesticated animals through the production of new and improved vaccines, growth-promoting hormones, and less expensive food additives. Seed crops will be produced that offer improved yields and better resistance to environmental conditions. Further applications have included the insertion of genes into plants or bacteria for production of toxins that can act as biochemical pesticides or allelophatic agents (chemicals that act as natural herbicides to prevent the growth of other plant species in the same geographical area).

### 12.4.1 General Safety Issues

Recombinant DNA technology represents one of the most innovative achievements in biology in the last century. Although the new technology has generated much enthusiasm for its potential applications, it has also raised concerns among both scientists and the public in general. Many of the early fears of the inadvertent development of an "Andromeda strain" during the genetic engineering of a specific microbe have long since vanished. However, other concerns remain. Can a gene cloned for toxic production from an rDNA microbe be transferred into normal bacterial flora? Could antibiotic-resistant genes be cloned and inadvertently inserted into clinically relevant pathogens not presently antibiotic-resistant? To reduce these possibilities, the National Institutes of Health has only certified nonconjugative plasmids (e.g., nonmating) for use in recombinant DNA microbes.

Studies by Levine et al. (1983) have addressed the issue of plasmid mobilizations, the movement of plasmids between different host cells. Human volunteers fed tetracycline along with *E. coli* HS-4 (typical of the normal intestinal flora of humans) bearing highly mobilized plasmids (e.g., pJBK5) that carried resistance to chloramphenicol and tetracycline became co-colonized with *E. coli* HS-4 bearing the antibiotic-resistant plasmid. However, the use of a poorly mobilizable plasmid (pBR325) did not result in plasmid transfer.

Taken as a whole, these studies establish the safety of recombinant DNA research when poorly mobilizable cloning vectors are used, while supporting the rationale for biologic containment of highly mobilizable plasmids. They also point out the need to protect laboratory workers on antibiotic therapy from potential exposure to recombinant DNA organisms carrying any sort of antibiotic-resistant genes. A reassuring point is the relatively poor survival of rDNA strains of *E. coli* in the intestinal environment. For example, in most successful studies, 50 billion *E. coli* HS-4 organisms were required to ensure survival within the harsh environment of a human's stomach.

### 12.4.2 Specific Toxicological Concerns

While rDNA techniques offer exciting possibilities, there are many unanswered questions about the potential toxicity that each new product represents. For example, acute clinical toxicities of interferons (IFNs) include flu-like syndrome, fever, chills, malaise, anorexia, fatigue, and headache. Chronic dose-limiting toxicities include neutropenia, thrombocytopenia, impairment of myeloid maturation, reversible dose-related hepatotoxicity, some neurological toxicity (stupor, psychosis, peripheral neuropathy) and gastrointestinal toxicity. Some of these toxicities would be difficult to ascertain in rodents, and, in fact, may be species-specific.

A particular toxicity associated with the administration of interferon to humans and experimental animals has been depression of the cytochrome P-450 monooxygenase (MFO) metabolizing enzymes. As a consequence of MFO inhibition following treatment with IFN, the sleep-time of mice treated with hexabarbital is increased, as is the toxicity of acetaminophen (Stebbing and Weck, 1984). Possible effects on the metabolism of chemotherapeutic agents or other drugs processed by the P-450 MFOs should be anticipated.

The *in vivo* antitumor effects of interferons are believed to be related to both augmentation of natural killer cell activity and antiproliferative effects. Antiproliferative activity probably also accounts for the bone marrow suppression observed in some individuals given IFN and could potentially produce effects in a routine preclinical reproduction or teratology evaluation. Dosing studies performed in newborn mice with homologous IFN have resulted in death at high doses and a marked wasting syndrome when given over an extended period (Gresser and Bourali, 1970). Both effects were attributed to the antiproliferative activity of IFNs. Inhibition of proliferation and metabolism represent potential dose-limiting toxicities of this family of rDNA molecules.

## 12.5. MONOCLONAL ANTIBODY TECHNOLOGY

Offering an impressive potential for human therapy, monoclonal antibodies have become the first commercialized products of the new biotechnology. They are now becoming widely used in diagnostic medicine and are proposed as potential therapeutic agents in cancer. In clinical diagnostic medicine they have provided us with the sensitivity not heretofore available for specific and rapid diagnosis of a particular drug level or infectious disease process.

Antibodies are important in the body as defense against infectious agents. They are extremely specific proteins that are produced in response to a foreign material, or antigen, by lymphoid cells of the immune system and share the property of being able to bind specifically to the inducing antigenic epitope (a single antigenic determinant; that portion of the antigen which combines with the antibody paratope). Unfortunately, under most conditions of antigenic stimulation, a family of antibodies is produced, each with a slightly different antigenic specificity.

In 1975, Kohler and Milstein observed that if an antibody-producing cell was fused with a myeloma tumor cell, a rapidly dividing hybrid was produced that synthesized a monospecific antibody. Each hybridoma formed then became a "factory," producing antibodies monospecific to a particular sensitizing antigenic epitope. Cell cloning allows selection of hybrids producing antibodies with the desired characteristics.

Monoclonal antibodies are thought to represent a major advance in cancer therapy because they have a very high therapeutic-to-toxic index when compared with anticancer drugs or radiation therapy, and should provide a greater degree of specificity for the tumor cell than other forms of therapy. The conjugation of toxins with monoclonal antibodies is theoretically very exciting because a high specific toxin activity could be achieved at the tumor target cell.

Clinically, monoclonal antibodies are also proposed as drug delivery vehicles in certain tumors where specific tumor-associated antigens are expressed. In this context, investigators have found that by conjugating toxins such as the A chain polypeptide of the plant protein ricin or the bacterial toxin from *Corynebacterium diphtheriae* to monoclonal antibodies specific for certain tumor type, as few as one or two molecules of antibody–toxin conjugate can destroy a tumor cell *in vitro*. Some success has also been obtained in clinical trials with monoclonal antibody-toxin conjugates.

Monoclonal antibodies have also been proposed for detoxification of individuals suffering from drug overdose or chemical intoxication, as well as for radioimaging of tumor burden or metastatic foci. In veterinary medicine, monoclonal antibodies are already being used to develop new rapid methods for diagnosis of infections in poultry, cattle and other animals.


### 12.5.1 Toxicological Concerns with Monoclonal Antibodies

It is already clear that there are certain problems implicit in the use of monoclonal antibodies in therapeutic trials. For example, there may be modulation of the antigenic determinant on the target cell, so that the monoclonal antibody cannot recognize its appropriate antigenic epitope. Second, the tumor cell may release free antigens so that the monoclonal antibody is effectively neutralized before it can reach the target cell. Third, antibodies to mouse epitopes on the monoclonal antibody could be induced (this may be overcome in the future by the use of human-human hybrids or the use of immunosuppressive agents to prevent the development of antibodies). Fourth, monoclonal antibodies have an extremely short half-life in systemic circulation, which would require that they be intermittently infused to provide the beneficial effect. Last, there may be an unwanted release of the toxin from its conjugate; or specificity problems may develop, whereby the antibody-toxin conjugates end up in an inappropriate organ.

The clinical toxicology findings associated with the use of monoclonal antibodies in therapeutic trials have included fever, chills, flushing, dyspnea, hypotension and tachycardia, anaphylactic and anaphylactoid reactions, urticaria, rash, nausea, elevated creatinine levels, headache, bronchial spasm, and serum sickness (Oldham, 1983). Few of these reactions might be predicted from safety evaluation in rodents. A major problem with using the intact ricin or diphtheria toxin molecule, containing both the A and B polypeptide chains, has been the dissociation of the parent molecule from the monoclonal antibody, leading to toxicity of the reticulo-endothelial system. A promising solution to this problem comes from separating the A chain (toxic moiety) from the B chain (cell association moiety) and preparing only A chain conjugates. This results in much lower toxicity if the A chain should become dissociated from the antibody conjugate because cellular association does not occur.

Since a monoclonal antibody is a fusion product of a malignant mouse cell and an antibody-producing cell, there is some concern about the safety of the production process itself (Petricciani, 1983). Methods for the production of monoclonal antibodies raise two general safety issues: (1) the theoretical risk of transferring in the product factors associated with malignancy (e.g., oncogene factors); and (2) the use of animals for antibody production that are known to harbor a number of microbial agents some of which can produce diseases in humans.

Preclinical studies should address the potential toxicity due to inappropriate release of the conjugated toxin. Preclinical toxicology of monoclonal antibodies may not require extensive animal studies but should be examined for cross-reactivity with antigenic epitopes present on normal cells *in vitro* and for the presence of human or rodent viruses. Early clinical trial should involve biodistribution studies with radiolabelled material.

## 12.6. BIOPROCESS TECHNOLOGY

In the chemical and pharmaceutical industry, recombinant DNA technology will allow the synthesis of chemicals that can only be practically achieved through a bioprocess. For example, methylation of a particular carbon in a chemical structure might be done quite easily with a recombinant-engineered bacteria. This technology will allow the synthesis of a family of isomers and the development of a synthetic process that cannot be achieved by strict physical chemical processes.

This area of recombinant DNA technology also has application in the degradation of solid waste materials: In waste water recovery, in leaching minerals from ore-containing rock, in improved oil recovery, and in the decontamination of chemical waste dumps through the engineering of microorganisms that can destroy specific toxic contaminants.

## 12.7. GENE THERAPY PRODUCTS

Gene therapy products, while holding tremendous promise, have so far delivered but limited (two cases as of this writing) positive outcomes. The concept involved—inserting functioning genes in place (or places) where nonfunctional or malfunctioning genes have produced a disease state—is stunning. But the public outcry over the death of Jesse Gelsinger, an 18-year-old, in a clinical trial at the University of Pennsylvania's Institute of Human Gene Therapy in 2000 has lead to a significant slowdown in the rate of evaluation. This tragic event, probably due to an innate immune response to a protein in the vector's protein coat (Stephenson, 2001), has led to increased restrictions.

Five aspects specific to gene therapy need to be evaluated to assess the safety of a therapy.

1. DNA/RNA biodistribution.
2. Gene transfer and biological activity.
3. Risk of vertical transmission of the gene.
4. The safety of the vector (the means of delivering the gene to the intended site).
5. The safety of the product protein.


1. *Evaluate DNA/RNA Biodistribution*
   Radiolabeling
   Southern Blot
   PCR
   Real time PCR
   *In situ* PCR

2. *Evaluate Gene Transfer and Biological Activity*

Immuno-histo-chemistry

Western Blot

ELISA (Enzyme-linked immunoabsorbant assay)

Flow cytometry

3. *Evaluate The Risk Of Vertical Transmission*

To gonads (If yes, then look at semen/germ cells), [If so, how long (persistence)?]

To circulating blood probably required anyway.

4. *Assess the Safety of the Vector*

Identify a suitable model species.

Assess the acute toxicity of the vector particle (in rabbits).
   At high dose, potential for an anaphylactic response (not seen in mice).
   Also look for neutrophil proliferation.

5. *Assess the safety of the product protein*

Use data from preclinical pharmacology toxicology ("safety") studies to support the safety of clinical trials.

Ones not appropriate for genotoxicity testing (instead, assess integration/ insertion frequency in a mammalian cell).

Standard rodent carcinogenicity *probably* not appropriate.

Regulatory authority for gene therapy products is unique in that overlapping responsibilities extend to both CBER and NIH.

CBER: Division of Cell and Gene Therapies

   Manufacturing

Division of Clinical Trial Design and Analysis

   Preclinical pharmacology and toxicology

   Clinical trial design, safety and efficacy

   20% of CBER clinical protocols are now for gene therapy.

   NIH: Recombinant DNA Advisory Committee (RAC)

   No authority for approval for clinical trials, but all adverse events must be reported

This duplicating of authority has led to both misunderstanding and problems in trials, as investigators must report adverse responses to both, but each has a different definition of what constitutes a reportable adverse response.

Currently, gene therapy is restricted to life-threatening and severely disabling diseases, but when a larger safety database has been accumulated there should be expanded opportunities for therapy. It is not possible or desirable to identify a uniform "recipe" for the safety studies that should be conducted with gene therapy products, to support either the first dose in humans or extended clinical evaluation. Each product should be treated on a case-by-case basis, taking into consideration a number of important factors, such as the clinical indication, the duration of expression of the gene, and whether DNA transfer will be *in vivo* or *ex vivo*. For example, elimination of a tumor may require short-term treatment such as the transient expression of a suicidal gene. On the other hand, treatment may be long-term, such as the replacement of a missing enzyme in the liver, where the goal may be life-time expression. Gene therapy is currently an area of limited but rapidly advancing knowledge, and a study design should be based on previous experience, together with ongoing feedback from the clinic throughout development. Considerable early thought should also be given to appropriate assays and their sensitivities. The choice of assay will need to be justified and the basic "tool kit" of assays properly considered and evaluated in advance.

## 12.7.1 Vectors

In gene therapy, genes typically are delivered using a vector which may be nonviral or viral. The complete construct should be tested; separate safety evaluation studies of vectors *per se* are not generally recommended except to explore mechanisms of action if potentially harmful effects have been demonstrated in a previous investigation, for example, red cell agglutination on intravenous administration. If a novel nonviral vector is to be used, evidence of its lack of toxicity and information on its basic pharmacokinetics will be an essential component of the preclinical package. The interaction between the vector and the gene is quite important, perhaps more so with the nonviral gene therapeutics, where the physicochemical properties of the particles themselves very much determine which tissues take up the gene. For viral vectors it is important to have sufficient knowledge of how they replicate, how to render the viruses replication-incompetent, any inherent pathogenicity and immunogenicity, and any risk of recombination with wild-type virus.

Conventional pharmaceutical quality assurance procedures should be applied to gene therapy products as well as appropriate infectivity tests for self-replicating, living vectors.

## 12.7.2 Studies to Support the First Dose in Humans

The most scientific approach is to replicate, in an appropriate animal, the type of dosing that would be expected to be used in humans, employing the "dose for dose: animal to human" principle. A single, suitable animal species should suffice. If viral vectors are used, the animal species should be sensitive to infection by the wild-type virus. Studies should not automatically be done in primates but, initially, the commonly used laboratory species should be utilized. Only if those are demonstrated to be unsuitable should the next step be to consider the use of a primate.

Based on these general principles, the first dose in humans should be supported by a single-dose study in an appropriate animal species by the intended clinical route. Several dose levels should be explored, as some gene therapy expression products have a narrow therapeutic index.

There are many circumstances when a single-dose intravenous (IV) study can provide useful information; for example, if the intended treatment route is intraperitoneal (i.p.), or if the product will be administered to an open wound or injected into a muscle or a tumor, it might accidentally enter a blood vessel, and the knowledge gained from an IV study would be of value as well as one by the clinical route. Hence, if the intended clinical route is not IV, the absence of an additional study with IV dosing would require specific justification.

The physiological consequences of the gene product should be explored in these studies, particularly with totally novel gene products. In addition, all the standard toxicological evaluations should be carried out, including examination of functional endpoints *in vivo* including cardiovascular and respiratory effects, and so on.

### 12.7.3  Distribution of the Gene and Gene Product

The distribution of the gene must be evaluated carefully in timepoint assays. The choice of assay used, with regard to their specificity and sensitivity, must be justified. The objectives are to identify the tissues in which the gene is present, demonstrate whether or not the gene product is expressed in particular tissues, and to demonstrate the time course of gene expression, that is, how long it persists.

Some regulatory authorities, including the U.K., are particularly concerned that the possibility of alteration to germ line cells should be excluded. Both male and female gonads should therefore be examined. If the gene is found there, then it is necessary to examine the gonads at a more detailed level to ascertain whether the gene is present in the actual germ cells. Where gene persistence is short as, for example, in nonintegrating nonreplicating vectors, assay of the gonads at an appropriate timepoint will minimize false positive findings.

### 12.7.4.  Studies to Support Multiple Doses in Humans

The animal studies should parallel the intended treatment regime in humans. At their present stage of development, a single dose of a gene therapeutic may not be totally curative, so multiple cycles of treatment may be used clinically rather than a single period of administration. It is appropriate to explore this in animal safety work, i.e. the cycle regimen should be paralleled in the animal, up to a maximum of three cycles. The duration of follow-up in the test animals after completion of the last test cycle should be based on the duration of gene expression, up to a maximum of 6 months. There may be situations, particularly if long-term gene expression is the goal, when there could be an argument for a longer follow-up but that should be considered on a case-by-case basis.

There should not be blind adoption of a checklist of assays and observations, but appropriate investigations should be selected, based on earlier findings in the single-dose studies. Increasing the number of doses raises more concern about the immune response. There may be indications of this, such as lymphocyte infiltration at the site of administration, and there are many markers from single-dose studies that would indicate when it might be appropriate to examine the immune response to the gene product and selection markers; for example, immunity to adenoviral vectors, or to expressed proteins, resulting in accelerated loss of the transgene.

### 12.7.5. Unnecessary Studies

Genotoxicity and carcinogenicity studies are not generally recommended or required. Eliminating the possibility of the gene being inserted in the germ line ensures that some elements of concern about reproduction toxicology have already been addressed; hence, classical reproduction and developmental toxicity studies are not generally recommended. They should be considered on a case-by-case basis; for example, if the treatment were to be intended to manage a long-term metabolic disease and the patients would then survive to reach reproductive competence.

Drug interaction studies are not generally appropriate, with the exception of gene-directed enzyme pro-drug therapy (involving a gene expressing an enzyme that activates a prodrug given subsequently). In the latter case, it is necessary to demonstrate the presence of the prodrug as well as the gene in the animal and to consider the potential toxicity of the active metabolite(s) both locally (which is the desired pharmacological effect) and systemically (the undesirable effects).

### 12.7.6. *Ex Vivo* Procedures

*Ex vivo* procedures involve removing cells and transfecting or transducing them. The cells should be checked to confirm that they are all healthy and that they are still expressing their normal surface markers, etc; observations of normal growth characteristics can also be reassuring. Animal studies are of limited value to test the safety of transfected or transduced human cells.

### 12.7.7. Change of Gene or Vector

Currently, only a limited number of vectors are available, although there is a large array of inserted genes. If the therapy involves developing a construct of a new gene in a well-characterized vector, it is important to use existing information on the vector. Rather than regenerating data on the vector itself, bridging studies of the construct should be carried out, that is, additional studies involving a limited toxicology evaluation to specifically characterize the nature of the new gene. Since the safety of the vector is already known, this should drive more exploration of the effects of the gene and the gene product, rather than the vector itself.

If the vector is changed, a full safety evaluation may be required. However, if the changes are minor compared to the structure of a fully evaluated vector, it is appropriate for safety to be addressed by bridging studies. For example, if there is only a minor change on one of the condensation peptides of a nonviral, self-assembling vector, then some simple bridging work, rather than a full evaluation, may be appropriate.

The possibility of abbreviated testing is referred to in *Points to Consider in Human Somatic Cell and Gene Therapy* (FDA, 1991), a guidance document on somatic cell and gene therapy published by the U.S. FDA. According to that guideline, if changes are made to the vector backbone which do not alter the safety properties of the vector, and the same route of administration and a similar dosing regimen is used to that employed previously, then truncated testing may be appropriate, depending upon the gene being expressed. When a promoter sequence or a targeting sequence in a viral or nonviral vector is changed, or the expression of viral gene products is considerably altered, the vector should be considered as a new vector, even though it may have the same gene as the previous version of that vector.

### 12.7.8  Change of Route

It is quite possible that a treatment may be initiated using, for example, intratumoral injections to deliver a gene, which may subsequently be administered systemically. As a considerable amount of relevant information will have already been generated to support the intratumoral route, this would be another case for doing bridging studies. Comparative distribution studies will help to identify how much more safety evaluation may be required.

### 12.7.9  Insertional Mutagenesis

The long-term management of genetic disorders will require integration of the therapeutic DNA into the host genome, or the maintenance of a stable episomal gene. The target of homologous recombination is still not achievable and until that time, the problem of insertional mutagenesis, that is, inappropriate insertion of DNA into the host genome, must be addressed. How can the risk be quantified? Characterization of gene expression over time is more important than the copy number of the gene. An increased copy number can equate to an increased risk of insertional mutagenesis, but on the other hand it also equates to an increase in the desired product. Insertional mutagenesis is a safety problem, and it is important to advise and warn patients who receive genes which will become integrated into the genome of this potential risk associated with their treatment.

### 12.8.  VACCINES

Vaccination against viral and bacterial diseases has been one of the success stories of human and veterinary medicine. Probably the most outstanding example of the effectiveness of vaccination is the eradication of smallpox. In 1967 between 10 and 15 million cases of smallpox occurred annually in some 33 countries. By 1977 the last naturally occurring case was reported in Somalia. Polio, too, has been controlled in developed countries, for example the number of cases in the USA was reduced from over 40,000 per year in the early 1950s, before a vaccine was available, to only a handful of cases in the 1980s. Diphtheria is now almost unheard of yet over 45,000 cases in 1940 led to 2480 deaths from diphtheria in the U.K. (similar numbers to those who died from AIDS in the U.K. in the entire 1980s). This has been reduced in the U.K. to only 13 cases and no deaths from the bacterium between 1986 and 1991. The scale of the problem is enormous: over 10 million deaths worldwide per year are due to infectious disease. UN figures suggest that cancers, circulatory problems, and injuries cause fewer deaths in developing countries than infectious diseases.

The process of developing vaccines is becoming increasingly complex due both to the nature of the infections being protected against and the nature of the cultures in which the affected individuals live. Kaufmann (1996) provided an excellent addressal of this process and the inherent problems.

## 12.8.1. Approaches to Vaccination

There are two classical strategies for vaccination. One involves vaccination with either killed pathogenic organisms or subunits of the pathogenic organism. The other utilizes live attenuated viruses or bacteria that do not cause disease but have been derived from the pathogenic parent organism.

Inactivated vaccines are made from virulent pathogens by destroying their infectivity usually with $\beta$-propiolactone or formalin to ensure the retention of full immunogenicity. Vaccines prepared in this way are relatively safe, and stimulate circulating antibody against the pathogens surface proteins, thereby conferring resistance to disease. Two or three vaccinations are usually required to give strong protection and booster doses are often required a number of years later to top up flagging immunity.

Subunit vaccines can be seen as a subcategory of inactivated vaccines because similar considerations apply to subunits and whole organisms. Doses, routes, duration of immunity, and efficacy of these vaccines are all very comparable. In this case a part of the pathogen, such as a surface protein, is used to elicit antibodies that will neutralize the infectivity of the pathogenic agent. The widespread use of hepatitis B virus surface antigen purified from the blood of carriers (or more recently from recombinant yeast) shows that this can be a very effective way to immunize. Hepatitis B virus surface antigen, the product of a single gene, assembles into a highly antigenic 22 nm particle which if used in three 40 µg doses at 0, 1, and 6 months gives virtually complete protection against infection with hepatitis B virus.

Another example that can be included in the subunit vaccine class is the use of bacterial toxoids. Many bacteria produce toxins which play an important role in the development of the disease caused by a particular organism. Thus, vaccines against some agents, for example tetanus and diphtheria, consist of the toxin inactivated with formaldehyde conjugated to an adjuvant. Immunization protects from disease by stimulating antitoxin antibody which neutralizes the effects of the toxin.

A further type of vaccine included in the subunit category is the capsular polysaccharide vaccines, for example, those against *Haemophilus influenzae* and meningococcal meningitis. In this case an extract of the polysaccharide outer capsule of the bacterium is used as a vaccine and is sometimes conjugated to protein to improve immunogenicity. Antibody persists for several years and is able to protect against the bacterium.

About half of all vaccines have traditionally been from live attenuated mutants of parent pathogenic organisms (Walker and Gingold, 1993). In effect, live vaccines mimic natural infection, yet produce subclinical symptoms and elicit long-lasting immunity, often giving rise to resistance at the portal of entry. Most of today's attenuated vaccine strains have been derived by a tortuous, often emperical, route involving passage in culture until the pathogen is found to lose its virulence. This loss of virulence is tested in animal model systems before being tested in human volunteers. For example the vaccine used to immunize against tuberculosis was derived after 13 years' passage in bile-containing medium by Calmette and Guerin (hence the name BCG (bacille Calmette–Guerin).

There has been much debate over the past 40 years as to the relative merits of live and killed vaccines, often generating more heat than light! The evidence is that both routes will give adequate vaccines that can be used to protect against disease under the appropriate conditions. Table 12.6 summarizes the major points of debate. Many

**TABLE 12.6  Relative Merits of Live versus Killed Vacines**

|  |  | Live | Killed/subunit |
| --- | --- | --- | --- |
| Production | Purification[a] | Relatively simple | More complex |
|  | Cost | Low[b] | Higher |
|  | Route | Natural or injection | Injection |
|  | Dose | Low, often single | High, multiple |
| Administration | Adjuvant | None | Required[d] |
|  | Heat lability | Yes | No |
|  | Need for refrigeration[c] | Yes | Yes |
|  | Antibody response | IgG; IgA | IgG |
| Efficacy | Duration of immunity | Many years | Often less |
|  | Cell mediated response | Good | Poor |
|  | Interference |  |  |
|  |  | Occasional OPV only[e] | No |
| Safety | Reversion to virulence | Rarely[f] |  |
|  | Side effects | Low level[g] | No |

[a] Increasing safety standards means that for new vaccines some of the older methodologies would not be acceptable.

[b] The price for new vaccines will approach that of killed subunit vaccines as safety standards are increased.

[c] The need for refrigeration increases the costs significantly.

[d] Very few adjuvants for human use are acceptable.

[e] Especially in the Third World.

[f] At very low levels (less than 1 case per $10^6$ vaccinations).

[g] This varies from occasional mild symptoms with rubella and measles vaccines to possible brain damage with pertussis vaccine.

factors including cost, safety, number of immunizations, ease of access to vaccines, politics, and social acceptance will determine whether there is a high uptake of a particular vaccine and whether it is ultimately successful in eradicating the target disease. Even if a perfectly viable, relatively safe vaccine is available, uptake may be limited. For example, it has been estimated that vaccination against measles within the WHO EPI has prevented over 60 million cases and 1.37 million deaths. Despite these efforts, there are still some 70 million cases of measles annually resulting in nearly 1.5 million deaths; consequently a recent WHO congress adopted the following goals:

(i)  Increasing immunization coverage;

(ii)  Improving surveillance;

(iii)  Developing laboratory services and improving vaccine quality;

(iv)  Training;

(v)  Promoting social mobilization;

(vi)  Developing rehabilitation services;

(vii)  Research and development.

This also serves to illustrate the importance of factors other than the efficacy of the vaccine itself in disease prevention.

The single most important issue in developed countries is the safety of a vaccine, a single death in a million vaccinations for a new vaccine would be unacceptable (except possibly if it were an effective AIDS vaccine). While this is obviously important in a Third World country, other issues such as cost and how to deliver the vaccine are of paramount importance.

## 12.8.2. Genetic Engineering and Vaccine Development

Not all protective antigens are as simple to identify, clone, and express as the surface antigen gene of hepatitis. The entire sequence of the hepatitis B virus genome became available and as it is less than 10 kb it was relatively simple to establish which open reading frame to express. It has been known for many years that irradiated malarial sporozoites protect against malaria. Because the sporozoite stage in the life cycle of the malarial parasite can only be grown in small quantities, it was left to recombinant DNA technology to identify, clone, and express components of the sporozoite that might be of use in vaccine production. The genome of the malarial parasite is many thousands of times larger than the genome of HBV and therefore provides a different scale of problem, not only was there little sequence data available but there was also no idea of which gene products may be protective.

The starting point of any recombinant DNA work is to generate a library of DNA in *E. coli* which is representative of the organism under study (Mackett, 1993). Once having a cDNA bank or a genomic library is developed, there are three basic ways of identifying and isolating a gene of interest.

***DNA/Oligonucleotide Hybridization.*** If there is some pre-existing knowledge of the nucleic acid sequence, or where purified mRNA is available, it is possible to detect recombinant clones by hybridization of $^{32}$P labeled DNA or RNA to bacterial colonies or bacteriophage plaques. Often a protein has been purified and some amino acid sequence is available which allows a corresponding nucleic acid sequence to be synthesized. Due to the degeneracy of the genetic code a complex mixture of oligonucleotides is required to ensure that all possible sequences are represented. Labeling this mixture of oligonucleotides yields a probe that can be used to screen a cDNA (or possibly genomic) library that might be expected to contain the gene of interest.

***Hybrid Selection and Cell Free Translation.*** A second approach is to use hybrid selection of mRNA coupled with cell free translation. DNA clones from a library, either individually or in pools of clones, can be immobilized by binding them to a solid support and mRNA hybridized to them. Only the mRNA that corresponds to the clones will bind and this can then be eluted and translated to protein in a cell free system. The protein can then be immunoprecipitated with antisera to the gene product of interest or assayed for activity. An example that encompasses both this approach and the sequence route is in the development of a vaccine for Epstein-Barr virus. It had been known since 1980 that antibody to the major membrane antigen of the virus (gp350/220) would neutralize the virus. Around 1983 a fragment of the virus genome was cloned and sequenced; using computer predictions, the gp340/220 gene was identified. The experimental evidence that confirmed this prediction was published in 1985 and came from experimental work that managed to hybridize select EBV mRNA using genomic DNA clones. This was followed by cell free translation of the eluted mRNA and immunoprecipitation of gm350/220 with a high titre antibody. The DNA clone that hybridized with the gm340/220 mRNA was the one predicted to encode the gp340/220 gene by computer analysis. The hybrid selection approach is rather labor intensive and has for the most part been superseded by one of the forms of expression cloning.

***Expression Cloning.*** This approach is invaluable when the only means of identification is an antisera against the protein or pathogen of interest. Probably the most laborious form of this approach is its use in conjunction with a biological assay. cDNA libraries are cloned into a plasmid that will allow expression in eukaryotic cells, for example, SV40 or EBV vectors. Clones or pools of clones are then transferred to appropriate cell types, for example, COS cells for SV40 vectors, and cell extracts or cell supernatant is assayed for biological activity. If a pool of clones gives the biological activity then the individual clones can be reassayed and the desired cDNA clone identified. This methodology, although tedious, has allowed many of the interleukin genes to be cloned, probably because the assays for these proteins are very sensitive.

Other gene products or vaccine antigens may require an enrichment step. For example, many genes expressed on the cell surface, that is, receptors, adhesion molecules, and so on have been cloned by "panning" techniques where the cells expressing the gene of interest are selected out either with antibody or by interaction with other cells. cDNA libraries are constructed in *E. coli* and the library is transferred to eukaryotic cells. Those cells expressing the gene of interest are enriched for the desired trait and the library transferred back to *E. coli*; this can be done for several rounds of expression and eventually individual clones conferring the selected phenotype will be isolated.

The most extensively used form of expression cloning involves the use of plasmid or bacteriophage vectors in *E. coli* and identification of DNA clones using antisera to the protein of interest. Here a vector such as the bacteriophage $\lambda$gt11 is set up so that when cDNA fragments are cloned into sites adjacent to the $\beta$-galactosidase gene, bacteria will express a $\beta$-galactosidase fusion protein containing epitopes present in the cDNA. Recombinant phage are detected with antisera. The cDNA insert is then sequenced and the whole gene can then be isolated in a more traditional way. The antisera used can be monoclonal antibodies, polyclonal monospecific antisera, or even polyclonal antisera with many antibody specificities present. A variation on this method allowed the initial cloning of the malarial sporozoite surface antigen. Malarial sporozoite stage cDNAs were introduced into the ampicillin resistance gene of the plasmid pBR322. Low levels of expression of the sporozoite surface antigen were detected by solid phase radioimmunoassay using a monoclonal antibody specific for the protein. In this way a cDNA clone coding for the antigen was isolated and subsequently sequenced. This information was then used to design peptide vaccines which have already been tested in humans.

The $\lambda$gt11 system is a more sophisticated bacteriophage version of the plasmid system described above and has been used to isolate many different antigens from various stages in the life cycle of the human malarial parasite using human immune sera as well as antigens from pathogens.

***Expression of Potential Vaccine Antigens.*** In general, in the future, eukaryotic cell culture is likely to be the method of choice for the production of subunit vaccine antigens where the organism to be vaccinated against replicates in eukaryotic cells. *E. coli* are unable to posttranslationally modify some vaccine candidates; for example, bacterial systems cannot add carbohydrate which is important in the antigenicity and structure of many protective antigens.

Since 1986, the USFDA has approved 22 vaccines (Table 12.7), half of them from a genetic engineering (and all, of course, from a biotechnology source). The cells used for such genetic engineering production of vaccine can be mammalian, insect or bacterial.

CBER has provided broad guidelines on the evaluation and production of vaccines (CBER, 1997). In general, the Center's requirements have paralleled those for other biotechnology products. Beyond establishing sterility, lack of pyrogenicity and of viral contaminants, a single GLP toxicity study in an appropriate species (one that has been established, if possible, to be immune responsive to the vaccine) is required. If the vaccine is to be used in pregnant women or women of childbearing potential, a segment I style reproductive study should be performed in an appropriate animal species.

**TABLE 12.7. Vaccines Approved by USFDA since 1986**

| Vaccine | Indication | Date approved | Company |
|---|---|---|---|
| Recombivax HB | Hepatitis B | June 23, 1986 | Merck, Chiron |
| ProHIBIT | Haemophilus influenza B | 1988 | Connaught |
| Pedvax | HIB | 1989 | Merck |
| Engerix-B | Hepatitis B | 1989 | SmithKlineBeecham |
| Tetramune, Hib TITR Haemophilis b, diphtheria CRM 197 protein conjugate | Bacterial Meningitus | Jan. 1991 | Lederle-Praxis Biologics/American Cyanamid |
| IPOL | Poliovirus vaccine inactivated-injected | 1991 | Inst. Merieux |
| Acel-Imune | Diphtheria, tetanus toxoids acellular pertussis vaccine | Jan. 6, 1992 | Takeda Chemical Industries/American Cyanamid |
| Tripedia | Diphtheria, tetanus toxoids and acellular pertussis | Aug. 20, 1992 | Connaught Laboratories Inc. |
| JE-VAX | Japanese encephalitis | Dec. 18, 1992 | Connaught/Biken |
| Enzon | Bubonic plague | 1994 | Green Labs |
| Typhim Vi | Typhoid | 1994 | Laboratories Inc. |
| Havrix | HAV | Mar. 1995 | SmithKlineBeecham |
| Varivax, Varicella Virus Vaccine Live | Chicken pox | Apr. 10, 1995 | Merck |
| VAQTA | Hepatitis A | Mar. 29, 1996 | Merck |
| COMVAX | Haeomophilis B and Hepatitis B | Oct. 2, 1996 | Merck |
| Infanivir | Diphtheria, tetanus and pertussis (DTP) | Jan. 27, 1997 | SmithKlineBeecham |
| Rabovert | Rabies (pre- and post-exposure) | Oct. 27, 1997 | Chiron/Behring |
| Certina | DTP | Jul. 29, 1998 | North American Vaccine |
| RotaShield[a] | Rotavirus | Aug. 31, 1998 | Wyeth |
| LYMEriv | Lyme Disease | Dec. 21, 1998 | SmithKlineBeecham |
| Prevnar | Pneumococcal disease | Feb. 17, 2000 | Lederle |
| TWINRIX | Hepatitis A and B | May 11, 2001 | SmithKlineBeecham |

[a]Subsequently withdrawn.

Regulatory guidance for the conduct of clinical trials on vaccines is specific. Traditional phase I trials in normal volunteers are not conducted. Rather, all trials assess not only safety but also efficacy (or at least immunogenicity). Trials may well be challenge trials, that is, after immunization subjects are purposely challenged with exposure to the infective agent of concern.

In any case, injection site responses (erythemia, edema, pain, and tenderness) and systemic responses are both evaluated in subjects (Mathieu, 1997). USFDA also has specific guidance on the tracking and reporting of adverse clinical responses to vaccines. Any adverse events or product problems with vaccines should not be sent to MedWatch but to the Vaccine Adverse Event Reporting System (VAERA), operated jointly by FDA and the national Centers for Disease Control and Prevention. For a copy of the VAERS form, call 1-800-822-7967, or download the form (in PDF format) from www.fda.gov/cber/vaers/vaers1.pdf on FDA's Website.

## 12.9. SPECIFIC CHALLENGES

The problem with using a classical toxicological approach for evaluating an rDNA product or species-specific protein is that standard protocols are probably inappropriate and nonrelevant in most cases. In the traditional approach to toxicology, a standard protocol or battery of tests is performed, followed by an estimation of the types of and degree of hazard or risk to humans. For example, conventional toxicity testing of a new rDNA product might lead to evaluation at excessively high doses in two rodent species. The production of antibody in the test species during preclinical toxicology testing may inactivate the test compound, and thus invalidate the toxicity evaluation.

This approach appears somewhat irrational and without much scientific merit, since many of these new molecules are minimally toxic or nontoxic by this sort of acute evaluation. As in the case of interferons or monoclonal antibodies, the toxic effects observed in humans might not be predicted from safety assessments in rodents. An appropriate test species should be selected. Is the rat or mouse the appropriate species to evaluate a species-specific rDNA protein such as human growth hormone or interferons, or would nonhuman primates be more suitable? Does the nonhuman primate really offer any advantages? There is some consensus that the nonhuman primate may be a more appropriate species for testing some rDNA human proteins.

In contrast, in the "pharmacological approach" to toxicology, the potential targets of toxicity are first identified (Zbinden, 1986). Then criteria for relevant effects are established, usually based on experience with reference substances, and appropriate *in vivo* or *in vitro* experimental models are selected to assess the pertinent toxicological responses.

Doses should be selected that are reasonable multiples of the proposed therapeutic dose to be employed, especially since in many cases the amount of material available for testing may be limited and not available in Kg amounts. Preclinical rodent or primate studies should merely provide the flags to monitor during Phase I clinical trials. Reason should prevail, not only in the selection of methods and models for assessing the potential toxicity of the new agents, but also in the use of these data for extrapolation to humans. Whether U.S. industry succeeds or fails in the biotechnology arena will depend on the quick resolution of issues such as selection of appropriate toxicologic tests, fermentation scale-up of the rDNA microbe, product purity, and expedition of regulatory pathways.

### 12.9.1. Purity and Homology

Major concerns in the production of a species-specific protein by rDNA technology are the purity of the product, the amount and type of contaminants present, and the homology of the product to the native molecule (Table 12.8). The toxicologist should be concerned about the acceptability and toxicity of intentional or inadvertent contaminants introduced during fermentation or isolation of the product (e.g., DNA, chemicals, *E. coli* proteins). Other issues concern the introduction of amino acid residues that might alter the three-dimensional structure or antigenicity of the molecule, partial denaturation of the product during isolation and recovery, genetic stability of the rDNA clone during production (mutation could result in altered amino acid sequence), and the level of foreign DNA present. Although these are issues of analytical biochemistry, their impact on the potential toxicity and overall safety of the finished product is of some toxicological concern.

### 12.9.2. Immunogenicity

The problem of the immunogenic nature of many human recombinant DNA proteins, and the potential to generate antibodies to a normal human protein, is of special interest to the immunotoxicologist. For example, 3 of 16 patients administered the rDNA-derived interferon-$\alpha$ (clone A) developed antibodies of the IgG class that were undetectable prior to or during therapy (Gutterman et al., 1982). These antibodies were capable of *in vitro* neutralization of interferon activity, although *in vivo* neutralization of interferon has not been documented. Since there are several different subtypes of interferon-$\alpha$'s, some contain epitopes not present on their own interferon subtype. Similarly, two patients treated with interferon-$\beta$ for many months developed high-titered antibody, which in one case was correlated with an inability of the patient's fibroblasts to produce interferon (Vallbracht et al., 1982).

**TABLE 12.8. Issues in the Safety Evaluation of Species-Specific rDNA Products**

Purity
Homology to native molecule
(Amino acid sequence, extra amino acids, three-dimensional structure)
Type and amounts of contaminants
(Chemicals, *E. coli* proteins, fermentation products, foreign DNA)

Stability of clone

Immunogenicity

Toxicities
(Direct or secondary to therapeutic effect)

Virtually all patients treated with conventional porcine insulin develop circulating anti-insulin antibodies (Klaff et al., 1978) that are less frequent and in lower titer in individuals treated with more highly purified porcine (Falholt, 1982) or rDNA human insulin (Fineberg et al., 1983). In the study by Fineberg and associates, 44% of the patients developed antibodies to rDNA human insulin over a 12-month period compared to a 60% antibody frequency with porcine insulin. Human growth hormone (HGH; Genentech, Inc.) prepared by rDNA technology was observed to produce a frequency of immunogenicity similar to that seen with human insulin (approximately 40% of the children developed antibody, according to the product insert). The ultimate goal is to develop rDNA products that will be less immunogenic than purified animal sources of these therapeutic agents.

The exact mechanism of the immunogenicity of species-specific rDNA proteins is unknown, but is believed to be attributable to (1) the addition of extra amino acid residues during synthesis, which the host reads as foreign; (2) denaturing of the native molecules or (3) contamination by *E. coli* polypeptides or lipopolysaccharides.

A second unanswered concern is whether the antibody induced by the recombinant protein has any discernible health effect. Other than some reports of neutralization of biological activity, little pathology has been attributed to the presence of antibodies in patients given recombinant protein therapy. It should also be noted that the question of antibody specificity has not been well studied, so that it is entirely conceivable that autoimmune pathology or even an anaphylaxis response could be induced. Equally important is the concern that induced antibody might neutralize the endogenous hormone or protein that it is intended to replace or supplement.

A third consideration is that certain routes of administration may favor immunogenicity of recombinant proteins. In early trials, rDNA proteins introduced by subcutaneous or intramuscular injections (procedures known to improve the immunogenicity of proteins) resulted in a higher frequency of antibody responses than in the intravenous route.

In summary, these are the clinically relevant questions about the immunogenicity of rDNA species-specific proteins: will antibody be induced in the recipient that will neutralize the therapeutic effect or lead to immune complex disease? What is the class (e.g., IgG or IgE) and specificity (i.e., reactivity against specific protein or contaminant) of the antibody induced? The former antibody type could potentially neutralize the product and produce immune complex disease, while the latter could result in an anaphylaxis response. It is possible that the antibody induced is of insignificant health consequence, and its presence is known only because of improvements made in the sensitivity of detection methods with the introduction of the enzyme-linked immunosorbent (ELISA) assay.


## 12.10. PLANNING A SAFETY EVALUATION PROGRAM

Safety evaluation of a candidate product should start with a consideration of specific nature and consequential hazards of the three P's:

- The producing system;
- The process;
- The product.

The need under each heading is to decide what data are required, then how to obtain them with the greatest efficiency and economy, and last, whether the toxicologist is necessarily the person with the appropriate skills and experimental techniques to do so. There will often be a trade-off between precise control by other means and possibly cheaper or more familiar, old-fashioned toxicological studies. The inventor of a new product or process, too, may often have to do a great deal of work to show safety by excluding hypothetical hazards, which subsequent manufacturers can afford to ignore.

***The Producing System.***    The questions of particular concern here are the nature of the system used to manufacture the desired substance, and the precision with which it is controlled. If the system consists of prokaryotic cells, then how well-defined is their provenance and how is their consistency demonstrated? If mammalian cells are employed, their lineage must be considered. In both instances, it is important to ensure that extraneous virus, infections, DNA and less well-defined factors such as "slow viruses" are excluded by the origins and history of the producer strain, or because the physical (e.g., filtration) or chemical (pH, solvents, affinity separation) nature of the production process can be relied upon to exclude passage of an infectious agent.

If the degree of safety arising from these factors is weak, the toxicologist should consider appropriate studies *in vivo* to exclude contaminating agents, oncogenic factors, and so on, but there is no point in doing short-term or prolonged animal experiments or other types of test unless the desired endpoint has first been clearly defined.

The aspect to which far more attention has been directed is the nature of the inserted gene(s) and promoters in rDNA products. Again, the toxicologist should ask how well the nucleotide sequence is known, whether there is only one reading frame, and how any introns are handled. Again, toxicity-type testing would appear to be an inefficient and expensive way to study molecular biology and biochemistry.

Last under this heading, for intact infectious organisms to be used directly in humans, assessment of pathogenicity to the range of individuals that make up our populations is needed, as well as consideration of the possibility of reversion to a wild and more dangerous strain, the hazard of an allergenic reaction to the organism (e.g., vaccinia) and the possibility of spread from subject to subject in a naïve or incompletely immune population.

There may be some role for animal experimentation here, if there is a suitable model, because it gives the chance to study the organism under intense pressure from commensals and the rising immune response.

Possible hazards in the manufacturing plant also need to be evaluated.

In general, conventional toxicity procedures seem to have little to offer here, except in specific instances of helping to exclude certain infection factors, perhaps ruling out oncogenicity and examining the stability of engineered organisms for direct infection of humans.

***The Process.*** Toxicologists have least to offer here. In fact, only their intellectual analysis and review of the literature should be required to asses the manufacturing process and any residues of its chemicals and so to set analytical limits on purity and residues in the final preparation.

***The Product.*** There are two distinct and probably divergent forces affecting the way in which toxicologists regard the final product. One is whether theirs is the first opportunity to learn about its biology and pharmacology, and the other is: What do scientific concern, clinical caution and industrial pace define as the minimum reasonable to do before clinical trial or marketing?

***Biology of Bioengineered Products.*** This may not be a useful concept scientifically, but it represents the practical point that the pace of development often forces the rapid sequence, (1) interesting biological property, (2) identification of the responsible molecule in very small amounts (e.g., tumor necrosis factor or erythropoietin), and (3) cloning, etc., resulting in large scale production, perhaps even before the full structure is known. The clinical interest in administering the substance to humans for investigative or therapeutic purposes must be balanced against the total lack of knowledge of its general effects on the body, or of the consequences of prolonged high level exposure to it of the function of interest.

As an example, there is the history of interferon, discovered through its antiviral actions, subsequently found to modulate mitosis and certain immune functions, capable of producing fever and probably ECG and EEG changes as evidence of membrane effects in excitable tissues, and so on. Were interferon a novel discovery, now just being produced for the first time, then investigation of its general biological effects on repeated administration to responsive animals would be important prior to a study in humans. The same arguments apply to the lymphokines, such as $\alpha$-IFN, IL-2, and so on.

The planning of this type of investigation as an empirical, open study of responses must be carefully related to the nature and what is known of the product concerned.

1. It is necessary to work in a species capable of responding to the principal activity. Interferons are notorious for their species specificity, but most other lymphokines at least are more generally active. Work in a primate may be required, but it depends on the substance to be tested. There may be no point in using more than one species in pivotal studies.

2. Any test should be as broad and as general as possible, that is, monitor many variables clinically, in the laboratory and by pathology, until enough is known for there to be confidence in a focused approach.

3. Relate any testing to the clinical circumstances of probable use. Thus, if a new synthetic antigen or engineered antigen is selected and is intended for testing,

for administration only a few times to humans, there would be no point in a multidose experiment. It should suffice to show that it was antigenic in the intended preparation. Unless there were a prior reason to do so, a special search for, say, auto-immune reactions seems unnecessary. Similarly, testing a monoclonal antibody for activity is likely to be difficult if not impossible, because of species specificity and the antigenicity of the preparation.

4. The toxicologist should be prepared to do nothing if the material is well-known, its properties are understood, and there is adequate characterization of the nature of the preparation supplied; for example, human insulin or growth hormone produced by genetic engineering should not be submitted to prolonged safety tests in animals, provided that the molecular forms present are sufficiently well understood.

It may be useful, however, to consider limited animal studies to examine the pharmacokinetics and duration of action even of a well-known material made by a new route, unless physiochemical analyses show that to be pointless.

## 12.10.1. Animal Models

Species selection is probably one of the most important considerations when designing a preclinical safety program; for a biotechnologically derived pharmaceutical, it requires an understanding of the biology of the product. Since most of these are either human proteins or target human receptors, they tend to be species-specific. Studies in rodents and dogs, the species commonly used in traditional toxicity studies, may not provide scientifically meaningful data. However, nonhuman primates are not necessarily the most appropriate species either, despite their phylogenetic similarity to human beings.

Some approaches that offer guidance in selecting relevant species include a literature review; determining the extent of homology between the endogenous animal protein and the human recombinant protein, determining the activity of the protein in pharmacological models and *in vivo* assays of the receptor/tissue binding.

A literature review may provide useful information about the physiological properties of the protein in animals and how they compare with those of the human protein. For example, prior to recombinant DNA technology, growth factors and/or hormones were purified from biological fluids. Although the quantities obtained were limited, they were nevertheless sufficient to allow investigation of the physiological properties of these proteins. Computer programs are now available for on-line searching of databases which hold information not only on the sequences of various animal and human proteins, but also the extent of homology between an animal protein and its human equivalent, including common amino acid sequences. It should be remembered, however, that a protein showing a high degree of monology to the human protein may not necessarily share similar pharmacological activities. Evaluation of activity or lack of activity in pharmacological animal models, if available, certainly would aid species selection. Finally, *in vitro* assays which analyze receptor and/or tissue binding are commonly used to determine the appropriate species for preclinical safety evaluation.

Some biotechnologically derived pharmaceuticals will cross-react with species that can be evaluated toxicologically, while others cross-react only with nonhuman primates such as the chimpanzee, a protected species. In this case, a well-designed "safety," or "Phase 0" study at doses higher than the proposed clinical dose may provide valuable safety information. However, a lack of cross-reactivity with any nonhuman species does not necessarily make preclinical safety evaluation impossible, not does it limit toxicity testing to species in which the protein lacks relevant pharmacological activity. Some alternative possibilities are summarized in Table 12.9.

Toxicity studies traditionally are conducted using "normal" animals. However, studies in animal disease models may provide additional safety information regarding the possibility of disease exacerbation. For example, the administration of human recombinant erythropoietin was associated with hypertension in patients with chronic renal failure, and also in uraemic dogs, but not in normal dogs.

Species differences must be considered when choosing a model and, in particular, species-specific immunological differences between the human and the test animal. For example, in humans, an anti-CD4 monoclonal antibody (MAb) will bind to CD4 expressed on monocytes, with subsequent fixing of complement and destruction of antigen-presenting cells. However, since CD4 molecules are not expressed on murine monocytes, these effects would not be evident in a murine model.

**TABLE 12.9. Alternative Models for Toxicity Assessment**

| Model | Example | Caveat |
|---|---|---|
| Nontraditional animal model | Transgenic mice carrying appropriate human receptor. | Antibody formation would need to be monitored, as it is probable that a large human protein would produce an immune response. |
| Homologous proteins and/or systems | Testing purified animal protein in the same species or, for monoclonal antibodies, testing an antibody directed against the receptor in the animal. | Data should be interpreted with caution as the biological properties of the animal protein may differ from those of the human protein. |
| *In vitro* methods | Tissue binding assays. | If no *in vivo* models are available, *in vitro* methods combined with *in vivo* testing in a pharmacologically nonreactive may suffice. |

### 12.10.2.  Study Design

It is questionable whether traditional toxicological paradigms are applicable to biological or protein agents. If they are not, then how can the clinician gain reassurance to administer the first dose to humans, to move into multidose trials and even assess the agent in combination with other established medicines or biological agents? Monoclonal antibodies, soluble cytokine receptors and growth factors have all been used in patients for nearly a decade, providing a wealth of experience in this area from which to learn. One of the most striking lessons is that pharmacodynamic effects may appear long after dosing of the agent has been discontinued.

As a class, biotechnologically derived pharmaceuticals share certain characteristics that have influenced their preclinical development. They are proteins and therefore toxicity was expected to be minimal and limited to an exaggeration of their desired pharmacological effects, a myth which was ultimately exploded. These agents are designed to perturb specific molecular or cell-to-cell interactions, sometimes with minimal effect on the pathophysiology of the target disease. Owing to the species-specific nature of these agents, preclinical toxicology is usually limited. For example, if a primatized anti-CD4 MAb cross-reacts only with chimpanzee and human CD4, the species of choice for toxicity tests is the chimpanzee, the use of which is restricted by its limited availability.

These characteristics of protein agents give rise to problems in clinical development, such that the traditional paradigm for preclinical testing may not be appropriate. The dose in animals may not be predictive of an appropriate starting dose for humans. A surrogate marker, for example, CD4 cell counts in the preclinical chimpanzee model, may be useful in setting the initial human dose, but may only serve to indicate a no-effect dose. Once in the clinic, trials conducted early in development are usually not sufficiently powered to distinguish effects due to the toxicity of the test agent from those due to, for example, the underlying disease, and concomitant or previous medications. Finally, short-term (3–6 months) preclinical studies do not necessarily predict the long-term effects of these agents.

The long-term toxicities of concern are opportunistic infections, lymphoproliferative disorders, and immunogenicity, manifesting as tachyphylaxis and/or allergic reactions. Preclinical approaches which serve to identify these as potential hazards to humans of a biologic drug moiety are thus needed.

The choice of toxicity studies, and the design of individual studies, will depend on the proposed clinical program. Important issues to consider are

- The frequency and route of administration, including the use of novel delivery systems.
- The duration of dosing.
- Special toxicity testing.

### 12.10.3.  Frequency and Route of Administration

Clinical trials for biotechnologically derived pharmaceuticals may be more complex than those for conventional pharmaceuticals and so the route and frequency of test drug administration should, if possible, mirror the proposed clinical use, even if that route employs a novel delivery system.

### 12.10.4. Duration

Traditionally, the duration of a toxicity study depends on the intended clinical use and disease duration. The potential immunogenicity of the human protein is a significant issue since antibody binding can partially or completely inhibit the biological activity of that protein, affect its catabolism or alter its distribution and clearance. Any multiple-dose study therefore should include evaluation of the impact of antibody formation, including their neutralizing capacity. However, antibody formation in itself should not be a reason for termination of a toxicity study, particularly if the antibodies are not neutralizing or do not alter the pharmaco-dynamics of the protein.

Multiple-dose toxicity studies are usually conducted before single-dose administration to volunteers. Many of the clinical trials for biological agents target life-threatening illnesses, and it has therefore been suggested that single-dose toxicity studies are sufficient to support single-dose "proof-of-concept" clinical studies. While this approach promotes faster introduction into the clinic, it may be of limited use since, once in many cases, there is a tendency to overlook the preclinical data. Clinical development may frequently not progress without interruption if relevant preclinical data are missing.

### 12.10.5. Special Toxicity Testing

In addition to multiple-dose studies, information on potential functional changes as obtained from safety pharmacology studies and the potential for genotoxicity, reproductive toxicity, and carcinogenicity may be required for registration. Once again, the species specificity of recombinant proteins may preclude the use of traditional animal species such as rodents and/or rabbits for safety pharmacology, reproductive toxicity and carcinogenicity studies. Functional evaluations of cardio-vascular and pulmonary systems could be incorporated into a nonhuman primate multidose toxicity study. If appropriate, potential reproductive toxicity can be evaluated in a nonhuman primate.

There may be situations which warrant an assessment of carcinogenic potential, but immunogenicity and species specificity may preclude a two-year rodent bioassay. It may be necessary to develop *in vitro* assays to address a particular concern. For example, growth factors which may have the potential to support or stimulate the growth of transformed cells should be assessed for their ability to promote growth of either malignant or normal cells.

Large molecular weight compounds are unlikely to react with DNA or other chromosomal material and therefore a genotoxicity evaluation may be of little value. However, genotoxicity studies may provide useful information about the safety of products containing organic linkers.

### 12.10.6. Program Design Considerations

The standard toxicological data package for any new drug entity typically evaluates

- Potential toxicity following single and multiple dosing.
- Genotoxic potential.
- Functional changes, that is, safety pharmacology studies.

In addition, depending on the proposed clinical plan, the following may need evaluation:

- Toxicity following chronic dosing.
- Carcinogenic potential.
- Possible reproductive toxicity.

Although biotechnologically derived pharmaceuticals often need customized preclinical development programs, certain issues are common to all. These include species specificity, potential immunogenicity and its impact on the duration of dosing, and the need for special toxicity testing.

## REFERENCES

CBER (1997). *Guidance for Industry for the Evaluation of Combination Vaccines for Preventable Diseases: Production, Testing and Clinical Studies.*

CBER (2000). *Guidance for Industry — Consideration for Reproductive Toxicity Studies for Preventive Vaccines for Infectious Disease Indications.*

CPMP (1989). Guidelines on the preclinical biological safety testing of medicinal products derived from biotechnology. *TIBTECH* 7: 613–617.

Dorato, M.A. and Vodicnik, M.J. (2001). The toxicological assessment of pharmaceutical and biotechnology products. In: *Principles and Methods of Toxicology*, (Hayes, A.W., Ed.). Taylor & Francis, Philadelphia, PA.

Falholt, K. (1982). Determination of insulin specific IgE in serum of diabetic patients by solid phase radioimmunoassay. *Diabetologia* 22: 254–257.

FDA (1996) Addendum to the points to consider in human somatic cell and gene cell therapy, *Human Gene Therapy* 1: 1181–1190.

Fent, K. and Zbinden, G. (1997). Toxicity of interferon and interleukin. *TIPS* 8: 100–105.

Fineberg, S.E., Galloway, J.A., Fineberg, N.S., Rathbun, M.J. and Hufferd, S. (1983). Immunogenicity of recombinant DNA human insulin. *Diabetologia* 25: 465–469.

Gresser, I. and Bourali, C. (1970). Development of newborn mice during prolonged treatment of interferon. *Eur. J. Cancer* 6: 553–556.

Gutterman, J.U., Fine, S., Quesada, J., Horning, S.J., Levine, J.F., Alexanian, R., Bernhardt, L., Kramer, M., Speigal, H., Colburn, W., Trown, P., Merigan, T. and Dziewanawska, Z. (1982). Recombinant leukocyte A interferon: Pharmacokinetics, single-dose tolerance, and biological effects in cancer patients. *Ann. Intern. Med.* 96: 549–556.

ICH (1997). *Preclinical Safety Evaluation of Biotechnology-Designed Pharmaceuticals.*

Kaufman, G.H.E. (1996). *Concepts in Vaccine Development*, Walter de Gruyter, New York.

Klaff, L.J., Vinik, A.I., Berelowitz, M. and Jackson, W.P.U. (1978). Circulating antibodies in diabetics treated with conventional and purified insulins. *S. Afr. Med J.* 54: 149–153.

Kohler, G. and Milstein, C. (1975). Continuous culture of fused cells secreting antibody of predefined specificity. *Nature* 256: 495–497.

Korwek, E.L. (1997). *United States Biotechnology Regulations Handbook.* FDLI, Washington, D.C.

Levine, M.M., Kaper, J.B., Lockman, H., Black, R.E., Clements, M.L. and Falkow, S. (1983). Recombinant DNA risk assessment studies in man: Efficacy of poorly mobilizable plasmids in biologic containment. *J. Infect. Dis.* 148: 699–709.

Mackett, M. (1993). Vaccination and Gene Manipulation. In: *Molecular Biology and Biotechnology*, 3rd ed. (Walker, J.M. and Gingold, E.B., Eds.). Royal Society of Chemists, Cambridge, U.K.

Malinowski, M.J. (1999). *Biotechnology: Law, Business and Regulation.* Aspen Law & Business, New York.

Mathieu, M. (1997). *Concepts in Vaccine Development*, Walter de Gruytor, New York.

Maulik, S. and Patel, S.D. (1997). *Molecular Biotechnology: Therapeutic Applications and Strategies.* Wiley-Liss, New York.

Oldham, R.K. (1983). Monoclonal antibodies in cancer therapy. *J. Clin. Oncol.* 1: 582–590.

Petricciani, J.C. (1983). An overview of safety and regulatory aspects of the new biotechnology. *Regulat. Toxicol. Pharmacol.* 3: 428–433.

Stebbing, N. and Weck, P.K. (1984). Preclinical assessment of biological properties of recombinant DNA-derived human interferons. In: *Recombinant DNA Products: Insulin, Interferon and Growth Hormone*, (Bollon, A.P., Ed.). CRC Press, Boca Raton, FL.

Stephenson, J. (2001). Studies Illuminate Cause of Total Reaction in Gene-Therapy Trial. *JAMA* 285: 2570–2571.

Thomas, J.A. and Myers, L.A. (1998). *Biotechnology and Safety Assessment.* Taylor & Francis, Philadelphia, P.A.

Vallbracht, A., Treuner, J., Manncke, K.H. and Niethammer, D. (1982). Autoantibodies against human *beta* interferon following treatment with interferon. *J. Interferon Res.* 2: 197.

Walker, J.M. and Gingold, E.B. (1993). *Molecular Biology and Biotechnology*, Royal Society of Chemists, Cambridge, U.K.

Weissinger, J. (1989). Nonclinical Pharmacologic and Toxicologic Considerations for Evaluating Biologic Products. *Regulatory Toxicol. Pharmacol.* 10: 255–263.

Zbinden, G. (1986). A toxicologist's view of immunotoxicology. In: *Proceedings of an International Seminar in the Immunological System as a Target for Toxic Damage*, CIJ, Everueax, France.

# 13

# FORMULATIONS, ROUTES, AND DOSAGE DESIGN

## 13.1. INTRODUCTION

Throughout the development process for pharmaceuticals, formulation development is proceeding with several objectives in mind. The importance of each of these factors changes over time (Monkhouse and Rhodes, 1998). Of first importence is optimizing the bioavailability of the therapeutic target organ site by the intended clinical route. Clinical route(s) are selected on a number of grounds (nature of the drug, patient acceptance, issues of safety). Second is minimizing any safety concerns. This means not just systemic toxicity but also local tissue tolerance at the site of application. Third is optimizing stability of the drug's active ingredient. Its activity and integrity must be maintained for long enough to be made effectively available to patients. Early on in preclinical development, simplicity and maximized bioavailability are essential. Early single-dose studies in animals are the starting place, and usually bear no relationship to the formulation used later.

Formulations used to administer potential drugs undergoing development occupy an unusual place in pharmaceutical safety assessment compared to the rest of industrial toxicology. Eventually, a separate function in the pharmaceutical company developing a drug will develop a specific formulation that is to be administered to people, a formulation that optimizes the conditions of absorption and stability for the drug entity (Racy, 1989). The final formulation will need to be assessed to see if it presents any unique local or short-term hazards, but as long as its nonactive constituents are drawn from the approved formulary lists, no significant separate evaluation of their safety is required preclinically. They can, of course, alter the toxicity of the drug under study.

442

Simultaneously with this development of an optimized clinical formulation, however, preclinical evaluations of the safety of the drug moiety must by performed. Separate preclinical formulations (which generally are less complex than the clinical ones) are developed, sometimes by a formulation group and other times by the toxicology group itself. These preclinical formulations will frequently include much higher concentrations of the drug moiety being tested than do any clinical formulations. The preclinical formulations are developed and evaluated with the aim of reproducibly delivering the drug (if at all possible by the route intended in humans), maintaining drug stability through an optimum period of time, and occluding the observed effects of the drug with vehicle effects to the minimum extent possible. These preclinical formulations are not restricted to materials that will (or even can) be used in final clinical formulations.

In pivotal studies, the actual blood levels of active moiety that are achieved will be determined so that correlations to later clinical studies can be made.

The formulations that are developed and used for preclinical studies are sometimes specific for the test species to be employed, but their development always starts with consideration of the route of exposure that is to be used clinically and, if possible, in accordance with a specified regimen of treatment (mirroring the intended clinical protocol. as much as possible). One aspect of both nonclinical and clinical formulation and testing which presents an important but often overlooked aspect of pharmaceutical safety assessment is the special field of excipients. These will be considered at the end of this chapter

Among the cardinal principles of both toxicology and pharmacology is that the means by which an agent comes in contact with or enters the body (i.e., the route of exposure or administration) does much to determine the nature and magnitude of an effect. However, a rigorous understanding of formulations, routes, and their implications to the design and analysis of safety studies is not widespread. And in the day-to-day operations of performing studies in animals, such an understanding of routes, their manipulation, means and pitfalls in achieving them, and the art and science of vehicles and formulations is essential to the sound and efficient conduct of a study.

As presented in Table 13.1 there are at least 26 potential routes of administration, of which 10 are commonly used in safety assessment and, therefore, are addressed here.


## 13.2. MECHANISMS

There are three primary sets of reasons why differences in formulations and the route of administration are critical in determining the effect of an agent of the biological system. These are (1) local effects, (2) absorption and distribution, and (3) metabolism.

1. *Local Effects*. Local effects are those that are peculiar to the first area or region of the body to which a test material gains entry or that it contacts. For the

**TABLE 13.1. Potential Routes of Administration**

A. Oral routes:
   1. Oral (PO)[a]
   2. Inhalation[a]
   3. Sublingual
   4. Buccal
B. Placed into a natural orifice in the body other than the mouth:
   1. Intranasal
   2. Intraauricular
   3. Rectal
   4. Intrafaginal
   5. Intrauterine
   6. Intraurethral
C. Parenteral (injected into the body or placed under the skin):
   1. Intravenous (IV)[a]
   2. Subcutaneous (SC)[a]
   3. Intramuscular (IM)[a]
   4. Intraarterial
   5. Intradermal (ID)[a]
   6. Intralesional
   7. Epidural
   8. Intrathecal
   9. Intracisternal
   10. Intracardial
   11. Intraventricular
   12. Intraocular
   13. Intraperitoneal (IP)[a]
D. Topical routes:
   1. Cutaneous[a]
   2. Transdermal (also called percutaneous)[a]
   3. Ophthalmic[a]

[a] Commonly used in safety assessment.

dermal route, these include irritation, corrosion, and sensitization. For the parenteral routes, these include irritation, pyrogenicity, sterility, and blood compatibility. In general, the same categories of possible adverse effects (irritation, immediate immune response, local tissue/cellular compatibility, and physicochemical interactions) are the mechanisms of, or basis for, concern.

In general, no matter what the route, certain characteristics will predispose a material to have local effects (and, by definition, if not present, tend to limit the possibility of local effects). These factors include pH, redox potential, high molar concentration, and the low flexibility and sharp edges of certain solids. These characteristics will increase the potential for irritation by any route and, subsequent to the initial irritation, other appropriate regional adaptive responses (for orally administered materials, for example, emesis and diarrhea).

2. *Absorption and Distribution.* For a material to be toxic, it must be absorbed into the organism (local effects are largely not true toxicities by this definition).

There are characteristics that influence absorption by the different routes, and these need to be understood by any person trying to evaluate and/or predict the toxicities of different moieties. Some key characteristics and considerations are summarized by route in the following list.

A. Oral and rectal routes (GI tract)
  1. Lipid-soluble compounds (nonionized) are more readily absorbed than water-soluble compounds (ionized).
     a. Weak organic bases are in the nonionized, lipid-soluble form in the intestine and tend to be absorbed there.
     b. Weak organic acids are in the nonionized, lipid-soluble form in the stomach and one would suspect that they would be absorbed there but absorption in the intestine is greater because of time and area of exposure.
  2. Specialized transport systems exist for some moieties: sugars, amino acids, pyrimidines, calcium, and sodium.
  3. Almost everything is absorbed, at least to a small extent (if it has a molecular weight below 10,000).
  4. Digestive fluids may modify the structure of a chemical.
  5. Dilution increases toxicity because of more rapid absorption from the intestine, unless stomach contents bind the moiety.
  6. Physical properties are important; for example, dissolution of metallic mercury is essential to allow its absorption.
  7. Age is important; for example, neonates have a poor intestinal barrier.
  8. Effect of fasting on absorption depends on the properties of the chemical of interest.

B. Inhalation (lungs)
  1. Aerosol deposition
     a. Nasopharyngeal: 5 μm or larger in humans, less in common laboratory animals.
     b. Tracheobronchial: 1 to 5 μm.
     c. Alveolar: 1 μm.
  2. If inhalant is a solid, mucociliary transport from lungs to GI tract may clear it out.
  3. Lungs are anatomically good for absorption.
     a. Large surface area (50–100 $m^2$).

    b. Blood flow is high.

    c. Close to blood ($10\,\mu m$ between gas media and blood).

4. Absorption of gases is dependent on solubility of the gas in blood.

    a. Chloroform, for example, has high solubility and is all absorbed, though respiration is limited.

    b. Ethylene has low solubility and only a small percentage is absorbed; blood flow limits absorption.

C. Parenteral routes

1. Irritation at the site of injection is influenced by solubility, toxicity, temperature, and pH of injected solution.

2. Pyrogenicity and blood compatibility are major concerns for intravenously administered materials.

3. Solubility of test material in an aqueous or modified aqueous solution is the chief limitation on how much material may be given intravenously.

D. Dermal routes

1. In general, any factor that increases absorption through the stratum corneum will also increase the severity of an intrinsic response. Unless this factor mirrors potential exposure conditions, it may, in turn, adversely affect the relevance of test results.

2. The physical nature of solids must be carefully considered both before testing and in interpreting results. Shape (sharp edges), size (small particles may abrade the skin by being rubbed back and forth under the occlusive wrap), and rigidity (stiff fibers or very hard particles will be physically irritating) of solids may all enhance an irritation response and alter absorption.

3. The degree of occlusion (in fact, the tightness of the wrap over the test site) also alters percutaneous absorption and therefore irritation. One important quality control issue in the laboratory is achieving a reproducible degree of occlusion in dermal wrappings.

4. Both the age of the test animal and the application site (saddle of the back versus flank) can markedly alter test outcome. Both of these factors are also operative in humans, of course, but in dermal irritation tests, the objective is to remove all such sources of variability. In general, as an animal ages, sensitivity to irritation decreases. Also, the skin on the middle of the back (other than directly over the spine) tends to be thicker (and therefore less sensitive to irritations) than that on the flanks.

5. The sex of the test animals can also alter study results, because both regional skin thickness and surface blood flow vary between males and females.

As a generalization, there is a pattern of relative absorption rates that characterizes the different routes that are commonly employed. This order of absorption (by rate from fastest to slowest and, in a less rigorous manner, by degree of absorption from most to least is IV (intravenous) > inhalation > IM (intramuscular) > IP (intraperitoneal) > SC (subcutaneous) > oral > ID (intradermal) > other.

3. *Metabolism.* Metabolism is directly influenced by both the region a material is initially absorbed into, and by distribution (both the rate and the pattern). Rate determines whether the primary enzyme systems will handle the entire xenobiotic dose, or if these are overwhelmed. Pattern determines which routes of metabolism are operative.

Absorption (total amount and rate, distribution, metabolism, and species similarity in response) are the reasons for selecting particular routes in toxicology in general. In safety assessment of pharmaceuticals, however, the route is usually dictated by the intended clinical route and dosing regimen. If this route of human exposure is uncertain, or if there is the potential for either a number of routes on the human absorption rate and pattern being greater than in animals, then the common practice becomes that of the most conservative approach. This approach stresses maximizing potential absorption in the animal species (within the limits of practicality) and selecting from among those routes commonly used in the laboratory that get the most material into the animal's system as quickly and completely as possible to evaluate the potential toxicity. Under this approach, many compounds are administered intraperitoneally in acute testing, though there is little or no real potential for human exposure by this route.

Assuming that a material is absorbed, distribution of a compound in early preclinical studies is usually of limited interest. In so-called heavy acute studies (Gad et al., 1984) where acute systemic toxicity is intensive and evaluated to the point of identifying target organs, or in range finder-type study results, for refining the design of longer-term studies, distribution would be of interest. Some factors that alter distribution are listed in Table 13.2.

The first special case is the parenteral route, where the systemic circulation presents a peak level of the moiety of interest to the body at one time, tempered only by the results of a single pass through the liver.

The second special case arises from inhalation exposures. Because of the arrangement of the circulatory system, inhaled compounds (and those administered via the buccal route) enter the full range of systemic circulation without any "first-pass" metabolism by the liver. Kerberle (1971) and O'Reilly (1972) have published reviews of absorption, distribution and metabolism that are relevant to acute testing.

## 13.3. COMMON ROUTES

Each of the ten routes most commonly used in safety assessment studies has its own peculiarities, and for each there are practical considerations and techniques ("tricks") that should be either known or available to the practicing toxicologist.

**TABLE 13.2. Selected Factors That May Affect Chemical Distribution to Various Tissues**

A. Factors relating to the chemical and its administration:
1. Degree of binding of chemical to plasma proteins (i.e., agent affinity for proteins) and tissues.
2. Chelation to calcium, which is deposited in growing bones and teeth (e.g., tetracyclines in young children).
3. Whether the chemical distributes evenly throughout the body (one-compartment model) or differentially between different compartments (models of two or more compartments).
4. Ability of chemical to cross the blood-brain barrier.
5. Diffusion of chemical into the tissues or organs and degree of binding to receptors that are and are not responsible for the drug's beneficial effects.
6. Quantity of chemical given.
7. Route of administration or exposure.
8. Partition coefficients (nonpolar chemicals are distributed more readily to fat tissues than are polar chemicals).
9. Interactions with other chemicals that may occupy receptors and prevent the drug from attaching to the receptor, inhibit active transport, or otherwise interfere with a drug's activity.
10. Molecular weight of the chemical.

B. Factors relating to the test subject:
1. Body size.
2. Fat content (e.g., obesity affects the distribution of drugs that are highly soluble in fats).
3. Permeability of membranes.
4. Active transport for chemicals carried across cell membranes by active processes.
5. Amount of proteins in blood, especially albumin.
6. Pathology or altered homeostasis that affects any of the other factors (e.g., cardiac failure, renal failure).
7. Presence of competitive binding substances (e.g., specific receptor sites in tissues bind drugs).
8. pH of blood and body tissues.
9. pH of urine.[a]
10. Blood flow to various tissues or organs (e.g., well-perfused organs usually tend to accumulate more chemical than less well perfused organs).

[a] The pH of urine is usually more important than the pH of blood.

### 13.3.2. Dermal Route

For all agents of concern in occupational toxicology (except therapeutics), the major route by which the general population is most frequently exposed is the percutaneous (dermal) route. Brown (1980) has previously reviewed background incidence data on pesticides, for example, that show such exposures to be common. Dermal (or topical) drugs are not as common, but are certainly numerous.

Percutaneous entry into the body is really by separate means (Marzulli, 1962; Scheuplein, 1965, 1967):

- Between the cells of the stratum corneum.
- Through the cells of the statum corneum.
- Via the hair follicles.
- Via the sweat glands.
- Via the sebacceous glands.

Certain aspects of the material of interest, as well as those of the test animals, including absorption (Blank and Scheuplein, 1964).

1. Small molecules penetrate skin better than large molecules.
2. Undissociated molecules penetrate skin better than do ions.
3. Preferential solubility of the toxicant in organic solvents indicates better penetration characteristics than preferential solubility in water.
4. The less viscous or more volatile the toxicant, the greater its penetrability.
5. The nature of the vehicle and the concentration of the toxicant in the vehicle both affect absorption (vehicles are discussed later in this chapter).
6. Hydration (water content) of the stratum corneum affects penetrability.
7. Ambient temperature can influence the uptake of toxicant through the skin. The warmer it is, the greater the blood flow through the skin and, therefore, the greater the percutaneous absorption.
8. Molecular shape (particularly symmetry) influences absorption (Medved and Kundiev, 1964).

There are at least two excellent texts on the subject of percutaneous absorption (Brandau and Lippold, 1982; Bronaugh and Maiback, 1985) that go into great detail.


### 13.3.3. Parenteral Route

The parenteral routes include three major ones: IV (intravenous), IM (intramuscular), and SC (subcutaneous) and a number of minor routes (such as intraarterial) that are not considered here. Administration by the parenteral routes raises a number of special safety concerns in addition to the usual systemic safety questions. These include irritation (vascular, muscular, or subcutaneous), pyrogenicity, blood compatibility, and sterility (Avis, 1985; Ballard, 1968). The background of each of these, along with the underlying mechanisms and factors that influence the level of occurrence of such an effect, are discussed in Chapter 11.

The need for a rapid onset of action (and/or clearance) usually requires that an IV route be used, although at a certain stage of cardiopulmonary resuscitation (for example), the need for an even more rapid effect may require the use of an intracardiac injection. The required site of action may influence the choice of route of administration (e.g., certain radiopaque dyes are given intraarterially near the site being evaluated; streptokinase is sometimes injected experimentally into the coronary arteries close to coronary vessel occlusion during a myocardial infarction to cause lysis of the thrombus and therefore re-establish coronary blood flow).

The characteristics of the fluid to be injected will also influence the choice of parenteral routes. The drug must be compatible with other fluids (e.g., saline, dextrose, Ringer's lactate) with which it may be combined for administration to the patient, as well as with the components of the blood itself.

There are certain clinical situations in which a parenteral route of administration is preferred to other possible routes. These include the following.

1. When the amount of drug given to a subject must be precisely controlled (e.g., in many pharmacokinetic studies), it is preferable to use a parenteral (usually IV) route of administration.

2. When the "first-pass effect" of a drug going through the liver must be avoided, a parenteral route of administration is usually chosen, although a sublingual route or dermal patch will also avoid the first-pass effect.

3. When one requires complete assurance that an uncooperative subject has actually received the drug and has not rejected it (e.g., via forced emesis).

4. When subjects are in a stupor, coma, or otherwise unable to take a drug orally.

5. When large volumes (i.e., more than a liter) of fluid are injected (such as in peritoneal dialysis, hyperalimentation, fluid replacement, and other conditions). Special consideration of fluid balance must be given to patients receiving large volumes, as well as careful consideration of the systemic effects of injection fluid components (e.g., amino acids and their nephrotoxicity).

Each of the three significant parenteral routes we are concerned with here has a specific set of either advantages and disadvantages or specific considerations that must be kept in mind.

***Intravenous Route.*** The IV route is the most common method of introducing a drug directly into the systemic circulation. It has the following advantages.

1. Rapid onset of effect.
2. Usefulness in situations of poor gastrointestinal absorption.
3. Avoidance of tissue irritation that may be present in IM or other routes (e.g., nitrogen mustard).
4. More precise control of levels of drug than with other routes, especially of toxic drugs, where the levels must be kept within narrow limits.
5. Ability to administer large volumes over time by a slow infusion.
6. Ability to administer drugs at a constant rate over a long period of time.

It also suffers from disadvantages.

1. Higher incidence of anaphylactic reactions than with many other routes.

2. Possibility of infection or phlebitis at site of injection.

3. Greater pain to patients than with many other routes.

4. Possibility that embolic phenomena may occur (either air embolism or vascular clot) as a result of damage to the vascular wall.

5. Impossibility of removing or lavaging drug after it is given, except by dialysis.

6. Inconvenience in many situations.

7. Possibility that rapid injection rates may cause severe adverse reactions.

8. Patient dislike of, and psychological discomfort with, the injection procedure.

For IV fluids, it must be determined how the dose will be given (i.e., by bolus or slow injection, intermittent or constant infusion, or by constant drip) and whether special equipment will be used to control and monitor the flow. Drugs with short half-lives are usually given by a constant drip or infusion technique. All IV fluids given immediately subsequent to an IV drug must be evaluated for their compatibility with the study drug. Suspensions are generally not given intravenously because of the possibility of blocking the capillaries.

In the IV route, anaphylactic reactions (caused by administration of an agent to an animal previously sensitized to it or to a particularly sensitive species such as a guinea pig) may be especially severe, probably because of sudden, massive antigen–antibody reactions. When the drug is given by other routes, its access to antibody molecules is necessarily slower; moreover, its further absorption can be retarded or prevented at the first sign of a serious allergic reaction.

Embolism is another possible complication of the IV route. Particulate matter may be introduced if a drug intended for intravenous use precipitates for some reason, or if a particular suspension intended for IM or SC use is inadvertently given into a vein. Hemolysis or agglutination of erythrocytes may be caused by injection of hypotonic/hypertonic solutions, or by more specific mechanisms (Gray, 1978).

*Bolus versus Infusion.* Technically, for all the parenteral routes (but in practice only for the IV route), there are two options for injecting a material into the body. The bolus and infusion methods are differentiated on the single basis of rate of injection, but they actually differ on a wide range of characteristics.

The most commonly exercised option is the bolus, "push," injection, in which the injection device (syringe or catheter) is appropriately entered into the vein and a defined volume of material is introduced through the device. The device is then removed. In this operation, it is relatively easy to restrain an experimental animal and the stress on the animal is limited. Though the person doing the injection must be skilled, it takes only a short amount of time to become so. And the one variable to be controlled in determining dosage is the total volume of material injected (assuming dosing solutions have been properly prepared). See Chapter 9 for a more complete discussion.

**Subcutaneous Route.** Drugs given by the SC route are forced into spaces between connective tissues, as with IM injections. Vasoconstrictors and drugs that cause local irritation should not be given subcutaneously under usual circumstances, since inflammation, abscess formation, or even tissue necrosis may result. When daily or even more frequent SC injections are made, the site of injection should be continually changed to prevent local complications. Fluids given subcutaneously must have an appropriate tonicity to prevent pain. Care must be taken to prevent injection of the drug directly into veins.

The absorption of drugs from a SC route is influenced by blood flow to the area, as with IM injections. The rate of absorption may be retarded by cooling the local area to cause vasoconstriction, adding epinephrine to the solution for the same purpose (e.g., with local anesthetics), decreasing blood flow with a tourniquet, or immobilizing the area. The opposite effect may be achieved by warming the injection region or by using the enzyme hyaluronidase, which breaks down mucopolysaccharides of the connective tissue matrix to allow the injected solution to spread over a larger area and thus increase its rate of absorption.

Absorption from SC injection sites is affected by the same factors that determine the rate of absorption from IM sites (Schou, 1971). Blood flow through these regions is generally poorer than in muscles, so the absorption rate is generally slower.

The rate of absorption from an SC injection site may be retarded by immobilization of the limb, local cooling to cause vasoconstriction, or application of a tourniquet proximal to the injection site to block the superficial venous drainage and lymphatic flow. In small amounts, adrenergic stimulants, such as epinephrine, will constrict the local blood vessels and, therefore, slow systemic absorption. Conversely, cholinergic stimulants (such as methacholine) will induce very rapid systemic absorption subcutaneously. Other agents may also alter their own rate of absorption by affecting local blood supply or capillary permeability.

A prime determinant of the absorption rate from an SC injection is the total surface area over which the absorption can occur. Although the subcutaneous tissues are somewhat loose and moderate amounts of fluid can be administered, the normal connective tissue matrix prevents indefinite lateral spread of the injected solution. These barriers may be overcome by agents that break down mucopolysaccharides of the connective tissue matrix; the resulting spread of injected solution leads to a much faster absorption rate.

In addition to fluids, solid forms of drugs may be given by SC injection. This has been done with compressed pellets of testosterone placed under the skin, which are absorbed at a relatively constant rate over a long period.

***Intramuscular Route.*** The IM route is frequently used for drugs dissolved in oily vehicles or for those in a microcrystalline formulation that are poorly soluble in water (e.g., procaine or penicillin G). Advantages include rapid absorption (often in under 30 min), the opportunity to inject a relatively large amount of solution, and a reduction in pain and local irritation compared with SC injections. Potential complications include infections and nerve damage. The latter usually results from the choice of an incorrect site for injection.

Although the time to peak drug concentration is often on the order of 1 to 2 h, depot preparations given by IM injection are absorbed extremely slowly. Numerous physiochemical properties of a material given intramuscularly will affect the rate of absorption from the site within the muscle (e.g., ionization of the drug, lipid solubility, osmolality of the solution, volume given). The primary sites used for IM injections in people are the gluteal (buttocks), deltoid (upper arm), and lateral vastus (lateral thigh) muscles, with the corresponding sites in test animals being species specific. The rate of drug absorption and the peak drug levels obtained will often differ between sites used for IM injections because of differences in blood flow between muscle groups. The site chosen for an IM injection in humans and some animals may be a critical factor in whether or not the drug exhibits an effect (Schwartz et al., 1974). Agents injected into the larger muscle masses are generally absorbed rapidly.

Blood flow through muscles in a resting animal is about $0.02$–$0.07\,\mathrm{ml\,min^{-1}\,g^{-1}}$ of tissue, and this flow rate may increase many times during exercise, when additional vascular channels open. Large amounts of solution can be introduced intramuscularly, and there is usually less pain and local irritation than is encountered by the SC route. Ordinary aqueous solutions of chemicals are usually absorbed from an intramuscular site within 10–30 min, but faster or slower absorption is possible, depending on the vascularity of the site, the ionization and lipid solubility of the drug, the volume of the injection, the osmolality of the solution, animal temperature, and other variables. Small molecules are absorbed directly into the capillaries from an intramuscular site, whereas large molecules (e.g., proteins) gain access to the circulation by way of the lymphatic channels. Radiolabeled compounds of widely differing molecular weights (maximum 585) and physical properties have been shown to be absorbed from rat muscle at virtually the same rate, about 16% per minute (i.e., the absorption process is limited by the rate of blood flow.)

Drugs that are insoluble at tissue pH, or that are in an oily vehicle, form a depot in the muscle tissue, from which absorption proceeds very slowly.

***Intraperitoneal Route.*** Kruger et al. (1962) demonstrated the efficiency of absorption of some chemicals injected IP, while Lukas et al. (1971) showed that compounds administered IP are absorbed primarily through the portal circulation.

A prime practical consideration in the use of the IP route for acute testing should be the utilization of aseptic techniques to preclude bacterial or viral contamination. If these are not exercised, the resulting infected and compromised animals cannot be expected to produce either valid or reproducible indications or actual chemical toxicity.

Compounds that are very lipophilic will be quickly absorbed systemically by the IP route, but not by the IM or SC route.

### 13.3.4. Oral Route

The oral route is the most commonly used route for the administration of drugs both because of ease of administration and because it is the most readily accepted route of administration. Although the dermal route may be as common for occupational exposure, it is much easier to accurately measure and administer doses by the oral route.

Enteral routes technically include any that will put a material directly into the GI tract, but the use of enteral routes other than oral (such as rectal) is rare in toxicology. Though there are a number of variations of technique and peculiarities of animal response that are specific to different animal species, there is also a great deal of commonality across species in methods, considerations, and mechanisms.

***Mechanisms of Absorption.*** Ingestion is generally referred to as oral or per oral (PO) exposure and includes direct intragastric exposure in experimental toxicology. The regions for possible agent action and absorption from PO absorption should, however, be considered separately.

Because of the rich blood supply to the mucous membranes of the mouth (buccal cavity), many compounds can be absorbed through them. Absorption from the buccal cavity is limited to nonionized, lipid-soluble compounds. Buccal absorption of a wide range of aromatic and aliphatic acids and basic drugs in human subjects has been found to be parabolically dependent on $\log P$, where $P$ is the octanol-water partition coefficient. The ideal lipophilic character ($\log P_0$) for maximum buccal absorption has also been shown to be in the range 4.2–5.5 (Lien et al., 1971). Compounds with large molecular weights are poorly absorbed in the buccal cavity, and, since absorption increases linearly with concentration and there is generally no difference between optical enantiomorphs of several compounds known to be absorbed from the mouth, it is believed that uptake is by passive diffusion rather than by active transport chemical moieties.

A knowledge of the buccal absorption characteristics of a chemical can be important in a case of accidental poisoning. Although an agent taken into the mouth will be voided immediately on being found objectionable, it is possible that significant absorption can occur before any material is swallowed.

Unless voided, most materials in the buccal cavity are swallowed. No significant absorption occurs in the esophagus and the agent passes on to enter the stomach. It is common practice in safety assessment studies to avoid the possibility of buccal absorption by intubation (gavage) or by the administration of the agent in gelatin capsules designed to disintegrate in the gastric fluid.

Absorption of chemicals with widely differing characteristics can occur at different levels in the GI tract (Schranker, 1960; Hogben et al., 1959; Schranker et al., 1957). The two factors primarily influencing this regional absorption are (1) the lipid-water partition characteristics of the undissociated toxicant and (2) the dissociation constant ($pK_a$) that determines the amount of toxicant in the dissociated form.

Therefore, weak organic acids and bases are readily absorbed as uncharged lipid-soluble molecules, whereas ionized compounds are absorbed only with difficulty, and nonionized toxicants with poor lipid-solubility characteristics are absorbed slowly. Lipid-soluble acid molecules can be absorbed efficiently through the gastric mucosa, but bases are not absorbed in the stomach.

In the intestines the nonionized form of the drug is preferentially absorbed and the rate of absorption is related to the lipid-water partition coefficient of the toxicant.

The highest $pK_a$ value for a base compatible with efficient gastric absorption is about 7.8 and the lowest $pK_a$ for an acid is about 3.0, although a limited amount of absorption can occur outside these ranges. The gastric absorption and the intestinal absorption of a series of compounds with different carbon chain lengths follow two different patterns. Absorption from the stomach increases as the chain lengthens from methyl to *n*-hexyl, whereas intestinal absorption increases over the range methyl to *n*-butyl and then diminishes as the chain length further increases. Houston et al. (1974) concluded that to explain the logic of optimal partition coefficients for intestinal absorption it was necessary to postulate a two-compartment model with a hydrophilic barrier and a lipoidal membrane and that if there is an acceptable optimal partition coefficient for gastric absorption it must be at least ten times greater than the corresponding intestinal value.

Because they are crucial to the course of an organism's response, the rate and extent of absorption of biologically active agents from the GI tract also have major implications for the formulation of test material dosages and also for how production (commercial) materials may be formulated to minimize potential accidental intoxications while maximizing the therapeutic profile.

There are a number of separate mechanisms involved in absorption from the gastrointestinal tract.

*Passive Absorption.* The membrane lining of the tract has a passive role in absorption. As toxicant molecules move from the bulk water phase of the intestinal contents into the epithelial cells, they must pass through two membranes in series, one layer of water and the other the lipid membrane of the microvillar surface (Wilson and Dietschy, 1974). The water layer may be the rate-limiting factor for passive absorption into the intestinal mucosa, but it is not rate-limiting for active absorption. The concentration gradient as well as the physiochemical properties of the drug and of the lining membrane are the controlling factors. Chemicals that are highly lipid soluble are capable of passive diffusion and they pass readily from the aqueous fluids of the gut lumen through the lipid barrier of the intestinal wall and into the bloodstream. The interference in the absorption process by the water layer increases with increasing absorbability of the substances in the intestine (Winne, 1978).

Aliphatic carbamates are rapidly absorbed from the colon by passive uptake (Wood et al., 1978) and it is found that there is a linear relationship between $\log k_a$ and $\log P$ for absorption of these carbamates in the colon and the stomach, whereas there is a parabolic relationship between these two values for absorption in the small intestine. The factors to be considered are

$$P = \text{octanol-buffer partition coefficient}$$

$$k_a = \text{absorption rate constant}$$

$$t = \text{time}$$

$$t^{1/2} = \text{half-life} = \frac{\ln 2}{k_a}$$

Organic acids that are extensively ionized at intestinal pH's are absorbed primarily by simple diffusion.

*Facilitated Diffusion.* Temporary combination of the chemical with some form of "carrier" occurs in the gut wall, facilitating the transfer of the toxicant across the membranes. This process is also dependent on the concentration gradient across the membrane, and there is no energy utilization in making the translocation. In some intoxications, the carrier may become saturated, making this the rate-limiting step in the absorption process.

*Active Transport.* As above, the process depends on a carrier, but differs in that the carrier provides energy for translocation from regions of lower concentration to regions of higher concentration.

*Pinocytosis.* This process by which particles are absorbed can be an important factor in the ingestion of particulate formulations of chemicals (e.g., dust formulations, suspensions of wettable powders, etc.); however, it must not be confused with absorption by one of the above processes, where the agent has been released from particles.

*Absorption via Lymphatic Channels.* Some lipophilic chemicals dissolved in lipids may be absorbed through the lymphatics.

*Convective Absorption.* Compounds with molecular radii of less than 4 nm can pass through pores in the gut membrane. The membrane exhibits a molecular sieving effect.

Characteristically, within certain concentration limits, if a chemical is absorbed by passive diffusion, then the concentration of toxicant in the gut and the rate of absorption are linearly related. However, if absorption is mediated by active transport, the relationship between concentration and rate of absorption conforms to Michaelis–Menten kinetics and a Lineweaver–Burk plot (i.e., reciprocal of rate of absorption plotted against reciprocal of concentration), which graphs as a straight line.

Differences in the physiological chemistry of gastrointestinal fluids can have a significant effect on toxicity. Both physical and chemical differences in the GI tract can lead to species differences in susceptibility to acute intoxication. The anti-helminthic pyrvinium chloride has an identical $LD_{50}$ value when administered intraperitoneally to rats and mice (approximately $4\,mg\,kg^{-1}$); when administered orally, however, the $LD_{50}$ value in mice was found to be $15\,mg\,kg^{-1}$, while for the rat, the $LD_{50}$ values were $430\,mg\,kg^{-1}$ for females and $1550\,mg\,kg^{-1}$ for males. It is thought that this is an absorption difference rather than a metabolic difference (Ritschel et al., 1974).

Most of any exogenous chemical absorbed from the GI tract must pass through the liver via the hepatic-portal system (leading to the so-called first-pass effect) and, as mixing of the venous blood with arterial blood from the liver occurs, consideration and caution are called for in estimating the amounts of chemical in both the systemic circulation and the liver itself.

Despite the gastrointestinal absorption characteristics discussed above, it is common for absorption from the alimentary tract to be facilitated by dilution of the toxicant. Borowitz et al. (1971) have suggested that the concentration effects they observed in atropine sulfate, aminopyrine, sodium salicylate, and sodium pentoparbital were due to a combination of rapid stomach emptying and the large surface area for absorption of the drugs.

Major structural or physiological differences in the alimentary tract (e.g., species differences or surgical effects) can give rise to modifications of toxicity. For example, ruminant animals may metabolize toxicants in the GI tract in a way that is unlikely to occur in nonruminants.

The presence of bile salts in the alimentary tract can affect absorption of potential toxicants in a variety of ways, depending on their solubility characteristics.

***Factors Affecting Absorption.*** Test chemicals are given most commonly by mouth. This is certainly the most convenient route, and it is the only one of practical importance for self-administration. Absorption, in general, takes place along the whole length of the gastrointestinal tract, but the chemical properties of each molecule determine whether it will be absorbed in the strongly acidic stomach or in the nearly neutral intestine. Gastric absorption is favored by an empty stomach, in which the chemical, in undiluted gastric juice, will have good access to the mucosal wall. Only when a chemical would be irritating to the gastric mucosa is it rational to administer it with or after a meal. However, the antibiotic griseofulvin is an example of a substance with poor water solubility, the absorption of which is aided by a fatty meal. The large surface area of the intestinal villi, the presence of bile, and the rich blood supply all favor intestinal absorption of griseofulvin and physiochemically similar compounds.

The presence of food can impair the absorption of chemicals given by mouth. Suggested mechanisms include reduced mixing, complexing with substances in the food, and retarded gastric emptying. In experiments with rats, prolonged fasting has been shown to diminish the absorption of several chemicals, possibly by deleterious effects upon the epithelium of intestinal villi.

Chemicals that are metabolized rapidly by the liver cannot be given for systemic effect by the enteral route because the portal circulation carries them directly to the liver. For example, lidocaine, a drug of value in controlling cardiac arrhythmias, is absorbed well from the gut, but is completely inactivated in a single passage through the liver.

The principles governing the absorption of drugs from the gastrointestinal lumen are the same as for the passage of drugs across biological membranes elsewhere. Low degree of ionization, high lipid-water partition coefficient of the nonionized form, and small atomic or molecular radii of water-soluble substances all favor rapid absorption. Water passes readily in both directions across the wall of the gastrointestinal lumen. Sodium ion is probably transported actively from lumen into blood. Magnesium ion is very poorly absorbed and therefore acts as a cathartic, retaining an osmotic equivalent of water as it passes down the intestinal tract. Ionic iron is absorbed as an amino acid complex, at a rate usually determined by the body's need for it. Glucose and amino acids are transported across the intestinal wall by specific carrier systems. Some compounds of high molecular weight (polysaccharides and large proteins) cannot be absorbed until they are degraded enzymatically. Other substances cannot be absorbed because they are destroyed by gastrointestinal enzymes: insulin, epinephrine, and histamine are examples. Substances that form insoluble precipitates in the gastrointestinal lumen or that are insoluble either in water or in lipid clearly cannot be absorbed.

*Absorption of Weak Acids and Bases.* Human gastric juice is very acid (about pH 1), whereas the intestinal contents are nearly neutral (actually very slightly acid). The pH difference between plasma (pH 7.4) and the lumen of the GI tract plays a major role in determining whether a drug that is a weak electrolyte will be absorbed into plasma, or excreted from plasma into the stomach or intestine. For practical purposes, the mucosal lining of the GI tract is impermeable to the ionized form of a weak acid or base, but the nonionized form equilibrates freely. The rate of equilibration of the nonionized molecule is directly related to its lipid solubility. If there is a pH difference across the membrane, then the fraction ionized may be considerably greater on one side than on the other. At equilibrium, the concentration of the nonionized moiety will be the same on both sides, but there will be more total drug on the side where the degree of ionization is greater. This mechanism is known as ion *trapping*. The energy for sustaining the unequal chemical potential of the acid or base in question is derived from whatever mechanism maintains the pH difference. In the stomach, this mechanism is the energy-dependent secretion of hydrogen ions.

Consider how a weak electrolyte is distributed across the gastric mucosa between plasma (pH 7.4) and gastric fluid (pH 1.0). In each compartment, the Henderson-Hasselbalch equation gives the ratio of acid-base concentrations. The negative logarithm of the acid dissociation constant is designated here by the symbol $pK_a$ rather than the more precisely correct $pK^1$.

$$pH = pK_aH = + \log \frac{(\text{base})}{(\text{acid})}$$

$$\log \frac{(\text{base})}{(\text{acid})} = pH - pK_a$$

$$\frac{(\text{base})}{(\text{acid})} = \text{antilog } (pH - pK_a)$$

The implications of the above equations are clear. Weak acids are readily absorbed from the stomach. Weak bases are not absorbed well; indeed, they would tend to accumulate within the stomach at the expense of agent in the bloodstream. Naturally, in the more alkaline intestine, bases would be absorbed better, acids more poorly.

It should be realized that although the principles outlined here are correct, the system is dynamic, not static. Molecules that are absorbed across the gastric or intestinal mucosa are removed constantly by blood flow; thus, simple reversible equilibrium across the membrane does not occur until the agent is distributed throughout the body.

Absorption from the stomach, as determined by direct measurements, conforms, in general, to the principles outlined above. Organic acids are absorbed well since they are all almost completely nonionized at the gastric pH; indeed, many of these substances are absorbed faster than ethyl alcohol, which had long been considered one of the few compounds that were absorbed well from the stomach (Share et al., 1971). Strong acids whose $pK_a$ values lie below 1, which are ionized even in the acid contents of the stomach, are not absorbed well. Weak bases are absorbed only negligibly, but their absorption can be increased by raising the pH of the gastric fluid.

As for bases, only the weakest are absorbed to any appreciable extent at normal gastric pH, but their absorption can be increased substantially by neutralizing the stomach contents. The quaternary cations, however, which are charged at all pH values, are not absorbed at either pH.

The accumulation of weak bases in the stomach by ion trapping mimics a secretory process; if the drug is administered systemically, it accumulates in the stomach. Dogs given various drugs intravenously by continuous infusion to maintain a constant drug level in the plasma had the gastric contents sampled by means of an indwelling catheter. The results showed that stronger bases ($pK_a > 5$) accumulated in stomach contents to many times their plasma concentrations; the weak bases appeared in about equal concentrations in gastric juice and in plasma. Among the acids, only the weakest appeared in detectable amounts in the stomach. One might wonder why the strong bases, which are completely ionized in gastric juice, and whose theoretical concentration ratios (gastric juice/plasma) are very large, should nevertheless attain only about a 40-fold excess over plasma. Direct measurements of arterial and venous blood show that essentially all the blood flowing through the gastric mucosa is cleared of these agents; obviously, no more chemical can enter the gastric juice in a given time period than is brought there by circulation. Another limitation comes into play when the base $pK_a$ exceeds 7.4; now a major fraction of the circulating base is cationic and a decreasing fraction is nonionized, so the effective concentration gradient for diffusion across the stomach wall is reduced.

The ion-trapping mechanism provides a method of some forensic value for detecting the presence of alkaloids (e.g., narcotics, cocaine, amphetamines) in cases of death suspected to be due to overdosage of self-administered drugs. Drug concentrations in gastric contents may be very high even after parenteral injection.

Absorption from the intestine has been studied by perfusing drug solutions slowly through rat intestine *in situ* and by varying the pH as desired. The relationships that emerge from such studies are the same as those for the stomach, the difference being that the intestinal pH is normally very near neutrality. As the pH is increased, the bases are absorbed better, the acids more poorly. Detailed studies with a great many drugs in unbuffered solutions revealed that in the normal intestine, acids with

$pK_a > 3.0$ and bases with $pK_a < 7.8$ are very well absorbed; outside these limits the absorption of acids and bases falls off rapidly. This behavior leads to the conclusion that the "virtual pH" in the microenvironment of the absorbing surface in the gut is about 5.3; this is somewhat more acidic than the pH in the intestinal lumen is usually considered to be.

Absorption from the buccal cavity has been shown to follow exactly the same principles as those described for absorption from the stomach and intestine. The pH of human and canine saliva is usually about 6. Bases in people are absorbed only on the alkaline side of their $pK_a$, that is, only in the nonionized form. At normal saliva pH, only weak bases are absorbed to a significant extent.

***Bioavailability and Thresholds.*** The difference between the extent of availability (often designated solely as bioavailability) and the rate of availability is illustrated in Figure 13.1, which depicts the concentration-time curve for a hypothetical agent formulated into three different dosage forms. Dosage forms A and B are designed so that the agent is put into the blood circulation at the same rate, but twice as fast as for dosage form C. The times at which agent concentrations reach a peak are identical for dosage forms A and B and occur earlier than the peak time for dosage form C. In general, the relative order of peak times following the administration of different dosage forms of the drug corresponds to the rates of availability of the chemical moiety from the various dosage forms. The extent of availability can be measured by using either chemical concentrations in the plasma or blood or amounts of

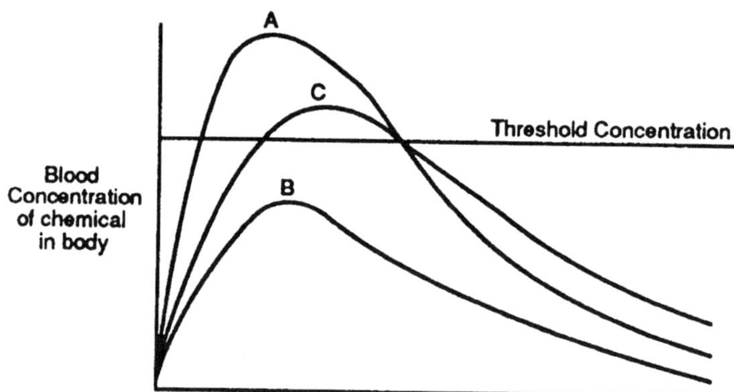


**FIGURE 13.1.** Blood concentration-time curves illustrating how changes in the rate and extent of chemical availability can influence the duration of action and the efficacy of a dose of an agent. The designated line indicates the threshold concentration ($T_c$) of the agent in the body that will evoke a response. Case A is absorbed rapidly and completely. This product produces a prompt and prolonged response. The agent in Case B is absorbed at the same rate as that in Case A, but is only 50% as available. There will be no response from this dose of the agent because the $T_c$ is not reached. The agent in Case C is absorbed at one-half the rate seen in Cases A and B, but is 100% available.

unchanged chemical in the urine. The area under the blood concentration-time curve for an agent can serve as a measure of the extent of its availability. In Figure 13.1, the areas under curves A and C are identical and twice as great as the area under curve B. In most cases, where clearance is constant, the relative areas under the curves or the amount of unchanged chemical excreted in the urine will quantitatively describe the relative availability of the agent from the different dosage forms. However, even in nonlinear cases, where clearance is dose dependent, the relative areas under the curves will yield a measurement of the rank order of availability from different dosage forms or from different routes of administration.

Because there is usually a critical concentration of a chemical in the blood that is necessary to elicit either a pharmacological or toxic effect, both the rate and extent of input or availability can alter the toxicity of a compound. In the majority of cases, the duration of effects will be a function of the length of time the blood-concentration curve is above the threshold concentration; the intensity of the effect for many agents will be a function of the elevation of the blood-concentration curve above the threshold concentration.

Thus, the three different dosage forms depicted in Figure 13.1 will exhibit significant differences in their levels of "toxicity." Dosage form B requires that twice the dose be administered to attain blood levels equivalent to those for dosage form A. Differences in the rate of availability are particularly important for agents given acutely. Dosage form A reaches the target concentration earlier than chemical from dosage form C; concentrations from A reach a higher level and remain above the minimum effect concentration for a longer period of time. In a multiple dosing regimen, dosage forms A and C will yield the same average blood concentrations, although dosage form A will show somewhat greater maximum and lower minimum concentrations.

For most chemicals, the rate of disposition or loss from the biological system is independent of rate of input, once the agent is absorbed. Disposition is defined as what happens to the active molecule after it reaches a site in the blood circulation where concentration measurements can be made (the systemic circulations, generally). Although disposition processes may be independent of input, the inverse is not necessarily true, because disposition can markedly affect the extent of availability. Agents absorbed from the stomach and the intestine must first pass through the liver before reaching the general circulation (Figure 13.2). Thus, if a compound is metabolized in the liver or excreted in bile, some of the active molecule absorbed from the GI tract will be inactivated by hepatic processes before it can reach the systemic circulation and be distributed to its sites of action. If the metabolizing or biliary excreting capacity of the liver is great, the effect on the extent of availability will be substantial. Thus, if the hepatic blood clearance for the chemical is large, relative to hepatic blood flow, the extent of availability for this chemical will be low when it is given by a route that yields first-pass metabolic effects. This decrease in availability is a function of the physiological site from which absorption takes place, and no amount of modification to dosage form can improve the availability under linear conditions. Of course, toxic blood levels can be reached by this route of administration if larger doses are given.

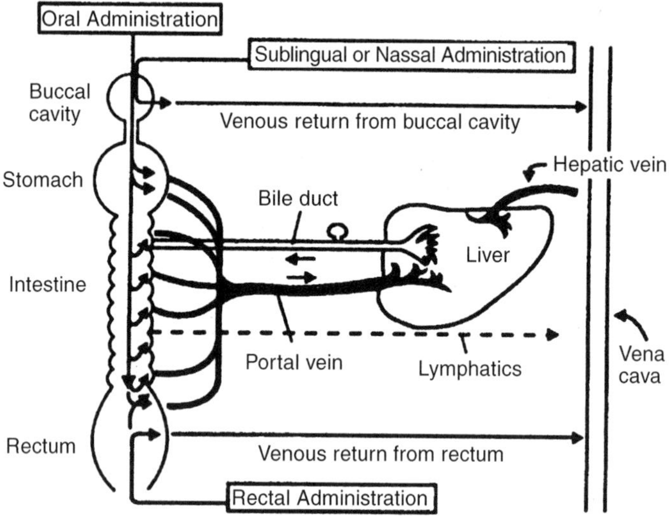


**FIGURE 13.2.** Diagrammatic representation of entry of drug moieties into the body from a variety of routes, with subsequent passage into the bloodstream and out of the body.

It is important to realize that chemicals with high extraction ratios (i.e., greater extents of removal by the liver during first-pass metabolism) will exhibit marked intersubject variability in bioavailability because of variations in hepatic function or blood flow or both. For the chemical with an extraction ratio of 0.90 that increases to 0.95, the bioavailability of the agent will be halved, from 0.10 to 0.05. These relationships can explain the marked variability in plasma or blood drug concentrations that occurs among individual animals given similar doses of a chemical that is markedly extracted. Small variations in hepatic extraction between individual animals will result in large differences in availability and plasma drug concentrations.

The first-pass effect can be avoided, to a great extent, by use of the sublingual route and by topical preparations (e.g., nitroglycerine ointment), and it can be partially avoided by using rectal suppositories. The capillaries in the lower and middle sections of the rectum drain into the interior and middle hemorrhoidal veins, which in turn, drain into the inferior vena cava, thus bypassing the liver. However, suppositories tend to move upward in the rectum into a region where veins that lead to the liver predominate, such as the superior hemorrhoidal vein. In addition, there are extensive connections between the superior and middle hemorrhoidal veins, and thus probably only about 50% of a rectal dose can be assumed to bypass the liver. The lungs represent a good temporary clearing site for a number of chemicals (especially basic compounds) by partition into lipid tissues, as well as serve a filtering function for particulate matter that may be given by intravenous injection. In essence, the lung may cause first-pass loss by excretion and possible metabolism for chemicals input into the body by the nongastrointestinal routes of administration.

Biological (test subject) factors that can influence absorption of a chemical from the gastrointestinal tract are summarized in Table 13.3.

There are also a number of chemical factors that may influence absorption from the GI tract. These are summarized in Table 13.4.

***Techniques of Oral Absorption.*** There are three major techniques for oral delivery of drugs to test animals. The most common way is by gavage, which requires that the material be in a solution or suspension for delivery by tube to the stomach. Less common materials may be given as capsules (particularly to dogs) or in diet (for longer-term studies). Rarely, oral studies may also be done by inclusion of materials in drinking water.

Test materials may be administered as solutions or suspensions as long as they are homogeneous and delivery is accurate. For traditional oral administration (gavage), the solution or suspension can be administered with a suitable stomach tube or feeding needle ("Popper" tube) attached to a syringe. If the dose is too large to be administered at one time, it can be divided into equal subparts with 2 to 4 h between each administration; however, this subdivided dosing approach should generally be avoided.

Test chemicals placed into any natural orifice exert local effects and, in many instances, systemic effects as well. The possibility of systemic effects occurring when local effects are to be evaluated should be considered.

For routes of administration in which the chemical is given orally or placed into an orifice other than the mouth, clear instructions about the correct administration of the chemical must be provided. Many cases are known of oral pediatric drops for ear infections being placed into the ear, and vice versa (ear drops being swallowed) in humans. Errors in test-article administration are especially prevalent when a chemical form is being used in a nontraditional manner (e.g., suppositories that are given by the buccal route).

Administration of a drug in capsules is a common means of dosing larger test animals (particularly dogs). It is labor intensive (each capsule must be individually prepared, though robotic systems are now available for this), but capsules offer the advantages that neat drug may be used (no special formulation need be prepared, and the questions of formulation or solution stability are avoided), the dogs are less likely to vomit, and the actual act of dosing requires less labor than using a gavage tube. Capsules may also be used with primates, though they are not administered as easily.

Incorporation of a drug in the diet is commonly used for longer-term studies (particularly carcinogenicity studies, though the method is not limited to these). Dosing by diet is much less labor intensive than any other oral dosing methodology, which is particularly attractive over the course of a long (13-week, 1-year, 18-month, or 2-year) study.

The most critical factor to dietary studies is the proper preparation of the test chemicals-diet admixtures. The range of physical and chemical characteristics of test materials requires that appropriate mixing techniques be determined on an individual basis. Standard practices generally dictate the preparation of a premix, to which is added appropriate amounts of feed to achieve the proper concentrations.

**TABLE 13.3. Test Subject Characteristics That Can Influence GI Tract Absorption**[a]

A. General and inherent characteristics:
   1. General condition of the subject (e.g., starved versus well-fed, ambulatory versus supine).
   2. Presence of concurrent diseases (i.e., diseases may either speed or slow gastric emptying).
   3. Age.
   4. Weight and degree of obesity.
B. Physiological function:
   1. Status of the subject's renal function.
   2. Status of the subject's hepatic function.
   3. Status of the subject's cardiovascular system.
   4. Status of the subject's gastrointestinal motility and function (e.g., ability to swallow).
   5. pH of the gastric fluid (e.g., affected by fasting, disease, food intake, drugs).
   6. Gastrointestinal blood flow to the area of absorption.
   7. Blood flow to areas of absorption for dose forms other than those absorbed through gastrointestinal routes.
C. Acquired characteristics:
   1. Status of the subject's anatomy (e.g., previous surgery).
   2. Status of the subject's gastrointestinal flora.
   3. Timing of drug administration relative to meals (i.e., presence of food in the gastrointestinal tract).
   4. Body position of subject (e.g., lying on the side slows gastric emptying).
   5. Psychological state of subject (e.g., stress increases gastric emptying rate, and depression decreases rate).
   6. Physical exercise of subject may reduce gastric emptying rate.
D. Physiological principles:
   1. Food enhances gastric blood flow, which should theoretically increase the rate of absorption.
   2. Food slows the rate of gastric emptying, which should theoretically slow the rate of passage to the intestines where the largest amounts of most agents are absorbed. This should decrease the rate of absorption for most agents. Agents absorbed to a larger extent in the stomach will have increased time for absorption in the presence of food and should be absorbed more completely than in fasted patients.
   3. Bile flow and secretion are stimulated by fats and certain other foods. Bile salts may enhance or delay absorption depending on whether they form insoluble complexes with drugs or enhance the solubility of agents.
   4. Changes in splanchnic blood flow as a result of food depend on direction and magnitude of the type of food ingested.
   5. Presence of active (saturable) transport mechanisms places a limit on the amount of a chemical that may be absorbed.

[a] The minimization of variability due to these factors rests on the selection of an appropriate animal model, careful selection of healthy animals, and use of proper techniques.

**TABLE 13.4. Chemical Characteristics of a Drug That May Influence Absorption**

A. Administration of chemical and its passage through the body:
  1. Dissolution characteristics of solid dosage forms, which depend on formulation in addition to the properties of the chemical itself (e.g., vehicle may decrease permeability of suspension or capsule to water and retard dissolution and diffusion).
  2. Rate of dissolution in gastrointestinal fluids. Chemicals that are inadequately dissolved in gastric contents may be inadequately absorbed.
  3. Chemicals that are absorbed into food may have a delayed absorption.
  4. Carrier-transported chemicals are more likely to be absorbed in the small intestine.
  5. Route of administration.
  6. Chemicals undergo metabolism in the gastrointestinal tract.
B. Physiochemical properties of chemicals:
  1. Chemicals that chelate metal ions in food may form insoluble complexes and will not be adequately absorbed.
  2. pH of dosing solutions: weakly basic solutions are absorbed to a greater degree in the small intestine.
  3. Salts used.
  4. Hydrates or solvates.
  5. Crystal form of chemical (e.g., insulin).
  6. "Pharmaceutical" form (e.g., fluid, solid, suspension).
  7. Enteric coating.
  8. Absorption of quaternary compounds (e.g., hexamethonium, amiloride) are decreased by food.
  9. Molecular weight of chemical (e.g., when the molecular weight of a drug is above about 1000, absorption is markedly decreased).
  10. $pK_a$ (dissociation constant).
  11. Lipid solubility (i.e., a hydrophobic property relating to penetration through membranes).
  12. Particle size of chemical in solid dosage form: smaller particle sizes will increase the rate and/or degree of absorption if dissolution of the chemical is the rate-limiting factor in absorption. Chemicals that have a low dissolution rate may be made in a micronized form to increase their rate of dissolution.
  13. Particle size of the dispersed phase in an emulsion.
  14. Type of disintegrating agent in the formulation.
  15. Hardness of a solid (granule, pellet, or tablet) (i.e., related to amount of compression used to make tablet) or capsule if they do not disintegrate appropriately.

Dietary preparation involving liquid materials frequently results in either wet feed in which the test article does not disperse or formation of "gumballs": feed and test material that form discernible lumps and chemical "hotspots." Drying and grinding of the premix to a free-flowing form prior to mixing the final diets may be required; however, these actions can affect the chemical nature of the test article.

Solid materials require special techniques prior to or during addition to diets. Materials that are soluble in water may be dissolved and added as described above for liquids. Non-water-soluble materials may require several preparatory steps. The test chemical may be dissolved in corn oil, acetone, or other appropriate vehicle prior to addition to the weighed diet. When an organic solvent such as acetone is used, the mixing time for the premix should be sufficient for the solvent to evaporate. Some solids may require grinding in a mortar and pestle with feed added during the grinding process.

Prior to study initiation, stability of the test chemical in the diet must be determined over a test period at least equivalent to the time period during which animals are to be exposed to a specific diet mix. Stability of test samples under the conditions of the proposed study is preferable. Labor and expense can be saved when long-term stability data permit mixing of several weeks (or a month) of test diet in a single mixing interval.

Homogeneity and concentration analysis of the test-article-diet admixture are performed by sampling at three or four regions within the freshly mixed diet (e.g., samples from the top, middle, and bottom of the mixing bowl or blender).

A variety of feeders are commercially available for rats and mice. These include various-sized glass jars and stainless steel or galvanized feed cups, which can be equipped with restraining lids and food followers to preclude significant losses of feed due to animals digging in the feeders. Slotted metal feeders are designed so that animals cannot climb into the feed, and they also contain mesh food followers to prevent digging.

Another problem sometimes encountered is palatability; the material may taste so strong that animals will not eat it. As a result, palatability, stability in diet, and homogeneity of mix must all be ensured prior to the initiation of an actual study.

Inclusion in drinking water is rarely used for oral administration of human drugs to test animals, though it sees more frequent use for the study of environmental agents.

Physiochemical properties of the test material should be a major consideration in selection of drinking water as a dosing matrix. Unlike diet preparation or preparation of gavage dose solutions and suspensions where a variety of solvents and physical processes can be utilized to prepare a dosable form, preparations of drinking water solutions are less flexible. Water solubility of the test chemical is the major governing factor and is dependent on factors such as pH, dissolved salts, and temperature. The animal model itself sets limitations for these factors (acceptability and suitability of pH and salt-adjusted water by the animals as well as animal environmental specifications such as room temperature).

Stability of the test chemical in drinking water under study conditions should be determined prior to study initiation. Consideration should be given to conducting stability tests on test chemical-drinking water admixtures presented to some test animals. Besides difficulties of inherent stability, changes in chemical concentrations may result from other influences. Chemicals with low vapor pressure can volatilize from the water into the air space located above the water of an inverted water bottle; thus, a majority of the chemical may be found in the "dead space," not in the water.

Certain test chemicals may be degraded by contamination with microorganisms. A primary source of these microorganisms is the oral cavity of rodents. Although rats and mice are not as notorious as the guinea pig in spitting back into water bottles, significant bacteria can pass via the sipper tubes and water flow restraints into the water bottles. Sanitation and sterilization procedures for water bottles and sipper tubes must be carefully attended to.

Many technicians may not be familiar with terms such as sublingual (under the tongue), buccal (between the cheek and gingiva), otic, and so on. A clear description of each of these nontraditional routes (i.e., other than gavage routes) should be discussed with technicians, and instructions may also be written down and given to them. Demonstrations are often useful to illustrate selected techniques of administration (e.g., to use an inhaler or nebulizer). Some chemicals must be placed by technicians into body orifices (e.g., medicated intrauterine devices such as Progesterset).

### 13.3.5. Minor Routes

The minor routes do see some use in safety assessment and at least three should be briefly presented here.

***Perocular Route.*** The administration of drugs or accidental exposure of chemicals to the eyes is not commonly a concern in systemic toxicity due to the small surface area exposed and the efficiency of the protective mechanisms (i.e., blink reflex and tears). As long as the epithelium of the eyes remains intact, it is impermeable to many molecules, but, if the toxicant has a suitable polar-nonpolar balance, penetration may occur (Kondrizer et al., 1959; Swan and White, 1972).

Holmstedt (1959) and Brown and Muir (1971) have reviewed perocular absorption of pesticides. More recently, Sinow and Wei (1973) have shown that the quarternary herbicide paraquat can be lethal to rabbits if applied directly to the surface of the eyes. Parathion, in particular, is exceedingly toxic when administered via the eye, a concern that must be kept in mind for the protection of pesticide applicators.

***Rectal Administration.*** Since a number of therapeutic compounds are given in the form of suppositories, an indication of the toxicity after rectal administration is sometimes required. Toxicity studies and initial drug formulations of such compounds are usually performed by the oral route and the rectal formulation comes late in development and marketing. In view of the difference between laboratory animals and humans in the anatomy and microflora of the colon and rectum, animal toxicity studies late in drug development are of limited value. However, in cases where an indication of potential rectal hazard or bioavailability are required, the compound may be introduced into the rectum of the rat using an oral dosing needle to prevent tissue damage. To avoid the rapid excretion of the unabsorbed dose, anesthetized animals should be used and the dose retained with an inert plug or bung (such as a cork).

Drugs (and, therefore, test chemicals) are occasionally administered by rectum, but most are not as well absorbed here as they are from the upper intestine. Aminophylline, used in suppository form for the management of asthma, is one of the few drugs routinely given in this way. Inert vehicles employed for suppository preparations include cocoa butter, glycerinated vehicles, gelatin, and polyethylene glycol. Because the rectal mucosa are irritated by nonisotonic solutions, fluids administered by this route should always be isotonic with plasma (e.g., 0.9% NaCl).

***Vaginal Administration.*** Though not a common one, some materials do have routine exposure by this route (spermicides, tampons, douches, and antibiotics, for example), and, therefore, must be evaluated for irritation and toxicity by this route. The older preferred models used rabbits and monkeys (Eckstein et al., 1969), but, more recently, a model that uses rats has been developed (Staab et al., 1987). McConnell (1973) clearly described the limitations, particularly of volume of test material, involved in such tests.

***Nasal Administration.*** A route that has gained increasing popularity of late for pharmaceutical administration in humans is the intranasal route. The reasons for this popularity are the ease of use (and, therefore, ready patient acceptance and high compliance rate), the high degree and rate of absorption of many substances (reportedly for most substances up to 1000 molecular weight; McMartin et al., 1987), and the avoidance of the highly acid environment in the stomach and first-pass metabolism in the liver (particularly important for some of the newer peptide moieties) (Attman and Dittmer, 1971). The only special safety concerns are the potential for irritation of the mucous membrane and the rapid distribution of administered materials to the CNS.

A number of means may be used to administer materials nasally, nebulizers and aerosol pumps being the most attractive first choices. Accurate dose administration requires careful planning, evaluation of the administration device, and attention to technique.

***Volume Limitations by Route.*** In the strictest sense, absolute limitations on how much of a dosage form may be administered by any particular route are determined by specific aspects of the test species or dosage form. But there are some general guidelines (determined by issues of humane treatment of animals, accurate deliver of dose and such) that can be put forth. These are summarized in Table 13.5. Section 13.8 and Section 13.4, "Formulation of Test Materials," should, of course, be checked to see if there is specific guidance due to the characteristics of a particular vehicle.

### 13.3.6. Route Comparisons and Contrasts

The first part of this chapter described, compared, and contrasted the various routes used in toxicology and presented guidelines for their use. There are, however, some exceptions to the general rules that the practicing toxicologist should keep in mind.

The relative ranking of efficacy of routes that was presented earlier in the chapter is not absolute; there can be striking exceptions. For example, though materials are usually much quicker acting and more potent when given by the oral route than by the dermal, this is not always the case. In the literature, Shaffer and West (1960)

**TABLE 13.5. General Guidelines for Maximum Dose Volumes by Route**

| Route | Volume ($ml\,kg^{-1}$) should not exceed | Notes |
|---|---|---|
| Oral | 20 | Fasted animals |
| Dermal | 2 | Limit is accuracy of dosing per available body surface. |
| Intravenous | 1 | Over 5 min |
| Intramuscular | 0.5 | At one site |
| Perocular | 0.01 ml | |
| Rectal | 0.5 | |
| Vaginal | 0.2 ml in rat | |
| | 1 ml in rabbit | |
| Inhalation | 2 mg $liter^{-1}$ | |
| Nasal | 0.1 ml per nostril in monkey or dog | |

(Baker et al., 1979; Garramone, 1986).

reported that tetram as an aqueous solution was more toxic when applied dermally than when given orally to rats. $LD_{50}$s reported were as follows [$LD_{50}$ ($mg\,kg^{-1}$) of tetram; 95% confidence limits]:

| Rat | Oral ($mg\,k^{-1}$) | Percutaneous ($mg\,k^{-1}$) |
|---|---|---|
| Male | 9 (7–13) | 2 (1–3) |
| Female | 8 (6–11) | 2 (1–3) |

The author has in the past, experienced this same phenomenon. Several materials that were found to be relatively nontoxic orally were extremely potent by the dermal route (differences in potency of more than an order of magnitude have been seen at least twice).

A general rule applicable to routes and vehicles should be presented here.

***Vehicles Can Mask the Effects of Active Ingredients.*** Particularly for clinical signs, attention should be paid to the fact that a number of vehicles (propylene glycol, for example) cause transient neurobehavioral effects that may mask similar short-lived (though not necessarily equally transient and reversible) effects of test materials.

## 13.4. FORMULATION OF TEST MATERIALS

One of the areas that is overlooked by virtually everyone in toxicology testing and research, yet is of crucial importance, is the use of vehicles in the formulation of test chemicals for administration to test animals. For a number of reasons, a drug of interest is rarely administered or applied as is ("neat"). Rather, it must be put in a form that can be accurately given to animals in such a way that it will be absorbed and not be too irritating. Most laboratory toxicologists come to understand vehicles and formulation, but to the knowledge of the author, guidance on the subject is limited to a short chapter on formulations by Fitzgerald et al. (1983). There is also a very helpful text on veterinary (Blodinger, 1982) and human (Levi, 1963) dosage forms.

Regulatory toxicology in the United States can be said to have arisen due to the problem of vehicles and formulation, in the late 1930s, when attempts were made to formulate the new drug sulphanilamide. This drug is not very soluble in water, and a U.S. firm called Massengill produced a clear, syrupy elixir formulation that was easy to take orally. The figures illustrate how easy it is to be misled. The drug sulphanilamide is not very soluble in glycerol, which has an $LD_{50}$ in mice of $31.5\,g\,kg^{-1}$, but there are other glycols that have the characteristic sweet taste and a much higher solvent capacity. Ethylene glycol has an $LD_{50}$ of $13.7\,g\,kg^{-1}$ in mice and $8.5\,g\,kg^{-1}$ in rats, making it slightly more toxic than diethylene glycol, which has an $LD_{50}$ in rats of $20.8\,g\,kg^{-1}$, similar to that for glycerol. The drug, which is itself inherently toxic, was marketed in a 75% aqueous diethylene glycol-flavored elixir. Early in 1937 came the first reports of deaths, but the situation remained obscure for about six months until it became clear that the toxic ingredient in the elixir was the diethylene glycol. Even as late as March 1937, Haag and Ambrose were reporting that the glycol was excreted substantially unchanged in dogs, suggesting that it was likely to be safe (Hagenbusch, 1937). Within a few weeks, Holick (1937) confirmed that a low concentration of diethylene in drinking water was fatal to a number of species. Hagenbusch (1937) found that the results of necropsies performed on patients who had been taking 60–70 ml of the solvent per day were similar to those of rats, rabbits, and dogs taking the same dose of solvent with or without the drug. This clearly implicated the solvent, although some authors considered that the solvent was simply potentiating the toxicity of the drug. Some idea of the magnitude of this disaster may be found in the paper of Calvary and Klumpp (1939), who reviewed 105 deaths and a further 2560 survivors who were affected to varying degrees, usually with progressive failure of the renal system. It is easy to be wise after the event, but the formulator fell into a classic trap, in that the difference between acute and chronic toxicity had not been adequately considered. In passing, the widespread use of ethylene glycol itself as an antifreeze has led to a number of accidental deaths, which suggests that the lethal dose in humans is around $1.4\,ml\,kg^{-1}$, or a volume of about 100 ml. In the preface to the first United States Pharmacopoeia, published in 1820, there is a the statement that "It is the object of the Pharmacopoeia to select from among substances which possess medical power, those, the utility of which is most fully established and best understood; and to form from them preparations and compositions, in which their powers may be exerted to the greatest advantage." This statement suggests that the influence that formulation and preparation may have on the biological activity of a drug (and on nonpharmaceutical chemicals) has been appreciated for a considerable time.

Available and commonly used vehicles and formulating agents are reviewed, along with basic information on their characteristics and usages, in Section 13.8 at the end of this chapter. There is a general presumption that those excipients and formulating agents listed in the Pharmacopoeia or in the *Inactive Ingredient Guide* prepared by the FDA are safe to use and without biological effect. This may not always be the case in either experimental animals (see Section 13.8) or humans (see Weiner and Bernstein, 1989), either directly or in how they alter absorption of and response to the active ingredient.

There are some basic principles to be observed in developing and preparing test material formulations. These are presented in Table 13.6.

*Bioavailability* is defined as the fraction of the dose reaching either the therapeutic target organ or tissue or the systemic circulation as unchanged compound following administration by any route. For an agent administered orally, bioavailability may be less than unity, for several reasons. The chemical may be incompletely absorbed. It may be metabolized in the gut, the gut wall, the portal blood, or the liver prior to entry into the systemic circulation (see Figure 13.2). It may undergo enterohepatic cycling with incomplete reabsorption following elimination into the bile. Biotransformation of some chemicals in the liver following oral administration is an important factor in the pharmacokinetic profile, as will be discussed further. Bioavailability measures following oral administration are generally given as the percentage of the dose available to the systemic circulation.

As the components of a mixture may have various physiochemical characteristics (solubility, vapor pressure, density, etc.), great care must be taken in preparing and administering any mixture so that what is actually tested is the mixture of interest.

Examples of such procedures are making dilutions (not all components of the mixture may be equally soluble or miscible with the vehicle) and generating either vapors or respirable aerosols (not all the components may have equivalent volatility or surface tension, leading to a test atmosphere that contains only a portion of the components of the mixture).

**TABLE 13.6. Desirable Characteristics of a Dosing Formulation and Its Preparation**

A. Preparation of the formulation should not involve heating of the test material anywhere near to the point where its chemical or physical characteristics are altered.

B. If the material is a solid and it is to be assessed for dermal effects, its shape and particle size should be preserved.

C. Multicomponent test materials (mixtures) should be formulated so that the administered form accurately represents the original mixture (i.e., components should not be selectively suspended or taken into solution).

D. Formulation should preserve the chemical stability and identity of the test material.

E. The formulation should be such as to minimize total test volumes. Use just enough solvent or vehicle.

F. The formulation should be easy to administer accurately.

G. pH of dosing formulations should be between 5 and 9, if possible.

H. Acids or bases should not be used to divide the test material (for both humane reasons and to avoid pH partitioning in either the gut or the renal tubule).

I. If a parental route is to be employed, final solutions should be as nearly isotonic as possible.

By increasing or decreasing the viscosity of a formulation, the absorption of a drug can be altered (Ritschel et al., 1974; Groves, 1966). Conversely, the use of absorbents to diminish absorption has been used as an antidote therapy for some forms of intoxication. Using the knowledge that rats cannot vomit, there have been serious attempts at making rodenticides safer to nontarget animals by incorporating emetics into the formulations, but this has had only a limited success. Gaines used *in vivo* liver perfusion techniques to investigate the apparent anomaly that the carbamate Isolan was more toxic when administered to rats percutaneously than when administered orally (Gaines, 1960). It has been shown that these results, a manifestation of different formulations, have been used for the two routes of exposure (oral and percutaneous) in estimating the $LD_{50}$ values using a common solvent, *n*-octanol. It was found that Isolan was significantly more toxic by the oral route than by the percutaneous route; by regression analysis it was found that at no level of lethal dose values was the reverse correct.

Although the oral route is the most convenient, there are numerous factors that make it unpredictable. Absorption by this route is subject to significant variation from animal to animal, and even in the same individual animal at different times. Considerable effort has been spent by the pharmaceutical industry to develop drug formulations with absorption characteristics that are both effective and dependable. Protective enteric coatings for pharmaceuticals were introduced long ago to retard the action of gastric fluids and then disintegrate and dissolve after passage of a tablet into the human intestine. The purposes of these coatings for drugs are to protect the active ingredient, which would be degraded in the stomach, to prevent nausea and vomiting caused by local gastric irritation (also a big problem in rodent studies, where over a long time period gastric irritation frequently leads to forestomach hyperplasia), to obtain higher local concentrations of the active ingredient intended to act locally in the intestinal tract, to produce a delayed biological effect, or to deliver the active ingredient to the intestinal tract for optimal absorption there. Such coatings are generally fats, fatty acids, waxes, or other such agents, and all of these intended purposes for drug delivery can readily be made to apply for some toxicity studies. Their major drawback, however, is the marked variability in time for a substance to be passed through the stomach. In humans, this gastric emptying time can range from minutes to as long as 12 h. One would expect the same for animals, as the limited available data suggest is the case. Similar coating systems, including microencapsulation (see Melnick et al., 1987), are available for, and currently used in, animal toxicity studies.

The test chemical is unlikely to be absorbed or excreted unless it is first released from its formulation. It is this stage of the process that is the first and most critical step for the activity of many chemicals. If the formulation does not release the chemical, the rest of the process becomes somewhat pointless.

It might be argued that the simplest way around the formulation problem is to administer any test as a solution in water, thereby avoiding the difficulties altogether. However, since multiple, small, accurately measured doses of a chemical are required repeatedly, reproducible dilutions must be used. Also, the water itself is to be regarded as the formulation vehicle, and the test substance must be water soluble and stable in solution, which many are not. If we take into account the need for accuracy, stability, and optimum performance *in vivo*, the problem can become complex.

Direct connections between observed toxicity and formulation components is uncommon and it is usually assumed that vehicles and other nontest chemical components are innocuous or have only transitory pharmacological effects. Historically, however, this has certainly not been the case. Even lactose may have marked toxicity in individual test animals (or humans) who are genetically incapable of tolerating it.

The initial stage of drug release from the formulation, both in terms of the amount and the rate of release, may exercise considerable influence at the clinical response level. A close consideration of the formulation parameters of any chemical is therefore essential during the development of any new drug, and, indeed, there are examples where formulations of established drugs also appear to require additional investigation.

The effects of formulation additives on chemical bioavailability from oral solutions and suspensions have been well reviewed by Hem (1973). He pointed out how the presence of sugars in a formulation may increase the viscosity of the vehicle. However, sugar solutions alone may delay stomach-emptying time considerably when compared to solutions of the same viscosity prepared with celluloses, which may be due to sugar's effect on osmotic pressure. Sugars of different types may also have an effect on fluid uptake by tissues and this, in turn, correlates with the effect of sugars such as glucose and mannitol on drug transport.

Surfactants have been explored widely for their effects on drug absorption, in particular using experimental animals (Gibaldi and Feldman, 1970; Gibaldi, 1976). Surfactants alter dissolution rates (of lipid materials), surface areas of particles and droplets, and membrane characteristics, all of which affect absorption.

Surfactants may increase the solubility of the drug via micelle formation, but the amounts of material required to increase solubility significantly are such that at least orally the laxative effects are likely to be unacceptable. The competition between the surfactant micelles and the absorption sites is also likely to reduce any useful effect and make any prediction of net overall effect difficult. However, if a surfactant has any effect at all, it is likely to be in the realm of agents that help disperse suspensions of insoluble materials and make them available for solution. Natural surfactants, in particular bile salts, may enhance absorption of poorly soluble materials.

The effective surface area of an ingested chemical is usually much smaller than the specific surface area that is an idealized *in vitro* measurement. Many drugs whose dissolution characteristics could be improved by particle-size reduction are extremely hydrophobic and may resist wetting by gastrointestinal fluids. Therefore, the gastrointestinal fluids may come in intimate contact with only a fraction of the potentially available surface area. The effective surface area of hydrophobic particle can often be increased by the addition of a surface-active agent to the formulation, which reduces the contact angle between the solid and the gastrointestinal fluids, thereby increasing effective surface area and dissolution rate.

Formulations for administering dermally applied toxicants present different considerations and problems. The extent of penetration and speed with which a biologically active substance penetrates the skin or other biological membrane depends on the effect that the three factors—vehicle, membrane, and chemical—exert on the diffusion process. It is now accepted that they together represent a functional unit that controls the penetration and location of the externally applied chemicals in the deeper layers of the skin or membrane layer. The importance of the vehicle for the absorption process has been neglected until recently. One of the few requirements demanded of the vehicle has been that it act as an inert medium that incorporates the test chemical in the most homogeneous distribution possible. In addition, chemical stability and good cosmetic appearance have been desirable. Most formulation in toxicology are based on empirical experience.

The chemical incorporated in a vehicle should reach the surface of the skin at a suitable rate and concentration. If the site of action lies in the deeper layers of the epidermis or below, the substance must cross the stratum corneum, if the skin is intact. Both processes, diffusion from the dosage form and diffusion through the skin barriers, are inextricably linked. They should be considered simultaneously and can be influenced by the choice of formulation.

The thesis that all lipid-soluble compounds basically penetrate faster than water-soluble ones cannot be supported in this absolute form. A lipophilic agent can penetrate faster or slower or at the same rate as a hydrophilic agent, depending on the vehicle used.

Disregarding such chemical-specific properties as dissociation constants (in the case of ionic compounds), particle size, and polymorphism, as well as side effects of viscosity, binding to vehicle components, complex formulation, and the like, the following formulation principles arise:

1. Optimization of the concentration of chemical capable of diffusion by testing its maximum solubility.
2. Reduction of the proportion of solvent to a degree that is adequate to keep the test material still in solution.
3. Use of vehicle components that reduce the permeability barriers.

These principles lead to the conclusion that each test substance requires an individual formulation. Sometimes different ingredients will be required for different concentrations to obtain the maximum rate of release. No universal vehicle is available for any route, but a number of approaches are. Any dosage preparation lab should be equipped with glassware, a stirring hot plate, a sonicator, a good homogenizer, and a stock of the basic formulating material, as detailed at the end of this chapter.

### 13.4.1. Dermal Formulations

Preparing formulations for application to the skin has special considerations associated with it, which, in the case of human pharmaceuticals, has even led to a separate book (Barry, 1983).

The physical state of the skin is considerable affected by external factors such as relative humidity, temperature, and air movement at the skin surface. If this contact is broken (for example, by external applications of ointments or creams), it is reasonable to assume that the new skin will change in some way, sometimes to an extent that creates new conditions of permeability for the test material. This would be the case, for example, if the stratum corneum becomes more hydrated than normal due to the topical delivery form. Temperature might also have an effect, as is the case when any constituents of the vehicle affect the inner structure of the skin through interactions with endogenous skin substances. Often several of these processes occur together.

Since this is a question of interactions between the vehicle and the skin (and the latter cannot be viewed as an inert medium), the composition of the vehicle itself, may be altered (e.g., by incorporation of skin constituents or through loss of volatile components).

The first contact between vehicle and skin occurs on the skin's surface. The first phase of interaction undoubtedly begins with the lipid mantle, in the case of so-called normal skin. If the skin has been damaged by wounds, the surface can form a moist milieu of serious exudate, resulting in abnormal wetting properties. Normally it is impregnated with oily sebaceous secretions and horny fat, presenting a hydrophobic surface layer. Water will not spread out as a film but will form droplets, while bases with a high affinity to the skin surface constituents spread spontaneously into a film and can wet. In the case of a base low viscosity, the degree of wetting can often be determined by measuring the angle of contact. If the preparation wets the skin surface, is drawn by capillary action from the visible area into the large inner surface of the stratum corneum, and is transported away into the interior, then it is said that the ointment or cream penetrates well. Spreading and wetting are purely surface phenomena, not penetration in the strict sense. If the skin shows a high content of its own lipids, spreading is limited. It is also reduced if the value of the surface tension of the skin ($o_s$) decreases compared to the value of the interfacial force between the skin and subject liquid ($y_{s/1}$) and the surface tension of the subject liquid ($0_1$), as is the case with aqueous bases. Addition of amphiphilic compounds decreases $o_1$ and $y_{s/1}$ and thus spreadability increases.

How much the endogenous emulsifying substances of the fatty film, such as cholesterol esters, and fatty acid salts, affect this spreading process is not clear. They can probably promote the emulsification of hydrophobic substances with water. Whether the sebaceous and epidermal lipids alone are sufficient to emulsify water and so form a type of emulsive film remains controversial. However, it is assumed that they, together with appropriate vehicle components, improve the spreading of the applied vehicle and that this effect can be potentiated by mechanical means such as intensive rubbing in. A good spreadability ensures that the active ingredient is distributed over a large area.

High local concentrations are avoided and, at the same time, close contact is made between the chemical and the upper layers of the skin.

In grossly simplified terms, hydrogels, suspensions, and oil-water emulsions behave on the skin surface similarly to aqueous solutions. By contrast, pastes and water-oil emulsions act like oil. The ability of an organic solvent to stick or wet depends on its specific properties (e.g., its viscosity and its surface tension).

At present, the information concerning alterations in vehicle composition on the skin surface is sparse. However, two possible extremes are conceivable. On the one hand, if the vehicle has a high vapor pressure, it often completely evaporates shortly after application. On the other hand, the vehicle may remain on the skin surface in an almost completely unchanged composition, (e.g., highly viscous Vaseline or similar thick covering systems). Between these two extremes lie the remaining types of vehicle.

The first situation applies for the short-chain alcohols, acetone, or ether. After their evaporation, the drug remains finely dispersed on or in the skin at 100% concentration.

If individual components evaporate, the structure of the vehicle changes and, under certain circumstances, also the effective drug concentration. Oil-water emulsions lose water rapidly, giving rise to the well-known cooling effect. If evaporation continues, the dispersed oil phase coalesces and forms a more or less occlusive film on the skin, together with the emulsifier and the drug. Of course, it is possible that a certain hydrophilic proportion of the drug is then present in suspended form or at least can react with charged molecules and is thus removed from the diffusion process at the start, at the same time, it is to be expected that soluble constituents of the skin are incorporated so that a new system can be formed on the surface and the adjoining layers of skin. Comparable transformations probably also occur after application of water-oil emulsions, providing one realizes that the water evaporates more slowly, the cooling effect is less strong and, due to the water-oil character of the molecule, the occlusive effect can be more marked because of the affinity of the oily components for the skin.

By contrast, Vaseline and similar highly viscous, lipid bases from the outset form an impenetrable layer, virtually unaffected by external factors or effects emanating from the skin itself. Interactions with the skin lipids are only likely at the boundary between ointment and skin.

The evaporation of the water from the skin into the atmosphere is a continuous process. It can be increased or decreased by the use of suitable vehicles. An evaporation increase will always occur if the water vapor from the vehicle is taken away more quickly than water can diffuse from the deeper layers into the stratum corneum. This applies in principle to all hydrophilic bases, particularly for systems with an oil-water character that, after loss of most of their own water, develop a true draining effect that can lead to the drying out of the underlying tissue. How much the penetration of hydrophilic drugs can be improved with the help of oil-water systems depends on the solution properties of the rest of the components in the skin. Generally, such compounds can only seldom reach deeper layers. It is equally difficult to show an adequate release of water from hydrophilic systems to a dry skin. If any such effects do occur, they are short term, and are quickly overtaken by opposing processes. The same seems to apply to most of the traditional moisturizers such as glycerin and propylene glycol (Powers and Fox, 1957; Rieger and Deems, 1974). They can also cause a large rise in the rate of evaporation, depending on the relative humidity, and thus increase the transepidermal loss of water. It is probably impossible to prevent this drying out without preparations having some occlusive properties.

In contrast, vehicle that are immiscible with water and those with a high proportion of oils have occlusive effects. They reduce both insensible perspiration and the release of sweat. The sweat collects as droplets at the opening of the glands, but does not spread as a film between the hydrophobic skin surface and the lipophilic base because the free surface energy of the vehicle-skin interface is smaller than that between water and skin. If a lipophilic layer of vehicle is present, this is not spontaneously replaced by the water-skin layer if sweat is secreted.

The horny layer consists of about 10% extracellular components such as lipids, proteins, and mucopolysaccharides. Around 5% of the protein and lipids form the cell wall. The majority of the remainder is present in the highly organized cell contents, predominantly as keratin fibers, which are generally assigned an $\alpha$-helical structure. They are embedded in a sulphur-rich amorphous matrix, enclosed by lipids that probably lie perpendicular to the protein axis. Since the stratum corneum is able to take up considerably more water than the amount that corresponds to its volume, it is assumed that this absorbed fluid volume is mainly located in the region of these keratin structures.

Some insight into where on the relative humidity continuum water molecules are absorbed can be gained from equilibrium isotherms (Ziegenmeyer, 1982) (Figure 13.3), which show a characteristic sigmoidal shape. At low relative humidity, water is first absorbed at specific skin sites, probably in the region of the peptide compounds and the various polar side chains. At higher moisture content, layers of water form on the skin. By using Zimm–Lundberg cluster theory (Zimm and Lundberg, 1956), additional information can be obtained about the nature of the absorbed water.

Because of thick intertwining protein fibers in the cell and in the area of the cell membrane, cell structure is rigid and remains so, but is altered by the osmotic effect of the penetrating water. The uptake of water entails a continual shifting of the cell

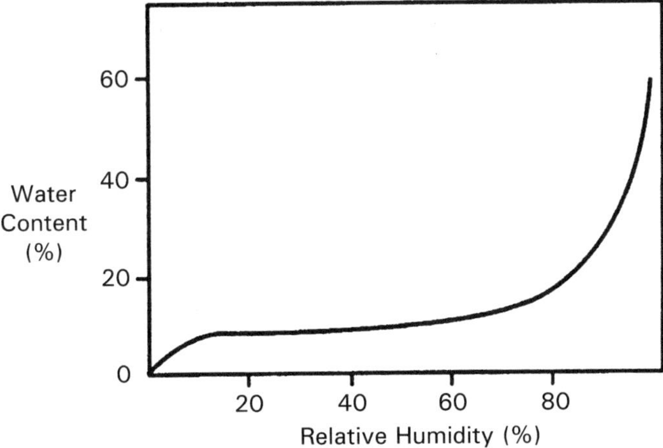


**FIGURE 13.3.** Sorption isotherms of water vapor as a function of the relative humidity, composition of constituents, and water content in the stratum corneum.

matrix, which gradually develops elastic opposing forces that increasingly resist further expansion. An equilibrium is reached if both forces balance each other. In the case of water, it takes quite a long time to completely hydrate the cell. This process can, however, be shortened if there are components present with a solvent effect diffusing out of a basic vehicle. The duration and degree of swelling depends on the affinity of all the dissolved substances for the tissue, and on the size of the maximum possible elastic reaction, which stabilizes cell structure.

### 13.4.2. Interactions Between Skin, Vehicle, and Test Chemical

The diffusion coefficient of the hydrated stratum corneum is larger than that of dry skin. Therefore, hydration increases the rate of passage of all substances that penetrate the skin. If the hydrated keratin complex is represented by a biphasix system, then it can be considered to exist as a continuous region covered with layers of water and intervening layers of lipids. Nonpolar compounds are predominantly dissolved in the nonpolar lipid matrix and diffuse through it. Polar substances, by contrast, pass through the aqueous layers. The diffusion of water and low molecular weight, hydrophilic molecules through these layers of water is more difficult than a corresponding free diffusion in an aqueous solution. This could, under certain circumstances, be due to a higher degree of organization of water in the protein structures (than in plasma or the free state), in the sense that this water is only available as the driving force of the diffusion process to a limited degree.

The degree of hydration can be controlled by the choice of vehicle. Lipophilic paraffin bases are available, but vehicles such as water-oil emulsions are more acceptable since they are less occlusive and offer ease of formulation.

In principle, temperature can also have an effect on penetration, which may be exerted on the basic vehicle if it contains temperature-sensitive components (e.g., nonionic tensides). Room and body temperatures can be enough to change the hydrophilic-lipophilic balance and thus possibly change the entire system. It has long been known that increasing temperature can considerably reduce diffusional resistance and thereby increase the rate of penetration of substances. In practice, however, this effect is of no importance. Of course, skin temperature will be increased a few degrees by occlusion because of the prevention of sweating and restriction of heat radiation. However, compared to the increase in penetration achieved by the simultaneous hydration process, this effect is insignificant.

Additives aimed at accelerating penetration always attempt to enable diffusion of pharmacologically active compounds into or through the stratum corneum without damaging it and without causing undesirable systemic effects. Although attempts have been made to limit these effects, this goal has not been achieved as yet. There are numerous substances that decrease the diffusional resistance of the skin, such as propylene glycol, tensides, parotic substances such as urea, DMSO (dimethyl sulfoxide), DMF (dimethyl formamide), and various other organic solvents, mostly of medium chain length. They all improve the penetration of dissolved agents, but only at the cost of the integrity of skin structure, raising the question of the degree of damage and reversibility.

If the substances have passed the stratum corneum, they also generally diffuse into the living part of the epidermis, reach the circulation, and then have systemic effects depending on the amount absorbed. Because these are often constituents of formulations, one generally expects them to have little direct influence on skin penetration. However, their amphiphilic properties allow them to form new systems with the body's constituents and even to change the physical state of water in the skin. By this means, a pathway is cleared for other hydrophilic substances to gain entry into the general circulation.

Most of a permeability enhancer (such as tenside) is bound to the stratum corneum. It is assumed that the underlying mechanism of the process involves interactions with keratin structures. Positively and negatively charged ionic groups of proteins have been suggested as binding sites for ionic substances. Ion pairs could also form. On the other hand, hydrophobic areas are present that bind with the uncharged part of the enhancers. The total free binding energy of molecules to keratin is made up of the contributions arising from electrostatic and nonpolar interactions. Nonpolar interactions increase with chain length of the molecule. This would be the reason why predominantly anionic molecules of medium chain length exert stronger effects on the keratin structure than those of shorter chain length (Dominguez et al., 1977).

In order to reach the interior of the tightly enmeshed keratin, the molecule must overcome the elastic energy of the polypeptide matrix. The energy necessary to do this is proportional to the volume of the penetrating molecule. The larger the volume, the more difficult it will be for the molecule to approach the various binding sites of proteins in the interior of the keratin complex. Thus, the size of the penetrating molecule is subject to certain limits. If more molecules are present than can become bound, it is possible that a few of them will reach the living layers of the epidermis, as has been described for several anionic, mostly medium-chain enhancer molecules such as tensides. It remains unclear whether this is a consequence of pure saturation or if other interactions are involved (e.g., with structural lipids or hydrophilic materials from the intercellular lipids).

The extent to which the vehicle can affect the entire diffusion process can be shown by an example. In a four-component system of 40% oil, 40% water, and 20% of an emulsifying agent and coemulsifier, alteration of only the proportion of emulsifier to coemulsifier leads to systems of completely different colloidal-chemical structures, which can be labeled as either creams, gels, or microemulsions.

Dermal administration presents fewer logistic difficulties than oral administration. Liquids can be administered as supplied and powders or solids can be moistened with saline to form a thick paste or slurry, or can be applied dry and moistened with saline. Solid materials (sheets or plastic, fabric, etc.) can also be administered dermally. Liquid materials or slurries are applied directly to the skin, taking care to spread the material evenly over the entire area or as much of the area as can reasonably be covered, and then covering with a strip of gauze. If a large amount of material is being administered and the abdominal skin will be exposed, it is sometimes necessary to apply material to the gauze and to the skin. Dry materials are weighed out, then placed on the gauze strip and moistened with physiological saline (generally 15 ml) so that they will adhere to the gauze. The gauze is then wrapped around the animal. This porous gauze dressing is then held in place by an additional wrapping, generally of an impervious material, to create an "occlusive" covering. This occlusion enhances penetration and prevents ingestion or evaporation of the test material.

Another recently developed approach is the use of plastic containment capsules (modified Hilltop Chambers) for administration of well-measured doses in a moisturized microenvironment (Derelanko et al., 1987).

Finally, it should be noted that for some agents (contrary to the general rule), decreasing the concentration of chemical in a vehicle may increase its apparent intrinsic toxicity.

### 13.4.3. Oral Formulations

The physical form of a material destined for oral administration often presents unique challenges. Liquids can be administered as supplied or diluted with an appropriate vehicle, and powders or particulates can often be dissolved or suspended in an appropriate vehicle. However, selection of an appropriate vehicle is often difficult. Water and oil (such as the vegetable oils) are used most commonly. Materials that are not readily soluble in either water or oil can frequently be suspended in a 1% aqueous mixture of methylcellulose. Occasionally, a more concentrated methylcellulose suspension (up to 5%) may be necessary. Materials for which appropriate solutions or suspensions cannot be prepared using one of these three vehicles often present major difficulties.

Limited solubility or suspendability of a material often dictates preparation of dilute mixtures that may require large volumes to be administered. The total volume of liquid dosing solution or suspension that can be administered to a rodent is limited by the size of its stomach. However, because rats lack a gagging reflex and have no emetic mechanism, any material administered will be retained. Guidelines for maximum amounts to be administered are given in Table 13.5.

Limitations on total volume, therefore, present difficulties for materials that cannot easily be dissolved or suspended. The most dilute solutions that can be administered for a limit-type test ($5000\,\mathrm{mg\,kg^{-1}}$), using the maximum volumes shown in Table 13.5, generally are 1% for aqueous mixtures and 50% for other vehicles.

Although vehicle control animals are not required for commonly used vehicles (water, oil, methylcellulose), most regulations require that the biological properties of a vehicle be known and/or that historical data be available. Unfortunately, the best solvents are generally toxic and, thus, cannot be used as vehicles. Ethanol and acetone can be tolerated in relatively high doses but produce effects that may complicate interpretation of toxicity associated with the test material alone. It is sometimes possible to dissolve a material in a small amount of one of these vehicles and then dilute the solution in water or in oil.

Gels and resins often present problems because of their viscosity at room temperature. Warming these materials in a water bath to a temperature of up to 50°C will frequently facilitate mixing and dosing. However, it is important to ascertain that no thermal degradation occurs and that actually administered formulations be at or near body temperature.

Other possibilities for insoluble materials are to mix the desired amount of material with a small amount of the animal's diet or to use capsules. The difficulty with the diet approach is the likelihood that the animal will not consume all of the treated diet or that it may selectively not consume chunks of test material. Use of capsules, meanwhile, is labor intensive. In rare cases, if all of these approaches fail, it may not be possible to test a material by oral administration. In capsules, particle size is generally inversely related to solubility and bioavailability. However, milling of solids may adversely affect their chemical nature and/or pose issues of safety.

If necessary, the test substance should be dissolved or suspended as a suitable vehicle, preferably in water, saline, or an aqueous suspension such as 0.5% methyl cellulose in water. If a test substance cannot be dissolved or suspended in an aqueous medium to form a homogenous dosage preparation, corn oil or another solvent can be used. The animals in the vehicle control group should receive the same volume of vehicle given to animals in the highest-dose group.

The test substance can be administered to animals at a constant concentration across all dose levels (i.e., varying the dose volume) or at a constant dose volume (i.e., varying the dose concentration). However, the investigator should be aware that the toxicity observed by administration in a constant concentration may be different from that observed when given in a constant dose volume. For instance, when a large volume of corn oil is given orally, gastrointestinal motility is increased, causing diarrhea and decreasing the time available for absorption of the test substance in the GI tract. This situation is particularly true when a highly lipid-soluble chemical is tested.

If an organic solvent is used to dissolve the chemical, water should be added to reduce the dehydrating effect of the solvent within the gut lumen. The volume of water or solvent-water mixture used to dissolve the chemical should be kept low, since excess quantities may distend the stomach and cause rapid gastric emptying. In addition, large volumes of water may carry the chemical through membrane pores and increase the rate of absorption. Thus, if dose-dependent absorption is suspected, it is important that the different doses are given in the same volume of solution.

Larger volumes than those detailed earlier may be given, although nonlinear kinetics seen under such circumstances may be due to solvent-induced alteration of intestinal function. The use of water-immiscible solvents such as corn oil (which are sometimes used for gavage doses) should be avoided, since it is possible that mobilization from the vehicle may be rate limiting. Magnetic stirring bars or homogenizers can be used in preparing suspensions. Sometimes a small amount of a surfactant such as Tween 80, Span 20, or Span 60 is helpful in obtaining a homogenous suspension.

A large fraction of such a material may quickly pass through the gastrointestinal tract and remain unabsorbed. Local irritation by a test substance generally decreases when the material is diluted. If the objective of the study is to establish systemic toxicity, the test substance should be administered in a constant volume to minimize gastrointestinal irritation that may, in turn, affect its absorption. If, however, the objective is to assess the irritation potential of the test substance, then it should be administered undiluted.

### 13.4.4. Parenteral Formulations

Parenteral dose forms include aqueous, aqueous organic, and oily solutions, emulsions, suspensions, and solid forms for implantation. These parenterals need to be sterile and pyrogen-free; they are, if possible, buffered close to normal physiological pH and preferably are isotonic with the body fluids.

The preparation of parenteral dosage forms of approved and potential drugs for animals is the same as for humans. Turco and King (1974) provide a comprehensive review of the subject, which, though written with human therapeutics in mind, contains very little that is not applicable to animals. Sterility, lack of pyrogenicity, blood compatibility, and low to no irritation at the point of injection are biological requirements; there are also a corresponding set of physicochemical requirements.

Parenteral products are usually given to humans when an immediate effect is needed, when a patient is unable to accept medication by the oral route, or when the drug will be ineffective by the oral route. These conditions apply to animals used in safety evaluation.

Parenteral products can be easily administered to confined or restrained animals, leaving no doubt that the animal received its medication.

To be acceptable, a subcutaneous or intramuscular formulation should cause only a minimum of irritation, no permanent damage to the tissues, and be systemically distributed and active when administered by this route. The ideal parenteral product is an aqueous solution isotonic with the body fluids with a pH between 7 and 8. When the drug lacks sufficient aqueous solubility, a suspension may be considered; however, in most cases, the bioavailability of the drug may be affected and encapsulation by the body at the site of injection is extremely likely. The solubility of the drug in water may be improved by the addition of cosolvents such as alcohol, propylene glycol, polyethylene glycol, dimethylacetamide, dimethylsulfoxide, or dimethylformamide. The resulting solution must have additional tolerance for water so that the drug will not precipitate at the site of injection when the solution is diluted by body fluids. If precipitation occurs at the site of injection, the absorption of the drug may be delayed or even completely inhibited.

Water-miscible solvents alone can be used when the drug is chemically unstable in the presence of any water. The number of solvents available for this purpose is extremely limited. The classic review of this subject was made in 1963 (Spiegel and Noseworthy), and some 30 years later, no additional solvents are available. This is unlikely to change in the near future due to the extensive effort necessary to determine the safety of a solvent used as a vehicle. When a nonaqueous vehicle is used, one can invariably expect some degree of pain upon injection, and subsequent tissue destruction is possible. This damage may be due to the heat of solution as vehicle mixes with body fluids; it may be associated with tissues rejecting the solvent; or, it may be an inherent property of the solvent.

Fixed oils of vegetable origin and their esters may be used as parenteral vehicles for some drugs, particularly steroidal hormones. While an oleaginous vehicle may delay or impair absorption of the drug, this characteristic has been used to advantage with some drugs where a small dose is desired over a long period of time. The formulator must know which species will receive the formulation and the type of equipment used in its administration. A product intended for a dog or primate is usually given to a single animal at a time. Conventional glass or disposable syringes will be used with a 20- or 22-gauge needle, which may impede the flow of the liquid, especially when an oleaginous vehicle is used. Impedance is usually compensated for by using small animals, since the volume of injection is small and no more than one injection is normally given at one time.

The viscosity of the solution will influence its acceptability when automatic injection equipment is used. If many animals are injected at one time, a viscous solution that requires a great deal of force to eject will rapidly tire the user. When the automatic injector is refilled from a reservoir, a viscous solution will be slow to fill the volumetric chamber. The subjective aspect of measuring the ease of expelling a dose can be eliminated by constructing an apparatus that will measure the pressure needed to expel a dose. An objective means of measuring ease will allow the formulator to vary the composition of the injection and measure any improvement in injectability. For example, the addition of a wetting agent can be investigated and, if improvement is seen, the level of use can be optimized.

A parenteral product in a multidose vial must contain a preservative to protect the contents of the vial against contamination during repeated withdrawal of dose aliquots.

## 13.5.  DOSING CALCULATIONS

One of the first things a new technician (or graduate student) must learn is how to calculate dose. Generally, administered doses in systemic toxicity studies are based on the body weight of the animal (expressed as either weight or volume, for liquids, of the test substance per kilogram of body weight of the animal), although some would maintain that surface area may be a more appropriate basis on which to gauge individual dose. The weight (or dose) of the test substance is often expressed in milligrams or grams of active ingredient if the test substance is not pure (i.e., if it is not 100% active ingredient).

Ideally, only the 100% pure sample should be tested; however, impurity-free samples are difficult to obtain and preparation of formulations (as previously discussed) is frequently essential. The toxicity of impurities or formulation components should be examined separately if the investigator feels that they may contribute significantly to the toxicity of the test substance.

If the test substance contains only 75% active ingredient and the investigator chooses a constant dose volume of $10\,\mathrm{ml\,kg^{-1}}$ body weight across all dose levels, it will be more convenient to prepare a stock solution such that when $10\,\mathrm{ml\,kg^{-1}}$ of this stock solution is given to the animal, the dose will be the desired one (say $500\,\mathrm{mg\,kg^{-1}}$ of active ingredient). The concentration of this stock solution would be $(500\,\mathrm{mg}/10\,\mathrm{ml})/0.75 = 66.7\,\mathrm{mg}$ of the test substance per milliliter of diluent.

Aliquots of the test substance for other dose levels can then be prepared by dilution of the stock solution. For example, the solution concentration for a

250 mg kg$^{-1}$ dose level is (200 mg/10 ml)/0.75 = 26.7 mg of the test substance per milliliter of diluent.

This solution can be prepared by diluting the stock solution 25 times; that is, for each ml of the 26.7 mg ml$^{-1}$ solution to be prepared,

$$\frac{(26.7 \text{ mg ml}^{-1})(1 \text{ ml})}{66.7 \text{ mg ml}^{-1}} = 0.400 \text{ ml of the stock solution}$$

This amount should be diluted to a final volume of 1 ml with the vehicle.

The other way to express a relative dose in animals or humans is to do so in terms of body surface area. There are many reasons for believing that the surface area approach is more accurate for relating doses between species (Schmidt-Nielson, 1984), and especially between test animals and humans, but this is still a less common approach in safety assessment, although it is the currently accepted norm in several areas: carcinogenesis and chemotherapy, for example.

## 13.6. CALCULATING MATERIAL REQUIREMENTS

One of the essential basic skills for the efficient design and conduct of safety assessment studies is to be able to accurately project compound requirements for the conduct of a study. In theory, this simply requires plugging numbers into a formula such as

$$(A \times B \times C \times D)1.1 = \text{total compound requirement}$$

where

A = number of animals in each study group
B = the sum of doses of the dose groups (such as 0.1 + 0.3 + 1.0 mg kg$^{-1}$ = 1.4 mg kg$^{-1}$
C = the number of doses to be delivered (usually the length of the study in days)
D = the average body weight per animal (assuming dosing is done on a per body weight basis).
1.1 = a safety factor (in effect, 10%) to allow for spillage, etc.

As an example of this approach, consider a study that calls for 10 dogs/sex/group (A = 10 × 2 = 20) to receive 0, 10, 50, or 150 mg kg$^{-1}$ day$^{-1}$ (B = 10 + 50 + 150 = 210 mg kg$^{-1}$) for 30 days (C = 30). On average, our dogs of the age range used weigh 10 kg (D = 10 kg). Our compound need is then (20 × 210 mg kg$^{-1}$ × 30 × 10 kg) 1.1 = 1.386 kg.

The real-life situation is a bit more complicated, since animal weights change over time, diet studies have doses dependent on daily diet consumption, the material may be a salt but dosage should be calculated on the basis of the parent compound, and not all animals may be carried through the entire study.

**TABLE 13.7. Standardized Total Compound Requirements for Rodent Diet Studies**[a]

| Length of Study | Total Compound Requirement (g) per dose (mg kg$^{-1}$ day$^{-1}$) | | | | | |
| --- | --- | --- | --- | --- | --- | --- |
| | 1 | 3 | 10 | 30 | 100 | 300 |
| Rat[b] | | | | | | |
| 2 wks | 0.2 | 0.4 | 1.2 | 4 | 10.6 | 32 |
| 4 wks | 0.43 | 0.7 | 2.5 | 7.5 | 25 | 75 |
| 13 wks | 0.8 | 2.6 | 8.5 | 25.5 | 85 | 260 |
| 52 wks | 7 | 21 | 70 | 210 | 0.7[c] | 2.1[c] |
| 2 yrs | 15 | 45 | 150 | 450 | 1.5[c] | 4.5[c] |
| Mouse | | | | | | |
| 2 wks | 0.03 | 0.06 | 0.22 | 0.65 | 2.2 | 6.4 |
| 4 wks | 0.08 | 0.14 | 0.8 | 1.4 | 8 | 14 |
| 13 wks | 0.14 | 0.42 | 1.4 | 4.2 | 14 | 42 |
| 18 mos | 0.85 | 2.5 | 8.5 | 25 | 85 | 250 |

[a] Based on 10 animals per sex per group for the length of the study that are 6–8 weeks old at study initiation. Animals are weighed to determine body weights.
[b] Sprague-Dawley rats (body weights and compound requirements for Fischers would be less).
[c] In kilograms.

For rats and mice (where weight change is most dramatic and diet studies most common), Table 13.7 presents some reliable planning values for compound requirements during diet studies.

## 13.7.  EXCIPIENTS

Excipients are usually thought of as inert substances (such as gum arabic and starch) that form the vehicle or bulk of the dosage form of a drug. They are, of course, both much more complicated than this and not necessarily inert. A better definition would be that of the USP and National Formulary, which defined excipients as any component, other than the active substances (that is, drug substances or DS) intentionally added to the formulation of a dosage form. These substances serve a wide variety of purposes: enhancing stability, adding bulking, increasing and/or controlling absorption, providing or masking flavor, coloring and serving as a lubricant in the manufacturing process. They are, in fact, essential for the production and delivery of marketed drug products. As will soon be made clear, they are regulated both directly and as part of the drug product (DP). For the pharmaceutical manufacturers, using established and accepted excipients (such as can be found in Smolinske, 1992 or APA, 1994, although these lists are not complete) is much preferred. However, both pharmaceutical manufacturers and the companies which supply excipients must from time to time utilize (and therefore develop, evaluate for safety and get approved) new excipients.

### 13.7.1. Regulation of Excipients

Table 13.8 lists the relevant sections of CFR 21 which govern excipients. Under Section 201(g)(1) of the Federal Food, Drug, and Cosmetic Act (FD&C Act; 1), the term *drug* is defined as:

(A) articles recognized in the official *United States Pharmacopeia*, official *Homeopathic Pharmacopeia of the United States*, or official *National Formulary*, or any supplement to any of them; and (B) Articles intended for use in the diagnosis, cure, mitigation, treatment, or prevention of disease in man or other animals; and (C) Articles (other than food) intended to affect the structure of any function of the body of man or other animals; and (D) Articles intended for use as a component of any articles specified in clause (A), (B), or (C).

An excipient meets the definitions as listed in (A) and (D) above.

In 21 CFR Section 210.3(b)(8)(2), an "inactive ingredient means any component other than an active ingredient." According to the CFR, the term "inactive ingredient" includes materials in addition to excipients. 21 CFR Section 201.117 states

Inactive ingredients: A harmless drug that is ordinarily used as an inactive ingredient, such as a coloring, emulsifier, excipient, flavoring, lubricant, preservative, or solvent in the preparation of other drugs shall be exempt from Section 502(f)(1) of the Act. This exemption shall not apply to any substance intended for a use which results in the preparation of a new drug, unless an approved new-drug application provides for such use.

Excipients also meet the definition of component in the Good Manufacturing Practice (GMP) regulations in 21 CFR Section 210.3(b)(3): "Component means any ingredient intended for use in the manufacture of a drug product, including those that may not appear in such drug product."

The *NF* Admissions Policy in the *United States Pharmacopeia 23/National Formulary 18* defines the word excipient (3): "An excipient is any component other than the active substance(s), intentionally added to the formulation of a dosage form. It is not defined as an inert commodity or an inert component of a dosage form."

Similar to all other drugs, excipients must comply with the adulteration and misbranding provisions of the FD&C Act. Under Section 501(a), an excipient shall be deemed to be adulterated if it consists in whole or in part of any filthy, putrid, or decomposed substance, or if it has been prepared, packed, or held under insanitary conditions whereby it may have been contaminated with filth, or whereby it may have been rendered injurious to health. An excipient is adulterated if the methods used in, or the facilities or controls used for its manufacture, processing, packing, or holding do not conform to or are not operated or administered in conformity with current Good Manufacturing Practice to assure that such drug meets the requirements of the act as to safety and has the identity and strength, and meets the quality and purity characteristics which it purports or is represented to possess. In addition, under Section 501(b), an excipient shall be deemed to be adulterated if it purports to

**TABLE 13.8. U.S. Code of Federal Register References to Excipients**

| Subject | Reference | Content |
|---|---|---|
| General | 21 CFR § 210.3(b)(8) | Definitions |
| | 21 CFR § 201.117 | Inactive ingredients |
| | 21 CFR § 210.3(b)(3) | Definitions |
| Over-the-counter drug products | 21 CFR § 330.1(e) | General conditions for general recognition as safe, effective, and not misbranded |
| | 21 CFR § 328 | Over-the-counter drug products intended for oral ingestion that contain alcohol |
| Drug Master Files | 21 CFR § 314.420 | Drug master files |
| Investigational New Drug Application | 21 CFR § 312.23(a)(7) | IND content and format |
| New Drug Application | 21 CFR § 312.31 | Information amendments |
| | 21 CFR § 314.50(d)(1)(ii)(a) | Content and format of an application |
| | 21 CFR § 314.70 | Supplements and other changes to an approved application |
| Abbreviated New Drug Application | 21 CFR § 314.94(a)(9) | Content and format of an abbreviated application |
| | 21 CFR § 314.127 | Refusal to approve an abbreviated new drug application |
| | 21 CFR § 314.127(a)(8) | Refusal to approve an abbreviated new drug application |
| Current Good Manufacturing Practice | 21 CFR § 211.84(d) | Testing an approval or ejection of components, drug product containers and closures |
| | 21 CFR § 211.165 | Testing and release for distribution |
| | 21 CFR § 211.180(b) | General requirements |
| | 21 CFR § 211.80 | General requirements |
| | 21 CFR § 211.137 | Expiration dating |
| Listing of drugs | 21 CFR § 207 | Registration of procedures of drugs and listing of drugs in commercial distribution |
| | 21 CFR § 207.31(b) | Additional drug listing information |
| | 21 CFR § 207.10(e) | Exceptions for domestic establishments |

*(continued)*

**TABLE 13.8.** (*continued*)

| Subject | Reference | Content |
| --- | --- | --- |
| Labeling | 21 CFR § 201.100(b)(5) | Prescription drugs for human use |
| | 21 CFR § 201.20 | Declaration of presence of FD&C Yellow No. 5 and/or FD&C Yellow No. 6 in certain drugs for human use |
| | 21 CFR § 201.21 | Declaration of presence of phenylalanine as a component of aspartame in over-the-counter and prescription drugs for human use |
| | 21 CFR § 201.22 | Prescription drugs containing sulfites; required warning statements |

be or is represented as a drug the name of which is recognized in an official compendium, and its strength differs from, or its quality or purity falls below, the standards set forth in such compendium.

U.S. Food and Drug Administration (FDA) compliance officials strongly encourage the use of inactive ingredients that meet compendial standards when standards exist. The FDA Center for Drug Evaluation and Research maintains an Inactive Ingredient Committee whose charter includes the evaluation of the safety of inactive ingredients on an as-needed basis, preparation of recommendations concerning the types of data needed for excipients to be declared safe for inclusion in a drug product, and other related functions (4).

From a regulatory standpoint, the FDA's concern regarding safety involves the toxicity, degradants, and impurities of excipients, as discussed in other chapters in this book. In addition, other chapters of this book address types of toxicity concerns, toxicity testing strategies, and exposure and risk assessment of excipients.

Excipients must be safe for their intended use. Under 21 CFR Section 330.1(e), over-the-counter (OTC) human drugs that are generally recognized as safe and effective and not misbranded, may only contain inactive ingredients if they are suitable and if the amounts administered are safe and do not interfere with the effectiveness of the drug or with required tests or assays. Color additives may be used in accordance with the provisions of the FD&C Act and the regulations of 21 CFR Parts 70–82. The FDA proposed that to make it clear that, to be considered as suitable within the meaning of 21 CFR Section 330.1(e), each inactive ingredient in an OTC human drug product should perform a specific function (5). The proposed regulation defined *safe and suitable* to mean that the inactive ingredient meets various conditions as mentioned in the foregoing. OTC drug manufacturers are responsible for assuring that these conditions are met. There is no formal approval mechanism.

In the United States, the safety and suitability of excipients used in new drugs are considered as part of the New Drug Application (NDA) process. There is no separate and independent review and approval system for excipients. There are no specific regulations or guidelines that specify the requirements needed to gain approval of a new drug that contains a new excipient. Generally, pharmaceutical companies choose excipients that previously have been approved for commercial use in other NDAs. The FDA's Inactive Ingredient Guide (6), discussed later in this chapter, contains a listing of inactive ingredients present in approved drug products. There is currently no way of gaining a listing for an excipient in the guide independent of the NDA route. The FDA reviews the status of an excipient in food as information to support its use in drug products. Factors relative to the use of an excipient, such as dosing regimen and route of administration, are also reviewed. Advances in excipient technology and drug dosage from technology have created a need for a separate regulatory approval process for new excipients. The *USP* published IPEC's Excipient Safety Evaluation Guidelines as Information Chapter ⟨1074⟩ Excipient Biological Safety Evaluation Guideline.

Information on existing or new excipients can be described and provided to the FDA in an NDA directly. Alternatively, the manufacturers of excipients may prepare and submit type IV Drug Master Files (DMF) to support the use of an excipient in one or more NDAs. The DMFs are discussed in FDA's regulations under 21 CFR Section 314.420 and the FDA-issued Guidance for Drug Master Files (8). When authorized by the DMF submitter (i.e., the excipient manufacturer) and cross-referenced by an NDA submitter, the FDA reviews the DMF to make determinations on the safety, manufacture, and quality of the excipient use in the new drug that is the subject of the then pending NDA. The DMF becomes active when reviewed in conjunction with the review and approval of an NDA.

The *USP/NF* provides a listing of excipients by categories in a table according to the function of the excipient in a dosage form, such as tablet binder, disintegrant, and such. An excellent reference for excipient information is the APA's *Handbook of Pharmaceutical Excipients* (1994).

Excipients have historically not been subjected to extensive safety testing because they have been considered *a priori* to be biologically inactive, therefore, nontoxic. Many, if not most, excipients used are approved food ingredients, the safety of which has been assured by a documented history of safe use or appropriate animal testing. Some of the excipients are Generally Recognized As Safe (GRAS) food ingredients. The excipient is an integral component of the finished drug preparation and, in most countries, is evaluated as part of this preparation. There has been no apparent need to develop specific guidelines for the safety evaluation of excipients, and most developed countries do not have specific guidelines. However, as drug development has become more complex and/or new dosage forms have developed, improved drug bioavailability has become more important. It was noted that the available excipients were often inadequate; new pharmaceutical excipients specifically designed to meet the challenges of delivering new drugs were needed, and these are being developed.

The proper safety evaluation of new excipients has now become an integral part of drug safety evaluation.

In the absence of official regulatory guidelines, the Safety Committees of the International Pharmaceutical Excipients Council (IPEC) in the United States, Europe, and Japan developed guidelines for the proper safety evaluation of new pharmaceutical excipients (IPEC, 1997). The Committees critically evaluated guidelines for the safety evaluation of food ingredients, cosmetics, and other products, as well as excipients, and other appropriate materials. Before initiating a safety evaluation program for a new pharmaceutical excipient, it is advisable to address the following:

1. Chemical and physical properties and functional characterization of the test material.
2. Analytical methods that are sensitive and specific for the test material and that can be used to analyze for the test material in animal food used in the feeding studies or in the vehicle used for other studies.
3. Available biological, toxicological, and pharmacological information on the test material and related materials (which involves a thorough search of the scientific literature).
4. Intended conditions of use, including reasonable estimates of exposure.
5. Potentially sensitive segments of the population.

As discussed in Chapter 1, a comprehensive and critical search of the scientific literature on the test material and related materials is essential before the start of any testing program.

As pharmaceutical excipients are assumed to be biologically nonreactive, dose-response relations cannot always be established. An acceptable alternative is to use a maximum attainable or maximum feasible dose. This is the highest dose possible that will not compromise the nutritional or health status of the animal. Table 13.9 summarizes the maximum or limit doses for various types of studies by different routes of exposure. For example, 2000 mg/kg body weight of an orally administered test material is the maximum dose recommended for a testing strategy that has been developed for new pharmaceutical excipients that takes into consideration the physical-chemical nature of the product and the potential route(s) and duration of exposures, both through its intended use as part of a drug product and through workplace exposure during manufacturing. The number and types of studies recommended in this tiered approach are based on the duration and routes of potential human exposure. Thus, the longer the exposure to the new pharmaceutical excipient, the more studies are necessary to assure safety. Table 13.10 summarizes the entire set of toxicological studies recommended for new pharmaceutical excipients (Weiner and Katkoskie, 1999; IPEC, 1997).

Tests have been outlined for each exposure category to assure safe use of the time period designated. The tests for each exposure category assure the safe use of the new pharmaceutical excipient for the time frame specified for the specific exposure category. Additional tests are required for longer exposure times.

**TABLE 13.9. Limit Doses for Toxicological Studies**

| Nature of Test | Species | Limit Dose[a] |
|---|---|---|
| Acute oral | Rodent | 2000 mg/kg bw |
| Acute dermal | Rabbit | 2000 mg/kg bw |
| | Rat | |
| Acute inhalation[b] | Rat | 5 mg/L air for 4 h or maximum attainable level under conditions of study |
| Dermal irritation | Rabbit | 0.5 mL liquid<br>0.5 g solid |
| Eye irritation | Rabbit | 0.1 mL liquid<br>100 mg solid |
| 14-day/28-day oral repeated dosing; 90-day subchronic | Rodent, Nonrodent | 1000 mg/kg bw/day |
| 14-day/28-day oral repeated dosing; 90-day subchronic | Rat, rabbit | 1000 mg/kg bw/day |
| Chronic toxicity, carcinogenicity | Rats, mice | 5% maximum dietary concentration for nonnutrients |
| Reproduction | Rats | 1000 mg/kg bw/day |
| Developmental toxicity (teratology) | Mice, rats, rabbits | 1000 mg/kg bw/day |

[a] mg/kg bw, milligrams of test material dosed per kilogram of body weight to the test species.
[b] Acute inhalation guidelines that indicate this limit dose are U.S. Environmental Protection Agency Toxic Substance Health Effect Test Guidelines, Oct., 1984; (PB82-232984) Acute Inhalation Toxicity Study; the OECD Guidelines of the Testing of Chemicals, Vol 2, Section 4; Health Effects, 403, Acute Inhalation Toxicity Study, May 12, 1982, and the Official Journal of the European Communities, L383A, Vol 35, Dec. 29, 1992, Part B.2 (adapted from Wiener and Katkoskie, 1999).

The base set required for all excipients is detailed in Table 13.11. These are sufficient, however, only for those excipients intended for use for up to two weeks in humans.

If exposure to the new pharmaceutical excipient is expected to occur for longer than two but no more than six weeks, additional toxicological studies are required, as shown in Table 13.12. The longer the expected human exposure, the more extensive will be the toxicological studies to assure safety. A tiered approach assures that those tests necessary to ensure safety for the expected duration of human exposure are conducted. Thus, to assure safe use for greater than two weeks, but no more than six weeks in humans, subchronic toxicity and developmental toxicity studies are required. To assure safe use for greater than six continuous weeks, chronic or oncogenicity studies are conditionally required, as per Table 13.12. This means long-term studies should be considered for prolonged human exposures, but may not be absolutely required. A thorough scientific review of the data generated in the base set and (Table 13.10) studies should be undertaken. From a critical evaluation by a competent toxicologist, the results of the physical–chemical properties of the test

**TABLE 13.10. Summary of Toxicological Studies Recommended for New Pharmaceutical Excipients Based on Route of Exposure[a]**

| Tests | Oral | Mucosal | Trans-dermal | Dermal/ topical | Paren-teral | Inhalation/ intranasal | Ocular |
|---|---|---|---|---|---|---|---|
| Appendix 1-base set | R | R | R | R | R | R | R |
|   Acute oral toxicity | R | R | R | R | R | R | R |
|   Acute dermal toxicity | C | C | C | C | C | R | C |
|   Acute inhalation toxicity | R | R | R | R | R | R | R |
|   Eye irritation | R | R | R | R | R | R | R |
|   Skin irritation | R | R | R | R | R | R | R |
|   Skin sensitization | R | R | R | R | R | R | R |
|   Acute parenteral toxicity | — | — | — | — | R | — | — |
|   Application site evaluation | — | — | R | R | R | R | — |
|   Pulmonary sensitization | — | — | — | — | — | R | — |
|   Phototoxicity/photoallergy | — | — | R | R | — | — | — |
|   Ames test | R | R | R | R | R | R | R |
|   Micronucleus test | R | R | R | R | R | R | R |
|   ADME-intended route | R | R | R | R | R | R | R |
|   28-day toxicity (2 species) intended route | R | R | R | R | R | R | R |
| Appendix 2 | | | | | | | |
|   90-day toxicity (most appropriate species) | R | R | R | R | R | R | R |
|   Developmental toxicity (rat and rabbit) | R | R | R | R | R | R | R |
|   Additional assays | C | C | C | C | C | C | C |
|   Genotoxicity assays | R | R | R | R | R | R | R |
| Appendix 3 | | | | | | | |
|   Chronic toxicity (rodent, nonrodent) | C | C | C | C | C | C | C |
|   Photocarcinogenicity | — | — | C | C | — | — | — |
|   Carcinogenicity | C | C | C | C | C | C | — |

[a] R: required; C: conditionally required.

material, the 28-day, and 90-day tests, the ADME-PK acute and repeated-dose tests, and the developmental toxicity test(s), a final determination can be made on the value of chronic toxicity or oncogenicity studies.

For example, if no toxicity is observed at a limit dose of 1000 mg/kg body weight per day following the 90-day toxicity study, no genotoxicity was found, and the ADME-PK profile indicates that the material is not absorbed and is completed excreted unchanged in the feces, then it is likely that a chronic study is not necessary. The decision to conduct chronic studies should be determined on a case-by-case basis using scientific judgement. It will be interesting to observe how this scheme may change in light of ICH.

**TABLE 13.11.  Base Set Studies for a Single Dose up to Two-Weeks Exposure in Humans**

| Test | Purpose |
| --- | --- |
| Acute oral toxicity | To determine the potential acute toxicity-lethality following a single oral dose |
| Acute dermal toxicity | To determine the potential acute toxicity-lethality following a single dermal dose |
| Acute inhalation toxicity | To determine the potential acute toxicity-lethality following a single 4-h inhalation exposure to a test atmosphere containing the new pharmaceutical excipient (aerosol, vapor or particles) |
| Eye irritation | To determine the potential to produce acute irritation or damage to the eye |
| Skin irritation | To determine the potential to produce acute irritation or damage to the skin |
| Skin sensitization | To determine the potential to induce skin sensitization reactions |
| Ames test | To evaluate potential mutagenic activity in a bacterial reverse mutation system with and without metabolic activation |
| Micronucleus test | To evaluate the clastogenic activity in mice using polychromatic erythrocytes |
| ADME, intended route | To determine the extent of absorption, distribution, metabolism, and excretion by the intended route of exposure following a single dose and repeated doses |
| 28-day toxicity, intended route | To assess the repeated-dose toxicity in male and female animals of two species following dosing for 28 days by the intended route of exposure |

**TABLE 13.12.  (From Table 13.10) Studies for Repeated Chronic Exposure in Humans**

| Test | Purpose |
| --- | --- |
| Chronic Toxicity | To assess the toxicity following chronic (lifetime) exposure by the route of intended exposure |
| Oncogenicity | To assess the potential to induce tumors by the intended route of exposure |
| One-generation reproduction | To assess the potential reproductive and developmental toxicity in males and females by the intended route of exposure |

## 13.8.  VEHICLES AND EXCIPIENTS*

(Budavari, 1989; Hawley, 1971)

   Common name: **Acetone**
   Chemical name: 2-Propanone

---

**Source*: APhA (1986).

Molecular weight: 58.08

Formula: $C_3H_6O$

Density: $0.780 \, g \, ml^{-1}$

Volatility: High

Solubility/miscibility: Miscible with water, ethanol, DMFO, vegetable oils

Biological considerations: Orally, will produce transient ($\sim 4\,h$) neurobehavioral intoxication. Repeated dermal use will lead to defatting of skin at application site. Oral $LD_{50}$ (rats) $= 10.7 \, ml \, kg^{-1}$. Higher doses can cause systemic acidosis

Chemical compatibility/Stability considerations: Highly flammable, colorless liquid

Uses (routes): Dermal and oral. Not preferred for oral: volume of instillation should be limited to $5 \, ml \, kg^{-1}$ by the oral route

Common name: **Carboxyl methyl cellulose; CMC**

Chemical name: NA

Molecular weight: 21,000–500,000

Formula: $R_nOCH_2COOH$

Density: $1.59 \, g \, ml^{-1}$

Volatility: NA

Solubility/miscibility: Soluble in both hot and cold water

Biological considerations: Practically inert polymer

Chemical compatibility/Stability considerations: White granules. Stable in pH range 2–10

Uses (routes): Orally, as a 0.1 to 5% mixture with water

Common name: **Corn oil/Mazola**

Chemical name: NA

Molecular weight: NA

Formula: Mixture of natural products

Density: $0.916–0.921 \, g \, ml^{-1}$

Volatility: Low

Solubility/miscibility: Miscible with chloroform, ether. Slightly soluble in ethanol

Biological considerations: Orally, serves as energy source (and therefore can alter food consumption and/or body weight). Prolonged oral administration has been associated with enhanced carcinogenesis

Chemical compatibility/Stability considerations: Thickens upon prolonged exposure to air

Uses (routes): Oral, dermal, vaginal, rectal, and subcutaneous

Common name: **DMFO**

Chemical name: *N*,*N*-Dimethylformamide

Molecular weight: 73.09

Formula: $HCON(CH_3)_2$

Density: $0.945\,g\,ml^{-1}$

Volatility: Low

Solubility/miscibility: Miscible with water and most common organic solvents

Biological considerations: Oral $LD_{50}$ (rats $7.6\,ml\,kg^{-1}$. Not cytotoxic to primary cells in culture

Chemical compatibility/Stability considerations: Colorless to very slightly yellow liquid

Uses (routes): Carrier for oral, dermal, intraperitoneal, or intravenous at concentrations up to 1%

Common name: **DMSO/Dimethyl sulfoxide**

Chemical name: Sulfinylbis [methane]

Molecular weight: 78.13

Formula: $C_2H_6OS$

Density: $1.100\,g\,ml^{-1}$

Volatility: Medium

Solubility/miscibility: Soluble in water, ethanol, acetone, ether

Biological considerations: Oral $LD_{50}$ (rats) $= 17.9\,ml\,kg^{-1}$. Repeated dermal exposure can defat skin. Repeated oral exposure can produce corneal opacities. Not cytotoxic to cells in primary culture. Intraperitoneal $LD_{50}$ (mice) $= 11.6\,ml\,kg^{-1}$

Chemical compatibility/Stability considerations: Very hydroscopic liquid

Uses (routes): All, as a carrier at up to 5% to enhance absorption

Common name: **Ethanol; ETOH**

Chemical name: Ethyl alcohol

Molecular weight: 46.07

Formula: $C_2H_6O$

Density: $0.789\,g\,ml^{-1}$

Volatility: High, but declines when part of mixture with water

Solubility/miscibility: Miscible with water, acetone, and most other vehicles

Biological considerations: Orally, will produce transient neurobehavioral intoxication. Oral $LD_{50}$ (rats) $= 13.0\,ml\,kg^{-1}$. Intravenous $LD_{50}$ (mice) $= 5.1\,ml\,kg^{-1}$

Chemical compatibility/Stability considerations: Flammable colorless liquid

Uses (routes): Dermal and oral, though can be used in lower concentrations for most other routes. Volume of oral instillation should be limited 5 ml kg$^{-1}$

Common name: **Glycerol; Glycerin**

Chemical name: 1,2,3-Propanetriol

Molecular weight: 92.09

Formula: $C_3H_8O_3$

Density: 1.264 g ml$^{-1}$

Volatility: Low

Solubility/miscibility: Miscible with water and ethanol. Soluble in water and ether

Biological considerations: Oral LD$_{50}$ (rats) greater than 20 ml kg$^{-1}$. Can serve as an energy source

Chemical compatibility/Stability considerations: Syrupy liquid, absorbs moisture from air. Contact with strong oxidizing agents (such as potassium permanganate) may cause an explosion

Uses (routes): Oral, dermal, vaginal, rectal, and intravenous (as part of an aqueous solution)

Common name: **Gum Arabic; Acacia**

Chemical name: NA

Molecular weight: Estimated 240,000–580,000

Formula: Mixture of natural products

Density: 1.35–1.49 g ml$^{-1}$

Volatility: NA

Solubility/miscibility: Insoluble in ethanol. Soluble to twice its weight (2 × grams) in water (×ml). Soluble in glycerol and propylene glycol

Biological considerations: Virtually biologically inert

Chemical compatibility/Stability considerations: None

Uses (routes): Orally, as diluent or viscosity increaser in solvents

Common name: **Lactose (milk sugar)**

Chemical name: 4-0-$\beta$-D-Galactopyranosyl-D-glucose

Molecular weight: 342.30

Formula: $C_{12}H_{22}O_{11}$

Density: NA

Volatility: None

Solubility/miscibility: One gram soluble in 5 ml water; slightly soluble in alcohol

Biological considerations: White powder. Energy source

Chemical compatibility/Stability considerations: None

Uses (routes): Orally, as a diluent for materials that may be excessively irritant if given pure

Common name: **Methyl cellulose/Methocel**

Chemical name: Cellulose methyl ether

Molecular weight: 40,000–180,000

Formula: NA

Density: Depends on concentration

Volatility: NA

Solubility/miscibility: Soluble in cold water; insoluble in hot water. Forms stable aqueous solution at room temperature. Insoluble in alcohol or ether

Biological considerations: Can act as a laxative

Chemical compatibility/Stability considerations: White granules or grayish white powder. Aqueous solutions are neutral to litmus. Combustible

Uses (routes): Orally, as a 0.1 to 5% mixture with water. Acts to increase viscosity of suspension, thereby reducing settling rate and improving homogeneity

Common name: **Methyl ethyl ketone; MEK**

Chemical name: 2-Butanone

Molecular weight: 72.10

Formula: $C_4H_8O$

Density: $0.805\,g\,ml^{-1}$

Volatility: Medium

Solubility/miscibility: 22.6% soluble in water, miscible with methanol and oils. Soluble in alcohol and ether

Biological considerations: Oral $LD_{50}$ (rats) $= 6.86\,ml\,kg^{-1}$. Repeated dermal use can lead to defatting of skin. CNS depressant by inhalation

Chemical compatibility/Stability considerations: Flammable, colorless liquid

Uses (routes): Dermal

Common name: **Mineral oil; Liquid petrolatum**

Chemical name: NA

Molecular weight: NA (mixture)

Formula: A mixture of light hydrocarbons from petroleum

Density: $0.83$–$0.90\,g\,ml^{-1}$

Volatility: Very low

Solubility/miscibility: Insoluble in water and ethanol. Soluble in ether and oils

Biological considerations: Aspiration may cause lipoid pneumonia

Chemical compatibility/Stability considerations: Flammable

Uses (routes): Oral, vaginal, rectal, dermal. Suspending agent

Common name: **Olive oil**
Chemical name: NA
Molecular weight: NA
Formula: Mixture of natural products
Density: $0.909–0.915\,\mathrm{g\,ml^{-1}}$
Volatility: Very low
Solubility/miscibility: Slightly soluble in ethanol; miscible with ether
Biological considerations: Can serve as an energy source
Chemical compatibility/Stability considerations: Pale yellow or light greenish-yellow oil. Becomes rancid upon exposure to air
Uses (routes): Oral

Common name: **Peanut oil/Arachis oil**
Chemical name: NA
Molecular weight: NA
Formula: Mixture of natural products
Density: $0.910–0.915\,\mathrm{g\,ml^{-1}}$
Volatility: Low
Solubility/miscibility: Miscible with ether and other oils. Slightly soluble in ethanol; slightly soluble in ether
Biological considerations: Orally, serves as an energy source
Chemical compatibility/Stability considerations: Clouds at room temperatures. Thickens upon prolonged exposure to the air
Uses (routes): Oral, dermal, vaginal, rectal, subcutaneous, and intramuscular

Common name: **Petroleum/Vaseline/Petroleum jelly**
Chemical name: NA
Molecular weight: NA
Formula: Mixture of petroleum fractions
Density: $0.820–0.869\,\mathrm{g\,ml^{-1}}$
Volatility: None
Solubility/miscibility: Practically insoluble in water, glycerol, or ethanol
Biological considerations: Practically inert
Chemical compatibility/Stability considerations: Yellowish, white or light amber semisolid
Uses (routes): Dermal, vaginal, rectal

Common name: **Polyethylene glycol-400 (Carbowax)**
Chemical name: NA
Molecular weight: 400 (approximate average, range 380–420)
Formula: $H(OCH_2CH_2)_n OH$

Density: $1.128\,\mathrm{g\,ml^{-1}}$

Volatility: Very low

Solubility/miscibility: Highly soluble in water. Soluble in alcohol and many organic solvents

Biological considerations: Employed as water-soluble emulsifying and dispersing agent. Oral $LD_{50}$ (mice) $= 23.7\,\mathrm{ml\,kg^{-1}}$. Oral $LD_{50}$ (rats) $= 30\,\mathrm{ml\,kg^{-1}}$

Chemical compatibility/Stability considerations: Does not hydrolyze or deteriorate on storage and will not support mold growth. Clear, viscous liquid

Uses (routes): For oral administration as a vehicle full strength or mixed with water. Total dosage of PEG-400 should not exceed $0.5$–$10\,\mathrm{ml}$

Common name: **Propylene glycol**

Chemical name: Propane-1,2-diol; 1,2-Propanediol

Molecular weight: 76.09

Formula: $C_3H_8O_2$

Density: $1.036\,\mathrm{g\,ml^{-1}}$

Volatility: Low

Solubility/miscibility: Miscible with water and acetone. Soluble in ether and ethanol

Biological considerations: Orally, causes transient (24 h) neurobehavioral intoxication. Oral $LD_{50}$ (rats) $= 25\,\mathrm{ml\,kg^{-1}}$. Subcutaneous $LD_{50}$ (mice) $= 20.0\,\mathrm{ml\,kg^{-1}}$

Chemical compatibility/Stability considerations: None

Uses (routes): Oral, dermal, vaginal, rectal, subcutaneous, and intradermal

Common name: **Saline**

Chemical name: Physiological saline

Molecular weight: 18.02

Formula: 0.9% NaCl in water (weight to volume)

Density: As water

Volatility: Low

Solubility/miscibility: As water

Biological considerations: No limitations. Preferable to water in parenteral applications

Chemical compatibility/Stability considerations: None

Uses (routes): All except dermal and periocular

Common name: **Tween 80/Polysorbate 80**

Chemical name: Sorbitan mono-9-octadecenoate poly (oxy-1,2-ethanediyl) derivatives

Molecular weight: NA (mixture)

Formula: A complex mixture of polyoxyethylene ethers of mixed partial oleic esters of sorbitol anhydrides

Density: 1.06–1.110 g ml$^{-1}$

Volatility: High

Solubility/miscibility: Generally very soluble or miscible in water. Soluble in ethanol, corn oil, and olive oil. Insoluble in mineral oil

Biological considerations: Surfactant. May cause micelle formation, with incumbent effects on bioavailability if included at concentrations of 1% or higher. May be associated with irritation if given intravenously or intramuscularly. Dogs have the peculiarity that Tweens injected parenterally induce the spontaneous systemic release of histamine. This response is particularly striking with IV injection, and therefore Tweens should not be used as components of IV vehicles in dogs

Chemical compatibility/Stability considerations: Acts as detergent in polar–nonpolar mixed solvent systems

Uses (routes): Wetting agent (at 0.1 to 0.5%) in the preparation of suspensions. Most commonly used in water

Common name: **Water**

Chemical name: Hydrogen oxide

Molecular weight: 18.02

Formula: $H_2O$

Density: 1.000 g ml$^{-1}$

Volatility: Low

Solubility/miscibility: Miscible with MEK, ethanol, acetone

Biological considerations: No limitations except high volumes via the IV route can disturb systemic electrolyte balance and cause hemolysis and hematuria

Chemical compatibility/Stability considerations: None

Uses (routes): All. The vehicle and solvent of first choice

# REFERENCES

APA (1994). *Handbook of Pharmaceutical Excipients*, 2nd edition. American Pharmaceutical Association, Washington, D.C.

Attman, P.L. and Dittmer, D.S., (Eds.) (1971). *Respiration and Circulation*. FASEB, Bethesda, MD, pp. 56–59.

Avis, K.E. (1985). Parenteral preparations. In: *Remington's Pharmaceutical Sciences* (Gennaro, A.R., Ed.). Mack Publishing Company, Easton, PA, pp. 1518–1541.

Baker, H.J., Lindsey, J.R. and Weisbroth, S.H. (1979). *The Laboratory Rat*, Vol. 1. Academic Press, New York, pp. 411–412.

Ballard, B.E. (1968). Biopharmaceutical considerations in subcutaneous and intramuscular drug administration. *J. Pharm. Sci.* 57: 357–378.

Barry, B.W. (1983). *Dermatological Formulations.* Marcel Dekker, New York.

Bates, T.R. and Gibaldi, M. (1970). Gastrointestinal absorption of drugs. In: *Current Concepts in the Pharmaceutical Sciences: Biopharmaceutics* (Swarbrick, J., Ed.). Lea & Febiger, Philadelphia, pp. 58–99.

Blank, I.H. and Scheuplein, R.J. (1964). The epidermal barrier. In: *Progress in the Biological Sciences in Relation to Dermatology*, Vol. 2. (Rook, W. and Champion, I., Eds.). Cambridge University Press, Cambridge, pp. 243–281.

Blodinger, J. (1982). *Formulation of Veterinary Dosage Forms.* Marcel Dekker, New York.

Borowitz, J.L., Moore, P.F., Yim, G.K.W. and Miya, T.S. (1971). Mechanism of enhanced drug effects produced by dilution of the oral dose. *Toxicol. Appl. Pharmacol.* 19: 164–168.

Brandau, R. and Lippold, B.H. (1982). *Dermal and Transdermal Absorption.* Wissenschaftliche, Verlagsgesellschaft mbH, Stuttgart.

Bronaugh, R.L. and Maibach, H.I. (1985). *Percutaneous Absorption.* Marcel Dekker, New York.

Brown, V.K. (1980). *Acute Toxicity in Theory and Practice.* Wiley, New York.

Brown, V.K. and Muir, C.M.C. (1971). Some factors affecting the acute toxicity of pesticides to mammals when absorbed through skin and eyes. *Int. Pest Control* 13: 16–21.

Budavari, S. (1989). *The Merck Index*, 11th ed. Merck & Co., Rahway, NJ.

Calvary, H.O. and Klump, T.G. (1939). The toxicity for human beings for diethylene glycol with sulfanilimide. *Southern Med. J.* 32: 1105.

Derelanko, M.J., Gad, S.C., Gavigan, F.A., Babich, P.C. and Rinehart, W.E. (1987). Toxicity of hydroxylamine sulfate following dermal exposure: Variability with exposure method and species. *Fund. Appl. Toxicol.* 8: 425–X31.

Dominguez, J.G., Parra, J.L., Infante, M.R., Pelejero, C.M., Balaguer, F. and Sastre, T. (1977). Physiocochemical Aspects of Skin Absorption. *J. Soc. Cosmet. Chem.* 28: 165.

Eckstein, P., Jackson, M.C.N., Millman, N. and Sobrero, A.J. (1969). Comparison of vaginal tolerance tests and spermicidal preparations in rabbits and monkeys. *J. Reprod. Fertil.* 20: 85–93.

Fitzgerald, J.M., Boyd, V.F. and Manus, A.G. (1983). Formulations of insoluble and immiscible test agents in liquid vehicles for toxicity testing. In: *Chemistry for Toxicity Testing* (Jameson, C.W. and Walters, D.B., Eds.). Butterworth, Boston, pp. 83–90.

Gad, S.C., Smith, A.C., Cramp, A.L., Gavigan, F.A. and Derelanko, M.J. (1984). Innovative designs and practices for acute systemic toxicity studies. *Drug Chem. Toxicol.* 7(5): 423–434.

Gaines, T.B. (1960). The acute toxicity of pesticides to rats. *Toxicol. Appl. Pharmacol.* 2: 88–99.

Garramone, J.P. (1986). *Vascular Access Port Model SLA Users Manual.* Norfolk Medical Products, Skokie, IL.

Gibaldi, M. (1976). *Biopharmaceutics in the Theory and Practice of Industrial Pharmacy*, 2nd ed. (Lachman, L., Lieberman, H.A. and Kanig, J.L., Eds.). Lea & Febiger, Philadelphia.

Gibaldi, M. and Feldman, S. (1970). Mechanisms of surfactant effects on drug absorption. *J. Pharm. Sci.* 59: 579.

Gray, J.E. (1978). Pathological evaluation of injection injury. In: *Sustained and Controlled Release Drug Delivery System* (Robinson, J., Ed.). Marcel Dekker, New York, pp. 35–105.

Groves, M. (1966). The influence of formulation upon the activity of thermotherapeutic agents. *Rep. Progr. Appl. Chem.* 12: 51–151.

Hagenbusch, O.E. (1937). Elixir of sulfanilamide massengill. *JAMA* 109: 1531.

Hawley, G.G. (1971). *The Condensed Chemical Dictionary.* Van Nostrand Reinhold, New York.

Hem, S.L. (1973). *Current Concepts in Pharmaceutical Sciences: Dosage Form, Design and Bioavailability* (Swarbrick, J., Ed.). Lea & Febiger, Philadelphia.

Hogben, C.A.M., Tocco, D.I., Brodie, B.B. and Schranker, L.S. (1959). On the mechanism of intestinal absorption of drugs. *J. Pharmacol. Exp. Therap.* T25: 275.

Holick, H.G.O. (1937). Glycerine, ethylene glycol, propylene glycol and diethylene glycol. *JAMA* 109: 1517.

Holmstedt, B. (1959). Pharmacology of organophosphorus cholinesterase inhibitors. *Pharmacol. Rev.* 11: 567–688.

Houston, J.B., Upshall, D.G. and Bridges, J.W. (1974). The re-evaluation of the importance of partition coefficients in the gastrointestinal absorption of nutrients. *J. Pharmacol. Exptl. Ther.* 189: 244–254.

IPEC (1997). Europe Safety Committee: The proposed new guidelines for safety evaluation of new excipients. *Eur. Pharm. Rev.* Nov. 1997: 13–20.

Kerberle, H. (1971). Physicochemical factors of drugs affecting absorption, distribution and excretion. *Acta Pharmacol. Toxicol.* 29 (Suppl 3): 30–47.

Kondrizer, A.A., Mayer, W.H. and Zviblis, P. (1959). Removal of sarin from skin and eyes. *Arch. Industr. Health* 20: 50–52.

Kruger, S., Greve, D.W. and Schueler, F.W. (1962). The absorption of fluid from the peritoneal cavity. *Arch. Int. Pharmacodyn.* 137: 173–178.

Levi, G. (1963). *Prescription Pharmacy* (Sprowls, J.B., Ed.). Lea & Febiger, Philadelphia.

Lien, E., Koda, R.T. and Tong, G.L. (1971). Buccal and percutaneous absorptions. *Drug Intel. Clin. Pharm.* 5: 38–41.

Lukas, G., Brindle, S.D. and Greengard, P. (1971). The route of absorption of intraperitoneally administered compounds. *J. Pharmacol. Exptl. Ther.* 178: 562–566.

Marzulli, F.N. (1962). Barriers to skin penetration. *J. Invest. Derm.* 39: 387–393.

McMartin, C., Hutchinson, L.E.F., Hyde, R. and Peters, G.E. (1987). Analysis of structural requirements for the absorption of drugs and macromolecules from the nasal cavity. *J. Pharm. Sci.* 76: 535–540.

Medved, L.L. and Kundiev, Y.I. (1964). On the methods of study of penetration of chemical substances through the intact skin (Russian). *Gig. Sanit.* 29: 71–76.

Melnick, R.L., Jameson, C.W., Goehl, T.J. and Kuhn, G.O. (1987). Application of micro-encapsulation for toxicology studies. *Fund. Appl. Toxicol.* 11: 425–431.

Monkhouse, D.C. and Rhodes, C.T. (1998). *Drug Products for Clinical Trials.* Marcel Dekker, New York.

O'Reilly, W.J. (1972). Pharmacokinetics in drug metabolism and toxicology. *Canad. J. Pharm. Sci.* 7: 6–77.

Powers, D.H. and Fox, C. (1957). A study of the effect of cosmetic ingredients, creams and lotions on the rate of moisture loss. *Proc. Sci. Sect. Toilet Goods from the Skin Ass.* 28: 21.

Racy, I. (1989). *Drug Formulation.* Wiley, New York.

Rieger, M.M. and Deems, D.E. (1974). Skin Moisturizers. II. The effects of cosmetic ingredients on human stratum corneum. *J. Soc. Cosmet. Chem.* 25: 253.

Ritschel, W.A., Siegel, E.G. and Ring, P.E. (1974). Biopharmaceutical factors influencing LDP: Pt. 1. Viscosity. *Arzneim.-Forsch.* 24: 907–910.

Scheuplein, R.J. (1965). Mechanism of percutaneous absorption. (i) Routes of penetration and the influence of solubility. *J. Invest. Derm.* 45: 334–346.

Scheuplein, R.J. (1967). Mechanism of percutaneous absorption. (ii) Transient diffusion and the relative importance of various routes of skin penetration. *J. Invest. Derm.* 48: 79–88.

Schmidt-Nielsen, K. (1984). *Scaling: Why Is Animal Size So Important?* Cambridge University Press, New York.

Schou, J. (1971). Subcutaneous and intramuscular injection of drugs. In: *Handbook of Experimental Pharmacology* (Brodie, B.B. and Gillette, J.R., Eds.). Springer, Berlin, Ch. 4.

Schranker, L.S. (1960). On the mechanism of absorption of drugs from the gastrointestinal tract. *J. Med. Pharm. Chem.* 2: 343–359.

Schranker, L.S., Shore, P.A., Brodie, B.B. and Hogben, C.A.M. (1957). Absorption of drugs from the stomach, I. The rat. *J. Pharmacol. Exp. Therap.* 120: 528.

Schwartz, M.L., Meyer, M.B., Covino, B.G. and Narang, R.M. (1974). Antiarrhythmic effectiveness of intramuscular lidocaine: Influence of different injection sites. *J. Clin. Pharmacol.* 14: 77–83.

Shaffer, C.B. and West, B. (1960). The acute and subacute toxicity of technical *o,o*-diethyl *s*-2-diethyl-aminoethyl phosphorothioate hydrogen oxalate (TETRAM). *Toxicol. Appl. Pharmacol.* 2: 1–13.

Share, P.A., Brodie, B.B. and Hogben, C.A.M. (1971). The gastric secretion of drugs: A pH partition hypothesis. *J. Pharmacol. Exp. Therap.* 119: 361.

Sinow, J. and Wei, E. (1973). Ocular toxicity of paraquat. *Bull. Environ. Contam. Toxicol.* 9: 163–168.

Smolinske, S.C. (1992). *Handbook of Food, Drug and Cosmetic Excipients*. CRC Press, Boca Raton, FL.

Spiegel, A.J. and Noseworthy, M.M. (1963). Use of nonaqueous solvents in parenteral products. *J. Pharm. Sci.* 52: 917–927.

Staab, R.J., Palmer, M.A., Auletta, C.S., Blaszcak, D.L. and McConnell, R.F. (1987). A relevant vaginal irritation/subacute toxicity model in the rabbit and ovariectomized rat. *Toxicologist* 7A: 1096.

Swan, K.C. and White, N.G. (1972). Corneal permeability: (1) factors affecting penetration of drugs into the cornea. *Amer. J. Ophthalmol.* 25: 1043–1058.

Theeuwes, F. and Yum, S.I. (1976). Principles of the design and operation of generic osmotic pumps for the delivery of semisolid or liquid drug formulations. *Ann. Biomed. Eng.* 4: 343–353.

Turco, S. and King, R.E. (1974). *Sterile Dosage Forms*. Lea & Febiger, Philadelphia.

Weiner, M. and Bernstein, I.L. (1989). *Adverse Reactions to Drug Formulation Agents*. Marcel Dekker, New York.

Wilson, F.A. and Dietschy, J.M. (1974). The intestinal unstirred layer—its surface area and effect on active transport kinetics. *Biochem. Biophys. Acta.* 363: 112–126.

Wiener, M.L. and Katkoskie, L.A. (1999). *Excipient Toxicity and Safety*. Marcel Dekker, New York.

Winne, D. (1978). Dependence of intestinal absorption *in vivo* in the unstirred layer. *Nauyn-Schmiedelberg's Arch. Pharmacol.* 304: 175–181.

Wood, S.G., Upshall, D.G. and Bridges, J.W. (1978). The absorption of aliphatic carbamates from the rat colon. *J. Pharm. Pharmac.* 30: 638–641.

Ziegenmeyer, J. (1982). The influence of the vehicle on the absorption and permeation of drugs. In: *Dermal and Transdermal Absorption* (Brandan, R. and Reisen, P., Eds.). Wissenschaftliche, Verlagsgesellschaft, Stuttgart, pp. 73–89.

Zimm, B.H. and Lundberg, J.L. (1956). Sorption of vapors by high polymers. *J. Phys. Chem.* 60: 425.

# 14

# OCCUPATIONAL TOXICOLOGY IN THE PHARMACEUTICAL INDUSTRY

## 14.1. INTRODUCTION

Most of the assessment of toxicology and safety of therapeutics is focused on the patients who are to benefit from the new medicine. However, there are two other groups of individuals (each of which has different exposure profiles) that one must be concerned about: the healthcare providers (nurses, pharmacists and physicians) who provide and/or administer the drugs and the individuals involved in manufacturing them. The concerns here are in the realm of occupational toxicology.

Modern toxicology has its roots in the occupational environment. The earliest recorded observations relating exposure to chemical substances and toxic manifestations were made about workers. These include Agricola's identification of the diseases of miners and Pott's investigation of scrotal cancer incidence among chimney sweeps. Occupational toxicology, as its name implies, concerns itself with the toxicological implications of exposure to chemicals in the work environment.

In this chapter we will examine occupational toxicology as it applies to and is currently practiced in the pharmaceutical industry. This industry, which by definition involves biologically active compounds, has been a driving force in the development of the science of toxicology. The need for a thorough safety evaluation of potential therapeutics prior to marketing approval has driven the continued evolution of toxicological testing methods and the identification of mechanisms of toxic action. The area of occupational toxicology has gained momentum in the pharmaceutical industry since the early 1980s. This is made clear by the increased number of companies that have implemented occupational toxicology programs during this period. Still, occupational-related activities generally represent only a small fraction of activity in safety assessment in the pharmaceutical and biotechnology industries. It is difficult to gauge the level of activity in this occupational area due to the paucity of publications on the subject (Teichman et al., 1988). This is probably the result of the fact that most occupational toxicologists function in an administrative environment and thus experience less pressure to publish, and that they in general deal with information relating to new chemical processes that may not be protected by patents. The lack of general knowledge about the function of the occupational toxicologist that has resulted could lead one to conclude that (1) the thorough evaluation of drugs to obtain marketing approval makes an investigation of their potential hazards to manufacturing employees unnecessary and (2) because they are used therapeutically, pharmaceutical agents are safe under any and all circumstances in occupational settings.

## 14.2. OCCUPATIONAL TOXICOLOGY VERSUS DRUG SAFETY EVALUATION

While pharmaceutical products are indeed created to treat disease, they cannot always be considered nonhazardous. The clinician must evaluate the benefits to the patient in light of any side effects or adverse reactions that may be associated with drug usage and any other toxicological properties uncovered in animal studies. Examples range from antibiotics, which have clastogenic properties in mice (for which, to the patient, their activity in suppressing lifethreatening infections presents a clear and overriding benefit), to an antineoplastic that has extreme renal toxicity but which effectively kills established tumors. The occupational toxicologist must look at pharmaceutical agents in a completely different light. These same risk/benefit analyses do not apply in an occupational setting. Even agents with minimal clinical adverse reactions and whose pharmacological activity could be considered generally beneficial in the clinical setting may present certain employees with health hazards in the manufacturing or healthcare provider settings.

Let us explore some of the basic differences in the way preclinical and occupational toxicologists must approach their work (Table 14.1). Preclinical development of a pharmaceutical product requires exhaustive testing of drug candidates under the requirements of the Federal Food and Drug Administration (FDA) or equivalent national agency to help predict and evaluate clinical findings and to preclude serious or chronic hazards that would not ordinarily be observed in clinical studies limited in duration and population (FDA, 1990). By contrast, the occupational toxicologist must evaluate the potential of a compound to cause toxicity from unintended exposures via a variety of routes of administration and a wide range of exposure levels of varying lengths. In drug safety evaluations, studies are designed to approximate the clinical setting, particularly in terms of routes of administration and dosage. Thus, most preclinical studies generally focus on oral and/or parenteral administration with dosages that either are comparable to or exceed therapeutic levels. However, neither oral nor parenteral administration is a likely route of exposure among employees. Rather, during manufacturing operations

**TABLE 14.1. Comparison of Occupational and Preclinical Toxicology**

|  | Occupational | Preclinical |
| --- | --- | --- |
| Purpose | Potential for effects from unintended exposure | Predict and evaluate clinical findings and preclude serious hazards from clinical use |
| Routes of administration | Inhalation, direct contact with skin or eyes | Oral and/or parenteral most likely |
| Dose level | Not really predictable | Relative to estimated therapeutic dose or maximum tolerated dose |
| Duration of exposure | Extremely variable; depends on campaign/batch, procedure, etc.; may be short daily exposure for working lifetime | Dependent on therapeutic use and test model |

employees are more likely to be exposed via inhalation or direct contact with the skin or eyes. In addition to the route of exposure itself, the effects occurring following direct contact or inhalation exposure may be of a nature not predictable by the studies undertaken for preclinical safety evaluation. Most important among these effects are irritation and sensitization. Dermal, ocular, and respiratory irritation potential generally cannot be predicted from preclinical studies utilizing oral or parenteral administration. Similarly, sensitization, which has the potential to significantly add to the difficulty of conducting manufacturing operations safely, is difficult to evaluate even with current specific methods and models. For most pharmaceutical agents, testing to ascertain the potential to induce dermal sensitization reactions is not conducted during a typical preclinical development program.

Other important differences lie in the length of treatment and the dosages involved. Therapeutic use of pharmacological agents may be of acute or limited duration, such as in the administration of anti-infectives, or chronic, as with antihypertensive agents. Occupational exposure may also be of varying length, limited by shift or batch manufacturing methods. It is possible, however, that the manufacture of certain high-volume products such as antibiotics may result in daily exposure, if only in limited doses, over a significant portion of a working lifetime. The levels to which employees may be exposed are, in general, potentially lower than those that are used therapeutically, although exposures will vary with the type of operations performed.

The area of occupational toxicology has received a great deal of attention in the chemical industry. Historically, the chemical industry has focused on the occupational environment and developed many of our current toxicological methods to address health and safety concerns. However, since the mid-1970s the chemical industry has increasingly become subject to testing requirements relevant to the protection of the environment and the public at large, as mandated by Environmental

Protection Agency (EPA) regulations in the United States (EPA, 1976, 1979). Data development for occupational health hazard evaluation has seldom been sought by the Occupational Safety and Health Administration (OSHA). Consequently, few new test methods have been developed and those in current use are generally modifications of methods introduced in the 1930s and 1940s. Some of the differences in the issues addressed by occupational toxicologists in the pharmaceutical and chemical industries are highlighted in Table 14.2. Among these, a major difference lies in the physical and functional nature of the substances involved. Pharmaceutical agents are generally handled as solids, while chemical industry products are generally processed as liquids or vapors. Although there is a greater focus on the consequences of occupational exposure, the occupational toxicologist in the chemical industry rarely has available the wealth of information that exists in the pharmaceutical industry. New drug dossiers include toxicological information as well as data on the pharmacology, pharmacokinetics, and mechanism of action, and, most important, much of this information has been gathered from clinical trials on human beings. Even though the data are not developed for the purpose of evaluating the occupational environment, they can be invaluable for this purpose. Clinical studies, even if the doses and routes of administration may be different from those used in clinical trials/therapeutically, provide insight into the unique responses of the human

**TABLE 14.2. Toxicological Testing Requirements under EC Seventh Amendment (Directive 92/32/EC-Notification of New Substances)**

| Quantity imported to, or Manufactured in, EC | Test Results to be Submitted |
| --- | --- |
| $<1000\,kg\,yr^{-1}$ or $<5000\,kg$ total | None needed unless the compound is considered toxic (oral $LD_{50}$ 25–200 mg kg$^{-1}$) or very toxic (oral $LD_{50}$ <25 mg kg$^{-1}$) |
| $>1000\,kg\,yr^{-1}$ or 5000 kg total | Acute oral/dermal $LD_{50}$<br>Acute inhalation $LC_{50}$<br>Skin irritation<br>Eye irritation<br>Skin sensitisation<br>28-day subacute toxicity<br>Mutagenicity (bacteriological and nonbacteriological tests)<br>Acute toxicity to fish ($LC_{50}$)<br>Acute toxicity to *Daphnia* |
| $>10,000\,kg\,yr^{-1}$ or 50,000 kg total | Additional tests may be required depending on results, including:<br>Fertility—1 or 2 generation (males or females)<br>Teratology—additional species<br>Subchronic or chronic—90 days to 2 years<br>Carcinogenicity<br>Acute and subacute on additional species |

body. Another important difference in the parameters involved in the chemical and pharmaceutical industries concerns biological activity. The chemical industry strives to minimize it, while pharmaceutical agents are specifically designed to be biologically active. Recent advances in our understanding of molecular and cellular processes have led to the development of agents with improved specificity for unique receptor or molecular targets. These potent agents may present increased hazards for employees and a great challenge to the occupational toxicologist in the pharmaceutical industry.

At the same time, several types of data necessary to ensure proper management of occupational risks associated with a drug substance are not generally useful in evaluating potential patient risks. So the necessary tests—eye and skin irritation, sensitization and inhalation toxicity, as well as assessment of the hazards of by-products and impurities that do not get incorporated into the final therapeutic product—are not performed in the normal course of development.

## 14.3. REGULATORY PRESSURES IN THE UNITED STATES AND THE EUROPEAN COMMUNITY

The safety and health of workers in the United States is regulated under the Occupational Health and Safety Act of 1970, which established OSHA. Since its inception, OSHA has promulgated a variety of health standards, including compound-specific regulations, permissible exposure limits (PELs) and rules for providing access to medical records (OSHA, 1986) and for communicating to employees the hazards of the materials they handle. This last regulation, the Hazard Communication Standard (OSHA, 1987) is a standard that specifically requires manufacturers or importers to carry out an evaluation of the toxicological properties of chemicals. This standard outlines specific criteria for evaluating substances as hazardous or nonhazardous. However, there still is no U.S. regulatory requirement for testing a compound of unknown toxicity (Gad, 2001). Rather, such a compound could be classified as nonhazardous, based on the unavailability of data. Pharmaceutical agents are generally considered hazardous under the standard since they meet the criterion of having a biological effect on humans. Any adverse reaction observed during clinical use will be construed as toxicity, however irrelevant to the occupational environment. The main result of classification as hazardous is a requirement to develop a Material Safety Data Sheet (MSDS) as the main vehicle for providing information to employees. The model MSDS suggested for use in complying with the OSHA Hazard Communication Standard contains a great deal of information about the physical properties and hazards and the procedures necessary to deal with the accidental spill, fire, explosion, or accidental contact with hazardous material. The Standard requires that all information regarding adverse effects in human beings and most animal toxicity data be included in the MSDS, however irrelevant this information may be to the work environment. The resulting MSDS can be a highly technical document that may not be the optimal vehicle for conveying this type of information to manufacturing employees handing pharmaceutical agents.

In the environmental area, the EPA's TSCA (Toxic Substances Control Act) (EPA, 1976) regulations for filing of premanufacture notification (PMN) (EPA, 1979) have resulted in the development of toxicological information on many new industrial chemicals. New chemical entities generated for use as pharmaceutical agents are exempted from PMN requirements. This exemption may also extend to all intermediates generated during chemical synthesis. Many pharmaceutical companies have instituted toxicological testing of these compounds even though there is no specific U.S. regulatory impetus to develop such information. The European Community (EC) has implemented several directives that parallel and exceed the OSHA Hazard Communication Standard and TSCA regulations. European Community Directive 80/1107 [European Economic Community (EEC), 1992] requires employee communication of hazards of chemical substances as well as biological materials. Another EC directive, which was the impetus for the development of Notification of New Substances regulations in several member nations, requires the development of toxicological data on new compounds and does not exempt pharmaceutical agents or isolated intermediates (EEC, 1979). Notification and testing must be conducted in accordance with the amount of the substance manufactured in, or imported into, Europe yearly (Table 14.2). These regulations will support the development of toxicological data on entities manufactured or processed in Europe that can in turn be applied to occupational health hazard evaluations. Pharmaceutical companies are, as demonstrated in Table 14.3, very different from chemical companies in their handling of occupational toxicology.

## 14.4 ORGANIZATIONAL STRUCTURE

The occupational toxicology function is organized and structured in very different ways across the industry. The function exists in many of the major PhRMA member companies. In most of these companies the occupational toxicology function is located within the employee safety/industrial hygiene area, while in some it resides within the research and development (R&D), toxicology, or employee health/medical services areas. How the function fits into the organization greatly depends on its mission. Occupational toxicology will function well with the R&D environment if the evaluation of occupational health hazards is considered an integral requirement in the development and approval process. In such an organization there would likely be a greater emphasis on developing toxicological data on novel compounds and their synthetic intermediates, rather than on existing processes, or such other activities as training. This organization provides great opportunity for interaction and cooperation with those disciplines that are charged with implementing the toxicologist's recommendations. Good interaction between the occupational toxicologist and the industrial hygienist can be particularly useful in developing and implementing solutions to potential health hazards. However, poor understanding of the limitations of scientific data by the more engineering-oriented

**TABLE 14.3. Comparison of Occupational Toxicology in Pharmaceutical and Chemical Industries**

|  | Pharmaceutical | Chemical |
| --- | --- | --- |
| Compounds |  |  |
|   Physical state | Generally solids | Liquids, vapors, polymers, solids |
|   Biological activity | Designed for biological activity | Strive for biological inertness |
| Toxicology data |  |  |
|   Development | Focus on preclinical evaluation | Focus on occupational and general environment |
|   Study length | Acute to chronic for final products; acute for intermediates | Acute to chronic (depending on volume) |
| Human data |  |  |
|   "ADME"[a] | Generally available for oral/parenteral routes | Not generally available |
|   Mechanism of action | Targeted during drug development | Not generally studied |
|   Adverse effects | Extensive clinical trial studies for final products from oral or parenteral route | Generally only known as a result of overexposure, accident, etc. |

[a]ADME: absorption, distribution, metabolism, and excretion.

safety specialists may lead to unrealistic expectations for easy solutions or answers. The last existing arrangement is for the occupational toxicologist to report into the Medical Services area. This arrangement provides perhaps the easiest interactions for the toxicologist, who shares a common language and understanding of biological systems with the occupational physician. However, in order to effect any changes in the work environment, it is necessary to enlist the aid of the Employee Safety/ Industrial Hygiene group, an act that may incur the potential problems just mentioned. Clearly, wherever the function is located, the occupational toxicologist must be able to interact well with a variety of disciplines, including R&D, Safety, Industrial Hygiene, Medical Services, Legal Services, Regulatory Affairs, Technical Services, and, of course, Operations Management.

Staffing of industrial toxicology programs varies among the different programs, including groups with two or three full-time Ph.D.'s who spend all of their time on occupational issues and those with one or two Ph.D. or masters-level staff members who may have part-time responsibility for occupational-related issues along with R&D responsibilities. The level of staffing depends, of course, on the activities assigned to the occupational toxicology group and these may vary from one organization to another. It is impossible to generalize or recommend an adequate staffing level, since that will be dictated by the emphasis placed on specific activities. Whatever the mission of the occupational toxicology function, a high level of education or professional credentials is desirable. A doctoral degree and/or board certification in toxicology should be imperative to enable effective interaction with many of the other disciplines mentioned above, particularly R&D management.

## 14.5. ACTIVITIES

The scope of activities of occupational toxicologists may be quite different from one organization to another, depending on its specific mission, resources available and corporate culture. In general, their activities can be divided into four broad areas: data development, data evaluation and dissemination, hazard assessment, and employee training.

### 14.5.1. Data Evaluation and Dissemination

It is important first to establish who will use the toxicological information provided and how this information will be applied. Unlike the preclinical toxicologist who provides information to other toxicologists, to the regulatory agencies, or to physicians for evaluation of potential therapeutic liabilities, the occupational toxicologist is providing information to a variety of individuals and functions. First, the information will be provided to the industrial hygienist or safety specialist who must evaluate the quality of the work environment and the appropriateness of personal protective equipment. Second, the information will be given to the occupational physician who must evaluate the potential causes of any symptoms reported by employees who may have been exposed to the material. Third, R&D, plant management, and/or manufacturing services must evaluate the need to implement engineering or other controls and weigh these costs against the commercial viability of the product. Last, but not least, the information must be provided to the production employees who will be handling the compound and who need to know of its hazards. Clearly, there is a need to provide the necessary information in such a way that it can be clearly understood by nonscientists. With an audience of such a potentially wide-ranging educational level and understanding, multiple communication vehicles may be necessary.

To be effective, the toxicology evaluation must meet several criteria: it must be (1) thorough, (2) clear and concise, (3) in a form appropriate to its target audience, and (4) include a conclusion or recommendation.

Thoroughness can be achieved through an exhaustive search of the published literature using the available computerized data bases. There is a risk, particularly when dealing with pharmaceutical agents, that the most relevant information to occupational toxicology can be overlooked in the great number of clinical case reports, many of which are not relevant to the work environment. In general, little information has been published on the occupational hazards of pharmaceutical agents. A thorough review does not mean a listing of every reported clinical adverse reaction. This type of information is more likely to confuse readers, and may lead them to ignore important occupational hazards. The toxicologist must, therefore, be extremely selective in performing this evaluation. A review of the available clinical information, however, may yield data that can be used in evaluation, particularly if the product has been tested for dermal administration. An integral part of assuring the thoroughness of the evaluation must be a process of updating the information on a regular basis. In general, it is unlikely that new clinical data will significantly change a review for an established pharmaceutical agent. However, new therapeutic entities should be reviewed more frequently since new data may be published on potential adverse reactions not identified in clinical trials, and these data may impact the occupational evaluation.

When providing information to technical personnel, it is best to use language that does not require the use of a medical dictionary. It is tempting to use medical terms, particularly when quoting from the clinical literature. However, use of these terms may result in poor understanding of the information and may also evoke unnecessary anxiety in the reader. A good rule of thumb is to think of what the reader will do with the information: If the biological effect will require more than a few words to be clearly explained in plain language and it is irrelevant or unimportant to the work environment, it is best left off any communication to the field.

It is not always possible to reach a conclusion regarding the degree of hazard of exposure to a compound, particularly if the data are not directly relevant to the work environment. There is often a temptation to provide a thorough evaluation, setting out all necessary information in plain language but leaving the formulation of a conclusion to the reader. However, if it is difficult for the trained toxicologist to reach such a conclusion, it must be even more difficult for the layperson. If an estimate of the hazard cannot be reached, then the evaluation must conclude with an advisory on the type of exposures that may increase hazard, or the type of effect that is most likely to occur should there be an overexposure. These may at least give the industrial hygienist or physician a useful reference point. At the same time, it is important to express to the reader the inherent limitations of such a conclusion. The audience may expect black-and-white answers; if this is not possible, they should be made to understand why.

Perhaps the most difficult part of the communication equation is matching the information to the audience. This may be best illustrated using an example. Over the past ten years one company has developed several vehicles for communicating information to various audiences. One instrument is the toxicology review. In general, this is a one- to two-page document that reviews the published literature on the compound. A reference list is prepared and maintained on file for future reference. This review is provided to safety, medical, and industrial hygiene personnel and, if appropriate, research chemists. These individuals have received training to help them understand the terms used and the effects outlined. A second method of communication involves a computerized data base. This personal computer based system, which provides only bottom-line information, is available on-line via a modem to safety, industrial hygiene, nursing, and research personnel (Sussman and Gáler, 1990). It includes only that information specifically relevant to the work environment and necessary for compliance with OSHA Hazard Communication Standard or EC Directive 80/1107. A third vehicle was developed jointly with an industrial hygiene department and consists of a short paragraph highlighting the specific hazards of the compound followed by safe handling recommendations.

A fourth commonly used method is the Material Safety Data Sheet. The toxicology department prepares the toxicology section of the MSDS. The appropriate other disciplines complete the remaining sections, and the completed MSDS is then reviewed and approved by a committee. Last, for certain compounds, an on-site training programs, such as those described below, can be presented by the toxicologist on the hazards of the chemical. These various formats for the same information were developed to serve the informational needs and educational levels of various audiences. This is one approach to filling the need to communicate toxicological information to a variety of groups. The appropriate vehicle for each company will, of course, depend on the available resources and corporate culture. Even a large number of formats may not suffice. The occupational toxicologist should determine, through discussions and follow-up communications, how the information is received and if it is understood. The communication of toxicological information may represent approximately 50% of the occupational toxicologist's responsibilities, thus indicating the level of commitment needed to develop appropriate formats. The MSDS alone is often insufficient for the successful communication of health hazard information to employees.

### 14.5.2. Data Development

The motivation for conducting toxicological tests for pharmaceutical, chemical intermediates and impurities arises from the need to ensure the health of employees by preventing adverse reactions from occupational exposure. Employers thus secondarily minimize the associated potential for work interruption. Programs in place at many larger companies routinely test new drug candidates and/or isolated synthetic intermediates for the purpose of occupational health hazard evaluation.

The development of a toxicological testing program for occupational health hazard evaluation requires consideration of (1) the compounds to be tested, (2) the stage of drug development at which testing occurs, (3) the specific tests to be conducted, and (4) the means for funding.

These four issues are, of course, interdependent, and it is not always possible to deal with one without affecting the others. As indicated previously, drug candidates undergo extensive toxicological testing to ensure an adequate margin of safety for patients. Additional tests are usually required to obtain information specific to the work environment. By contrast, synthetic intermediates are generally not subject to testing for drug safety evaluation. These compounds, if they have the potential to present an exposure hazard to employees, may warrant evaluation. Clearly, it is neither feasible nor necessary to conduct the same level of testing required for drug marketing approval. However, a toxicological assessment can often be developed to determine whether these isolated intermediates have the potential to elicit toxicity from exposures that could occur during work.

Compounds should be selected for testing on the basis of an evaluation of potential exposure and likelihood of their causing adverse effects. The first evaluation is best achieved by including the research chemist, industrial hygienist, and/or safety specialist in the decision-making process. They are in the best possible position for judging potential sources of employee exposure. Including these disciplines in the pretesting stage ensures not only their commitment to the program, but also that the studies will be designed with careful consideration of the work experience. The second evaluation, an estimate of toxic effects, may be obtained from a comparison of the compounds in question to known toxic agents, also known as a structure-activity relationship (SAR) evaluation. There are, currently, software programs available for obtaining a quantitative estimate of toxicity using SAR models. However, it is most likely that an SAR evaluation will be achieved by simple comparison to the final product, similar pharmacological agents, or raw materials that have known toxic properties. Information on potential exposures and toxic effects can, thus, be utilized to decide which compounds to test or to assign priorities to compounds selected for testing.

The timing of these studies depends greatly on the developmental track for the test compounds and may vary for intermediates and final products. Discovery early in the development process that an isolated intermediate poses a significant health hazard may prompt a change in the chemical synthesis or process, or in the implementation of engineering controls or personal protective equipment. Thus it is generally useful to test intermediates at an early stage. This approach presents several practical problems. First, in a long development program, such as occurs in the pharmaceutical industry, there are many opportunities for changing the synthetic route for reasons other than toxicity. Thus, a large percentage of the intermediates tested during the early development stages may be replaced in the ultimate manufacturing process. Second, only a fraction of new drug candidates actually reach the drug approval process. Therefore, the majority of intermediates tested early in development process will likely never reach large-scale manufacture. Conducting a toxicological assessment of intermediates at a later stage in the development process presents a comparable set of advantages and disadvantages: It is more likely that the compounds tested will be manufactured on a large scale, but the ability to make fundamental changes in the chemical process will be greatly diminished. Testing of new drug candidates for occupational health hazards can be an integral part of the drug safety evaluation process. Acute oral toxicity is frequently evaluated as the first step in the drug's safety assessment. Adding acute dermal toxicity and, thus, skin irritation evaluation at the same time can often be accomplished with a minimum impact on the development schedule. This additional information can then be used not only to protect employees manufacturing supplies of the chemical, but also those laboratory employees handling test doses of the substance. Eye irritation testing requires minimal amounts of test compounds and could also be accomplished at the same time. Sensitization testing requires a greater commitment in terms of time and the quantity of compounds needed. Therefore, investigation of a compound's allergenic properties is often postponed until sufficient toxicological information is available to permit a decision as to whether the compounds will advance to the next stage in the development process.

Practical considerations of funding and the selection of the testing laboratory need to be addressed when developing an occupational toxicology testing program.

The actual program will vary depending on the organizational structure of the occupational toxicology function. As indicated above, if the activity is located within the R&D department, it may be simple to include the cost of conducting these tests within the new drug's development budget. There is a possible risk in this situation, however, that the safety and industrial hygiene communities may be inadvertently omitted from the prioritization process and the information loop. Explaining the necessity of testing programs to nonscientific management personnel may be challenging. Solutions to these barriers may be found with R&D funding of testing or designation of testing cost, thus possibly including these programs in research funds.

The occupational toxicology community in the pharmaceutical industry is currently trying to develop a consensus approach to toxicological testing for health hazard evaluation. The types of toxicological tests utilized are selected by individual toxicologists, since there are no specific regulatory requirements. While there is as yet no consensus on what tests should be done or when these should be conducted, there is general agreement as to the type of effects that need to be addressed: skin and eye irritation, sensitization, and acute oral and dermal toxicity. Testing for these effects generally involves studies of short duration. Thus, results can often be obtained relatively quickly. Additional tests for inhalation toxicity and/or sensory irritation and mutagenicity are conducted by several companies.

Although there is general agreement on the effects to be investigated, the methods used have not necessarily been consistent. Several companies have developed protocols uniquely tailored to the needs of their workplace health hazard evaluation and their in-house testing resources. The most common protocols utilized for occupational health hazard evaluation are briefly described on Table 14.4 (Gad and Chengelis, 1988). Any one company's program is an example of a program that has developed specifically modified protocols over a period of several years to meet particular needs (Gáler, 1989). These modifications included a combined protocol to assess acute dermal toxicity as well as skin irritation in rabbits and a stepwise approach to acute oral toxicity determination rather than a classic $LD_{50}$ (Gáler, 1989). Doses are selected based on regulatory criteria, such as those that are required for classification as a toxic under the OSHA Hazard Communication Standard and/or EC 80/1107 (Cook, 1987). Testing for eye irritation involves a modification of current methods using rabbits. While in some views there is no justification for testing cosmetic products in live animals, eye irritation information pertaining to unique pharmacological chemicals is important to protect employees from accidental exposures. There are currently no acceptable alternatives to the rabbit eye irritation test (Society of Toxicology, 1989); therefore, the rabbit eye irritation test is used by the occupational toxicologist. Current protocols include refinements to the original method, including a reduction in the number of animals used, the application of topical anesthetics to decrease animals' sensation, and rinsing with distilled water following the instillation of the test compound to allow evaluation of the benefits of washing the eye as a first aid measure. Another refinement that may be utilized is a reduction in the amount of material instilled into the eye (Griffith and Yam, 1989). In general, modifications of this type have not affected the reliability of this test

(Hatoum et al., 1990) and may, in fact, better simulate possible workplace accidents and provide additional information.

The battery of tests shown in Table 14.4 can provide useful information to complete a workplace hazard assessment. However, they are not the only tools that may be used to determine the toxic potential of a workplace contaminant. Additional tests may be required to provide more rigorous recommendations. Depending on the results of initial tests, a second stage of testing may be initiated to address specific needs. For example, sensory irritation tests may be conducted for compounds that are found to have irritant properties. The sensory irritation tests, developed by Alarie (1966), is used to develop a parameter, the $RD_{50}$, that has been directly correlated with threshold limit values (TLVs) for a certain class of compounds (Kane et al., 1979; Alarie, 1981). However, the usefulness of this test for solid compounds, which include most pharmaceutical agents, has not been determined. Results of genotoxicity tests may present a need for testing in additional systems to assess genotoxic potential. Mechanistic studies may also be appropriate for certain compounds, such as intermediates, in the synthesis of inhibitors of specific enzymes or receptor agonists/antagonists. The information available from clinical, pharmacology, or pharmacokinetic studies on the final drug can be useful in determining possible avenues for investigation. A particularly interesting type of study, yet to be developed, might involve determination of the absorption and the bioavailability of compounds from occupational exposures that could then be related to similar parameters developed in clinical or preclinical pharmacokinetic studies. The need to conduct additional testing will depend on the application of the information by the individual toxicologist and the resources available. The cost of additional tests should be weighed against the cost of applying the most conservative interpretation of the data to the work environment. In some cases implementing stricter controls based on preliminary tests may be less costly than conducting more extensive confirmatory testing.

There has recently been increasing pressure from governmental agencies and animal rights advocates to reduce the number of animals used in toxicological testing. As alternative toxicological methods become more accurate and sophisticated, they should be considered for incorporation into the occupational toxicology battery. Additional tools such as computer-aided quantitative structure-activity relationship (QSAR) evaluations may also be considered as additions or alternatives to animal tests (Jurs et al, 1985; Klopman, 1985; Frierson et al., 1986; Enslein, 1988). As indicated previously, QSAR methods may be particularly well suited to aid in the selection and/or prioritization of chemicals for testing, particularly in the case of intermediates. Alternative test methods currently under investigation, such as those being proposed for replacement of the Draize eye irritation test, do not appear to be well suited to the testing of pharmaceuticals or their synthetic intermediates (Booman et al., 1988, 1989). An intensive program of testing the available alternative models with compounds in this class is required to determine the ultimate usefulness of these alternative testing methods.

Occupational toxicologists from several companies initiated a program to evaluate several experimental models as alternatives to the rabbit eye irritation test

**TABLE 14.4. Summary of Protocols Used for Current Test Methods**

| Test | Species | Method | Dose | Data application | Additional data |
|---|---|---|---|---|---|
| Acute toxicity | | | | | |
| Oral | Rat or mouse | $N = 5$/se/dose; 14-day observation period; necropsy with/without histopathology | Chosen as limit (0.5 or $5\,\mathrm{g\,kg^{-1}}$) or for $LD_{50}$ | Classify compounds as Harmful/Toxic/Highly toxic | |
| Dermal | Rabbit | $N = 5$/sex/dose; 24-h dermal application under occlusion; 14-day observation period; necropsy with/without histopathology; dermal irritation scores | Chosen as limit ($2\,\mathrm{g\,kg^{-1}}$) or for $LD_{50}$ | Classify compounds as Harmful/Toxic/Highly toxic; selection of protective equipment | Irritation potential class; target organ information |
| Inhalation | Rat or mouse | $N = 5$/sex/dose; 4 h nose only or whole-body exposure; 14-day observation period; necropsy with/without histopathology | Chosen as limit ($20\,\mathrm{g/m^3}$) or for $LD_{50}$ | Classify compounds as Harmful/Toxic/Highly toxic; selection of protective equipment | Respiratory irritation potential; target organ information |
| Skin irritation | Rabbit | $N = 3$; 4-h application under semiocclusive binder to abraded and nonabraded skin; irritation scores at $\frac{1}{2}$, 1, 24, 48, and 72 h | 500 mg/site | Classify irritation potential | |

| Eye irritation | Rabbit | $N = 3–6$/group; into right eye, compare to untreated eye; test only compounds with pH<11 or >2; score at 1, 24, 48, and 72 h and up to 21 days for corneal opacity, conjunctivitis, iritis: may use a rinse with some animals | 100 mg or 0.1 ml in standard protocol or 10 mg or 0.01 ml in low-volume protocol | Classify eye irritation potential; selective equipment | Evaluate first aid methods; ocular toxicity |
|---|---|---|---|---|---|
| Sensitization Buehler method | Guinea pigs | $N = 10–15$; topical applications 1–3 times per week for 3 weeks, 2-week rest then challenge at a naïve site; concurrent negative/vehicle and positive controls | Up to 500 mg or 0.5 ml per dose | Classify as sensitizer— most sensitive for moderate to strong sensitizers; selection of protective equipment; evaluation of allergic reactions | Repeated dermal dosing; additional data on skin irritation and dermal absorption |
| Maximization | Guinea pigs | $N = 10–15$; combines 2 intradermal $+/-$ adjuvant and 1 topical occlusive administration for induction, 2-week rest then topical application for challenge at naïve site; concurrent positive and negative/vehicle controls | 0.1 ml of compound in solution for induction; nonirritating concentration for challenge | May be sensitive to mild sensitizing agents, but may also overpredict severity | |
| Local Lymph node | Mouse (female) | $N = 5$; combines dermal exposure on ear with IV challenge by tail vein on sixth day with tritiated methyl thymidine. | 25 µL of compound in solvent on each ear for three days | Does produce some false positives | No rechallenge possible |

(Gáler et al., 1993; Sina et al., 1995). As a result of this cooperative study, several of the participating companies have implemented the routine use of several of these alternative models in their test batteries (R. G. Sussman and J. Sina, personal communications), thus effectively increasing the number and classes of compounds evaluated in alternative models.

### 14.5.3. Hazard Assessment

This is quite possibly the most difficult and controversial activity for the occupational toxicologist. Just as there is no blueprint for conducting toxicological testing, there is no formula for performing an occupational risk assessment. I have indicated (Section 14.5.2) the need to include an indication of the degree of hazard from occupational exposure in informational communications. A more specific form of hazard assessment is the development of occupational exposure limits (OELs). Occupational exposure limits, such as the American Conference of Governmental Industrial Hygienists (ACGIH, 1995) threshold limit values (TLVs), have been available for approximately 50 years (Cook, 1987). Similar workplace limits developed by OSHA are known as permissible exposure limits (PELs) (OSHA, 1987). The majority of the substances for which TLVs or PELs have been developed are large-volume industrial chemicals, often encountered in the workplace as vapors. The process of developing TLVs and PELs has been documented by ACGIH and OSHA, respectively (ACGIH, 1995; OSHA, 1987). Unfortunately, the process is not always consistent or straightforward. Some TLVs or PELs are intended to prevent chronic effects yet are developed using acute reactions as reference points. Others are based on an existing TLV developed for a third compound. Clearly, these are not examples that can be easily followed by the pharmaceutical industry.

Individual companies have, nonetheless, developed methodologies for formulating OELs based on the type of data available and other resources available. One method involves a formula for extrapolating to an 8-h time-weighted average from the therapeutic dose of the drug using safety factors (Sargent and Kirk, 1988). A group composed of occupational toxicologists from several companies presented a monograph at the second annual Occupational Toxicology Roundtable, held in November 1989, regarding the development of occupational exposure limits (Gáler et al., 1989, 1992). The authors reviewed the data considerations, methodologies, and implications of developing occupational exposure limits. In summary, they concluded that toxicological and pharmacokinetic data are necessary to develop OELs and determine the most appropriate method of developing them. Furthermore, there is significant uncertainty in any OEL developed, resulting from questions of the relevance of the available data and the sophistication of the risk assessment model applied. The authors also cautioned against the use of OELs as though they were inherent toxicological properties of the chemical substance.

Several methods are available for developing OELs: analogy, correlation, safety and uncertainty factors, and low-dose extrapolation (Table 14.5). The appropriate method must be selected on the basis of the appropriateness of the available data. For example, low-dose extrapolation may be appropriate only if sufficient pharmaco-

**TABLE 14.5. Methods for Setting Occupational Exposure Limits (OELs)**

| Method | Formula[a] |
| --- | --- |
| Analogy | $OEL_i = OEL_j$ |
| Correlation | $OEL_i = (PP_i/PP_j) \times OEL_j$ |
| Safety factors | $OEL = \text{reference dose}/UF_1 \times UF_2 \times SF \times BR$ |
| Low-dose extrapolation | $OEL = [\text{rodent RSD} \times (BW_H/BW_R)^{-1/3}]/BR$<br>Or, if PB-PK available,<br>$OEL = (\text{human reference dose})/BR$ |

[a]OEL, Occupational exposure limit; PP, physical property; $UF_1$, uncertainty in extrapolation to NOEL; $UF_2$, uncertainty from interspecies extrapolation; SF, safety factor; BR, breathing rate for 8-h workday; PB-PK, physiologically based pharmacokinetic model; RSD, risk specific dose; BW, body weight.
*Source:* Adapted from Gáler *et al.*, 1989.

kinetic data are available to build a suitable physiologically based pharmacokinetic (PB-PK) model. Analogy is a method by which the OEL for one compound is adopted for a second, based on the two compounds' structural and functional similarity. This method is suitable only if the two compounds are similar in every aspect, including therapeutic or toxic dose, physical properties, and the like. Correlation is similar to analogy in that it compares similar compounds. However, the OEL is chosen based on a key property of the chemical that influences its toxicological properties. An example would be the use of the relative potency of two drugs as the key property used to adjust the reference OEL. The most commonly used method is that of applying safety and/or uncertainty factors to a reference dose, which may be the lowest therapeutic dose. In using this method, it is important to choose the reference dose and endpoint with great care. In general, the most sensitive endpoint should be chosen. Uncertainty factors are selected to approximate levels from effective doses and to account for interspecies differences. A safety factor is selected based on the overall toxicological evaluation of the compound. Because it is necessary to look at the complete toxicological profile, it is generally inappropriate to assign specific values to each type of toxic effect.

There are diverse opinions as to whether one company's OEL can be used when evaluating another's workplace. However, it is likely that as more pharmaceutical manufacturers begin to establish OELs, the process will essentially become an industry standard. Furthermore, while U.S. OSHA regulations do not require that manufacturers establish OELs, European governmental agencies have begun the process. The first country to require this activity was the United Kingdom, under its Control of Substances Hazardous to Health (COSHH) regulations (Health and Safety Executive, 1988; Agius, 1989). A similar requirement is included in the EC Directive 80/1107, which may be promulgated into law by other EC member nations.

In creating a program for establishing OELs, several disciplines will generally be included in the development or approval process. In those programs that are currently in place, Safety, Industrial Hygiene, Manufacturing or Technical Services, Medical Services, Legal Services, Research and Development, and, of course, Occupational Toxicology may take part in the process. While the ability to make the OEL level in the workplace does not drive the process, the OEL may often be issued as an interim guideline to provide manufacturing locations an opportunity to bring their operations into compliance and for the development of a suitable industrial hygiene sampling and analysis method.

### 14.5.5. Employee Training

The ultimate client for the services of the occupational toxicologist is the manufacturing or research employee, who must be informed of and protected from the potential hazards of chemicals present in the work environment. However, most of the work of the occupational toxicologist is directed to other disciplines such as Safety or Medical Services. There can often be little opportunity to interact directly with manufacturing employees. However, this can be a most effective way of preventing occupational disease and may also be a most rewarding activity. Providing employees with health hazard information directly through presentations or training programs not only accomplishes this task better than most written communications, but also provides an excellent way to build confidence in the organization and its safety and health programs. The trust gained in this manner can be an invaluable asset when a company is challenged with the manufacture of especially toxic or potent compounds. Face-to-face communication will also promote discussions with plant employees and give the occupational toxicologist the opportunity to learn of those adverse health effects that might otherwise go unnoticed or uninvestigated.

There are several areas for which it may be useful to consider developing specific training programs. The Hazard Communication Standard requires that employees be trained to understand the hazards of chemicals as they are outlined in the MSDS. There is an obvious need for the occupational toxicologist to be involved in the development of an internal training program or the selection of a commercial program to address this need. In addition to this required training, it may be useful to consider a more in-depth program on basic concepts involved in health hazard evaluation, particularly the dose-response relationship and the different types of chronic health hazards. It may be particularly important to promote an understanding of health hazard information obtained at work as well as through the news media. There are several commercial training programs available that may be useful for this purpose, including computerbased self-training programs and videos.

Specific training on compounds of interest can also be useful, particularly before the beginning of a manufacturing campaign, and is particularly effective if coupled with industrial hygiene training on appropriate safe handling techniques. If a testing program is in place, it is good policy to present an evaluation of the information gained in the compound's testing program to the research or manufacturing chemists involved in the project.

Another area in which it is useful to provide training is in the activities of the occupational toxicology function itself. Though this might seem unnecessary, it is an especially useful activity not only to ensure good understanding of the abilities and limitations of this function, but also to create and enhance lines of communication with those disciplines that need access to the information and that can provide useful information to the toxicologist. It may be particularly useful to provide this type of training to plant and divisional management.

Training programs also provide the occupational toxicologist with an opportunity to exercise some creativity. There are now many methods available to conduct training programs. The most traditional method, lecturing, is probably also the least effective. Media such as video, slides, computer-based training, and games can be used to accomplish training objectives with fun and flair.

## 14.6. FUTURE ISSUES IN OCCUPATIONAL TOXICOLOGY IN THE PHARMACEUTICAL INDUSTRY

As the area of occupational toxicology develops and grows, we will be faced with many new challenges. Among the most important will be the development of an industry consensus in the areas of toxicological testing programs and protocols and toxicological methods for establishing occupational exposure limits. It is not surprising that these two subjects recur year after year as topics for discussion at the Occupational Toxicology Roundtable.

Issues that will gain in importance for pharmaceutical industry occupational toxicologists will be those relating to the new, more potent drugs currently being designed. While, for the most part, we have up till now dealt with drugs with dose levels ranging down to the microgram levels, it is likely that in the not-so-distant future dose levels of new drugs will be several orders of magnitude smaller. Hazard assessment and OEL development may be nearly impossible or inappropriate when dealing with drugs active at pico- or femtogram levels. Alternative methods of evaluating occupational exposures and assuring a safe work environment may need to be developed. Similar considerations may be required when dealing with products of biotechnology.

The biotechnology pipeline has yielded an increasing number of products, most commonly peptides and proteins with significant allergenic potential in an occupational setting. The potential occupational health hazards of this class of potent but large molecular weight products have not been fully evaluated. Because of the inherent functional and structural differences, the extrapolation of testing methods from traditional pharmaceutical products to biotechnology derived compounds may be fraught with many difficulties. Hypersensitivity and other immunologically based toxicities are particularly of concern for protein- and peptide-based therapeutics.

## 14.7. CONCLUSION

The field of occupational toxicology in the pharmaceutical industry presents continuing challenges to the industry. Occupational toxicologists find that they must become "experts" in several fields, and not be limited to the scientific area. Unlike the preclinical toxicologist, the occupational practitioner functions under less stringent regulatory requirements and minimal precedents. Additionally, as new classes of therapeutic agents enter development and commerce, new concerns and challenges will accompany them.

## REFERENCES


ACGIH (American Conference of Governmental Industrial Hygienists). (1995). *Documentation of Threshold Limit Values and Biological Exposure Indices*, 6th ed. With 1996, 1997 and 1998 supplements. American Conference of Governmental Industrial Hygienists, Cincinnati, OH.

Agius, R. (1989). Occupational exposure limits for therapeutic substances. *Ann. Occup. Hyg.* 33: 555–562.

Alarie, Y. (1981) Bioassay for evaluating the potency of airborne sensory irritants and predicting acceptable levels of exposure in man. *Fd. Cosmet. Toxic.* 19: 623–626.

Alarie, Y. (1966). Irritating properties of airborne materials to the upper respiratory tract. *Arch. Environ. Health* 13: 433–449.

Booman, K.A., Cascieri, T.M., Demetrulias, J., Diedger, A., Griffith, J.F., Grochosky, G.T., Kong, B., McCormick, W.C., North-Root, H., Rozen, M.G., and Sedlak, R.I. (1988). *In vitro* methods for estimating eye irritancy of cleaning products. Phase I: Preliminary assessment. *J. Toxicol.—Cut. & Ocular Toxicol.* 7: 173–185.

Booman, K.A., DeProspo, J., Demetrulias, J., Diedger, A., Griffith, J.F., Grochosky, G., Kong, B., McCormick, W.C., North-Root, H., Rozen, M.G., and Sedlak, R. I. (1989). The SDA alternatives program: Comparison of *in vitro* data with Draize test data. *J. Toxicol.—Cut. & Ocular Toxicol.* 8: 35–49.

Cook, W.A. (1987). *Occupational Exposure Limits—Worldwide.* American Industrial Hygiene Association, Cincinnati, OH.

Enslein, K. (1988). An overview of structure-activity relationships as an alternative to testing in animals for carcinogenicity, mutagenicity, dermal and eye irritation and acute oral toxicity. *Toxicol. and Indust. Health* 4: 479–498.

Environmental Protection Agency (EPA). (1976). Toxic Substances Control Act, Public Law 94–469, 94th Congress.

Environmental Protection Agency (EPA). (1979). Toxic Substances Control Act: Premanufacture testing of new chemical substances. Guidance for premanufacture testing: Discussion of policy issues, alternative approaches and tests methods. 44 *FR* 16240–16292.

European Economic Community (EEC). (1979). Council Directive 67/548/EEC as amended by Directive 79/831/EEC. *Official Journal of the European Communities* No. L259, 10.

European Economic Community (EEC). (1992). Council Directive 92/32/EC of 27 November, 1980, on the protection of workers from the risks related to exposure to chemical, physical, and biological agents at work. *Official Journal of the European Communities* No. L327, 8.

Food and Drug Administration. (1990). (FDA) Applications for FDA approval to market a new drug or an antibiotic drug. 21 CFR Part 314.

Frierson, M.R., Klopman, G., and Rosenkranz, H.S. (1986). Structure-activity relationships (SARs) among mutagens and carcinogens: A review. *Env. Mutagen.* 8: 283–327.

Gad, S.C. (2001). *Regulatory Toxicology*, 2nd ed. Taylor & Francis, Philadelphia, PA.

Gad, S.-C., and Chengelis, C.P. (1998). *Acute Toxicology Testing*, 2nd ed. Academic Press, San Diego, CA.

Gáler, D.M. (1989). A testing battery for evaluating occupational health hazards. *J. Amer. Coll. Toxicol.* 8: 1215.

Gáler, D. M., Leung, H.-W., Sussman, R.G. and Trzos, R.J. (1989). *Scientific and practical considerations for developing occupational exposure limits for chemical substances.* Presentation to the Second Annual Occupational Toxicology Roundtable, November 21, 1989, Rahway, New Jersey.

Gáler, D.M., Leung, H.W., Sussman, R.G., and Trzos, R.J. (1992). Scientific and practical considerations for the development of occupational exposure limits (OELs) for chemical substances. *Regulatory Toxicol. & Pharmacol.* 15: 291–306.

Gáler, D.M., Curren, R., Gad, S.C., Gautheron, P., Leong, B., Miller, K., Sargent, E., Shah, P.V., Sina, J. and Sussman, R.G. (1993). A 10-company collaborative evaluation of alternatives to the eye irritation test using chemical intermediates. *Alternative Methods Toxicol.* 9: 237.

Griffith, J.F., and Yam, J. (1989). The low-volume eye irritation test. Current status of use and acceptance. *J. Amer. Coll. Toxicol.* 8: 1215.

Hatoum, N.S., Leach, C.L., Talmsa, D.M., Gibbons, R.D., and Garvin, P.F. (1990). A statistical basis for using fewer rabbits in dermal irritation testing. *J. Amer. Coll. Toxicol.* 9: 49–59.

Health and Safety Executive, U.K. (1988). The control of substances hazardous to health regulations 1988. *Statutory Instruments* 1988, No. 1657.

Jurs, P.C., Stouch, T.P., Czerwinski, M., and Narvaez, J.N. (1985). Computer-assisted studies of molecular structure-activity relationships. *J. Chem. Inf. Comput. Sci.* 25: 296–308.

Kane, L.E., Barrow, C.S., and Alarie, Y. (1979). A short-term test to predict acceptable levels of exposure to airborne sensory irritants. *Am. Ind. Hyg. J.* 40: 207–229.

Klopman, G. (1985). Predicting toxicity through a computer automated structure evaluation program. *Environ. Health Perspect.* 61: 269–274.

Occupational Safety and Health Administration (OSHA). (1986). Administrative Rule concerning OSHA access to employee medical records. 29 *Code of Federal Regulations* (CFR) Part 1913.

OSHA. (1987). Hazard Communication Standard. 29 *Code of Federal Regulations* (CFR) Part 1910, Subpart Z, Section 1910.1200.

Sargent, E.V., and Kirk, G.D. (1988). Establishing airborne exposure control limits in the pharmaceutical industry. *Amer. Ind. Hyg. Assoc. J.* 49: 309–313.

Sina, J. F., Gáler, D.M., Sussman, R.G., Gautheron, P.D., Sargent, E.V., Leong, B., Shah, P.V., Curren, R. and Miller, K. (1995). A collaborative evaluation of seven alternatives to the

Draize eye irritations test using pharmaceutical intermediates. *Fundam. Appl. Toxicol.* 26: 20–31.

Society and Toxicology. (1989). SOT Position Paper, comments on the $LD_{50}$ and acute eye and skin irritation tests. *Fundam. Appl. Toxicol.* 13: 621–623.

Sussman, R. and Gáler, D. (1990). A database for communicating toxicology information to safety personnel. *Toxicologist* 10: 87.

Teichman, R.F., Fallon, L.F. and Brandt-Rauf, P. (1988). Health effects of workers in the pharmaceutical industry: A review. *J. Soc. Occup. Med.* 38: 55–57.

# 15

# IMMUNOTOXICOLOGY IN PHARMACEUTICAL DEVELOPMENT

## 15.1. INTRODUCTION

The immune system is a highly complex system of cells involved in a multitude of functions including antigen presentation and recognition, amplification, and cell proliferation with subsequent differentiation and secretion of lymphokines and antibodies. The end result is an integrated system responsible for defense against foreign pathogens and spontaneously occurring neoplasms that, if left unchecked, may result in infection and malignancy. To be effective, the immune system must be able both to recognize and to destroy foreign antigens. To accomplish this, cellular and soluble components of diverse function and specificity circulate through blood and lymphatic vessels, thus allowing them to act at remote sites and tissues. For this system to function in balance and harmony requires regulation through cell-to-cell communications and precise recognition of self versus nonself. Immunotoxicants can upset this balance if they are lethal to one or more of the cell types or alter membrane morphology and receptors. There are several undesired immune system responses that may occur upon repeated therapeutic administration of a pharmaceutical that may ultimately present barriers to its development, including

- Down-modulation of the immune response (immunosuppression), which may result in an impaired ability to deal with neoplasia and infections. This is of particular concern if the therapeutic agent is intended to be used in patients with preexisting conditions such as cancer, severe infection, or immunodeficiency diseases.
- Up-modulation of the immune system (i.e., autoimmunity).

527

- Direct adverse immune responses to the agent itself in the form of hypersensitivity responses (anaphylaxis and delayed contact hypersensitivity).
- Direct immune responses to the agents that limit or nullify its efficacy (i.e., the development of neutralizing antibodies).

Immune modulated responses to drugs ("drug allergies") are a major problem and cause of discontinuance of use by patients who do need access to the therapeutic benefits (Patterson et al., 1986), and there remains no adequate preclinical methodology for identifying/predicting these responses to orally administered small molecule drugs (Hastings, 2001). The most common drug allergy (to penicillin) not only is limiting in itself, but also due to cross-reactivity to antibiotics of similar structure, can be severely limiting (Batchelor et al., 1965).

It is the intent of this chapter to provide an understanding of these adverse immunological effects, the types of preclinical tests that may be used to detect them, and approaches for testing and interpreting test results.

Immunotoxicology has evolved over the last 20 years as a specialty within toxicology that brings together knowledge from basic immunology, molecular biology, microbiology, pharmacology, and physiology. As a discipline, immunotoxicology involves the study of adverse effects that xenobiotics have on the immune system. As listed above, several different types of adverse immunological effects may occur, including immunosuppression, autoimmunity, and hypersensitivity. Although these effects are clearly distinct, they are not mutually exclusive. For example, immunosuppressive drugs that suppress suppressor-cell activity can also induce autoimmunity (Hutchings et al., 1985), and drugs that are immunoenhancing at low doses may be immunotoxic at high doses. Chemical xenobiotics may be in the form of natural or man-made environmental chemicals; pharmaceuticals and biologicals that are pharmacologically, endocrinologically, or toxicologically active. Although, in general, xenobiotics are not endogenously produced, immunologically active biological response modifiers that naturally occur in the body should also be included, since many are not known to compromise immune function when administered in pharmacologically effective doses (Koller, 1987; Steele, et al., 1989).

Although the types of immunological responses to various xenobiotics may be similar, the approach taken for screening potential immunological activity will vary depending on the application of the compound. Thus, this chapter will primarily focus on the immunotoxicology of pharmaceuticals. In contrast to potential environmental exposures, pharmaceuticals are developed with intentional but restricted human exposure and their biological effects are extensively studied in surveillance. Pharmaceuticals are developed to be biologically active, and, in some cases, intentionally immunomodulating or immunosuppressive. Many will react with biological macromolecules or require receptor binding in order to be pharmacologically active. By their nature, these interactions may result in toxicity to the cells of the immune system, may adversely alter the appearance of "self" to produce an autoimmune response, or may form a hapten, which may then elicit a hypersensitivity response. Because of the fast-expanding development of new drugs that can potentially impact the immune responsiveness of humans, immunotoxicity testing of new pharmaceutical products has become a growing concern.

Until recently, immunotoxicology in pharmaceutical safety assessment has been poorly addressed by both regulatory requirements/guidelines and by existing practice. Notable exceptions are the testing requirements for delayed contact hypersensitivity for dermally administered agents and antigenicity/anaphylaxis testing for drugs to be registered in Japan. The most recently announced regulatory expectation for parenterally administered protein or peptide agents produced by biotechnology is that the development of antibodies (neutralizing and otherwise) should be evaluated in at least one (preferably two) of the animal models used to assess general systemic toxicity.

Unanticipated immunotoxicity is infrequently observed with drugs that have been approved for marketing. With the exception of drugs that are intended to be immunomodulatory or immunosuppressive as part of their therapeutic mode of action, there is little evidence that drugs cause unintended functional immunosuppression in humans (Gleichman et al., 1989). However, hypersensitivity (allergy) and autoimmunity are frequently observed and are serious consequences of some drug therapies (DeSwarte, 1986; Patterson et al., 1986; Choquet-Kastylevsky and Descotes, 2001; Pieters, 2001). An adverse immune response in the form of hypersensitivity is one of the most frequent safety causes for withdrawal of drugs that have already made it to the market (see Table 15.3) and accounts for approximately 15% of adverse reactions to xenobiotics (deWeck, 1983). In addition, adverse immune responses such as this (usually urticaria and frank rashes) are the chief "unexpected" finding in clinical studies. These findings are unexpected in that they are not predicted by preclinical studies because there is a lack of good preclinical models for predicting systemic hypersensitivity responses, especially to orally administered agents. As a consequence, the unexpected occurrence of hypersensitivity in the clinic may delay, or even preclude, further development and commercialization. Thus, a primary purpose for preclinical immunotoxicology testing is to help us detect these adverse effects earlier in development, before they are found in clinical trials.


## 15.2. REGULATORY POSITIONS

The pharmaceutical and medical device industries are increasingly concerned with whether preclinical testing of their products should include routine immunotoxicologic screening or be done on an "as needed" basis, triggered by the toxicological profile of the xenobiotic established in routine preclinical safety testing (Bloom et al., 1987). Although the FDA has not as yet officially released guidelines for immunotoxicity testing of pharmaceuticals, recent drug development efforts in the areas of biotechnology, prostaglandins, interleukins, and recombinant biological modifiers have elicited the expectation that the development of antibodies (neutralizing and otherwise) should be evaluated in at least one of the animal models used to assess general systemic toxicity. And more to the point, draft guidelines have been released for devices (CDRH, 1997). The other available guidance has been the draft guidelines in the revision of the "Redbook" (FDA, 1993). However, CDER (2001) released draft guidelines for evaluation of investigational new drugs.

Federal attention and efforts to identify and control substances that may harm the immune system are discussed in a background paper by the Congressional Office of Technology Assessment (U.S. Congress, 1991). The National Academy of Science has convened a panel of immunotoxicologists to discuss the importance of immunotoxicology testing. The chemical industry has been a proponent of using a battery of assays to assess chemical-induced immunotoxicity, hence guidelines for a two-tiered screen approach have been proposed by the National Toxicology Program (NTP) (Luster et al., 1988). This strategy, which was developed for nontherapeutic chemicals and environmental contaminants that have different safety standards, does not address some of the safety issues and test strategy issues that are unique to pharmaceuticals. The FDA has drafted a similar two-leveled approach (Hinton, 1992) for assessing immunotoxicity of food colors and additives; however, these guidelines are likewise not necessarily relevant for testing pharmaceuticals. However, since direct food additives are meant for human consumption and are tested thoroughly in animal toxicology tests, this strategy may be more applicable to pharmaceuticals than the strategy of the NTP. In all of these testing schemes, the initial tier generally includes a fundamental histopathologic assessment of the major components of the immune system. Additional tiers are then added to more precisely evaluate the functionality of the components that appeared to be adversely affected in the first tier of tests. These test strategies are primarily geared toward the detection of chemical-induced immunosuppression, thus the effectiveness of these test schemes for detecting immunostimulation has not yet been determined (Spreafico, 1988).

The NTP defines the first tier of assays (Table 15.1) to include an assessment of immunopathology: humoral, cell-mediated, and nonspecific immunity such as natural killer cell activity. The second tier (Table 15.2) includes a more comprehensive battery that should be used once functional changes are observed in the Tier I assays. The Tier II assays focus on mechanisms of immunotoxicity such as depletion of specific cell subsets by flow cytometry analysis or evaluation of secondary immune responses by examining IgG response. Cell-mediated immunity is assessed through a functional assay that looks at the ability of cytotoxic T cells to kill target cells, and nonspecific immunity is evaluated by examining various function of macrophages: (1) the ability to phagocytize inert fluorescent beads or radiolabeled chicken erythrocytes and (2) the ability to produce cytokines such as IL-1 or macrophage activation factor. The ultimate immune test would be to examine the effects of xenobiotics on the intact animal's response to challenge by viral, bacterial, or parasitic pathogens, or neoplastic cells. The ability of the immune system to compensate or, conversely, its inability to compensate for loss or inhibition of its components is fully examined through host resistance mechanisms. This tiered test approach has been validated with 50 selected compounds, and results from these studies have shown that the use of only two or three immune tests are sufficient to predict known immunotoxic compounds in rodents with a >90% concordance

**TABLE 15.1. Tier I Screen**

| Parameter | Procedures |
|---|---|
| Immunopathology | Routine hematology—complete and differential count; routine toxicology information—weights of body, immune organs (spleen and thymus), liver, and kidney; histopathology of immune organs. |
| Humoral-mediated immunity | LPS (lipopolysaccharide) mitogen response or $F(ab)_2$ mitogenic response; enumeration of plaques by IgM antibody-forming cells to a T-dependent antigen (sheep red blood cells; serum IgM concentration |
| Cell-mediated immunity | Lymphocyte mitogenic response to concanavalin A and mixed lymphocyte response to allogeneic lymphocytes; local lymph node assay. |
| Nonspecific immunity | Natural killer cell activity |

*Source:* Adapted from Luster et al., 1988, and Vos et al., 1989.

**TABLE 15.2. Tier II Screen**

| Parameter | Procedures |
|---|---|
| Immunopathology | Enumeration of T and B cells and subsets; immunocytochemistry of lymphoid tissues; inumeration of cell types and numbers in the bone marrow |
| Humoral-mediated immunity | Enumeration of secondary antibody (IgG) response to sheep red blood cells |
| Cell-mediated immunity | Cytotoxic T lymphocyte killing; delayed type hypersensitivity response; mouse ear swelling test (MEST; Gad et al., 1986); guinea pig maximization test (Magnusson and Kligman, 1969). |
| Nonspecific immunity | Macrophage function—*in vitro* phagocytosis of fluorescent covaspheres, killing of *Listeria monocytogenes* or of tumor cells [basal and activated by macrophage activating factor (MAF)]. |
| Host resistance | Bacterial models—*Listeria monocytogenes* (mortality or spleen clearance); Streptococcus species (mortality); Viral models—influenza (mortality); Parasitic models—*Plasmodium yoelii* (parasitemia) or *Trichinella spiralis* (muscle larvae counts and worm expulsion); Syngeneic tumor models—PYB6 sarcoma (tumor incidence); B16F10 melanoma (lung burden). |

*Source:* Adapted from Luster et al., 1988, and Vos et al., 1989, unless otherwise indicated.

(Luster et al., 1992a, b). Specifically, the use of either a humoral response assay for plaque-forming colonies (PFC response) or determination of surface marker expression in combination with almost any other parameter significantly increased the ability to predict immunotoxicity when compared to the predictivity of any assay alone.

The FDA guidelines for immunotoxicity testing of food additives start with a Type 1 battery of tests. Type 1 tests can be derived from the routine measurements and examinations performed in short-term and subchronic rodent toxicity studies, since they do not require any perturbation of the test animals (immunization or challenge with infectious agents). These measurements include hematology and serum chemistry profiles, routine histopathologic examinations of immune-associated organs and tissues, and organ and body weight measurements including thymus and spleen. If a compound produces any primary indicators of immunotoxicity from these measurements, more definitive immunotoxicity tests, such as those indicated in the preceding paragraph, may be recommended on a case-by-case basis.

The following is a brief explanation of some of the indicators that may be used to trigger additional definitive testing and a description of some of the most commonly used assays to assess humoral, cell-mediated, or nonspecific immune dysfunction, which are common to most immunotoxicology test strategies.

### 15.2.1. CDRH Testing Framework

The CDRH draft document (1997) actually sets forth a concise and stepwise approach to evaluating the potential immunotoxicity risks of devices and is likely to serve as a basis for approaches by other FDA centers.

### 15.2.2. CDER Guidance for Investigational New Drugs

CDER's recently (2001) promulgated draft guidance for pre-INDA immunotoxicity is open for comment and certain to be modified somewhat, but clearly establishes the framework for the FDA's approach. It begins by characterizing five adverse event categories:

- Immunosuppression;
- Antigenicity;
- Hypersensitivity;
- Autoimmunity;
- Adverse immunostimulation.

Specific tests are proposed for each of these categories. It notes that immune system effects in noclinical toxicology studies are often attributed and written off as due to stress (Aden and Cohen, 1993). Such effects are frequently reversible with repeat dosing and tend not to be dose-related. It is also proposed that when possible

**TABLE 15.3. Drugs Withdrawn from the Market Due to Dose- and Time-Unrelated Toxicity Not Identified in Animal Experiments**

| Compound | Adverse Reaction | Year of Introduction | Years on the Market |
| --- | --- | --- | --- |
| Aminopyrine | Agranulocytosis | Approx 1900 | 75 |
| Phenacetin | Interstitial nephritis | Approx 1900 | 83 |
| Dipyrone | Agranulocytosis | Approx 1930 | 47 |
| Clioquinol | Subacute myelo-optic neuropathy | Approx 1930 | 51 |
| Oxyphenisatin | Chronic active hepatitis | Approx 1955 | 23 |
| Nialamide | Liver damage | 1959 | 19 |
| Phenoxypropazine | Liver damage | 1961 | 5 |
| Mebanazine | Liver damage | 1963 | 3 |
| Ibufenac | Hepatotoxicity | 1966 | 2 |
| Practolol | Oculo-mucocutaneous syndrome | 1970 | 6 |
| Alcolofenace | Hypersensitivity | 1972 | 7 |
| Azaribine | Thrombosis | 1975 | 1 |
| Ticrynafen | Nephropathy | 1979 | 1 |
| Benoxaprofen | Photosensitivity, hepatotoxicity | 1980 | 2 |
| Zomepirac | Urticaria, anaphylactic shock | 1980 | 3 |
| Zirnelidine | Hepatotoxicity | 1982 | 2 |
| Temafloxacin | Hepato- and renal toxicity | 1990 | 2 |
| Tronan | Hepato- and renal toxicity | 1997 | 3 |
| Renzalin | Hepatotoxicity | 1996 | 4 |

*Source:* Adapted from Bakke et al., 1984.

dose extrapolations to those in clinical use be based on relative body area. Specific recommendations are made for when to conduct specific testing (as opposed to the broader general evaluations integrated into existing repeat-dose testing) (Figure 15.1) and for follow-up studies for exploring mechanisms (Figure 15.2).

## 15.3. OVERVIEW OF THE IMMUNE SYSTEM

A thorough review of the immune system is not the intent of this chapter, but a brief description of the important components of the system and their interactions is necessary for an understanding of how xenobiotics can affect immune function. A breakdown at any point in this intricate and dynamic system can lead to immuno-pathology.

The immune system is divided into two defense mechanisms: nonspecific, or innate, and specific, or adaptive, mechanisms that recognize and respond to foreign substances. Some of the important cellular components of nonspecific and specific immunity are described in Table 15.4. The nonspecific immune system is the first line of defense against infectious organisms. Its cellular components are the

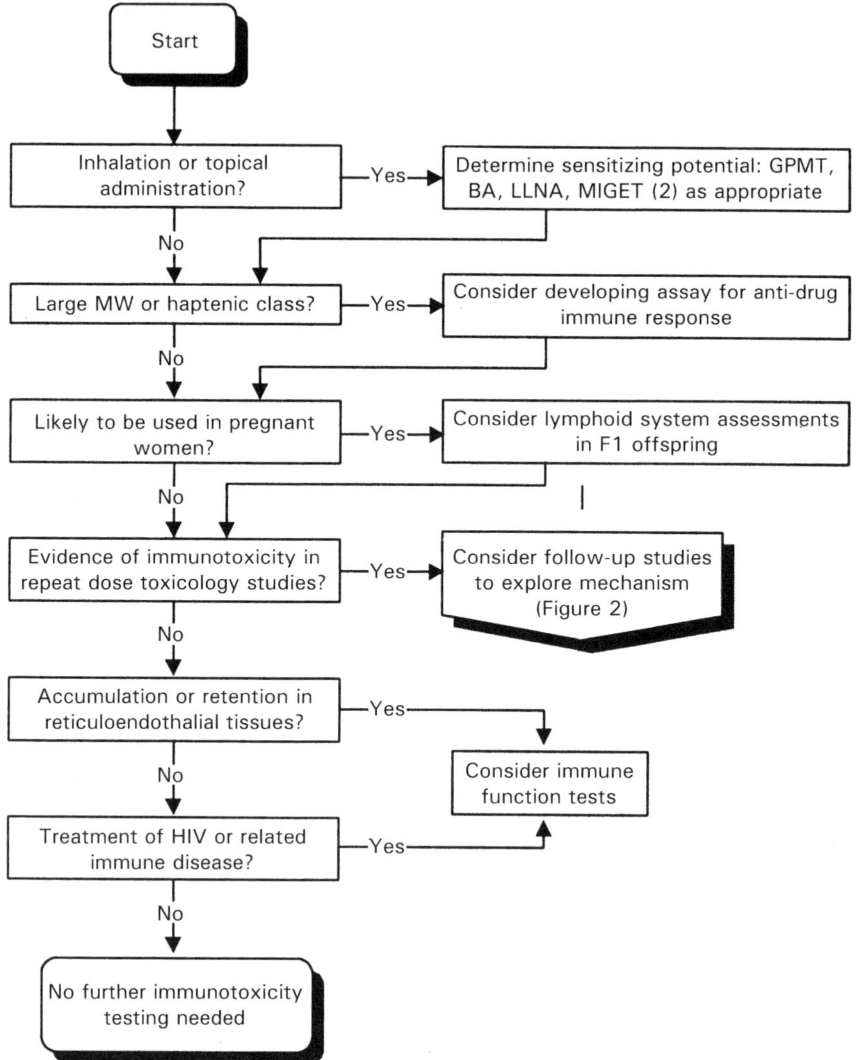


**FIGURE 15.1.** CDER flowchart for determining when to conduct specific immunotoxicity testing. GPMT: guinea pig maximization test; BA: Buehler assay (Buehler patch test); LLNA: local lymph node assay; MIGET: mouse IgE test. (There is only a relatively small database available for assessing the usefulness of the MIGET for drug regulatory purposes.)

phagocytic cells such as the monocytes, macrophages, and polymorphic neutrophils (PMNs).

The specific, or adaptive, immune system is characterized by memory, specificity, and the ability to distinguish "self" from "nonself." The important cells of the adaptive immune system are the lymphocytes and antigen-presenting cells that are

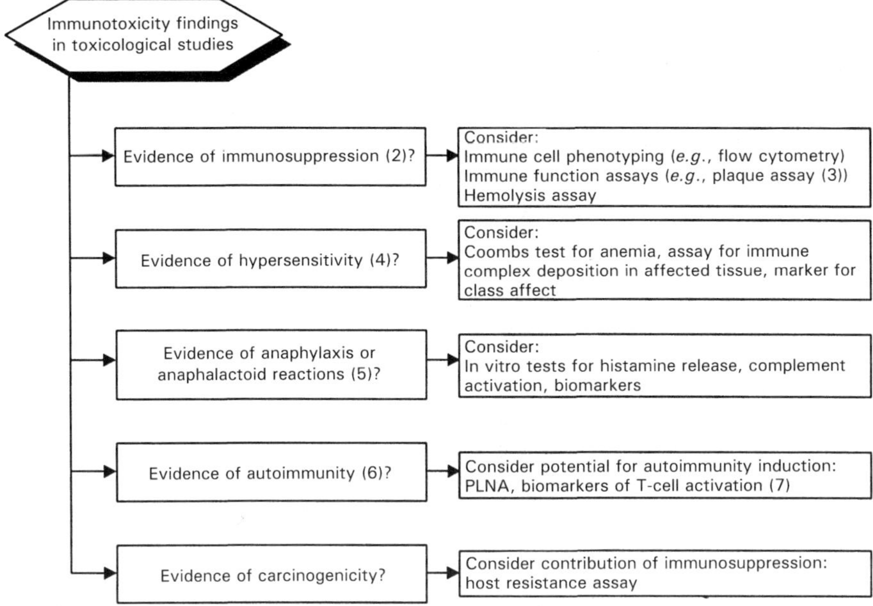


**FIGURE 15.2.** Follow-up studies to consider for exploring mechanisms of immunotoxicity.

1. Examples include myelosuppression, histopathology in immune associated tissues, increased infection, tumors, decreased serum Ig, phenotypic changes in immune cells.

2. Other acceptable assays include drug effect on NK cell function *in vitro* bastogenesis, cytotoxic T cell function, cytokine production, delayed-type hypersensitivity, host resistance to infections or implanted tumors.

3. Examples include anemia, luekopenia, thrombocytopenia, pnuemonitis, vasculitis, lupus-like reactions, glomerulonephritis.

4. Examples include cardiopulmonary distress, rashes, flushed skin, swelling of face or limbs.

5. Examples include vasculitis, lupus-like reactions, glomerulonephritis, hemolytic anemia.

6. There are no established assays that reliably assess potential for autoimmunity and acute systemic hypersensitivity. The popliteal lymph node assay (PLNA) has only a relatively small database available for assessing its usefulness for drug regulatory purposes.

part of nonspecific immunity. The lymphocytes, which originate from pluripotent stem cells located in the hematopoietic tissues of the liver (fetal) and bone marrow, are composed of two general cell types; T and B cells. The T cells differentiate in the thymus and are made up of three subsets: helper, suppressor, and cytotoxic. The B cells, which have the capacity to produce antibodies, differentiate in the bone marrow or fetal liver. The various functions of the T cells include presenting antigen to B cells, helping B cells to make antibody, killing virally infected cells, regulating the level of the immune response, and stimulating cytotoxic activity of other cells such as macrophages (Male et al., 1987).

**TABLE 15.4. Cellular Components of the Immune System and Their Functions**

| Cell Subpopulations | Markers[a] | Functions |
| --- | --- | --- |
| *Nonspecific immunity* | | |
| Granulocytes | | Degranulate to release mediators |
|   Neutrophils (blood) | | |
|   Basophils (blood) | | |
|   Eosinophils (blood) | | |
|   Mast cells (connective tissue) | | |
| | | Nonsensitized lymphocytes; directly kill target cells |
| Natural killer cells (NK) | | |
| Reticuloendothelial | CD14; HLA-DR | Antigen processing, presentation, and phagocytosis (humoral and some cell-mediated responses) |
|   Macrophage (peritoneal, pleural, alveolar spaces) | | |
|   Histiocytes (tissues) | | |
|   Monocytes (blood) | | |
| *Specific immunity* | | |
| Humoral immunity | | |
|   Activated B cells | CD19; CD23 | Proliferate; form plasma cells |
|   Plasma cells | | Secrete antibody; terminally differentiated |
|     Resting | | Secrete IgM antibodies (primary response) |
|     Memory | | Secrete IgG antibodies (secondary response) |
| *Cell-mediated immunity* | | |
|   T-Cell types: | | |
|     Helper ($T_h$) | CD4; CDE25 | Assists in humoral immunity; required for antibody production |
|     Cytotoxic ($T_k$) | CD8; CD25 | Target lysis |
|     Suppressor ($T_s$) | CD8; CD25 | Suppresses/regulates humoral and cell-mediated responses |

[a]Activation surface markers detected by specific monoclonal antibodies; can be assayed with flow cytometry.

Activation of the immune system is thought to occur when antigen-presenting cells (APCs) such as macrophages and dendritic cells take up antigen via $F_c$ or complement receptors, process the antigen, and present it to T cells (see Figure 15.3). Macrophages release soluble mediators such as interleukin 1 (IL-1), which stimulate T cells to proliferate. Antigen-presenting cells must present antigen to T cells in conjunction with the class II major histocompatibility complex (MHC) proteins that are located on the surfaces of T cells. The receptor on the T cell is a complex of the Ti molecule that binds antigen, the MHC proteins, and the T3 molecular complex, which is often referred to as the CD3 complex. Upon stimulation, T cells proliferate, differentiate, and express interleukin-2 (IL-2) receptors. T cells also produce and secrete IL-2, which, in turn, acts on antigen-specific B cells, causing them to proliferate and differentiate into antibody-forming (plasma) cells.

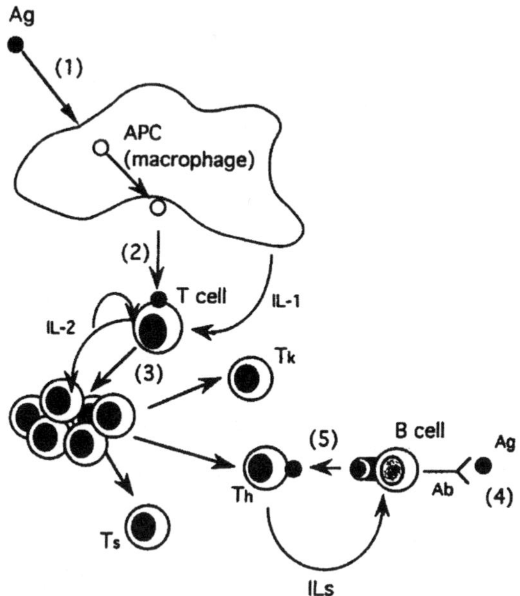


**FIGURE 15.3.** A simplified schematic of the immunoregulatory circuit that regulates the activation of T cells and B cells involved in humoral (T-cell dependent) and cell-mediated immunity. (1) Antigen (Ag) is processed by the APCs expressing class II MHC molecules. (2) Antigen plus class II MHC is then presented to antigen-specific T helper cells (CD4[+]), which stimulates secretion of IL-2. (3) IL-2 in turn stimulates proliferation (clonal expansion) of T cells and differentiation into T suppressor ($T_s$), T killer ($T_k$), and T helper ($T_h$) effector cells. The expanded clone has a higher likelihood of finding the appropriate B cell that has the same antigen and class II molecules on its surface. (4) Next, the antigen binds to an antibody (Ab) on the surface of a specific B cell. (5) The B cell, in turn, processes the antigen and presents it (plus class II MHC) to the specific $T_h$ cell. The $T_h$ cell is then stimulated to secrete additional interleukins (ILs) that stimulate clonal expansion and differentiation of the antigen-specific B cell.

Antibodies circulate freely in the blood or lymph and are important in neutralizing foreign antigens. The various types of antibodies involved in humoral immunity and their functions are described in Table 15.5. There are multiple genes (polymorphisms) that encode diversity to the variable region of the antibody. B cells are capable of generating further diversity to antibody specificity by a sequence of molecular events involving somatic mutations, chromosomal rearrangements during mitosis, and recombination of gene segments (Roitt, 1985).

The immune system is regulated in part by feedback inhibition involving complex interactions between the various growth and differentiation factors listed in Table 15.6. Since antigen initiates the signal for the immune response, elimination of antigen will decrease further stimulation (Male et al., 1982). T suppressor cells ($T_s$) also regulate the immune response and are thought to be important in the development of tolerance to self-antigens. In addition to the humoral immune system or the branch that is modulated by antibody, cell-mediated immunity and cytotoxic cell types play a major role in the defense against virally infected cells, tumor cells, and cells of foreign tissue transplants. Cytotoxic $T_k$ cells (T killer cells) recognize antigen in association with class I molecules of the MHC, while natural killer cells (NK cells) are not MHC restricted. Cell-killing results in a sequence of events following activation of the effector cell, lysosomal degranulation, and calcium influx into the targeted cell. The various types of cells involved in cell-mediated cytotoxicity and their mechanisms of action are outlined in Table 15.7.

## 15.4. IMMUNOTOXIC EFFECTS

The immune system is a highly integrated and regulated network of cell types that requires continual renewal to achieve balance and immunocompetence. The delicacy of this balance makes the immune system a natural target for cytotoxic drugs or their metabolites. Since renewal is dependent on the ability of cells to proliferate and differentiate, exposure to agents that arrest cell division can subsequently lead to reduced immune function or immunosuppression. This concept has been exploited in the development of therapeutic drugs intended to treat leukemias, autoimmune disease, and chronic inflammatory diseases and to prevent transplant rejection. However, some drugs may adversely modulate the immune system secondarily to their therapeutic effects.

Two broad categories of immunotoxicity have been defined on the basis of suppression or stimulation of normal immune function. Immunosuppression is a down-modulation of the immune system characterized by cell depletion, dysfunction, or dysregulation that may subsequently result in increased susceptibility to infection and tumors. By contrast, immunostimulation is an increased or exaggerated immune responsiveness that may be apparent in the form of a tissue-damaging allergic hypersensitivity response or pathological autoimmunity. However, as knowledge of the mechanisms involved in each of these conditions has expanded, the distinction between them has become less clear. Some agents can cause immunosuppression at one dose or duration of exposure, and immunostimulation at others.

**TABLE 15.5. Antibodies Involved in the Humoral Immune Response**

| Antibodies | Serum conc.<br>$Mg\,ml^{-1}$ (%) | Characteristics/functions |
| --- | --- | --- |
| IgG | 10–12 (80%) | Monomeric structure ($\gamma$-globulin); secreted from B cells during secondary response; binds complement; can cross placenta |
| IgM | 1–2 (5–10%) | Pentameric structure; secreted from B cells during primary response; potent binder of complement; high levels indicative of systemic lupus erythematosus or rheumatoid arthritis; cannot cross placenta |
| IgA | 3–4 (10–15%) | Dimeric or monomeric structures; found in seromucous secretions (breast milk); secreted by B cells associated with epithelial cells in GI tract, lung, etc. |
| IgD | 0.03 (<1%) | Monomer; extremely labile; functions not well known |
| IgE | <0.0001 | Reaginic antibody involved in immediate hypersensitivity; antihelminthic; does not bind complement |

*Source:* Extracted and modified from Clark, 1983.

**TABLE 15.6. Growth and Differentiation Factors of the Immune System**

| Factors | Cell of origin | Primary immune functions |
| --- | --- | --- |
| *Interleukins*[a] | | |
| IL-1 | Macrophage, B and T cells | Lymphocyte-activating factor; enhances activation of T and B cells, NK cells, and macrophages |
| IL-2 | T cells ($T_h$) | T-cell growth factor; stimulates T-cell growth and effector differentiation; stimulates B-cell proliferation/differentiation |
| IL-3 | T cells ($T_h$) | Mast-cell growth factor; stimulates proliferation/differentiation of mast cells, neutrophils, and macrophages |
| IL-4 | T cells ($T_h$), mast cells, B cells | B-cell growth factor; induces proliferation/differentiation of B cells and secretion of IgA, $IgG_1$, and IgE; promotes T-cell growth; activates macrophages |
| IL-5 | T cells ($T_h$) | Stimulates antibody secretion (IgA), proliferation of B cells, and eosinophil differentiation |
| IL-6 | T cells, fibroblasts, monocytes | Stimulates growth/differentiation of B cells and secretion of IgG; promotes IL-2-induced growth of T cells |
| IL-7 | Bone marrow stromal cells | Stimulates pre-B- and pre-T-cell growth/differentiation; enhances thymocyte proliferation |
| IL-8 | Monocytes, fibroblasts | Neutrophil chemotaxis |
| IL-9 | T cells | Stimulates T cells and mast cells |
| IL-10 | T cells | Stimulates mast cells and thymocytes; induction of class II MHC |
| *Interferons (INF)* | | |
| A-INF | Leukocytes and mast cells | Antiviral; increases NK-cell function, B-cell differentiation, potentiates macrophage production of IL-1 |

| | | |
|---|---|---|
| B-INF | Fibroblasts, epithelial cells | Antiviral; potentiates macrophage production of IL-1; increases NK-cell function |
| Γ-INF | T cells (T$_h$), cytotoxic T cells | Antiviral; activates macrophages; induces MHC class II expression on macrophages, epithelial, and endothelial cells |
| *Tumor necrosis factors (TNF)* | | |
| TNFα | Macrophage, B and T cells | Catectin; promotes tumor cytotoxicity; activates macrophages and neutrophils; enhances IL-2 receptor expression on T cells; inhibits antibody secretion |
| TNF$\beta$ | T cells (T$_h$) | Lymphotoxin; promotes T-cell-mediates cytotoxicity |
| | NK cells | B cell activation |
| *Colony stimulating factors (CSF)* | | |
| | *Stem cells:* | *Promotes growth and differentiation of:* |
| Granulocyte CSF | Myeloid | Granulocytes and macrophages |
| Macrophage CSF | Myeloid | Macrophages and granulocytes |
| Granulocyte-macrophage CSF | Myeloid | Granulocytes, macrophages, eosinophils, mast cells, and pluripotent progenitor cells |

[a]Includes lymphokines, monokines, and cytokines produced by T cells, macrophages, and other cells, respectively.

*Source:* Extracted and modified from Golub and Green, 1991.

**TABLE 15.7. Cells and Mechanisms Involved in Cell-Mediated Cytotoxicity**

| Cell type | Mechanism of cytotoxicity |
|---|---|
| $T_k$ cells | $T_k$ cells that are specifically sensitized to antigens on target cells interact directly with target cells to lyse them. |
| $T_D$ | Cells involved in delayed hypersensitivity that act indirectly to kill target cells; $T_D$ cells react with antigen and release cytokines that can kill target cells. |
| NK cells | Nonspecific T cells that react directly with target cells (tumor cells) without prior sensitization. |
| Null cells | Antibody-dependent cell-mediated cytotoxicity (ADCC) involving non-T/non-B cells (null cells) with $F_c$ receptors specific for antibody-coated target cells. |
| Macrophages | Nonspecific, direct killing of target by phagocytosis; also involved in presenting antigen to specific $T_k$ cells that can then mediate cytotoxicity as described above. |

For instance, the chemotherapeutic drug cyclophosphamide is in most cases immunosuppressive; however, it can also induce autoimmunity (Hutchings et al., 1985). Likewise, dimethylnitrosamine, a nitrosamine detected in some foods, has been shown to have both suppressing and enhancing effects on the immune system (Yoshida et al., 1989).

## 15.5. IMMUNOSUPPRESSION

The various cells of the immune system may differ in their sensitivity to a given xenobiotic. Thus, immunosuppression may be expressed as varying degrees of reduced activity of a single cell type of multiple populations of immunocytes. Several lymphoid organs such as the bone marrow, spleen, thymus, and lymph nodes may be affected simultaneously or the immunodeficiency may be isolated to a single tissue, such as the Peyer's patches of the intestines. The resulting deficiency may in turn lead to an array of clinical outcomes of varying ranges of severity. These outcomes include increased susceptibility to infections, increased severity or persistence of infections, or infections with unusual organisms (e.g., systemic fungal infections). Immunosuppression can be induced in a dose-related manner by a variety of therapeutic agents at dose levels lower than those required to produce overt clinical signs of general toxicity. In addition, immunosuppression can occur without regard to genetic predisposition, given that a sufficient dose level and duration of exposure has been achieved.

Humoral immunity is characterized by the production of antigen-specific antibodies that enhance phagocytosis and destruction of microorganisms through opsonization. Thus, deficiencies of humoral immunity (B lymphocytes) may lead to reduced antibody titers and are typically associated with acute gram-positive bacterial infections (i.e., *Streptococcus*). Although chronic infection is usually associated with dysfunction of some aspect of cellular immunity, chronic infections can also occur when facultative intracellular organisms such as *Listeria* or *Mycobacterium* evade antibodies and multiply within phagocytic cells.

Since cellular immunity results in the release of chemotactic lymphocytes that in turn enhance phagocytosis, a deficiency in cellular immunity may also result in chronic infections. Cellular immunity is mediated by T cells, macrophages, and NK cells involved in complex compensatory networks and secondary changes. Immunosuppressive agents may act directly by lethality to T cells, or indirectly by blocking mitosis, lymphokine synthesis, lymphokine release, or membrane receptors to lymphokines. In addition, cellular immunity is involved in the production and release of interferon, a lymphokine that ultimately results in blockage of viral replication (Table 15.4). Viruses are particularly susceptible to cytolysis by T cells since they often attach to the surface of infected cells. Thus, immunosuppression of any of the components of cellular immunity may result in an increase in protozoan, fungal, and viral infections as well as opportunistic bacterial infections.

Immune depression may result unintentionally as a side effect of cancer chemotherapy or intentionally from therapeutics administered to prevent graft rejection. In fact, both transplant patients administered immunosuppressive drugs and cancer patients treated with chemotherapeutic agents have been shown to be at high risk of developing secondary cancers, particularly of lymphoreticular etiology (Penn, 1977). Most of these drugs are alkylating or cross-linking agents that by their chemical nature are electrophilic and highly reactive with nucleophilic macromolecules (protein and nucleic acids). Nucleophilic sites are quite ubiquitous and include amino, hydroxyl, mercapto, and histidine functional groups. Thus, immunotoxic agents used in chemotherapy may induce secondary tumors through direct genotoxic mechanisms (i.e., DNA alkylation).

Reduced cellular immunity may result in increased malignancy and decreased viral resistance through indirect mechanisms as well, by modulating immune surveillance of aberrant cells. T lymphocytes, macrophage cells, and NK cells are all involved in immunosurveillance through cytolysis of virally infected cells or tumor cells, each by a different mechanism (Table 15.5) (Burnet, 1970). In addition to the common cell types described in Table 15.5, at least two other types of cytotoxic effector cells of T-cell origin have been identified, each of which has a unique lytic specificity phenotype, and activity profile (Merluzzi, 1985). Of these, both LAK and TIL cells have been shown to lyse a variety of different tumor cells. However, TIL cells have 50–100 times more lytic activity than LAK cells. Most tumor cells express unique surface antigens that render them different from normal cells. Once detected as foreign, they are presented to the T helper cells in association with MHC molecules to form an antigen-MHC complex. This association elicits a genetic component to the immunospecificity reaction. T helper cells subsequently direct the antigen complex toward the cytotoxic T lymphocytes, which possess receptors for antigen-MHC complexes. These cells can then proliferate, respond to specific viral antigens or antigens on the membranes of tumor cells, and destroy them. (Yoshida et al, 1989).

In contrast, the macrophages and natural killer (NK) cells are involved in nonspecific immunosurveillance in that they do not require prior sensitization with a foreign antigen as a prerequisite for lysis, and are not involved with MHC molecules. The enhancement of either NK cell function or macrophage function has been shown to reduce metastasis of some types of tumors. Macrophage cells accumulate at the tumor site and have been shown to lyse a variety of transformed tumor cells (Volkman, 1984). Natural killer cells are involved in the lysis of primary autochthonous tumor cells. Migration of NK cells to tumor sites has been well documented. Although not clearly defined, it appears that they can recognize certain proteinaceous structures on tumor cells and lyse them with cytolysin.

### 15.5.1. Immunosuppressive Drugs

Table 15.8 lists numerous types of drugs that are immunosuppressive and describes their immunotoxic effects. Several classes of drugs that characteristically depress the immune system are further discussed in the next section.

***Antimetabolites.*** This class of drugs includes purine, pyrimidine, and folic acid analogs that have been successfully used to treat various carcinomas, autoimmune diseases, and dermatological disorders such as psoriasis. Because of their structural similarities to normal components of DNA and RNA synthesis, they are capable of competing with the normal macromolecules and alkylating biological nucleophiles.

Thioguanine and mercaptopurine are purine analogs structurally similar to guanine and hypoxanthine that have been used to treat malignancies. Azathioprine, an imidazolyl derivative of mercaptopurine, has been used as an immunosuppressive therapeutic in organ transplants and to treat severe refractory rheumatoid arthritis (Hunter et al., 1975) and autoimmune disorders including pemphigus vulgaris and bullous pemphigoid. These drugs act as antimetabolites to block *de novo* purine synthesis through the erroneous incorporation of thioinosinic acid into the pathway in place of inosine. The antimetabolite can bind to the inosine receptor, which in turn will inhibit the synthesis of DNA, RNA, protein synthesis, and ultimately T-cell differentiation (Hadden et al., 1984). For example, both thioguanine and mercaptopurine can act as substrates for the HGPRT enzyme to produce T-IMP (thioinosine monophosphate) and T-GMP (thioguanine monophosphate), respectively. Thioinosine monophosphate is a poor substrate for guanylyl kinase, which would normally catalyze the conversion of GMP to GDP (Calabresi and Chabner, 1990). Thus T-IMP can accumulate in the cell and inhibit several vital metabolic reactions. At high doses, these drugs can suppress the entire immune system. However, at clinical dosages, only the T-cell response is affected, without an apparent decrease in T-cell numbers (Spreafico and Anaclerio, 1977).

Pentostatin (2′-deoxycoformycin) is an adenosine analog that is a potent inhibitor of adenosine deaminase. Pentostatin is particularly useful for treating T-cell leukemia since malignant T cells have higher levels of adenosine deaminase than most cells. Similar to individuals that are genetically deficient in adenosine deaminase, treatment with pentostatin produces immunosuppression of both T and B lymphocytes, with minimal effect on other tissues. As a result, severe opportunistic infections are often associated with its clinical use.

5-Fluorouracil (5-FU), adenosine arabinoside (AraA) and cytosine arabinoside (AraC) are pyrimidine analogs to uracil, adenine, and cytosine, respectively. 5-FU is used primarily to treat cancer of the breast and gastrointestinal tract as well as severe recalcitrant psoriasis (Alper et al., 1985). AraC is predominantly indicated for the treatment of acute leukemia and non-Hodgkin's lymphomas. Although high-dose therapy with AraC has a good likelihood of producing complete remission, it is often accompanied by severe leukopenia, thrombocytopenia, and anemia (Barnett et al., 1985). Likewise, myelosuppression is the major toxicity associated with bolus-dose regimens of 5-FU.

***Glucocorticosteroids.*** Corticosteroids are commonly used to reduce inflammation, treat autoimmune diseases such as systemic lupus erythematosus (SLE), and as a prophylactic measure to prevent transplant rejection. The adrenocorticosteroid prednisone is often coadministered with other immunosuppressives such as cyclosporine and azathioprine (Elion and Hitchings, 1975). Glucocorticosteroids act pharmacologically by modulating the rate of protein synthesis. The molecule reacts with specific receptors to form a complex that crosses into the nucleus of the cell and regulates transcription of specific mRNA. The corticosteroid complex releases inhibition of transcription, thus enhancing protein synthesis (Hollenberg et al., 1987). This may lead to the initiation of *de novo* synthesis of the phospholipase A2 inhibiting protein, lipocortin, which blocks the synthesis of arachidonic acid and its prostaglandin and leukotriene metabolites (Wallner et al., 1986). Glucocorticosteroids induce immunosuppression and anti-inflammation as a result of the inhibition of specific leukocyte functions such as lymphokine activity. Glucocorticoids can also inhibit recruitment of leukocytes and macrophages into the site of inflammation. In addition, amplification of cell-mediated immunity can be suppressed by inhibiting the interaction of IL-2 with its T-cell receptors. However, the immunosuppression is reversible and immune function recovers once therapy has ceased.

***Cyclosporine.*** Cyclosporin A (cyclosporine) is an 11 amino acid cyclic peptide residue of fungal origin isolated from the fermentation products of *Trichoderma polysporum* and *Cylindrocarpon lucidum*. In addition to having a very narrow range of antibiotic activity it was also found to inhibit proliferation of lymphocytes, which made it unsuitable as an antibiotic. Cyclosporine inhibits the early cellular response of helper T cells to antigens (Kay and Benzie, 1984) primarily by inhibiting production of IL-2 (Elliot et al., 1984), and at higher doses it may inhibit expression of IL-2 receptors (Herold et al., 1986). Cyclosporine does not prevent the stimulation of helper T cell clonal expansion by IL-2, only its activation. Since it is not myelosuppressive at therapeutic dosages, the incidence of secondary infection is lower than that induced by other classes of immunosuppressives. Thus, cyclosporine is ideal as an immunosuppressive agent to prevent transplant rejection and graft-host disease (Kahan and Bach, 1988). Cyclosporine has also been used as an anti-

**TABLE 15.8. Immunosuppressive Drugs and Their Effects**

| Drugs | Biological Activity and Indications | Immunotoxic Effects |
|---|---|---|
| *Hormones and antagonists* | | |
| Corticosteroids (prednisone) | Anti-inflammatory; systemic lupus erythematosus; leukemias; rheumatoid arthritis; breast cancer | Depresses T- and B-cell function; reduces lymphokines; alters macrophage function; increases infections |
| Diethylstilbestrol | Synthetic estrogen; cancer chemotherapy | Depletes or functionally impairs T cells; enhances macrophage suppressor cell; increases infections and tumorigenesis |
| Estradiol | Synthetic estrogen; dysmenorrhea; osteoporosis | Decreases $T_h$ cells and IL-2 synthesis; increases $T_s$ cell function, infections, and tumorigenesis |
| *Antibiotics* | | |
| Cephalosporins | $\beta$-lactam antimicrobial | Granulocytopenia; cytopenia |
| Chloroamphenol | Wide-spectrum antimicrobial | Pancytopenia, leukopenia (idiosyncratic) |
| Penicillins | $\beta$-lactam antimicrobial | Granulocytopenia; cytopenia |
| Rifampin | Macrocyclic antibiotic | Suppresses T-cell function |
| Tetracyclines | Antimicrobial | Decreased migration of granulocytes |
| *Chemotherapeutics and Immunomodulators* | | |
| Arabinoside (AraA and AraC) | Antimetabolites; antivirals; leukemias; lymphomas | Leukopenia; thrombocytopenia |
| Azathioprine | Antimetabolite; leukemia; arthritis; transplant rejection | Inhibits protein synthesis; bone marrow suppression |
| Busulfan | Alkylating agent; chronic granulocytic leukemia | Leukopenia; myelosuppressive; granulocytopenia |
| Carmutin and Lomustin (BCNU and CCNU) | Alkylating agents; Hodgkin's disease; lymphomas | Delayed hematopoietic depression; leukopenia; thrombocytopenia |
| Chlorambucil | Alkylating agent; leukemia; lymphomas; vasculitis | Bone marrow suppression; myelosuppressive |

| Cyclophosphamide (Cytotoxin) | Alkylating agent; cancer chemotherapy; transplant rejection; rheumatoid arthritis | Decreased $T_s$ cells, B cells, and NK cells |
| --- | --- | --- |
| Cyclosporin A | Transplant rejections | Depresses T cells; inhibits IL-2 production |
| Interferon | Immunomodulator; antiviral, hairy cell leukemia | Bone marrow suppression; granulocytopenia; leukopenia |
| Melphalan (L-PAM) | Alkylating agent; breast and ovarian cancer | Leukopenia; bone marrow suppression; granulocytopenia; pancytopenia |
| 6-Mercaptopurine | Antimetabolite; acute leukemias; arthritis | Decreased T-cell function; bone marrow suppression |
| Methotrexate | Folic acid analog; cancer chemotherapy, arthritis | Inhibits proliferation; T-cell suppression; granulocytopenia; lymphocytopenia |
| Penostatin | Adenosine analog; T-cell leukemia | Inhibits adenosine deaminase; suppresses T and B cells |
| Zidovudine (AZT) | Antiviral (HIV) | Decreases $T_h$ cells and granulocytes |
| *Miscellaneous* | | |
| Colchicine | Antimitotic; gout; anti-inflammatory | Inhibits migration of granulocytes; leukopenia; agranulocytosis |
| Diphenylhydantoin (Phenytoin) | Antiepileptic | Leukocytopenia; neutrapenia |
| Indomethacin (Indocin) | Nonsteroidal anti-inflammatory; analgesic; antipyretic | Neutrapenia |
| Procainamide | Antiarrhythmic | Agranulocytosis; leukopenia (rare) |
| Sulfasalazine | Antimicrobial anti-inflammatory; ulcerative colitis/inflammatory bowel diseases | Suppresses NK cells; impaired lymphocyte function |

*Source:* Extracted and modified primarily from Gilman et al., 1990.

helminthic and as an anti-inflammatory agent to treat rheumatoid arthritis and other autoimmune-type diseases.

***Nitrogen Mustards.*** Nitrogen mustards characteristically consist of a bis(2-chloroethly) group bonded to nitrogen. These molecules are highly reactive bifunctional alkylating agents that have been successfully used in cancer chemotherapy. Included in this group are mechlorethamine, L-phenylalanine mustard (melphalan), chlorambucil, ifosfamide, and cyclophosphamide. The cytotoxic effects of each on the bone marrow and lymphoid organs are similar; however, their pharmacokinetic and toxic profiles can vary on the basis of the substituted side group. For example, the side group may consist of a simple methyl group, as is the case of mechlorethamine, or substituted phenyl groups, in the cases of melphalan and chlorambucil.

Cyclophosphamide, which contains a cyclic phosphamide group bonded to the nitrogen mustard, is representative of this class. The parent compound itself is not active *in vitro* unless treated in conjunction with an exogenous P450 microsomal enzyme system (Colvin, 1982) such as rat liver S9 homogenate, which metabolizes it to a highly reactive alkylating agent (4-hydroxy-cyclophosphamide). Thus, *in vivo*, cyclophosphamide is not toxic until it is metabolically activated in the liver. Cyclophosphamide has been the most widely used nitrogen mustard; it has been effective as a cancer chemotherapeutic and to treat autoimmune-type diseases including SLE, multiple sclerosis, and rheumatoid arthritis (Calabresi and Parks, 1985). Treatment with cyclophosphamide suppresses all classes of lymphoid cells, which may result in reduced lymphocyte function as well as lymphopenia and neutropenia (Webb and Winkelstein, 1982). Thus, it has also been administered as a large single dose prior to bone marrow transplants to suppress cellular immunity and subsequently inhibit rejection (Shand, 1979).

***Estrogens.*** $\beta$-estradiol (Luster et al., 1984; Pung et al., 1984) and therapeutics with estrogenic activity, such as diethylstilbestrol (DES), have also been shown to be immunosuppressive (Luster et al., 1985). Estrogens have been shown to increase T suppressor cell activity in splenocytes, decrease numbers of T helper cells, inhibit IL-2 synthesis, and modulate production of immunoregulatory factors (Luster et al., 1987). These effects have been particularly characterized in studies with DES, a nonsteroidal synthetic estrogen used widely in the treatment of prostate and breast cancers, as well as administered to pregnant women as a "morning after" contraceptive. Decreased mitogenicity of human peripheral blood lymphocytes has been observed in men treated with DES for prostate cancer and women exposed *in utero* (Haukass et al., 1982; Ways et al., 1987). In mice, thymic involution and atrophy with depletion of the cortical lymphocytes have been observed histologically. Function is also modulated, as evident by depressed mixed lymphocyte responses, mitogenicity, and T-cell release of IL-2 (Pung et al., 1985). Dean et al. (1980) speculated that DES treatment selectively depletes or functionally impairs T cells and/or the induction of suppressor macrophages, resulting in immunosuppression. Macrophage suppressor cell activity is enhanced (Luster et al., 1980) and PMN cells accumulate following bacterial challenge. Although macrophage functions of phagocytosis and tumor growth inhibition are potentiated, defects in macrophage migration and decreased bactericidal activity contribute to decreased host resistance with resulting increased susceptibility to bacterial infections.

***Heavy Metals.*** Some heavy metals such as gold and platinum are used pharmacologically as immunomodulators to treat rheumatoid arthritis and as antineoplastic drugs, respectively. Most heavy metals inhibit mitogenicity, antibody responses, and host resistance to bacterial or viral challenge, and tumor growth. Platinum has been shown to suppress humoral immunity, lymphocyte proliferation, and macrophage function (Lawrence, 1985). Clinically, mild to moderate myelosuppression may also be evident with transient leukopenia and thrombocytopenia.

Likewise, injectable gold salts such as gold sodium thiomalate affect a variety of immune responses in humans (Bloom et al., 1987). Severe thrombocytopenia occurs in 1% of patients as a result of an immunological disturbance that accelerates the degradation of platelets. Leukopenia, agranulocytosis, and fatal aplastic anemia may also occur. Although better tolerated than parenteral preparations, the organic gold compound, auranofin, administered orally is also immunosuppressive. In a dog study, auranofin was shown to produce thrombocytopenia similar to that described in humans administered parenteral preparations (Bloom et al., 1985a). Long-term toxicity studies with these compounds in dogs show evidence of immune-modulating activity, possible drug-induced immunotoxicity, and treatment-related changes in immune function (e.g., lymphocyte activation).

***Antibiotics.*** $\beta$-lactam-containing antibiotics such as the cephalosporins may also induce significant immunosuppressive effects (Caspritz and Hadden, 1987) in a small percentage of human patients. Adverse effects including anemia, neutropenia, thrombocytopenia, and bone marrow depression were observed in dogs administered high doses of cefonicid for six months (Bloom et al., 1985b). A similar syndrome has been characterized in cefazedone-treated dogs expressing an agglutinating red cell antibody. Further studies with this drug indicated that both cytopenia (Bloom et al., 1985b) and suppression of bone marrow stem cell activity appear to be antibody-mediated (Deldar et al., 1985).

### 15.5.2. Immunostimulation

A variety of drugs as well as environmental chemicals have been shown to have immunostimulatory or sensitizing effects on the immune system and these effects are well documented in humans exposed to drugs (DeSwarte, 1986). The drug or metabolite can act as a hapten and covalently bind to a protein or other cellular constituent of the host to appear foreign and become antigenic. Haptens are low molecular weight substances that are not in themselves immunogenic but will induce an immune response if conjugated with nucleophilic groups on proteins or other macromolecular carriers. In both allergy and autoimmunity, the immune system is stimulated or sensitized by the drug conjugate to produce specific pathological responses. An allergic hypersensitivity reaction may vary from one which results in an immediate anaphylactic response to one which produces a delayed hypersensitivity reaction or immune complex reaction. Allergic hypersensitivity reactions result in a heightened sensitivity to nonself antigens, whereas autoimmunity results in an altered response to self antigens. Unlike immunosuppression, which nonspecifically affects all individuals in a dose-related manner, both allergy and autoimmunity have a genetic component that creates susceptibility in those individuals with a genetic predisposition. Susceptible individuals, once sensitized, can respond to even minute quantities of the antigen. Several examples of drugs that can stimulate the immune system are presented in Table 15.9.

***Hypersensitivity.*** The four types of hypersensitivity reactions as classified by Coombs and Gell (1975) are outlined in Table 15.10. The first three types are immediate antibody-mediated reactions, whereas the fourth type is a cellular-mediated delayed-type response that may require 1–2 days to occur after a secondary exposure. Type I reactions are characterized by an anaphylaxis response to a variety of compounds, including proteinaceous materials and pharmaceuticals such as penicillin. Various target organs may be involved depending on the route of exposure. For example, the gastrointestinal tract is usually involved with food allergies, the respiratory system with inhaled allergens, the skin with dermal exposure, and smooth muscle vasculature with systemic exposure. The type of response elicited often depends on the site of exposure and includes dermatitis and urticaria (dermal), rhinitis and asthma (inhalation), increased gastrointestinal emptying (ingestion), and systemic anaphylactic shock (parenteral).

*Type I Hypersensitivity.* During an initial exposure, IgE antibodies are produced and bind to the cell surface of mast cells and basophils. Upon subsequent exposures to the antigen, reaginic IgE antibodies bound to the surface of target cells at the $F_c$ region (mast cells and basophils) become cross-linked (at the $F_{ab}$ regions) by the antigen. Cross-linking causes distortion of the cell surface and IgE molecule, which, in turn, activates a series of enzymatic reactions, ultimately leading to degranulation of the mast cells and basophils. These granules contain a variety of pharmacological substances (Table 15.11), such as histamines, serotonins, prostaglandins, bradykinins, and leukotrienes (SRS-A and ECR-A). Upon subsequent challenge exposures, these factors are responsible for eliciting an allergic reaction through vasodilation and increased vascular permeability. The nasal passages contain both mast cells and plasma cells that secrete IgE antibodies. Allergic responses localized in the nasal mucosa result in dilation of the local blood vessels, tissue swelling, mucus secretion, and sneezing. Reactions localized in the respiratory tract, also rich in mast cells and IgE, result in an allergic asthma response. This condition is triggered by the release of histamine and SRS-A, which induce constriction of the bronchi and alveoli, pulmonary edema, and mucous secretions that block the bronchi and alveoli, together resulting in severe difficulty in breathing. In the case of a challenge dose of a drug administered systemically, the reactive patient may have difficulty breathing within minutes of exposure and may experience convulsions, vomiting, and low blood pressure. The effects of anaphylactic shock and respiratory distress, if severe, may ultimately result in death.

**TABLE 15.9. Drugs That Produce Immunostimulation**

| Drug | Type of response |
| --- | --- |
| *Antibiotics* | *Hypersensitivity* |
| Cephalosporins | Anaphylaxis, urticaria, rash, granulocytopenia |
| Chloramphenicol | Rash, dermatitis, urticaria |
| Neomycin | Dermal exposure-rash, dermatitis |
| Sulfathiazole | Rash, dermatitis, urticaria |
| Spiramycin | Rash, dermatitis, urticaria |
| Quinolones | Photosensitivity |
| Tetracyclines | Photosensitivity, anaphylaxis, asthma, dermatitis |
| | |
| *Others* | |
| Allopurinol | Rash, urticaria, fever, eosinophilia |
| Avridine | Delayed-type hypersensitivity; increases NK cells, T cells, IL-1, and IL-2 |
| Isoprinosine | Delayed-type hypersensitivity; increases T-lymphocytes |
| Indomethacin | Rash, urticaria, asthma, granulocytopenia |
| Quinidine | Fever, anaphylaxis, asthma |
| Salicylates | Rash, urticaria |
| | |
| | *Autoimmunity* |
| Amiodarone | Thyroiditis |
| Captopril | Autoimmune hemolytic anemia, pemphigus, granulocytopenia |
| Chlorpromazine | Granulocytopenia |
| Halothane | Autoimmune chronic active hepatitis |
| Hydralizine | Autoimmune hemolytic anemia, drug-induced SLE, myasthenia gravis, pemphigus, glomerulonephritis, Goodpasture's disease |
| Methyldopa | Autoimmune hemolytic anemia, leukopenia, drug-induced SLE, pemphigus |
| Nitrofurantion | Peripheral neuritis |
| D-Penicillamine | Autoimmunity; drug-induced SLE, myasthenia gravis, pemphigus, glomerulonephritis, Goodpasture's disease |
| Propranolol | Autoimmunity |
| Procainamide | Autoimmunity, drug-induced SLE, rash, vasculitis, myalgias |
| Pyrithioxine | Pemphigus |
| | |
| *Antibiotics* | *Hypersensitivity and Autoimmunity* |
| Isoniazid | Rash, dermatitis, vasculitis, arthritis, drug-induced SLE |
| Penicillins | Anaphylaxis, dermatitis; vasculitis, serum sickness, hemolytic anemia |
| Sulfonamides | Dermatitis, photosensitivity; pemphigus, hemolytic anemia, serum sickness, drug-induced SLE |
| | |
| *Others* | |
| Acetazolamide | Rash, fever, autoimmunity |
| Lithium | Dermatitis; autoimmune thyroiditis, vasculitis |
| Thiaazides | Hypersensitivity, photosensitivity; autoimmunity (diabetes) |
| Phenytoin | Rash; drug-induced SLE, hepatitis |

**TABLE 15.10. Types of Hypersensitivity Responses**

| Type and Designation[a] | Agents: Clinical Manifestations | Components | Effects | Mechanism |
|---|---|---|---|---|
| I, Immediate (reaginic) | Food additives (GI allergies; anaphylactic)<br><br>Penicillin: uticaria and dermatitis | Mast cells; IgE | Anaphylaxis, asthma, urticaria, rhinitis, dermatitis | IgE binds to mast cells to stimulate release of humoral factors |
| II, Cytotoxic | Cephalosporine: hemolytic anemia<br><br>Quinidine: thrombocytopenia | IgG, IgM | Hemolytic anemia, Goodpasture's disease | IgG and IgM bind to cells (e.g., RBCs), fix complement (opsinization), then lyse cells |
| III, Immune complex (arthus) | Methicillin: chronic glomeruleno-phritis | Antigen-antibody complexes (Ag-Ab) | SLE, rheumatoid arthritis, glomerular nephritis, serum sickness, vasculitis | Ag-Ab complexes deposit in tissues, and may fix complement |
| IV, Delayed hypersensitivity | Penicillin: contact dermatitis | $T_D$ cells; macrophages | Contact dermatitis, tuberculosis | Sensitized T cells induce a delayed-hypersensitivity response upon challenge |

*Source:* Based on classification system of Gell and Coombs, 1967.

**TABLE 15.11. Proteins and Soluble Mediators Involved in Hypersensitivity**

| Factor | Origin | Characteristics/Functions |
|---|---|---|
| Histamine | Mast cells, basophils | Contraction of smooth muscle; increases vascular permeability |
| Serotonin | Mast cells, basophils | Contraction of smooth muscle; leukotriene |
| SRS-A | Lung tissue | (Slow-reacting substance of anaphylaxis); Contraction of smooth muscle; acidic polypeptide |
| ECF-A | Mast cells | (Eosinophilic chemotactic factor of anaphylaxis); attracts eosinophils; small peptide |
| Prostaglandins | Various tissues | Modifies release of histamine and serotonin from mast cells and basophils |

*Source:* Extracted and modified from Clark, 1983.

Antibiotics containing $\beta$-lactam structures, such as penicillin and cephalosporins, are the most commonly occurring inducers of anaphylactic shock and drug hypersensitivity in general. Other hypersensitivity reactions may include urticarial rash, fever, bronchospasm, serum sickness, and vasculitis with reported incidences of all types varying from 0.7 to 10% (Idsøe et al., 1968) and the incidence of anaphylactoid reactions varying from 0.04 to 0.2%. when the $\beta$-lactam ring is opened during metabolism, the penicilloyl moiety can form covalent conjugates with nucleophilic sites on proteins. The penicilloyl conjugates can then act as haptens to form the determinants for antibody induction. Although most patients that have received penicillin produce antibodies against the metabolite benzylpenicilloyl, only a fraction experience allergic reaction (Garraty and Petz, 1975), which suggests a genetic component to susceptibility.

*Type II Hypersensitivity.* Type II cytolytic reactions are mediated by IgG and IgM antibodies that can fix complement, opsonize particles, or induce antibody-dependent cellular cytolysis reactions. Erythrocytes, lymphocytes, and platelets of the circulatory system are the major target cells that interact with the cytolytic antibodies causing depletion of these cells. Hemolytic anemia (penicillin, methyldopa), leukopenia, thrombocytopenia (quinidine), and/or granulocytopenia (sulfonamide) may result. Type II reactions involving the lungs and kidneys occur through the development of antibodies (autoantibodies) to the basement membranes in the alveoli or glomeruli, respectively. Prolonged damage may result in Goodpasture's disease, an autoimmune disease characterized by pulmonary hemorrhage and glomerulonephritis. Several other autoimmune-type diseases have been associated with extended treatments with D-penicillamine and other pharmaceuticals. Various types of autoimmune responses and examples of drug-induced autoimmunity are discussed in further detail in the next section.

*Type III Hypersensitivity.* Type III reactions (arthus) are characterized as an immediate hypersensitivity reaction initiated by antigen-antibody complexes that form freely in the plasma instead of at the cell surface. Regardless of whether the antigens are self or foreign, complexes mediated by IgG can form and settle into the tissue compartments of the host. These complexes can then fix complement and release C3a and C5a fragments that are chemotactic for phagocytic cells. Polymorphonuclear leukocytes are then attracted to the site, where they phagocytize the complexes and release hydrolytic enzymes into the tissues. Additional damage can be caused by the binding to and activating of platelets and basophils, which, in the end, results in localized necrosis, hemorrhage, and increased permeability of local blood vessels. These reactions commonly target the kidney, resulting in glomerulonephritis through the deposition of the complexes in the glomeruli.

Some antibiotics ($\beta$-lactam) have been reported to produce glomerular nephritis in humans that has been attributed to circulating immune complexes. These complexes have also been observed in preclinical toxicology studies with baboons treated with a $\beta$-lactam antibiotic, prior to the appearance of any biochemical or clinical changes (Descotes and Mazue, 1987). In addition, immunoglobulin complexes have been observed in rats treated with gold and autologus immune complex nephritis has been observed in guinea pigs (Ueda et al., 1980). Similar evidence of immunomediated nephrotoxicity has been reported in rheumatoid arthritis patients administered long-term treatments with gold compounds; proteinuria has been observed in approximately 10% of these patients.

Other target organs such as the skin with lupus, the joints with rheumatoid arthritis, and the lungs with pneumonitis may be affected. The deposition of antigen-antibody complexes through the circulatory system results in a syndrome referred to as serum sickness, which was quite prevalent prior to 1940 (Clark, 1983), when serum therapy for diphtheria was commonly used. Serum sickness occurs when the serum itself becomes antigenic as a side effect from passive immunization with heterologous antiserum produced from various sources of farm animals. The antitoxin for diphtheria was produced in a horse and administered to humans as multiple injections of passive antibody. As a consequence, these people often became sensitized to the horse serum and developed a severe form of arthritis and glomerulonephritis caused by deposition of antigen-antibody complexes. Clinical symptoms of serum sickness present as urticarial skin eruptions, arthralgia or arthritis, lymphadenopathy, and fever. Drugs such as sulfonamides, penicillin, and iodides can induce a similar type of reaction. Although uncommon today, transplant patients receiving immunosuppressive therapy with heterologous antilymphocyte serum or globulins may also exhibit serum sickness.

*Type IV Delayed-type Hypersensitivity (DTH).* Delayed-type hypersensitivity reactions are T-cell mediated with no involvement of antibodies. However, these reactions are controlled through accessory cells, suppressor T cells, and monokine-secreting macrophages, which regulate the proliferation and differentiation of T cells. The most frequent form of DTH manifests itself as contact dermatitis. The drug or metabolite binds to a protein in the skin or the Langerhans cell membrane (class II MHC molecules) where it is recognized as an antigen and triggers cell proliferation. After a sufficient period of time for migration of the antigen and clonal expansion (latency period), a subsequent exposure will elicit a dermatitis reaction. A 24–48 h delay often occurs between the time of exposure and onset of symptoms to allow time for infiltration of lymphocytes to the site of exposure. The T cells (CD4$^+$) that react with the antigen are activated and release lymphokines that are chemotactic for monocytes and macrophages. Although these cells infiltrate to the site via the circulatory vessels, an intact lymphatic drainage system from the site is necessary since the reaction is initiated in drainage lymph nodes proximal to the site (Clark, 1983). The release (degranulation) of enzymes and histamines from the macrophages may then result in tissue damage. Clinical symptoms of local dermal reactions may include a rash (not limited to sites of exposure), itching, and/or burning sensations. Erythema is generally observed in the area around the site, which may become thickened and hard to the touch. In severe cases, necrosis may appear in the center of the site followed by desquamation during the healing process. The immune-enhancing drugs isoprinosine and avridine have been shown to induce a delayed-type hypersensitivity reaction in rats (Exon et al., 1986).

A second form of delayed-type hypersensitivity response is similar to that of contact dermatitis in that macrophages are the primary effector cells responsible for stimulating CD4$^+$ T cells; however, this response is not necessarily localized to the epidermis. A classical example of this type of response is demonstrated by the tuberculin diagnostic tests. To determine if an individual has been exposed to tuberculosis, a small amount of fluid from tubercle bacilli cultures is injected subcutaneously. The development of induration after 48 h at the site of injection is diagnostic of prior exposure.

Shock, similar to that of anaphylaxis, may occur as a third form of a delayed systemic hypersensitivity response. However, unlike anaphylaxis, IgE antibodies are not involved. This type of response may occur 5–8 h after systemic exposure and can result in fatality within 24 h following intravenous or intraperitoneal injection.

A fourth form of delayed hypersensitivity results in the formation of granulomas. If the antigen is allowed to persist unchecked, macrophages and fibroblasts are recruited to the site to proliferate, produce collagen, and effectively "wall off" the antigen. A granuloma requires a minimum of one to two weeks to form.

***Photosensitization.*** Regardless of the route of exposure, some haptens (photoantigens) that are absorbed locally into the skin, or reach the skin through systemic absorption, can be photoactivated by ultraviolet (UV) light between 320–400 nm. Once activated, the hapten can bind to the dermal receptors to initiate sensitization (photoallergy). Subsequent exposures to the hapten in the presence of UF light can result in a hypersensitivity response. Clinical symptoms of photoallergy may occur within minutes (immediate hypersensitivity) of exposure to sunlight, or 24 h or more after exposure (DTH). Symptoms may range from acute urticarial reactions to eczematous or papular lesions. Although both phototoxic and photoallergic reactions require the compound to be exposed to sunlight in order to elicit a response, their mechanisms of action are quite different. Since photosensitization is an immune-mediated condition, repeated exposures with a latency period between the initial exposure and subsequent exposures is required, the response is not dose related (small amounts can produce a response once sensitized), and not all individuals exposed to the compound will necessarily respond (genetic component to susceptibility). Although both conditions can present similar symptoms (erythema), phototoxicity is limited mainly to erythema, whereas photoallergy can result in erythema, edema, and dermatitis as just described.

Several drug classes, including tetracycline, sulfonamide, and quinolone antibiotics, as well as chlorothiazide, chlorpromazine, and amiodarone hydrochloride, have been shown to be photoantigens. Photosensitivity may persist even after withdrawal of the drug, as has been observed with the antiarrhythmic drug amiodarone hydrochloride, since it is lipophilic and can be stored for extended periods in the body fat (Unkovic et al., 1984). In addition, it is quite common for cross-reactions to occur between structurally related drugs of the same class.

***Autoimmunity.*** In autoimmunity, as with hypersensitivity, the immune system is stimulated by specific responses that are pathogenic, and both tend to have a genetic component that predisposes some individuals more than others. However, as is the case with hypersensitivity, the adverse immune response of drug-induced autoimmunity is not restricted to the drug itself, but also involves a response to self-antigens.

Autoimmune responses directed against normal components of the body may consist of antibody-driven humoral responses and/or cell-mediated, delayed-type hypersensitivity responses. T cells can react directly against specific target organs, or B cells can secrete autoantibodies that target "self." Autoimmunity may occur spontaneously as the result of a loss of regulatory controls that initiate or suppress normal immunity, causing the immune system to produce lymphocytes reactive against its own cells and macromolecules such as DNA, RNA, or erythrocytes.

Although autoantibodies are often associated with autoimmune reactions, they are not necessarily indicative of autoimmunity (Russel, 1981). Antinuclear antibodies can occur normally with aging in some healthy women without autoimmune disease, and all individuals have B cells with the potential of reacting with self antigens through Ig receptors (Dighiero et al., 1983). The presence of an antibody titer to a particular immunogen indicates that haptenization of serum albumin has occurred as part of a normal immune response. However, if cells are stimulated to proliferate and secrete autoantibodies directed against a specific cell or cellular component, a pathological response may result. The tissue damage associated with autoimmune disease is usually a consequence of type II or III hypersensitivity reactions that result in the deposition of antibody-antigen complexes.

Several diseases have been associated with the production of autoantibodies against various tissues. For example, an autoimmune form of hemolytic anemia can occur if the antibodies are directed against erythrocytes. Similarly, antibodies that react with acetylcholine receptors may cause myasthenia gravis, those directed against glomerular basement membranes may cause Goodpasture's syndrome, and those that target the liver may cause hepatitis. Other forms of organ-specific autoimmunity include autoimmune thyroiditis (as seen with amiodarone) and juvenile diabetes mellitus, which can result from autoantibodies directed against the tissue-specific antigens thyroglobulin and cytoplasmic components of pancreatic islet cells, respectively. In contrast, systemic autoimmune diseases may occur if the autoantibodies are directed against an antigen that is ubiquitous throughout the body, such as DNA or RNA. For example, systemic lupus erythematosus (SLE) occurs as the result of autoimmunity to nuclear antigens that form immune complexes in the walls of blood vessels and basement membranes of tissues throughout the body.

The etiology of drug-induced autoimmunity is not well established and is confounded by factors such as age, sex, and nutritional state, as well as genetic influences on pharmacological and immune susceptibility. Unlike idiopathic auto-immunity, which is progressive or characterized by an alternating series of relapses and remissions, drug-induced autoimmunity is thought to subside after the drug is discontinued. However, this is not certain since a major determining factor for diagnosis of a drug-related disorder is dependent on the observation of remission upon withdrawal of the drug (Bigazzi, 1988).

One possible mechanism for xenobiotic-induced autoimmunity involves xeno-biotic binding to autologus molecules, which then appear foreign to the immuno-surveillance system. If a self antigen is chemically altered, a specific T helper ($T_h$) cell may see it as foreign and react to the altered antigenic determinant portion, allowing an autoreactive B cell to react to the unaltered hapten. This interaction results in a carrier-hapten bridge between the specific $T_h$ and autoreactive B cell, bringing them together for subsequent production of autoantibodies specific to the self antigen that was chemically altered (Weigle, 1980). Conversely, a xenobiotic may alter B cells directly, including those that are autoreactive. Thus, the altered B cells may react to self antigens independent from $T_h$-cell recognition and in a nontissue-specific manner.

Another possible mechanism is that the xenobiotic may stimulate nonspecific mitogenicity of B cells. This could result in a polyclonal activation of B cells with subsequent production of autoantibodies. Alternatively, the xenobiotic may stimulate mitogenicity of T cells that recognize self, which in turn activate B-cell production of antibodies in response to "self" molecules. There is also evidence to suggest that anti-DNA autoantibodies may originate from somatic mutations in lymphocyte precursors with antibacterial or antiviral specificity. For example, a single amino acid substitution resulting from a mutation in a monoclonal antibody to polyphor-ylcholine was shown to result in a loss of the original specificity and an acquisition of DNA reactivity similar to that observed for anti-DNA antibodies in SLE (Talal, 1987).

The mechanisms of autoimmunity may also entail interaction with MHC structures determined by the HLA alleles. Individuals carrying certain HLA alleles have been shown to be predisposed to certain autoimmune diseases, which may account in part for the genetic variability of autoimmunity. In addition, metabolites of a particular drug may vary between individuals to confound the development of drug-induced autoimmunity. Dendritic cells, such as the Langerhans cells of the skin and B lymphocytes that function to present antigens to $T_h$ cells, express class-II

MHC structures. Although the exact involvement of these MHC structures is unknown, Gleichmann et al. (1989) have theorized that self antigens rendered foreign by drugs such as D-penicillamine may be presented to $T_h$ cells by MHC class-II structures. An alternate hypothesis is that the drug or a metabolite may alter MHC class-II structures on B cells, making them appear foreign to $T_h$ cells.

A number of different drugs have been shown to induce autoimmunity in susceptible individuals. A syndrome similar to that of SLE was described in a patient administered sulfadiazine in 1945 by Hoffman (see Bigazzi, 1988). Sulfonamides were one of the first classes of drugs identified to induce an autoimmune response, while to date, over 40 other drugs have been associated with a similar syndrome.

Autoantibodies to red blood cells and autoimmune hemolytic anemia have been observed in patients treated with numerous drugs, including procainamide, chlorpropaminde, captopril, cefalexin, penicillin, and methyldopa (Logue et al., 1970; Kleinman et al., 1984). Hydralazine- and procainamide-induced autoantibodies may also result in SLE. Approximately 20% of patients administered methyldopa for several weeks for the treatment of essential hypertension developed a dose-related titer and incidence of autoantibodies to erythrocytes, 1% of which presented with hemolytic anemia. Methlydopa does not appear to act as a hapten but appears to act by modifying erythrocyte surface antigens. IgG autoantibodies then develop against the modified erythrocytes.

D-penicillamine is used to treat patients with rheumatoid arthritis, to reduce excess cystine excretion in patients with cystinurias, and as a chelating agent for copper in patients with Wilson's disease. D-penicillamine can cause multiple forms of autoimmunity including SLE, myasthenia gravis, pemphigus, and autoimmune thyroiditis. This drug is thought to act as immunomodulator in patients by initiating or even potentiating anti-DNA antibody synthesis (Mach et al., 1986). The highly reactive thiol group may react with various receptors and biological macromolecules to induce autoantibodies. Long-term (many months) treatment has been shown to induce autoimmunity resulting in myasthenia gravis in 0.5% of patients (Bigazzi, 1988) and SLE in approximately 2% of patients as exhibited by varying degrees of joint pain, synovitis, myalgia, malaise, rash, nephritis, pleurisy, and neurological effects. In patients exhibiting myasthenia gravis, D-penicillamine may act to alter the acetylcholine receptors. Autoantibodies to acetylcholine receptors have been detected in these patients and have been shown to decrease gradually after drug withdrawal concomitant with reversibility of the clinical syndrome. However, myasthenia gravis may persist for long periods of time after D-penicillamine therapy has ceased.

Although rare, cases of renal lupus syndrome and pemphigus blisters have also been reported as a consequence of D-penicillamine-induced immune complexes (Ntoso et al., 1986; Bigazzi, 1988), as well as with other drugs. With renal lupus syndrome, secondary glomerulonephritis may result if granular IgG antibodies are produced and deposited on the basement membranes. In patients with pemphigus blisters, autoantibodies to the intercellular substance of the skin have been recovered from the sera, and dermal biopsies have demonstrated intracellular deposits or immunoglobulin deposits on the basement membranes. Pemphigus has also been observed in patients treated with sulfhydryl compounds such as captopril and pyrithioxine (Bigazzi, 1988).

Some metals that are used therapeutically have also been shown to induce autoimmune responses. Gold salts used to treat arthritis may induce formation of antiglomerular basement membrane antibodies, which may lead to glomerulonephritis similar to that seen in Goodpasture's disease (see "Type II Hypersensitivity" in Section 15.5.2.). Since gold is not observed at the site of the lesions (Druet et al., 1982) it has been hypothesized that the metal elicits an antiself response. Lithium, used to treat manic-depression, is thought to induce autoantibodies against thyroglobulin, which in some patients results in hypothyroidism. In studies with rats, levels of antibodies to thyroglobulin were shown to increase significantly in lithium-treated rats compared to controls immediately after immunization with thyroglobulin; however, rats that were not immunized with thyroglobulin did not produce circulation antithyroglobulin antibodies upon receiving lithium, and there was no effect of lithium on lymphocytic infiltration of the thyroid in either group (Hassman et al., 1985).

Some drugs such as penicillin have been shown to induce autoimmunity as well as anaphylaxis (Gleichman et al., 1989). The carbonyl of the $\beta$-lactam ring of penicillin can form a covalent penicilloyl conjugate with nucleophilic sites on proteins, particularly the amino groups of lysine residues. This conjugate, which acts as the major immunogenic determinant, may become biotransformed to other isomeric forms of clinical relevance (Batchelor et al., 1965).

A genetic predisposition to drug-induced development of SLE has been shown to occur in some individuals treated with the drugs hydralazine, isoniazid, procainamide, and sulphamethazine. A polymorphism, which is known to exist for the genes responsible for expression of hepatic $N$-acetyl transferase enzymes, determines the rate of acetylation of these drugs to regulate the rate of drug inactivation. Individuals that are relatively slow acetylators of these drugs are more likely to develop antinuclear antibodies and are at a higher risk for developing SLE (Perry et al., 1970). Other predisposing factors, such as HLA phenotype (HLA-DR4 and/or C4 allele), may also play a genetic role in determining susceptibility to hydralazine-induced SLE (Spears and Batchelor, 1987).

In addition, silicone-containing medical devices, particularly breast prostheses, have been reported to cause serum-sickness-like reactions, scleroderma-like lesions, and an SLE-like disease termed "human adjuvant disease" (Kumagai et al., 1984; Guillaume et al., 1984). Some patients may also present with granulomas and autoantibodies. Human adjuvant disease is a connective tissue or autoimmune disease similar to that of adjuvant arthritis in rats and rheumatoid arthritis in humans. Autoimmune disease-like symptoms usually develop 2–5 yr after implantation in a small percentage of people that receive implants, which may indicate that there is a genetic predisposition similar to that for SLE. An early hypothesis is that the prosthesis or injected silicone plays an adjuvant role by enhancing the immune response through increased macrophage and T-cell helper function. There is currently controversy as to whether silicone, as a foreign body, induces a nonspecific inflammation reaction, a specific cell-mediated immunological reaction, or no reaction at all. However, there is strong support to indicate that silicone microparticles can act as haptens to produce a delayed hypersensitivity reaction in a genetically susceptible population of people.

## 15.6. EVALUATION OF THE IMMUNE SYSTEM

The FDA guidelines for immunotoxicity testing of food additives start with a Type I battery of tests. Type I tests can be derived from the routine measurements and examinations performed in short-term and subchronic rodent toxicity studies, since they do not require any perturbation of the test animals (immunization or challenge with infectious agents). These measurements include hematology and serum chemistry profiles, routine histopathologic examinations of immune-associated organs and tissues, and organ and body weight measurements including thymus and spleen. If a compound produces any primary indicators of immunotoxicity from these measurements, more definitive immunotoxicity tests, such as those indicated in the preceding paragraph, may be recommended on a case-by-case basis.

The following is a brief explanation of some of the indicators that may be used to trigger additional definitive testing and a description of some of the most commonly used assays to assess humoral, cell-mediated, or nonspecific immune dysfunction, which are common to most immunotoxicology test strategies.

### 15.6.1. Immunopathologic Assessments

Various general toxicological and histopathologic evaluations of the immune system can be made as part of routine preclinical safety testing to obtain a preliminary assessment of potential drug-related effects on the immune system. At necropsy, various immunological organs of the immune system such as thymus, spleen, and lymph nodes are typically observed for gross abnormalities and weighed in order to detect decreased or increased cellularity. Bone marrow and peripheral blood samples are also taken to evaluate abnormal types and/or frequencies of the various cellular components. Table 15.12 summarizes the observations and interpretations.

***Organ and Body Weights.***   Changes in absolute weight, organ-to-body weight ratios, and organ-to-brain weight ratios of tissues such as thymus and spleen are useful general indicators of potential immunotoxicity. However, these measures are nonspecific for immunotoxicity since they may also reflect general toxicity and effects on endocrine function that can indirectly affect the immune system.

***Hematology.***   Hemacytometers or electronic cell counters can be used to assess the numbers of lymphocytes, neutrophils, monocytes, basophils, and eosinophils in the peripheral blood, while changes in relative ratios of the various cell types can be assessed by microscopic differential evaluation. Similar evaluations can be

**TABLE 15.12. Examples of Antemortem and Postmorten Findings That May Include Potential Immunotoxicity if Treatment Related**

| Parameter | Possible Observation (cause) | Possible State of Immune Competence |
|---|---|---|
| | *Antemortem* | |
| Mortality | Increased (infection) | Depressed |
| Body weight | Decreased (infection) | Depressed |
| Clinical signs | Rales, nasal discharge (respiratory infection) | Depressed |
| | Swollen cervical area (sislodacryoadenitis virus) | Depressed |
| Physical examinations | Enlarged tonsils (infection) | Depressed |
| Hematology | Leukopenia/lymphopenia | Depressed |
| | Leukocytosis (infection/cancer) | Enhanced/depressed |
| | Thrombocytopenia | Hypersensitivity |
| | Neutropenia | Hypersensitivity |
| Protein electrophoresis | Hypogammaglobulinemia | Depressed |
| | Hypergammaglobulinemia (ongoing immune response or infection) | Enhanced/activated |
| | *Postmortem* | |
| Organ weights: | | |
| Thymus | Decreased | Depressed |
| Histopathology: | | |
| Adrenal glands | Cortical hypertrophy (stress) | Depressed (secondary) |
| Bone marrow | Hypoplasia | Depressed |
| Kidney | Amyloisosis | Autoimmunity |
| | Glomerulonephritis (immune complex) | |
| Lung | Pneumonitis (infection) | Depressed |
| Lymph node | Atrophy | Depressed |
| Spleen | Hypertrophy/hyperplasia | Enhanced/activated |
| | Depletion of follicles | Depressed B cells |
| | Hypocellularity of periateriolar sheath | Depressed T cells |
| | Active germinal centers | Enhanced/activated |
| Thymus | Atrophy | Depressed |
| Thyroid | Inflammation | Autoimmunity |

performed with bone marrow aspirates, where changes may reflect immunotoxicity to the pluripotent stem cells and newly developing lymphoid precursor cells. Potential hematological indicators of immunotoxicity include altered white blood cell counts or differential ratios, lymphocytosis, lymphopenia, or eosinophilia. Changes in any of these parameters can be followed up with more sophisticated flow cytometric analyses or immunostaining techniques that are useful for phenotyping the various types of lymphocytes (B cell, T cell) and the T-cell subsets (CD4$^+$ and CD8$^+$) on the basis of unique surface markers. Decreases or increases in the percentages of any of the cell populations relative to controls, or in the ratios of B cells/T cells, or CD$^{4+}$/CD8$^+$ cells may be indicators of immunotoxicity.

***Clinical Chemistry.*** Nonspecific clinical chemistry indicators of potential immune dysfunction include changes in serum protein levels in conjunction with changes in the albumin-to-globulin (A/G) ratio. Immunoelectrophoretic analysis of serum proteins can then be performed to quantify the relative percentages of albumin and the $\alpha$-, $\beta$-, and $\gamma$-globulin fractions. To perform these assays, a drop of serum (antigen) is placed into a well cut in a gel, then the gel is subjected to electrophoresis so that each molecule in the serum moves in the electric field according to its charge. This separation is then exposed to specific antiserum, which is placed in a trough cut parallel to the direction in which the components have moved. By passive diffusion, the antibody reaches the electrophoretically separated antigen and reacts to form Ag-Ab complexes. The $\gamma$-globulin fractions can be separated and further quantified for the relative proportions of IgG, IgM, IgA, and IgE using similar techniques.

Serum concentrations of immunoglobulin classes and subclasses can also be measured using various techniques such as radioimmunoassays (RIAs) or enzyme-linked immunosorbent assays (ELISAs). In the ELISA, antigens specific for each class of immunoglobulin can be adsorbed onto the surfaces for microtiter plates. To determine the quantity of each antibody in a test sample, an aliquot of antiserum is allowed to react with the adsorbed antigens. Unreacted molecules are rinsed off and an enzyme-linked anti-Ig is then added to each well. Next, substrate is added and the amount of color that develops is quantified using a spectrophotometric device. The amount of antibody can then be extrapolated from standard curves since the amount of color is proportional to the amount of enzyme-linked antibody that reacts. Variations in levels of a given antibody may indicate the decreased ability of B cells of decreased numbers of B cells producing that antibody. In addition, serum autoantibodies to DNA, mitochondria, and parietal cells, can be used to assess autoimmunity. Serum cytokines (IL-1, IL-2, and $\gamma$-interferon) can also be evaluated using immunochemical assays to evaluate macrophage, lymphocyte, and lymphokine activity; prostaglandin $E_2$ can also be measured to evaluate macrophage function.

CH50 determinations can be used to analyze the total serum complement and are useful for monitoring immune complex diseases (Sullivan, 1989); activation of complement (Table 15.13) in the presence of autoantibodies is indicative of immune complex diseases and autoimmunity. The various components of the complement system (C3, C4) can also be measured to assess the integrity of the system. For instance, low serum concentrations of C3 and C4, with a concomitant decrease in CH50 may indicate activation of complement, while a low C4 alone is a sensitive indicator of reduced activation of the complement system. Since C3 is used as an alternate complement pathway, it usually measures high. Therefore, a low C3 with a normal C4 may indicate an alternate pathway of activation.

**TABLE 15.13. The Complement System**

| Response Factors | Origin | Characteristics/Functions |
| --- | --- | --- |
| Complement fixation | Serum | Critical component of humoral immune response leading to lysis of cell membranes, chemotaxis, and phagocytosis |
| C1 | | Binds with IgG or IgM on membrane of the target cell to initiate activation of complement cascade |
| C4 and C2 | | Activated by C1; act together as a complex to activate C3; exposes a membrane site recognizable to granulocytes and macrophages resulting in opsinization |
| C3 and C5 | Liver, macrophage | C3 binds to C42 complex to form C423; C5 binds to C423 to form C4235; provides sites for C6 and C7 |
| C6 and C7 | | C6 and C7 bind to C5 site to result in C567 |
| C8 | | One molecule of C567 binds with C8 to result in C5678 |
| C9 | | Up to six C9 molecules can bind with C5678 to trigger lysis by disrupting the lipid layer of the cell membrane |

***Histopathology.*** Histopathologic abnormalities can be found in lymphoid tissues during gross and routine microscopic evaluations of the spleen, lymph nodes, thymus, bone marrow, and gut-associated lymphoid tissues such as Peyer's patches and mesenteric lymph nodes. Microscopic evaluations should include descriptive qualitative changes such as types of cells, densities of cell populations, proliferation in known T- and B-cell areas (e.g., germinal centers), relative numbers of follicles and germinal centers (immune activation), and the appearance of atrophy or necrosis. In addition, unusual findings such as granulomas and scattered, focal mononuclear cell infiltrates in nonlymphoid tissues may be observed as indicators of chronic hypersensitivity or autoimmunity. A complete histopathologic evaluation should also include a quantitative assessment of cellularity through direct counts of each cell type in the various lymphoid tissues. In addition, changes in cellularity of the spleen can be more precisely quantitated from routine hematoxylin-eosin (H&E) sections using morphometric analysis of the germinal centers (B cells) and periarteriolar lymphocyte sheath (T cells). Similar morphometric measurements can be made of the relative areas of the cortex and medulla of the thymus. If changes in cellularity are apparent from routinely stained histopathology sections, special immunostaining (immunoperoxidase or immunofluorescence) of B cells in the spleen and lymph nodes using polyclonal antibodies to IgG or immunostaining of the T cells and their subsets in the spleen using mono- or polyclonal antibodies to their specific surface markers, can be used to further characterize changes in cellularity.

Numerous physiological and environmental factors such as age, stress, nutritional deficiency, and infections may affect the immune system (Sullivan, 1989). Thus, adverse findings in animal studies may reflect these indirect immunotoxic effects rather than the direct immunotoxic potential of a chemical or drug. Indirect immunotoxic effects may be assessed through histopathologic evaluations of endocrine organs such as the adrenals and pituitary.

It is also well known that the functional reserves of the immune system can allow biologically significant, immunotoxic insults to occur without the appearance of morphological changes. In addition, there is some built-in redundancy in the system in that several mechanisms may produce the same outcome. For instance, cytotoxic T cells may alone be sufficient to protect the organism against a bacterial infection; however, the body will also produce antibodies for future protection. Thus, if one mechanism is insufficient to fight off infection, the second mechanism can serve as a back-up. Because of this functional reserve, adverse effects may remain subclinical until the organism is subjected to undue stress or subsequent challenge (Bloom et al., 1987). Therefore, routine immunopathologic assessments as part of standard preclinical toxicity tests may not be sufficient to detect all immunotoxins. Although changes detected in routine toxicological and pathological evaluations are non-specific, and of undetermined biological significance to the test animal, they can be invaluable as flags for triggering additional testing.

### 15.6.2. Humoral Immunity

As described previously, the humoral immune response results in the proliferation, activation, and subsequent production of antibodies by B cells following antigenic exposure and stimulation. The functionality and interplay between the three primary types of immune cells (macrophage, B cells, and T cells) required to elicit a humoral response can be assessed through various *in vitro* assays using cells from the peripheral blood or lymphoid tissues.

***Antibody Plaque-Forming Cell (PFC) Assay.*** The number of B cells producing antibody (PFC) to a T-dependent antigen such as sheep red blood cells (SRBCs) can be assessed *in vitro* following *in vivo* exposure to the test article and antigen (*ex vivo* tests). The PFC response to a T-dependent antigen is included as a Tier I test by the NTP since it appears to be the most commonly affected functional parameter of exposure to immunosuppressants. However, this test is designated as a Type 2 test in the FDA *Redbook* since it requires an *in vivo* immunization of the animals with antigen, and thus cannot be evaluated as part of an initial toxicity screen.

Although this assay requires that B cells be fully competent in secreting antibodies, T cells and macrophage cells are also essential for the proper functioning of humoral immunity. However, this assay is nonspecific in that it cannot determine which cell type(s) is responsible for dysfunction. Macrophage cells are needed to process antigen and produce IL-1. T cells are needed for several functions including antigen recognition of surface membrane proteins and B-cell maturation through the production of various lymphokines that stimulate growth and differentiation. SRBCs are most commonly used as the T-dependent antigen, although T-cell independent antigens may also be useful to rule out T helper dysfunction as a cause of immunodysfunction.

The PFC assay has evolved from methodology originally developed as a hemolytic plaque assay (or Jerne plaque assay) by Nils Jerne to quantitate the number of antibody-forming cells in a cell suspension plated with RBCs onto agar plates (Jerne and Nordin, 1963). In its present form, animals are treated *in vivo* with the test compound, immunized with approximately $5 \times 10^8$ SRBCs administered intravenously within two to three days posttreatment, and then sacrificed four days (IgM) or six days (IgG) later. Antibody-producing spleen cell suspensions are then mixed *in vitro* with SRBCs, placed onto covered slides, and incubated for a few hours in the presence of complement. During incubation, antibody diffuses from the anti-SRBC-producing cells and forms Ag-Ab complexes on the surfaces of nearby SRBCs. In the presence of complement, the Ag-Ab complexes cause lysis of the SRBCs, resulting in the formation of small, clear plaques on the slide. Plaques are then counted and expressed as PFCs/$10^6$ spleen cells. A dose-related reduction in PFCs is indicative of immunosuppression.

***B-cell Lymphoproliferation Response.*** The NTP has classified this assay as a Tier I test since mitogenesis can be performed easily in tandem with other tests to provide an assessment of the proliferative capacity of the cells (Luster et al., 1988). Since this assay is performed *ex vivo* with peripheral blood (or spleen) and is well characterized for use in various animal species, it has also been included as an Expanded Type I test in the revised *Redbook*.

The proliferation of peripheral blood or splenic B cells following stimulation with lipopolysaccharide (LPS) or other mitogens (pokeweed mitogen extract) is another measurement of humoral immunity. LPS (a bacterial lipopolysaccharide) is a B-cell-specific mitogen that stimulates polyclonal proliferation (mitosis) as part of the natural sequence of antigen recognition, activation, and clonal expansion. The mitogen does not interact with just one particular antigen-specific clone, but with all cells bearing the carbohydrate surface marker for which it is specific. Since mitogens are both polyclonal and polyfunctional, they can stimulate a wider spectrum of antigenic determinants than antigens, which can only stimulate a low number ($10^{-6}$) of specific cells.

In this assay, lymphocytes from animals are treated *in vivo* and cultured *in vitro* in microtiter plates in the presence of tritiated [$^3$H]thymidine (or uridine) using a range of at least three concentrations of mitogen to optimize the response. Lymphocytes can be obtained aseptically from peripheral blood or from single cell suspensions of spleen cells that are prepared by pushing the tissue through sterile gauze or 60-mesh wire screens. A decrease in DNA synthesis (incorporation of $^3$H) as compared to the unexposed cells of control animals may indicate that the B cells were unable to respond to antigenic stimulation. Alternative methodology employs a 18–20 h incubation with $^{125}$I-labeled iododeoxyuridine ([$^{125}$I]IudR) and fluorodeoxyuridine (FudR) (White et al., 1985). After incubation, the cells are collected onto filter disks and then counted with a gamma counter.

Assays such as this that use polyclonal mitogens for activation may not be as sensitive as specific antigen-driven systems (Luster et al., 1988). In addition, suppression of the mitogen response does not always correlate with the PFC response. Since mitogenesis represents only a small aspect of B-cell function and maturation, this endpoint is not sensitive to early events that may affect activation, or later events that may affect differentiation of B cells into antibody-secreting cells (Klaus and Hawrylowicz, 1984).

### 15.6.3. Cell-Mediated Immunity

***T-cell Lymphoproliferation Response.*** This assay is analogous to the B-cell lymphoproliferative response assay described in the preceding paragraph. Thus, this assay is also classified as a Tier I test by the NTP and as an Expanded Type I test in the revised draft of the *Redbook*.

T cells from the peripheral blood or spleen undergo blastogenesis and proliferation in response to specific antigens that evoke a cell-mediated immune response. T-cell proliferation is assessed using T-cell-specific mitogens such as the plant lectins, concanavalin A (Con A), and phytohemagglutinin (PHA) or T-cell-specific antigens (i.e., tuberin, *Listeria*). Uptake of $^3$H as an indicator of DNA synthesis is used as described in 13.6.2 for evaluating B-cell proliferation. T-cell mitogens do not just stimulate synthesis of DNA but, in fact, they also stimulate the expression of cell-specific functions. For instance, Con A can trigger the expression of T helper, suppressor, and cytotoxic effector cells, and either mitogen may induce the expression (or re-expression of memory cells) of differentiated function (Clark et al, 1983). Since cell populations responsive to Con A are thought to be relatively immature compared to those that are stimulated with PHA, the parallel usage of both mitogens may be useful for distinguishing the affected subset (Tabo and Paul, 1973). A secondary response to T-cell antigens such as purified protein derivative of tuberculin (PPD) or tetanus toxoid can also be assessed.

***Mixed Lymphocyte Response (MLR) Assay.*** This assay has been shown to be sensitive for the detection of chemical-induced immunosuppression and is a recommended Tier I assay by the NTP (Luster et al., 1988). In addition, it has been shown to be predictive of host response to transplantation and of general immunocompetence (Harmon et al., 1982).

The mixcd lymphocyte response assay assesses the ability of T cells to recognize foreign antigens on allogenic lymphocytes and, thus, is an indirect measure of the cell-mediated ability to recognize graft or tumor cells as foreign. Responder lymphocytes from animals treated *in vivo* with the test compound are mixed with allogenic stimulator lymphocytes that have been treated *in vitro* with mitomycin C or irradiated to render them unable to respond (Bach and Voynow, 1966). Both cell types are cultured *in vitro* for three to five days, then incubated with $^3$H for an additional 6 h. Once the radiolabel is incorporated into the DNA of the responding cells, the DNA is extracted and the amount of radioactive label is measured to quantitate proliferation of the responder cells of drug-treated animals compared to those of the controls.

***Cytotoxic T lymphocyte (CTL) Mediated Assay.*** This assay is similar to the MLR assay and can be performed in parallel or as a Tier II follow-up to the MLR assay.

The CTL assay ascertains the ability of cytotoxic T cells to lyse an allogenic target cell or the specific target cell type with which they were immunized. In general, the cytolytic response of activated effector cells is assessed by measuring the amount of radioactivity ($^{51}$Cr) that is released from the target cell. When performed in conjunction with the MLR assay, lymphoid cells of the two strains are cultured together *in vitro* as described; however, $^{51}$Cr is added to the culture after four to five days (instead of $^{3}$H). Both responder and target cells are labeled with the $^{51}$Cr, which is taken up rapidly by the cells through passive diffusion but is released slowly as long as the cell membrane is intact. Furthermore, since chromium is reduced from $Cr^{6+}$ to $Cr^{3+}$, and since $Cr^{3+}$ enters the cells at a much slower rate than $Cr^{6+}$, the $^{51}$Cr released from the damaged target cells is not significantly reincorporated into undamaged cells (Clark, 1983), which would reduce the sensitivity of the assay. Thus, the amount of chromium released into the medium and recovered in the supernatant of the mixture of the cells is directly proportionate to the extent of lysis of the target cells by the sensitized responder cells.

In a capillary tube assay developed in 1962 by George and Vaughan, the inhibition of migration of macrophage cells can be used to access normal T-cell function (see Clark, 1983). T cells are obtained from the peripheral blood of animals treated *in vivo* with a test article and injected with antigen (e.g., tuberculin). If these T cells are functioning normally, they should release migration inhibition factor (MIF). As a consequence, the macrophages, which generally show a propensity for migration upon stimulation with the antigen, should show a MIF-induced reduction in migratory behavior.

***Delayed-type Hypersensitivity (DTH) Response.*** The DTH response assay is considered by the NTP to be a comprehensive Tier II assay for cell-mediated immunity.

To express a DTH inflammatory response, the immune system must be capable of recognizing and processing antigen, blastogenesis and proliferation of T cells, migration of memory T cells to the challenge site of exposure to antigen, and subsequent production of inflammatory mediators and lymphokines that elicit the inflammatory response. Thus, by measuring a DTH response to an antigen, these assays assess the functional status of both the afferent (antigen recognition and processing) and efferent (lymphokine production) arms of cellular immunity. Various antigens have been used for assessing DTH, including keyhole limpet hemocyanin (KLH), oxazolone, dinitrochlorbenzene, and sheep red blood cells (SRBCs) (Vos, 1977; Godfrey and Gell, 1978; Luster et al., 1988).

In one such assay described by White et al. (1985), mice previously treated with the test article are sensitized to SRBCs by inoculation of SRBCs into the hind footpad and four days later challenged in the same footpad. Seventeen hours following challenge, they are injected intravenously with [125]I-labeled human serum albumin (HSA), then sacrificed 2 h later. Both hind feet are then radioassayed in a gamma counter (the second foot serves as a control for background infiltration of the label). With a normal functioning cell-mediated response, [125]I-labeled HSA will extravasate into the edematous area produced by the DTH response (Paranjpe and Boone, 1972). In general, a decrease in the extravasation of [125]I-labeled HSA is indicative of immunosuppression of the efferent arm of the cell-mediated immune system.

To assay specifically the afferent arm of the DTH response, the proliferation of the popliteal lymph node cells to SRBCs can also be measured (White et al., 1985). As described, mice treated with the test article are sensitized to SRBCs by inoculation of SRBCs into the hind footpad. However, 1.5 h later they are challenged intraperitoneally with FUdR and 2 h later they are administered [[125]I]IUdR intravenously (instead of [125]I-labeled HSA). Mice are sacrificed 24 h after challenge and both popliteal lymph nodes are removed and counted in a gamma counter.

Similar assays for DTH have been traditionally performed with the antigen *Mycobacterium tuberculosis*, which preferentially elicits a cell-mediated response. In this assay a small amount of antigen contained in the supernatant fluid from the medium in which the pathogen was grown is injected into the footpad. Upon challenge, a visible and palpable lump should appear by 48 h. The amount of swelling is then measured and compared with the footpad that did not receive the challenge. Alternatively, methods used by the NTP employ a modified [125]I-labeled uridine (UdR) technique to measure the monocyte influx at the challenge site (ear) injected with keyhole limpet hemocyanin antigen. This assay has been shown to correlate well with decreased resistance to infectious disease (Luster et al., 1988). However, one should note that regardless of which technique is used, anti-inflammatory drugs may produce false-positive results in this type of assay.

### 15.6.4. Nonspecific Immunity

***Natural Killer Cell Assays.*** This assay is a Tier I test for nonspecific immunity in the NTP testing scheme (Luster et al., 1988) and is proposed as an additional Type I test in the draft *Redbook*.

Natural killer (NK) cells, like cytotoxic T cells, have the ability to attack and destroy tumor cells or virus-infected cells. However, unlike T cells, they are not antigen specific, do not have unique, clonally distributed receptors, and do not undergo clonal selection. In *in vitro* or *ex vivo* tests, target cells (e.g., YAC-1 tumor cells) are radiolabeled *in vitro* or *in vivo* with [51]Cr and incubated *in vitro* with effector NK cells from the spleens of animals that had been treated with a xenobiotic. This assay can be run in microtiter plates over a range of various ratios of effector/target cells. Cytotoxic activity is then measured by the amount of radioactivity released from the damaged tumor cells as was previously described for cytotoxic T cells. This assay can also be performed *in vivo*, where YAC-1 cells labeled with [[125]I]IUdR are injected directly into mice and NK cell activity is correlated with its level of radioactivity (Riccardi et al., 1979). Immunotoxicity observed as reduced NK cell activity is correlated with increased tumorigenesis and infectivity.

***Macrophage Function.*** Several assays are available to measure various aspects of macrophage function, including quantitation of resident peritoneal cells, antigen presentation, cytokine production, phagocytosis, intracellular production of oxygen free radicals (used to kill foreign bodies) and direct tumor-killing potential. Techniques for quantitation of peritoneal cells and functional assays for phagocytic ability are classified as comprehensive Tier II tests by the NTP and as additional Type 1 tests in the draft *Redbook*.

Macrophage cells and other polymorphonuclear cells (PMNs) contribute to the first-line defense of nonspecific immunity through their ability to phagocytize foreign materials, including pathogens, tumor cells, and fibers (e.g., silica, asbestos). Xenobiotics can affect macrophage function by direct toxicity to macrophages or by modulating their ability to become activated. Differential counts of resident peritoneal cells can be made as a rapid, preliminary assessment of macrophage function for xenobiotics that are not administered parenterally.

Numerous *in vitro* assays can be employed to assess common functions of macrophages and PMNs including adherence to glass, migration inhibition, phagocytosis, respiratory activity (chemiluminescent assays or nitroblue tetrazolim), and target cell killing. In one such assay, the chemotactic response to soluble attractants is evaluated using a Boyden chamber with two compartments that are separated by a filter. Macrophage cells or PMNs from treated animals are placed in one side and a chemotactic agent in the other. Chemotaxis is then quantified by counting the number of cells that pass through the filter. In another assay, the ability of the macrophages to phagocytize foreign materials can be evaluated by adding fluorescent latex beads to cultures containing macrophage cells, then determining the proportion of cells that have phagocytized the beads using a fluorescent microscope or by flow cytometry (Duke et al., 1985). Similar functions can be evaluated by incubating the cells with known amounts of bacteria. The cells are then removed by filtration or centrifugation, the remaining fluid is plated onto bacterial nutrient agar, and, after a few days of incubation, the bacterial colonies are counted. Furthermore, the efficiency of the cells to kill the bacteria once phagocytized can be assayed by lysing the cells and plating the lysate onto bacterial agar.

Various *in vivo* assessments of macrophage function have also been used. For example, peritoneal exudate cell (PEC) recruitment can be assessed using eliciting agents such as *Corynebacterium parvum*, MVE-2, or thioglycolate (Dean et al., 1984). In one such assay (White et al., 1985), mice are injected intraperitoneally with thioglycolate, sacrificed five days later, and the peritoneal cavity is flushed with culture medium. The cell suspension is then counted, the cell concentration is adjusted to a known density ($2 \times 10^5$ ml$^{-1}$), and the cells are cultured for 1 h in 24-well culture dishes. Adherent cells are then washed with medium and aliquots of $^{51}$Cr-labeled SRBCs that were opsonized with mouse IgG are added to each well and incubated for various times. This same system can be used to assess adherence and chemotaxis of the PECs (Laskin et al., 1981). Phagocytosis can also be evaluated *in vivo* by measuring the clearance of injected particles from the circulation and the accumulation of the particles in lymphatic tissues such as the spleen.

***Mast Cell/Basophil Function.*** The function of mast cells and basophils to degranulate can be evaluated using a passive cutaneous anaphylaxis test (Cromwell et al., 1986). Serum containing specific anaphylactic (IgE) antibodies from donor animals previously exposed to a known antigen is first administered by intradermal (or subcutaneous) injection into unexposed host animals. After a sufficient latency period to allow binding of the donor IgE to the host tissue mast cells, the animals are administered a second intravenous injection of the antigen. The anaphylactic antibodies present in the serum will stimulate normally functioning mast cells to degranulate (release histamines) and produce a marked inflammatory response. Using similar *in vitro* assays with mast cells and basophils, the quantities of histamines that are released from the cells can be measured directly in the culture medium.

### 15.6.5. Host-Resistance Assays

Host-resistance assays can be used to assess the overall immunocompetence of the humoral or cell-mediated immune systems of the test animal (host) to fend off infection with pathogenic microbes, or to resist tumorigenesis and metastasis. These assays are performed entirely *in vivo* and are dependent on all of the various components of the immune system to be functioning properly. Thus, these assays may be considered to be more biologically relevant than *in vitro* tests that only assess the function of cells from one source and of one type. Since these assays require that the animal be inoculated with a pathogen or exogenous tumor cell, they cannot be performed as part of a general preclinical toxicity assessment, and are thus classified as Type 2 tests in the revised *Redbook*. These assays are also included as Tier II tests by the NTP.

Several host-resistance assays have been developed using various infectious agents, including bacteria (*Listeria monocytogenes*, *Streptococcus*, and *Escherichia coli*), viruses (influenza, cytomegalovirus, and herpes), yeast (*Candida albicans*), and parasites (*Trichinella spiralis* and *Plasmodium berghei*). These assays have been described in the NTP guidelines (Luster et al., 1988). In general, animals previously treated with a xenobiotic are injected with the pathogen at a target dose that is estimated to kill 10 to 30% of control animals ($LD^{10-30}$). After a period of time, the animals receive a challenge dose at a much higher concentration ($LD^{60-80}$) and by a different route to determine if animals are resistant to reinfection. Although these assays are similar in their mechanisms of resistance to different pathogens, they have been shown to differ with regard to varying degrees of susceptibility by the same drug (Morahan et al., 1979). Thus, for screening purposes, it is recommended that at least two tests be used (Descotes and Mazue, 1987). Although these tests are relatively easy to perform, those involving the use of pathogens require special handling, containment, and decontamination procedures to prevent infection to humans and throughout the animal colony.

Similar host-resistance assays are used to evaluate the immunosurveillance of spontaneous tumors, which is assessed as the capacity of the organism to reject grafted syngeneic tumors. Various animal-bearing tumor models (Pasten et al., 1986) and host-resistance models have been used to assess immunotoxicity. Several of the host-resistance assays utilize cultured tumor cell lines such as PYB6 sarcoma and B16F10 melanoma cells that are used with C57/BL/6 mice, or the MADB106 lung tumor cell lines that are used with Fischer 344 rats. For example, the PYB6 sarcoma model uses death as an endpoint. In this assay, syngeneic mice are injected with the PYB6 sarcoma cells and death due to tumor is recorded daily. In another routinely used assay, animals that have been treated with a xenobiotic are injected with either B16F10 melanoma cells or Lewis lung carcinoma cells, then approximately 20 days later they are sacrificed and pulmonary tumors are measured and counted.

### 15.6.6. Hypersensitivity

***Type I Hypersensitivity.*** Although there are acceptable systems for evaluating Type I (immediate) reactions following systemic exposure, there are no reliable animal models for predicting Type I reactions following dermal applications or oral administrations of drug. Repeated exposure of a xenobiotic is required to produce a Type I response. A drug in the form of a hapten must covalently bind to macromolecules (proteins, nucleic acids) before it can initiate a primary antibody response. Once sensitized, even the smallest exposure to the xenobiotic can elicit a rapid, intensive IgE antibody-mediated inflammatory response. With the exception of antivirals and chemotherapeutic drugs, most drugs should not be reactive with biological nucleophiles since these drugs are usually screened out as mutagens or carcinogens in preclinical safety studies. However, Type I hypersensitivity is a particular problem with biotechnology products themselves (e.g., insulin, growth hormones, interleukins), trace impurities from the producing organisms (e.g., *E coli* proteins, mycelium), or the vehicles used to form emulsions (Matori et al., 1985).

The production of neutralizing antibodies to recombinant DNA protein products or their contaminants may be assayed using ELISAs or RIAs. A suitable animal model used to evaluate the potential for a Type I response to protein hydrolysates is detailed in the U.S. Pharmacopoeia. This test is very sensitive for testing proteins administered by the parenteral route, but is of little value for low molecular weight drugs and those that are administered orally (Descotes and Mazue, 1987). Active systemic anaphylaxis can be assessed in guinea pigs following systemic exposure to the test compound. For dermal exposures, however, rabbits or guinea pigs must be exposed to the test article by intradermal injections and then evaluated for their ability to mount a systemic anaphylactic response. The passive cutaneous anaphylaxis test (as described above for mast cells) can also be used to assess a potential anaphylactic response to a test compound. The serum containing potential anaphylactic (IgE) antibodies from donor animals previously exposed to the test compound is first administered by intradermal (or subcutaneous) injection into unexposed host animals. After a latency period, the animals are administered an intravenous injection of the test compound together with a dye. If anaphylactic antibodies are present in the serum, the subsequent exposure to the test compound will cause a release of vasoactive amines (degranulation of mast cells), ultimately resulting in the migration of the dye to the sites of the intradermal serum injections.

***Types II and III Hypersensitivity.*** No simple animal models are currently available to assess Type II (antibody-mediated cytotoxicity) hypersensitivity reactions. IgE antibodies and immune complexes in the sera of exposed animals can be assayed using ELISA or RIA techniques that require the use of specific antibodies to the drug.

Type III (immune complex related disease) reactions have been demonstrated by the presence of proteinuria and immune complex deposits in the kidneys of the Brown-Norway, Lewis, and PVG/C rat strains. However, susceptibility to the deposition and the subsequent lesions (glomerularnephritis) are often variable and dependent on the strain (Bigazzi, 1985). For example, despite the appearance of clinical signs and proteinuria, after two-months administration of mercuric chloride, detectable levels of circulating antinuclear autoantibodies can no longer be observed in the Brown-Norway strain (Bellon et al., 1982). By contrast, in PVG/C rats administered mercuric chloride, immune complex deposition and antinuclear auto-antibodies are present for longer periods of time; however, proteinurea is not observed (Weeping et al., 1978).

***Type IV Hypersensitivity.*** There are several well-established preclinical models for assessing Type IV (delayed-type) hypersensitivity reactions following dermal exposure, but not for predicting this response after systemic exposure.

Type IV hypersensitivity responses are elicited by T lymphocytes and are controlled by accessory cells and suppressor T cells. Macrophages are also involved in that they secrete several monokines, which results in proliferation and differentiation of T cells. Thus, there are numerous points along this intricate pathway in which drugs may modulate the final response. To achieve a Type IV response, an initial high-dose exposure or repeated lower-dose exposures are applied to the skin; the antigen is carried from the skin by Langerhans cells and presented to cells in the thymus to initiate T-cell proliferation and sensitization. Once sensitized, a second "challenge" dose will elicit an inflammatory response. Thus, before sensitivity can be assessed, each of the models used to evaluate dermal hypersensitivity requires as a minimum:

- an initial induction exposure;
- a latency period for expression;
- a challenge exposure.

A preliminary test for acute irritancy is also required to ensure that the initial dose is sufficient to stimulate sensitization, and that the challenge dose is sufficient to ensure expression of the response without producing irritation, which would confound the response. To confirm suspected sensitization or determine a threshold dose, each assay may also include a second challenge dose one to two weeks after the first challenge, at the same or lower concentrations. To increase penetration of the test article, various methods of abrasion (e.g., tape stripping) and occlusive coverings may also be used.

Several systems are used routinely to test compounds for dermal hypersensitivity. The two most commonly used, the modified Buehler test and the guinea pig maximization test (GPMT), are briefly reviewed. More detailed methodology and a description of alternative test systems can be found in Gad and Chengelis (1988). Although either rabbits or guinea pigs are sensitive test species, guinea pigs have traditionally been the animal of choice. Guinea pig models of skin sensitization are widely used and have been valuable in assessing human risk (Andersen and Maibach, 1985).

***Modified Buehler.*** Buehler (1964) developed the first test system to use an occlusive patch to maximize dermal exposure and to increase the test sensitivity (Buehler, 1964). Although, this assay is still insensitive for some xenobiotics that may not sufficiently traverse the epidermis, it is particularly useful for compounds that are either highly irritating by intradermal injection or cannot be dissolved or suspended in a form that is conducive to injection. Other advantages are that the test produces few false positives, rarely overpredicts the potency of sensitizers, and is less likely to produce limiting system toxicity or ulceration at the induction sites. Figure 15.4 shows the test design in its current (OECD) form.

During the induction phase, the test compound is applied to a cotton patch (1 × 1 in. or placed in a Hilltop-style occlusive chamber. The patch is then placed onto a shaven area of epidermis on the left flank of a guinea pig and secured firmly in place for 24 h, after which time the patch is removed and the area is observed and scored for irritation (i.e., edema, erythema). A fresh patch is then reapplied for 6 h every other day during the induction period for a total of ten treatments, while the scoring of the application site is continued at 24 and 48 h from the start of each treatment. Two weeks after the last induction exposure, the animals receive a challenge exposure for 24 h in the form of a patch applied to a shaven area of epidermis on the other flank (opposite the one used for induction). The challenge dose should be the highest concentration that does not produce dermal irritation after a single, 24-h exposure. The challenge site is observed for evidence of inflammation 24, 48, and 72 h after the patch is removed. Both the intensity and duration of a response to the test article compared to that of the vehicle are used to determine the potential and severity of sensitization.

***Guinea pig Maximization Test.*** This assay, as developed by Magnusson and Kligman (1969), differs from the Buehler test in that the compound is administered by intradermal injection during the first stage of induction and coadministered with an adjuvant (Freund's complete adjuvant) during the induction phase to further stimulate the immune system. This test system is more sensitive (fewer false negatives) than the Buehler test; however, it may overpredict the potency for many sensitizers. Figures 15.5 and 15.6 illustrate the study design.

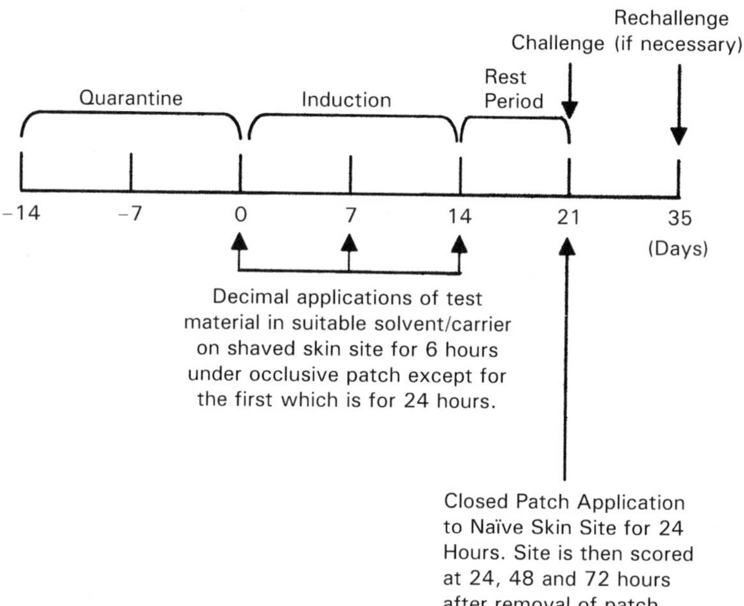



**FIGURE 15.4.** Line chart for modified Buehler test for delayed contact dermal sensitization in the guinea pig.

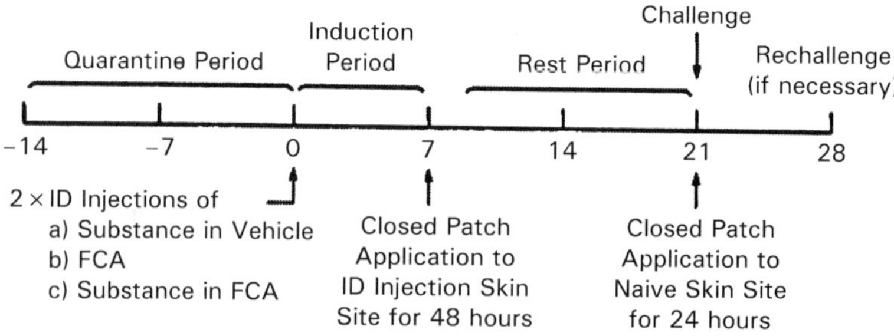



**FIGURE 15.5.** Line chart for guinea pig maximization test for dermal sensitization.

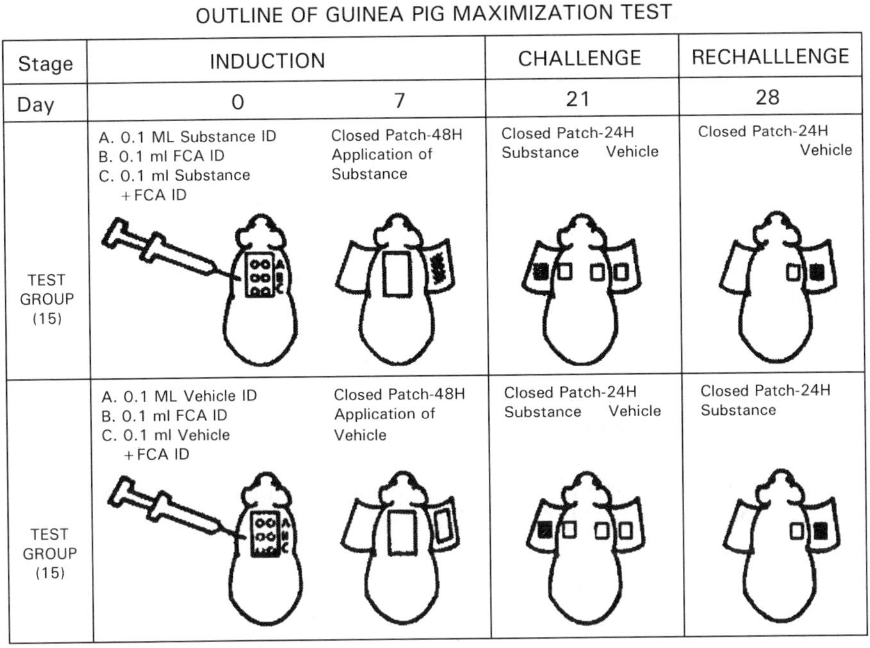

**OUTLINE OF GUINEA PIG MAXIMIZATION TEST**



**FIGURE 15.6.** Illustrative figures for injection and patching of animals in GPMT.

Prior to induction, a $4\times6$-cm area of fur is clipped from the shoulder region of each guinea pig. On Day 0, three pairs of intradermal injections are made along opposite sides of the dorsal midline of the animal. The first pair (closest to the head) are administered as test substance in vehicle, the second pair are administered proximal to the first pair and consists only of Freund's complete adjuvant (FCA), and the third pair (spaced most posteriorly) are administered as the test substance in FCA. Seven days later (Day 7), a mild to moderately irritating dose of the test article is spread onto a $1\times2$-in. filter paper patch, secured, and occluded for 48 h on the epidermal site that received the initial injections. On Day 21, an area of fur on each flank is shaved and a $1\times1$-in. patch containing a nonirritating concentration of the test article is applied to one flank and a patch containing vehicle alone is applied to the other flank. The patches are secured and occluded for 24 h, and the challenge sites are scored for inflammation 24 and 48 h after removal of the patches. The incidence of animals that respond as well as the intensity and duration of a response to the test article are used to determine the potential and severity of sensitization.

### 15.6.7. Local Lymph Node Assay (LLNA)

This method has developed out of the work of Ian Kimber and associates (Kimber et al., 1986, 1994; Kimber and Weisenberger, 1989; Basketter and Scholes, 1991). It has the advantage over the other methods discussed in this chapter in that it provides an objective and quantifiable endpoint. The method is based on the fact that dermal sensitization requires the elicitation of an immune response. This immune response requires proliferation of a lymphocyte subpopulation. The local lymph node assay (LLNA) relies on the detection of increased DNA synthesis via tritiated thymidine incorporation. Sensitization is measured as a function of lymph node cell proliferative responses induced in a draining lymph node following repeated topical exposure of the test animal to the test article. Unlike the other tests discussed in this chapter, this assay looks only at induction because there is no challenge phase.

The typical test (illustrated in Figure 15.7) is performed using mice, normally female CBA mice 6–10 weeks of age. Female BALB/c and ICR mice have also been used. After animal receipt, they are typically acclimated to standard laboratory husbandry conditions for 7–10 days. The usual protocol will consist of at least two groups (vehicle control and test article treated) of five mice each. They are treated on the dorsal surface of both ears with 25 µl (on each ear) of test article solution for three consecutive days. Twenty-four to forty-eight hours after the last test article exposure, the animals are given a bolus (0.25 ml) dose of [$^3$H]thymidine (20 µCi with a specific activity of 5.0–7.0 Ci/mmol) in phosphate buffered saline via a tail vein. Five hours after the injection, the animals are euthanized by $CO_2$ asphyxiation and the auricular lymph nodes removed.

After removal, the lymph nodes can either be pooled by group or processed individually. Single cell suspensions are prepared by gentle mechanical disaggregation through a nylon (100 $\mu_m$) mesh. Cells are washed twice by centrifugation in an excess of PBS. After the final supernatant wash is removed, the cells are precipitated with cold 5% trichloroacetic acid (TCA) and kept at 4°C for 12–18 hours. The precipitate is then pelleted by centrifugation and resuspended in 1 ml 5% TCA, and the amount of radioactivity is determined by liquid scintillation counting, using established techniques for tritium.

The data are reduced to the stimulation index (SI):

$$SI = \frac{H \text{ (dpm) treated group}}{H \text{ (dpm) control group}}$$

An SI of 3 or greater is considered a positive response; that is, the data support the hypothesis that the test material is a sensistizer.

The test article concentration is normally the highest nonirritating concentration. Several concentrations could be tested at the same time should one wish to establish a dose-response curve for induction. The test is easiest to perform if the vehicle is a standard nonirritating organic, such as acetone, ethanol, or dimethylformamide, or a solvent-olive oil blend. Until a laboratory develops its own historical control base, it is also preferable to include a positive control group. Either 0.25% dinitricholorobenzene or 0.05% oxazalone are recommended for positive controls. If the vehicle for the positive control is different than the vehicle for the test material, then two vehicle control groups may be necessary.

This method has been extensively validated in two international laboratory exercises (Basketter et al., 1991; Loveless et al., 1996). In the earlier work (Basketter

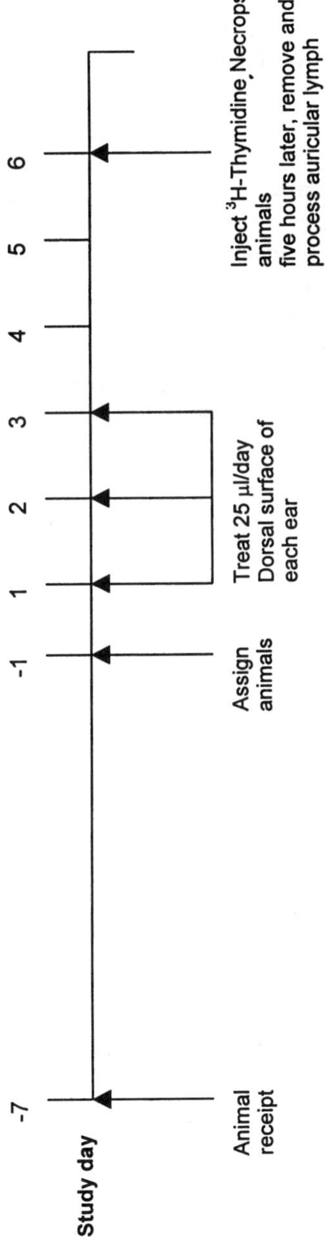


FIGURE 15.7. The mouse local lymph node assay.

et al., 1991), there was good correlation between the results obtained with guinea pig tests and those obtained with the LLNA. In the recent report, for example, five laboratories correctly identified dinitrochlorobenzene and oxazalone as sensitizers and the fact that *p*-aminobenzoic acid was not (Loveless et al., 1996). Arts and colleagues (1996) demonstrated that rats could be used as well as mice. Interestingly, they validated their assay (for both rats and mice) using BrDU uptake and immunohistochemical staining (rather than [3H] thymidine) to quantitated lymph node cell proliferation.

This method is relatively quick and inexpensive because it uses relatively few mice (which are much less expensive than guinea pigs) and takes considerably less time than traditional guinea pig assays. It has an advantage over other methods in that it does not depend on a somewhat subjective scoring system and produces an objective and quantifiable endpoint. It does require a radiochemistry laboratory. Unless one already has an appropriately equipped laboratory used for other purposes (most likely metabolism studies), setting one up for the sole purpose of running the LLNA does not make economic sense. The standard version of the test has been adopted by OECD and ICVAM (see Figure 15.8), but also has been shown to have a modest false positive rate (misidentifying strong irritants as sensitizers).

### 15.6.8. Photosensitization

Some compounds can act as photoantigens that require exposure to ultraviolet (UV) light to become photoactive haptens. The physiochemical characteristics of compounds can sometimes reveal them as potentially photoactive, particularly if they are photo-unstable to light in the UV range. There are several *in vivo* tests that are used for determining photosensitization. The two assays described here are similar to those previously described for DTH with the primary exception that the dermal test sites are exposed to a light source during the induction and challenge phases. Like the DTH assays, these assays may also include a second challenge dose, or the use of various methods of abrasion and occlusion to increase dermal penetration of the test article. The methods outlined in the following sections are more thoroughly described in Gad and Chengelis (1988).

***Harber and Shalita Method.*** This method (Harber and Shalita, 1975) is similar to the Buehler test in that the compound is applied topically to guinea pigs without the use of adjuvants; however, the test site is not occluded during exposure. During the induction phase, the compound is applied on alternate days during a 12-day period for a total of six applications. Thirty minutes after each application, the test sites are exposed to a sunlamp for 30 min and then to a black light for 30 min. The challenge dose is applied 21 days after the last induction exposure. Thirty minutes after application, the challenge site is shielded with a 3-mm thick piece of glass, while the site is exposed to the black light for an additional 30 min. The glass filters out erythrogenic (causing redness) radiation of less than 320 nm that may confound scoring the reaction. The challenge sites are observed and scored for inflammatory reactions 24 h later.

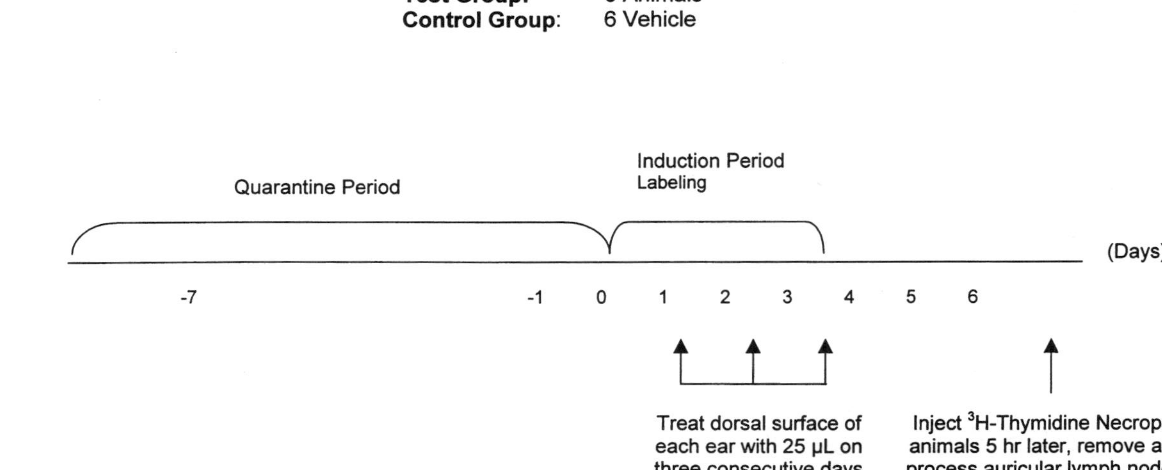



**FIGURE 15.8.** Mouse local lymph node assay (LLNA) (ICVAM protocol). Modification using flow cytometry instead of radiolabeling is preferable.

***Armstrong Method.*** This test (Ichikawa, 1981) resembles the guinea pig maximization test in that the Freund's complete adjuvant (FCA) is injected intradermally at the test sites; however, covered Hilltop chambers are used to apply and occlude the test article at the test site as was described for the Buehler test. During induction, four intradermal injections of FCA are administered at the test site; the test article is applied to the Hilltop chamber, which is then applied over the test site and occluded. After 4 h, the patches are removed and the test site is exposed to UV-A light (320 to 400 nm) for 30 min. Five additional applications of the test article (without FCA) with subsequent exposure to light are made on alternate days throughout the 11-day induction period. Nine to 13 days after the last induction exposure, the animals are challenged for 2 h with a nonirritating concentration of the test article on an occluded Hilltop chamber. The patches are then removed, and the sites are exposed to the UV-A light. Each site is graded for inflammation 24 and 48 h after challenge.

## 15.7. APPROACHES

### 15.7.1. Suggested Approaches to Testing

As outlined above, there are numerous assays available to assess the various endpoints that are relevant to immunotoxicity. Early in the development process, a new compound should be evaluated with regard to various factors that may flag it as a potential immunotoxin, including chemical structural or physiochemical properties (e.g., photoallergin) and therapeutic class (i.e., immunomodulators, anti-inflammatories, and antimetabolites). Compounds from therapeutic or structural classes that are known to be potential immunotoxins or immunomodulators should be evaluated for the effects in question on a case-by-case basis. With the exception of immunomodulators, protein products, and products of biotechnology, the majority of pharmaceuticals can be assessed for most forms of immunotoxicity during routine preclinical toxicity tests. In general, a well-conducted preclinical toxicity study can detect most serious immunotoxins in the form of altered clinical, hematologic, or histological endpoints. For example, possible effects on humoral immunity may be indicated from clinical observation of gastrointestinal or respiratory pathology, changes in serum total protein and globulin, and by histological changes in lymphoid cellularity. Likewise, effects on the cell-mediated response may be observed as increases in infections and tumor incidences, and by changes in the T-cell compartments of lymphoid tissues. In the case of immunosuppressive drugs such as cyclophosphamide and cyclosporin A, the immune effects seen in rodents are similar to those observed in the clinic (Dean et al., 1987).

If perturbations are observed in any hematologic or histopathologic indicators of immunotoxicity, it is then prudent to follow up these findings with one or more of the following:

- Use of special immunochemical and cytological assays that can be performed retrospectively on samples taken from the animals in question;

- Use of more specific *in vitro* assays to further assess effects on the pertinent target system and potential mechanism of activity;
- Use of more specific *in vitro* and *ex vivo* assays to determine toxicological significance;
- Inclusion of additional nonroutine parameters for immunotoxicity assessment in subsequent (longer-term) toxicity assays. Can also include additional satellite groups for functional tests that may require coadministration of adjuvants, pathogens, or tumor cells.

***Use of* in vivo *Tests.*** *In vivo* tests are more relevant indicators than are *in vitro* tests of immunotoxicity since the dynamic interactions between the various immunocomponents, as well as the pertinent pharmacokinetic (absorption, distribution, plasma concentrations) and metabolic factors, are taken into consideration. However, it is important to select the appropriate animal model and to design the protocol such that it will accurately reflect drug (or relevant metabolite) exposure to humans. For example, one should consider species variability when selecting the animal model, since biological diversity may further obscure the ability to accurately predict human toxicity.

***Species Selection.*** When possible, the species selected should demonstrate similar pharmacology and toxicity profiles to those anticipated in the clinic. Thus, the test animals should metabolize the drug and express the same target organ responses and toxic effects as humans. Although the rat and dog are the most common species used in preclinical safety tests, they are not as well characterized and validated as the mouse for assessing effects on immune function. For most immunosuppressive drugs, rodent data on target organ toxicities and comparability of immunosuppressive doses have been reflective of what was later observed in the clinic. Immunosuppressive effects and the doses that produced them have been shown to be similar in the various species that are typically used in preclinical safety tests (Dean and Thurmond, 1987). An exception has been seen with glucocorticosteroids, which are lympholytic in rodents but not in primates (Claman, 1972; Haynes and Murad, 1985). Although some compounds may show different pharmacokinetics and pharmacological effects in rodents than in humans, rodents still appear to be the most appropriate animals for assessing immunotoxicity of non-species-specific compounds (Dean and Thurmond, 1987).

The appropriate animal model is also important when performing follow-up testing or additional mechanistic tests to further investigate findings observed as part of the routine preclinical safety tests. When possible, these studies should employ the same animals or animal model in which the change was initially observed for several reasons, as outlined by Bloom et al. (1987), including:

- The incidence of adverse effect may be low and not easy to reproduce.
- Another species may not be genetically susceptible to the toxic effect.
- The biological significance of the change is well defined in that model.

- If the change follows long-term exposure to the drug, reproducing the effect in another model may be costly and impractical.

***Route and Treatment Regimen.*** When possible, it is important to administer the compound by the route and treatment regimen most appropriate for demonstrating the specific response and/or reflecting the intended clinical route of administration. It is also necessary for the compound to be in the same dosage form (i.e., salt form, excipients, solubilizers) that will be used clinically. With the exception of tests for contact hypersensitivity, most of the *in vivo* tests can be carried out with a minimum of three dose levels, which are needed to assess a dose-response relationship. Dose levels should range from the proposed clinical dose, or one that approximates the no-effect level, to a maximum-tolerated (or limit) dose that is lower than the $LD_{10}$ but that produces some evidence of general toxicity (e.g., reduced body weight). A wide dose interval may be necessary to detect immune changes that show a nonlinear dose response. Proper dose selection is crucial for a meaningful interpretation of test results since severe stress and malnutrition may produce indirect immunotoxic effects that would confound a clear interpretation of the data.

For compounds such as antibiotics, with a relatively short duration of therapeutic exposure, a short treatment period of 1–2 weeks in the animal model is generally appropriate. Longer treatments may not be suitable for these drugs since animals can adapt to toxic doses or develop a tolerance by inducing enzymes that increase metabolism of the drug. However, for compounds with intended chronic or prolonged usage, animals should be treated at least daily for at least a month, to assess the cumulative effects of the drug.

***Use of* in vitro *Tests.*** *In vitro* tests are useful as sensitive follow-up tests to determine potential effects or mechanisms of effects on specific cell types at the cellular and molecular levels. In addition, most are relatively simple to perform and *ex vivo* tests can be performed in conjunction with preclinical *in vivo* tests. There are several advantages to using *in vitro* tests:

- Specific cell types of humoral components of the immune system can be isolated and studied.
- Cells can be stimulated with various mitogens to assess their proliferative functions *in vitro*.
- For mechanistic studies, cells and their secretory products can be systematically studied in isolation and in various combinations to assess their interactions and cell-to-cell communications.

However, for general preclinical assessments and screening purposes, *in vitro* tests should be well validated and used cautiously for several reasons.

- They may over- or underestimate an effect or give contradictory results compared to *in vivo* tests.

- Most immunotoxic responses express a clear dose-response relationship that can be used for human risk assessment. However, it is more difficult to extrapolate *in vitro* concentrations than *in vivo* animal doses (plasma concentrations) to the clinical dose.

- It is difficult to simulate *in vitro* the interaction of all of the various cell types and modulators of immune function that make up the *in vivo* system.

- Cells can be harvested from a variety of sources and each source may have a different sensitivity since they may be at various stages of maturation or activation.

### 15.7.2. Suggested Approaches to Evaluation of Results

Several rodent toxicity studies have shown impaired host resistance to infectious agents or tumor cells at exposure levels of drugs that did not cause overt signs of toxicity (Vos, 1977; Dean et al., 1982). One serious limitation to the incorporation of specific immunotoxicological evaluations into general use in safety assessment for pharmaceuticals is a lack of clarity in how to evaluate and use such findings. This problem is true for all new diagnostic techniques in medicine and for all the new and more sensitive tools designed to evaluate specific target organ toxicities. Ultimately, as we have more experience and a reliable data base that allows us to correlate laboratory findings with clinical experience, the required course of action will become clearer. However, some general suggestions and guidance can be offered.

1. First, it is generally agreed that adverse effects observed above a certain level of severity should be given the same importance as any other life-threatening events when assessing biological significance. These are effects that are so severe that they are detected as part of the routine evaluations made in safety assessment studies. Such findings may include death, severe weight loss, early appearance of tumors, and the like. Findings such as significantly increased mortalities in a host-resistance assay would also fit into this category.

Second, there are specific endpoint assays for which an adverse outcome clearly dictates the action to be taken. These endpoints include either immediate or delayed hypersensitivity reactions, because once the individual is sensitized, a dose-response relationship may not apply.

Third, as with most toxicological effects, toxic effects to the immune system are dependent upon dose to the target site. The dose-response curve can be used to determine no-effect and low-effect levels for immunotoxicity. These levels can then be compared to the therapeutic levels to assess whether there is an adequate margin of safety for humans.

If we consider both the specific immunotoxicity assays surveyed earlier in this chapter and the arrays of endpoints evaluated in traditional toxicology studies, which may be indicative of an immune system effect, these guidelines leave many potential questions unanswered. As additional data on individual endpoints indicative of immune system responses are collected, the pharmaceutical toxicologist is challenged with various issues regarding assay interpretation and relevance to proposed (or future) clinical trials. For example, what do significant, but non-life-threatening, decreases in antibody response, lymphocyte numbers, macrophage functions, or host resistance in an animal mean about the clinical use of a drug in a patient? The intended patient population is clearly relevant here; if the disease is one in which the immune system is already challenged or incorrectly modulated, any immune system effect other than an intended one should be avoided. There are several additional considerations and questions that should be answered when evaluating the biological and clinical significance of a statistically significant immune response:

1. *Is there a dose response?* The dose response should be evaluated as a dose-related trend in both incidence and severity of the response. If there is a dose-related response, is the lowest dose (preferably plasma level) at which the effect is seen near or below the target clinical dose (plasma level), and is there an adequate therapeutic margin of safety?

2. *Does the finding stand alone?* Is a change observed in only one parameter, or are there correlated findings that suggest a generalized, biologically significant effect? For example, are there changes in lymph node and spleen weights and morphological changes in these tissues to accompany changes in lymphocyte numbers?

3. *Is the effect a measure of function or a single endpoint measurement?* Functional measures such as host resistance of phagocytosis involve multiple cells and immunocomponents and, therefore, are considered to be more biologically relevant than a significant change in a single endpoint measurement (e.g., T-cell number).

4. *Is the effect reversible?* Reversibility of a response is dependent on the drug itself, exposure levels/duration, and factors related to the test animal (metabolic capability, genetic susceptibility, etc.). Most effects produced by immunosuppressive drugs have been shown to be reversible after cessation of therapy, such as those produced during cancer chemotherapy. However, if a tumor develops before the immune system is restored, the effect is not reversible, as is the case of secondary tumors related to chemotherapy.

5. *Is there sufficient systematic toxicity data available at levels that demonstrate adequate exposure?* If a study was designed such that there was insufficient exposure or duration of exposure to potential lymphoid target tissues, the test protocol may not be adequate to demonstrate an adverse effect.

In general, a well-conducted long-term study in two species, with no indication of immunotoxicity, based on the considerations outlined above, should be adequate to evaluate the potential for drug-induced immunotoxicity. If the results from these studies do not produce evidence of immune-specific toxicity after examination of standard and/or additional hematologic, serum chemical, and histopathologic parameters, then additional testing should not be indicated. However, if there are structure-activity considerations that may indicate a potential for concern, of if significant abnormalities are observed that cannot be clearly attributed to other toxicities, then it is important to perform additional tests to fully assess the biological significance of the findings.


## 15.7. PROBLEMS AND FUTURE DIRECTIONS

There are some very pressing problems for immunotoxicology, particularly in the context of pharmaceuticals and biological therapeutics and the assessment of their safety. Unlike industrial chemicals, environmental agents, or agricultural chemicals, pharmaceutical products are intended for human exposure, are usually systemically absorbed, and have intentional biological effects on humans, some of which are intentionally immunomodulating (interleukins, growth factors) or immunotoxic (cyclosporine, cyclophosphamide).

1. *Data Interpretation.* The first major issue was presented and explored in the preceding section. This is how to evaluate and utilize the entire range of data that current immunotoxicological methodologies provide to determine the potential for immunotoxicity, and how to interpret the biological significance of minor findings.

2. *Appropriate Animal Models.* As previously addressed, most routine preclinical toxicology tests are performed with rats and dogs; therefore, toxicity, pharmacokinetic, and pharmacology data are most abundant for these species. However, most immunological parameters are best characterized and validated with mice. In addition, the NTP test battery was developed for the mouse, and some of these assays cannot be readily transferred to the rat. Over the last few years, several laboratories have begun adapting tests to both the rat and the dog (Bloom et al., 1987; Thiem et al., 1988); however, efforts need to continue along these lines to further our understanding of the immune responses in these species and how they correlate with other animal models and man.

3. *Indirect Immunotoxic Effects.* A problem related to data interpretation is how to distinguish secondary effects that may indirectly result in immunotoxicity from the primary effects of immunotoxicity in preclinical toxicity studies. Various factors may produce pathology similar to that of an immunotoxin:

- Stress in a chronically ill animal as related to general toxicity, such as lung or liver damage, can result in immune suppression.
- Malnutrition in animals with drug-induced anorexia or malabsorption can trigger immune suppression.
- Infections and/or parasites may also modulate immune parameters.

These indirect factors must be systematically ruled out, and additional mechanistic studies may be necessary to address this problem. The potential for some indirect effects may be assessed through histopathologic evaluation of endocrine organs such as the adrenals and pituitary.

4. *Hypersensitivity Tests.* Probably the largest immunotoxicity concern in clinical studies is unexpected hypersensitivity reactions. While the available guinea pig- and mouse-based tests for delayed contact hypersensitivity resulting from dermal exposure are generally good predictors, there are currently no well-validated models for either immediate or delayed hypersensitivity responses resulting from either oral ingestion or parenteral administration. Yet these two situations are the largest single cause for discontinuing clinical trials.

One assay that may hold some promise for delayed hypersensitivity is an adoptive transfer-popliteal lymph node assay (Klinkhammer et al., 1988). This assay, based on the techniques previously described for the popliteal lymph node assay (section 15.6.7) allows assessment of hypersensitivity following systemic exposure of the drug. Donor mice are first injected with drug for five consecutive days. After a four-week latency period, potentially sensitized T cells obtained from the spleen are injected into the footpad of a syngenic mouse together with a subcutaneous challenge dose of the drug. Two to five days after the cell transfer, the popliteal lymph nodes are measured and observed for evidence of a response (enlargement). Once this assay is validated, it should allow for a more relevant assessment of hypersensitivity for drugs that are administered systemically (Gleichman et al., 1989).

5. *Autoimmunity.* Traditional methods for assessing immunotoxicity as part of routine preclinical toxicity tests are primarily geared toward the detection of immunosuppressive effects. Although it is possible to incorporate clinical methods for detecting immune complexes and autoantibodies into the preclinical test protocols, the significance of adverse findings is ambiguous. Since these effects have a genetic component to their expression, the relevance of findings in animals is of questionable significance, particularly since these findings in the clinic do not always correlate with pathological effects.

6. *Functional Reserve Capacity.* As previously discussed, the immune system has a tremendous reserve capacity that offers several levels of protection and backups to the primary response. As a consequence, this functional reserve can allow biologically significant, immunotoxic insults to occur without the appearance of morphological changes. Furthermore, adverse effects may remain subclinical until the organism is subjected to undue stress or subsequent challenge. Thus, there is some concern that routine immunopathological assessments by themselves may not be sufficiently sensitive to detect all immunotoxins, particularly when testing is conducted in a relatively pathogen-free, stress-free laboratory environment.

7. *Significance of Minor Perturbations.* Although the immune system has a well-developed reserve capacity, some of these systems may act synergistically rather than independently. For instance, a macrophage can recognize and kill bacteria coated with antibodies more effectively than can either the macrophage or antibodies alone. Thus, even minor deficiencies and impairments may have some impact on the organism's ability to fend off infection or tumors, particularly if the organism is very young, old, ill, stressed, genetically predisposed to certain cancers, or otherwise

immunocompromised. These considerations lead to some additional questions that must be addressed:

- What level of immunosuppression will predispose healthy or immunocompromised individuals to increased risk of infections or tumors?
- Will slight disturbances or immunosuppression lead to a prolonged recovery from viral or bacterial infections?
- Will slight up-modulation for extended periods result in autoimmune diseases or increased susceptibility to allergy?
- Are individuals that are slightly immunosuppressed at higher risk of developing AIDS after exposure to HIV?

8. *Biotechnology Products.* Immunotherapeutics such as interferons and interleukins hold tremendous promise for those diseases where malfunctioning of the immune system is not the root of pathogenesis. Likewise, many of the new approaches to therapy of yet untreatable diseases are aimed at modulating the body's own immune system. Many of the new therapeutics coming from biotechnology are proteins of human origin. As such, they can evoke antibody responses in nonhuman species that are not indicative of what will be seen in patients. Meaningful evaluations must allow the toxicologist to discriminate between those responses that are relevant to clinical development/utilization and those that are not. In summary, it is the role of preclinical immunotoxicology testing to allow us to identify potential immune hazards early in development, before they are found in the clinic, and to provide us with a mechanistic understanding for the basis of these effects so that we may direct the development of alternative agents and/or treatment regimens to avoid them. The challenge for the toxicologist is to determine the appropriate course of action for evaluating each unique drug and to differentiate the desired therapeutic effects from the undesired and potentially adverse effects.

# REFERENCES


Ader, R. and Cohen, N. (1993). Psychoneuroimmunology: conditioning and stress. *Ann. Rev. Psychol.* 44: 53–85.

Alper, J.C., Wieman, M.C., Rueckl, F.S., McDonald, C.J. and Calabresi, P. (1985). Rationally designed combination chemotherapy for the treatment of patients with recalcitrant psoriasis. *J. Am. Acad. Dermatol.* 13: 567–577.

Andersen, K.E. and Maibach, H.I., (Eds.) (1985). Contact allergy predictive test in guinea pigs. *Current Problems in Dermatology.* Vol. 14. S. Karger, Basel.

Arts, J.H.E., Droge, S.C.M., Bloksma, N. and Kuper, C.F. (1996). Local lymph node activation in rats after application of the sensitizers 2,4-dinitrochlorobenzene and trimellic anhydride. *Fd. Chem. Toxicol.* 34: 55–62.

Bach, F.H. and Voynow, N.K. (1966). One-way stimulation in mixed leukocyte cultures. *Science* 153: 545–547.

Bakke, O.M., Wardell, W.M. and Lasagna, L. (1984). Drug discontinuations in the United Kingdom and United States, 1964–1983: Issues of safety. *Clin. Pharmacol. Therapy* 35: 559–567.

Barnett, M.J., Waxman, J.H., Richards, M.A., Ganesan, T.S., Bragman, K.S., Rohatiner, A.Z.S. and Lister, T.A. (1985). High-dose cytosine arabinoside in the initial treatment of acute leukemia. *Semin. Oncol.* 12: 133–138.

Basketter, D.A., Scholes, E.W., Kimber, I., Botham, P.A., Hilton, J., Miller, K., Robbins, M.C., Harrison, P.T.C. and Waite, S.J. (1991). Interlaboratory evaluation of the local lymph node assay with 25 chemicals and comparison with guinea pig test data. *Toxicol. Methods* 1: 30–43.

Basketter, D.A. and Scholes, E.W. (1991). Comparison of the local lymph node assay with the guinea pig maximization test for the detection of a range of contact allergens. *Food Chem. Toxical.* 30: 65–69

Batchelor, F.R., Dewdney, J.M. and Cazzard, D. (1965). Penicillin allergy: the formation of penicilloyl determinant. *Nature (London)* 206: 362–364.

Bellon, B., Capron, M., Druet, E., Verroust, P., Wial, M.C., Sapin, C., Girard, J.F., Foidart, J.M., Mahieu, P. and Druet, P. (1982). Mercuric chloride induced autoimmune disease in Brown-Norway rats: Sequential search for anti-basement membrane antibodies and circulating immune complexes. *Eur. J. Clin. Invest.* 12: 127–133.

Bigazzi, P.E. (1985). Mechanisms of chemical-induced autoimmunity. *Immunotoxicology and Immunopharmacology* (Dean, J.H., Luster, M.I., Munson, A.E. and Amos, H., Eds.). Raven Press, New York, p. 277.

Bigazzi, P.E. (1988). Autoimmunity induced by chemicals. *Clin. Toxicol.* 26: 125–126.

Bloom, J.C., Thiem, P.A., Sellers, T.S., Deldar, A. and Lewis, H.B. (1985a). Cephalosporin-induced immune cytopenia in the dog: Demonstration of cell-associated antibodies. *Blood* 66: 1232.

Bloom, J.C., Blackmer, S.A., Bugelski, P.J., Sowinski, J.M. and Saunders, L.Z. (1985b). Gold-induced immune thrombocytopenia in the dog. *Vet. Pathol.* 22: 492–499.

Bloom, J.C., Thiem, P.A. and Morgan, D.G. (1987). The role of conventional pathology and toxicology in evaluating the immunotoxic potential of xenobiotics. *Toxicol. Path.* 15: 283–293.

Buehler, E.V. (1964). A new method for detecting potential sensitizers using the guinea pig. *Toxicol. Appl. Pharmacol.* 6: 341.

Burnet, F.M. (1970). The concept of immunological surveillance. *Progr. Exper. Tumor. Res.* 13: 1–27.

Calabresi, P. and Parks, R. (1985). Antiproliferative agents and drugs used for immunosuppression. In: *Goodman and Gilman's The Pharmacological Basis of Therapeutics*, 7th ed. (Gilman, A.G., Goodman, L.S., Rall, T.W. and Murad, F., Eds.) Macmillan, New York, pp. 1247–1306.

Calabresi, P. and Chabner, B.A. (1990). Antineoplastic agents. In: *The Pharmacological Basis of Therapeutics* Goodman, A.G., Rall, T.W., Nies, A.S. and Taylor, P., Eds.). Pergamon Press, New York, pp. 1209–1263.

Caspritz, G. and Hadden, J. (1987). The immunopharmacology of immunotoxicology and immunorestoration. *Toxicol. Path.* 15: 320–322.

CDER (2001). *Guidance for Industry: Immunotoxicology Evaluation of Investigational New Drugs.* U.S. Department of Health and Human Services. Washington, D.C.

CDRH (1997). *Immunotoxicology Testing Framework*, Draft Document., U.S. Department of Health and Human Services, Washington, D.C.

Choquet-Kastylevsky, G. Vial, T. and Descotes, J. (2001). Drug allergy diagnosis in humans: possibilities and pitfalls. *Toxicology* 158: 1–10.

Claman, H. (1972). Corticosteroids and lymphoid cells. *New Engl. J. Med.* 287: 388–397.

Clark, W.R. (1983). *The Experimental Foundations of Modern Immunology*, 2nd ed. Wiley, New York, pp. 1–453.

Colvin, M. (1982). The alkylating agents. In: *Pharmacologic Principles of Cancer Treatment* (Chabner, B.A., Ed.). W.B. Saunders, Philadelphia, pp. 276–308.

Coombs, R.R.A. and Gell, P.G.H. (1975). Classification of allergic reactions responsible for clinical hypersensitivity and disease. In: *Clinical Aspects of Immunology*. (Gell, P.G.H., Coombs, R.R.A. and Lachman, D.J., Eds.). Blackwell Scientific Publications, Oxford, p. 761.

Cromwell, O., Durham, S.R., Shaw, R.J., Mackay, J.A. and Kay, A.B. (1986). Provocation tests and measurements of mediators from mast cells and basophils in asthma and allergic rhinitis. In: *Handbook of Experimental Immunology* (Weir, D.M., Herzenberg, L.A. and Blackwell, C., Eds.). 4th ed. Blackwell, Oxford, pp. 127.1–127.51.

Dean, J.H. and Thurmond, L.M. (1987). Immunotoxicology: An overview. *Toxicol. Path.* 265–271.

Dean, J.H., Luster, M.I., Boorman, G.A., Luebke, R.W. and Lauer, L.D. (1980). The effect of adult exposure to diethylstilbestrol in the mouse: Alterations in tumor susceptibility and host resistance parameters. *J. Reticuloendothelial. Soc.* 28: 571–583.

Dean, J.H., Luster, M.I. and Boorman, G.A. (1982). Immunotoxicology. In: *Immunopharmacology* (Sirois, P. and Rola-Pleszczynski, M., Eds.). Elsevier Biomedial Press, Amsterdam, pp. 349–397.

Dean, J.H., Boorman, G.A., Luster, M.I., Adkins, B.J., Lauer, L.D. and Adams, D.O. (1984). Effect of agents of environmental concern on macrophage functions. In: *Mononuclear Phagocyte Biology* (Volkman, A., Ed.). Marcel Dekker, New York, pp. 473–485.

Dean, J.H., Thurmond, L.M., Lauer, L.D. and House, R.V. (1987). Comparative toxicology and correlative immunotoxicology in rodents. In: *Environmental Chemical Exposure and Immune System Integrity* (Burger, E.J., Tardiff, R.G. and Bellanti, J.A., Eds.). Princeton Scientific Publishing, Princeton, pp. 265–271.

Deldar, A., Lewis, H.B., Bloom, J.C., Apostoli, A. and Weiss, L. (1985). Residual stem cell defects associated with cephalosporin therapy in dogs. *Blood* 66: 1202.

Descotes, G. and Mazue, G. (1987). Immunotoxicology. *Adv. Veterinary Science Comparative Med.* 31: 95–119.

DeSwarte, R.D. (1986). Drug allergy: An overview. *Clin. Rev. Allergy* 4: 143–169.

DeWeck, A.L. (1983). Immunopathological mechanisms and clinical aspects of allergic reactions to drugs. In: *Handbook of Experimental Pharmacology: Allergic Reactions to Drugs* (deWeck, A.L. and Bundgaard, H., Eds.). Springer-Verlag, New York, pp. 75–133.

Dighiero, G., Lymberi, J., Marie, J.C., Rouyse, S., Butler-Browne, G.S., Whalen, R.G. and Avrameas, S. (1983). Murine hybridomas secreting natural monoclonal antibodies reacting with self antigens. *J. Immunol.* 135: 2267–2271.

Druet, P., Bernard, A., Hirsch, F., Weening, J.J., Gengoux, P., Mahieu, P. and Brikenland, S. (1982). Immunologically mediated glomerulonephritis induced by heavy metals. *Arch. Toxicol.* 50: 187–194.

Duke, S.S., Schook, L.B. and Holsapple, M.P. (1985). Effects of *N*-nitrosodimethylamine on tumor susceptibility. *J. Leukocyte Biol.* 37: 383–394.

Elion, G.B. and Hitchings, G.H. (1975). Azathioprine. In: *Antineoplastic and Immunosuppressive Agents* (Sartorelli, A.C. and Johns, D.G., Eds.). Springer, Berlin, pp. 403–425.

Elliot, J.F., Lin, Y., Mizel, S.B., Bleackley, R.C., Harnish, D.G., and Peaettian, V. (1984). Induction of interleukin 2 messenger RNA inhibited by cyclosporin A. *Science* 226: 1439–1441.

Exon, J.H., Koller, L.D., Talcott, P.A., O'Reilly, C.A. and Henningsen, G.M. (1986). Immunotoxicology testing: An economical multiple assay approach. *Fund. Appl. Toxicol.* 7: 387–397.

FDA (Food and Drug Administration), Center for Safety and Applied Nutrition. (1993). Draft: Toxicological Principles for the Safety Assessment of Direct Food Additives and Color Additives Used in Food. *Federal Register* 58: 10536.

Gad, S.C., and Chengelis, C.P. (1998). *Acute Toxicology Testing*, 2nd ed. Academic Press, San Diego, CA.

Gad, S.C., Dunn, B.J., Dobbs, D.W. and Walsh, R.D. (1986) Developmental and validation of an alternative dermal sensitization test: The Mouse Ear Swelling Test (MEST), *Topical Appl. Pharmacol.* 84: 93–114.

Garratty, G. and Petz, L.D. (1975). Drug-induced immune hemolytic anemia. *Am. J. Med.* 58: 398–407.

Gell, P.G.H. and Combs, R.R.A. (1963) *Clinical Aspects of Immunology*, Blackwell, Oxford.

Gilman, A.G., Rall, T.W., Nies, A.S., and Taylor, P. (1990). *The Pharmacological Basis of Therapeutics*, 8th ed. Pergamon Press, New York, pp. 1–1811.

Gleichmann, E., Kimber, I. and Purchase, I.F.H. (1989). Immunotoxicology: suppressive and stimulatory effects of drugs and environmental chemicals on the immune system. *Arch. Toxicol.* 63: 257–273.

Godfrey, H.P. and Gell, P.G.H. (1978). Cellular and molecular events in the delayed-onset hypersensitivities. *Revs. Physiol. Biochem. Pharmacol.* 84: 2.

Golub, E.S. and Green, D.R. (1991). *Immunology: a Synthesis*. Sinauer, Sunderland, Massachusetts, pp. 1–744.

Guillaume, J.C., Roujeau, J.C. and Touraine, R. (1984). Lupus systémique après protheses mammaires. *Ann. Derm. Verner.* 111: 703–704.

Hadden, J.W., Cornaglia-Ferraris, P. and Coffey, R.G. (1984). Purine analogs as immunomodulators. In: *Progress in Immunology IV* (Yamamura, Y. and Tada, T., Eds.). Academic Press, London, pp. 1393–1407.

Harber, L.C., and Shalita, A.R. (1975). The guinea pig as an effective model for the demonstration of immunologically-mediated contact photosensitivity. In: *Animal Models in Dermatology* (Maibach, H., Ed.). Churchill Livingstone, New York, pp. 90–102.

Harmon, W.E., Parkman, R., Gavin, P.T., Grupe, W.E.,, Ingelfunger, J.R., Yunis, E.J. and Levey, R.H. (1982). Comparison of cell-mediated lympholysis and mixed lymphocyte culture in the immunologic evaluation for renal transplantation. *J. Immunol.* 129: 1573–1577.

Hassman, R.A., Lazarus, J.H., Dieguez, C., Weetman, A.P., Hall, R. and McGregor, A.M. (1985). The influence of lithium chloride on experimental autoimmune thyroid disease. *Clin. Exp. Immunol.* 61: 49–57.

Hastings, K.L. (2001). Pre-clinical methods for detecting the hypersensitivity potential of pharmaceuticals: regulatory consideration. *Toxicology* 158: 85–89.

Haukaas, S.A., Hoisater, P.A. and Kalland, T. (1982). *In vitro* and *in vivo* effects of diethylstilbestrol and estramustine phosphate (Estracyte) on the mutagen responsiveness of human peripheral blood lymphocytes. *Prostate* 3: 405–414.

Haynes, R.C., and Murad, F. (1985). Adrenocorticotropic hormone; adrenocortical steroids and their synthetic analogs; inhibitors of adrenocortical steroid biosynthesis. In: *Goodman and Gilman's The Pharmacological Basis of Therapeutics* (Goodman, A.G., Goodman, L.S., Rell, T.W. and Murad, F., Eds.). Macmillan, New York, pp. 1459–1489.

Herold, K.C., Lancki, D.W., Moldwin, R.L. and Fitch, F.W. (1986). Immunosuppressive effects of cyclosporin A on cloned T cells. *J. Immunol.* 136: 1315–1321.

Hinton, D.M. (1992). Testing guidelines for evaluation of the immunotoxic potential of direct food additives. *Critical Rev. in Food Sci. Nutrition* 32: 173–190.

Hollenberg, S.M., Giguere, V., Segui, P. and Evans, R.M. (1987). Colocalization of DNA-binding and transcriptional activation functions in the human glucocorticoid receptor. *Cell* 49: 39–46.

Hunter, T., Urowitz, M.B., Gordon, D.A., Smythe, H.A. and Ogryzlo, M.A. (1975). Azathio-prine in rheumatoid arthritis. A long-term follow-up study. *Arthr. Rheum.* I 8: 15–20.

Hutchings, P., Nador, D., and Cooke, A. (1985). Effects of low doses of cyclophosphamide and low doses of irradiation on the regulation of induced erythrocyte autoantibodies in mice. *Immunology* 54: 97–104.

Ichikawa, H., Armstrong, R.B. and Harber, L.C. (1981). Photoallergic contact dermatitis in guinea pigs: improved induction technique using Freund's complete adjuvant. *J. Invest. Dermatol.* 76: 498–501.

Idsøe, O., Guthe, T., Willcox, R.R., and DeWeck, A.L. (1968). Nature and extent of penicillin side-reactions, with particular reference to fatalities from anaphylactic shock. *Bull. WHO* 38: 159–188.

Jerne, N.K. and Nordin, A.A. (1963). Plaque formation in agar by single antibody-producing cells. *Science* 140: 405.

Kahan, B.D. and Bach, J.F. (1988). Proceedings of the Second International Congress on Cyclosporine. *Transplant. Proc.* 20 (Suppl.): 11131.

Kay, J.E. and Benzie, C.R. (1984). Rapid loss of sensitivity of mitogen-induced lymphocyte activation to inhibition by cyclosporin A. *Cell Immunol.* 87: 217–224.

Kimber, I. and Weisenberger, C. (1989). A murine local lymph node assay for the identification of contact allergens: Assay development and result of an initial validation study. *Arch Toxicol.* 63: 274–282.

Kimber, I., Mitchell, J.A. and Griffin, A.C. (1986). Development of murine local lymph node assay for the determination of sensitising potential. *Fd. Chem. Toxicol.* 24: 585–586.

Kimber, I., Dearman, R.J., Scholes, E.W. and Basketter, D.A. (1994). The local lymph node assay: Developments and applications. *Toxicology* 93: 13–31.

Klaus, G.G.B. and Hawrylowicz, C.M. (1984). Cell-cycle control in lymphocyte stimulation. *Immunol. Today* 5: 15–19.

Kleinman, S., Nelson, R., Smith, L. and Goldfinger, D. (1984). Positive direct antiglobulin tests and immune hemolytic anemia in patients receiving procainamide. *New Engl. J. Med.* 311: 809–812.

Klinkhammer, C., Popowa, P. and Gleichmann, H. (1988). Specific immunity to the diabetogen streptozotocin: cellular requirements for induction of lymphoproliferation. *Diabetes* 37: 74–80.

Koller, L.D. (1987). Immunotoxicology today. *Toxicol. Path.* 15: 346–351.

Kumagai, Y., Shiokawa, Y., Medsger, T.A.J. and Rodnan, G.P. (1984). Clinical spectrum of connective tissue disease after cosmetic surgery. Observations of eighteen patients and a review of the Japanese literature. *Arthr. Rheum.* 27: 1–12.

Laskin, D.L., Laskin, J.D., Weinstein, I.B. and Carchman, R.A. (1981). Induction of chemotaxis in mouse peritoneal macrophages by phorbolester tumor promoters. *Cancer Res.* 41: 1923.

Lawrence, D.A. (1985). Immunotoxicity of heavy metals. In: *Immunotoxicology and Immunopharmacology.* (Dean, J.H., Luster, M.I., Munson, A.E. and Amos, H.A., Eds.). Raven, New York, pp. 341–353.

Logue, G.L., Boyd, A.E., and Rosse, W.F. (1970). Chlorpropamide-induced immune hemolytic anemia. *New Engl. J. Med.* 283: 900–904.

Loveless, S.E., Ladics, G.S., Greberick, G.F., Ryan, C.A., Basketter, D.A., Scholes, E.W., House, R.V., Hilton, J., Dearman, R.J. and Kimber I. (1996). Further evaluation of the local lymph node assay in the final phase of the international collaborative trial. *Toxicology* 108: 141–152.

Luster, M.L., Boorman, G.A., Dean, J.H., Luebke, R.W. and Lawson, L.D. (1980). The effect of adult exposure to diethylstilbestrol in the mouse. Alterations in immunological function. *J. Reticuloendothel. Soc.* 28: 561–569.

Luster, M.L., Hayes, H.T., Korach, K., Tucker, A.N. and Dean, J.H. (1984). Estrogen immunosuppression is regulated through estrogenic responses in the thymus. *J. Immunol.* 133: 110–116.

Luster, M.L., Pfeifer, R.W. and Tucher, A.N. (1985). Influence of sex hormones on immunoregulation with specific reference to natural and synthetic estrogens. In: *Endocrine Toxicology.* (McLachlin, J.A., Korach, K. and Thomas, J., Eds.). Raven, New York, pp. 67–83.

Luster, M.L., Blank, J.A., and Dean, J.H. (1987). Molecular and cellular basis of chemically induced immunotoxicity. *Ann. Rev. Pharmacol. Toxicol.* 27: 23–49.

Luster, M.L., Munson, A.E., Thomas, P.T., Holsapple, M.P., Fenters, J.D., White, K.L., Jr., Lauer, L.D., Germolec, D.R., Rosenthal, G.J. and Dean, J.H. (1988). Development of a testing battery to assess chemical-induced immunotoxicity: National Toxicology Program's Guidelines for Immunotoxicity Evaluation in Mice. *Fund. Appl. Toxicol.* 10: 2–19.

Luster, M.L., Pait, D.G., Portier, C., Rosenthal, G.J., Dermolec, D.R., Comment, C.E., Munson, A.E., White, K. and Pollock, P. (1992a). Qualitative and quantitative experimental models to aid in risk assessment for immunotoxicology. *Toxicol. Lett.* 64/65: 71–78.

Luster, M.L., Portier, C., Pait, D.G., White, K.L., Jr., Gennings, C., Munson, A.E. and Rosenthal, G.J. (1992b). Risk assessment in Immunotoxicology. I. Sensitivity and predictability of immune tests. *Fund. Appl. Toxicol.* 18: 200–210.

Mach, P.S., Brouilhet, H. and Smor, B. (1986). D-penicillamine: a modulator of anti-DNA antibody production. *Clin. Exp. Immunol.* 63: 414–418.

Magnusson, B. and Kligman, A.M. (1969). The identification of contact allergens by animal assay. *J. Invest. Dermatol.* 52: 268–276.

Male, D., Champion, B. and Cooke, A. (1982). *Advanced Immunology.* J.B. Lippincott, Philadelphia.

Matory, Y.L., Chang, A.E., Lipford, E.H., Braziel, R., Hyatt, C.L., McDonald, H.D. and Rosenberg, S.A. (1985). Toxicity of recombinant human interleukin-2 in rats following intravenous infusion. *J. Biol. Response Mod.* 4: 377–390.

Merluzzi, V.J. (1985). Comparison of murine lymphokine, activated killer cells, natural killer cells, and cytotoxic T lymphocytes. *Cell Immunol.* 95: 95–104.

Morahan, P.S., Klykken, P.C., Smith, S.H., Harris, L.S. and Munson, A. (1979). *Infect. Immunol.* 53: 670–674.

Ntoso, K.A., Tomaszewski, J.E., Jimenez, S.A. and Neilson, E.G. (1986). Penicillamine-induced rapidly progressive glomerulonephritis in patients with progressive systemic sclerosis: successful treatment of two patients and a review of the literature. *Amer. J. Kidney Dis.* 8: 159–163.

Paranjpe, M.S. and Boone, C.W. (1972). Delayed hypersensitivity to simian virus 40 tumor cells in BALB/c mice demonstrated by a radioisotopic footpad assay. *J. Natl. Cancer Inst.* 48: 563.

Pastan, L, Willingham, M.C. and FitzGerald, D.J. (1986). Immunotoxins. *Cell* 47: 641–648.

Patterson, R., De Ewarte, R.D., Greenberger, P.A., and Grammer, L.C. (1986). Drug Allergies and Protocols for Management of Drug Allergies. *NER Allergy Proc.* 7: 325–342.

Penn, I. (1977). Development of cancer as a complication of clinical transplantation. *Transplant. Proc.* 9: 1121–1127.

Perry, H.M., Tane, M. and Camody, S. (1970). Relationship of acetyl transferase activity to antinuclear antibodies and toxic symptoms in hypertensive patients treated with hydralazine. *J. Lab. Clin. Med.* 76: 114–125.

Pieters, R. (2001). The popliteal lymph node assay: a tool for predicting drug allergies. *Toxicology* 158: 65–69.

Pung, O.J., Luster, M.L, Hayes, H.T. and Rader, J. (1984). Influence of steroidal and nonsteroidal sex hormones on host resistance in the mouse: Increased susceptibility to *Listeria monocytogenes* following exposure to estrogenic hormones. *Infect. Immun.* 46: 301–307.

Pung, O.J., Tucker, A.N., Yore. S.J. and Luster, M.I. (1985). Influence of estrogen on host resistance: Increased susceptibility of mice to *Listeria monocytogenes* correlates with depressed production of interleukin 2. *Infect. Immun.* 50: 91–96.

Riccardi, C., Puccetti, P., Santoni, A. and Herberman, R.B. (1979). Rapid *in vivo* assay of mouse natural killer cell activity. *J. Natl. Cancer Inst.* 63: 1041–1045.

Roitt, I.M., Brostoff, J., and Male, D.K. (1985). *Immunology.* C.V. Mosby, St. Louis.

Russel, A.S. (1981). Drug-induced autoimmune disease. *Clin. Immun. Allergy* 1: 57.

Shand, F.L. (1979). Review/Commentary: The immunopharmacology of cyclophosphamide. *Int. J. Immunopharm.* 1: 165–171.

Spears, C.J. and Batchelor, J.R. (1987). Drug-induced autoimmune disease. *Adv. Nephrol.* 16: 219–230.

Spreafico, F. (1988). Immunotoxicology in 1987: Problems and challenges. *Fund. Clin. Pharmacol.* 2: 353–367.

Spreafico, F., and Anaclerio, A. (1977). Immunosuppressive agents. In: *Immunopharmacology 3* (Hadden, J., Coffey, R. and Spreafico, R., Eds.). Plenum, New York, pp. 245–278.

Steele, R.W., Williams, L.W., and Beck, S.A. (1989). Immunotoxicology. *Ann. Allergy* 63: 168–174.

Sullivan, J. (1989). Immunological alterations and chemical exposure. *Clin. Toxicol.* 27: 311–343.

Tabo, J.D. and Paul, W.E. (1973). Functional heterogeneity of murine lymphoid cells. III. Differential responsiveness of T cells to phytohemagglutinin and concanavalin A for T cell subsets. *J. Immunol.* 110: 362–369.

Talal, N. (1998). Autoimmune mechanisms in patients and animal models. *Toxicol. Path.* 15: 272–275.

Thiem, P.A., Halper, L.K. and Bloom, J.C. (1988). Techniques for assessing canine mononuclear phagocyte function as part of an immunotoxicologic evaluation. *Int. J. Immunopharm.* 10: 765–771.

Ueda, S., Wakahim, Y., Takei, L, Mori, T. and Lesato, K. (1980). Autologous immune complex nephritis in gold injected guinea pigs. *Nippon Jinzo Gakkai Shi* 22: 1221–1230.

Unkovic, J., Combes, M., Mazue, G. and Roncucci, R. (1984). Poster. *Annual Meeting of the American Society of Dermatology.* Washington, D.C.

U.S. Congress, Office of Technical Assessment. (1991). *Identifying and Controlling Immunotoxic Substances—Background Paper.* U.S. Government Printing Office, Washington, D.C., pp. 1–93.

Volkman, A. (1984). *Mononuclear Phagocyte Function.* Marcel Dekker, New York.

Vos, J.G. (1977). Immune suppression as related to toxicology. *CRC Crit. Rev. Toxicol.* 5: 67.

Vos, J., Van Loveren, H., Wester, P. and Vethaak, D. (1989). Toxic effects of environmental chemicals on the immune system. *TIPS* 10: 289–292.

Wallner, B.P., Mattaliano, R.J., Hession, C., Cate, R.L., Tizard, R., Sinclair, L.K., Foeller, C., Chow, E.P., Browning, J.L., Ramachandran, K.L. and Pepinsky, R.B. (1986). Cloning and expression of human lipocortin, a phospholipase A2 inhibitor with potential anti-inflammatory activity. *Nature* 320: 77–80.

Ways, S.C., Mortola, J.F., Zvaifler, N.J., Weiss, R.J. and Yen, S.S.C. (1987). Alterations in immune responsiveness in women exposed to diethylstilbestrol in utero. *Fertil. Steril.* 48: 193–197.

Webb, D.R. and Winkelstein, A. (1982). Immunosuppression, immunopotentiation and anti-inflammatory drugs. In: *Basic and Clinical Immunology* 4th ed. (Stites, D.P., Stobo, J.D., Fudenberg, H.H. and Wells, J.V., Eds.). Lange Medical, Los Altos, CA, pp. 277–292.

Weeping, J.J., Fleuren, G.J. and Hoedemaeker, J. (1978). Demonstration of antinuclear antibodies in mercuric chloride-induced glomerulopathy in the rat. *Lab. Invest.* 39: 405–411.

Weigle, W.O. (1980). Analysis of autoimmunity through experimental models of thyroiditis and allergic encephalomyelitis. *Adv. Immunol.* 30: 159–275.

White, K.L., Jr., Sanders, V.M., Barnes, D.W., Shopp, J.G.M. and Munson, A.E. (1985). Immunotoxicological investigations in the mouse: General approach and methods. *Drug. Chem. Toxicol.* 8: 299–331.

Yoshida, S., Golub, M.S. and Gershwin, M.E. (1989). Immunological aspects of toxicology: Premises not promises. *Regul. Toxicol. Pharmacol.* 9: 56–80.

# 16

# NONRODENT ANIMAL STUDIES

## 16.1. INTRODUCTION

Most safety assessment studies are conducted in rodents (rats, mice, and hamsters) or their close "cousins," rabbits and guinea pigs. Outside of the pharmaceutical, medical device, and veterinary product industries, it has become rare for the practicing toxicologist to have close familiarity with the nonrodent animal species addressed in this chapter. Indeed, it is unlikely that a toxicologist has received any significant academic experience or training with these species. Yet, the proper use of nonrodent species is essential in the evaluation of potential new therapeutic entities, on both scientific and regulatory grounds. Indeed, there are now studies showing significantly better concordance between man and nonrodents than man and rodents for detection of adverse responses to pharmaceuticals (Olson et al., 2000). This has long been recognized in regulation informally by the use of a five-fold safety factor for nonrodent to human extrapolation as compared to a ten-fold for rodent data.

In addition to rodent studies, regulatory guidelines for pharmaceuticals require that repeated dose safety studies of up to nine months (in the United States, six months elsewhere) in duration be conducted in a nonrodent species. The most commonly used nonrodent species is the dog, followed by the monkey and pig. Another nonrodent model used to a limited extent in systemic safety evaluation is the ferret. The major objectives of this chapter are (1) to discuss differences in rodent and nonrodent experimental design, (2) to examine the feasibility of using the dog, monkey, pig, and ferret in safety assessment testing, and (3) to identify the advantages and limitations associated with each species.

## 16.2. COMPARISON BETWEEN RODENT AND NONRODENT EXPERIMENTAL DESIGN

### 16.2.1. Number of Animals

One of the main differences in experimental design between rodent and nonrodent safety studies is the number of animals used (Table 16.1). In general, approximately 4–11 times as many rodents are used in toxicity studies as nonrodents. This difference is reflected in the 1998 estimates of overall usage of animals in the United States as published by the National Research Council (NRC) (1998), which showed that only about 14% of the animals used in general research for that year were either nonhuman primates (3%), pigs (2%), or dogs (9%). The fewer number of nonrodents used is related in part to the higher costs associated with their purchase, housing, and maintenance, and in part to their limited use in other areas of research.

### 16.2.2. Differences in Study Activities

***Blood Collection.*** In rodent studies, large numbers of satellite animals (often close to the number used in the main study phase) are usually needed for pharmacokinetic blood sampling, whereas with most nonrodent species, blood samples can be collected from the main study animals without compromising their health status.

***Dosing.*** Dietary administration is a commonly used oral dosing route for long-term rodent studies, but not for nonrodents. Reasons for this include the potential for excessive feed spillage by nonrodents due to excitability (especially when humans are present) and finicky eating habits, which can result in erratic and variable daily blood levels of test compound and/or metabolites. Capsule dosing is probably the most appropriate route of oral administration for dogs, and gavage for monkeys and ferrets.

***Handling of Animals.*** Once rodents are acclimated to handling, they are generally relatively easy to work with. In contrast, some nonrodent species, such as nonhuman primates, are often difficult to handle because of their size, strength, emotionality,

**TABLE 16.1. Comparison of Rodent and Nonrodent Experimental Design**

| Duration of Study | Total Numbers of Animals on Study (no./group/sex) | | | |
|---|---|---|---|---|
| | Rat | Dog | Pig | Monkey |
| 4 weeks | 360(20)[a] | 40(4) | 40(4) | 32(4) |
| 13 weeks | 280(20)[a,b] | 48(6)[b] | 48(6)[b] | 48(6)[b] |
| 52 weeks/9 months | 360(10)[a,b] | 64(8)[b] | 64(8)[b] | 48(6)[b] |

[a]Includes satellite animals for pharmacokinetic evaluation.
[b]Number of animals/group includes several animals.

and aggressiveness. This can make the conduct of routine study activities (such as dosing, blood collection, and recording electrocardiograms) relatively time-consuming, as well as stressful to the animals.

***Behavioral Evaluation.*** Behavioral assessment of nonrodents is generally more difficult than evaluation of rodents because of their larger size, difficulties associated with handling and manipulation, and their greater awareness of and reactivity to the experimenter. Such factors can confound detection and/or interpretation of more subtle test compound-related behavioral changes.

## 16.3. NONRODENT MODELS

This section is devoted to the definition and comparison of the three nonrodent animal models (dog, ferret, and monkey) in terms of experimental procedures, environmental and dietary requirements, as well as advantages and disadvantages of use in safety assessment testing.

### 16.3.7. Dog

***Environmental and Dietary Requirements.*** Typical housing for laboratory dogs consists of stainless steel or fiberglass cages (of dimensions appropriate to the dog's size) or indoor pens (typical dimensions are three feet eight inches wide, eight feet high, and ten feet long). Two important aspects of the laboratory dog's environment are the need for exercise and socialization. Recent amendments to the United States Department of Agriculture's Animal Welfare Act require that an exercise program be established for dogs maintained in a laboratory environment. Difficulty often arises in establishing a program that will be truly beneficial to the animals. One important consideration is whether dogs should be group or individually exercised. Studies have demonstrated that dogs exercised alone tend to spend most of their time walking or investigating the area rather than jumping or running (Campbell et al., 1988), which suggests that group exercise is more beneficial.

The need for a certain degree of socialization is also important, both in terms of dog–dog and dog–human contact. If at all possible, dogs should share a cage or pen with another animal. One on-study approach undertaken by some laboratories has been to allow dogs of the same sex and treatment group to have daily contact with each other, usually from early evening to early morning. If study dictates do not make this approach feasible, efforts should be made to ensure the animals are housed in such a way that they have visual, auditory, and olfactory access to each other.

Recommended dry-bulb temperatures and relative humidity ranges for dogs are 64.4–84.2°F (16–27°C) and 30–70%, respectively (*Guide for the Care and Use of Laboratory Animals*, 1985). Increases in temperature and high humidity are of particular concern because of the dog's limited capacity to dissipate heat (primarily through panting and, to a lesser extent, through radiation and conduction). Dogs would likely not survive exposure for extended periods of time to environments where the temperature is in excess of 40°C and 40% relative humidity (Norris et al., 1968).

While the dog is a carnivore, it is able to adapt to an omnivorous diet. Requirements for dietary sources of energy, amino acids, glucose precursors, fatty acids, minerals, vitamins, and water have been established based on recommendations by the National Research Council (NRC, 1985). Adult beagles maintained in a laboratory environment function well with one feeding of standard laboratory chow per day. In safety assessment testing, however, some compounds may induce serious dietary deficiencies through induced loss of appetite, malabsorption, or vomiting, and, in these cases, it may be advisable to provide a dietary supplement.

The dog's requirement for water appears to be self-regulated and depends on factors such as the type of feed consumed, ambient temperature, amount of exercise, and physiological state; therefore, in most cases, dogs should have free access to water.

***Common Study Protocols.***  The dog is the most commonly used nonrodent species in safety assessment testing (i.e., acute, subchronic, and chronic studies). The exception to this is its use in developmental toxicity and reproductive studies. For developmental toxicity studies, the dog does not appear to be as sensitive an indicator of teratogens as other nonrodent species such as the monkey (Earl et al., 1973) or the ferret (Gulamhusein et al., 1980), and, for reproductive studies, the dog is not the species of choice because fertility testing is difficult to conduct (due to prolonged anestrus and the unpredictability of the onset of proestrus) and there is no reliable procedure for induction of estrus or ovulation.

Examples of experimental designs and suggested timing of various study activities for 4- and 13-week dog studies are shown in Tables 16.2 and 16.3,

**TABLE 16.2. Four-Week Dog or Cynomolgus Monkey Toxicity Study**

*Experimental design*
Four to five groups (including a control group)—4/sex/group
Repeated daily dosing for 29 or 30 days
Necropsy starting on day 29

*Study activities*
Daily observations: Pretreatment and twice daily during the study period
Physical examinations: Pretreatment and after dosing during Weeks 2 and 4
ECG: Pretreatment and after dosing during Weeks 2 and 4
Ophthalmic examinations: Pretreatment and during Week 4
Body weight: Pretreatment, weekly, and prior to scheduled necropsy
Feed consumption: Pretreatment and weekly
Clinical lab: Twice before the first dosing day, before dosing on Day 2, during Week 2, and prior to scheduled necropsy
Urine collection: Pretreatment and during Weeks 2 and 4
Pharmacokinetic: Blood collected at specified times after dosing on Days 1 and 28

*Source:* Adapted from a table in *Animal Models in Toxicology* (Gad and Chengelis, 1992).

**TABLE 16.3. Thirteen-Week Dog Toxicity Study**

*Experimental design*
Four groups (including a control group)—6/sex/group
Repeated daily dosing for 91–93 days
Necropsy of main group (4/sex/group) on Week 14
Necropsy of reversal group (2/sex/group) on Week 18

*Study activities*
Daily observations: Pretreatment, twice daily during treatment, and once daily during reversal
Physical examinations: Pretreatment, after dosing during Weeks 4, 8, and 13 of treatment, and during Week 4 of reversal
ECG: Pretreatment, after dosing during Weeks 4, 8, and 13 of treatment, and during Week 4 of reversal
Ophthalmic examinations: Pretreatment, during Weeks 6 and 13 of treatment, and during Week 4 of reversal
Body weight: Pretreatment (3 times), weekly during the treatment and reversal periods, and prior to scheduled necropsy
Feed consumption: Pretreatment, weekly through first month, bimonthly during the remainder of treatment period, and weekly during reversal
Clinical lab: Pretreatment, during Weeks 4 and 8 of treatment, prior to scheduled necropsy, and during Weeks 1 and 4 of reversal
Urine collection: Pretreatment, monthly during treatment, and during Week 4 of reversal
Pharmacokinetic samples: Blood collected at specified times after dosing on Day 1 and during Weeks six and 12

*Source:* Adapted from a table in Animal Models in Toxicology (Gad and Chengelis, 1992).

respectively. Beagles are generally in the age range of six to nine months at study start, and the number of animals per sex per treatment group ($N$) will depend on the duration of the study. For a two- to four-week study without a reversal phase, $N$ will likely be four, whereas for a 26-week or one-year study, $N$ will be larger (e.g., $N$ may be nine including three/sex/group for the reversal phase).

Dogs should be selected for study use on the basis of acceptable body weights, urinalysis, and clinical pathology findings, as well as physical, ophthalmic, and electrocardiographic evaluations. To minimize familial effects, efforts should be made to ensure that no two littermates of the same sex are assigned to the same treatment group.

Because most, if not all, study-related activities are conducted in the same dogs, the stress induced by repeated manipulation of dogs for activities such as blood collection, ECG, and physical examinations needs to be taken into consideration. Efforts should be made wherever possible to separate study activities by several days.

### General Study Activities

*Dosing Techniques.* The most frequently used route of administration in dog safety assessment studies is oral. Dosing by capsule is usually the preferred oral route in the dog. Gavage is also used, but is a more labor intensive technique, and there is always the possibility of gavage error or aspiration. Since dogs have a natural tendency to vomit, it is recommended that they be sham dosed with empty capsules or gavaged with a water solution for several days prior to starting a study so that they can become acclimated to the dosing procedure.

Next to oral dosing, the most common dosing route for dogs is intravenous. For bolus or limited infusion intravenous dosing, the femoral, cephalic, and saphenous veins are commonly used. For continuous infusion, the jugular is often the vein of choice, and the procedure will require surgical preparation either for a direct line catheterization or subcutaneous insertion of a vascular access port (a rigid, multi-puncturable reservoir equipped with an indwelling catheter).

Other routes of administration used less commonly in dog safety studies are subcutaneous, intramuscular, intraperitoneal, rectal, and vaginal.

*Clinical Observations and Physical Examinations.* Daily clinical observations in dog safety studies, usually conducted pretreatment (prior to cage cleaning) and at a specified time(s) after dosing, consist of a home cage observation with notation of clinical signs indicative of poor health (such as salivation, weight loss, abnormal feces and vomitus) or abnormal behavior (such as reduced activity or increased aggression).

Physical examinations are conducted less frequently and generally involve the evaluation of gait, mobility, demeanor, and reflexes (pupillary light, corneal patellar, wheelbarrowing, and hopping, etc.), as well as an examination of the head (eyes, ears, mouth, teeth, gums, and tongue), body (palpation for signs of masses and nodal swellings), and urogenital and anal regions.

*Feed Consumption.* Feed consumption is relatively easy to measure in the dog, since dogs do not usually spill much of their feed. The full feed bowl is weighed at the beginning and the empty bowl at the end of the feeding period (usually a 4-h period). This is repeated over two or three consecutive days and the average daily feed consumption calculated.

*Electrocardiograms (ECGs).* A ten-lead system, consisting of the bipolar leads (I, II, III), the augmented unipolar leads (aVR, aVL, and aVF), and the unipolar precordial leads [V10, CV6LL(V2), CV6LU(V4), CV5RL(rV2)], has been recommended for dogs in the conscious state (Detweiler, Patterson, Buchanan, and Knight, 1979; Detweiler, 1980). For toxicity studies, dog ECGs are usually recorded by technical personnel and read at a later time by a cardiologist. Depending on the length of the study and the pharmacological-toxicological profile of the test compound, ECGs may be recorded as frequently as every day or as infrequently as every three months. Dog ECGs can also be highly variable. Factors that can affect the quality of the tracing include the positioning of the electrodes, the positioning of the dog, and the degree of nervousness and excitability of the animal. Conditioning the dogs to the electrode clips and the recording position (usually sphinx or right-lateral recumbency) during the pretreatment period will help improve the quality of the recording.

*Blood and Urine Collection.*  As mentioned previously, serial blood samples can be fairly easily collected from the dog. The jugular vein is probably the most commonly used vein because of its size and accessibility. Other veins used less frequently are the cephalic, femoral, brachial, and saphenous.

Due to the difficulty in obtaining sufficient volumes of urine in dogs over short collection periods, urine is usually collected overnight (approximately a 16- to 17-h period) in metabolism cages. It is recommended that a sample for urinalysis be taken early in the collection process, and that all samples be collected in light-resistant containers to help avoid problems such as dissolution of urine casts, increased bacterial activity, and breakdown of bilirubin with exposure of the sample to light.

***Advantages and Disadvantages.***  Some of the advantages and disadvantages of using the dog in safety assessment studies are listed in Table 16.4. With respect to its medium size and even temperament, the beagle is certainly a desirable nonrodent model. The relative ease in handling beagles makes them suitable for activities such as serial collection of blood samples and recording of electrocardiograms.

Disadvantages include an often wide variation in size and body weight and a loud, penetrating bark. The large amount of space required to house dogs and the current emphasis on regular exercise may also be disadvantages. Test compound requirements are generally higher for the dog than for many other nonrodents used in safety testing. This may be a problem in the early period of drug development when compound availability is often limited. Other problems center around the dog's tendency to vomit, which can be a disadvantage when compounds are orally administered, and the fact that, unlike rodents, studies requiring large numbers of dogs need careful advance planning to ensure that sufficient numbers of animals of the appropriate age can be obtained in a timely manner.

**TABLE 16.4.  Use of the Beagle in Safety Assessment Studies**

*Advantages*
Medium size
Moderate length of hair coat
Adaptability to living in group housing
Ease of handling (e.g., dosing, blood collection, ECG)

*Disadvantages*
Variation in size and body weight
Loud, penetrating bark
Greater test compound requirements than smaller nonrodent species
Availability
Exercise and housing requirements

*Source:* Adapted from a table in Animal Models in Toxicology (Gad and Chengelis, 1992).

### 6.3.2. The Ferret

The ferret, *Mustela putorius furo,* is a small carnivore that has become an increasingly popular species in various areas or research including anatomy, virology, bacteriology, physiology (gastrointestinal, pulmonary, and cardiovascular), pharmacology, neurology, teratology, and to some extent, toxicology. The reader is referred to the excellent reviews by Thornton et al. (1979) and Fox (1988) on the biology and diseases of the ferret, and to the chapter in Gad and Chengelis (1992) or the recent paper by Gad (2000a) on the ferret as an animal model in toxicology. Since 1990, the literature has reported on work done by Pfizer, Hoffman LaRoche, Gilead, Bristol Myers Squibb, Merck, Yamanouchi, Proctor and Gamble, Abbot and Glaxo Wellcome using ferrets in pharmaceutical development.

***Environmental and Dietary Requirements.*** For reasons of environmental control, ferrets used in safety assessment studies should be housed indoors. It has been suggested that an optimal temperature range for the ferret is 40–65°F (4–18°C), while relative humidity should be maintained in the range of 40 to 65% (Fox, 1988). The ferret does not tolerate heat well due to its lack of well-developed sweat glands; the primary method of regulating heat loss appears to be through panting (Moody et al., 1985).

Since ferrets are seasonal breeders, the female being monestrus and an induced ovulator, the breeding cycle can be controlled by varying the length of exposure to artificial light. For safety studies, it is desirable to prevent both estrus in females and increased sexual activity in males; thus it has been recommended that the light period be kept short (Fox, 1988). A 9-h light/15-h dark cycle has been used successfully for this purpose.

Ferrets should be housed in well-ventilated rooms that provide at least 10–15 air changes per hour. Good ventilation is important, since ferrets are susceptible to respiratory viral infections. Additionally, there is a need to dissipate the musky odor of the animals. While housing standards for ferrets are not specified in the NIH *Guide to the Care and Use of Laboratory Animals* (1985), space requirements of 49×46×46 cm have been defined by other groups (Wilson and Donnoghue, 1982). Stainless steel cat or rabbit cages equipped with a drop pan to catch feces and urine are a suitable form of primary housing for ferrets. Ferrets are more content when they have access to a small secluded nesting area within their cage in which they can sleep. The use of paper to line the cage or drop pan is not recommended, since the ferrets arc likcly to cat it. For socialization purposes, ferrets should be housed as a group, or have visual access to neighboring ferrets if housed individually.

Since ferrets eat only their caloric requirements, and since their gastrointestinal transit time is short (3–5 h), it is recommended that they receive diet *ad libitum*. Dry cat food was previously recommended for ferrets; however, there are now at least two standardized ferret chows commercially available. The most important dietary variable is the quality of the protein, and ferrets appear to do best with a high percentage of animal protein in their diet (Morton and Morton, 1985). Feed consumption will be higher in the fall and winter and lower in the spring and summer. Hairball laxative is essential during the spring and summer months when the animals experience considerable hair loss. Water should be available at all times.

***Study Protocols.*** Historically, the ferret has been used more often in teratology (Hoar, 1984), reproductive (Hoar, 1984), and acute safety studies than in repeated dose studies (4–52 weeks in duration). More consideration, however, is now being given to the use of the ferret in pivotal repeated-dose safety assessment testing (Thornton et al., 1979; Hart, 1986; Haggerty et al., 1989).

An example of the experimental design for a four-week pivotal study in ferrets is shown in Table 16.5. Young adult ferrets are usually in the age range of 9–11 months at study start, and there should be sufficient numbers of animals in each group for statistical confidence (generally in the range of six to eight animals per sex per group). For longer-term studies, the number of animals per group would be increased to include reversal group animals (three to four animals per sex per dose group).

Assignment of ferrets to a study should be based on evaluation of pretreatment clinical signs and body weights, as well as physical, electrocardiographic, and opthalmological findings.

For longer-term studies, females should be spayed to avoid the development of aplastic anemia, which will occur if the animals go into heat and are not bred (Morton and Morton, 1985).

As with dogs, efforts should be made to separate study activities as much as possible to minimize the stress of multiple activities being performed in the same animals.

### General Study Activities

*Dosing Techniques.* Oral dosing of ferrets is usually done by gavage. One method is to hold the ferret perpendicular to the floor, insert the appropriate size stainless steel

**TABLE 16.5. Four-Week Ferret Toxicity Study**

---

*Experimental design*
Five groups (including a control group)—7/sex/group
Repeated daily dosing for 29 or 30 days
Necropsy starting on day 29

*Study activities*
Daily observations: Pretreatment and twice daily during the study period
Physical examinations: Pretreatment and after dosing during Weeks 1, 2, and 4
ECG: Pretreatment and after dosing during Weeks 2, and 4
Ophthalmic examinations: Pretreatment and during Week 4
Body weight: Pretreatment, twice weekly, and prior to scheduled necropsy
Feed consumption: Pretreatment and weekly during the study
Clinical lab: Pretreatment, Week 2, and prior to scheduled necropsy
Urine collection: Pretreatment and during Weeks 2 and 4
Pharmacokinetic samples: Blood collected at specified times after dosing on Days 1 and 28

---

gavage needle into the animal's mouth, back into the esophagus and down toward the stomach. Confirmation of correct positioning of the tube can be determined by visual inspection of the aspirate. As with dogs, ferrets have a tendency to retch or vomit, and daily gavaging with a water solution for several days prior to starting a study (for adaptation purposes) is recommended.

Repeated daily intravenous dosing in the ferret is generally considered to be technically difficult and time-consuming; the use of an indwelling catheter is recommended (Moody et al., 1985). There are, however, reports in the literature of subchronic intravenous dosing (three times weekly for three months) of the ferret via the caudal vein (Mclain et al., 1987).

Dosing techniques, such as intramuscular, intradermal, subcutaneous, and intraperitoneal administration, can be used for the ferret. Care needs to be taken, however, when administering lipophilic compounds by the subcutaneous or intradermal routs, to avoid inadvertently injecting compounds into the ferret's thick layer of subcutaneous fat, which can result in poor absorption (Moody et al., 1985).

*Clinical Observations and Examinations.* Daily clinical observations will usually begin the week prior to study start and continue twice daily (pre- and postdosing) throughout the study. Ferrets are observed in their home cage for signs of physical debilitation (such as abnormal feces or vomitus), behavioral abnormalities, hair loss, swelling of the vulva (females), and testicular prominence (males). A physical examination should periodically be made and should include measurement of rectal temperature, observation of general demeanor and activity, palpation of the head, thorax, and abdomen, examination of eyes, ears, and body orifices, and testing of the pupillary and patellar reflexes.

*Feed Consumption.* Feed consumption can be measured over two to three consecutive days, and the average daily intake calculated. A problem with measuring feed intake in ferrets is their tendency to dig through their feed bowl, which often results in an unacceptable amount of spillage. Use of a feed follower may help reduce the spillage.

*Electrocardiograms.* Most electrocardiographic evaluation in the ferret is done in the anesthetized animal. This allows electrocardiograms to be recorded using the limb (I, II, and III) and augmented (aVR, aVL, and aVF) leads. Fairly good quality ECGs in the conscious ferret have been obtained using leads I, II, and III. The standard position used for recording ECGs in the conscious or anesthetized ferret is right-lateral incumbency. ECGs have also been measured in the ferret using surface electrodes placed between two points on the chest, with the signals being led off to an amplifier by a long, flexible cable and recorded on magnetic tape for later analysis (Andrews et al., 1979). The advantage of such a system is that the animals are allowed to move freely during the recording.

*Blood and Urine Collection.* About 5–10 ml of blood can be collected from adult ferrets using retroorbital blood collection techniques. Other methods of blood collection include cephalic and jugular veins and caudal tail venipuncture, as well as bleeding via the ventral tail artery. Cardiac puncture is also used but in the opinion of some (Hart, 1986) laboratories, the procedure is traumatic and can cause myocardial scarring. Blood collection from the tail can be difficult, because the ferret tail is short and the tail veins and arteries cannot be seen. For all the above-mentioned collection techniques, some form of pharmacological or mechanical restraint is required. To facilitate serial blood collection, methodology has been developed for a tethered restraint system with an implanted indwelling venous jugular catheter, which does not interfere with the normal activities of the ferrets and allows blood sampling to occur from outside the cage (Jackson et al., 1988).

For urine collection, rat metabolism cages work well for short-term or overnight collection. Care needs to be taken to avoid contamination of the urine with feces.

***Advantages and Disadvantages.*** Two advantages to using the ferret are its cost and its size (Table 16.6). The cost of the ferret is approximately one-tenth that of the dog. The ferret's smaller size means that it is easier to maintain and more economically housed and fed than the dog (Hart, 1986). Smaller size also means that test compound requirements for the ferret will be considerably less than those for larger nonrodent species (e.g., on the order of one tenth of that needed for the dog). Another advantage is that if exercise requirements are ever established for the ferret, it will be an easier species than the dog for which to design an acceptable exercise program.

Disadvantages associated with the ferret include its pervading musky odor and its background disease profile. While the scent glands can be removed, 90% of the animal's odor is derived from sebaceous secretions onto the skin. However, neutering the males and spaying the females, in addition to de-scenting, will markedly reduce the odor. Rats should be housed as far away from ferrets as possible because of their inherent fear of ferrets (triggered by olfactory stimulation), which can interrupt breeding cycles or disturb other physiological functions (Fox, 1988). Ferrets, which are generally less docile than dogs, can be difficult to handle and prone to bite,

**TABLE 16.6. Use of the Ferret in Safety Assessment Studies**

*Advantages*
Small size
Significantly lower cost than most other nonrodents
Lower test material requirements (relative to larger nonrodents)
Adaptability to an exercise program

Disadvantages
Pervading musky odor
Rodents' inherent fear of ferrets
Can be difficult to handle
Background disease profile with resulting "background noise" and increased variability in
    clinical and anatomical pathology

especially when restrained for activities such as ophthalmic and ECG examinations. The lack of easily accessible veins for intravenous dosing and serial blood collection is also a disadvantage.

The major disadvantage in the use of the ferret in safety studies is the profile of diseases associated with the species and the resulting variability in background clinical and anatomical pathology. Pneumonitis and hepatic lymphoid accumulation, associated with chronic parvovirus infection, have been observed in ferrets (Haggerty et al., 1989). Submucosal lymphoid nodules of the intestines are also a common finding (Hart, 1986). Additionally, a relatively high incidence of electrocardiographic (atrial or ventricular premature depolarization, atrial and ventricular extrasystoles) and ophthalmological (optic nerve hypoplasia and cataracts) anomalies have been found in ferrets. While it may be possible to work with the animal suppliers to reduce the chances of receiving animals with background ECG or ocular abnormalities, at the present time there is no supplier of a disease- and viral-free ferret.

### 16.3.3.  The Pig

***Background.*** The use of pigs (*Sus scrufa*) in biomedical research is well established. In toxicology, the use of pigs in the United States is largely limited to dermal studies, whereas in Europe they have become very popular for pharmaceutical studies in place of dogs and primates. They have been extensively used for surgical (Swindle, Smith and Hepburn, 1988) and physiological (primarily cardiovascular, renal, and digestive) research (Khan, 1984; Clausing et al., 1986) for years. Until relatively recently, their use in toxicity testing was uncommon except in the testing of veterinary or herd-management drugs intended for use in swine or in dermal toxicity and absorption studies. Because of their well-accepted physiological similarities to humans, minipigs are becoming increasingly attractive toxicological models (Table 16.7). In fact, they are already more frequently used in nutritional toxicology studies (Clausing et al., 1986). Among the more common experimental animals, pigs are the only ones whose use is on the increase (Khan, 1984). Their expense (both in procurement and maintenance) and their relatively large size have mitigated against their use in more general toxicity testing. The development of

**TABLE 16.7.  The Minipig in Toxicity Testing**

---

Due to the many advantages, mini- and micropigs are real alternatives to the use of nonrodents
(dogs, ferrets and primates)
Minnesota minipig introduced in 1949
Body weights at age 2 years
    Yucatan minipig: 70–90 kg
    Yucatan micropig 40–45 kg
    Göttinger micropig: 35–40 kg
Use in general toxicity testing and reproduction, teratological and behavioral toxicity (aspects
of public acceptance as a species for testing)

---

**TABLE 16.8. Main Advantages of the Minipig**

Similarity to humans in:
   Cardiovascular anatomy and physiology
      Ventricular performance
      Electrophysiology
      Coronary artery distribution
   Human skin
      Thickness and permeability
      Pigmentation
      Allergic reaction
      Reaction to burning and distress
   Gastrointestinal system and digestion
   Renal system
   Immune system (FDA: "…better than rodents")
   P450 total enzyme activity (especially CYP2E1, CYP3A4)

minipigs has resulted in a strain of more manageable size. In addition, the increase in expense in the use of dogs, as well as the perceived lay opposition to their uses, make minipigs even more attractive as a nonrodent species for general toxicity studies. The dog is a far more common companion animal and many of the recent developments in animal care and use laws have made specific provisions about the care of dogs. Minipigs have been shown to be more sensitive to a wide variety of drugs and chemicals (e.g., carbaryl, methylmercury) than dogs (Khan, 1984). The Food and Drug Administration (FDA) has kept its own breeding colony of minipigs since the early 1960s. In short, there are scientific, economic, and sociological reasons that make minipigs good toxicological models. The reader is referred to an excellent short review by Phillips and Tumbleson (1986) that puts the issue of minipigs in biomedical research into the context of modeling in general. Table 16.8 presents the advantages of the minipig.

Several breeds of miniature swine have been developed. These include in the United States, the Yucatan micro- and minipigs, the Handford, the Sinclair, the Pitman-Moore, and the Hormel. The Yucutan and the Sinclair tend to be the most commonly used, though the Göttinger (widely used in Europe) is seeing increasing use (Ellegaard et al., 1995). Panepinto and Phillips (1986) have discussed the characteristics, advantages, and disadvantages of the Yucatan minipig in some detail. In Europe, the Göttinger minipig is extensively used. At sexual maturity (4–6 months) the typical minipig weighs 20 to 40 kg, as compared to 102 kg for the more common pig, 8 to 15 kg for the dog. Micropigs weigh about 14 to 20 kg at sexual maturity. The minipig and the dog have comparable life spans; for example, Peggins, Shipley and Weiner (1984) reported that the average life span for miniature swine is 15 to 17 years. The average beagle dog may have a life span of 8 to 12 years. Most of this discussion will focus on the purpose-bred minipigs, primarily the Yucatan and the Sinclair.

***Housing.*** A general review of handling and husbandry have been described by Panepinto (1986) and Swindle, Smith and Hepburn (1988). Young weanling pigs can be kept for short periods of time (up to one month) in standard dog cages with the floor modified with narrow mesh to account for the smaller foot of the pig. After that, however, their rapid growth generally makes such caging inappropriate. Larger stainless steel cages would be extremely expensive. Standard dog runs could have enough floor space to be converted for pigs, but smooth flooring does not provide appropriate footing for pigs and needs to be covered with wood chip bedding (Swindle, Smith and Hepburn, 1988). Although pigs are very social, they do not have to be group housed, as discussed by Barnett and Hensworth (1986); individually housed swine show little evidence of a chronic stress response. Insufficient space, on the other hand, can cause chronic stress in pigs. Hunsaker, Norden and Allen (1984) have described an inexpensive caging system for miniature swine that is appropriate for toxicology studies. The flooring and walls are constructed of 0.50-cm welded wire coated with polyvinyl chloride polymer. As described, the unit has sufficient room for two pigs, separated by a partition. These units are relatively inexpensive and provide more than sufficient floor space (about $17\,\mathrm{ft}^2$ per pig) to meet the recommendations for pigs.

***Water and Feed.*** Like all animals, pigs should be permitted free access to potable water, preferably from a municipal water supply intended for human consumption. Drinking water intended for pigs does not have to be filtered or deionized. Various diets have been described. Because of their size (i.e., high maintenance charges and test articles demand), pigs have seldom been used for chronic studies where the possibility of waterborne envinronmental contaminants could influence a study.

For miniature swine, the consistent use of a certified chow from a major manufacturer is recommended (Swindle, Smith, and Hepburn, 1988). Free access to feed is not recommended as pigs will eat to excess. Available feed should be restricted to approximately 4% of body weight per day to prevent the animals from becoming obese.

***Restraint and Dosing.*** In general, minipigs are docile, and easily socialized and trained. Barnett and Hensworth (1986) recommended a socialization regimen of two minutes of gentle interaction (e.g., stroking, etc.). Pigs, like most experimental animals, are rarely simply kept and fed, but have to be occasionally restrained so samples can be taken and other measurements made. Restraint methods designed for commercial swine should not be used for laboratory swine. Panepinto et al. (1983) have described a sling method that provides restraint with minimal stress. The most frequently mentioned dosing routes in the literature are dietary admix, dermal (topical), gavage, and intravenous injections. Generally, minipigs are restrained in a sling while being dosed by the active route such as gavage. If the experiment requires the implantation of, for example, an indwelling catheter, minipigs can be anesthetized with ketamine (20 mg/kg IM) as described by Swindle, Smith and Hepburn (1988).

***Clinical Laboratory.*** Clinical chemical and hematological parameters for minipigs have been studied. Ranges for some of the more commonly examined parameters from Yucatan minipigs are summarized in Tables 16.9 and 16.10 (from Radin, Weiser and Frettman, 1986). Parson and Wells (1986) have published similar data on the Yucatan minipig. Brechbuler, Kaeslin and Wyler (1984), Oldigs (1986),

**TABLE 16.9. Minipig Clinical Chemistry Parameters in Different Strains**

| Parameter | Yucatan | Göttinger |
|---|---|---|
| Glucose (mmol/l) | $3.75 \pm 0.64$ | $5.98 \pm 1.01$ |
| Urea (mmol/l) | $7.84 \pm 2.64$ | $3.19 \pm 1.15$ |
| Creatinine (µmol/l) | $115 \pm 16$ | $52.2 \pm 11.1$ |
| Total protein (g/l) | $74 \pm 9$ | $54.0 \pm 4.6$ |
| Albumin (g/l) | $50 \pm 6$ | $26.2 \pm 6.0$ |
| Bilirubin total (µmol/l) | $3.42 \pm 1.37$ | — |
| Triglycerides (mg/l) | $267 \pm 134$ | $565 \pm 250$ |
| Total cholesterol (mmol/l) | $1.85 \pm 0.38$ | $1.65 \pm 0.38$ |
| $\gamma$-Glutamyl transpeptidase (U/l) | $61.6 \pm 11.2$ | — |
| Alanine aminotransferase (U/l) | $72.5 \pm 13.6$ | — |
| Aspartate aminotrasnferase (U/l) | $40.3 \pm 5.9$ | — |
| $Na^+$ (mmol/l) | $140.5 \pm 4.2$ | $142.3 \pm 3.00$ |
| $K^+$ (mmol/l) | $4.1 \pm 0.3$ | $3.94 \pm 0.32$ |
| $CL^-$ (mmol/l) | $103.1 \pm 4.3$ | $101.3 \pm 3.6$ |
| $Ca^{++}$ (mmol/) | $2.62 \pm 0.18$ | $2.58 \pm 0.16$ |
| $PO_4^=$ (mmol/l) | $2.41 \pm 0.26$ | $1.61 \pm 0.30$ |

[a]Data are mean $\pm$ SD.
*Source:* Parson and Wells 1986; Brechbuler, Kaeslin, and Wyler, 1984; Odigs, 1986.

**TABLE 16.10. Minipig Hematological Parameters in Different Strains**

| Parameter | Yucatan | Göttinger |
|---|---|---|
| Red blood cell ($10^6$/mm$^3$)$10^6$/mm$^3$) | $7.61 \pm 0.15$ | $7.0 \pm 0.80$ |
| Hemoglobin (g/dl) | $14.87 \pm 0.18$ | $14.9 \pm 1.20$ |
| Hematocrit (%) | $44 \pm 0.5$ | $44.6 \pm 4.1$ |
| Mean corpuscular volume (fl) | $58.5 \pm 0.8$ | $64.4 \pm 3.7$ |
| Mean corpuscular hemoglobin (pg) | $19.8 \pm 0.3$ | $21.4 \pm 1.3$ |
| Mean corpuscular hemoglobin concentration (g/dl) | $33.9 \pm 0.3$ | $33.2 \pm 0.8$ |
| White blood cell ($10^3$/mm$^3$) | $12.73 \pm 0.41$ | $12.6 \pm 3.0$ |
| Lymphocytes ($10^3$/mm$^3$) | $7.25 \pm 0.24$ | $5.75 \pm 1.52$ |
| Neutrophil (per mm$^3$) | $4.47 \pm 0.24$ | $5.27 \pm 1.29$ |
| Eosinophils (per mm$^3$) | $534 \pm 57$ | $517 \pm 31$ |
| Monocyte (per mm$^3$) | $422 \pm 35$ | $945 \pm 71$ |
| Basophils (per mm$^3$) | $89 \pm 15$ | $63 \pm 1.3$ |
| Platelets ($10^3$/mm$^3$) | — | $441 \pm 119$ |

*Source:* Burks et al. 1977 (12-month-old, sexes pooled); Radin, Weiser and Frettman, 1986.

Ellegaard et al. (1995) and Koch et al. (2001) have published on the Göttinger minipig. Middleton and coworkers have published extensive lists (organized by age and sex) on the hematological parameters (Burks et al, 1977) and serum electrolytes (Hutcheson, Tumbleson and Middleton, 1979) for the Sinclair minipig. In general, the clinical laboratory picture of the various strains are quite similar. No real differences between sexes have been identified, but age can be very much a factor. For example, serum creatinine can be 33% higher in a three-month-old as compared to 18-month-old Sinclair minipigs (based on data reported by Burks et al., 1977). As with other species, health status, feed composition, feeding regimen, fasting state, season, time of day, and the like, can affect clinical laboratory results in the minipig. Toxicological experiments should not be run without concurrent controls.

***Xenobiotic Metabolism.*** Some critical parameters of hepatic microsomal drug metabolism in the minipig, common swine, and rats are given in Table 16.11. As most investigators tend to use younger minipigs the values reported in this table are for young (less than four-years-old) minipigs. Relatively few papers have examined the MMFO in a broad age range (10 months to 12 years) of Hanford minipigs. They identified definite age-related differences. The amounts of cytochrome P-450, the mitochondrial mixed functional oxidases (MMFO) activity with aniline and *p*-chloro-*N*-methylaniline, and glucoronosyl transferase activity were all significantly higher in middle-aged (5–8 years) versus young (less than four years) minipigs. Freudanthal et al. (1976) examined Hanford minipigs in the two- to eight-months age range, and obtained somewhat different cytochrome P-450 (approximately

**TABLE 16.11. Comparison of Xenobiotic Metabolism Systems in Rat and Pig**

| Enzyme | Rat[a] | Minipig[b] | Common Swine[a] |
|---|---|---|---|
| Cytochrome P-450[c] | $0.59 \pm 0.04$ | $0.95 \pm 0.02$ | $0.30 \pm 0.04$ |
| MMFO activity[a] | | | |
|   Ethylmorphine | $5.09 \pm 0.34$ | $8.53 \pm 0.51$ | $1.39 \pm 0.16$ |
|   Ethoxyresorufin | $0.134 \pm 0.022$ | | $0.88 \pm 0.02$ |
| Epoxide hydrolase | $8.36 \pm 2.48$ | — | $11.4 \pm 1.67$ |
| UDP-glucoronosyl transferase | | | |
|   1-Naphthol | $6.43 \pm 1.66$ | — | $5.50 \pm 0.89$ |
|   4-Nitrophenol | $4.51 \pm 0.50$ | $5.5 \pm 1.5$ | $9.38 \pm 1.07$ |
| Glutathione *S*-transferase | | | |
|   DNCB | $2659 \pm 168$ | | $2746 \pm 499$ |
|   DCNB | $118 \pm 8.8$ | — | $2.44 + 0.23$ |
| PAPS sulfotransferase | $0.785 \pm 0.066$ | — | $0.095 \pm 0.025$ |
|   2-Naphthol | | | |
| Acetyltransferase | | | |
|   *p*-Aminobenzoate | $0.77 \pm 0.23$ | — | $0.621 \pm 0.111$ |

[a]All enzyme activities; nmol/min/mg (either microsomal or cytosolic) protein.
[b]nmol/mg microsomal protein.
[c]*Source:* Smith et al., 1984; Watkins and Klaassen, 1986.
[d]*Source:* Freundenthal et al., 1976; Peggins, Shipley, and Weiner, 1984.

0.95 nmol/mg) values than did Peggins, Shupley, and Weiner (1984) (approximately 0.50 nmol). The reported ranges for aniline hydroxylase (about 0.70 nmol/min/mg) and UDP-glucoronosyl transferase (about 50 nmol/min/mg) were similar in the two papers. Hence, the available data on the MMFO of young Hanford minipigs are fairly consistent.

Little work has been reported on isozomic cytochrome P-450 characteristics, the response to inducers, or the specificity of metabolic function of the pig. Work by Mueller et al. (1980) comparing the effects of arochlor induction on the subsequent responses in the Ames *Salmonella* mutagenicity test of seven different species with five different known mutagens is an exception. Animals were treated with a single dose of arochlor 1254 (500 mg/kg IP in sesame oil) and sacrificed five days later. The minipig responded in the same fashion as rats and mice, with large increases (3.9-fold) in ethylmorphine demethylase activity. Liver fractions from untreated minipigs had low activation in the Ames assay with benzo(a)pyrene, cyclophosphamide, and dethylnitrosamine. In contrast, liver preparations from induced animals add greatly increased activity (5- to 10-fold) in the Ames assay with these mutagens. This is a pattern very similar to that seen in the rat. Thus, the MMFO of the minipig is inducible and the resulting changes in metabolism may not be dissimilar from those produced by the rat.

The flavin adenosine dinucleotide (FAD) containing monooxygenase (FMFO) has traditionally been studied in hog liver obtained from slaughterhouses (Tynes and Hodgson, 1984). Interestingly, when FMFO activity is compared between species, substrate specificites are found to be generally very similar (Tynes and Hodgson, 1984). Rettie et al. (1990) isolated and studied the FMDO from Yucatan minipig liver. As with the enzyme studied from other species, the hepatic enzyme exists as a single isozymic species, is active with both dimethylanaline (*N*-oxide formation) and alkyl *p*-tolyl sulfides (sulfoxidation), and is enantioselective in metabolite formation. It would thus appear that the minipig does not differ appreciably from regular swine in the presence or activity of FMFO.

Perhaps some aspects of minipig xenobiotic metabolism can be inferred from studies in regular swine. For example, Rendic et al. (1984) demonstrated that cimetidine and ranitidine are excellent inhibitors of the porcine MMFO *in vitro*, and is probably also inhibitory in microsomal preparations from minpigs. Walker, Bentley, and Oesch (1978) reported on epoxide hydratase activity in various species, including the pig. Depending on the substrate, the pig had activities equivalent to or greater than that of the rat. This was confirmed by Smith et al. (1984) and Watkins and Klaasen (1986). The MMFO, epoxide hydrolase, UDP-glucoronosyl transferase, *N*-acetyl transferase, glutathione *S*-transferase, and sulfotransferase activities in regular swine may be used to help infer the expected activity in minipigs until more complete and specific information appears in the literature on minipigs.

There are relatively few papers that compare *in vivo* pharmacokinetic behavior of a specific chemical in the minipig versus another animal. Schneider, Bradley and Andersen (1977) reported on the toxicology and pharmacokinetics of cyclotrimethylenetrinitramine in the rat and minipig. Rats convulsed within the first several hours after receiving this chemical, whereas minipigs convulsed 12 to 14 hours later. This is consistent with the observation that at 24 hours postdosing (100 mg/kg p.o.), the plasma levels were 3.0 µg/ml in rats and 4.7 µg/ml in minipigs. Other differences in pharmacokinetics and metabolism between the two species were described. The latent period for convulsion development was more similar between minipigs and humans than between rats and humans. The implication in this paper is that the minipig is a more suitable model for the study of the toxicity and metabolism of the nitramines than rats.

***General Toxicity Testing.*** Are minipigs an appropriate species for the general toxicity testing of new drugs and chemicals? This question is perhaps best addressed by comparing the toxicity of known chemicals in minipigs with that observed in other animals. Unfortunately, relatively few examples of the use of minipigs in a safety assessment package have been published. In one of the few such examples, Van Ryzin and Trapold (1980) published on the toxicity of proquazone (a nonsteroidal anti-inflammatory drug [NSAID]) in rats, dogs and minipigs. Rats in general are exquisitely sensitive to NSAIDs, and proquazone was no exception; dosages of 25 mg/kg/day (13 weeks) and above caused evidence of gastrointestinal (GI) toxicity. In dogs, dosages as high as 75 mg/kg were without effect, and higher dosages caused emesis, anorexia, and anemia, but no GI lesions. In a longer-term study, however, evidence of gastric damage was produced in the dog. In minipigs, dosages ranged from 6 to 94 mg/kg/day (26 weeks). Dosage-related mortality, diarrhea, and gastric ulceration was observed at all levels. In this particular example, if the minipig had been used in place of the dog, somewhat different conclusions regarding the safety of proquazone would have been reached. Generalizing from this single case, minipigs may be more similar to rats than to human beings in their response to NSAIDs.

***Dermal Toxicity.*** Although rabbits are commonly used for the assessment of primary dermal irritation, pigs have generally been considered to be better models for the more sophisticated study of dermal permeability and toxicity. As reviewed by Sambuco (1985), human and porcine skin are similar with regard to sparsity of the pelage, thickness and general morphology, epidermal cell turnover time, and size, orientation, and distribution of vessels in the skin. The particularly thin haircoat and lack of pigments of the Yucatan minipig makes it particularly ideal for dermal studies. The size of the animal also provides the additional practical advantage of abundant surface area for multiple site testing.

Sambuco (1985) has described the sunburn response of the Yucatan minipig to ultraviolet (UV) light, suggesting that this species would also make a good model in phototoxicity as well as photocontact dermatitis studies. Thirty 12-cm sites were demarcated, permitting the study of 15 different dermal dosages of UV radiation.

Mannisto and coworkers (1984) have published a series of articles on the dermal toxicity of the anthralins in the minipig. In one experiment, 24 sites per minipig were used to assess the acute dermal irritation of various concentrations to four different chemicals per site. The range of concentrations tested permitted them to calculate the median erythema concentration and median irritation concentrations with relatively few animals. They were able to show clear differences between anthralin congeners (antipsoriatic drugs) with regard to irritation. When compared to other species (mouse and guinea pig) the response of the minipig was the most similar to humans in that in both species these chemicals are delayed irritants, and several days postexposure may pass before the maximal irritant response is presented.

In a second experiment (Hanhijarvi, Nevalainen, and Mannisto, 1985), the chronic, cumulative dermal effects of anthralin chemicals were studied in minipigs. Using only 12 animals, they were able, by having 32 sites per animal, to study the effects of two different chemicals (dithranol and butantrone; both anthralins) in three different formulations at three different concentrations each. The protocol also included observations for systemic toxicity, clinical laboratory measurements, plasma drug analyses, and gross and histopathological examinations.

In a third report (very similar to the second), Hanhijarvi, Nevalainen and Mannisto (1985) clearly demonstrated that the type of vehicle can greatly influence irritation, in that dithranol was clearly more irritating when applied in paraffin that when applied in a gel. They were also able to demonstrate that although dithranol was less acutely irritating than butantrone, the cumulative irritations (mean scores at the end of six months of six times per week applications) were quite similar (Mannisto et al., 1984). There was no evidence of systemic toxicity nor of test article in plasma with either species.

***Cardiovascular Toxicity.*** In general, the published literature consistently maintains that the cardiovascular sytsems of swine and humans are very similar. For example, as reviewed by Lee (1986), swine, including minipigs, have a noticeable background incidence of atherosclerotic lesions, and that swine fed high lipid diets will develop even more extensive atherosclerotic lesions. High lipid diets will produce lesions similar to advanced atheromatous lesions seen in humans. Although few drugs or chemicals have been shown to cause atherosclerosis, this information has three general applications to toxicology and pharmacology. First, the feeding regimen of minipigs should be carefully controlled in general toxicity studies to minimize the incidence of arterial disease, especially in long-term studies. Second, the pathologist should be aware of the natural background of this disease when preparing a diagnosis. Third, the minipig could provide a convenient model for the study of atherosclerotic disease and the screening of potential therapies.

The minipig has been used to study cardiotoxicity. Van Vleet, Herman, and Ferrans (1984) reported that minipigs were the only species studied other than dogs to develop cardiac damage in response to large doses of minoxidil. In both pig and the dog, minoxidil cardiotoxicity is characterized by vascular damage (with hemorrhage in the arterial epicardium) and myocardial necrosis (mostly of the left ventricular papillary muscles). Interestingly, in the dog the atrial lesion is largely restricted to the right atrium, whereas in the pig it is restricted to the left atrium. These lesions can be produced in roughly 50% of the minipigs given 10 mg/kg of minoxidil for two days and sacrificed 48 hours after the last dose (Herman et al., 1989; Herman, Ferrans, and Young, 1988). Herman and colleagues have published extensive descriptions of minoxidil-induced lesions in minipigs in comparison to those produced in dogs (Herman, Ferrans, and Young, 1988; Herman et al., 1989). The right versus left arterial difference is believed to be due to differences in the anatomical pattern of coronary circulation between two species (Herman, Ferrans, and Young, 1988).

Minipigs are also sensitive to the cardiotoxic effect of doxorubicin. When given six intravenous injections of either 1.6 or 2.4 mg/kg of doxorubicin at 3-week intervals, minipigs develop cardiac lesions similar to those seen in dogs, rabbits and other experimental animals (Herman et al. 1989). The lesion is characterized by cytoplasmic vacuolation and varying degrees of myofibrillar degeneration and loss. Thus, the minipig is sensitive to the cardiotoxic effect of two well-known and extensively studied chemicals. Therefore, it is a suitable nonrodent species for the general assessment of cardiotoxicity.

***Advantages and Disadvantages.*** There are two disadvantages to the use of minipigs. The first is their size. Although minipigs are smaller than regular swine, at maturity they are generally larger than beagle dogs. The second is their expense: they are not only larger than dogs, but currently carry higher purchasing costs. Among the advantages are the facts that they are long-lived, cooperative animals with well-defined physiological and metabolic characteristics. As they are not popular companion animals (like dogs) or do not physically resemble humans (like monkeys), minipigs are not specifically discussed in animal "welfare" laws like the other two species. Depending on their final form, new animal welfare regulations could make the space and maintenance costs for dogs and monkeys very prohibitive. This may make minipigs increasingly more attractive as a nonrodent species for general toxicity testing.

### 16.3.4. Nonhuman Primates

Nonhuman primates are often the nonrodent species of choice for safety assessment studies. There are over 500 species of nonhuman primates that differ widely from each other in size and physical characteristics. Most of the monkeys used in experimental research belong to the suborder Anthropoidea and especially to the superfamilies of Ceboidea (marmoset, squirrel monkey) and Cercopitcoidea (macaque, papio species, rhesus). These have been popular because of (1) assumed better concordance of effects seen to those in man and (2) smaller weights (and therefore reduced compound requirement). However, predominant factors leading to a decision whether or not to select primates as the nonrodent species for safety evaluation are summarized as follows (Hobson, 2000).

### Primates are Selected for Safety Studies Because

- They are the only species which exhibit the human response to the test article.
- Due to smaller body size, they conserve rare or expensive test articles.
- They do not form neutralizing antibodies to the test article.
- They are physiologically more similar to humans than other test animals.

- Regulatory agencies require their use.
- Prior development history dictates species choice.
- Known class effects have previously been seen in primates.

**Primates are Not Selected for Safety Studies Because of**

- Perceived expense;
- Facility and logistic concerns;
- Limited supplies;
- Biosafety concerns;
- Perceived animal rights or animal welfare concerns or pressures;
- Tradition and prior development history;
- Regulatory agency direction;
- Data suggesting that other animal models are the "most sensitive species".

Tradition and cost are the two most frequently quoted reasons for selecting dogs as the second toxicology species instead of nonhuman primates. Many pharmaceutical companies, especially those that primarily work with small molecules, have many years of background data in dogs and do not choose to venture into primate research without a compelling reason to do so. Secondary concerns often center on perceived biosafety or animal rights issues. Contrary to conventional wisdom, primate studies are often more cost efficient than studies in dogs. Although the purchase cost for primates is approximately twice that of dogs, many other factors suggest that the total cost of a primate safety study may be less than the cost for a similar-sized dog study. Husbandry costs are higher in dogs because of the United States Department of Agriculture (USDA) requirement for exercise. Approximately fourfold more building space is required for a dog study due to the larger cages needed. Perhaps most important, the smaller body size of macaques means that the requirement for expensive or scarce test article in a primate study is approximately a third of that of a dog study.

**Comparison of Costs for Typical 90-Day Studies Conducted with Nonhuman Primates or Dogs**

Animal Cost (assume 40 animals)
    Cost of dogs        $40 \times \$900 = \$36,000$
    Cost of primates    $40 \times \$2200 = \$88,000$
Per diem
    Dogs           $90 \text{ days} \times \$11 \times 40 = \$39,600$
    Primates      $90 \text{ days} \times \$7 \times 40 = \$25,200$
Test article (at \$400/mg)
    Dogs           $10 \text{ kg} \times 90 \text{ days} \times 40 \text{ animals}$
                      $\times 100 \text{ µg/kg/day} = \$1,440,000$
    Primates      $4 \text{ kg} \times 90 \text{ days} \times 40 \text{ animals}$
                      $\times 100 \text{ µg/kg/day} = \$576,000$

Clearly, the amount and cost of test article and the length of the study determine which species is most cost efficient.

Because nonhuman primates are phylogenetically closer to humans than other species, there is less chance that they will recognize human protein, peptide or antibody-based biopharmaceuticals as foreign. Thus, they are often selected for safety studies of these materials. Although highly conserved proteins may not be immunogenic in lower species, clearly the formation of neutralizing antibodies to less conserved proteins during a safety study can confound experimental results (Dean et al., 1990). The formation of neutralizing antibodies to human biopharmaceuticals almost never occurs in chimpanzees, but occurs more and more frequently as the primate phylogenetic tree is descended. It is generally believed that nonhuman primates' phylogenetic difference from man is ranked as follows: great apes, baboons, other old-world primates (including macaques), and new-world primates. Clearly, as proteins are modified, they can become immunogenic in all primate species, including humans (Konrad et al., 1987).

The physiological similarity and phylogenetic proximity of nonhuman primates to humans are often cited as rationale for primate selection for safety studies; especially when mechanisms of toxicity or pharmacologic action are expected to be closely related to potential physiological reactions in humans. Likewise, species selection is often based on the demonstration of pharmacologic activity of the test article. Many biopharmaceuticals do not exhibit their intended activity in nonprimate species, whereas small molecules may have activity across all species.

Regulatory agencies sometimes suggest (read "dictate") use of primates for certain study designs or drug classes. These requirements are often a surprise to companies when they are first presented. Usually they are derived from confidential data that the regulatory agencies have reviewed. Often the regulatory bodies are privy to data that suggest that a class effect is seen in primates and not in other species, or that primates are the most sensitive species. A recent example was regulatory agency encouragement to perform cardiovascular evaluations of oligonucleotide pharmaceutical candidates in primates (Black et al., 1993, 1994). This was based on background information that suggested that oligonucleotides induced complement activation and the attendant hemodynamic and cardiovascular changes in primates but not in other species (Galbraith et al., 1994).

Animal welfare and conservative issues have frequently led to decisions to avoid primate use. Through the mid-1980s many nonhuman primates used in medical research came from wild populations. This led to strong conservationist concerns with the use of monkeys in research. Now, however, almost all nonhuman primates used in research are purpose-bred and the conservationist concern has abated. Although there is some animal rights pressure specifically directed against primate use, it is not as formidable as the well-financed and sophisticated efforts to prevent the use of cats and dogs in research. As a consequence, a few pharmaceutical companies are considering switching to nonhuman primates for their second toxicology species.

***Environmental and Dietary Requirements.*** For most nonhuman primate species, room temperatures should be maintained in the range of $75 \pm 5°F$ with a relative humidity of 40% or greater. These temperature and humidity ranges have been found to be beneficial to the prevention of pneumonia and bloody nose syndrome. A 14-h light/10-h dark cycle is used for all species of monkey (such as rhesus, cynomolgus, squirrel, and marmoset). Rooms in which monkeys are housed should have 10–15 air changes per hour and be kept under negative pressure in relation to other parts of the building. Where there is significant risk of airborne infection, it is necessary to contain infected animals in units designed to remove the air away from personnel (Mazue and Richez, 1982).

Physical comfort should be an important consideration when determining the appropriate housing for nonhuman primates. For individually housed monkeys, the floor area and height of cages should be about $0.28 \text{ cm}^2 \times 76.20$ cm for animals in the weight range of 1–3 kg and $0.40 \text{ cm}^2 \times 76.20$ cm for monkeys weighing 3–10 kg (*Guide*, 1985). Probably the most common form of commercially available housing is mobile stainless steel rack-mounted cages. Group housing of nonhuman primates used in safety studies is likely to become more common in the future as a result of the United States Department of Agriculture's new animal welfare regulations, which require that nonhuman primates have the opportunity for socialization.

Another requirement of the new animal welfare regulations is that any cage or pen in which nonhuman primates are housed must also contain toys, food, or other objects that animals can manipulate, as they would objects in their natural environment. From experience, laboratories have found that toys in themselves are not sufficient since the animals quickly lose interest. Effective enrichment materials include foraging boards (fur-covered objects under which food is buried) and puzzle feeders for more complex foraging.

In many laboratories, monkeys are often fed commercial pelleted chow *ad libitum* supplemented with fresh fruits and bread. Like humans and guinea pigs, the monkey cannot synthesize vitamin C and, thus, has a dietary requirement for this vitamin. Powdered chow is an inefficient form for feeding nonhuman primates, because a high percentage of the diet is wasted. Also, dust associated with the chow can cause respiratory problems in some species (NRC, 1978). Even with pelleted or extruded food, monkeys will waste about 50% of the ration sorting through the pellets (Mazue and Richez, 1982). Monkeys should have *ad libitum* access to water, and it is important that the device (either a water bottle equipped with a sipper tube or an automatic watering system) be fixed securely to the cage to avoid detachment by the animal.

***Common Study Protocols.*** Group sizes and numbers of animals per group for nonhuman primate toxicology studies vary slightly from country to country and from company to company; however, with the movement for international harmonization there is trend toward less variation in study design. Selection of group size is a compromise among regulatory guidelines, cost, statistical power, and conservation of animals.

An example of a protocol for a four-week safety study in cynomolgus monkeys is shown in Table 16.12. Depending on availability, cynomolgus monkeys are generally in the age range of one to three years at study start. A two- or four-week study will usually have about four animals per sex per group. For the longer-

**TABLE 16.12. Permissible Dosing Volumes for Nonhuman Primates**

| Route | Maximum Permissible Dose[a] |
| --- | --- |
| Intravenous | Varies with duration of administration and character of test article |
| Subcutaneous | 1.5 ml/site and 2–3 ml/kg |
| Intramuscular | 0.5 ml/site and 1–2 ml/kg |
| Oral/Nasogastric | 2–3 ml/kg |

[a]Values are given for single or infrequent administration. Smaller volumes are appropriate for repeated dosing.

term studies, the number of animals per group will be larger in order to include reversal animals. As with dogs and ferrets, monkeys should be selected for study use based on acceptable pretreatment body weights, clinical laboratory profiles, and physical, ECG, and ophthalmic examinations.

One aspect of study design in nonhuman primates that is not well understood is caused by the variability in the age at which monkeys undergo puberty. Although age at the onset of puberty is highly variable within macaque species, there is a remarkable correlation between body weight and sexual maturity in macaques. Rhesus females undergo menarche at $3000\pm200$ g irrespecive of age, whereas males tend to become sexually mature around 4500 g. This means that a "typical" study is initiated with sexually mature females and sexually immature males. This practice is debatable and is certainly not universally adopted. A few pharmaceutical companies require mature animals of both sexes, because sexual maturation in males occurs many months later than in females. Rearing costs are higher for males and animal numbers may be limited because the younger males may have already been sold with their female birth-year counterparts.

### General Study Activities

*Common Dosing Techniques.*  Dosing routes and permissible volumes for nonhuman primates vary between laboratories. The volume limitations from one laboratory are presented in Table 16.12.

Primates offer all of the possible dosing routes available in humans, but body size often limits dosing volumes. If volumes for subcutaneous or intramuscular injections exceed those suggested above, enzyme elevations [particularly alanine aminotransferase (ALT) and aspartate aminotransferase (AST)] are frequently observed (unpublished results). Continuous infusion techniques in alert animals are available in some laboratories either through use of programmable backpack pumps or jacket-and-tether systems (Perkin and Stejskal, 1994).

Probably the most common oral route is gavage. This procedure usually requires some degree of physical restraint of the animal (by one or more persons) while a stomach tube for dosing is inserted either orally or intranasally. Other oral dosing methods include buccal, capsule, or addition of the test compound to the drinking water. It is also possible to prepare a modified diet admixture consisting of test compound, diet meal, water, agar, and a jelling agent. This type of preparation will reduce both the feed spillage and the dust normally associated with powdered chow; however, it is susceptible to microbial growth and must be kept frozen or refrigerated (NRC, 1978).

Bolus intravenous, intramuscular, or subcutaneous injections can be administered by a single person by securing the animal's arm through the cage bars (Mazue and Richez, 1982). For safety considerations, many investigators prefer to have the animal physically restrained by a second person before the injection is given. Arterial injections (via the femoral artery) as well as limited or continuous intravenous infusion (via catheterization of the femoral or jugular vein) are other less commonly used parenteral routes in the monkey.

Other routes of administration sometimes used in monkey safety assessment studies are intravaginal dosing, topical application, inhalation, and nasal administration.

*Clinical Observations and Examinations.* As with other species, it is important to have a good understanding of the types of behaviors and clinical signs that can be seen in normal, untreated monkeys before attempting to make observations in drug-treated animals. Cage-side observations in the monkey should be conducted at least two times daily to monitor general health and behavior. The first observation should be made before cages are cleaned in the morning, and the floors of the cages should be critically examined for signs of blood, abnormal feces, or vomitus. Clinical signs to which investigators should pay particular attention include reduced activity and lethargy, excessive excitation, reduced feed consumption, vomiting, and abnormal feces. If at all possible, the same people should work on a study for its entirety. The behavior of more timorous monkeys can be affected by the presence of unfamiliar personnel, resulting in undesirable clinical signs such as a loss of appetite and lethargy (Evans et al., 1982). To circumvent these kinds of problems, isolated observation using a video camera system may be a preferable approach.

Physical examinations of monkeys are usually conducted no more than once a week and generally consist of the measurement of rectal temperature, observation of general demeanor, palpation of the head, thorax, and abdomen, examination of eyes, ears, and bodily orifices, as well as testing of the pupillary and patellar reflexes.

*Feed Consumption.* As mentioned previously, monkeys tend to scatter their feed, which can make feed consumption difficult to measure. In one laboratory feed consumption in monkeys was successfully monitored by using the larger chow biscuits and counting the number of biscuits (or fractions of biscuits) consumed over two consecutive 24-h periods.

*Electrocardiograms and Cardiovascular Measurements.* The availability of excellent GLP-validated telemetry systems has led to recent increases in the number of cardiovasular safety pharmacology studies conducted in primates. In addition, telemetry is now sometimes included as a design element in standard safety studies. Because of the ability to collect large amounts of high quality data over an extended time, total numbers of animals can often be reduced by appropriate application of telemetry. Indeed, it is often difficult to avoid statistical and reporting problems caused by the temptation to collect too much data using telemetry. Implanted transmitters can function continuously for up to a year without battery replacement while providing data such as blood pressure, heart rate, electrocardiogram (ECG), body temperature, and activity.

For safety assessment studies, it is preferable to record monkey ECGs in the conscious animal, which, if using standard ECG techniques, requires chairing the animal. Electrocardiographic leads used include II, aVL and V10. To help reduce emotional tachycardia, it is recommended that there be pretreatment habituation (no more than 10–30 minutes at least twice before study start) to the chairing and attachment of the surface electrodes. Probably the best and least stressful approach to monitoring ECG activity in conscious monkeys is automatic monitoring using a biotelemetry system. With this system, a transmitter, surgically implanted subcutaneously along the dorsal midline, broadcasts a radio signal encoding the ECG to a receiver mounted on top of the animal's cage, and a computer records the signal at 2-min intervals (Line et al., 1989).

*Blood and Urine Collections.* For blood collection, the rhesus can be bled from the saphenous or femoral vein. For female rhesus monkeys, it may not be possible to use the saphenous vein because of the swelling of the sex skin (i.e., the edematous thickening and reddening of the skin over the external genital region, rump, and tail that often extends down the leg to the knee). For the cynomolgus and squirrel monkeys, the veins are very small, and the femoral vein is usually the one of choice. Depending on the species, 5 to 20 ml may be collected. However, experimental designs in primates are often constrained by the limitations in the amount of blood that can be safely and humanely obtained during the course of a study (Fuller et al., 1992). With increasing emphasis on obtaining toxicokinetic data during safety studies, these constraints have become more vexing. One laboratory uses a guideline for maximum blood withdrawal of 10 ml/kg/day (Heiser, 1970). More blood can be collected, but hematocrits should be monitored (Schalm, 1975). These amounts do not approach maximum amounts allowable for humane considerations, but do represent the maximum that can be collected without causing more than slight decreases in hematologic parameters (notably hematocrit, hemoglobin, and red cell count). Recently, new catheter material and vascular access ports have been developed which permit long-term frequent blood collection without the catheter clotting and emboli problems experienced in the past. We have found that the new vascular access ports remain patent for over a year with routine maintenance. Vascular access ports are particularly useful in primates where frequent samples are required because blood sample collection through ports appears to be far less stressful than collection by needle stick. They have also been found useful when evaluating anticoagulant test articles because venipuncture is contraindicated. Sample quality is also superior with ported collections.

Urine collection in nonhuman primates can be measured using either a metabolism cage or a collection pan (equipped with a screen to catch the feces), which is inserted under the floor grid of the home cage. The advantage of the latter system is that the animals do not need to be removed from their home cage; however, care needs to be taken to avoid contamination of the urine with drinking water.

***Advantages and Disadvantages.*** Advantages of using monkeys in safety assessment studies include their phylogenetic proximity, as well as their physiological, behavioral, and, often, metabolic similarities, to humans (Table 16.13). An example is the similarity between the ovarian cycle of female monkeys and women (Mazue and Richez, 1982), which makes the monkey the ideal animal model for reproductive studies. Another advantage associated with most species of monkeys used in safety assessment studies is that they are much smaller than nonrodents such as the dog and, thus like the ferret, require less test compound.

Disadvantages associated with the use of monkeys include their availability and cost. Nonhuman primates are either wild caught or laboratory bred, and there are limitations as to the number of animals that will be available from either source at any given time. Even more so than with the dog, careful advance planning is needed to ensure adequate animals will be available to the investigator. Monkeys are also considerably more expensive than many other nonrodent species; for example, the cost of a cynomolgus monkey is at least 10 to 100 times more expensive than the dog and ferret, respectively. Other disadvantages are the great strength and emotionality of monkeys, which make them more difficult to work with than other nonrodent species such as the dog.

Finally, the most significant disadvantage to working with monkeys is the serious spontaneous diseases they can carry that are transmissible, and often life-threatening, to humans. An example of one such disease is *Herpesvirus simiae* (B-virus). B-virus is widespread, especially amongst wild-caught, and to some extent laboratory-bred, rhesus monkeys, including cynomolgus monkeys. Human exposure to B-virus occurs during handling of monkeys and monkey tissues (via contact with tears, blood, or saliva of infected animals) and is associated with a high incidence of human mortality (DiGiacomo and Shah, 1972). Other serious-to-very-serious diseases that can be transmitted from monkeys to humans are Marburg disease, viral hepatitis, tuberculosis, and monkeypox.

**TABLE 16.13. Use of the Nonhuman Primate in Safety Assessment Studies**

*Advantages*
Small size of many species
Less test material needed than for other nonrodent species
Physiological, behavioral, and often, metabolic similarities to man

*Disadvantages*
Limited availability
Cost
Need to develop environmental enrichment program
High potential for spontaneous diseases

## 16.4. STATISTICS IN LARGE ANIMAL STUDIES

Large animal toxicology studies, typically ranging from 14 days to generally a maximum of 26 weeks, pose different types of statistical problems and open up new possibilities in terms of statistical evaluations. Standard statistical methods used for chronic toxicology studies, such as one-way designs, often do not provide any meaningful insights because of small sample sizes used in large animal studies. The designs for such studies are, generally speaking, nonoptimal. As a consequence, an investigator must attempt to use optimal statistical methods to evaluate such studies. Fortunately, for many of the relevant parameters for such studies, there are fewer-to-none dropouts (if one is careful) and there are repeated measurements on the same parameters of interest, both pre- and posttreatment intervals. Optimality of statistical methods for such studies is then achieved by making use of the longitudinal observations in the analysis. The optimality can be further enhanced by introducing sex as a factor in the evaluation of the data in many such studies.

Many of the standard assumptions in both parametric and distribution-free statistical methods cannot be meaningfully tested in large animal studies because of extremely small sample sizes (which is not necessarily dictated by scientific doctrine, but by economic and minimum regulatory requirements). Fortunately, by making use of solid biological as well as statistical judgements, we seem to have made many discoveries in terms of human safety and efficacy in large animal toxicology.

Instead of conventional textbook-type layout, this discussion will try to focus on various issues in large animal toxicology experiments with plausible examples. One word of caution before we get deeper into our discussion: as in most areas of applied statistics, there really is no gospel in what we will be discussing. Many statisticians may have variations of the theme to be brought out here.

### 16.4.1. Reasons For Small Sample Sizes in Large Animal Toxicology

The following are some of the main reasons for having only three to five dogs or monkeys per sex in a typical large animal study:

1. These studies are very expensive. A typical full-fledged study may cost as much as $30,000 to $500,000 (for 13 weeks).
2. There is tremendous pressure from the animal rights groups to look for alternatives, rather than using dogs and monkeys for investigating purposes.
3. Regulatory agencies throughout the world recognize these two facts and recommend small sample sizes as minimum requirements. As a consequence, the pharmaceutical and chemical industries are reluctant to expand the scopes of such studies.

### 16.4.2. Cross Sectional or Longitudinal Analysis?

Many of the studies we deal with have various parameters, such as body weight, food consumption, clinical chemistry, and hematology, that are collected repeatedly at various pretreatment and posttreatment intervals. Unfortunately, many investigators in the field do not take advantage of this important design feature in such studies. Instead, one finds the literature is full of simple parametric or distribution-free one-way techniques such as Student's $t$-test, Wilcoxon–Mann–Whitney Rank Test, one-way analysis of variance (ANOVA) methods, and the like being used widely, sometimes without satisfaction. The argument is given that "although there is apparent biological effect (or lack of it), because of small sample sizes and poor statistics, no significant effects can be determined from these data," or something like that. If truth be known, the small sample size part of this argument may be correct; however, no attempts were made to optimize on the statistical methods above using the various pieces of the particular design. The repeated-sampling part of the design (repeated measures) is very important for such studies and therefore should be incorporated in the analysis of the data. After all, design of experiment and analysis of data are inseperable. There are advantages and disadvantages of such analyses (the advantages generally outweigh the disadvantages) as described in the following lists.

### 16.4.3. Repeated Measures: Advantages

1. Between-subject variations are excluded from the experimental and stochastic errors.
2. Only the within-subject variation is included in the mean square error (MSE) term.
3. Each subject becomes its own control.
4. Economizes on the number of subjects in an experiment.
5. Minimizes both type I (false positive) and type II (false negative) error rates, thereby increasing power of the test statistic to be employed while decreasing inconsistent significant effects.

### 16.4.4. Repeated Measures: Disadvantages

1. Order of the treatment may cause interference which can be avoided by appropriate randomization.
2. There is the possibility of carry-over effects. This is more crucial in Latin square and other cross-over designs. Knowledge of pharmacokinetics and metabolism of a compound under study generally helps in avoiding this problem.
3. Exact permutation and distribution-free techniques are not as widely developed as in the cases of one-way methods.
4. Power and sample size computations are a little more difficult to compute than for one-way designs.
5. Generally requires computers for performing the analyses using specialized software (not a major issue in most societies nowadays).
6. It is a little more difficult to interpret the results than their one-way counterparts.

### 16.4.5. Common Practices in Large Animal Toxicology

As mentioned earlier, older (and some newer) literature in large animal toxicology is full of two-sample, one-way parametric, and distribution-free techniques. Some of the newer works use repeated-measures and even multivariate techniques. The following is a brief exposé of various methods used in the field.

1. One-way analysis of variance/covariance/regression and preplanned and *post hoc* group comparisons.
2. Two-sample Student's *t* test, Wilcoxian–Mann–Whitney Rank Test, and so on.
3. Graphical display of response over time (as two- or three-dimensional plots).
4. Univariate repeated measures analysis of variance–covariance techniques.
5. Multivariate analysis of variance–covariance (MANOVA/MANCOVA) techniques.

We will skip (1) and (2) above as methods not to be preferred as global analyses. Graphical displays have tremendous values as exploratory data analysis (EDA) techniques with the type of data one encounters in these studies. For formal analyses, one could weigh univariate repeated and other factorial designs against their true multivariate counterparts.

### 16.4.6. Univariate (Repeated-Measures) Techniques: Advantages

1. Easier to compute.
2. Less susceptible to violation of normality.
3. Exact and distribution-free tests are easier to compute.
4. Require smaller sample sizes; there is more power.
5. Very few test statistics to deal with: classical ANOVA $F$; Greenhouse–Geisser and Huynh–Feldt adjusted $df$, and ANOVA $F$.
6. Biologically meaningful and easier to resolve contrasts and multiple comparison tests.
7. Missing values are easily handled.

### 16.4.7. Univariate (Repeated Measures) Techniques: Disadvantages

1. Susceptible to heteroscedasticity (heterogencity of variances).
2. Less fancy! (compared to multivariate techniques).

### 16.4.8. Multivariate Techniques: Advantages

1. Less susceptible to heteroscedasticity.
2. Handles multiple dependent variables.
3. Real fancy! (compared to univariate ANOVA/ANCOVA techniques).

### 16.4.9. Multivariate Techniques: Disadvantages

1. More susceptible to violation of normality.
2. Less power than univariate ANOVA, particularly with small sample sizes.
3. Contrasts and multiple comparisons are difficult to construct.
4. Missing values are more difficult to handle.
5. Computationally more difficult (a mute point nowadays with personal computers).
6. Too many test statistics, sometimes giving contradictory answers, to deal with.

### 16.4.10. Some Other Design Factors to be Considered in Analysis

Most of the toxicological studies are designed to evaluate efficacy and safety in both sexes. With small sample sizes, one can increase the power-efficiency of the particular test statistic by including sex as a factor in a full factorial analysis (not combining the two sexes) where appropriate. The factorial analysis will reveal whether there is any need to separate the two sexes. The other design fact that should be weighed carefully is the presence of any concomitant variables or covariates. For example, most large animal studies will involve collection of data both prior to the beginning of the experiments as well as after. Thus pretreatment values and other characteristic control variables (body weights, for example) may be important covariates in the analysis of the data. There are both advantages and disadvantages in including covariates in the analysis.

### 16.4.11. Covariates: Advantages

1. Increases precision of an analysis (indirect or statistical control of variability).
2. Correction of bias.
3. Elimination of extraneous variation in the data.

### 16.4.12. Covariates: Disadvantages

1. Unequal intra- and intergroup covariate slopes may actually introduce bias as a consequence.
2. Nonlinearity of covariate slopes may have the same effect as in (1).
3. In some cases the covariates may be affected by treatment.

An example is shown in Table 16.14. A two-factor analysis of variance for the covariate, as shown in Table 16.15, clearly indicates that the two sexes started with approximately the same means ($p = 0.5598$). Moreover, there were no differences between the group means in either sex as indicated by the large tail probabilities for treatment ($p = 0.8823$) and sex$\times$treatment interaction ($p = 0.6532$). These facts justify using sex as a factor in the analysis, as was done here.

**TABLE 16.14. Example 1**

| Sex | Control | | Treatment 1 | | Treatment 2 | |
|---|---|---|---|---|---|---|
| | Covariate | Variate | Covariate | Variate | Covariate | Variate |
| Male | 40 | 95 | 30 | 85 | 50 | 90 |
| | 35 | 80 | 40 | 100 | 40 | 85 |
| | 40 | 95 | 45 | 85 | 40 | 90 |
| | 50 | 105 | 40 | 90 | 30 | 80 |
| | 45 | 100 | 40 | 90 | 40 | 85 |
| Raw mean | 42.0 | 95.0 | 39.0 | 90.0 | 40.0 | 86.0 |
| SD | 5.7 | 9.4 | 5.8 | 6.1 | 7.1 | 4.2 |
| Female | 50 | 100 | 50 | 100 | 45 | 95 |
| | 30 | 95 | 30 | 90 | 30 | 85 |
| | 35 | 95 | 40 | 95 | 25 | 75 |
| | 45 | 110 | 45 | 90 | 50 | 105 |
| | 30 | 88 | 40 | 95 | 35 | 85 |
| Raw Mean | 38.0 | 97.6 | 41.0 | 94.0 | 37.0 | 89.0 |
| SD | 9.1 | 8.1 | 7.4 | 4.2 | 10.4 | 11.4 |

There are various other ways of examining the variate in question in this case. Let us first examine simple one-way ANOVA of the variate by sex as in Table 16.16. In neither of the two cases was there any indication of significant treatment differences at any reasonable level. Because the two sexes did not show any pretreatment differences based on the two-factor analysis of the covariate, let us combine the two sexes and analyze the data by one-way ANOVA as in Table 16.17. In this case, because of the increased sample sizes for combining the two sexes, there was indication of some treatment differences ($p = 0.0454$). Unfortunately, this analysis assumes that because there were no pretreatment differences between the two sexes, that pattern will hold during the posttreatment period. That often may not be the case because of biological reasons.

Let us now investigate whether there is any major sex difference in the effect on the variate by a two-factor ANOVA as in Table 16.18.

**TABLE 16.15. Two-factor Analysis of Variance for the Covariate**

| Source | Sum of Squares | *DF* | Mean Squares | *F* | Tail Probability |
|---|---|---|---|---|---|
| Mean | 46807.50000 | 1 | 46807.50000 | 785.58 | 0.0000 |
| Sex | 20.83333 | 1 | 20.83333 | 0.35 | 0.5598 |
| Treatment | 15.00000 | 2 | 7.50000 | 0.13 | 0.8823 |
| Sex×Treatment | 51.66667 | 2 | 25.83333 | 0.43 | 0.6532 |
| Error | 1430.00000 | 24 | 59.58333 | | |

**TABLE 16.16. One-Way Analysis of Variance of the Variate of Sex**

| Source | Sum of Squares | DF | Mean Squares | F | Tail Probability |
|---|---|---|---|---|---|
| | | | Males | | |
| Mean | 122,401.66667 | 1 | 122,401.66667 | 2576.88 | 0.0000 |
| Treatment | 203.33333 | 2 | 101.66667 | 2.14 | 0.1603 |
| Error | 570.00000 | 12 | 47.50000 | | |
| | | | Females | | |
| Mean | 131,227.26667 | 1 | 131,227.26667 | 1841.36 | 0.0000 |
| Treatment | 186.53333 | 2 | 93.26667 | 1.31 | 0.3061 |
| Error | 855.20000 | 12 | 71.26667 | | |

**TABLE 16.17. One-way Analysis of Variance for Combined Sexes**

| Source | Sum of Squares | DF | Mean Squares | F | Tail Probability |
|---|---|---|---|---|---|
| Mean | 253,552.13333 | 1 | 253,552.13333 | 4549.999 | 0.0000 |
| Treatment | 387.26667 | 2 | 193.63333 | 3.47 | 0.454 |
| Error | 1504.60000 | 27 | 55.72593 | | |

**TABLE 16.18. Two-Factor Analysis of Variance with Sex as a Factor**

| Source | Sum of Squares | DF | Mean Squares | F | Tail Probability |
|---|---|---|---|---|---|
| Mean | 253,552.13333 | 1 | 253,552.13333 | 4269.75 | 0.0000 |
| Sex | 76.80000 | 1 | 76.80000 | 1.29 | 0.2667 |
| Treatment | 387.26667 | 2 | 193.63333 | 3.26 | 0.0559 |
| Sex × Treatment | 2.60000 | 2 | 1.30000 | 0.02 | 0.9784 |
| Error | 125.20000 | 24 | 59.38333 | | |

The above analysis establishes that there was no significant sex difference, as indicated by the tail probabilities for sex ($p = 0.2667$) and sex × treatment interaction ($p = 0.9784$). There was also some indication that there may have been some treatment effect across the treatment groups in both sexes ($p = 0.0559$). Examination of the variate means indicated that both sexes seemed to have lower means than their respective controls. The picture was clouded by the fact that there was a similar slightly lower tendency, though not very consistent, in the covariate means as well. Under this circumstance, it is more appropriate to take both the covariate and the variate into any optimal analysis. Table 16.19 shows an analysis of covariance for the factorial model.

As the ANCOVA table indicates, there was definite significant treatment effect ($p = 0.0104$), but this effect was not sex specific because there was no significant

**TABLE 16.19. Analysis of Covariance of the Factorial Model**

| Source | Sum of Squares | DF | Mean Squares | F | Tail Probability |
|---|---|---|---|---|---|
| Mean | 147.42310 | 1 | 147.42310 | 5.65 | 0.0262 |
| Sex | 292.81064 | 2 | 146.40532 | 5.61 | 0.0104 |
| Treatment | 14.41235 | 2 | 7.20617 | 0.28 | 0.7613 |
| Sex × Treatment | 824.75245 | 1 | 824.75245 | 31.59 | 0.0000 |
| Error | 600.44755 | 23 | 26.10642 | | |

| | Control | Treatment 1 | Treatment 2 |
|---|---|---|---|
| | Adjusted cell means and standard errors (males) | | |
| Mean | 93.10140 | 90.37972 | 85.62028 |
| Standard error | 2.30985 | 2.28601 | 2.28601 |
| | Adjusted cell means and standard errors (females) | | |
| Mean | 98.73916 | 92.86084 | 90.89860 |
| Standard error | 2.29398 | 2.29398 | 2.30985 |

sex × treatment interaction ($p = 0.7613$). Furthermore, there was a significant difference between the two sexes in terms of magnitude but not in the direction of the effect. These findings are apparent in the covariate-adjusted means in all groups in both sexes. The magnitude of the treatment effect became amplified by introducing the covariate in the model. As can be seen from the two ANOVA and ANCOVA tables above, despite the fact that the ANCOVA error term lost one degree of freedom ($df = 23$) as opposed to the ANOVA error term ($df = 24$), the former gains some edge over the latter because of increased precision. Precision in this context is defined as the ratio between the MSEs of ANOVA and ANCOVA. For this example,

$$\text{Precision}(1/\text{MSE}_{\text{ANCOVA}})/(1/\text{MSE}_{\text{ANOVA}})$$
$$= (\text{MSE}_{\text{ANOVA}}/\text{MSE}_{\text{ANCOVA}})$$
$$= 59.38333/26.10642 \sim 2.3$$

In other words, we have gained about 2.3-fold precision by ANCOVA over ANOVA in resolving treatment effect.

With the advent of powerful personal computers and the availability of sophisticated "do-it-all" statistical packages, there is a trend among nonstatisticians (even some statisticians) to accept the results from these packages without contemplating twice. Many of these packages have flexible features that allow one to perform different types of analyses with the same data set, inappropriately or appropriately sometimes. What popular statistical packages give is not necessarily correct statistics, or they may not be correct under specific designs. Some programs, for example BMDP's 2V (1992), have "intelligence" built into them whereby they can identify the design based on the data matrix. By following the data matrix setup specified in the manual correctly, one can simply press the button and get the appropriate analysis needed. On the other hand, incorrect specification of the data matrix will produce incorrect results (although some programs, such as 2V, will often give an error message or prompt to make sure one wants what one is asking for; some, such as SAS's PROC GLM, may not, and give results that are not even remotely related to the design). In other words, one must know some statistics and must be well versed in the features of the particular package before using them. The one-time famous mathematician-statistician-composer-pianist-singer-producer-recording artist Tom Leher (1959), in one of his famous monologues, said, "Life is a sewer; what one gets out of it depends on what one puts into it." Statistical packages are exactly like that.

### 16.4.13. Missing Values

All investigators know that missing values are a nuisance. They also create statistical nightmares. Classical statistical techniques were not geared towards having missing values in experiments. Unfortunately, in real life situations, it just happens. Animals may die, or are censored for various reasons. There are various techniques of calculating missing values for specific designs (Miller, 1981) just as there are for extreme values or outliers (SAS, 1996). In neither case is there any unique way of handling them that is completely agreed upon by statisticians. One should remember that every time a missing value is computed and used in statistical analyses, one looses a degree of freedom. In large animal toxicology, with small sampling sizes, one must be very careful about dealing with missing values. In a repeated-measures analysis, if one observation is missing from an animal during one interval, classical techniques automatically will exclude observations from that animal for all remaining intervals. Newer techniques based on regression or imputation have been developed in recent years and have been implemented in popular packages such as BMDP (5V) or SAS (PROC MIXED). Within a single package, there may be various techniques based on assumptions on covariance structures (unstructured, compound symmetry, etc.) and statistical algorithms (maximum likelihood, restricted minimum likelihood, etc.). The results sometimes could be very different under the same assumptions and algorithms. As a result, given the same compound symmetry assumption and using the same restricted maximum likelihood (REML) algorithm, two well-known programs give different quantitative results. These methods are still experimental in nature and should not be taken for granted. Actually, the BMDP manual clearly warns users about the nature of this method. Consequently, the best way to avoid confusion is to try to make sure that missing values do not occur in key parameters in large animal studies (Thakur, 2000).

## 16.5. SUMMARY

While there are advantages and disadvantages associated with all three nonrodent species, the dog is probably the nonrodent species most frequently used in safety assessment studies. This is because dogs are relatively docile and even tempered, they are generally more easy to obtain and relatively less expensive than monkeys, they carry fewer serious diseases than the ferret and the monkey, and they have a more extensive historical data base in safety studies. It should be noted, however, that if the technical and health problems associated with the ferret can be overcome, its small size in terms of compound requirements, cost, and housing may make it an ideal nonrodent species for future use in safety assessment studies.


## REFERENCES

Andrews, P.L.R., Bower, A.J. and Illman, O. (1979). Some aspects of the physiology and anatomy of the cardiovascular system of the ferret, *Mustela putorius furo. Lab. Anim.* 13: 215–220.

Barnett, J. and Hensworth, P. (1986). The impact of handling and environmental factors on the stress response and its consequences in swine. *Lab. Anim. Sci.* 36: 366–369.

Black, L.E., DeGeorge, J.J., Cavagnaro, J.A., Jordan, A. and Ahn. C.H. (1993). Regulatory considerations for evaluating the pharmacology and toxicology of antisense drugs. *Antisense Res. Dev.* 3: 399–404.

Black, L.E., Farrelly, J.G., Cavagnero, J.A., Ahn, C.H., DeGeorge, J.J., Taylor, A.S., DeFelice, A.F. and Jordan, A. (1994). Regulatory considerations for oligonucleotide drugs: Updated recommendations for pharmacology and toxicology studies. *Antisense Res. Dev.* 4: 299–301.

Brechbuler, T., Kaeslin, M. and Wyler, F. (1984). Reference values of various blood constituents in young minipigs. *J. Clin. Chem. Clin. Biochem.* 22: 301–304.

Burks, M., Tumbleson, M., Hicklin, K., Hutcheson, D. and Middleton, C. (1977). Age and sex related changes of hematologic parameters in Sinclair (S-1) miniature swine. *Growth* 41: 51–62.

Campbell, S.A., Hughes, H.C., Griffin, H.E., Landis, M.S. and Mallon, F.M. (1988). Some effects of limited exercise on purpose-bred beagles. *Amer. J. Vet. Res.* 49: 1298–1301.

Clausing, P., Beitz, H., Gericke, S. and Solecki, S. (1986). On the usefulness of minipigs in toxicology testing of pesticides. *Arch Toxicol.* 9 (Suppl.): 225–271.

Dean, J.H., Cornacoff, J.B., Labrie, T. and Barbolt, T.A. (1990). Assessment of immune responses in rodents and non-human primates—Implications in preclinical evaluation of proteins. In *Preclinical Evaluation of Peptides and Recombinant Proteins*, (Sundwall, A. et al., Eds.) Malmo. Skogs Grafiska AB, Stockholm, Sweden, pp. 23–34.

Detweiler, D.K. (1980). The use of electrocardiography in toxicological studies with beagle dogs. In: *Cardiac Toxicity*, CRC Press, Boca Raton, FL.

Detweiler, D.K., Patterson, D. F., Buchanan, J.N. and Knight, D.H. (1979). The cardiovascular system. In: *Canine Medicine*, Vol. 2 (Catcott, E.J., Ed.). American Veterinary Publications, Santa Barbara, CA.

DiGiacomo, R.F. and Shah, K.V. (1972). Virtual absence of infection with *Herpesvirus simiae* in colony-reared rhesus monkeys (*Macaca mulatta*) with a literature review on antibody prevalence in natural and laboratory populations. *Lab. Anim. Sci.* 27: 61–67.

Earl, F.L., Miller, E. and Van Loon, E.J. (1973). Teratogenic research in beagle dogs and miniature swine. *The Laboratory Animal in Drug Testing: Fifth Symposium*, Internal Committee on Laboratory Animals (Spiegel, H., Ed.). pp. 233–247.

Ellegaard, L., Jorgensen, K.D., Klastbruck, S., Hansen, A.K. and Svendsen, O. (1995). Haematologic and clinical chemical values in three- and six-month old Göttinger minipigs. *Scand J. Lab Anim. Sci.* 22: 239–248.

Evans, R.H. (1982). *Nonhuman Primates.* Ralston Purina Co., St. Louis, MO.

Fox, J.G. (1988). *Biology and Diseases of the Ferret.* Lea and Febiger, Philadelphia.

Freudenthal, R., Leber, P., Emmerling, D., Kerchner, G. and Campbell, D. (1976). Characterization of the hepatic microsomal mixed-function oxidase system in miniature pigs. *Drug Metab. Dispos.* 4: 25–27.

Fuller, G.B., Hobson, W.C., Renquist, D.M., Port, C.D. and Chengelis, C.P. (1992). Nonhuman primates. In: *Animal Models in Toxicology,* (Gad, S.C. and Chengelis, C.P., Eds.), Marcel Dekker, New York, pp. 675–735.

Gad, S.C. (2000a). Pigs and ferrets as models in toxicology and biological safety assessment. *Int. J. Toxicol.* 19: 149–168.

Gad, S.C. (2000b). Large animal toxicology: Introduction and general principles. *Int. J. Toxicol.* 19: 129–132.

Gad, S.C. and Chengelis, C.P. (1992). *Animal Models in Toxicology.* Marcel Dekker, New York.

Galbraith, W.M., Hobson, W.C., Giclas, P.C., Schechter, P.J. and Agrawal, S. (1994). Complement activation and hemodynamic changes following intravenous administration of phosphorothioate oligonucleotides in the monkey. *Antisense Res. Dev.* 4: 201–206.

*Guide for the Care and Use of Laboratory Animals.* (1985). U.S. Department of Health and Human Services, NIH Publication No. 86–23. Washington, D.C.

Gulamhusein, A.P., Harrison–Sage, C., Beck, F. and Al-Alousi, A. (1980). Salicylate-induced teratogenesis in the ferret. *Life Sci.* 27: 1799–1805.

Haggerty, G.C., Miller, G., Port, C. and Gad, S. (1989). *Four–week oral toxicity study of diclofenac in the ferret.* Presented at the National Meeting of the American College of Toxicology, Williamsburg, Virginia.

Hanhijarvi, H., Nevalainen, T. and Mannisto, P. (1985). A six–month dermal irritation test with anthralins in the Göttinger miniature swine. *Arch. Toxicol,* 8 (Suppl.): 463–468.

Hart, J.E. (1986). The ferret as a replacement for the dog in toxicity studies. *Anim. Technol.* 37: 201–206.

Heiser, H.J. (1970). *Atlas of Comparative Hematology.* Academic Press, New York.

Herman, E., Ferrans, V. and Young, R. (1988). Examination of minoxidil-induced acute cardiotoxicity in miniature swine. *Toxicology* 48: 41–51.

Herman, E., Ferrans, V., Young, R. and Balazs, T. (1989). A comparative study in minoxidil-induced myocardial lesions in beagle dogs and miniature swine. *Toxicol. Pathol.* 17: 189–191.

Hoar, R.M. (1984). Use of ferrets in toxicity testing. *J. Amer. Coll. Toxicol.* 3: 325–329.

Hobson, W. (2000). Safety assessment studies in nonhuman primates. *Int. J. Toxicol.* 19: 141–147.

Hunsaker, H., Norden, S. and Allen, K. (1984). An inexpensive caging method for miniature swine suitable for trace-element studies. *Lab Animal Sci.* 2: 386–387.

Hutcheson, D., Tumbleson, M, and Middleton, C. (1979). Serum electrolyte concentrations in Sinclair (S-1) miniature swine from 1 through 36 months of age. *Growth* 43: 62–70.

Jackson, R.K., Kieffer, V.A., Sauber, J.J. and King, G.L. (1988). A tether-restraint system for blood collection from ferrets. *Lab. Anim. Sci.* 38: 625–628.

Khan, M. (1984). Minipig: Advantages and disadvantages as a model in toxicity testing, *J. Am. Coll. Toxicol.* 3: 337–342.

Koch, W., Windt, H., Walles, M., Borlak, J. and Clausing, P. (2001). Inhalation Studies with the Göttinger Minipig, *Inhalation Toxicology* 13: 249–259.

Lee, K. (1986). Swine as animal models in cardiovascular research, *Swine Biomed. Res.* 3: 1481–1496.

Lehrer, T. (1959). *An Evening Wasted with Tom Lehrer.* Lehrer Records TL202.

Line, S.W., Morgan, K.N., Markowitz, H. and Strong, S. (1989). Influence of cage size on heart rate and behavior in rhesus monkeys. *Amer. J. Vet. Res.* 50: 1523–1526.

Mannisto, P., Havas, A., Haasio, K., Hahnijarvi, H. and Mustakallio, K. (1984). Skin irritation by dithranol (anthralin) and its 10-aceyl analogues in three animal models. *Contact Dermatitis* 10: 140–145.

Mazue, G. and Richez, P. (1982). Problems in utilizing monkeys in toxicology. In: *Animals in Toxicological Research* (Bartosek, I., Ed.) Raven Press, New York, pp. 147–163.

Mclain, D., McCartney, M., Giovanetto, S., Martis, L., Greener, Y. and Youkilis, E. (1987). Assessment of the subchronic intravenous toxicity and disposition of ($^{14}$C) Acrolein in the rat and the acute and subchronic toxicity in ferrets. *Toxicologist* 7: 208.

Miller, R.G., Jr. (1981). *Simultaneous Statistical Inference*, 2nd ed. Springer, New York.

Moody, K.D., Bowman, T.A. and Lang, C.M. (1985). Laboratory management of the ferret for biomedical research. *Lab. Anim. Sci.* 35: 272–279.

Morton, C. and Morton, F. (1985). *Ferrets: A Complete Pet Owner's Manual* (Vriends, M.M., Consult. Ed.). Barron's Educational Series, Hauppauge, NY.

Mueller, D., Nelles, J., Deparde, E. and Arni, P. (1980). The activity of S-9 liver fractions from seven species in salmonella/mammalian-microsome mutagenicity tests. *Mutat. Res.* 70: 279–300.

National Research Council (NRC). (1978). *Nutrient Requirements of Nonhuman Primates.* Panel on Nonhuman Primate Nutrition, National Research Council, Washington, D.C.

National Research Council (NRC). (1985). *Nutrient Requirements of Dogs.* Subcommittee on Dog Nutrition, National Research Council, National Academy Press, Washington, D.C.

National Research Council (NRC). (1998). *Use of Laboratory Animals in Biomedical and Behavioral Research.* Commission on Life Sciences, National Research Council, National Academy Press, Washington, D.C.

Norris, W. P., Poole, C.M., Frye, R.J. and Kretz, N.D. (1968). *A Study of Thermoregulatory Capabilities of Normal, Aged and Irradiated Beagles.* Argonne National Laboratory, IL, pp. 166–169.

Oldigs, B. (1986). Effects of internal factors upon hematological and clinical chemical parameters in the Göttinger miniature pig. *Swine Biomed. Res.* 2: 809–813.

Olson, H., Betton, G., Robinson, D., Karluss, T., Monro, A., Kolaja, G., Lilly, P., Sanders, J., Sipes, G., Bracken, W., Dorato, M., Van Deun, K., Smith, P., Berger, B. and Heller, A. (2000). Concordance of the toxicity of pharmaceuticals in humans and in animals, *Reg. Tox. Pharmacol.* 32: 56–67.

Panepinto, L. (1986). Laboratory methodology and management of swine in biomedical research. *Swine Biomed. Res.* 1: 97–109.

Panepinto, L. and Phillips, R. (1986). The Yucatan miniature pig: Characterization and utilization in biomedical research. *Lab. Animal Sci.* 36: 344–347.

Parsons, A. and Wells, R. (1986). Serum biochemistry of healthy Yucatan miniature pigs. *Lab. Animal Sci.* 36: 428–430.

Peggins, J., Shipley, L. and Weiner, M. (1984). Characterization of age-related changes in hepatic drug metabolism in miniature swine. *Drug Metab. Dispos.* 12: 379–381.

Perkin, C.J. and Stejskal, R. (1994). Intravenous infusion in dogs and primates. *J. Am. Col. Toxicol.* 13: 40–47.

Phillips, R. and Tumbleson, M. (1986). Models. *Swine Biomed. Res.* 1: 437–440.

Radin, M., Weiser, M. and Frettman, M. (1986). Hematologic and serum biochemical values for Yucatan miniature swine. *Lab Anim. Sci.* 36: 425–427.

Rendic, S., Ruf, S., Weber, P. and Kajfez, F. (1984). Cimetidine and ranitidine: Their interaction with human and pig liver microsomes and with purified cytochrome P-450. *Eur. J. Drug Metab. Pharmacokinet.* 9: 195–200.

Rettie, A., Bogucki, B., Lim, I. and Meier, P. (1990). Steroselective sulfadioxidation of a series of alkyl P-tolyl sulfides by microsomal and purified flavin-containing monooxygenases. *Mol. Pharmacol.* 37: 643–651.

Sambuco, P. (1985). Miniature swine as an animal model in photodermatology: Factors influencing sunburn cell formation. *Photodermatology* 2: 144–150.

Schalm, D.W. (1975). Materials and methods for the study of the blood including brief comments on factors to be considered in interpretation. In *Veterinary Hematology* (Jain, N.C. Carroll, E.J., Eds.), Lea and Febiger, Philadelphia, p. 24.

Schneider, N., Bradley, S. and Andersen, M. (1977). Toxicology of cyclomethylenetrinitramine: Distribution and metabolisms in the rat and the miniature swine. *Toxicol. Appl. Pharmacol.* 39: 531–541.

Smith, G., Watkins, J., Thompson, T., Rozman, K. and Klassen, C. (1984). Oxidative and conjugative metabolism of xenobiotics by livers of cattle, sheep, swine and rats. *J. Anim. Sci.* 58: 386–395.

Statistical Analysis System (SAS). (1996). SAS Institute, Cary, NC.

Swindle, M., Smith, A. and Hepburn, B. (1988). Swine as models in experimental surgery. *J. Invest. Surg.* 1: 65–79.

Thakur, A.K. (2000). Statistical issues in large animal toxicology. *Int. J. Toxicol.* 19: 133–140.

Thornton, P.C., Wright, P.A., Sacra, P.J. and Goodier, T.E.W. (1979). The ferret, *Mustela putorius furo*, as a new species in toxicology. *Lab. Anim.* 13: 119–124.

Tynes, R. and Hodgson, E. (1984). The measurement of FAD-containing oxygenase activity in microsomes containing cytochrome P-450. *Xenobiotica* 14: 515–520.

Van Ryzin, R. and Trapold, J. (1980). The toxicology profile of the anti-inflammatory drug proquazone in animals. *Drug Chem. Toxicol.* 3: 361–379.

Van Vleet, J., Herman, E. and Ferrans, V. (1984). Cardiac morphologic alterations in acute minoxidil cardiotoxicity in miniature swine. *Exp. Mol. Pathol.* 41: 10–25.

Walker, C., Bentley, P. and Oesch, P. (1978). Phylogenetic distribution of epoxide hydratase in different vertebrate species, strains and tissues measured using three substrates. *Biochem. Biophys. Acta.* 539: 427–434.

Watkins, J. and Klaassen, C. (1986). Xenobiotic biotransformation in livestock: Comparison to other species commonly used in toxicity testing. *J. Anim. Sci.* 63: 933–942.

Wilson, M.S. and Donnoghue, P.N.D. (1982). A mobile rack of cages for ferrets (*Mustela putorius furo*). *Lab. Anim.* 16: 278–288.

# 17

# THE APPLICATION OF *IN VITRO* TECHNIQUES IN DRUG SAFETY ASSESSMENT

## 17.1. INTRODUCTION

*In vitro* toxicology simply describes a field of endeavor that applies technologies inclusive of isolated organs, isolated tissues, cell culture, biochemistry, and chemistry to the study of toxic or adverse reactions to xenobiotics. An extensive number of reviews and books have been written on this topic; thus, the objective of this chapter is not to provide a comprehensive report of all the activities and approaches in this field. Rather, it is to provide a perspective of the evolution of *in vitro* toxicology, particularly as it applies to the pharmaceutical industry. In discussing this evolutionary process, we begin with a brief historical perspective on *in vitro* techniques in toxicology, followed by industrial applications. A discussion of the philosophical and scientific considerations in *in vitro* test development, as well as the safety assessment process itself, precedes the illustration of several examples of *in vitro* models utilized in toxicologic assessment.

## 17.2. HISTORICAL PERSPECTIVE

The decade of the 1980s was marked by prominent interest and activity in the applications of *in vitro* techniques in toxicology, both in the academic and industrial sectors. This activity was manifested by the appearance of a number of journals

634

devoted to *in vitro* biochemical or molecular approaches to toxicology, the establishment of laboratories focused on the search for alternatives, and the conduct of numerous symposia and workshops devoted to the topic of *in vitro* toxicology. Most important, the past decade was associated with a growing commitment of industry to *in vitro* test development. This commitment was reflected by the formation of groups within many industrial safety assessment components that focused on investigational research often involving *in vitro* techniques. Several factors have impacted on these parallel developments in an additive fashion. The first of these factors concerns the status of technological developments in science itself. Consider that the application of *in vitro* or biochemical techniques, in general, to related disciplines such as pharmacology is a relatively recent development in this century. For example, the applied aspects of sciences such as biochemistry and cell biology, spawned at the turn of the century, have only recently been made available to pharmacologists and toxicologists. The advent of two such applied sciences, virology and receptor pharmacology, occurred in the 1950s and 1970s, respectively. As an outgrowth of these technological developments, toxicologists educated in the 1970s brought to the industrial setting new skills and techniques to perform investigative research, as well as enthusiasm to participate in toxicology's evolution as a science. In addition, the application of microbiological and cell biology techniques to monitor genotoxic or mutagenic events occurred in the late 1970s. The incorporation of these *in vitro* tests in drug safety testing provided perhaps the earliest indication that these new techniques were to join the toxicologist's armamentarium. Thus, the availability of the applied technologies themselves, and the personnel trained to perform them, blossomed in the 1970s and 1980s. The contribution of the public sector in the developments of the 1980s must also be recognized. Toxicology, particularly as an industrial activity, has always been strongly influenced by public opinion and pressure. The impetus for the formation of the Food and Drug Administration (FDA), and the issuance of regulatory laws commencing with the Food, Drug, and Cosmetic Act of 1938, can largely be attributed to public reaction to tragedies such as those caused by sulfanilamide in 1937 and thalidomide in 1961. So, too, has public pressure for animal welfare concerns in the last decade played a significant role in solidifying the commitment to investigate and utilize *in vitro* techniques whenever possible.

Last, in viewing the progression of *in vitro* toxicology in the pharmaceutical industry, it is relevant to note that the advent of toxicology itself as a profession is a recent development in this century. This development can be gauged by the formation of the Society of Toxicology in 1961 and the establishment of drug safety units distinct from pharmacology departments within the industry in the 1950s and 1960s. Toxicology can therefore be regarded as a relatively young profession when compared to pharmacology, whose professional society, the American Society for Pharmacology and Experimental Therapeutics (ASPET), was established in 1908. Industrial laboratories have, therefore, been in the forefront in the incorporation of *in vitro* techniques in toxicology.

## 17.3. INDUSTRIAL APPLICATIONS

The number and types of *in vitro* toxicological models utilized in the pharmaceutical industry encompass virtually every major target organ of toxicological interest. A partial listing of representative test methods is provided in Table 17.1. The breadth of the systems available is impressive, and again signifies a relatively rapid progression of *in vitro* test development in toxicology.

**TABLE 17.1. *In Vitro* Toxicity Models**

| Organ | Models(s) | Applications |
| --- | --- | --- |
| Liver | Hepatocytes | Hepatotoxicity |
| | Enzymes | Peroxisomal proliferation |
| | Isolated perfused liver | Enzyme inhibition/induction |
| Kidney | Tissue slices | Nephrotoxicity |
| | Cells | Renal transport |
| | Tubules | |
| | Membranes | |
| Brain | Slices | Receptor interactions |
| | Homogenates | Neurotoxicity |
| | Cells | |
| Heart | Myocytes | Cardiotoxicity |
| | Isolated atria | Receptor interactions |
| | Isolated perfused heart | |
| Muscle | Cells | Muscle irritation |
| | Smooth muscles | Receptor interactions and smooth muscle effects |
| | Skeletal muscle | Neuromuscular blockade |
| | Phrenic nerve/diaphragm | |
| Blood | RBC | Hemolytic potential |
| | Mast cells | Histamine release |
| | Platelets | Aggregation |
| Reproductive/Endocrine | Sperm | Fertility |
| | Limb bud growth | Teratogenic potential |
| | Whole embryo culture | Teratogenic potential |
| | Pituitary cultures | Prolactin, LH, FSH release |
| | Testicular cultures | Reproductive toxicity |
| Immune | Mitogen assay | Immunomodulation |
| | Mixed lymphocyte response | Immunomodulation |
| | Plaque-forming cell assay | Immunomodulation |
| | Macrophage phagocytosis assay | Immunomodulation |
| | Bone marrow CFU assay | Myelosuppression |
| Other | Yeast | Phototoxicity |
| | Bacterial/mammalian cells | DNA/chromosome damage |
| | Ocular cells/organ systems | Ocular irritation |
| | Dermal cells/organ systems | Dermal irritation |

*Source*: (Gad, 2001).

The fact that many of the *in vitro* test systems listed in Table 17.1 are utilized in toxicology underscores the commitment of industry to the principles of reduction, refinement, and replacement of whole animal *in vivo* tests whenever possible. However, the industrial toxicologist must appropriately balance this commitment with a fourth "R": responsibility (Figure 17.1), originally discussed by Gad (1990). The ethical and legal responsibility of the toxicologist is to assess the safety of new products, and to protect, to the best of his or her ability, the public from harm. Thus, current test procedures cannot be abandoned unless the new tools can be adopted with the assurance that adverse properties will be reliably detected. A key factor in the application of *in vitro* techniques in toxicology involves the degree of correlation between events occurring *in vitro* and those that the toxicologist evaluates in the intact animal. This correlation determines the ultimate scientific value of the techniques, and the level of confidence associated with a particular test in terms of its predictability from a safety perspective.

The criteria that determine the degree of correlation or level of confidence in a given test are summarized in Table 17.2. The first of these is predictability, both qualitative and quantitative. Qualitatively, do the rankings or order of toxicities *in vitro* correlate with the order of toxicities *in vivo*? From a quantitative aspect, what are the dose-response characteristics from which potency estimates and comparisons can be made? Finally, how do drug concentrations *in vitro* compare with those achieved *in vivo*? The second criterion to examine is that of test system identity. To what degree does the *in vitro* system structurally and functionally mimic the *in vivo* organ? Third, the area of mechanisms of cellular injury is a key criterion to consider in the utilization of *in vitro* models for toxicological evaluation. The variety of mechanisms that can play a central role in cell injury underscores the need to recognize specifically how the response of the *in vitro* test system correlates with the response in the intact organ or organism. Last, the topic of compensatory factors needs to be considered. How does the ability of the *in vitro* system to scavenge toxic reaction products compare with *in vivo* abilities? What detoxification or toxification pathways relevant to the *in vivo* fate of toxins or chemicals are present in the *in vitro* test system? These questions must be addressed prior to utilization of *in vitro* procedures to establish a clear understanding of the assumptions and/or limitations of the data to be generated. While, to be useful, *in vitro* systems need not fulfill all

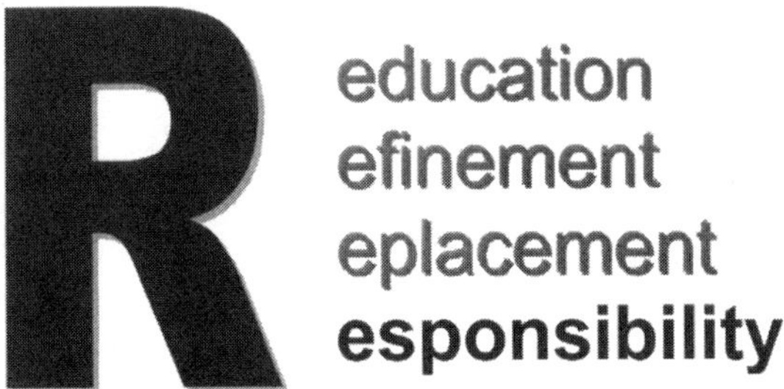


**FIGURE 17.1.** The four R's of *in vitro* testing.

**TABLE 17.2. Criteria for Establishing *In Vitro–In Vivo* Correlations**

Predictability
  Qualitative:  Rankings (% maximum response)
  Quantitative:  Dose-response characteristics
  Relative drug concentrations *in vitro–in vivo*
Identity
  Structure:  Morphological correlates
  Function:  Tissue specificity (e.g., transport characteristics, metabolic pathways)
Mechanisms of injury
  Membrane damage (structural, functional)
  Synthetic activity (protein, RNA, DNA)
  Metabolic poisoning ($O_2$ utilization/consumption, glycolysis, gluconeogenesis)
Compensatory factors
  Biochemical scavengers (glutathione, metalloproteins)
  Detoxification pathways (oxidation/reduction/hydrolysis/conjugation)
  Toxification pathways (oxidation/reduction/hydrolysis/conjugation)

the correlative criteria outlined, the successful achievement of these criteria will be required to replace current whole animal tests.

### 17.3.1. *In Vitro* Testing in Pharmaceutical Safety Assessment

The preclinical assessment of the safety of potential new pharmaceuticals and new devices represents a special case of the general practice of toxicology (Gad, 1999; Meyer, 1989), possessing its own peculiarities and special considerations and differing in several ways from the practice of toxicology in other fields, for some significant reasons. Because of the economics involved and the essential close interactions with other activities (e.g., clinical trials, chemical process optimization, formulation development, regulatory reviews), the development and execution of a crisp and flexible, yet scientifically sound, program is a prerequisite for success. The ultimate aim of preclinical safety and biocompatibility assessment also makes them different. A good safety assessment program seeks to efficiently and effectively move safe potential therapeutic agents or devices into clinical evaluation, then to registration, and finally to market, and to support them through this process. This requires the quick identification of those agents that are not safe so that effort (and limited resources) are not wasted on them.

Pharmaceuticals are intended to have human exposure. Furthermore, pharmaceuticals are intended to have biological effects on the people that receive them. Frequently, the interpretation of results and the formulation of decisions about the continued development and eventual use of a drug are based on an understanding of both the potential adverse effects of the agent and its likely benefits, as well as the dose separation between these two. This makes a clear understanding of dose-response relationship critical, so that the actual risk/benefit ratio can be identified. It is also essential that the pharmacokinetics be understood and that "doses" (plasma tissue levels) at target organ sites be known (Scheuplein et al., 1990). Integral pharmacokinetics are essential to such a safety program, especially now that there is wider recognition of the existence and importance of subpopulations with different metabolic competencies. As we have come to understand that pharmacogenetics underlie many of the subpopulation effects we see in both the safety and efficacy of drugs, we have also come to recognize that *in vitro* methods also offer some of the best and most efficient means of understanding the basis for these differences and for identifying members of specific subpopulations.

The development and safety evaluation of pharmaceuticals and medical devices have many aspects broadly or tightly specified by regulatory agencies (Gad, 2001). An extensive set of defined safety evaluations is required before a product is ever approved for market. For pharmaceuticals, regulatory agencies have increasingly come to require not only the establishment of a "clean dose" in two species with adequate safety factors to cover potential differences between species, but also an elucidation of the mechanisms underlying those adverse effects that are seen at higher doses and are not well understood. These regulatory requirements are compelling to the pharmaceutical toxicologist (Traina, 1983). There is not, however, a set menu of what must be done. Rather, much (particularly in terms of the timing of testing) is open to professional judgement.

The discovery, development and registration of a pharmaceutical or biologic is an immensely expensive operation and represents a rather unique challenge. For every 9000 to 10,000 compounds specifically synthesized or isolated as potential thera-peutics, one (on average) will actually reach the market. The overall cost for each successful compound is currently estimated to be between 250 and 320 million dollars (though those figures are, of course, burdened with the cost of all the unsuccessful compounds), with each successive stage in the development process being more expensive. This dynamic makes it of great interest to identify as early as possible those agents that are likely not to go the entire distance, allowing a concentration of effort on the compounds that have the highest probability of reaching the market (and of possessing therapeutic utility) to do so.

Compounds "drop out" of the process primarily for three reasons: (1) toxicity or (lack of) tolerance, (2) (lack of) efficacy, (3) (lack of) bioavailability of the therapeutic active moiety in humans. Early identification of "losers" in each of these three categories is thus extremely important (Fishlock, 1990), forming the basis for the use of screening in pharmaceutical discovery and development. How much and which resources to invest in screening, and each successive step in support of the development of a potential drug are matters of strategy and phasing that are detailed elsewhere (Gad, 2000). A range of test systems is available to be used in screening and in the definitive testing that follows for selected promising compounds. Table 17.3 presents a summary of the levels of available model systems. Those test systems that involve *in vitro* methods are now providing new tools for use in both early screening and in understanding the mechanisms of observed toxicity in preclinical and clinical studies (Gad, 1988, 1989, 1992, 1993, 1996, 1998). Devices are generally less complicated in design and in their testing procedures, and have a

**TABLE 17.3. Levels of Models for Safety Assessment and Toxicological Research**

| Level/Model | Advantages | Disadvantages |
| --- | --- | --- |
| *In vivo* (intact higher organism) | Full range of organismic responses similar to target species | Cost<br>Ethical/animal welfare concerns<br>Species-to-species variability |
| Lower organisms (earth worms, fish) | Range of integrated organismic responses | Frequently lack responses typical of higher organisms<br>Animal welfare concerns |
| Isolated organisms | Intact yet isolated tissue and vascular system<br>Controlled environment and exposure conditions | Donor organism still required<br>Time-consuming and expensive<br>No intact organismic responses<br>Limited duration of viability |
| Cultured cells | No intact animals directly involved<br>Ability to carefully manipulate system<br>Low cost<br>Ability to study a wide range of variables | Instability of system<br>Limited enzymatic capabilities and viability of system<br>No (or limited) integrated multicell and/or organismic responses |
| Chemical/biochemical systems | No donor organism problems<br>Low cost<br>Long-term stability of preparation<br>Ability to study wide range of variables<br>Specificity of response | No *de facto* correlation to *in vivo* systems<br>Limited to investigation of a single defined mechanism |
| Genomics and proteomics | Speed and broad scope | Much effort is still required to correlate to intact organism effects |
| Computer simulations | No animal welfare concerns<br>Speed and low per-evaluation cost | May not have predictive value beyond a narrow range of structures<br>Expensive to establish |

much lower rate of failure in the qualification and approval stages that precede going to market. The trend in devices, however, is for regulatory authorities to require more testing, to be more critical of results, and to take longer in the review and approval process.

The entire safety assessment process that supports new product research and development is a multistage effort in which none of the individual steps is overwhelmingly complex, but for which the integration of the whole process involves fitting together a large and complex pattern of pieces. This paper proposes an approach in which integration of *in vitro* test systems calls for a modification of the approach to the general safety assessment problem. This modification can be addressed by starting with the current general case and progressing to a means of changing the process in an itcrative fashion as new tools become available. Particularly with an understanding of mechanisms of toxicity becoming increasingly important in both candidate drug selection and the design and evaluation of the relevance of findings, the integration of *in vitro* methodologies particularly into the pharmaceutical safety assessment process, has become essential. Determining what information is needed calls for an understanding of the way in which the device or pharmaceutical is to be made and used, as well as an understanding of the potential health and safety risks associated with exposure of humans who will be either using the drug or device or associated with the processes involved in making it. This is on the basis of a hazard and toxicity profile. Once such a profile is established, the available literature is searched to determine what is already known. Much of the necessary information for support of safety claims in registration of a new drug or device is regulatorily mandated. This is not the case at all, however, for those safety studies done (1) to select candidate products or materials for development, or (2) to design pivotal safety studies to support registration, or (3) to pursue mechanistic questions about materials and products in development.

Taking into consideration this literature information and the previously defined exposures profile, investigators have traditionally used a tier approach to generate a list of tests or studies to be performed based on regulatory requirements. What goes into a tier system is determined by (1) regulatory requirements imposed by government agencies, (2) the philosophy of the parent organization, (3) economics, and (4) available technology. How such tests are actually performed is determined on one of the two bases. The first (and most common) is the menu approach, which involves selecting a series of standard design tests as "modules" of data. This assumes that all drugs or devices are alike except for route and duration of administration. The second is an interactive/iterative approach, where strategies are developed and studies are designed based both on needs and on what has been learned to date about the product.

## 17.4. DEFINING TESTING OBJECTIVE

The initial and most important aspect of a product safety evaluation program is the series of steps that leads to an actual statement of the problem or of the objectives of testing and research programs. This definition of objectives is essential and, as proposed here, consists of five steps: (1) defining product or material use, (2) estimating or quantitating exposure potential, (3) identifying potential hazards, (4) gathering baseline data, and (5) designing and defining the actual research program to answer outstanding questions.

### 17.4.1. Objectives Behind Data Generation and Utilization

To understand how product safety and toxicity data are used and how the data generation process might be changed to better meet the product safety assessment needs of society, it is essential to understand that different regulatory organizations have different answers to these questions. The ultimate solution is in the form of a multidimensional matrix, with the three major dimension of the matrix being (1) the toxicity or biocompatibility data type (lethality, sensitization, corrosion, irritation, photosensitization, phototoxicity, etc.), (2) exposure characteristics (extent, population size, population characteristics, etc.), and (3) the stage in the research and development process we are dealing with.

What is called for is a careful zero-based consideration of what the optimum product safety assessment strategy for a particular development problem should be. Before formulating such a strategy and deciding what mix of tests should be used, it is first necessary to decide criteria for what would constitute an ideal (or at least acceptable) test system.

The ideal test should have an endpoint measurement that provides data such that dose-response relationships can be obtained where possible or necessary (and such are almost always necessary). Furthermore, any criterion of effect must be sufficiently accurate in the sense that it can be used to reliably resolve the relative toxicity of two compounds that produce distinct (in terms of hazard to humans) yet similar responses. In general, it may not be sufficient to classify compounds into generic toxicity categories, such as "intermediate" toxicity, since a candidate chemical that falls in a given category yet is borderline to the next more severe toxicity category should be treated with more concern than a second candidate that falls at the less toxic extreme of the same category. Therefore it is useful for a test system to be able to rank compounds with potentially similar uses accurately within any common toxicity category.

The endpoint measurement of the "ideal" test system must be objective, so that a given compound will give similar results when tested using the standard test protocol in different laboratories. If it is not possible to obtain reproductive results in a given laboratory over time or between various laboratories, then the historical database against which new compounds are evaluated will be time- and laboratory-dependent. Along these lines, it is important for the test protocol to incorporate internal standards to serve as quality controls. Thus, test data could be represented utilizing a reference scale based on the test system response to the internal controls. Such normalization, if properly documented, could reduce intertest variability.

The test results from any given compound should be reproducible both intrinsically (within the same laboratory over time) and extrinsically (between laboratories). If these conditions are not satisfied, then there will be significant limitations on the application of the test system because it could potentially produce conflicting results at different times and places. Such a possibility would significantly reduce confidence in the outcome of any single assay or assay set. From a regulatory point of view, this possibility would be highly undesirable (and perhaps indefensible). Alternatives to current *in vivo* test systems basically should be designed to evaluate the subject toxic response in a manner as closely predictive of that occurring in humans as possible while also reducing animal use and avoiding inhumane treatments where possible.

From a practical point of view, several additional features of the "ideal" test should be satisfied. The test should be rapid so that the turnaround time for a given compound is reasonable. Obviously, the speed of the test and the ability to conduct tests on several candidate drugs or materials simultaneously will determine the overall productivity. The test should be inexpensive, so that it is economically competitive with current testing practices (in the pharmaceutical industry, any reduction in critical path time for decisions has great economic value, so speed is generally preferable to lower cost, within limits). And finally, the technology should be easily transferred from one laboratory to another without excessive capital investment specific to test implementation. Although some of these practical considerations may appear to present formidable limitations for a given test system at the present time, the possibility of future developments in testing technology could overcome these obstacles.

This brief discussion of the characteristics of the "ideal" test system provides a general framework for evaluation of alternative test systems in general. No test system is likely to be ideal, of course. Our current armamentarium of tests, primarily *in vivo* tests using mammals, has developed and been maintained because (1) the tests have generally performed well in preventing dangerous drugs and materials from reaching the marketplace (Gad, 1996a, b) and (2) we are comfortable with them. A significant number of rationales exist for the use of current *in vivo* test systems:

1. They provide evaluation of actions and effects on intact animal and organ/tissue interactions.
2. Either pure chemical entities or complete formulated products (complex mixtures) can be evaluated.
3. Either concentrated or diluted products can be tested.
4. They yield data on the recovery and healing processes.
5. They are required statutory tests for agencies such as the Food and Drug Administration (for "pivotal" safety studies) and the European Economic Community (EEC).
6. They are quantitative and qualitative tests with scoring systems generally capable of ranking materials as to relative hazard.
7. They are amenable to modifications to meet the requirements of special situations (such as multiple dosing or exposure schedules).
8. They have extensive available database and cross-reference capability for evaluation of relevance to human situations.
9. They are easy to perform and relatively low in capital costs in many cases.
10. They are generally both conservative and broad in scope, providing for maximum protection by erring on the side of overprediction of hazard to humans.
11. They can be either single endpoint (such as lethality and pyrogenicity) or shotgun (also called multiple endpoint, including such test systems as a 13-week oral toxicity study).

At the same time, progress and critical examination over the last 15 years has led to the formulation of an equally impressive list of reasons for pursuing the development of *in vitro* test systems:

1. They avoid the complications (and potential confounding or masking findings) of animal and tissue/organ *in vivo* evaluation.

2. *In vivo* systems may assess only short-term site of application or immediate structural alterations produced by agents. Note, however, that tests may be intended to evaluate only local effects.

3. Technician training and monitoring are critical in *in vivo* testing (particularly if the evaluation called for is subjective by nature).

4. If our objective is either the total exclusion of a particular type of agent or the identification of truly severe acting agents on an absolute basis (that is, without false-positives or false-negatives), then *in vivo* tests in animals do not perfectly predict results in humans.

5. Structural and biochemical differences exist between test animals and humans that make extrapolation from one to the other difficult.

6. *In vivo* systems are not standardized.

7. *In vitro* tests provide variable correlation with human results.

8. Large biological variability exists between more complex experimental units (i.e., individual animals).

9. Large, diverse and fragmented databases (which are not readily comparable) are generated by *in vivo* studies.

Therefore, it will be necessary to weigh the strengths and weaknesses of each proposed test system in order to reach a conclusion on how "good" any particular test is. The next section presents the basis for specific test evaluations.


## 17.5. DESIGNING THE TESTING PROGRAM AND BUILDING THE LIBRARY

The next step, given that no relevant data can be found from any literature sources or from any internal files (and that it has been determined what data are needed or most likely to allow selection of desirable candidate compounds), is to perform appropriate predictive tests. The bulk of this section addresses the specifics of performing such evaluations using *in vitro* models. Before considering how to design, develop the components of, and conduct such a testing program, we must first consider how the practice of safety assessment came to its current state of acceptance and utilization of such tests.

To understand how product safety and toxicity data are used and how the data generation process might be changed to better meet the safety assessment needs of both industry and society, it is essential to understand that different commercial and regulatory organizations have different questions to address and operate in different cultures. The ultimate answer as to whether a drug, biologic, or device is safe requires consideration of a multidimensional matrix, whose four major dimensions are (1) the toxicity data type (lethality, sensitization, irritation, photosensitization, genetic toxicity, liver toxicity, etc.), (2) exposure characteristics (extent of use and routes of exposure, patient population size, patient population characteristics, etc.), (3) the benefit to be derived from the marketing and use of the drug, device, or biologic, and (4) the type of commercial organization (what do they make and who regulates them; that is, what is the community of interest?).

Medical devices and pharmaceuticals are two closely related communities. Their materials of concern are agents intended as therapeutics or as components of devices to be used in healthcare, where the production worker or healthcare provider (doctor, nurse, or pharmacist) may have a significant chance of exposure, but the major concern is for those patients who receive or use the drug or device. Various centers of the Food and Drug Administration (FDA) are the primary U.S. regulators.

What is needed is a careful consideration of what the optimum product safety assessment (including safety pharmacology assessments for pharmaceuticals and biologics) strategy would be. The framework for such a strategy calls for considering each of the issues to be resolved or data points to be generated as a separate box or compartment in a flowchart. As in any flowchart, the individual components need to be arranged in a logical order so that work is not duplicated and that the data from earlier "cells" (studies) is available and utilized to help better design, execute and evaluate the results from subsequent cells. These component studies can each be considered a tool for generating required data, and the entire collection as arranged can be thought of as a data-generation toolbox. Many (most) of the components that constitute each of the data-generation toolboxes (screens, confirmatory tests, higher-tier tests, and mechanistic evaluations) are common to all safety assessment programs in some form. But what is actually used for each of these tasks is not common to all of these programs, nor is how the decision points or notes in the chart operate (acceptance criteria and risk/benefit judgement for proceeding with the development of the candidate drug or device). The selection of these details is what constitutes the actual formulation of a strategy. Before formulating such a strategy and deciding what mix of tests should be used, it is first necessary to decide criteria for what would constitute an ideal (or acceptable) test program.

### 17.5.1. Considerations in Adopting New Test Systems

Conducting toxicological investigations in two or more species of laboratory animals is generally accepted as a benign, prudent and responsible practice in developing a new chemical entity, especially one that is expected to receive widespread use and to have exposure potential over human lifetimes. Adding a second or third species to the testing regimen offers an extra measure of confidence to the toxicologists and the other professionals who will be responsible for evaluating the associated risks, benefits, and exposure limitations or protective measures (Gad, 2000; Smith, 1992). Although it undoubtedly broadens and deepens a compound's profile of toxicity, the practice of enlarging on the number of test species is, as has been demonstrated in multiple points in the literature (Gad and Chengelis, 1999), an indiscriminate scientific generalization. Moreover, such a tactic is certain to generate the problem of species-specific toxicoses; that is, a toxic response or an inordinately low biological threshold for toxicity is evident in one species or strain, whereas all other species examined are either unresponsive or strikingly less sensitive. The investigator confronting such findings must be prepared to address the all-important question: Are humans likely to react positively or negatively to the test agent under similar circumstances?

Assuming that numerical odds prevail and that humans automatically fit into the predominant category, whether on the side of being safe or at risk, would be scientifically irresponsible. Far from being an irreconcilable nuisance, however, such a confounded situation can be an opportunity to advance more quickly into the heart of the search for predictive information. Species-specific toxicosis can frequently contribute toward better understanding of the general case if the underlying biological mechanism either causing or enhancing toxicity is defined, especially if it is discovered to uniquely reside in the sensitive species.

A mention of species-specific toxicoses usually implies that either different metabolic pathways for converting and excreting xenobiotics or anatomical differences are involved. The design of our current safety evaluation tests appear to serve society reasonably well (i.e., significantly more times than not) in identifying hazards in a confirmatory manner that would be unacceptable. However, the process can just as clearly be improved from the standpoints of both protecting society and performing necessary screening and exploratory research in a manner that uses fewer animals and uses these fewer animals in a more humane manner.


### 17.5.2. *In Vitro* Models

*In vitro* models, at least as screening test, have been with us in toxicology for some 25 years now. The last 10 to 15 years have brought a great upsurge of interest in such models. This increased interest is due to economic and animal welfare pressures and technological improvements (Rowan and Stratmann, 1980; Tyson and Fraizer, 1993; Salem and Baskin, 1993), and has led to the development and (in some cases) successful utilization of numerous new test methods.

In addition to potential advantages, *in vitro* systems also have a number of limitations that can contribute to their not being acceptable modes.

1. The chemical is not absorbed at all or is poorly absorbed in *in vivo* studies.
2. The chemical is well absorbed but is subject to "first-pass effect" in the liver.
3. The chemical is distributed so that less (or more) reaches the target tissue than would be predicted on the basis of its absorption.
4. The chemical is rapidly metabolized to an active or inactive metabolite that has a different profile of activity and/or different duration of action than the parent drug.

5. The chemical is rapidly eliminated (e.g., through secretory mechanisms).

6. Species of the two test systems used are different.

7. Experimental conditions of the *in vitro* and *in vivo* experiments differed and may have led to different effects than expected. These conditions include factors such as temperature or age, sex, and strain of animal.

8. Effects elicited *in vitro* and *in vivo* by the particular test substance in question differ in their characteristics.

9. Tests used to measure responses may differ greatly for *in vitro* and *in vivo* studies, and the types of data obtained may not be comparable.

10. The *in vitro* study may not use adequate controls (e.g., pH, vehicle used, volume of test agent given, samples taken from sham-operated animals), resulting in "artifacts" of methods rather than results.

11. *In vitro* data cannot predict the volume of distribution in central or in peripheral compartments.

12. *In vitro* data cannot predict the rate constants for chemical movement between compartments.

13. *In vitro* data cannot predict the rate constants of chemical elimination.

14. *In vitro* data cannot predict whether linear or nonlinear kinetics will occur with specific dose of a chemical *in vivo*.

15. Pharmacokinetic parameters (e.g., bioavailability, peak plasma concentration, half-life) cannot be predicted based solely on *in vitro* studies.

16. *In vivo* effects of a chemical are due to an alteration in the higher-order integration of an intact animal system, which cannot be reflected in a less complex system.

At the same time, as pointed out in this chapter, there are substantial potential advantages in using *in vitro* systems. Using cell or tissue culture in toxicological testing results in (1) isolation of test cells or organ fragments from homeostatic and hormonal control, (2) accurate dosing, and (3) quantitation of results. It is important to devise a suitable model system that is related to the mode of toxicity of the compound. Tissue and cell culture have the immediate potential to be used in two very different ways by industry: (1) to examine a particular aspect of the toxicity of a compound in relation to its toxicity *in vivo* (i.e., mechanistic or explanatory studies), and (2) as a form of rapid screening to compare the toxicity of a group of compounds for a particular form of response. Indeed, the pharmaceutical industry has used *in vitro* test systems in these two ways for years in the search for new potential drug entities.

The author has already addressed the theory and use of screens in toxicology (Gad, 1988 and Chapter 4) and the general concepts associated with their integration into the pharmaceutical and device development process (Gad, 1995). Mechanistic and explanatory studies are generally called for when a traditional test system gives a result that is unclear or whose relevance to the real-life human exposure is doubted. *In vitro* systems are particularly attractive for such cases because they can focus on defined single aspects of a problem or pathogenic response, free of the confounding influence of the multiple responses on an intact higher-level organism. Note, however, that first one must know the nature (indeed the existence of) the questions to be addressed.

### 17.5.3. Current Case: A Mixed Battery

The current situation reflects the significant advances made in toxicology since 1985 (Gad, 1996 and 2001). It is rare to see a pharmaceutical or device researched and developed with the use of other than an extensively commingled *in vivo* and *in vitro* test battery. This is reflected in the use of what may be termed a "mixed test battery." The principles behind the development of these batteries are as follows.

1. Pharmaceutical and device development (particularly the product safety assessment aspects of it) cannot continue to be performed as it has been traditionally (on ethical, economic, or competitive grounds).

2. While there are no generally accepted *in vitro* test systems immediately available to completely replace all (or, indeed, any) of the regulatorily mandated *in vivo* testing requirements, there are test systems that can replace distinct components *in vivo* tests (or, just as important, preclude their having to be performed by providing information quickly that makes difficult "go/no go" decisions viable at an earlier (and cheaper) stage of development.

3. Some steps can be taken to move development and acceptance of additional *in vitro* systems along, including wider industry utilization of available test methodologies, increased public regulatory acceptance of *in vitro* data where appropriate and continued multilab validation/evaluation studies of alternatives. The single most helpful step, however, would be the clear definition of what constitutes acceptance criterion for new test designs by regulatory authorities.

4. Some modifications to current *in vivo* testing methods both can and should be adopted. A current example of this would be in medical devices where a substantial portion of the requirements under the governing regulatory (ISO 10993) can be met with *in vitro* alternatives (cytogenicity, muscle cell implantation, the limulus test for pyrogens, and *in vitro* mutagenicity assays).

### 17.5.4. Continuing Incremental Advances: How to Get Them

Great progress has been made in conducting safety assessment tests in intact animals and in developing an array of promising *in vitro* replacements, supplements, and candidates for replacement of the *in vivo* test. We would like to have in place (that is, accepted and used by industry and accepted without question by regulatory agencies) a battery of *in vitro* systems that would preclude or reduce the need for intact animal testing to necessary cases. And we would also like duplicate or unnecessary testing of materials to be reduced to a minimum. These goals are dictated as much by economic reasons and the need to do better science as they are by ethical and humane concerns. The efficient and effective safety assessment or toxicology laboratory of the very near future will have as its "front door" an *in vitro* screening shop that will draw validated specific target organ screens from a library, as needed to perform the initial go/no go evaluations on new compounds (or at least provide guidance as to where further evaluation is required). This same shop would also provide (again, from its established collection) *in vitro* system models to elucidate mechanistic questions later in the assessment process.

Some would say that this is the current state of the art. Much of the necessary library could be assembled from test systems that have been extensively evaluated and have already undergone extensive validation (Gad, 2000, 2001). Three critical steps must be taken for the eventual fulfillment of these objectives: (1) acceptance of a scientific approach to the problem of safety assessment; (2) development of an operative validation and acceptance process for new test procedures; (3) clear enunciation of an acceptance criterion for new test designs by regulatory authorities.

A scientific approach to safety assessment, such as the one presented in this chapter, does have proponents and adherents. Such an approach requires those involved in both the management and conduct of the safety assessment process to continually question (and test) both the efficacy and the validity of their evaluation systems and processes. More to the point, it requires recognition of the fact that "we have always done it this way" is not a reason for continuing to do so. This approach asks first what is the objective behind the testing, and then it asks how well our testing is meeting this objective.

Currently, the second step, a collaborative process involving industrial, academic, and regulatory agencies for the validation and "acceptance" for new test systems, is totally absent. The general model of peer recognition leading to acceptance by the scientific community is not working in this case, as should have been expected from a situation where politics, social policy, and litigation have as much influence as science itself.

## 17.6. SUMMARY OF PRINCIPLES

The first principle in hazard assessment is to have the data correspond as closely as possible to the real-life situation; that is, the nearer the model to humans, the better the quality of the prediction of any potential hazards. The second principle should now also be clear: to be able to translate toxicity to hazard, and to be able to manage such hazards, it is essential to know how the agent is to be used and the marketplace it is to be part of. It is hoped that this section has made these relationships clear.

Finally, alternatives of both *in vitro* and *in vivo* types are in the process of development for almost all the different endpoints of concern in safety assessment. Many of these have promise and could be used as screens for many of the uses presented here or as mechanistic tools, but complete replacement is clearly not near at hand, particularly for the more complicated endpoints. How these tests can (and should) be integrated into strategies for product safety assessment is the key scientific and managerial challenge for the next decade. Not only are there strong reasons against continuing where we are, there is also the possibility of tremendous competitive advantage to those who successfully manage to integrate *in vitro* tools as both efficient screens and effective means of isolating and understanding the mechanistic underpinning for toxic and pathogenic processes. These advantages are not primarily a matter of each piece of testing (data generation point) being less expensive, but rather that multitudes of information can be on hand much earlier in the research (discovery) and development process (before the bulk of expenses associated with individual compounds has been incurred) to allow the elimination of noncompetitive candidates. At the same time, each practicing toxicologist should feel both a moral and ethical compulsion to reduce the number of animals used in research and testing to the fullest extent possible, and to ensure that those that are used are maintained and used in as humane a manner possible.

## 17.7. EXAMPLES OF *IN VITRO* MODELS

### 17.7.1. The Hepatocyte

The liver extensively metabolizes and biotransforms xenobiotics, and the subsequent hepatotoxicity due to exposure to a parent compound or its metabolites is a common clinical event. Isolated hepatocytes, either in suspension or monolayer culture, have been utilized to study the hepatotoxicity of many compounds (Klaasen and Stacy, 1982; Suolinna, 1982; Holme, 1985; Guillouzo, 1986; Castell et al., 1988). The utilization of monolayer cultures has several advantages: (1) monolayer cultures consist of viable cells, while suspensions typically contain a mixed population of viable and dead cells; (2) monolayer cells can be maintained for a longer period of time, which is an important factor in studying chronic exposure of a compound; (3) monolayer cultures allow cell-to-cell contact, which is important for studying the processes necessary for cellular organization. The following section discusses the methods employed in the establishment of primary hepatocyte cultures and provides insights as to how hepatocyte cultures are a valuable model for short-term studies involving the safety assessment of xenobiotics.

*Methods.* The utility of primary hepatocyte cultures is most aptly illustrated by the number of species from which primary cultures can be derived. Isolation of hepatocytes from livers of small animals such as mice, hamsters, guinea pigs, and rats is generally performed *in situ* (Williams, 1976a, b; Dougherty et al., 1980; McQueen and Williams, 1981). In large animals such as rabbits, dogs, and monkeys, and even in human tissue, isolation of hepatocytes is performed by perfusion of biopsy liver specimens (Reese and Byard, 1981; Strom et al., 1982; Smolarek et al., 1990a, b).

*Preparation of Hepatocytes.* In general, the harvesting of hepatocytes from the liver or liver specimen is performed by tissue perfusion using a peristaltic pump with two solutions: one consisting of 0.5 mM ethylene glycol bis ($\beta$-aminoethyl ether) $N,N'$-tetraacetic acid (EGTA) in Hank's balanced salt solution without $Ca^{2+}$ or $MG^{2+}$, and the other consisting of 100 units collagenase per milliliter Williams medium E (WME) buffered with 10 mM $N$-2-hydroxy-ethylpiperazine-$N$-1-ethanesulfonic acid (HEPES) and adjusted to pH 7.35 with 1 N sodium hydroxide (Maslansky and Williams, 1985; McQueen and Williams, 1985). The solutions are filter-sterilized and kept at 37°C. *In situ* perfusion involves cannulation of the portal, or of the biopsy liver specimen; perfusion involves implantation of a large-gauge needle into the sinus cavities of the lobe, followed by perfusion at a slow rate with the solution containing EGTA. The rate of perfusion and the volume of perfusate will vary depending on the size of the tissue. In the *in situ* method, the subhepatic inferior vena cava is severed to prevent excessive swelling of the tissue and to allow the perfusate to leave as waste. In the tissue specimen, perfusate diffuses freely out of the tissue. After uniform blanching of the liver is observed with the first solution, the solution containing collagenase is perfused through the tissue at a rate dependent of the size of the tissue. The liver is covered to keep it moist and a lamp is positioned above the liver to keep it warm. The liver is removed and placed into a sterile petri dish containing cold WME. Hepatocytes are dispersed into the medium by gentle teasing of the tissue. The cell suspension is then washed several times in WME containing 5–10% calf serum and 50 μg ml$^{-1}$ gentamycin sulfate. The viability is determined by trypan blue exclusion, and suspensions having viabilities of 9–100% are plated.

*Culture Conditions.* As previously noted, the viability of freshly isolated hepatocytes in suspension does not usually exceed 5–6 h (Gugen-Guillouzo et al., 1988). Thus, the extended viability of hepatocytes requires culture techniques initially involving cell attachment to a support structure (Gugen-Guillouzo et al., 1988). There are a number of matrices that have been used to maintain primary hepatocyte cultures: laminin (Ledbetter et al., 1984); collagen type IV derived from rat tail tendons (Seglen and Fossa, 1978); a preparation of collagen type IV and laminin in a solubilized basement membrane derived from a transplantable mouse tumor (Kleinman et al., 1986); commercially prepared plastic flasks that incorporate amide and amino function groups (Pittner et al., 1985; Hockin and Paine, 1983; Seglen et al., 1980); and cocultivation of hepatocytes with undifferentiated epithelial cells (Ratanasavanh et al., 1988). The success in maintaining primary hepatocyte cultures from different species on these matrices may vary considerably. In general, freshly derived hepatocytes are most easily maintained on collagen type IV coated tissue culture flasks.

The tissue culture medium is another important factor in supporting survival and proliferation of primary hepatocyte cultures. Typically, hepatocytes are incubated at 37°C, 5% $CO_2$/95% air in either WME media containing 50 μg ml$^{-1}$ gentamycin and 1–10% fetal calf serum (McQueen and Williams, 1985) or Eagle's minimum essential medium supplemented with Earle's salts, nonessential amino acids, 50 μg ml$^{-1}$ gentamycin and 5% fetal calf serum (Seglen, 1976). The initial culture medium is removed 2 to 4 h postplating and replenished with fresh media with serum or without serum. Due to the significant losses of cytochrome P-450 content during the first day in culture, much effort has been devoted to developing culture media devoid of fetal calf serum and supplemented with a variety of substances. Supplements such as aminolevulinic acid (Hockin and Paine, 1983), ascorbic acid (Guzelian and Bissell, 1974), adenine (Guzelian and Bissell, 1974), nicotinamide (Decad et al., 1977), dimethylsuphoxide (Isom et al., 1985), and selenium (Paine and Hockin, 1980) are reportedly important for the maintenance of P-450 activities in primary hepatocyte cultures. In addition, long-term exposure of the hepatocyte cultures to fetal calf serum has been found to be deleterious by inhibiting expression of liver-specific functions, being cytostatic at all plating densities, and being cytotoxic at low seeding densities (Enat et al., 1984).

### Specific Applications

*Cytotoxicity.* The liver is the primary target organ for a variety of drugs and chemicals (Hasemen et al., 1984; Farland et al., 1985). The prevalence of drug- and chemical-induced liver injury is of concern because some xenobiotics can produce liver damage at dose levels that are magnitudes below that which causes cell death (Plaa, 1976). Environmental and commercial chemicals can increase this effect by as much as 100-fold (Plaa and Hewitt, 1982; Plaa, 1976). Studies of early cell injury caused by exposure to a toxicant can be undertaken easily in monolayer cultures of hepatocytes, whereas early cell injury is very difficult to assess *in vivo*.

The methods that have been used to determine cytotoxicity in primary hepatocyte cultures include morphological changes, assessment of enzyme leakage, and membrane blebbing (Jewell et al., 1982; Story et al., 1983; McQueen et al., 1984). Together, these endpoints depend on the compound tested and, in general, at least two endpoints should be monitored. Commonly used indicators of hepatocyte toxicity that suggest impaired cell function, but not necessarily cell death, include leakage of lactate dehydrogenase (Story et al., 1983), changes in cell morphology (McQueen et al., 1984), and inhibition of protein or DNA synthesis (Shaw et al., 1975; Seglen et al., 1980). Indicators of cell death include exclusion of neutral red dye, inclusion of trypan blue (McQueen et al., 1984), and the loss of cell attachment (Simmerman et al., 1974). Gomez-Lechon et al., (1988) studied the use of primary hepatocyte cultures in predicting the hepatotoxicity of xenobiotics. Four well-documented indirect hepatotoxins ($\alpha$-amanitin, D-galactosamine, thioacetamide, and acetaminophen) were studied in cultured rat hepatocytes, and the results compared with the toxicity *in vivo* (Gomez-Lechon et al., 1988). The data indicated that when functional parameters were utilized, toxicity occurred *in vitro* at concentrations at which no effects were seen *in vivo*. These results indicate the sensitivity of the assay and the necessity of selecting the correct indicators of toxicity.

Primary hepatocyte cultures have been used as a tool to predict the hepatotoxicity of many compounds such as nonsteroidal anti-inflammatory drugs (Castell et al., 1988), psychotropic drugs (Boelsterli et al., 1987), immunosuppressant drugs (Boelsterli et al., 1988), and salicylates (Tolman et al., 1978). Rat primary hepatocyte cultures have also been shown to be a good model for examining the mechanisms of metallothionein-induced tolerance to cadmium toxicity (Liu et al.,

1990). Guillouzo et al. (1988) developed a coculture system of rat or human hepatocytes with rat liver epithelial cells that maintains the hepatocytes in a differentiated state for extended periods of time, thereby allowing studies involving chronic treatment with the test substance to be conducted. Primary cultures of hepatocytes can therefore provide a useful model for short- and long-term studies involving the safety assessment of xenobiotics.

*Comparative Metabolism.* Since the liver is the major organ involved in the biotransformation of xenobiotics, primary hepatocyte cultures provide an excellent model for *in vitro* metabolism studies. Primary hepatocyte cultures provide useful tools with which to study the comparative metabolism of xenobiotics by both humans and laboratory animals.

Primary hepatocyte cultures undergo a significant decrease in the activities of phase I and II enzymes that correlates with time in culture. Croci and Williams (1985) compared, during the first 24 h in culture, representative phase I and phase II biotransformation pathways in hepatocyte primary cultures isolated from male and female rats to freshly isolated hepatocytes. Hepatocytes lost 50% of cytochrome P-450 activity during the first 24 h in culture, but maintained high mixed-function activities; 75% of aryl hydrocarbon hydroxylase and 65% of benzphetamine demethylase activities were preserved in hepatocytes from male rates. Uridine $5'$-diphosphate (UDP)-glucuronosyl transferase activities were slightly increased during 24 h of culture to levels higher than present in liver tissue before perfusion. Glutathione transferase activity after 24 h diminished to 20% of the initial enzyme activity for one form while another form was stable. Donata et al. (1990) showed that in human hepatocytes, 3-methylcholanthrene, phenobarbital, and ethanol can increase the activity of cytochrome P-450 monooxygenases, aryl hydrocarbon hydroxylase, and 7-ethoxycoumarin $0$-de-ethylase.

Hepatocyte cultures are not affected by some of the variables that influence *in vivo* studies such as absorption and distribution; accordingly, the exact concentration of the parent compound is known, and the total number and amount of each metabolite formed over time can be accurately determined. Species-specific differences in the metabolism of xenobiotics may, in fact, play a major role in determining relative susceptibilities to chemical toxicants. As an example, studies were recently conducted utilizing primary hepatocyte cultures derived from the perfusion of livers from rats, dogs, and monkeys to determine if the species-specific differences in acetaminophen- (APAP) induced cytotoxicity were correlated with species-specific differences in the amounts of APAP metabolized and the formation of APAP conjugates (Smolark et al., 1990a). *In vivo* studies on the hepatotoxicity of APAP have shown a species-specific difference in susceptibility to its hepatotoxic effects (Davis et al., 1974). The dog, hamster, and mouse are very sensitive, but the rabbit, guinea pig, and rat are resistant. Rat, rabbit, dog, and monkey hepatocyte cultures were exposed to 2 mM APAP for 24 h (Smolarek et al., 1990a). Aliquots of hepatocyte culture media containing APAP and its metabolites were analyzed by reverse-phase high-pressure liquid chromatography (HPLC). The sensitivity of the dog hepatocytes to APAP was directly related to low conjugating enzyme activity. In contrast, monkey hepatocyte cultures had a very large capacity to transform APAP to glucuronide conjugates, and a very high level of glutathione *S*-transferase activity, which correlated with their resistance to cytotoxicity. These studies indicate that the competing pathways of APAP conjugation in hepatocyte cultures from different species explain the differences observed in APAP-induced cytotoxicity (Smolarek et al., 1990a). Similar comparisons have also been made relating species-specific tetrahydroaminoacridine- (THA) induced hepatotoxicity to differences in the rate and the extent of THA biotransformation in cultured hepatocytes from rat, dog, and monkey (Smolarek et al., 1990b). These studies demonstrated that the hepatocytes from these three species differed in their sensitivity to concentration-dependent cytotoxicity, with the monkey cells being most sensitive and the canine cells least sensitive to THA-associated cytotoxicity. Tetrahydroaminoacridine biotransformation also differed among the three species, with the canine hepatocytes most effective and monkey hepatocytes least effective in the conversion of THA to most polar metabolites (Smolarek et al., 1990b). These *in vitro* studies correlate differences in the cytotoxicity of THA to its biotransformation. They also suggest that the monkey would be a good animal model for *in vivo* THA toxicity testing (Smolarek et al., 1990b).

Green et al. (1986) compared the metabolism of amphetamine in isolated hepatocyte suspensions from rat, dog, squirrel, monkey, and human livers. The metabolite profile of hepatocytes from each species corresponded to the profile of urinary metabolites identified previously. These results indicate that species-specific differences in the metabolic activation of compounds seen *in vivo* can be reproduced *in vitro* by the utilization of primary hepatocyte cultures.

Primary hepatocyte cultures have been used *in vitro* to metabolically activate toxins for evaluation with target tissues. Cocultures of rat embryos with hepatocytes have been used to study the role of metabolism in teratogenesis (Oglesby et al., 1986). Lindahl-Kiessling et al., (1989), in an attempt to bring test conditions closer to *in vivo* conditions, developed an assay utilizing primary rat hepatocytes and human peripheral lymphocytes to detect metabolism-mediated mutagenesis.

***Genotoxicity.***   The genotoxicity of drugs and chemicals can be detected by measurement of their interactions with cellular DNA. Many test chemicals are not genotoxic by themselves and thus may require metabolic activation to a DNA-reactive metabolite. Primary hepatocyte cultures function (1) as metabolic activating systems for chemicals and (2) as target cells for the interaction of reactive metabolites with hepatocellular DNA. Indirect assessment of human genotoxicity can be implemented when primary human hepatocytes are used to assess a chemical genotoxicity. In primary hepatocyte cultures, studies to resolve the extent of xenobiotic-DNA interaction products formed as a result of exposure to a test chemical determine the total amount of xenobiotic bound per milligram DNA (Poirier et al., 1980) and quantify the number of single-strand beaks in DNA by alkaline elution (Bradley et al., 1982). An indirect method for determining the genotoxicity of xenobiotics from a wide variety of structural classes in primary hepatocyte cultures is to measure DNA repair by autoradiography (Williams 1976a). McQueen and Williams (1983) tested a large number of chemicals utilizing this technique and reported that all of the known noncarcinogens tested were negative in eliciting DNA repair, while approximately 90% of the known carcinogens were positive. The suggested reasons for 10% of the carcinogens not eliciting DNA repair are that many carcinogens are of the epigenetic type and therefore will not produce DNA damage and, second, that the carcinogen may inhibit DNA repair. Audioradiographic measurement of DNA repair allows cells undergoing replicative DNA synthesis to be readily distinguished from those in repair, and it allows DNA repair to be studied at concentrations of compound that are not cytotoxic.

Species-specific differences in DNA repair by primary hepatocyte cultures have been demonstrated by McQueen and Williams (1983). The relative resistance of the mouse to aflatoxin $\beta_1$-induced carcinogenesis was shown by the 10–100 times higher concentration of aflatoxin $\beta_1$ necessary to cause maximum DNA repair in the mouse than in other species tested. Administration of safrole to primary hepatocytes cultures elicited a positive response in DNA repair for the hamster and mouse hepatocyte cultures, but was negative in the rat hepatocyte cultures, suggesting the importance of multispecies genotoxicity testing of a compound (McQueen and Williams, 1987). With respect to the toxicological testing tier, genotoxicity testing contributes to the overall safety assessment of new drug candidates, and it can also be applied at the preproject stages of evaluation.

***Summary.*** It is clear from the proceeding discussions that the primary hepatocyte in culture represents a versatile *in vitro* tool in the safety assessment process. The applications of the hepatocyte are summarized in Table 17.4. First, they provide a useful model for studying drug- and chemical-induced hepatotoxicity. Second, they afford the potential to generate and examine the toxicity of phase I and phase II metabolites to liver cells or other target organs *in vitro*. Third, they provide a mechanism to examine potential species differences in metabolism of drug candidates prior to *in vivo* studies. Early in the drug discovery process, primary hepatocyte cultures can therefore aid in the selection of a chemical series, based on favorable metabolic and toxicological profiles. The choice of the animal species appropriate for *in vivo* toxicology studies could also be based on data obtained from primary hepatocyte cultures of several species. Last, utilization of primary hepatocyte cultures derived from livers of humans is becoming more commonplace. The toxicologist's ultimate goal of determining hepatoxic (and genetoxic) risk to humans should be greatly enhanced through the utilization of primary human hepatocyte cultures.

**TABLE 17.4. *In Vitro* Testing Utilizing Hepatocyte Cultures**

| | |
|---|---|
| Cytotoxicity mechanisms | Cellular damage and necrosis |
| Comparative metabolism | Species specificity |
| Teratogenic mechanisms | Proteratogens |
| Genotoxic mechanisms | DNA repair |

***Needs for the Future.*** Primary hepatocyte is a well-established technology for studying the pharmacology and toxicology of different classes of xenobiotics. However, since there are currently no well-defined experimental conditions for establishing primary hepatocyte cultures, it is difficult to compare experimental results from different laboratories. The major variable consists of the cell culture media used for maintaining hepatocytes. Although each specialized medium has been shown to be useful for a specific application, a real need exists to establish an optimal medium that can be standardized. A common objective of most of the varieties of cell culture media is to define a system that maintains cytochrome P-450 activity and the hepatocellular differentiated state. Conventional cell culture conditions have only maintained approximately 20 to 40% of cytochrome P-450 activity in rodent hepatocytes cultured for two days, while human hepatocyte cultures seemed to be more stable and maintained approximately 50 to 60% of their initial P-450 activity after five to six days in culture (Guguen-Guillouzo et al., 1988). Development of a well-defined matrix upon which to grow primary hepatocytes also needs further consideration. The greater degree of loss of P-450 activity in primary hepatocytes in suspension relative to monolayer cultures suggests that cell-to-cell contact is an important issue. A procedure that should contribute some degree of uniformity to primary hepatocyte culture as a test system is to verify the status of the cultures prior to utilization in a particular way in a particular assay. This could be accomplished by routinely checking standard cytotoxic parameters such as leakage of cytoplasmic enzymes or cell survival, as well as metabolic parameters such as protein synthesis and gluconeogenesis.

In light of the interest and value of studying the responses of human hepatocytes relative to other species, an important need for the future is to develop successful techniques to culture and freeze preparations of human hepatocytes which, upon thawing, maintain their viability and metabolic capabilities. Typically, human liver tissue is obtained in large quantities. Since only a small portion of the total tissue is needed to provide sufficient material for a given experiment, the remaining portion could be frozen for future use if the proper freezing techniques were established. As previously noted, there has been some success in coculturing human hepatocytes with liver epithelial cells for long-term cultures useful in chronic toxicity testing (Guillouzo et al., 1988), and for maintaining the viability of previously frozen human hepatocytes (Li et al., 1990). Recent advances in culturing techniques should provide a well-defined experimental system for culturing primary hepatocytes in the near future. The role of primary human hepatocytes cultures in safety assessment will become increasingly important, and therefore successful efforts in freezing hepatocytes will help to meet the increasing needs in pharmacological and toxicological studies.

### 17.7.2 Ocular Alternatives

In recent years, much attention and effort have been directed toward the search for non-whole-animal tests to predict ocular irritation by drugs and chemicals. A variety of *in vitro* assays, as well as "nonexperimental" approaches, have been proposed. These model systems run the gamut of responses observed *in vivo* using biological systems encompassing a range of organization (from cells to whole eye) and measure a multitude of responses. In addition to these experimental tests, one may also think about prediction of ocular irritation by means that require no additional animal work. The use of literature or computer data bases, computer modeling, prediction from physical or chemical parameters or other toxicity data (such as dermal or acute toxicity), are examples of such an approach. Given a plethora of possibilities, where does one begin in trying to develop a program for establishing ocular irritation potential without the use of live animals? What are the general strengths and weaknesses of the existing techniques, and what developmental work needs to be done? How does one "validate" a model system and use it in the decision-making process? These issues are addressed in the next section.

### Methods

*"Nonexperimental" Techniques.* Perhaps the most obvious and practical starting point for irritation potential to the eye is to ask what is already known about a compound or related structures. If enough data exist, perhaps further experimental work will be unnecessary. Such data might include (1) information from the literature or other data bases, (2) data generated by computer modeling, (3) physical and chemical characteristics of the test compound, or (4) previously obtained toxicity data such as acute and/or dermal toxicity. The use of each of these approaches has its advantages and disadvantages, which are discussed as follows:

1. *Published Data.* One might assume that previously collected data appearing in the literature should be quite useful and reliable in evaluating potential ocular irritancy. In practice, however, two basic issues detract from the utility of the literature data bases. The first is illustrated in a paper by Weil and Scala (1971). In their study, a number of laboratories tested the same set of compounds for ocular irritation potential in both a standard protocol and in the routine protocol of the particular laboratory. Comparisons of the results showed considerable variability between laboratories, and to some degree within the laboratories, in the ranking of test compounds. These findings are not surprising in light of the subjective nature of the scoring systems, which makes it difficult to achieve consistent results among individuals and laboratories. How then, does one determine which literature data to accept and which to reject?

The second issue involves the nature of published material itself. Due to journal space limitations and/or other factors, it is rare to find enough detail presented for a reader to make an independent evaluation of the value of the irritation data. Sometimes the test methodology is not defined, making direct comparisons to results obtained in other laboratory situations tenuous at best. Often raw data are lacking, and the results are reduced to either a plus–minus score or a broad categorization (mild, moderate, severe), so that a more specific appraisal cannot be made. These factors preclude the resolution and evaluation of seemingly conflicting data that one often finds in the literature.

A possible means of overcoming these problems is to use information generated within one's own company. In-house data are usually more consistent since the methodology generally does not change substantially over time, and one usually has the further advantage that the original raw data are available. The in-house data base is also more likely to contain information on compounds whose chemistry is similar to the unknowns to be tested. However, irrespective of the source of background data on related substances, such information can only provide a starting point for the investigation of an unknown compound. While the data may be potentially useful in raising a warning flag, they are unlikely to be sufficient for a definitive judgement.

2. *Computer Modeling.* Computer modeling shares essentially the same problems as literature data. A computer simulation can only be as reliable as the data used in its construction. A model system called TOPKAT is available commercially from Health Designs, Inc. According to their own literature (HDI *Newsletter*, 1987; TOPKAT manual), eye irritation has been quite difficult to model due to the inherent variability of classification of compounds. Health Designs has, in fact, had to design two sets of equations; one to separate nonirritants from all other compounds, and the second to separate severe irritants from the rest, leaving a fair number of compounds broadly classified between these extremes. Furthermore, the model is predicted to be unsuitable for approximately 30% of chemical structures, and the number of indeterminates is higher than the developers would like. It appears that computer modeling, while promising, is somewhat limited as a definitive predictive tool. As with data from the literature, one can probably use the computer model to obtain a rough idea of irritation potential, but more definitive categorization will likely require further testing.

3. *Physical and Chemical Parameters.* Knowledge of the physical and chemical parameters of a compound should be a useful point of reference in predicting irritation potential. In fact, many companies have already reduced animal testing by using a rule of thumb with regard to the pH of a material. Compounds with an exceedingly high or low pH (for instance $<3$ or $>12$) are presumed to be irritants, and would simply be labeled as such without further testing. This practice has some support in the literature (Guillot et al., 1982b), and further work in this area is ongoing in a study sponsored by the Soap and Detergent Association (SDA). A preliminary finding in the SDA study is that the alkalinity of a compound (i.e., the strength of the acid or base) may be more important than the simple measure of pH (Booman et al., 1989).

The correlation (or lack of correlation) of other physiochemical characteristics has not yet been established. For instance, are all surfactants irritants? Can one classify severity by the size of the molecule? Can octanol : water partition coefficients predict irritation potential; does a propensity to partition out of the ocular fluid mean that a compound presents more of an irritation hazard than one which is more water soluble? Theoretically, these data should reflect the ability of a compound to penetrate the eye and cause an irreversible lesion. However, until definitive data are available, physical and chemical parameters will probably have limited utility in an overall assessment of irritation.

4. *Data from Other Toxicological Testing.* Another question under study has been whether dermal or systemic (acute) toxicity is predictive of ocular irritant potential. Little work has been reported in the literature regarding the correlation

between ocular irritation and acute toxicity, so one can only speculate as to this relationship. When one considers the multiplicity of physiological mechanisms involved in acute lethal reactions (e.g., at the cardiovascular and CNS levels), it is difficult to envision homology with equally complex responses of tissue damage and inflammation observed at the ocular site. Thus, from a correlative viewpoint, it is unlikely that mechanisms of lethality operating in acute toxicity tests would also occur in ocular injury, thereby making any predictive analysis strictly fortuitous.

However, more extensive information is available comparing dermal and ocular irritation. Gillman et al. (1983), for example, examined dermal and ocular irritation data on selected petrochemicals and consumer products, and reported no reliable correlation between ocular and dermal irritation scores. Guillot et al. (1982a, b) examined ocular and dermal irritation of 56 compounds, comparing different protocols. If one combines the data from both papers, one finds that of 11 dermal irritants, all showed ocular irritation, but the extent of irritation was not predictable. Of the 45 compounds that were nonirritating to slightly irritating dermally, only 18 were non- or slightly irritating to the eye. The remaining 27 compounds ranged from mild or moderate to extremely irritating upon ocular exposure. Similar results were reported by Williams (1984, 1985), who examined 60 severe dermal irritants and found 39 to be severe ocular irritants, while 6 were moderate irritants and 15 mild to nonirritant in the eye. Last, in a study by Gad et al. (1986), it was revealed that correlations between dermal and ocular data differed dramatically depending on the scale of irritation used for the comparison. When the compounds were classified simply as positive or negative in both dermal and ocular irritation, the correlation was better than when one attempted to predict a specific classification (i.e., negligible, mild, moderate, severe). The only generalization that can be made is that if a compound is a severe dermal irritant, it is likely to be a strong ocular irritant. However, as alluded to previously, severe irritancy can be predicted, in many cases, on the basis of chemical properties alone (e.g., pH). Nonetheless, it appears that dermal irritancy data can be predictive of ocular irritation for severe dermal irritants. However, as cited earlier in this paragraph, a number of false positives will occur. Caution is therefore advised in the use of this parameter.

To summarize the utility of "nonexperimental" methods, it is obvious that the more available information there is about a compound, the more likely one will be able to substantially reduce the amount of testing involved in prediction of ocular irritation potential. However, at this point in time, none of the individual methods, alone or in combination, are sufficiently predictive to provide a definitive assessment of *in vivo* ocular irritation. There is definitely a place, however, for consideration of the above factors in a battery of tests, as well as for prioritizing compounds to be tested further.

*In Vitro Methods.* In view of the limitations of extrapolation of irritancy by nonexperimental methods, it is clear that in most cases new experimental data will need to be generated. This new information can be obtained using *in vitro* approaches in conjunction with *in vivo* data, when necessary. In selecting an *in vitro* procedure, the first step would be to evaluate what processes one is attempting to model, followed by the development of a methodology to mimic that particular biochemical effect. However, while the broad processes of inflammation, opacity, and the like, are known to be involved in ocular injury and irritation, a detailed understanding of the underlying mechanisms of these processes in the eye is lacking. As previously mentioned, in examining criteria for *in vitro* test systems, it is extremely useful to know enough about the underlying mechanism(s) to identify and measure a specific endpoint that is (preferably) causal to the *in vivo* effect. For instance, is the process of opacification due to osmotic imbalances, protein coagulation, necrosis of cells within the epithelial organization, stromal swelling due to ionic interference with cell-to-cell junctional complexes, or (more likely) does the mechanism differ with the compound being tested? And what is really known about inflammation at the cellular and molecular levels? Which components of the arachidonic acid cascade are involved? Do these components act synergistically or antagonistically, and what about specificity of cell response? Should corneal epithelial or endothelial cells, conjunctivae, or stroma be examined as the primary tissue affected? Some of the answers are known, but our deficiencies in knowledge and understanding highlight the complexity of modeling ocular responses to toxins.

Given the mechanistic complexity of the ocular response to xenobiotics, attempting to predict irritation with one assay may not be realistic at this time. The type of approach more likely to be immediately fruitful, as suggested by a number of people (Fielder et al., 1987; ECETOC, 1988), is to use a tiered approach, taking advantage of as wide a diversity of methods as is practical to get a comprehensive picture of irritation potential. Indeed, various regulatory agencies have unofficially stated that they would like to see all components of the Draize score addressed before they would consider *in vitro* data in lieu of animal data. Thus, a logical approach would be to examine an assay(s) for each component of ocular irritation (i.e., opacity, inflammation, necrosis, or toxicity).

Because the materials tested for ocular irritancy in the pharmaceutical industry are diverse and many are novel chemical entities, it is advantageous to identify an *in vitro* assay that closely mirrors the target tissue biochemistry and physiology and monitors the specific endpoint of interest. The expectation of such a system would be that the methodology applied would detect compounds exerting toxic effects by a variety of mechanisms. An extensive list of proposed alternatives has been compiled and categorized by Frazier et al. (1987). While this listing can serve as a starting point as to the available technology, many of these methods do not possess any obvious correlation with the target tissue of interest and/or are not well validated. The following sections provide an overview of one or two representative methodologies for each component of the Draize system, along with reported advantages and disadvantages.

1. *Opacity.* Corneal opacity is the most heavily weighted of the components of the Draize eye score (80 out of 110 possible points) (Conquet et al., 1977). Thus, an *in vitro* system that provides an accurate measure of opacification should contribute substantially toward *in vitro* modeling of the classical Draize test. Two assays attempting to model this process are discussed.

A bovine corneal opacity (BCO) assay described by Muir (1984, 1985) seems to be quite promising as a model for studying opacification. Recently, this technology has been further developed for the prediction of drug- and chemical-induced ocular irritation (Gautheron and Sina, 1990; Gautheron et al., 1992). Basically, the BCO assay uses freshly isolated bovine eyes obtained from an abattoir. Alternatively, whole corneas may be obtained for experimental purposes from other species such as the rabbit (Elgebaly, personal communication, 1990) or pig (Igarashi et al., 1989). Corneas are removed, allowed to equilibrate in medium for a period of time, then mounted in a special chamber in which both sides of the cornea are bathed in fluid. Test compound is added to the epithelial side of the cornea for a defined period of time and opacity is measured at intervals using an opacitometer. An evaluation of commercially available compounds (Table 17.5), as well as a substantial number of pharmaceutical candidates and process intermediates, has shown an excellent correlation between the BCO assay and *in vivo* irritation scores. A few severe ocular irritants give a false-negative reading in this test because they cause the entire epithelial layer to slough from the cornea, thereby producing a lower opacity reading than expected. This difficulty can be overcome by simple examination of the cornea

**TABLE 17.5. Comparison between *In Vivo* Ocular Irritancy and Opacity Induced in Bovine Cornea**

| Compound | *In vivo* irritancy | Opacity at 100% |
|---|---|---|
| Tween 20 | Mild[b] | 1.7 |
| DMSO | Mild | 11.7 |
| Ethanol | Mild/Moderate[b] | 20.0 |
| Ethylene glycol | Mild/Moderate[b] | 24.0 |
| Isopropyl alcohol | Mild/Moderate[b,c] | 30.1 |
| Methanol | Mild/Moderate[b] | 32.1 |
| Ethylene glycol | Mild/Moderate[d] | 33.2 |
| Carbitol | Mild/Moderate[b] | 36.5 |
| Formamide | Mild/Moderate[b] | 51.8 |
| Acetone | Mild/Moderate[b] | 65.5 |
| Tetrahydrofurfuryl | Moderate[c] | 71.2 |
| Ethylene glycol | Moderate[d] | 72.3 |
| Tetramethyl | Severe[b] | 80.7 |
| Solketal | Moderate[c] | 87.7 |
| Acetonitrile | Severe[e] | 88.5 |
| Pyridine | Severe[b] | 92.3 |
| Allyl alcohol | Severe[b,c] | 123 |
| Trichloroacetic acid | Severe[b] | 219 |

*Sources*:
[a] Opacity scaling described in Gautheron et al. (1992).
[b] Grant (1986).
[c] Clayton and Clayton (1981).
[d] Smyth et al. (1951).
[e] Smyth et al. (1949).

postexposure. The only other drawback encountered has been observed with some insoluble compounds. These materials are generally not a problem (although the highest dose texted is limited), since the corneas can be washed prior to obtaining an opacity reading. However, in a few cases compound can adhere too tightly for effective rinsing, thus giving an artificially high opacity reading. Overall, the BCO assay has been found to be an excellent first-line test in a battery of alternatives, and interlaboratory evaluation studies are currently being initiated in Europe.

A commercially available methodology (Eytex$^{TM}$) has recently been put forth as an alternative corneal opacification assay. The method, based upon the presumption that opacification is due to coagulation or denaturation of protein, measures the precipitation caused in a protein matrix by the introduction of a test compound (Gordon and Kelly, 1989). The developers have tested a number of materials, a substantial number of which are surfactants or surfactant-based products, and claim a high level of correlation with ocular irritation. However, evaluation of the methodology has been undertaken by various researchers with mixed results. For instance, on the one hand, Lawrence-Beckett and James (1990) and Soto et al. (1989) found the test useful for evaluating industrial chemicals. On the other hand, Bruner and Parker (1990) found that the Eytex$^{TM}$ assay was not very predictive of household product irritancy compared with five other *in vitro* assays. One potential reason for this type of discrepancy may be found in the evaluation performed by Thomson et al. (1989a). These researchers tested a series of compounds within a variety of groups of formulations, and found good correlations with *in vivo* data when the Eytex$^{TM}$ assay was used for surfactant blends and eye-area-use products. However, the correlation was not acceptable when alcohol-containing formulations were tested. This illustrates a recurring caveat in the field of *in vitro* toxicology: a technique must be evaluated with materials from a variety of chemical classes, and preferably with compounds that are likely to be tested as unknowns, before it can be considered a "validated" assay.

*2. Cytotoxicity Testing.* The majority of proposed alternative tests are assays for cytotoxicity in which a target cell is exposed to test compound and some endpoint of viability is measured. The advantages of such tests are that these methods are usually very easily and rapidly performed, and can be readily transferred among different laboratories. Furthermore, some investigators report that the choice of target cell is relatively unimportant to the predictivity of the assay (Borenfreund and Borrero, 1984), suggesting that the choice of the target cell-ending combination is essentially unlimited. However, despite these advantages, cytotoxicity assays cannot, in general, be considered mechanisticaly based, and may not be appropriate for every situation. While it is likely that a number of compounds, particularly severe to extreme irritants, damage the eye through overt cellular toxicity, it is equally clear that a number of compounds exert their effects by different mechanisms. The need for judicious use of the cytotoxicity endpoint, preferably as part of a battery of approaches, is borne out by a number of evaluations reported in the literature (Bracher et al., 1987; Flower, 1987; Kennah et al., 1989).

Consider, for example, the neutral red assay developed by Borenfreund and Peurner (1984, 1987). This test has been evaluated with a number of surfactants and cosmetic ingredients and has reportedly given good correlations with *in vivo* ocular irritation data (Bracher et al., 1987; Shopsis, 1989; Bruner and Parker, 1990). However, Thomson et al. (1989b) used this assay to examine a variety of products and found high correlations with some types of materials and poor correlations with others. Again, the basis for this variation in assay performance seems to be the class of chemical being evaluated.

Recently, the cytotoxicity of various drug candidates and process intermediates, as well as commercially available compounds, was examined in the presumed target cell, rabbit corneal epithelium, and a nontarget cell, V79 fibroblasts (Sina and Gautheron, 1990; Sina et al., 1992). Two endpoints of toxicity were monitored; leucine incorporation into protein, a general measure of toxicity, and the tetrazolium dye assay (MTT), a measure of mitochondrial dysfunction. An $IC_{50}$ (concentration necessary to reduce endpoint to 50% of control value) was determined for each cell-endpoint combination, and correlations were drawn with the *in vivo* classifications (i.e., mild, mild/moderate, moderate, severe). The data showed such a broad overlapping of the $IC_{50}$ values that no definitive cutoff could be established between classifications (Figure 17.2). Subsequently, an $IC_{50}$ threshold was established simply to distinguish severe *in vivo* irritants. Again, such a value was difficult to determine. If one evaluates commercially available and in-house products separately, a threshold value that allows approximately 70–75% predictivity between these two broad categories can be established. However, this value changes dramatically with the types of compounds as well as with the different target cell-endpoint combinations. It is, therefore, of limited value in testing unknowns.

Thus, cytotoxicity assays are unlikely to provide an adequate predictor of *in vivo* irritation in every case. There is no doubt that some type of compounds (such as surfactants) will give (and have given) acceptable correlations with *in vivo* data. However, for the diversity of compounds common in the pharmaceutical industry, cytotoxicity assays alone are inadequate predictors of ocular irritation, though they may have a place in a battery of tests. For instance, if one is interested in a very quick assessment that will be corroborated later, cytotoxicity assays may be indicated. But each laboratory needs to make its own evaluation of the utility and value of these methods.

3. *Inflammation.* To complete the examination of the major components of the Draize score, one also needs to examine inflammation. Although inflammation is not a large portion of the Draize score (20 of 110 total points), most people appear to put a great deal of weight on this component due to the subjectivity inherent in the scoring. Furthermore, an evaluation of in-house historical data [Sina, 1994 (unpublished)] indicates that of those compounds that cause opacity, the majority show moderate to severe inflammation first. This suggests that inflammation may be a more important and predictive component of ocular irritation that the Draize scoring system would suggest.

One approach to examining inflammation is the assay reported by Elgebaly et al. (1987) for the release of chemotactic factors. Earlier work has elegantly shown that neutrophil or macrophage infiltration from either the endothelial or epithelial surface

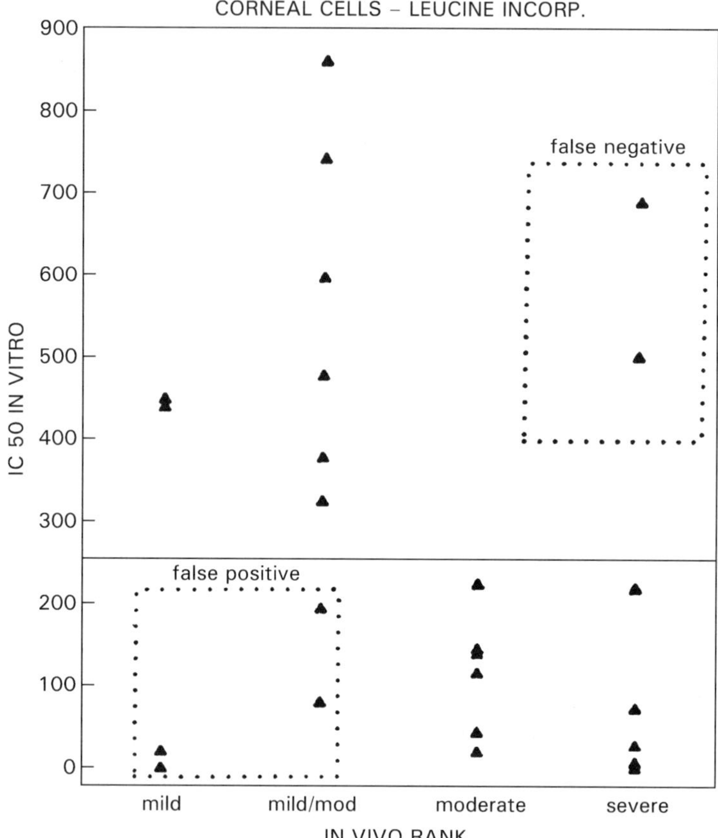


**FIGURE 17.2.** Comparison of cytotoxicity in corneal cells (leucine incorporation) and ocular irritancy *in vivo*.

can cause substantial damage to the eye (Elgebaly et al., 1985). Thus, it seems likely that release of inflammatory mediators will correlate with ocular irritation or, more important, with the potential for ocular damage. Briefly, the methodology involves the exposure of the isolated bovine cornea (or cornea from other species) to a compound, with the intact structure serving as a cup to contain the test material. After an indicated time, the exposure medium is harvested and analyzed for the release of chemotactic mediators by means of a chemotaxis assay. Conceptually, this assay is quite attractive and validation is currently underway.

Another approach that has been proposed under the category of inflammation assays [though it has been suggested (Lawrence, 1987) that the assay measures necrosis rather than the true inflammation] is the chick chorioallantoic membrane (CAM) test and its modifications (Leighton et al., 1983; Leupke, 1985; Kong et al, 1987; Bagley et al., 1989). Basically the assay scores alterations (vascularity, necrosis, etc.) in the chorioallantoic membrane of chicken eggs upon exposure to test compounds. As with most of the other assays discussed here, the CAM assay has proven useful in some applications, but inadequate in others. For instance, Bagley et al. (1989) report good predictivity of ocular irritation for surfactant-based materials with a CAM modification, the CAMVA method. By contrast, Price et al. (1986) and Lawrence et al. (1986) found the assay inadequate for their purposes. The reason(s) for these discrepancies may be due to the compound classes tested, or to various methodological differences between laboratories. Another point worth mentioning with regard to this assay is that since a viable chicken embryo is part of the model, the CAM may not be truly considered an *in vitro* model, particularly in Europe (Lawrence, 1987).

***Specific Applications.*** How are the above-proposed tests integrated into the safety assessment process? An important issue that arises (and impinges upon the number of assays or types of data required) relative to answering this question is the scheme for decision making. Some approaches have been suggested (Fielder et al., 1987; ECETOC, 1988). For instance, the most straightforward approach would be to gather as much data as possible by nonexperimental methods such as those described above, then proceed to *in vitro* testing, and finally, if required, perform an animal assay. But, do all steps in the tier need to be performed? Will nonexperimental methods be sufficient? If *in vitro* assays are needed, how many should be performed? And if different assays are inconsistent, how does one decide which data are more accurate? Unfortunately, the answers to questions such as these are elusive. The manner in which alternative methods will be used in decision making will likely depend both on the individual company, and, within a company, on the reason for testing (i.e., how precise a measure of irritation is required, and does the answer need to be definitive, subjective, or conservative?).

For example, if testing is to be done on a new entity about which little is known, one would need to perform more assays than if testing a material that is essentially a reformulation of previously tested components. Additionally, if the reason for developing *in vitro* assays is to completely replace animals in irritation testing, then an extensive battery of methods examining a range of endpoints and potential mechanisms of action becomes essential since no confirming animal data will be obtained. If, on the other hand, the alternative methods are used as a prescreen to reduce the number of animals used, then fewer tests would be required, since one is only attempting to approximate the irritation potential. A decision would then be made whether to simply label a compound as irritating or to proceed with animal testing for a more accurate assessment.

In addition, the type and number of assays developed may depend on why the testing is being done. If, on the one hand, the testing is to be done for worker safety within the industrial or pharmaceutical environment, where eye protection is mandatory for all employees, it may only be necessary to establish an irritant–nonirritant label rather than a qualitative ranking (nonirritating, slight, mild, moderate, severe, extreme). In these circumstances, only a single *in vitro* test or reliance on a data base of information on similar compounds may be required to achieve this level of information. However, because the information obtained would provide a simple "yes/no," irritant versus nonirritant label, the methods used must be highly conservative; that is to say, false positives, while undesirable, would be more acceptable than false negatives, which could have drastic consequences upon accidental exposure. If, on the other hand, the testing is to be done on an ocular product where exposure to the eye would be deliberate, or on a consumer product, where a large, unprotected population may be potentially exposed, a more extensive and definitive irritancy evaluation would be necessary. Thus, it seems likely that no one approach to alternative testing can be consistently applied, but that the objectives of each laboratory and situation need to be considered in deciding on an appropriate test battery.

Whatever the specific need or application, the use of a tier testing scheme can significantly reduce, and in some cases eliminate, the use of animals. An example of a decision-making tree and its applications in ocular testing is provided in Figure 17.3. First, all available data about a test material (or related compounds), including chemical characteristics, historical data, other known toxicity, and the like, are collected. Analysis of these data could provide a strong indication of irritation potential, in which case the material would be labeled a presumed positive and

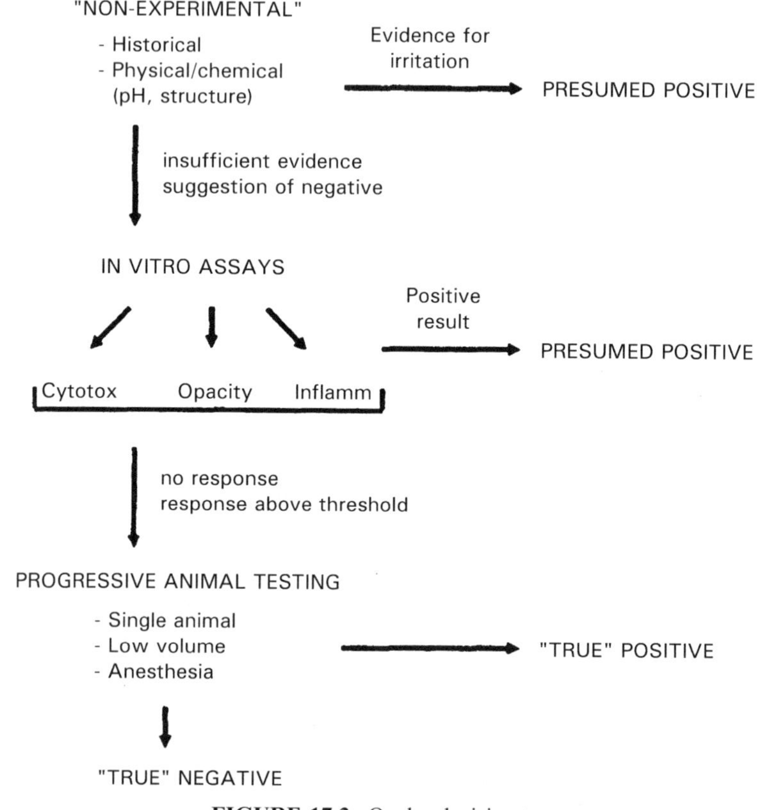


**FIGURE 17.3.** Ocular decision tree.

handled as such. Alternatively, the data may be equivocal or insufficient, in which case a battery of *in vitro* assays could be performed.

The *in vitro* battery would ideally include measures of opacity, cytotoxicity, and inflammation. The actual test method(s) will vary depending upon the experience of the laboratory, types of compounds to be tested, and so on. If the measured endpoint(s) indicates that the test material is approximately equipotent with known irritants, one would presume the unknown to be an irritant and further testing would not generally be required. One should keep in mind, however, that in many cases *in vitro* assays are more sensitive than whole-animal testing, so a positive response *in vitro* may not always indicate an *in vivo* irritant. If the assays give equivocal results or responses similar to those seen with non- or mild irritants, some type of animal testing may be indicated as confirmation.

If animal testing is required, a full-scale Draize test may not be necessary given the background established in the beginning of the tier approach. For instance, the compound could be tested in a single sentinel animal to obtain confirmation of *in vitro* data. In addition, other modifications could be used, such as the administration of appropriate anesthetics to the test animals, or the use of the low-volume Draize modification (Falahee et al., 1982; Freeberg et al., 1984; Griffith, 1987).

***Needs for the Future.*** One significant need in the area of ocular alternatives is for the validation of current *in vitro* assays. The key point is that users of the assay(s) need to have confidence in their ability to interpret and reliably use the data generated. This confidence level can only be achieved by parallel testing in one's own laboratory with compounds similar to those likely to be evaluated as unknowns. The validation process will be a long, somewhat tedious project, but will be necessary before *in vitro* alternatives can be used responsibly.

Another area where advances need to be made is in facing certain common technical issues in the *in vitro* methods themselves. A number of these potential pitfalls have been outlined by Frazier and Bradlaw (1989). One of the chief issues is the testing of water-insoluble materials. Many assay methods are based on material maintained in aqueous media; therefore, dosing the target cells with insoluble or immiscible test agents is difficult or impossible. Agar overlays or partitioning of test compound from a membrane have been used in some cases, but these are not universally applicable. Application of test material in various solvents may or may not allow adequate doses to be achieved. However, the toxicity of the solvents alone and in combination with test compounds must be carefully examined. Until adequate solutions to these solubility problems are found, some materials will simply not be able to be tested with *in vitro* methodologies.

Finally, as previously stated, if *in vitro* models are to be fully effective, the underlying mechanisms of ocular irritation need to be identified. Many of the *in vitro* assays proposed as alternatives to *in vivo* testing are based on correlations rather than mechanisms of irritation. The scoring or ranking of substances utilizing the *in vitro* endpoint may correlate with the severity of the *in vivo* response, but the reason for the agreement may be unclear and strictly fortuitous for the compounds evaluated. The ideal assay would monitor several biochemical or biological events specifically evoked in the whole animal by irritants. If events that are actually causal to irritation are measured, the probability of false results would decrease. Until we fully understand the mechanisms of the irritant response seen in the whole eye, a battery of tests aimed at evaluating as many biological events as possible is likely to be the best approach.

### 17.7.3. Nephrotoxicity *In Vitro*

The kidney is a frequent site of toxic insult due to drug and chemical exposure in experimental animals and man. Broad classes of drugs and industrial chemicals are implicated in nephrotoxic reactions (Cohen and Barac Neito, 1973; Smith et al., 1983). The use of various *in vitro* models in studying renal toxicology is well documented in the literature (Ware et al., 1979; Kacew and Hirsch, 1981; Hassall et al., 1983; Hook and Hewitt, 1986; Smith et al., 1987; Tay et al., 1988; Williams, 1989). A listing of the available *in vitro* models is provided in Table 17.6. Each model system possesses its own advantages and disadvantages, and all have demonstrated their usefulness and application in renal toxicology.

### *Methods*

**Isolated Perfused Kidney**. As the name implies, the isolated perfused kidney consists of the intact organ maintained in a tissue bath apparatus. An excellent review of the methods involved in preparing this model has been published by Newton and Hook (1981). With respect to functional integrity of the model, proximal tubule transport processes such as glucose uptake (Bowman and Maack, 1972), protein reabsorption (Maak, 1975), and amino acid uptake (De Mello and Maack, 1976) have been shown to be maintained. While this model has been used widely to examine renal physiological and drug disposition issues, it has not been extensively utilized as a toxicological tool (Bekersky, 1983). Cojocel et al. (1983) have used the isolated perfused rat kidney to examine the mechanisms of proteinuria induced by various aminoglycosides, while several other investigators have studies brush-border and basolateral aspects of renal accumulation and toxic reactions to aminoglycosides in the isolated perfused kidney (Collier et al., 1979; Williams et al., 1984). In another series of investigations, Newton et al. (1982a, b) examined the

**TABLE 17.6. *In Vitro* Nephrotoxicity Models**

| |
|---|
| Isolated perfused kidney |
| Isolated tubules |
| Renal cells |
| Cell lines |
| Primary cells |
| Kidney slices |
| Isolated organelles |

metabolism of acetaminophen in relationship to the nephrotoxicity of this agent. Using the isolated perfused kidney, they were able to show that the kidney was capable of metabolizing acetaminophen to the toxic chemical species, *para*-aminophenol, and of generating electrophilic intermediates capable of depleting glutathione.

*Kidney Slices.* Renal tissue slice technology has been extensively exploited for renal pharmacology and toxicology assessments. This methodology involves the removal of longitudinal sections of kidney tissue of varying thickness and weight with a razor guided either free-hand or through the use of an apparatus known as a Stadie–Riggs microtome (Stadie and Riggs, 1944). Kidney slices from virtually all species can be prepared; however, rat and rabbit have been the most frequently utilized models. Renal slices maintain the architecture and cellular heterogeneity of the intact kidney, with tubular segments and surrounding interstitial and vascular elements present. Functionally, renal slices also exhibit organic ion transport, gluconeogenesis, and active maintenance of cellular sodium and potassium balance through the enzymatic activity of $Na^+K^+$-ATPase (Cross and Taggart, 1950; Berndt et al., 1984).

Typically, the functional and morphological integrity of renal slices has a relatively short life span of approximately 2 h. However, one laboratory has succeeded in prolonging the viability of tissue slices for as long as 24 h (Ruegg et al., 1987a, b).

It is contended that the renal slice technique measures primarily basolateral uptake of substrates or nephrotoxins, based on histological evidence of collapsed tubular lumens. This results in the inaccessibility of brush-border surfaces for reabsorptive transport (Burg and Orloff, 1969; Cohen and Kamm, 1976). This observation limits the ability of this model to accurately reflect reactions to nephrotoxins that occur as the result of brush-border accumulation of an injurious agent. Ultrastructurally, a number of alterations, particularly in the plasma membrane and mitochondrial compartments, have been shown to occur over a 2-h incubation period (Martel-Pelletier et al., 1977). This deterioration in morphology is very likely a consequence of the insufficient diffusion of oxygen, metabolic substrates, and waste products in the innermost regions of the kidney slice (Cohen and Kamm, 1976). Such factors also limit the use of slices in studying renal metabolism and transport functions.

Renal cortical slices have been used to study numerous nephrotoxins including gentamicin (Hsu et al., 1977; Johnson and Maack, 1977; Kluwe and Hook, 1978), cisplatin (Goldstein et al., 1981; Safirstein et al., 1981; Phelps et al., 1987), cephaloridine (Goldstein et al., 1986, 1987), chloroform (Smith and Hook, 1983; Smith et al., 1983), potassium dichromate (Kacew and Hirsch, 1981; Ruegg et al., 1987b), and the mycotoxin citrinin (Berndt et al., 1984; Baggett and Berndt, 1984), to name a few. While congruence between biochemical effects of nephrotoxins on *in vitro* and *ex vivo* renal slice function has been achieved, correlations of morphological features of nephrotoxin-induced damage in kidney slices with *in vivo* effects are largely lacking.

*Isolated Tubules.* Isolated renal proximal tubule segments are most commonly prepared from either rats or rabbits by collagenase digestion of the kidneys followed by dispersion of the tissue into an appropriate buffer and filtration through sieves. Although this technique yields a tubule suspension that is highly contaminated with cellular debris, glomeruli, and distal tubules, the preparation can be further purified in a number of ways (Balaban et al., 1980; Vinay et al., 1981; Taub, 1984; Hatzinger and Stevens, 1989).

Renal tubular fragments appear to retain most of their *in vivo* functions and morphology. An important feature of this preparation was that the tubular lumina were open. (Balaban et al., 1980) reported that less than 3% of the tubular cells had any structural pathology except for the removal of the basement membrane. Functionally, isolated proximal tubular fragments transport *para*-aminohippurate, tetra-ethylammonium, $\alpha$-methylglucoside, phosphate, and $^{86}$Rb in a fashion similar to that reported *in vivo*, demonstrating the functional integrity of membrane processes of the preparation (Vinay et al., 1981; Dantzler and Brokl, 1984; Tessitore et al., 1986; Dantzler et al., 1989). With respect to renal cortical glutathione (GSH), isolated tubules are approximately 50–70% GSH depleted when compared to control tissue. However, suspensions of isolated rabbit tubules will synthesize GSH from the constituent amino acids: glutamate, cysteine, and glycine.

Isolated proximal tubules have been utilized to study the mechanisms of nephrotoxicity induced by antibiotics (Sina et al., 1985, 1986), radiocontrast dyes (Humes et al., 1987), metals (Rylander et al., 1985), anoxia (Weinberg, 1985; Weinberg et al., 1987), cellular oxidants (Messana et al., 1988), cysteine conjugates (Rylander et al., 1985; Schnellman et al., 1987; Zhang and Stevens, 1989), and a variety of nephrotoxic bromobenzene metabolites (Schnellman and Mandel, 1986; Schnellman et al., 1987).

*Renal Cells.* A variety of isolated cellular models exist for studying renal function and injury. These models can generally be divided into two categories: models derived from permanent renal cell lines and cellular models derived from freshly isolated renal tissue.

1. *Cell Lines.* Cell lines, derived from tissue of various species, are commercially available from tissue culture banks. These cell populations are "immortalized" in that they possess the capacity to permanently proliferate in culture. Such cellular models can be studied in short-term suspension (hours) or longer-term monolayer culture (days, weeks, months). Since cell lines have been extensively cultured or passaged for multiple generations, the degree or retention (or loss) of kidney-specific morphology and function is an important limitation that is not thoroughly addressed for a number of renal cell lines. One renal cell line that has been relatively well characterized is the pig kidney cell line, LLC-PK$_1$.

The LLC-PK$_1$ (porcine kidney) cell line (Hull et al., 1976) exhibits a range of morphological and functional properties of proximal tubule epithelium. For example, Na$^+$-dependent glucose and amino acid transport have been demonstrated in LLC-PK$_1$ cells (Rabito and Ausiello, 1980; Rabito and Karish, 1982, 1983). LLC-

PK$_1$ cells have also demonstrated the ability to transport organic cations such as tetraethylammonium (TEA) (Inui et al., 1985), but do not appear to possess the capacity for organic anion transport (Rabito, 1986). Morphologically, LLC-PK$_1$ cells have been shown to be polarized with apical microvilli, apical junctional complexes, desmosomes, and basolateral unfoldings (Cereijido et al., 1978), which is typical of transporting epithelial cells. The expression of brush-border morphology is striking in LLC-PK$_1$ cells, although the amount of brush border is less than that observed in the proximal tubule *in vivo*. High activities of proximal tubule brush-border membrane enzymes have also been observed in LLC-PK$_1$ cells (Gstraunthaler et al., 1985). LLC-PK$_1$ Cells also possess significant levels of the basolateral enzyme marker Na$^+$K$^+$-ATPase, which is thought to result in the formation of fluid-filled "blisters" or domes in monolayer culture via transepithelial sodium and water transport (Gstraunthaler et al., 1985).

Renal cell lines have been utilized to a limited extent for evaluation nephrotoxins. A rabbit kidney cell line (LLC-RK$_1$) has been utilized for evaluating nephrotoxic antibiotics (Viano et al., 1983; Hottendorf et al., 1987; Williams et al., 1988). LLC-PK$_1$ cells have by far been the most widely employed cell line for studying drug-induced nephrotoxicity, specifically in the evaluation of aminoglycoside antibiotics (Hori et al., 1984; Schwertz et al., 1986; Williams et al., 1986b; Holohan et al., 1988). The morphological alterations induced by aminoglycosides in LLC-PK$_1$ cells correlated well with *in vivo* histological findings in the kidney, including the formation of secondary lysosomal inclusions referred to as myeloid bodies.

2. *Primary Cells*. Cells from freshly isolated renal tissue can be obtained by explant cultures, cultures of isolated renal tubules discussed in the previous section, and by digestion and isolation of individual renal cells. Cultures of isolated renal fragments such as the proximal tubule (Fine and Sakhrani, 1986) and collecting tubule (Grenier, 1986) have been the most extensively characterized models to date. Primary cultures of proximal tubules have been isolated from rabbit (Chung et al., 1982), dog (Goligorsky et al., 1986), rat (Bellemann, 1980; Hatzinger and Stevens, 1989), and human kidneys (Detrisac et al., 1984; Wilson et al., 1985). Primary cultures prepared from rabbit proximal tubules have been shown to exhibit polarity and transport characteristics consistent with proximal tubule function. As with certain renal cell lines such as the LLC-PK$_1$ and MDCK, primary cultures also possess tight junctions and basolateral Na$^+$K$^+$-ATPase activity that results in the formation of fluid-filled "blisters" or domes in monolayer culture. Transport functions including phlorizin-sensitive Na$^+$-dependent glucose uptake (Sakhrani et al., 1984) and organic anion and cation transport (Yang et al., 1988) are present in rabbit primary cultures. Primary cultures of rabbit proximal tubules have also been shown to be responsive to parathyroid hormone (Chung et al., 1982), to maintain cellular glutathione levels (Aleo et al., 1990), and to exhibit brush-border enzyme activity (Ford et al., 1987).

Primary renal cell culture has been utilized to study a number of nephrotoxic agents including mercuric chloride (Inamoto et al., 1976), cadmium (Cherian, 1982), lead (McLachlin et al., 1980), cisplatin (Tay et al., 1988), aminoglycoside antibiotics

(Chatterjee et al., 1984; Sens et al., 1988), and cyclosporine (Trifillis et al., 1984). Studies reported by Tay et al. (1988) in rabbit proximal tubule cultures with cisplatin revealed biochemical effects upon DNA synthetic activty that correlated with *in vivo* histochemical effects of this antitumor agent in animals. With respect to studies involving mercuric chloride and aminoglycoside antibiotics in primary renal cultures, light and electron microscopy revealed similar patterns of cellular pathology *in vitro* as compared to *in vivo* exposure in animals (Chatterjee et al., 1984; Aleo et al., 1987).

Suspensions rather than cultures of renal cell lines and primary cells are also available for short-term evaluations. Procedures for the isolation and purification of specific renal cell types include density gradient centrifugation, flow cytometry, free flow electrophoresis, enzymatic digestion, and monoclonal antibodies (Dworzack and Grantham, 1975; Kreisberg et al., 1977; Heidrich and Dew, 1977; Eveloff et al., 1980; Endou et al., 1982; Smith and Garcia-Perez, 1985). While primary renal cell suspensions possess the advantage of being freshly isolated and derived from intact kidney tissue, a major disadvantage is their lack of cellular polarity that is exhibited with cells in culture. Relatively few reports of renal suspension cultures being used in nephrotoxic evaluations are in the literature at this time (Holohan et al., 1988).

One of the unique advantages of renal cell culture rests in making possible the study of the directional aspects of drug exposure and cellular injury that operate *in vivo*. The technology to grow renal epithelial cells on filter inserts for this purpose has recently been made available (Figure 17.4). This potential provides the opportunity to study compounds that interact or accumulate within the renal tubular epithelium *in vivo* via tubular reabsorption from the luminal surface or extraction

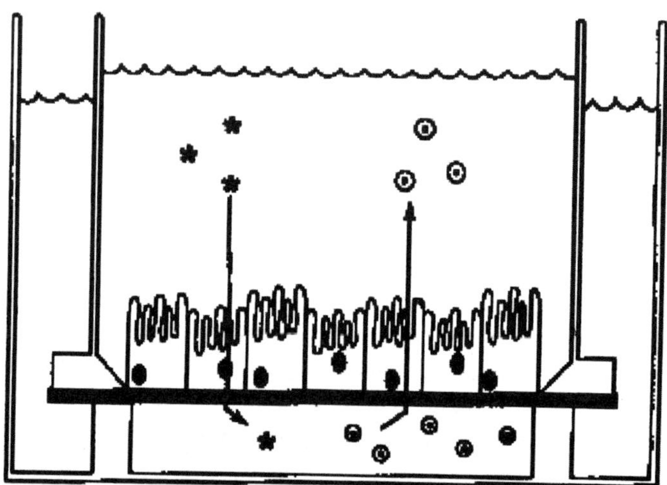

**FIGURE 17.4.** Developing technology for bidirectional exposure/transport in polarized epithelial cells. Shown are kidney cells grown on porous membrane filters. Symbols represent chemical exposure from basolateral (☉) and brush border (*) surfaces.

from the basolateral or blood surface. Preliminary data involving the directional aspects of antibiotic toxicity to LLC-PK$_1$ cells have recently been obtained, indicating that LLC-PK$_1$ cells are significantly more sensitive to the nephrotoxin cephaloridine when the antibiotic was applied to the basolateral surface of the kidney cell (Williams et al., 1993). These data are consistent with the evidence that cephaloridine is accumulated in renal cells predominantly through basolateral transport. This cellular accumulation is then presumed to precipitate cellular injury and death.

*Biochemical Systems.* In addition to the isolated organ, tubule, and cellular models just described, biochemical systems derived from renal tissue represent valuable resources for *in vitro* evaluations of nephrotoxins. Particularly, the use of isolated cellular organelles such as mitochondria and plasma membranes has been applied to the study of nephrotoxins (Williams and Hottendorf, 1985, 1986; Tune et al., 1988, 1989). The examination of mechanisms of accumulation of nephrotoxins in the kidney has been accomplished utilizing purified renal brush-border and basolateral membrane vesicles for aminoglycosides (Williams and Hottendorf, 1986; Williams et al., 1987), cephalosporins (Kasher et al., 1983; Williams et al., 1985), and cisplatin (Williams and Hottendorf, 1985). Williams and coworkers (1987) reported that the affinity for renal membrane binding sites correlated well with the nephrotoxic potential of aminoglycosides. Thus, this membrane model could be utilized to assess the relative nephrotoxic potential of new aminoglycosides. Furthermore, isolated renal membranes were successfully employed in the identification of *in vivo* nephrotoxicity inhibitors for aminoglycosides (Williams et al., 1986a). The correlation between the ability of polyamino acids to inhibit *in vitro* binding and *in vivo* nephrotoxicity of aminoglycosides with aminoglycosides coadministered with polyamino acids demonstrated the utility of *in vitro* models to contribute to the drug discovery process.

**Needs for the Future.** Challenges for the future involve the continued development of current *in vitro* models to provide psychological and morphological characteristics that correlate more closely with the kidney *in vivo*. These challenges will include, for example, defining conditions that facilitate and optimize the retention of renal transport and metabolizing capabilities in cell culture. Perhaps most challenging is the need to establish *in vitro* systems that reproduce the dynamic features of the nephron *in vivo*. The kidney, like other organs, exists in a dynamic rather than static environment. The fluid dynamics and vasculature of the renal nephron most certainly play a role in the sensitivity of the kidney in terms of both dose and time responses to nephrotoxins.

## 17.8. VALIDATION

Perhaps one of the biggest issues in developing alternative test strategies is the validation of the test methods. One reason that this topic has become controversial is that validation has different meanings to different people. In the strictest scientific and linguistic sense, validation is the process of proving adherence to principles, logic, and facts, free from error or superficiality. As applied to *in vitro* test procedures designed to mimic *in vivo* responses, this definition would require adherence to the principles and facts of *in vivo* toxicity, according to the criteria previously outlined (Table 17.2). However, test reproducibility, simplicity, and transferability are frequently viewed as the critical ingredients to test validation, at the expense of any mechanistic or scientific validity. It can be argued that such components, though important in test standardization and acceptance, may have little bearing on the true scientific validation and rigor of new test procedures. Despite divergent opinions on validation, much has been written about this topic, and a number of validation or evaluation projects are currently underway within various organizations such as the Soap and Detergent Association (Booman et al., 1988), the Fund for the Replacement of Animals in Medical Experiments (FRAME), the German Federal Health Office (Kalweit et al., 1987), and the Cosmetics, Toiletries, and Fragrances Association, as well as within the laboratories of individuals working with specific assays.

What constitutes acceptable validation? Suggested in the preceding paragraph, there is no general agreement on this point; the answer is likely to be different for each company or individual performing the tests. If one generalization is to be made concerning validation, it would be that one needs to test enough compounds with different characteristics and mechanisms of action to develop confidence in the *in vitro* data. And this, in turn, will depend upon the individual user. If one simply requires a toxicity classification for purposes of prescreening, the validation process may be less involved than if a more definitive classification is required of a test system. Stated in another way, the more one expects in terms of predictability from the *in vitro* data, the more testing needs to be done to develop confidence in the methods. The cornerstone to this confidence lies in the fulfillment of the scientific criteria previously outlined (Table 17.2).

Additionally, the test materials used in the validation process should be as closely related as possible to the characteristics of the unknowns to be tested. It is clear from the literature, for instance, that many cytotoxicity assays give good correlations with the *in vivo* ocular irritancy data for surfactants, but the correlations fail when compounds from other chemical classes are tested. Since any particular assay may be used differently by individual safety assessment programs, users must evaluate potential methods under conditions likely to be encountered in their own situations.


## 17.9. THE FUTURE

The future of *in vitro* techniques in toxicological assessment takes us back to our introductory discussion of the philosophical and scientific considerations operating in the evolution of alternative methods.

Scientifically, the future will depend on the level of confidence achieved that *in vitro* systems provide information that is representative of the *in vivo* processes the toxicologist seeks to model and predict. The degree to which this level of confidence will evolve is directly proportional to the fulfillment of the scientific criteria outlined in Table 17.2, which determine the strength of the *in vitro–in vivo* correlations obtained. Because gaps remain in our knowledge with respect to these important criteria, the future will also depend on advancements in available knowledge and technology with respect to biochemical or *in vitro* toxicological events. Specifically, challenges for the future involve the continued development of current *in vitro* models to provide psychological and morphological characteristics that correlate more closely with target organs *in vivo*. These challenges will include defining media constituents that will facilitate the retention of normal morphology and metabolizing capabilities *in vitro*, as well as the establishment of systems that reproduce the dynamic features or organs *in vivo*. With *in vitro–in vivo* correlations playing a key role in *in vitro* test development, the growth of technologies that focus on differentiated functions, cellular relationships, human models, and other *in vivo* properties, such as fluid dynamics, will be critical to the future applications of *in vitro* techniques in toxicology. An example of a scientific and technological advancement that promises to contribute to the field of *in vitro* pharmacology and toxicology is the development of a human skin equivalent model. This commercially available material possesses the qualities of differentiation, cellular relationship, and the incorporation of human tissue, and has already shown usefulness in the study of dermal absorption and irritancy (Bell et al., 1981, 1983, 1989).

Philosophically, where will the future lead us? Assuming that the industrial toxicologist continues to play a central role in the evaluation and prediction of product safety, one can envision continuing involvement in performing extrapolations from animal data to potential human risk. At the same time, one may also expect increasing public pressure to reduce animal testing. With these toxicological and societal goals in mind, the value and application of human tissue in predicting human metabolism and target organ effects is likely to grow. This approach not only reduces animal use, but may significantly enhance our correlative abilities with the ultimate species of concern: humans. Perhaps challenges in risk assessment in the future will involve extrapolations from human tissues to human safety. However, the ultimate value of using human tissues *in vitro* relies on the technological and intellectual advances in performing and interpreting *in vitro* biochemical data. Thus, the challenges in extrapolating *in vitro* data from human tissues to human responses *in vivo* are identical to current issues in the use of *in vitro* models to predict toxicity to animals. As predictability and correlation of *in vitro* models with specific *in vivo* events is achieved, toxicologists can look forward to performing meaningful species comparisons *in vitro*, involving direct preclinical assessments in humans (Figure 17.5).

## 17.10. CONCLUSIONS

In summary, an examination of the current state of the art in the pharmaceutical industry illustrates exciting and important roles that *in vitro* systems can play in

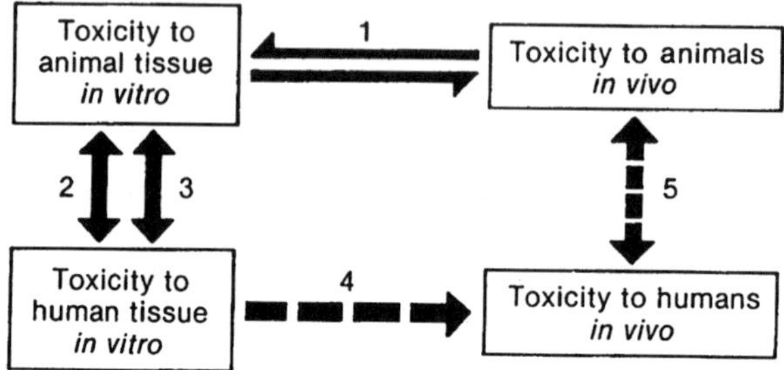



**FIGURE 17.5.** The use of *in vitro* techniques in performing interspecies comparisons. 1, correlation of *in vitro* with *in vivo* observations; 2, development of parallel *in vitro* systems in man; 3, comparison of *in vivo* sensitivity of different species; 4, potential toxicity *in vivo*; 5, comparison of *in vivo* sensitivity of different species.

toxicological assessments. With the development of *in vitro* models more closely representing organ function and dynamics, the ability to accurately predict toxic reactions *in vivo* will be enhanced. As time and experience build scientific confidence and validation of these *in vitro* models, one can envision the toxicologist utilizing *in vitro* models more extensively in the assessment of toxicity. However, in order to advance alternative methodology to this stage, it is clear that the toxicologist must continue to take an active role in the research of toxic mechanisms and the development of the tools to study them. Without such a commitment, the field of *in vitro* toxicology might be expected to remain static. Thus, while the current uses of *in vitro* techniques have significantly reduced animal use, and advanced our understanding of toxic mechanisms, the full potential of *in vitro* models to further reduce, refine, and replace whole-animal tests has certainly not been realized. The future, in fact, is only limited by the amount of energy and creativity we, as scientists, can apply to *in vitro* test development.

For the present, the utilization of *in vivo* toxicological models is imperative for responsible risk assessment of new chemical entities. At the same time, the use of the many *in vitro* models currently available can serve as valuable adjuncts to these *in vivo* assessments, not only reducing the number of animals used in risk assessment, but providing unique information and possibilities for scientists involved in the drug discovery and development process.

It is not clear how the immense base of knowledge generated under the various rubrics of "genomics" will ultimately be utilized to improve drug safety and the drug development process. What is clear, however, is that it will be some years before such studies displace the current paradigm of testing.

# REFERENCES


Aleo, M.D., Wyatt, R.D. and Schnellmann, R.G. (1991). The role of altered mitochondrial function in citrinin-induced toxicity to rat renal proximal tubule suspensions. *Toxicol. Appl. Pharmacol.* 109: 455–463.

Baggett, J.M. and Berndt, W.O. (1984). Interaction of potassium dichromate with the nephrotoxins, mercuric chloride and citrinin. *Toxicology* 33(2): 157–169.

Bagley, D.M., Dong, B.M. and De Salva, S.J. (1989). Assessing the eye irritation potential of surfactant-based materials using the chorioallantoic membrane vascular assay (CAMVA). In: *Alternative Methods in Toxicology*, Vol. 7 (Goldberg, A.M., ed.) Mary Ann Liebert, New York, pp. 265–272.

Balaban, R.S., Soltoff, S.P., Storey, J.M. and Mandel, L.J. (1980). Improved renal cortical suspension: spectrophotometric study of $O_2$ delivery. *Am. J. Physiol.* 238: F50–F59.

Bekersky, I. (1983). The isolated perfused kidney as a pharmacological tool. *TIBS* 4: 6–7.

Bell, E., Ehrlich, H.P., Buttle, D.J. and Nakatusuji, T. (1981). Living tissue formed *in vitro* and accepted as skin-equivalent tissue of full thickness. *Science* 211: 1052–1054.

Bell, E., Sher, S., Hull, B., Merrill, C., Rosen, S., Chamson, A., Asselineau, D., Dubertret, L., Coulomb, B., Lapiere, C., Nusgens, B. and Neveus, Y. (1983). The reconstitution of living skin. *J. Invest. Dermatol.* 81: 2s–10s.

Bell, E., Gay, R., Swiderek, M., Class, T., Kemp, P., Green, G., Haimes, H. and Bilbo, P. (1989). *Use of fabricated living tissue and organ equivalents as defined higher order systems for the study of pharmacologic responses to test substances.* Presented at NATO Advanced Research Workshop, September 4–9, Bandol, France.

Bellemann, P. (1980). Primary monolayer culture of liver parenchymal cells and kidney cortical tubules as a useful new model for biochemical pharmacology and experimental toxicology. Studies *in vitro* on hepatic membrane transport, induction of liver enzymes, and adaptive changes in renal cortical enzymes. *Arch. Toxicol.* 44: 63–84.

Berndt, W.O., Hayes, A.W. and Baggett, J.M. (1984). Effects of fungal toxins on renal slice calcium balance. *Toxicol. Appl. Pharmacol.* 74(1): 78–85.

Boelsterli, U.A., Bouis, P. and Donatsch, P. (1987). Relative cytotoxicity of psychotropic drugs in cultured rat hepatocytes. *Cell Biol. Toxicol.* 3: 231–250.

Boelsterli, U.A., Bouis, P., Brouillard, J.F. and Donatsch, P. (1988). *In vitro* toxicity assessment of cyclosporin A and its analogs in a primary rat hepatocyte culture model. *Toxicol. Appl. Pharmacol.* 96: 212–221.

Booman, K.A., Cascieri, T.M., Demetrulias, J., Driedger, A., Griffith, J.F., Grochoski, G.T., Kong, B., McCormick, W.C., North-Root, H., Rozen, M.G. and Sedlak, R.I. (1988). *In vitro* methods for estimating eye irritancy of cleaning products phase I: preliminary assessment. *J. Toxicol. – Cut. Ocular Toxicol.* 7: 173–185.

Booman, K.A., DeProspo, J., Demetrulias, J., Driedger, A., Griffith, J.F., Grochoski, G., King, B., McCormick, W.C., North-Root, H., Rozen, M.G. and Sedlak, R.I. (1989). The SDA alternatives program: comparison of *in vitro* data with Draize test data. *J. Toxicol. – Cut. Ocular Toxicol.* 8: 35–49.

Borenfreund, E. and Borrero, O. (1984). *In vitro* cytotoxicity assays: potential alternatives to the Draize ocular irritancy test. *Cell Biol. Toxicol.* 1: 33–39.

Borenfruend, E. and Puerner, J.A. (1984). A simple quantitative procedure using monolayer cultures for cytotoxicity assays. *J. Tissue Culture Meth.* 9: 7–9.

Borenfruend, E. and Puerner, J.A. (1987). Short-term quantitative *in vitro* cytotoxicity assay involving an S-9 activating system. *Cancer Lett.* 34: 243–248.

Bowman, R.H. and Maack, T. (1972). Glucose transport by the isolated perfused rat kidney. *Am. J. Physiol.* 222: 1499–1504.

Bracher, M., Faller, C., Spengler, J. and Reinhardt, C.A. (1987). Comparison of *in vitro* cell toxicity with *in vivo* eye irritation. *Molec. Toxicol.* 1: 561–570.

Bradley, M.O., Dysart, G., Fitzsimmons, K., Harback, P., Lewin, J. and Wolf, G. (1982). Measurement by filter elution of DNA single- and double-strand breaks in rat hepatocytes: Effects of nitrosamines and $\gamma$-irradiation. *Cancer Res.* 42: 2569–2597.

Bruner, L.H. and Parker, R.D. (1990). Evaluation of six *in vitro* alternatives for ocular irritancy testing. *Toxicologist* 10: 258.

Burg, M.B. and Orloff, J. (1969). *Para*-aminohippurate uptake and exchange by separated renal tubules. *Amer. J. Physiol.* 217: 1064–1068.

Castell, J.V., Larrauri, A. and Gomez-Lechon, M.J. (1988). A study of the relative hepatotoxicity *in vitro* of the non-steroidal anti-inflammatory drugs ibuprofen, flurbiprofen and butibufen. *Xenobiotica* 18: 737–745.

Cereijido, M., Robbins, E.S., Doland, W.J., Rotunno, C.A. and Sabatini, D.D. (1978). Polarized monolayers formed by epithelial cells on a permeable and translucent support. *J. Cell Biol.* 77: 853–880.

Chatterjee, S., Trifillis, A. and Regec, A. (1984). Morphological and biochemical effects of gentamicin on cultured human-kidney renal tubular cells. *Human Toxicology* 3: 455.

Cherian, M.G. (1982). Studies on toxicity of metallothionein in rat kidney epithelial cell culture. *Dev. Toxicol. Environ. Sci.* 9: 193–202.

Chung, S.D., Alavi, N., Livingston, D., Hiller, S. and Taub, M. (1982). Characterization of primary rabbit kidney cultures that express proximal tubule functions in a hormonally defined medium. *J. Cell Biol.* 95: 118–126.

Clayton, G.D. and Clayton, F.E., (Eds.). (1981). *Patty's Industrial Hygiene and Toxicology.* Wiley, New York.

Cohen, J.J. and Barac Neito, M. (1973). Renal metabolism of substrates in relation to renal function. In: *Handbook of Physiology* (Orloff, J. and Berliner, R.W., Eds.). American Physiological Society, Washington, D.C., pp. 909–926.

Cohen, J.J. and Kamm, D.E. (1976). Renal metabolism: Relation to renal function. In: *The Kidney* (Brenner, B.M. and Rector, F.C., Eds.). Saunders, Philadelphia, pp. 126–214.

Cojocel, C., Dociu, N., Maita, K., Sleight, S.D. and Hook, J.B. (1983). Effects of aminoglycosides on glomerular permeability, tubular reabsorption, and intracellular catabolism of the cationic low molecular weight protein lysozyme. *Toxicol. Appl. Pharm.* 39: 129–139.

Collier, V., Lietman, P. and Mitch, W. (1979). Evidence for luminal uptake of gentamicin in the perfused rat kidney. *J. Pharmacol. Exp. Ther.* 210: 247–251.

Conquet, P., Durand, G., Lailler, J. and Plazonnet, B. (1977). Evaluation of ocular irritation in the rabbit: Objective versus subjective assessment. *Toxicol. Appl. Pharm.* 39: 129–139.

Croci, T. and Williams, G.M. (1985). Activities of several phase I and phase II xenobiotic biotransformation enzymes in cultured hepatocytes from male and female rats. *Biochem. Pharm.* 17(34): 3029–3035.

Cross, R.J. and Taggart, J.L. (1950). Renal tubular transport: Accumlation of *p*-aminohippurate by rabbit kidney slices. *Amer. J. Physiol.* 161: 181–190.

Dantzler, W.H. and Brokl, O.H. (1984). Effects of low $[Ca^{2+}]$ and $La^{3+}$ on PAH transport by isolated perfused renal tubules. *Am. J. Physiol.* 246: F175–F187.

Dantzler, W.H., Brokl, O.H. and Wright, S.H. (1989). Brush-border TEA transport in intact proximal tubules and isolated membrane vesicles. *Am. J. Physiol.* 256: F290–F297.

Davis, D.C., Potter, W.Z., Jollow, D.J. and Mitchell, J.R. (1974). Species differences in hepatic glutathione depletion, covalent binding and hepatic necrosis after acetaminophen. *Life Sci.* 14: 2099–2109.

Decad, G.M., Hsieh, D.P.H. and Byard, J.L. (1977). Maintenance of cytochrome P-450 and metabolism of aflatoxin $B_1$ in primary hepatocyte cultures. *Biochem. Biophys. Res. Comm.* 78: 279–287.

De Mello, G. and Maack, T. (1976). Nephron function of the isolated perfused rat kidney. *Am. J. Physiol.* 231: 1699–1707.

Detrisac, C.J., Sens, M.A., Garvin, A.J., Spicer, S.S. and Sens, D.A. (1984). Tissue culture of human kidney epithelial cells of proximal tubule origin. *Kidney Int.* 25: 383–390.

Donata, M.T., Gomez-Lechon, M.J. and Castell, J.V. (1990). Effect of xenobiotics on monooxygenase activities in cultured human hepatocytes. *Biochem. Pharmacol.* 8(39): 1321–1326.

Dougherty, K.K., Spilman, S.D., Green, C.E., Steward, A.R. and Byard, J.L. (1980). Primary cultures of adult mouse and rat hepatocytes for studying the metabolism of foreign compounds. *Biochem. Pharmacol.* 29: 2117–2124.

Dworzack, D.L. and Grantham, J.J. (1975). Preparation of renal papillary collecting duct cells for study *in vitro*. *Kidney Int.* 8: 191–194.

ECETOC (1988). Eye irritation testing. Monograph No. 11, Brussels, pp. 1–65.

Elgebaly, S.A., Gillies, C., Forouhar, F., Hahem, M., Baddour, M., O'Rourke, J. and Dreutzer, D.L. (1985). An *in vitro* model of leukocyte mediated injury to the corneal epithelium. *Curr. Eye Res.* 4: 31–41.

Elgebaly, S.A., Forouhar, F. and Kreutzer, D.L. (1987). *In vitro* detection of cornea-derived leukocytic chemotactic factors as indicators of corneal inflammation. In: *Alternative Methods in Toxicology*, Vol. 5 (Goldberg, A.M., Ed.). Mary Ann Liebert, Inc., New York, pp. 257–268.

Enat, R., Jefferson, D.M., Ruiz-Opazo, N., Gatmaitan, Z., Leinwand, L.A. and Reid, L.M. (1984). Hepatocyte proliferation *in vitro*: Its dependence on the use of serum-free hormonally defined medium and substrata of extracellular matrix. *Proc. Natl. Acad. Sci U.S.A.* 81: 1411–1415.

Endou, H., Koseki, C., Kimura, K., Yokokura, Y., Fukida, S. and Sakai, F. (1982). Use of a flow cytometer for the separation of isolated kidney cells. In: *Biochemistry of Kidney Functions* (Morel, F., ed.). Elsevier Biomedical Press, Amsterdam, pp. 69–78.

Eveloff, J., Haase, W. and Kinne, R. (1980). Separation of renal medullary cells: isolation of cells from the thick ascending limb of Henle's loop. *J. Cell Biol.* 87: 672–681.

Falahee, K.J., Rose, C.S., Seifried, H.F. and Sawhney, D. (1982). Alternatives in toxicity testing. In: *Product Safety Evaluation* (Goldberg, A.M., Ed.). Alternative Methods in Toxicology, Vol. 1. Mary Ann Liebert, New York, pp. 137–162.

Farland, W.H., Tyson, C.A. and Sawhney, D.S. (1985). Rationale and use of functions tests in toxicity testing: a review. In: *Organ Function Tests in Toxicity Evaluation* (Tyson, C.A. and Sawhney, D.S., Eds.). Noyes Publications, Park Ridge, NJ, pp. 1–22.

Fielder, R.J., Gaunt, I.F., Rhodes, C., Sullivan, F.M. and Swanston, D.W. (1987). A hierarchical approach to the assessment of dermal and ocular irritancy: a report by the British Toxicological Society working party on irritancy. *Human Toxicol.* 6: 269–278.

Fine, L.G. and Sakhrani, L.M. (1986). Proximal tubular cells in primary culture. *Mineral Electrolyte Metab.* 12: 51–57.

Fishlock, D. (1990). Survival of the fittest drugs. *Financial Times.* 24 April: 16–17.

Flower, C. (1987). Some problems in validating cytotoxicity as a correlate of ocular irritancy. In: *Alternative Methods in Toxicology,* Vol. 5. (Goldberg, A.M., Ed.). Mary Ann Liebert, New York, pp. 269–274.

Ford, S.M., Bennett, D., Laska, D.A., Tay, L.K. and Williams, P.D. (1987). Biochemical comparison of fresh kidney homogenates, rabbit primary proximal tubule cultures (RPT), and a rabbit kidney epithelial cell line (LLC-RK$_1$). *FASEB J.,* April, 1987.

Frazier, J.M. and Bradlow, J.A. (1989). *Technical Problems Associated with In Vitro Toxicity Testing Systems.* Technical Report 1. Johns Hopkins Center for Alternatives to Animal Testing, Baltimore, MA.

Frazier, J.M., Gad, S.C., Goldberg, A.M. and McCulley, J.P. (1987). *A Critical Evaluation of Alternatives to Acute Ocular Irritation Testing. Alternative Methods in Toxicology,* Vol. 4. Mary Ann Liebert, New York.

Freeberg, F.E., Griffith, J.F., Bruce, R.D. and Bay, P.H.S. (1984). Correlation of animal test methods with human experience for household products. *J. Toxicol. – Cut. Ocular Toxicol.* 1: 53–64.

Gad, S.C. (1988). Principles of screening in toxicology: with special emphasis on applications to neurotoxicology. *J. Am. Coll. Toxicol* 8: 21–27.

Gad, S.C. (1988). A tier testing strategy incorporating *in vitro* testing methods for pharmaceutical safety assessment. *Humane Innovations Alternatives Anim. Exp.* 3: 75–79.

Gad, S.C. (1989). A Tier Testing Strategy Incorporating *In Vitro* Testing Methods for Pharmaceutical Safety Assessment. *Humane Innovations Alternatives Anim. Exp.* 3: 75–79.

Gad, S.C. (1990). Recent developments in replacing, reducing, and refining animal use in toxicologic research and testing. *Fund. Appl. Toxicol.* 15: 8–16.

Gad, S.C. (1992). Industrial application for *in vitro* toxicity testing methods: A tier testing strategy for product safety assessment. In: *In Vitro Toxicity Testing* (Frazier, J., Ed.). Marcel Dekker, New York, pp. 253–279.

Gad, S.C. (1993). *In Vivo* and *In Vitro* Tox, in *Biotechnology and Safety Assessment* (Thomas, J.A. and Myers, L.A., Eds.). Raven Press, New York, 97–129.

Gad, S.C. (1995a). Integration of alternative methods into the safety evaluation process in the United States. *Comments in Toxicol.* 5: 301–314.

Gad, S.C. (1995b). Challenges and needs in the safety assessment of new therapeutics. *Toxicol. Meth.* 5: viii–x.

Gad, S.C. (1996). Strategies for the application and interpretation of *in vitro* methods to the development of new pharmaceuticals and medical devices. *Toxicol. Methods* 6: 1–12.

Gad, S.C. (1996a). Histologic and clinical pathology in the safety assessment and development of new therapeutic agents. *Scand. J. Lab. Anim. Sci.*

Gad, S.C. (1996b). Preclinical toxicity testing in the development of new therapeutic agents. *Scand. J. Lab. Anim. Sci.*

Gad, S.C. (1998). Strategies and application of *in vitro* methods to the development of pharmaceuticals and devices. In: *Advances in Animal Alternatives for Safety and Efficacy Testing* (Salem, H., Ed.). Taylor & Francis, Philadelphia, PA, pp. 293–302.

Gad, S.C. (1999). *Product Safety Evaluation Handbook,* 2nd ed. Marcel Dekker, New York.

Gad, S.C. (2000). *In Vitro Toxicology,* 2nd ed. Taylor & Francis, Philadelphia, PA.

Gad, S.C. (2001). *Regulatory Toxicology,* 2nd ed. Taylor & Francis, Philadelphia, PA.

Gad, S.C. (2001). Alternatives to *in vivo* studies in toxicology. In: *General & Applied Toxicology*, 2nd ed. (Ballantyne, B., Marvis, T. and Turner, P., Eds.). Macmillan, New York, pp. 401–424.

Gad, S.C. and Chengelis, C.P. (1999). *Acute Toxicology*, 2nd ed. Academic Press, San Diego, CA.

Gad, S.C., Walsh, R.D. and Dunn, B.J. (1986). Correlation of ocular and dermal irritancy of industrial chemicals. *J. Toxicol. – Cut. Ocular Toxicol.* 5: 195–213.

Gautheron, P.D. and Sina, J.F. (1990). The bovine corneal opacity, an *in vitro* assay of ocular irritancy. *Toxicologist* 10: 258.

Gautheron, P.D., Dukic, M., Alix, D. and Sina, J.F. (1992). Bovine corneal opacity and permeability test: An *in vitro* assay of ocular irritation. *Fund. Appl. Toxicol. – Cut. Ocular Toxicol.* 2: 107–117.

Gillman, M.R., Jackson, E.M., Cerven, D.R. and Moreno, M.T. (1983). Relationship between the primary dermal irritation index and ocular irritation. *J. Toxicol. – Cut. Ocular Toxicol.* 2: 107–117.

Goldstein, R.S., Noordewier, B., Bond, J.T., Hook, J.B. and Mayor, G.H. (1981). *Cis*-diaminedichloroplatinum nephrotoxicity: Time course and dose response of renal functional impairment. *Toxicol. Appl. Pharmacol.* 60: 163–175.

Goldstein, R.S., Pasino, D.A., Hewitt, W.R. and Hook, J.B. (1986). Biochemical mechanisms of cephaloridine nephrotoxicity: Time and concentration dependence of peroxidative injury. *Toxicol. Appl. Pharmacol.* 83(2): 261–270.

Goldstein, R.S., Contardi, L.R., Pasino, D.A. and Hook, J.B. (1987). Mechanisms mediating cephaloridine inhibition of renal gluconeogenesis. *Toxicol. Appl. Pharmacol.* 87(2): 297–305.

Goligorsky, M.S., Menton, D.M. and Hruska, K.A. (1986). Parathyroid hormone-induced changes of the brush border topography and cytoskeleton in cultured renal proximal tubular cells. *J. Membr. Biol.* 92: 151–162.

Gomez-Lechon, M.J., Montoya, A., Lopez, P., Donato, T., Larrauri, A. and Castell, J.V. (1988). The potential use of cultured hepatocytes in predicting the hepatotoxicity of xenobiotics. *Xenobiotica* 18: 725–735.

Gordon, V.C. and Kelly, C.P. (1989). An *in vitro* method for determining ocular irritation. *Cosmetics & Toiletries* 104: 69–73.

Grant, W.M. (1986). *Toxicology of the Eye*. Charles C. Thomas, Springfield, IL.

Green, C.E., LeValley, S.E. and Tyson, C.A. (1986). Comparison of amphetamine metabolism using isolated hepatocytes from five species including human. *J. Pharm. Exp. Ther.* 237: 931–936.

Grenier, F.C. (1986). Characteristics of renal collecting tubule cells in primary culture. *Mineral Electrolyte Metab.* 12: 58–63.

Griffith, J.F. (1987). The low-volume eye irritation test: A case study in progress toward validation. *Chemical Times and Trends*, July, pp. 19–40.

Gstraunthaler, G., Pfaller, W. and Kotanko, P. (1985). Biochemical characterization of renal epithelial cell cultures (LLC-PK$_1$ and MDCK). *Am. J. Physiol.* 248 (Renal Fluid Electrolyte Physiol.) 17: F536–544.

Guguen-Guillouzo, C., Gripon, P., Vandenbughe, Y., Lamballe, F., Rataanasavanh, D. and Guillouzo, A. (1988). Hepatotoxicity and molecular aspects of hepatocyte function in primary culture. *Xenobiotica* 18: 773–783.

Guillot, J.P., Gonnet, J.F., Clement, C., Caillard, L. and Truhaut, R. (1982a). Evaluation of the cutaneous-irritation potential of 56 compounds. *Food Chem. Toxicol.* 20: 563–572.

Guillot, J.P., Gonnet, J.F., Clement, C., Caillard, L. and Truhaut, R. (1982b). Evaluation of the ocular-irritation potential of 56 compounds. *Food Chem. Toxicol.* 20: 573–582.

Guillouzo, A. (1986). Use of isolated and cultured hepatocytes for xenobiotic metabolism and cytotoxicity studies. In: *Isolated and Cultured Hepatocytes* (Guillouzo, A. and Guguen-Guillouzo, C., Eds.). John Libbey, London, pp. 313–332.

Guillouzo, A., Begue, J.M., Ratanasavanh, D. and Chesne, C. (1988). Drug metabolism and cytotoxicity in long-term cultured hepatocytes. In: *Liver Cells and Drugs* (Guillouzo, A., Ed.). Colloque Inserm, John Libbey Eurotext Ltd., Paris, France, 164. pp. 235–244.

Guzelian, P.S. and Bissell, D.M. (1974). Metabolic factors in the regulation for cytochrome P-450. Studies in rat hepatocyte monolayer culture. *Fed Proc.* 33: 1246.

Haseman, J.K., Crawford, D.D., Huff, J.E., Boorman, G.A. and McConnell, E.E. (1984). Results from 86 two-year carcinogenicity studies conducted by the National Toxicology Program. *J. Toxicol. Environ. Health* 14: 621–639.

Hassall, C.D., Gandolfi, A.J. and Brendel, K. (1983). Correlation of the *in vivo* and *in vitro* renal toxicity of *S*-(1,2-dichlorovinyl)-L-cysteine. *Drug. Chem. Toxicol.* 6: 507–520.

Hatzinger, P.B. and Stevens, J.L. (1989). Rat kidney proximal tubule cells in defined medium: the roles of cholera toxin, extracellular calcium and serum in cell growth and expression of $\gamma$-glutamyltransferase. *In Vitro Cell. Dev. Biol.* 25(2): 205–212.

HDI *Toxicology Newsletter* (1987). HDI develops rabbit eye irritation model. No. 6 (Enslein, K., Ed.) Health Designs, Inc., Rochester, New York.

Heidrich, H.G. and Dew, M.E. (1977). Homogeneous cell populations from rabbit kidney cortex. *J. Cell Biol.* 74: 780–788.

Hockin, L.J. and Paine, A.J. (1983). The role of 5-aminolevulinate synthetase, haem oxygenase and ligand formation in the mechanism of maintenance of cytochrome P-450 concentration in hepatocyte culture. *Biochem. Pharmacol.* 210: 855–857.

Holme, J. (1985). Xenobiotic metabolism and toxicity in primary monolayer cultures of hepatocytes. *NIPH Ann.* 8: 49–63.

Holohan, P.D., Sokol, P.P., Ross, C.R., Coulson, R., Trimble, M.E., Laska, D.A., Kracke, M.J. and Williams, P.D. (1988). Gentamicin-induced increases in cytosolic calcium in pig kidney cells (LLC-PK$_1$). *J. Pharmacol. Exp. Ther.* 247: 349–354.

Hook, J.B. and Hewitt, W.R. (1986). Toxic responses of the kidney. In: *Casarett & Doull's Toxicology. The Basic Science of Poisons*, 3rd Ed. (Klaassen, C.D., Amdur, M.O. and Doull, J., Eds.). Macmillan, New York, pp. 310–329.

Hori, R., Yamamoto, S., H., Kohno, M. and Inui, K. (1984). Effect of aminoglycoside antibiotics on cellular functions of kidney epithelial cell line (LLC-PK$_1$): a model system for aminoglycoside nephrotoxicity. *Pharmacol. Exp. Ther.* 230: 742–748.

Hottendorf, G.H., Laska, D.A., Ford, S.M. and Williams, P.D. (1987). The role of desacetylation in the detoxification of cephalothin in renal cells in culture. *J. Toxicol. Environ. Health* 22: 101–111.

Hsu, C.H., Kurtz, T.W. and Weller, J.M. (1977). *In vitro* uptake of gentamicin by rat renal cortical tissue. *Antimicrob. Ag. Chemother.* 12: 192–194.

Hull, R.N., Cherry, W.R. and Weaver, G.W. (1976). The origin and characteristics of a pig kidney cell strain LLC-PK$_1$. *In Vitro* 12: 670–677.

Humes, H.D., Hunt, D.A. and White, M.D. (1987). Direct toxic influence of the radiocontrast agent diatrizoate on renal proximal tubule cells. *Am. J. Physiol.* 252: F246–F255.

Igarashi, H., Katsuta, Y., Matsumo, H., Nakazoto, Y. and Kawasaki, T. (1989). Opacification test by using the pig isolated cornea and its application to a test of corneal opacity induced by befunolol hydrochloride. *J. Toxicol. Sci. (Japan)* 14: 91–103.

Inamoto, H., Ino, Y., Inamoto, N., Wada, T., Kihara, H., Watanabe, I. and Asano, S. (1976). Effect of $HgCl_2$ on rat kidney cells primary culture. *Lab. Invest.* 34: 489–493.

Inui, K., Saito, H. and Hori, R. (1985). $H^+$ gradient-dependent active transport of tetaethylammonium cation in apical-membrane vesicles isolated from kidney epithelial cell line LLC-$PK_1$. *Biochem. J.* 227: 199–203.

Isom, H.C., Secott, T., Georgoff, I., Woodworth, C. and Mummaw, J. (1985). Maintenance of differentiated rat hepatocytes in primary culture. *Proc. Natl. Acad. Sci. U.S.A.* 82: 3252–3256.

Jewell, S.A., Bellomo, G., Thor, H., Orrenius, S. and Smith, M.T. (1982). Bleb formation in hepatocytes during drug metabolism is caused by disturbances in thiol and calcium ion homeostasis. *Science* 217: 1257–1258.

Johnson, V. and Maack, T. (1977). Renal extraction, filtration, absorption, and catabolism of growth hormone. *Am. J. Physiol.* 233(2): F185–196.

Kacew, S. and Hirsch, G.H. (1981). Evaluation of nephrotoxicity of various compounds by means of *in vitro* techniques and comparison to *in vivo* methods. In: *Toxicology of the Kidney* (Hook, J.B., Ed.). Raven Press, New York, pp. 77–98.

Kalweit, S., Gerner, I. and Spielmann, H. (1987). Validation project of alternatives for the Draize eye test. *Mol. Toxicol.* 1: 597–603.

Kasher, J.S., Holohan, P.D. and Ross, C.R. (1983). Effect of cephaloridine on the transport of organic ions in dog kidney plasma membrane vesicles. *J. Pharmacol. Exp. Ther.* 225(3): 606–610.

Kennah, H.E., Albulescu, D., Hignet, S. and Barrow, C.S. (1989). A critical evaluation of predicting ocular irritancy potential form an *in vitro* cytotoxicity assay. *Fundam. Appl. Toxicol.* 12: 281–290.

Klaasen, C.D. and Stacey, N.H. (1982). Use of isolated hepatocytes in toxicity assessment. In: *Toxicology of the Liver* (Plaa, G. and Hewitt, W.R., Eds.). Raven Press, New York, pp. 147–179.

Kleinman, H.K., McGarvey, M.L., Hassell, J.R., Star, V.L., Cannon, F.B., Laurie, G.W. and Martin, G.R. (1986). Basement membrane complexes with biological activity. *Biochemistry* 25: 312–318.

Kluwe, W.M. and Hook, J.B. (1978). Functional nephrotoxicity of gentamicin in the rat. *Toxicol. Appl. Pharmacol.* 45: 163–175.

Kong, B.M., Viau, C.J., Rizvi, P.Y. and De Salva, S.J. (1987). The development and evaluation for the chorioallantoic membrane (CAM) assay. In: *Alternative Methods in Toxicology*, Vol. 5. (Goldberg, A.M., Ed.). Mary Ann Liebert, New York, pp. 59–73.

Kreisberg, J.I., Pitts, A.M. and Pretlow, T.G. (1977). Separation of proximal tubule cells from suspensions of rat kidney cells in density gradients of Ficoll in tissue culture medium. *Am. J. Pathol.* 86: 591–601.

Lawrence, R.S. (1987). The choriollantoic membrane in irritancy testing. In: *In Vitro Methods in Toxicology* (Atterwill, C.K. and Steele, C.E., Eds.), Cambridge University Press, New York, pp. 263–278.

Lawrence, R.S., Groom, M.H., Ackroyd, D.M. and Parish, W.E. (1986). The chorioallantoic membrane in irritation testing. *Food Chem. Toxicol.* 24: 497–502.

Lawrence-Beckett, E.M. and James, J.T. (1990). Initial experience with the Eyetex *in vitro* eye irritation test system. *Toxicologist* 20: 259.

Ledbetter, S.R., Kleinman, H.K., Hassell, J.R. and Martin, G.R. (1984). Isolation of laminin. In: *Methods for Preparation of Media, Supplements and Substrata for Serum-Free Animal Cell Culture* (Barnes, D.W., Sirbasku, D.A. and Sato, G.H., Eds.). A.R. Liss, New York, pp. 231–238.

Leighton, J., Nassauer, J., Tchao, R. and Verdone, J. (1983). Development of a procedure using the chick egg as an alternative to the Draize rabbit test. In: *Alternative Methods in Toxicology*, Vol. 1 (Goldberg, A.M., Ed.). Mary Ann Liebert, New York, pp. 165–177.

Li, A.P., Merrill, J.C. and Beck, D.J. (1990). Future optimization of the cryopreservation procedures for rat and human hepatocytes. *Toxicologist* 10: 63.

Lindahl-Kiessling, K., Karlberg, I. and Olofsson, A.M. (1989). Induction of sister-chromatid exchanges by direct and indirect mutagens in human lymphocytes, co-cultured with intact rat liver cells: Effect of enzyme induction and preservation of the liver cells by freezing in liquid nitrogen. *Mutat. Res.* 211: 77–87.

Liu, J., Kershaw, W.C. and Klaasen, C.D. (1990). Rat primary hepatocyte cultures are a good model for examining metallothionein-induced tolerance to cadmium toxicity. *In Vitro Cell. Dev. Biol.* 26: 75–79.

Luepke, N.P. (1985). Hen's egg chorioallantoic membrane test for irritation potential. *Food. Chem. Toxicol.* 23: 287–291.

Maack, T. (1975). Renal handling of low molecular weight proteins. *Am. J. Med.* 58: 57–64.

Martel-Pelletier, J., Guerette, D. and Bergeron, M. (1977). Morphologic changes during incubation of renal slices. *Lab Invest.* 36(5): 509–518.

Maslansky, C.J. and Williams, G.M. (1985). Methods for the initiation and use of hepatocyte primary cultures from various rodent species to detect metabolic activation of carcinogens. In: *In vitro Models for Cancer Research* (Webber, M. and Sekely, L., Eds.). CRC Press, Boca Raton, FL, pp. 43–60.

McLachlin, J.R., Goyer, R.A. and Cherian, M.G. (1980). Formation of lead-induced inclusion bodies in primary rat kidney epithelial cell cultures: effect of actinomycin D and cycloheximide. *Toxicol. Appl. Pharmacol.* 56: 418–431.

McQueen, C.A. and Williams, G.M. (1981). Characterization of DNA repair elicited by carcinogens and drugs in the hepatocyte primary culture/DNA repair test. *J. Toxicol. Environ. Health* 8: 463–477.

McQueen, C.A. and Williams, G.M. (1983). The use of cells from rat, mouse, hamster, and rabbit in the hepatocyte primary culture/DNA repair test. *Ann. N.Y. Acad. Sci.* 407: 119–130.

McQueen, C.A. and Williams, G.M. (1985). Methods and modifications of the hepatocyte primary culture/DNA repair test. In: *Handbook of Carcinogenic Testing* (Milman, H.A. and Weisburger, E.K., Eds.). Noyes Publications, Park Ridge, NJ, pp. 116–129.

McQueen, C.A. and Williams, G.M. (1987). Toxicology studies in cultured hepatocytes from various species. In: *The Isolated Hepatocyte: Use in Toxicology and Xenobiotic Biotransformation* (Rauckman, E.J. and Padilla, G.M., Eds.). Academic Press, Orlando, FL, pp. 51–67.

McQueen, C.A., Merrill, B.M. and Williams, G.M. (1984). Comparison of several indicators of cytotoxicity in rat hepatocytes in primary culture. *Toxicologist* 4: 134.

Messana, J.M., Cieslinski, D.A., O'Connor, R.P. and Humes, H.D. (1988). Glutathione protects against exogenous oxidant injury to rabbit renal proximal tubules. *Amer. J. Physiol.* 255: F874–F884.

Meyer, D.S. (1989). Safety evaluation of new drugs. In: *Modern Drug Research* (Martin, Y.C., Kutter, E. and Austel, V., Eds.). Marcel Dekker, New York, pp. 355–399.

Muir, C.K. (1984). A simple method to assess surfactant-induced bovine corneal opacity *in vitro*: preliminary findings. *Toxicol. Lett.* 22: 199–203.

Muir, C.K. (1985). Opacity of bovine cornea *in vitro* induced by surfactants and industrial chemicals compared with ocular irritancy *in vivo*. *Toxicol. Lett.* 24: 157–162.

Newton, J.F. and Hook, J.B. (1981). Isolated perfused rat kidney. In: *Methods in Enzymology*, Vol. 77 (Jacoby, W.B., Ed.). Academic Press, New York.

Newton, J.F., Kuo, C.H., Gemborys, M.W., Mudge, G.H. and Hook, J.B. (1982a). Nephrotoxicity of *p*-aminophenol, a metabolite of acetaminophen, in the Fisher 344 rat. *Toxicol. Appl. Pharmacol.* 65: 336–344.

Newton, J.F., Braselton, W.E., Kuo, Kluwe, W.M.C.H., Gemborys, M.W., Mudge, G.H. and Hook, J.B. (1982b). Metabolism of acetaminophen by the isolated perfused kidney. *J. Pharmacol. Exp. Ther.* 221: 76–79.

Oglesby, L.A., Ebron, M.T., Beyer, P.E., Carver, B.D. and Kavlock, R.J. (1986). Co-culture of rat embryos and hepatocytes: *In vitro* detection of a proteratogen. *Teratogen. Carcinogen. Mutagen.* 6: 129–138.

Paine, A.J. and Hockin, L.J. (1980). Nutrient imbalance causes the loss of cytochrome P-450 in liver cell culture: formulation of culture media which maintain cytochrome P-450 at *in vivo* concentrations. *Biochem. Pharmacol.* 29: 3215–3218.

Phelps, J.S., Gandolfi, A.J., Berndel, K. and Dorr, R.T. (1987). Cisplatin nephrotoxicity: *in vitro* studies with precision-cut rabbit renal cortical slices. *Toxicol. Appl. Pharmacol.* 90: 501–512.

Pittner, R.A., Fears, R. and Brindley, D.N. (1985). Effects of glucocorticoids and insulin on activities of phosphatidate phosphohydrolase, tyrosine aminotransferase and glycerol kinase in isolated rat hepatocytes in relation to the control of triacyglycerol synthesis and gluconeogenesis. *Biochem. J.* 225: 455–462.

Plaa, G.L. (1976). Quantitative aspects in the assessment of liver injury. *Environ. Health Perspect.* 15: 39–46.

Plaa, G.L. and Hewitt, W.R. (1982). Quantitative evaluation of indices of hepatotoxicity. In: *Toxicology of the Liver* (Plaa, G.L. and Hewitt, W.R., Eds.). Raven, New York, pp. 103–120.

Poirier, M.C., Williams, G.M. and Yuspa, S.H. (1980). Effect of culture conditions cell type and species of origin on the distribution of acetylated and deacetylated deoxyguanosine C-8 adducts of *N*-acetoxy-2-acetylaminofluorene. *Mol. Pharmacol.* 18: 581–587.

Price, J.B., Barry, M.P. and Anderws, I.J. (1986). The use of the chick chorioallantoic membrane to predict eye irritants. *Food. Chem. Toxicol.* 24: 503–505.

Rabito, C.A. (1986). Occluding junctions in a renal cell line (LLC-PK$_1$). The basolateral systems. *J. Biol. Chem.* 257: 6802–6808.

Rabito, C.A. and Ausiello, D.A. (1980). Na$^+$-dependent sugar transport in a cultured epithelial cell line from a pig kidney. *J. Membr. Biol.* 54: 31–38.

Rabito, C.A. and Karish, M.V. (1982). Polarized amino acid transport by an epithelial cell line of renal origin (LLC-PK$_1$). The basolateral systems. *J. Biol. Chem.* 257: 6802–6808.

Rabito, C.A. and Karish, M.V. (1983). Polarized amino acid transport by an epithelial cell line of renal origin (LLC-PK$_1$). The apical systems. *J. Biol. Chem.* 258: 2543–2547.

Ratanasavahn, D., Baffet, G., Latinier, M.F., Fissel, M. and Guillouzo, A. (1988). Use of hepatocyte co-cultures in the assessment of drug toxicity from chronic exposure. *Xenobiotica* 18: 765–771.

Reese, J.A. and Byard, J.L. (1981). Isolation and culture of adult hepatocytes from liver biopsies. *In Vitro* 17: 935–940.

Rowan, A.N. and Stratmann, C.J. (1980). *The Use of Alternatives in Drug Research.* University Park, Baltimore, MD.

Ruegg, C.E., Gandolfi, A.J., Brendel, K., Nagle, R.B. and Krumdieck, C.L. (1987a). Preparation of positional renal slices for study of cell-specific toxicity. *J. Pharmacol. Methods* 12: 111–123.

Ruegg, C.E., Gandolfi, A.J., Nagle, R.B. and Brendel, K. (1987b). Differential patterns of injury to the proximal tubule of renal cortical slices following *in vitro* exposure to mercuric chloride, potassium dichromate or hypoxic conditions. *Toxicol. Appl. Pharmacol.* 90: 261–273.

Rylander, L.A., Gandolfi, A.J. and Brendel, K. (1985). Inhibition of organic acid/base transport in isolated rabbit renal tubules by nephrotoxins. In: *In Vitro Toxicology.* A progress report from Johns Hopkins Center for Alternatives to Animal Testing. Vol. 3 (Goldberg, A.M., Ed.). Mary Ann Liebert, New York, pp. 235–247.

Safirstein, R., Miller, P., Dikman, S., Lyman, S. and Shapiro, H. (1981). Cisplatin nephrotoxicity in rats. *Kidney Int.* 25: 753–758.

Sakhrani, L.M., Badie-Dezfooly, B., Trizna, W., Mikhails, N., Lowe, A., Taub, M. and Fine, L.G. (1984). Transport and metabolism of glucose by renal proximal tubular cells in primary culture. *Amer. J. Physiol.* 246: F757–F764.

Salem, H. and Baskin, S.I. (1993). *New Technologies and Concepts of Reducing Drug Toxicities.* CRC Press, Boca Raton, FL.

Scheuplein, R.J., Schoal, S.E. and Brown, R.N. (1990). Role of pharmacokinetics in safety evaluation and regulatory considerations. *Ann. Rev. Pharmacol. Toxicol.* 30: 197–218.

Schnellman, R.G. and Mandel, L.J. (1986). Cellular toxicity of bromobenzene and bromobenzene metabolites to rabbit proximal tubules: The role and mechanism of 2-bromohydroquinone. *J. Pharmacol. Exp. Ther.* 237: 456–461.

Schnellman, R.G., Lock, E.A. and Mandel, L.J. (1987). A mechanism of S-(1,2,3,4,4-Pentachloro-1,3-butadienyl)-L-cysteine toxicity to rabbit proximal tubules. *Toxicol. Appl. Pharmacol.* 90: 513–521.

Schwertz, D.W., Dreisberg, J.I. and Venkatachalam, M.A. (1986). Gentamicin-induced alterations in pig kidney epithelial (LLC-PK$_1$) cells in culture. *J. Pharmacol. Exp. Ther.* 236(1): 254–262.

Seglen, P.O. (1976). Preparation of isolated rat liver cells. *Methods Cell Biol.* 13: 29–83.

Seglen, P.O. and Fossa, J. (1978). Attachment of rat hepatocytes *in vitro* to substrate of serum protein collagen, or concanavalin A. *Exp. Cell Res.* 116: 199–206.

Seglen, P.O., Solheim, A.E., Grinde, P.B., Schwarze, P.E., Gjessing, R. and Poli, A. (1980). Amino acid control of protein synthesis and degradation in isolated rat hepatocytes. *Ann. N.Y. Acad. Sci.* 349: 1–17.

Sens, M.A., Hennigar, G.R., Hazen-Martin, D.J. and Sens, D.A. (1988). Cultured human proximal tubule cells as a model for aminoglycoside nephrotoxicity. *Ann. Clin. Lab. Sci.* 18: 204–214.

Shaw, J.L., Blanco, J. and Mueller, G.C. (1975). A simple procedure for isolation of DNA, RNA and protein factions from cultured animal cells. *Anal. Biochem.* 65: 125–131.

Shopsis, C. (1989). Validation study: ocular irritancy prediction with the total cell protein, uridine uptake, and neutral red assays applied to human epidermal keratinocytes and mouse 3t3 cells. In: *Alternative Methods in Toxicology*, Vol. 7 (Goldberg, A.M., Ed.). Mary Ann Liebert, New York, pp. 273–287.

Simmerman, H.J., Kendler, J., Libber, S. and Lukacs, L. (1974). Hepatocyte suspensions as a model for demonstration of drug hepatoxicity. *Biochem. Pharmacol.* 23: 2187–2189.

Sina, J.F. and Gautheron, P.D. (1990). Assessment of *in vivo* ocular irritation using *in vitro* cytotoxicity assays. *Toxicologist* 10: 259.

Sina, J.F., Bean, C.L., Noble, C. and Bradley, M.O. (1985). An *in vitro* nephrotoxicity assay utilizing proximal tubule suspensions from rabbit kidney. In: *In Vitro Toxicology*, Vol 3. Mary Ann Liebert, New York, pp. 683–693.

Sina, J.F., Bean, C.L., Bland, J.A., MacDonald, J.J., Noble, C., Robertson, R.T. and Bradley, M.O. (1986). An *in vitro* assay for cytotoxicity to proximal tubule suspensions from rabbit kidney. *In Vitro Toxicol.* 1(1): 12–22.

Sina, J.F., Ward, G.J., Laszek, M.A. and Gautheron, P.D. (1992). Assessment of cytotoxicity assays as predictors of ocular irritation of pharmaceuticals. *Fund. Appl. Toxicol.* 18: 515–521.

Smith, C.G. (1992). *The Process of New Drug Discovery and Development*. CRC Press, Boca Raton, FL.

Smith, J.H. and Hook, J.B. (1983). Mechanism of chloroform nephrotoxicity. II. *In vitro* evidence for renal metabolism of chloroform in mice. *Toxicol. Appl. Pharmacol.* 70: 480–485.

Smith, J.H., Maita, K., Sleight, S.D. and Hook, J.B. (1983). Mechanism of chloroform nephrotoxicity. I. Time course of chloroform toxicity in male and female mice. *Toxicol. Appl. Pharmacol.* 70: 467–479.

Smith, M.A., Hewitt, W.R. and Hook, J. (1987). *In vitro* methods in renal toxicity. In: *In Vitro Methods in Toxicology* (Atterwill, C.K. and Steele, C.E., Eds.). Cambridge University Press, Cambridge, pp. 13–35.

Smith, W.L. and Garcia-Perez, (1985). A. Immunodissection: use of monoclonal antibodies to isolate specific types of renal cells. *Am. J. Physiol.* 248: F1–F7.

Smolarek, T.A., Higgings, C.V. and Amacher, D.E. (1990a). Metabolism and cytotoxicity of acetaminophen in hepatocyte cultures from rat, rabbit, dog and monkey. *Drug Metabolism and Disposition* 18: 659–663.

Smolarek, T.A., Higgings, C.V. and Amacher, D.E. (1990b). The biotransformation of tetrahydroaminoacidine in cultured hepatocytes as the cause for relative cytotoxicity in 3 species. *Toxicologist* 10: 329.

Smyth, H.F., Carpenter, C.P. and Weil, C.S. (1949). Range-finding toxicity data, List III. *J. Industr. Hygiene* 31: 60–62.

Smyth, H.F., Carpenter, C.P. and Weil, C.S. (1951). Range-finding toxicity data, List IV. *Arch. Industr. Hygiene* 4: 119–122.

Soto, R.J., Servi, M.J. and Gordon, V.C. (1989). Evaluation of an alternative method for ocular irritation. In: *Alternative Methods in Toxicology*, Vol. 7 (Goldberg, A.M., Ed.). Mary Ann Liebert, New York, pp. 289–296.

Stadie, W.C. and Riggs, B.C. (1944). Microtome for the preparation of tissue slices for metabolic studies of tissues *in vitro*. *J. Biol. Chem.* 154: 687–690.

Story, D.L., Gee, S.J., Tyson, C.A. and Gould, D.H. (1983). Response of isolated hepatocytes to organic and inorganic cytotoxins. *J. Toxicol. Environ. Health* 11: 483–501.

Strom, S.C., Jirtle, R.L., Jones, R.S., Novicki, D.L., Rosenberg, M.R., Novotny, A., Irons, G.P., McLain, J.R. and Michalopoulous, G. (1982). Isolation, culture, and transplantation of human hepatocytes. *J. Natl. Cancer Inst.* 68: 771–778.

Suolinna, E. (1982). Isolation and culture of liver cells and their use in the biochemical research of xenobiotics. *Medical Biol.* 60: 237–254.

Taub, M. (1984). Growth of primary and established kidney cell cultures in serum-free media. In: *Methods for Serum-Free Culture of Epithelial and Fibroblastic Cells* (Barnes, D.W., Sirbasku, D.A.A. and Sato, G.H., Eds.). Alan R. Liss, New York, pp. 3–24.

Tay, L.K., Bregman, D.L., Maters, B.G. and Williams, P.D. (1988). Effects of *cis*-diaminedichloroplatinum (I) on rabbit kidney *in vivo* and on rabbit renal proximal tubule cells in culture. *Cancer Res.* 48: 2538–2543.

Tessitore, N., Sakhrani, L.M. and Massary, S.G. (1986). Quantitive requirement for ATP for active transport in isolated renal cells. *Am. J. Physiol.* 251: C120–C127.

Thomson, M.A., Dickens, M.S. and Gordon, V.C. (1989a, April). Evaluation of the Eytex biochemical assay for use in determining cosmetic product ocular irritancy. CAAT Symposium Poster, Baltimore, MD.

Thomson, M.A., Hearn, L.A., Smith, K.T., Teal, J.J. and Dickens, M.S. (1989b). Evaluation of the neutral red cytotoxicity assay as a predictive test for the ocular irritancy potential of cosmetic products. In: *Alternative Methods in Toxicology*, Vol. 7 (Goldberg, A.M., Ed.). Mary Ann Liebert, New York, pp. 297–305.

Tolman, K.G., Peterson, P., Gray, P. and Hammar, S.P. (1978). Hepatotoxicity of salicylates in monolayer cell cultures. *Gastroenterology* 74: 205–208.

Traina, V.M. (1983). The role of toxicology in drug research and development. *Med. Res. Rev.* 3: 43–72.

Trifillis, A., Regec, A., Hallcraggs, M. and Trump, B. (1984). Effects of cyclosporine on cultured human renal tubular cells. *Human Toxicology* 3: 454.

Tune, B.M., Sibley, R.K. and Hsu, C.Y. (1988). The mitochondrial respiratory toxicity of cephalosporin antibiotics. An inhibitory effect on substrate uptake. *J. Pharmacol. Exp. Ther.* 245: 1054–1059.

Tune, B.M., Fravert, D. and Hsu, C.Y. (1989). Oxidative and mitochondrial toxic effects of cephalosporin antibiotics in the kidney: A comparative study of cephaloridine and cephaloglycine. *Biochem. Pharmacol.* 38: 795–802.

Tyson, C.A. and Frazier, J.M. (1993). *Methods in Toxicology: In Vitro Biological Systems*. Academic Press, San Diego, CA.

Viano, I., Eandi, M. and Santiano, M. (1983). Toxic effects of some antibiotics on rabbit kidney cells. *Int. J. Tiss. Reac.* 2: 11–186.

Vinay, P., Gougoux, A. and Lemieux, G. (1981). Isolation of a pure suspension of rat proximal tubules. *Am. J. Physiol.* 241: F403–F411.

Ware, R.A., Burkholder, P.M. and Chang, L.W. (1975). Ultrastructural changes in renal proximal tubules after chronic organic and inorganic mercury intoxication. *Environ. Res.* 10: 121–140.

Weil, C.S. and Scala, R.A. (1971). Study of intra- and interlaboratory variability in the results of rabbit eye and skin irritation tests. *Toxicol. Appl. Pharm.* 19: 276–360.

Weinberg, J.M. (1985). Oxygen deprivation-induced injury to isolated rabbit kidney tubules. *J. Clin. Invest.* 76: 1193–2108.

Weinberg, J.M., Davis, J.A., Abarzua, M. and Rajan, T. (1987). Cytoprotective effects of glycine and glutathione against hypoxic injury to renal tubules. *J. Clin. Invest.* 80: 1446–1454.

Williams, G.M. (1976a). Carcinogen-induced DNA repair in primary rat liver cell cultures; a possible screen for chemical carcinogens. *Cancer Lett. (Shannon, Ire.)* 1: 231–236.

Williams, G.M. (1976b). The detection of chemical carcinogens by unscheduled DNA synthesis in rat liver primary cell cultures. *Cancer Res.* 37: 1845–1851.

Williams, P.D. (1989). The application of renal cells in culture in studying drug-induced nephrotoxicity. *In Vitro* 25: 800–805.

Williams, P.D. and Hottendorf, G.H. (1985). Effects of *cis*-dichlorodiamineplatinum-II (Cisplatin) on organic ion transport in membrane vesicles from rat kidney cortex. *Cancer Treat. Rep.* 69: 875–880.

Williams, P.D. and Hottendorf, G.H. (1986). $^3$H-Gentaminicin uptake in brush border and basolateral membrane vesicles from rat kidney cortex. *Biochem. Pharmacol.* 35: 2253–2256.

Williams, P.D., Trimble, M.E., Crespo, L., Holohan, P.D., Freedman, J.C. and Ross, C.R. (1984). Inhibition of renal $Na^+$, $K^+$-adenosine triphosphatase by gentimicin. *J. Pharmacol. Exp. Ther.* 231(2): 919–925.

Williams, P.D., Hitchcock, M.J.M. and Hottendorf, G.H. (1985). Effects of cephalosporins on organic ion transport in renal membrane vesicles from rat and rabbit kidney cortex. *Res. Comm. Chem. Pathol. Pharmacol.* 47(3): 357–371.

Williams, P.D., Hottendorf, G.H. and Bennett, D.B. (1986a). Inhibition of renal membrane binding and nephrotoxicity of aminoglycosides. *J. Pharmacol. Exp. Ther.* 237: 919–925.

Williams, P.D., Laska, D.A. and Hottendorf, G.H. (1986b). Comparative toxicity of aminoglycoside antibiotics in cell cultures derived from human and pig kidney. *In Vitro Toxicol.* 1: 23–32.

Williams, P.D., Bennett, D.B., Gleason, C.R. and Hottendorf, G.H. (1987). Correlation between renal membrane binding and nephrotoxicity of aminoglycosides. *Antimicrob. Ag. Chemother.* 31(4): 570–574.

Williams, P.D., Laska, D.A., Tay, L.K. and Hottendorf, G.H. (1988) Comparative toxicity of cephalosporin antibiotics in a rabbit kidney cell line (LLC-RK$_1$). *Antimicrob. Ag. Chemother.* 32(3): 314–318.

Williams, P.D., Laska, D.A., Heim, R.A. and Rush, G.F. (1993). Differential toxicity of parenteral antibiotic drugs in renal cells (LLC-PK$_1$) grown on permeable membrane filters. *Toxicol. Methods* 3(2): 130–141.

Williams, S.J. (1984). Prediction of ocular irritancy potential from dermal irritation test results. *Food. Chem. Toxicol.* 22: 157–161.

Williams, S.J. (1985). Changing concepts of ocular irritation evaluation: pitfalls and progress. *Food. Chem. Toxicol.* 23: 189–193.

Wilson, P.D., Dillingham, M.A., Breckon, R. and Anderson, R.J. (1985). Defined human renal tubular epithelia in culture: growth, characterization, and hormonal response. *Am. J. Physicol.* 248: F436–F443.

Yang, I.S., Goldinger, J.M., Hong, S.K. and Taub, M. (1988). Preparation of basolateral membranes that transport *p*-aminohippurate from primary cultures of rabbit kidney proximal tubule cells. *J. Cell. Physicol.* 135: 481–487.

Zhang, G. and Stevens, J.L. (1989). Tansport and activation of *S*-(1,2-dichlorovinyl)-L-cysteine and *N*-acetyl-S-(1,2-dichlorovinyl)-L-cysteine in rat kidney proximal tubules. *Toxicol. Appl. Pharmacol.* 100: 51–61.

# 18

# PHARMACOKINETICS AND TOXICOKINETICS IN DRUG SAFETY EVALUATION

## 18.1. INTRODUCTION

Among the cardinal principles of both toxicology and pharmacology is that the means by which an agent comes in contact with or enters the body (i.e., the route of exposure or administration) does much to determine the nature and magnitude of its effects. Accordingly, an understanding of route(s) of administration and their implications for absorption is essential. The fundamental therapeutic index is the ratio between what levels in the plasma (or at the target organ tissue) cause adverse effects to those levels that have the desired therapeutic effect.

Safety assessment studies usually involve a control group of animals (untreated and/or formulation treated) and at least three treated groups receiving "low," "intermediate," and "high" dose levels of the chemical entity of interest via a route approximately that used in humans (as closely as possible). Occasionally there also may be recovery groups to determine if any observed effects are reversible (and if so, to what extent). In most instances, the high dose level is expected to elicit some toxic effects in the animals, often expressed as decreased food consumption and/or below-normal body weight gain, and has been selected after consideration of earlier data, perhaps from dose range-finding studies, or at least to dose as high as possible by the intended route. The other two dose levels are anticipated not to cause toxic effects. Generally, but not always (e.g., nonsteroidal anti-inflammatory drugs in rodents), the "low" dose level is a several-fold multiple of the expected human therapeutic or exposure level (preferably five-fold for nonrodent and ten-fold for rodents). However, without knowing the true relationship of these dose levels to each other with respect to the absorption, distribution, and elimination of the new chemical entity as reflected by its pharmacokinetics, it is difficult to see how meaningful extrapolations concerning safety margins can be made from the toxicity data obtained. Also, without pharmacokinetic data from the positive control group, its inclusion is of limited value and the results obtained could lead to erroneous conclusions.

Pharmacokinetic studies can provide information on several aspects, knowledge of which greatly facilitates assessment of the safety of the chemical entity. Six such aspects can be mentioned.

1. Relationship between the dose levels used and the relative extent of absorption of the test compound.
2. Relationship between the protein-binding of the test compound and the dose levels used.
3. Relationship between pharmacological or toxicological effects and the kinetics of the test compound.
4. Effect of repeated doses on the kinetics of the test compound.
5. Relationship between the age of the animal and the kinetics of the test compound.
6. Relationship between the dose regimens of the test compound used in the toxicity studies and those employed clinically in humans.

ICH guidelines (ICH, 2000) dictate a clearly defined set of objectives for toxicokinetic studies.

- **Primary**
  To describe the systemic exposure achieved in animals and its relationship to dose level and the time course of toxicity studies.
- **Secondary**
  (i)   To relate the exposure achieved in toxicity studies to toxicological findings and contribute to the assessment of the relevance of these findings to clinical safety.
  (ii)  To support the choice of species and treatment regimen in nonclinical toxicity studies.
  (iii) To provide information which, in conjunction with the toxicity findings, contributes to the design of subsequent nonclinical toxicity studies.

These data may be obtained from all animals on a toxicity study, or from representative subgroups, from satellite groups, or from separate studies.

If toxicology can be described as the study of the effects of a chemical on an organism, metabolism can be described as the opposite: the effects of the organism on the chemical. Metabolism refers to a process by which a drug (xenobiotic) is chemically modified by an organism. It is part of the overall process of disposition of xenobiotic (ADME)—the process by which a chemical gains access to the inner working of an organism (absorption), how it moves around inside an organism (distribution), how it is changed by the organism (metabolism) and how it is eventually eliminated from the organism (elimination). The EPA definition of biotransformation or metabolism is "...the sum of processes by which a xenobiotic (foreign chemical) is handled by a living organism". The mathematical formulas used to describe and quantify these processes are collectively known as pharmacokinetics. The EPA definition of pharmacokinetics is "...quantitation and determination of the time course and dose dependency of the absorption, distribution, biotransformation and excretion of chemicals." The acronym ADME has been used to describe the multifaceted biological process. The term "metabolism" has also come into the profession as jargon to describe the entire process. This science has long played a central role in pharmaceutical development but has had a lesser role in the development of other types of products. The purpose of this chapter is to introduce the basic concepts of ADME and practices of studies conducted to study it, as described the regulations under EPA and OECD that require such data for nonpharmaceutical products and to give some real world examples.

## 18.2. REGULATIONS

The FDA believes that data from studies on the adsorption, distribution, metabolism, and excretion of a chemical can provide insight into mechanisms of toxicity and are essential in evaluating the design and results from other toxicity studies. Such data should be provided for all drugs and significant impurities. Recommendations for obtaining data on the metabolism and pharmacokinetics of these substances are presented in ICH guidelines and the FDA *Redbook II* (2000). In general, it is required that this information be obtained as part of initial and subsequent repeat dose studies with a drug.

## 18.3. PRINCIPLES

An understanding of the design and analysis of pharmacokinetic studies requires a broad understanding of the underlying concepts and principles inherent in the ADME process and in our current technology for studying such (Caldwell *et al.*, 1994; Connally and Anderson, 1991; Gabrielsson and Weiner, 1997). In the following sections, each of these four principle areas is overviewed from a practical basis as it relates to toxicology. First, however, one should consider the fundamental terminology used in pharmacokinetic studies (Table 18.1).

### 18.3.1. Absorption

Absorption is the process by which a chemical crosses a biological membrane to gain access to the inner workings of an organism. For mammals, this process results

**TABLE 18.1.** Fundamental Terms Used in Pharmacokinetic Studies

| | |
|---|---|
| Absolute bioavailability | The bioavailability of a dosage form relative to an intravenous administration. |
| Absorption | The process by which a xenobiotic and its metabolites are transferred from the site of absorption to the blood circulation. |
| Accumulation | The progressive increase of chemical and/or metabolites in the body. Accumulation is influenced by the dosing interval and half-life of the chemical. The process can be characterized by an "accumulation factor," which is the ratio of the plasma concentration at steady state to that following the first dose in a multiple dosing regimen. |
| Analyte | The chemical entity assayed in biological samples. |
| Area under curve (AUC) | The concentration of chemical and/or metabolites in the blood (or plasma/serum) integrated over time. This is typically considered the best indicator of exposure. |
| Bioavailability | The rate and extent to which a xenobiotic entity enters the systemic circulation intact, following oral or dermal administration. It is sometimes expanded to include therapeutically active metabolites. Also known as the comparative bioavailability. |
| Biotransformation | The process by which a xenobiotic is structurally and/or chemically changed in the body by either enzymatic or nonenzymatic reactions. The product of the reaction is a different composition of matter or different configuration than the original compound. |
| Clearance | The volume of biological fluid which is totally cleared of xenobiotic in a unit time. |
| $C_{max}$ | The maximum mean concentration of the chemical in the plasma. Also known as the peak plasma concentration. |
| Concomitant toxicokinetics | Toxicokinetic measurements performed in the toxicity study, either in all animals or in representative subgroups or in satellite groups. |
| Disposition | All processes and factors which are involved from the time a chemical enters the body to the time when it is eliminated from the body, either intact or in metabolite form. |
| Distribution | The process by which an absorbed xenobiotic and/or its metabolites partition between blood and various tissues and organs in the body. |
| Dosage form | The formulation (diet, lotion, capsule, solution, etc.) administered to animals or humans. |
| Dose proportionality | The relationship between doses of a chemical and measured parameters, usually including tests for linearity. |
| Enterohepatic circulation | The process by which xenobiotics are emptied via the bile into the small intestine and then reabsorbed into the hepatic circulation. |

**TABLE 18.1.** (*continued*)

| | |
|---|---|
| Enzyme induction | The increase in enzyme content (activity and/or amount) due to xenobiotic challenge, which may result in more rapid metabolism of a chemical. |
| Enzyme inhibition | The decrease in enzymatic activity due to the effect of xenobiotic challenge. |
| Excretion | The process by which the administered compound and/or its biotransformation product(s) are eliminated from the body. |
| Exposure | Exposure is represented by pharmacokinetic parameters demonstrating the local and systemic burden on the test species with the test compound and/or its metabolites. The area under the matrix level concentration-time curve (AUC) and/or the measurements of matrix concentrations at the expected peak-concentration time $C_{max}$, or at some other selected time $C_{(time)}$, are the most commonly used parameters. Other parameters might be more appropriate in particular cases. |
| First-order kinetics | Kinetic processes, the rate of which is proportional to the concentration. |
| First-pass effect | The phenomenon whereby xenobiotics may be extracted or metabolized following enteral absorption before reaching the systemic circulation. |
| Flux | Term (that takes area into consideration) used to describe the movement of a chemical across a barrier. Most typically used to describe the absorption of a chemical across the skin as $\mu g/cm^2/hr$. |
| Half-life | The time elapsed for a given chemical entity concentration or amount to be reduced by a factor of two. |
| Hepatic clearance | The rate of total body clearance accounted for by the liver. |
| Kel | The elimination constant for a chemical in plasma. Typically calculated using the formula $Kel = -\ln[10] \times b$ where $b$ is the slope of the linear regression line of the log of the mean plasma concentrations vs. time from the $t_{max}$ to 24 hours. |
| Lag time | The interval between compound administration and when the compound concentration is measurable in blood. |
| Metabolite characterization | The determination of physiochemical characteristics of the biotransformation product(s). |
| Metabolite identification | The structural elucidation of the biotransformation product(s). |
| Metabolite profile | The chromatographic pattern and/or aqueous/nonaqueous partitioning of the biotransformation products of the administered compound. |
| Monitor | To take a small number of matrix samples (e.g., 1 to 3) during a dosing interval to estimate $C_{(time)}$ and/or $C_{max}$. |
| Nonlinear kinetics (saturation kinetics) | Kinetic processes, the rate of which is not directly proportional to the concentration. |

(continued)

**TABLE 18.1.** (*continued*)

| | |
|---|---|
| Presystemic elimination | The loss of that portion of the dose that is not bioavailable. This would include, among others, loss through intestinal and gut-wall metabolism, lack of absorption, and first-pass hepatic metabolism. |
| Profile | To take (e.g., 4 to 8) matrix samples during a dosing interval to make and estimate of $C_{max}$ and/or $C_{(time)}$ and area under matrix concentration time curve (AUC). |
| Protein binding | The complexation of a xenobiotic and/or its metabolite(s) with plasma or tissue proteins. |
| Relative bioavailability | The bioavailability relative to a reference or standard formulation or agent. |
| Renal clearance | The rate of total body clearance accounted for by the kidney. Its magnitude is determined by the net effects of glomerular filtration, tubular secretion and reabsorption, renal blood flow, and protein binding. |
| Satellite | Groups of animals included in the design and conduct of a toxicity study, treated and housed under conditions identical to those of the main study animals, but used primarily for toxicokinetics. |
| Steady state | An equilibrium state where the rate of chemical input is equal to the rate of elimination during a given dose interval. |
| Support | In the context of a toxicity study: to ratify or confirm the design of a toxicity study with respect to pharmacokinetic and metabolic principles. This process may include 2 separate steps:<br><br>a. confirmation using toxicokinetic principles that the animals on a study were exposed to appropriate systemic levels of the administered compound and/or its metabolite(s).<br><br>b. confirmation that the metabolic profile in the species used was acceptable, data to support this will normally be derived from metabolism studies in animals and in humans. |
| $T_{max}$ | The sampling time point at which $C_{max}$ occurs. |
| Total clearance | The volume of biological fluid totally cleared of xenobiotic per unit time and usually includes hepatic clearance and renal clearance. |
| Toxicokinetics | The study of the kinetics of absorption, distribution, metabolism and excretion of toxic or potentially toxic chemicals. |
| Validate | In the context of an analytical method: to establish the accuracy, precision, reproducibility, response function and the specificity of the analytical method with reference to the biological matrix to be examined and the analyte to be quantified. |
| Volume of distribution ($V_d$) | A hypothetical volume of body fluid into which the chemical distributes. It is not a "real" volume, but is a proportionality constant relating the amount of chemical in the body to the measured concentration in blood or plasma. |

in the entry of the chemical into the blood stream, or systemic circulation. In this case the process is also called systemic absorption. Pharmaceutical products, procedures and devices, such as hypodermic needles or catheters, can be used to bypass biological barriers. Other products gain access to the systemic circulation via the oral, dermal, buccal, or inhalatory route of administration.

For a material to be toxic (local tissue effects are largely not true toxicities by this definition), the first requirement is that it be absorbed into the organism [for which purpose being in the cavity of the gastrointestinal (GI) tract does not qualify]. Most pharmaceuticals are intended to gain such access.

There are characteristics which influence absorption by the different routes, and these need to be understood by any person trying to evaluate and/or predict the toxicities of different moieties. Some key characteristics and considerations are summarized here by route.

A. Oral and rectal routes (gastrointestinal tract):
   1. Lipid-soluble compounds (nonionized) are more readily absorbed than water-soluble compounds (ionized).
      (a) Weak organic bases are in the nonionized, lipid-soluble form in the intestine and tend to be absorbed there.
      (b) Weak organic acids are in the nonionized, lipid-soluble form in the stomach and one would expect they would be absorbed there, but the intestine is more important because of time and area of exposure.
   2. Specialized transport systems exist for some moieties: sugars, amino acids, pyrimidines, calcium, and sodium.
   3. Almost everything is absorbed, at least to a small extent, if it has a molecular weight below 10,000.
   4. Digestive fluids may modify the structure of a chemical.
   5. Dilution increases toxicity by causing more rapid absorption from the intestine, unless stomach contents bind the moiety.
   6. Physical properties are important: for example, dissolution of metallic mercury is essential to allow absorption.
   7. Age: neonates have a poor intestinal barrier.
   8. Effect of fasting on absorption depends on the properties of the chemical of interest.

B. Inhalation (lungs):
   1. Aerosol deposition
      (a) Nasopharyngeal: 5 μm or larger in humans, less in common laboratory animals.
      (b) Tracheobronchiolar: 1–5 μm.
      (c) Alveolar: 1 μm.
   2. If a solid, mucociliary transport may serve to clear from lungs to GI tract.

3. Lungs are anatomically good for absorption.
    (a) Large surface area ($50$–$100\,\mathrm{m}^2$).
    (b) Blood flow is high.
    (c) Close to blood ($10\,\mu\mathrm{m}$ between gas media and blood).
4. Absorption of gases is dependent on solubility of the gas in blood.
    (a) Chloroform, for example, has high solubility and is all absorbed; respiration rate is the limiting factor.
    (b) Ethylene has low solubility and only a small percentage is absorbed; blood flow limited absorption.
    (c) Parenteral routes.
    (d) Dermal routes.

As a generalization, there is a pattern of relative absorption rates which extends between the different routes that are commonly employed. This order of absorption (by rate from fastest to slowest and, in a less rigorous manner, in degree to absorption from most to least) is intravenous > inhalation > intramuscular > intraperitoneal > subcutaneously > oral > intradermal > other dermal.

Absorption (total amount and rate), distribution, metabolism, and species similarity in response are the reasons for selecting particular routes in toxicology. In acute studies, however, these things are rarely known. So the cardinal rule for selecting routes of use in acute testing is to use those routes which mirror the intended route for human exposure. If this route of human exposure is uncertain, or if there is the potential for either a number of routes or the human absorption rate and pattern being greater, then the common practice becomes that of the most conservative approach. This approach stresses maximizing potential absorption in the animal species (within the limits of practicality) and selecting from among those routes commonly used in the laboratory that which gets the most material into the animal's system as quickly and completely as possible to evaluate the potential toxicity.

In general, chemicals cross biological barriers by one of three mechanisms: active transport, facilitative transport, and passive transport. In active transport, the chemical is specifically recognized by the organism, which then expends energy to take the chemical up, even against a concentration gradient. In facilitative transport, the organism produces a carrier molecule which reacts with the target molecule to form a complex which more easily traverses the membrane, but no energy is expended to take up the complex. Such complexes do not flow against a concentration barrier. The simplest mechanism is passive transfer or diffusion. Here, a chemical flows down a concentration gradient (from high concentration to a lower concentration) and must passively (no energy expended by organism) cross a biological membrane. Passive transfer or diffusion is the most common (if not the only) mechanism involved in the absorption of the vast majority of chemicals in commerce. The other mechanisms involved in absorption will not be further discussed here.

Drugs in solution have a natural tendency (more rigorously defined by the laws of thermodynamics) to move down a concentration gradient. That is to say, the individual molecules of solute tend to move from a region of high concentration toward regions of lower concentration. Also, the movement of a chemical across a permeable barrier, such as a biological membrane, is a process called diffusion, as illustrated by Figure 18.1. For most products, these biological barriers are either the wall of the gastrointestinal tract, the lining of the pulmonary system, and/or the skin.

Absorption from the GI tract is controlled by a variety of factors. These include the acid–base characteristics of the chemical (called the pKa), the solubility, the nature of the delivery (e.g., diet vs. gavage), the nature of any vehicle (suspensions vs. solution, or aqueous vs. nonaqueous), and the gastrointestinal tract of the species under study.

Ionized or charged organic moieties do not readily pass through the lipophilic cell membranes of the epithelial cells that line the GI tract. Thus more acidic molecules tend to be more readily absorbed from the stomach while more alkaline materials tend to be absorbed from the small intestine. This is because at the acidic pH of the stomach, acidic chemicals tend to be nonionized. More alkaline chemicals tend to be more ionized in the stomach and less ionized in the gut. The equilibrium reaction for acidic dissociation can be represented by this equation:

$$X-\underset{\underset{O}{\|}}{C}-OH + H_2O = X-\underset{\underset{O}{\|}}{C}-O + H_3O^+$$

Like all chemical equations, this one has an equilibrium constant. The discussion of basic chemistry is outside the purview of this book. Readers who may need a refresher are referred to Tse and Jaffe (1991). For every chemical, a pKa can be calculated, based on its equilibrium constant, which represents the proportion of ionized and unionized material in solution. The lower the pKa of a chemical, the more likely it is to be nonionized in the stomach.

***Absorption from the Pulmonary System.*** Of the three routes discussed here, absorption from the pulmonary system is perhaps the most rapid. Systemic absorption of inhaled materials is highly dependent on the physical properties of the inhaled materials, which dictate how easily the materials reach the alveoli of the deep lung. Gases and vapors easily penetrate into the deep lung. For mists and dusts, absorption will be highly dependent on particle size. In general, the larger the particles, the less they will penetrate the pulmonary system. The term "impaction" describes the deposition of particles in the respiratory tract. Particles of less than 0.2 μm are preferentially deposited in the pulmonary portion of the respiratory system and particles over 2 μm do not reach the alveolar epithelium in great number. Particles from 1 to 4 μm tend to be distributed over the length of the system and particles over 4 μm tend to be deposited in the nasal region. Aerosolized particles of greater than 20 μm do not commonly occur in nature. Tidal volume will also influence impaction. In general, the larger the tidal volume, and thus the more forceful the inhalatory process, the more deeply particles of all sizes tend to be driven into the lung.

Once deposited, materials must be in solution before they can be absorbed. Hence, materials in an aerosolized solution will be more readily absorbed than materials that are delivered as solid particles (e.g. dusts). Solid materials must be able to go into solution *in situ* in order to be absorbed. Particle size influences dissolution rate. Large particles dissolve more slowly (for any given material) than small particles due to the differences in surface area. Once in solution, the same laws of passive diffusion apply to materials in the lung as apply to material in the GI tract. The large surface area and the rich blood flow at the alveoli make for ideal conditions for rapid absorption into the systemic circulation. Absorption across the mucosa lining the upper airways is less rapid. Materials that do not dissolve are ingested by pulmonary macrophages and either broken down there or moved out of the lungs by the upward movement of the bronchociliary tree.

For gases and vapors, the amount absorbed is highly dependent on the partial pressure of the gas and the solubility of the gas in blood. Let's take the simple case of a gas that is not metabolized and is excreted by exhalation (e.g., an anesthetic gas or a Halon-type fire-extinguishing agent). At any given concentration (or partial pressure) in the atmosphere, the concentration in the blood will reach a steady state in the blood. Accordingly, prolonged exposure does not lead to continual buildup.

At equilibrium, the concentration in the blood is depicted by the formula (also known as the Ostwald coefficient) $X_b/X_a = S$, where $X_b$ is the concentration in the blood and $X_a$ is the concentration in the inspired air. Thus, if one knows the $S$ for a given chemical and the target concentration for a given exposure, one can predict what the resulting concentration may be at equilibrium. Additionally, the lower the $S$ value (i.e., the lower the solubility in blood) the more rapidly the chemical will achieve equilibrium.

***Absorption Across the Skin.*** An aqueous carrier may be used for a variety of dermal products. In fact, carriers can be designed to limit the transportation of the penetration of the active ingredient (such as an insect repellent), if the desired effect is to keep the activity on the surface of the skin. Once again, however, only those materials that are dissolved will be available for penetration across the skin to gain access to the systemic circulation. For almost all chemicals in or about to enter commerce, dermal penetration is a passive process. The relative thickness of the skin makes absorption (into the systemic circulation) slower than the absorption across the GI or pulmonary barriers. This is compounded by the fact that the stratum corneum function is to be impervious to the environment. One of the skin's major functions is protection from infection. Once a chemical penetrates into the dermis, it may partition into the subcutaneous fat. Essentially, absorption across the skin is a two-step process with the first being penetration and deposition into the skin and the second being release from the skin into the systemic circulation. The pattern of blood levels obtained via dermal penetration is generally one with a delayed absorption, a slow buildup to more of a plateau than a peak. Blood levels of chemicals absorbed via the dermal route are generally low.

Given the overwhelming influence of the physical properties of skin in determining bioavailabilities via the dermal route, assessment of dermal penetration is one area in metabolism and toxicology where *in vitro* methods can be effectively used to predict *in vivo* results and to screen chemicals. Apparatus and equipment exist that one can use to maintain sections of skin (obtained from euthanized animals or from human cadavers or surgical discard) for such experiments (Holland *et al.*, 1984). These apparatus are set up to maintain the metabolic integrity of the skin sample between two reservoirs: the one on the stratum corneum side, called the application reservoir and the one on the subcutaneous side, called the receptor reservoir. One simply places radiolabeled test material in the application reservoir and collects samples from the receptor fluid at various time points.

The rate of penetration can be presented by the traditional kinetic formulas to obtain a penetration rate constant. Given that exposed surface area also plays a role in the amount of material absorbed, the concept of flux is also important.

The three major considerations in determining the quantity of material that is absorbed into the skin, and eventually released into the systemic circulation, is primarily dependent upon three factors: the surface area exposed, the volume of material applied (and the concentration of the material applied) and the nature of the vehicle (Gad and Chengelis, 1997).

> Surface area: all things being equal, it is clear that the greater the surface exposed, the higher the achieved internal dose.
>
> Volume: the volume of material will obviously play a role in total dose, but it is not as straightforward as the relationship to surface area. Theoretically, the maximum absorption is obtained when the material is spread as thinly and uniformly as possible; piling material on so that it is literally rolling off the animal serves no practical purpose. In fact, it is not a sound practice when dealing with an *in vivo* animal experiment as it makes it more likely for the material to be available for oral ingestion.

***Parameters Controlling Absorption.*** The absorption of a chemical into the skin is a function of the nature of the molecule, the behavior of the vehicle, and the status of the skin. Three major variables account for differences in the rate of absorption or flux of different topical chemicals or of the same molecule in different vehicles: the concentration of the molecule in the vehicle, the partition coefficient of chemical between the stratum corneum and the vehicle, and the diffusion coefficient of molecule in the stratum corneum (Garner and Matthews, 1998).

The rate of diffusion is proportional to the concentration of molecule in the vehicle. The relationship is linear only at low molecule concentrations and only applies to soluble molecule in the vehicle. The latter factor may explain the variable therapeutic effects of different formulations of the same drug molecule. The partition coefficient is a measure of the molecule's ability to escape from the vehicle and is defined as the equilibrium solubility of molecule in the surface of the stratum corneum relative to its solubility in the vehicle. Increased lipid solubility favors penetration of molecule through the skin by increasing the solubility in the relatively lipophilic stratum corneum. The diffusion coefficient indicates the extent to which the matrix of the barrier restricts the mobility of the molecule. Increases in molecular size of the molecule will increase frictional resistance and decrease the diffusion coefficient (Bronaugh, 1998); molecules over 1000 daltons usually will not be absorbed easily into normal adult skin.

Finally, intact stratum corneum is an excellent barrier, but in disease states the resistance to absorption is rapidly lost and absorption can be facilitated.

### 18.3.2. Distribution

Once the chemical gains access to the body, it is carried by the bloodstream and distributed to the different organs. The preferential organ of deposition is determined by a variety of factors: the two most important are blood flow to the organ and the affinity of the chemical for that organ. Affinity is governed by two general characteristics. First, the product may be designed to have a specific affinity for a specific molecular entity in a target cell. For example, an anticholinesterase insecticide will tend to accumulate in the cells that have the highest concentration of cholinesterase. Secondly, the product may have a nonspecific or general chemical attraction for a specific cell type. The more highly lipophilic a chemical, the more likely it is to distribute and remain in adipose tissue. Blood flow will also have a major impact on distribution, as chemicals will be distributed more readily to those organs that are more highly perfused. A highly lipophilic chemical may first be deposited in the brain because it is richly perfused, and then be distributed to body fat with time.

Once a material is absorbed, distribution of a compound in most toxicology studies is usually of limited interest. Some factors which can serve to alter distribution are listed in Table 18.2.

For most drugs, the rate of disposition or loss from the biological system is independent of rate and input, once the agent is absorbed. "Disposition" is defined as what happens to the active molecule after it reaches a site in the blood circulation where concentration measurements can be made (the systemic circulations, generally). Although disposition processes may be independent of input, the inverse is not necessarily true because disposition can markedly affect the extent of availability. Agents absorbed from the stomach and the intestine must first pass through the liver before reaching the general circulation (Figure 18.1). Thus, if a compound is metabolized in the liver or excreted in bile, some of the active molecule absorbed from the gastrointestinal tract will be inactivated by hepatic processes before it can reach the systemic circulation and be distributed to its sites of action. If the metabolizing or biliary excreting capacity of the liver is great, the effect on the extent of availability will be substantial. Thus, if the hepatic blood clearance for the chemical is large, relative to hepatic blood flow, the extent of availability for this

**TABLE 18.2. Selected Factors that may Affect Chemical Distribution to Various Tissues**

Factors relating to the chemical and its administration
  Degree of binding of chemical to plasma proteins (i.e., agent affinity for proteins) and tissues.
  Chelation to calcium, which is deposited in growing bones and teeth (e.g., tetracyclines in young children).
  Whether the chemical distributes evenly throughout the body (one compartment model) or differentially between different compartments (two- or more compartment model).
  Ability of chemical to cross the blood-brain barrier.
  Diffusion of chemical into the tissues or organs and degree of binding to receptors that are and are not responsible for the drug's beneficial effects.
  Quantity of chemical given.
  Route of administration/exposure.
  Partition coefficients (nonpolar chemicals are distributed more readily to fat tissues than are polar chemicals).
  Interactions with other chemicals that may occupy receptors and prevent the drug from attaching to the receptor, inhibit active transport, or otherwise interfere with a drug's activity.
  Molecular weight of the chemical.

Factors relating to the test subject
  Body size.
  Fat content (e.g., obesity affects the distribution of drugs that are highly soluble in fats).
  Permeability of membranes.
  Active transport for chemicals carried across cell membranes by active processes.
  Amount of proteins in blood, especially albumin.
  Pathology or altered homeostasis that affects any of the other factors (e.g., cardiac failure and renal failure).
  The presence of competitive binding substances (e.g., specific receptor sites in tissues bind drugs).
  pH of blood and body tissues.
  pH of urine.[a]
  Blood flow to various tissues or organs (e.g., well-perfused organs usually tend to accumulate more chemical than less well-perfused organs).

[a] The pH of urine is usually more important than the pH of blood.

chemical will be low when it is given by a route that yields first-pass metabolic effects.

Likewise, metabolism is generally of only limited concern in most acute studies. There are some special cases, however, in which metabolic considerations must be factored in seeking to understand differences between routes and the effects which may be seen.

The first special case is parenteral routes, where the systemic circulation presents a peak level of the moiety of interest to the body at one time, tempered only by the

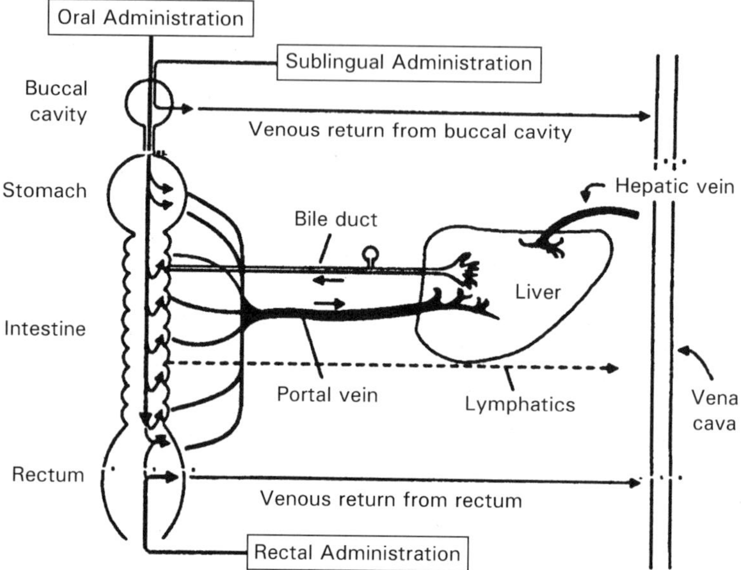


**FIGURE 18.1.** Passage of chemical moieties from the gastrointestinal tract into the blood-stream, shown in a diagrammatic fashion.

results of a single pass through the liver (Goldstein et al., 1974; Keberle et al., 1971; La Du et al., 1972).

The second special case arises from inhalation exposures. Because of the arrangements of the circulatory system, inhaled compounds enter the full range of systemic circulation without any "first-pass" metabolism by the liver. Keberle et al. (1971), O'Reilly (1972) and Pratt and Taylor (1990) have published relevant reviews of absorption, distribution, and metabolism.

***Protein Binding.*** The degree to which a chemical binds to plasma proteins will highly influence its distribution. Albumin, the most prominent of the many proteins found in mammalian plasma, carries both positive and negative charges with which a polar compound can associate by electrostatic attraction. As with all such reactions, it can be described by the following equations. The more avidly bound the material, the less will be distributed to surrounding fluids as part of a solution and only that portion that is free in solution will be available for diffusion into the tissues.

***Water Solubility.*** The solubility of a chemical has a direct bearing on its distribution. Recall that only molecules that are in solution will be available for absorption.

As mentioned, only that portion that is free in solution will be available for diffusion into the tissues. Hence, the more material that is in solution the more that will be available for diffusion.

***Volume of Distribution.*** If one takes the dose administered (mgs) and divides it by the plasma concentration of the test material (mg/ml), the result is a volume number.

$$\frac{\text{Dose}}{\text{Concentration}} = \text{Volume}$$

One can take this process a step further and extrapolate back from a plasma time curve to the $y$ axis. This is theoretically the plasma concentration ($C_0$) that would occur if, upon being administered, the material is instantly distributed throughout the body. The volume number obtained with the above equation becomes

$$\frac{\text{Dose}}{C_0} = V_D$$

where $V_D$ represents the apparent volume of distribution, a proportionality constant that reflects the relation of the concentration of a xenobiotic in plasma to the total amount of the entity in the body. Materials that are avidly bound to plasma proteins will have a high, while materials that are avidly taken by the tissues (deposit fat, for example) will have a low volume of distribution. The $V_D$ is a parameter that is simple to calculate yet gives one important information about the distribution of the chemical under investigation.

The available volumes and masses for distribution vary from species to species, as summarized in Tables 18.3 and 18.4.

### 18.3.3. Metabolism/Biotransformation

Metabolism is the process by which chemicals are changed by the body. In fact, very few foreign chemicals that enter the body are excreted unchanged. Most are chemically modified. In general, metabolism results in chemicals that are more polar and water soluble, and more easily excreted. Examples of the more common metabolic conversions are shown in Table 18.5. In general, the vast majority of

**TABLE 18.3. Volume and Half-Life of Body Water in Selected Species**

| Species | Sex | Exchangeable Body Water (% of body weight) | Half-Life (days) |
| --- | --- | --- | --- |
| Mouse | F | 58.5 | 1.13 |
| Rat | M | 59.6 | 2.53 |
| Rabbit | F | 58.4 | 3.87 |
| Dog | M | 66.0 | 5.14 |
| Cynomolgus monkey | M | 61.6 | 7.80 |
| Rhesus monkey | M | 61.6 | 7.80 |
| Humans | M, F | 55.3 | 9.46 |

**TABLE 18.4. Typical Organ Weights in Adult Laboratory Animals**

| | Percent of Body Weight | | | | |
|---|---|---|---|---|---|
| Organ | Rat | Mouse | Dog | Rabbit | Monkey |
| Liver | 3.5 | 6 | 3.5 | 3 | 2.5 |
| Kidney | 0.8 | 1.6 | 0.5 | 0.8 | 0.5 |
| Heart | 0.4 | 0.4 | 0.8 | 0.3 | 0.4 |
| Spleen | 0.3 | 0.5 | 0.3 | 0.04 | 0.1 |
| Brain | 0.5 | 0.6 | 0.8 | 0.4 | 3 |
| Adrenals | 0.02 | 0.01 | 0.01 | 0.02 | 0.03 |
| Lung | 0.6 | 0.6 | 1 | 0.6 | 0.7 |

lipophilic chemicals are first oxidized via the cytochrome P-450 dependent mixed function oxidase system of the liver. This is the process classically called phase I metabolism. Cytochrome P-450 exists as a family of isozymes (the CYP gene superfamily) with varying but overlapping substrate affinity and responses to different inducing agents. For a review of the molecular biology of the CYP gene superfamily the reader is referred to Meyer (1994). Induction is the process whereby exposure to a chemical leads to increased activity of the MMFO due to an increase in cytochrome P-450. The isoenzymes induced by a variety of different chemicals are given in Table 18.6. In a practical sense, a chemical can induce its own metabolism. Hence, repeated dosing with a chemical may lead to lower blood levels at the end, for example, of a thirteen week study than at the beginning. There could also be alterations in the spectrum of metabolites produced, such that an agent could become more, or less, toxic with repeated dosing, depending on the nature of the metabolites. It is not unusual during a subchronic or chronic toxicity test for tolerance to occur. There may be signs of toxicity early in the study but even with continued daily dosing, the signs abate. This phenomenon, particularly in rodents, is frequently due to microsomal induction, whereby the chemical has induced its own metabolism, and more rapid clearance of the parent chemical occurs.

After the chemical has been metabolically oxidized, it can in fact be further metabolized. In fact, it is possible for the metabolites to also be substrates of the MMFO and to be metabolized themselves.

The route of metabolic activation of the classic carcinogen benzo[a]pyrene is due to such a mechanism. The biology of these reactive intermediates has been extensively studied. Glutathione is among the most common organic intracellular chemical in all mammalian species, being present at a concentration of up to 10 mm and glutathione *S*-transferase is very active. Glutathine is a tripeptide (glutamine-cysteine glycyne). The sulfhydryl group of cysteine is the business end of the molecule where the reaction with the nucleophilic reactive intermediate takes place. After that, the glutamine conjugate is further metabolized to a cytinyl-acetyl moiety. These moieties are called mercapturic acids, and are generally found in the urine.

**TABLE 18.5. Summary of Prominent Phase I Biotransformation Reactions**

| Reaction | Enzyme | Location | Example/Comments |
|---|---|---|---|
| Hydrolysis | Carboxylesterase | Ubiquitous | vinyl acetate to acetate and acetaldehyde |
| | Peptidase | Blood, lysomesq | Amino-, carboxy- and endo peptidase which cleave peptides at specific amino acid linkages |
| Reductions | Epoxide hydroplase | Microsomes, cytosol | Cytosol conversion of styrene 7,8 epoxide to styrene 7,8 glycol |
| | Azo and nitro reduction | Gut microflora | Sequential conversion of nitrobenzene to aniline |
| | Carbonyl reductase | Cytosol | Conversion of haloperidol to reduced haloperidol (a secondary alcohol) |
| | Disulfide reduction | Cytosol | Glutathine dependent reduction of disulfiram to deithyldithiocarbamate |
| | Sulfoxide reduction | Cytosol | Thioredoxin dependent of sulindac to sulindac sulfide |
| | Quinone reduction | Cytosol, microsomes | DT diaphorase reduction of menadione to hydroquinone |
| | Reductive dehalogenation | Microsomes | Conversion of pentabromoethane to tetra bromoethane (releasing free bromide ion) |
| Oxidation | Alcohol dehydrogenase | Cytosol | Conversion of ethanol to acetaldehyde (DAD/DADH dependent reversible reaction) |
| | Aldehyde dehydrogenase | Mitochondria/cytosol | Conversion of acetaldehyde to acetate |
| | Aldehyde oxidase | Liver cytosol | FAD dependent metalloenzyme, oxidation of benzaldehyde to benzoic acid |
| | Xanthene oxidase | Cytosol | Oxidation of purine derivative, oxidation of allopurinol to alloxanthene |
| | Monamine oxidase | Mitochondria | FAD dependent oxidative deamination of monoamines, e.g. primaquine |
| | Diamine oxidase | Cytosol | Pyridoxal dependent, copper containing enzyme. Conversion of allylamine to acrolein |
| | Prostaglandin oxidase | Microsomes | Cooxidation reaction, can "activate" chemical in tissues low in cytochrome P-450, e.g., nephrotoxicity of acetaminophen, oxidation of phenylbutazone |
| | Flavin-mono-oxygenase | Microsomes | FAD dependent oxidation of nucleophilic nitrogen, sulfur and phosphorus heteroatoms, e.g. conversion of nicotine to nicotine $1'$-$N$-oxide, cimetidine to cimetidine $S$-oxide |
| | Cytochrome P-450 | Microsomes | |

**TABLE 18.6. Examples of Xenobiotics Activated by Human P-450**

CYP1A1
  Benzo[a]pyrene and other polycyclic aromatic hydrocarbons
CYP1A2
  Acetaminophen
  2-Acetylaminofluorene
  4-Aminobiphenyl
  2-Aminofluorene
  2-Naphthylamine
  NNK*
  Amino acid pyrolysis products
  (DiMeQx, MeIQ, MeIQx, Glu P-1, Glu P-2, IQ, PhIP, Trp P-1, Trp P-2)
CYP2A6
  $N$-nitrosodiethylamine
  NNK*
CYP2B6
  6-Aminochrysene
  Cyclophosphamide
  Ifosphamine
CYP2C8, 9, 18, 19
  None known
CYP2D6
  NNK*
CYP2E1
  Acetaminophen
  Acrylonitrile
  Benzene
  Carbon tetrachloride
  Chloroform
  Dichloromethane
  1,2-Dichloropropane
  Ethylene dibromide
  Ethylene dichloride
  Ethyl carbamate
  $N$-Nitrosodimethylamine
  Styrene
  Trichloroethylene
  Vinyl chloride
CYP3A4
  Acetaminophen
  Aflatoxin $B_1$ and $G_1$
  6-Aminochrysene
  Benzo[a]pyrene 7,8-dihydrodiol
  Cyclophosphamide
  Ifosphamide
  1-Nitropyrene
  Sterigmatocystin
  Senecionine
  *Tris*(2,3-dibromopropyl) phosphate
CYP4A9/11
  None known

The relative predominance of mercapturic acid over other metabolites may be considered a rough indication of how "reactive" the intermediates may have been. Teleologically, it is tempting to speculate that it is a very well designed protective mechanism. As long as intracellular glutathione concentrations remain above a critical level, the destructive actions of active metabolites can be held in check. Thus, a small dose of a chemical (bromo-benzene is a good example) may cause no liver damage while a large dose may. This is also a good example of one of the aspects of toxicokinetics versus pharmacokinetics where a high dose of a chemical will become toxic due to saturation of a detoxification pathway.

The glutathione $S$-transferase pathway is sometimes in biochemical competition with the epoxide hydratase pathway, in that both deactivate intermediates of the MMFO. Epoxide hydratase is a microsomal enzyme that acts specifically to deactivate epoxide intermediates, by the addition of water across the C—O bond to form a diol. As a very broad generality, the glutathione $S$-transferase pathway tends to be more prominent in rodents, while the epoxide hydratase pathway tends to be more dominant in nonrodents.

The hydroxyl or diol containing metabolites of the MMFO can be further metabolized by so-called phase II (synthetic) metabolism whereby they are conjugated to or from glucuronides and/or sulfates (so-called etherial sulfates). Amines can also be substrates. The net effect of phase II reactions is to create a more polar molecule that is more readily excretable. While there are species differences, glucuronides are actively transported and excreted in the bile into the GI tract. Sulfates are excreted more predominantly in the urine. Both glucuronides and sulfates, however, can be found in both the urine and the feces. Like the MMFO pathway, glutathione 3-transferase, UDP-glucuronyl transferase and eopoxide hydratase are inducible; that is, treatment with exogenous chemicals will increase the amount of enzyme protein present.

Beside the MMFO mediated (phase I) reactions there are a few other major reactions that are worthy of note. The two major ones involve ester hydrolysis and alcohol and aldehyde dehydrogenases. All mammalian species have an extensive ability to hydrolyze the ester bond. The products of the reactions then can go on to be further metabolized. In the pharmaceutical industry, this property has been utilized to synthesize prodrugs; that is, chemicals that have desirable pharmaceutical properties (generally increased water solubility) that are not converted to their active moiety until hydrolyzed in the body.

The activity of alcohol dehydrogenase is one with which we should all be familiar. It oxidizes alcohols to aldehydes. The aldehydes produced by this reaction can go on to be further metabolized to a carbocylic acid, if they are not sterically hindered. Sidechain constituents of aromatic compounds can also be a substrate for this reaction sequence, producing sidechain carboxylates. The oxidation of alcohols to aldehydes can also be a form of metabolic activation as aldehydes can have potent physiological actions. Fortunately, aldehyde dehydrogenase has a very high activity when compared to alcohol dehydrogenase, so that the aldehydes do not accumulate. Inhibition of aldehyde dehydrogenase by disulfiram (Antabuse) leads to the accumulation of acetaldehyde, causing nausea, dizziness, and flushing. Like disulfiram, some pesticides contain dithiocarbamates and have the potential of causing this type of reaction.

It is hoped that this little description of the major metabolic pathways has given some appreciation of the richness of the processes. The different sites of oxidation, the possibility of additional oxidative metabolism of metabolites, differences in phase II reactions all lead to a multiplicity of possible metabolites. Over 100 different metabolites of the human pharmaceutical chlorpromazine have been isolated and identified. When analyzed by HPLC, for example, the parent chemical and the different (detectable) metabolites will form a pattern of different peaks. This is referred to as the metabolic fingerprint or profile of a chemical. Different species will have different profiles. Ideally, in doing a risk assessment, one would like to know the similarity in this pattern between the animals used in the toxicology studies and that produced by human beings. This is only infrequently available for most nonpharmaceutical products, as pesticides (for example) are rarely given intentionally to human subjects for the purposes of study. The technology now exists, however, to address this potential problem. Cell lines with human cytochrome P-450 have been developed that can provide some indication of the similarities of human metabolism of a chemical to that of experimental animals. At least they may be able to assist in identifying the major oxidative metabolites. For nonpharmaceutical products, it would be an unusual circumstance that would require one to identify potential human metabolites as part of a marketing application; however, it may be useful to know that the technology exists to do so.

The processes of metabolic conversion are frequently involved in the mechanisms of toxicity and carcinogenicity.

***Metabolic Activation.*** As mentioned, most nonnutritive chemicals pass through the GI tract by passive absorption and then enter the mesenteric circulation. The venous circulation from the mesentery flows through the portal vein into the liver. The metabolic action of the liver literally sits between the GI tract and the general systemic circulation. Thus, even chemicals that may be highly absorbed from the GI tract could appear only sparingly in systemic circulation if they are highly metabolized by the liver. The combination of absorption from the GI tract and metabolism from the liver leads to what is called the first-pass effect. An extension of this is the fact that the gut flora contain glucuronidases, which can cleave glucuronides of chemicals and/or metabolites that are then available to be re-absorbed. This process is called entero-hepatic circulation.

***Induction of P-450 Metabolism and Isoenzymes.*** When organisms are exposed to certain xenobiotics their ability to metabolize a variety of chemicals is increased. This phenomenon can produce either a transitory reduction in the toxicity of a drug or an increase (if the metabolite is the more toxic species). However, this may not be the case with compounds that require metabolic activation. The exact toxicological outcome of such increased metabolism is dependent on the specific xenobiotic and its specific metabolic pathway. Since the outcome of a xenobiotic exposure can depend on the balance between those reactions that represent detoxication and those that represent activation, increases in metabolic capacity may at times produce unpredictable results.

The ability of different drugs to differentially inhibit and/or induce individual cytochrome P-450 isoenzymes has become critical in assessing the potential safety of drug molecules. Table 18.7 presents an overview of some of what we have come

**TABLE 18.7. Examples of Xenobiotics Activated by Human Cytochrome P-450 Isoenzymes**

| | |
|---|---|
| CYP1A1 | CYP2D6 |
|   Benzo[*a*]pyrene and other |   buforolol |
|     polycyclic aromatic hydrocarbons |   codeine |
| |   timolol |
| CYP1A2 |   metoprolol |
|   acetaminophen | |
|   2-Acetylaminofluorine | CYP2E1 |
|   4-Aminobiphenyl |   acetaminophen |
|   2-Aminofluorene |   acrylonitrile |
|   2-Naphthylamine |   benzene |
| |   carbon tetrachloride |
| CYP2A6 |   chloroform |
|   *N*-nitrosodiethylamine |   dichloromethane |
|   butadiene |   1,2-dichloropropane |
|   coumarin |   ethylene dibromide |
| |   ethylene dichloride |
| CYP2B6 |   ethyl carbamate |
|   6-Aminochrysene |   *N*-Nitrosodimethylamine |
|   Cyclophosphamide |   styrene |
|     ifosphamine |   trichloroethylene |
| |   Vinyl chloride |
| CYP2C8 | |
|   taxol | CYP3A4 |
| |   acetaminophen |
| CYP2C9 |   aflatoxin $B_1$ and $G_1$ |
|   diclofenac |   6-aminochrysene |
|   phenytoin |   benzo[*a*]pyrene 7,8-dihydrodiol |
|   piroxicam |   cyclophosphamide |
|   tolbutamide |   Ifosphamide |
| |   1-Nitropyrene |
| CYP2C19 |   sterigmatocystin |
|   diazepam |   senecionine |
|   diphenylhydantoin |   tris(2,3-dibromopropyl) phosphate |
|   hexabarbitol | |
|   propanolol | CYP4A9/11 |
| |   none known |

*Source:* Adapted in part from Parkinson (1996).

to know about differential metabolism by P-450 isoenzymes. Draper et al. (1998) have published on the use of human liver microsomes for determining the levels of activity or inhibition a chemical has or the formation of 6--testosterone as a model for CYP3A activity (1) and chlorzoxazone for CYP2E1 activity (2). If, for example, a chemical under study competitively inhibits the metabolism of the model substrates in these systems, then it is a substrate for that human isozyme. Using these more recently available *in vitro* systems it is much easier to perform cross-species comparisons with regard to biotransformation. It is now easier to determine how similar the routes of metabolism are in the experimental animals to those in humans without having to administer the chemical to human subjects. Human and animal model microsome preparations may be used as models to identify patterns of metabolites *in vitro*, allowing for better selection of model species for safety studies and competition, or inhibition activation of specific isoenzymes can be evaluated to identify potential problems of drug–drug interaction in patients.

It should always be kept in mind, particularly in humans that there can be significant gender based differences in metabolism (Mugfor and Kidderis, 1998). Particularly for drugs where there is a significant potential for disproportionate use by women, FDA expects early evaluation of this aspect.

***Species Differences.*** Species differences in metabolism are amongst the principal reasons that there are species differences in toxicity. Differences in cytochrome P450 is one of the most common reasons for differences in metabolism. For example, Monostory et al. (1997) recently published a paper comparing the metabolism of panomifene (a tamoxifen analog) in four different species. These data serve to address that the rates of metabolism in the non-human species was most rapid in the dog and slowest in the mouse. Thus, one should not *a priori* make any assumptions about which species will have the more rapid metabolism. Of the seven metabolites, only one was produced in all four species. Both the rat and the dog produced the two metabolites (M5 and M6) produced by human microsomes. So how does one decide which species best represents humans? One needs to consider the chemical structure of the metabolites and the rates at which they are produced. In this particular case, M5 and M6 were relatively minor metabolites in the dog, which produced three other metabolites in larger proportion. The rat produced the same metabolites at a higher proportion, with fewer other metabolites than the dog. Thus, in this particular instance, the rat, rather than the dog, was a better model. Table 18.8 offers a comparison of excretion patterns between three species for a simple inorganic compound.

A more thorough review on species differences in pharmacokinetics has been presented by Smith (1991) and in Gad and Chengelis (1992).

***Sex-Related Differences in Rodents.*** Not only are there differences in absorption, distribution, biotransformation and metabolism between species, there may also be differences between sexes within a species. Griffin et al. (1997), for example, has demonstrated sex-related differences in the metabolism of 2,4-dichlorophenoxyace-tic acid (Table 18.8). They noted that while there were differences between sexes,

**TABLE 18.8. Differences in the Disposition of 2,4-dichlorophenoxyacetic Acid[a]**

| Species | Sex | Urine | Feces |
|---|---|---|---|
| Rat | M | 31.2 | 2.7 |
| | F | 16.5 | 1.1 |
| Mouse | M | 12.7 | 2.8 |
| | F | 26.8 | 6.7 |
| Hamster | M | 4.9 | 2.5 |
| | F | 33.9 | 14.5 |

[a] All animals dosed orally with radiolabeled 2,4-D, 200 mg/kg. Results are expressed as percent of $^{14}C$ dose recovered. Urine was collected for 8 hours and feces for 24 hours.

they tended to be quantitative (rates), not qualitative (metabolites). Differences between species were greater than sex-related differences. With regard to sex-related differences, it is noteworthy that males do not always have the higher rates, as Griffen et al. have shown; in hamsters, the female metabolizes 2,4-D more rapidly than males. In general, male rats tend to have higher activity than female rats, especially with regard to CYP-dependent activity. In the case of 2,4-D, the only urinary metabolite is 2,4-D glucuronide, but the half-life of 2,4-D was 138 min in males and 382 in females.

***Excretion.*** Excretion encompasses the process by which chemicals or their metabolites are transported out of the body. There are three possible major routes of excretion, and a handful of minor ones. The major routes of excretion for chemicals, and in particular their metabolites, are as follows.

*Urine.* The kidneys filter the entire cardiac output multiple times each day, and thus provide a large opportunity for the removal of chemicals from the bloodstream. How much of a xenobiotic is actually excreted is dependent on three factors or processes.

1. The glomerular membrane has pores of 70–80 Å; under the positive hydrostatic conditions in the glomerulus, all molecules smaller than about 20,000 Da are filtered. Proteins and protein-bound compounds thus remain in the plasma, and about 20% of the nonbound entity is carried with 20% of the plasma water into the glomular filtrate.

2. Because the glomerular filtrate contains many important body constituents (e.g., glucose), there are specific active uptake processes for them. Also, lipid-soluble chemicals diffuse back from the tubule into the blood, especially as the urine becomes more concentrated because of water reabsorption. The pH of the urine is generally lower than that of the plasma, and therefore pH partitioning tends to increase the reabsorption of weak acids. The pH of the urine can be altered

appreciably by treatment with ammonium chloride (decreases pH) or sodium carbonate (increases pH); the buffered plasma shows little change.

3. Xenobiotics may be secreted actively into the renal tubule against a concentration gradient by anion and cation carrier processes. These processes are saturable and of relatively low specificity; many basic or acidic compounds and their metabolites (especially conjugation products) are removed by them. Because the dissociation rate for the chemical–albumin complex is rapid, it is possible for highly protein-bound compounds to be almost completely cleared at a single passage through the kidney.

***Feces.*** The most important mechanism allowing circulating foreign compounds to enter the gut is in the bile. The biological aspects of this mechanism have been reviewed (Pratt and Taylor, 1990), and certain pertinent points have emerged. The bile may be regarded as a complementary pathway to the urine, with small molecules being eliminated by the kidney and large molecules in the bile. Thus the bile becomes the principal excretory route for many drug conjugates. Species differences exist in the molecular weight requirement for significant biliary excretion, which has been estimated as $325 \pm 50$ in the rat, $440 \pm 50$ in the guinea pig, and $475 \pm 50$ in the rabbit. In the rat, small molecules (less than 350 Da) are not eliminated in the bile or large molecules (more than 450 Da) in the urine, even if the principal excretory mechanism is blocked by ligation of the renal pedicles or bile duct, respectively. Compounds of intermediate molecular weight (350–450 Da) are excreted by both routes, and ligation of one pathway results in increased use of the other.

Foreign compounds may also enter the gut by direct diffusion or secretion across the gut wall, elimination in the saliva, pH partitioning of bases into the low pH of the stomach, and elimination in the pancreatic juice.

***Expired Air.*** Volatile compounds or metabolites can be extensively excreted by passage across pulmonary membranes into the airspace of the lungs, then by expulsion from the lungs in expired air.

Minor routes for excretion can include tears, saliva, sweat, exfoliated keratinocytes, hair, and nasal discharge. These are of concern or significance only in rare cases. Accordingly, quantitation of excretion typically requires collection of urine, feces (and occasionally expired air) over a period of time.

### 18.3.4. Pharmacokinetics

The interplay of the processes of absorption, distribution, metabolism and excretion result in changes in concentration of the test chemical in different organs with time. With regard to the practical concerns of monitoring human exposure, the organ of interest is the blood. Blood can be considered a central compartment. Determining the concentration of the chemical in plasma gives one an assessment of exposure. Mathematical formulas are used to quantitatively describe this exposure.

***Physiologically Based Pharmacokinetic Modeling.*** Pharmacokinetic parameters are descriptive in nature. They quantitatively describe the manner in which a test material is absorbed and excreted, such that a specific blood or tissue level is achieved or maintained. In the past, experiments had to be done by every route of administration to gather the data appropriate for describing the pharmacokinetic behavior of a chemical administered by different routes. The development of more sophisticated and readily accessible computers has lead to the development of a different approach, that of pharmacokinetic modeling. In this computerized model, different compartments are represented as shown in boxes and the movement of the material in and out of the compartments is defined by the rate constants. These can be determined either *in vivo* or *in vitro*. Other physiological parameters are brought into play as well, such as octanol–water partition coefficient, blood flow through an organ, respiration rate (for the inhalation route of exposure), rate of microsomal metabolism, and so on.

## 18.4. LABORATORY METHODS

The actual means by which pharmacokinetic information is collected is through the conduct of one or more specific studies, employing a wide range of available analytical techniques. Administered therapeutic molecules can be identified and quantified in relevant samples collected in accordance with carefully designed and executed protocols.

### 18.4.1. Analytical Methods

There are three broad categories of analytical techniques now available: instrumental (cold chemical), radiolabeled and immunological. Each of these have advantages and disadvantages. Only an overview of these techniques will be given here; detailed explanations are beyond the scope of this text. These methodologies are all directed at being able to identify and/or quantify a chemical (and/or its metabolites) in various biological matrices.

***Instrumental Methods.*** These bioanalytical methods are also sometimes called cold chemistry methods. These generally start from a place of isolating the compound or compounds of interest, for which the workhorse methodology is high pressure liquid chromatography (HPLC). A wide variety of specialized columns are used to achieve desired separation. At the end of the column, where separation of molecular entities has been achieved, the outflow of the column can be directed to any of a wide variety of detection instruments, including various forms of detectors intrinsic to the HPLC. In general, all of the cold chemistry methodologies have less sensitivity (higher detection limits) than do radiochemical or immunological methods.

Mass spectrometry (MS), nuclear magnetic resonance (NMR) spectrography, electron skin resonance (ESR) spectrography, ultraviolet, infrared and visible spectrophotometry and mass spectroscopy are all well-established detection methodologies.

***Radiochemical Methods.*** The massive expansion of our understanding of toxico-kinetics since the late 1970s is to a large degree a reflection of the wide use of radioactive isotopes as tracers of chemical and biological processes. Appropriately, radiolabeled test compounds are commonly used in toxicokinetic studies, providing a simple means of following the administered dose in the body. This is particularly important when specific analytical methods are unavailable or too insensitive. The use of total radioactivity measurements allows an estimation of the total exposure to drug-related material and facilitates the achievement of material balance.

The most commonly used radionuclides in drug metabolism and disposition studies are carbon-14 ($^{14}$C) and tritium ($^{3}$H), both of which are referred to as beta emitters. Since these beta-emitting isotopes have relatively long half-lives, their radioactive decay during an experiment is insignificant. Additionally, they provide sufficient emission energy for measurement and are relatively safe to use, as indicated by the data in Table 18.9. Although individual beta particles can have any energy up to the maximum, $E_{max}$, the basic quantity in determining the energy imparted to tissues by beta emitters is the average energy, $E_{\beta}$. The range is the maximum thickness the beta particles can penetrate. Beta particles present virtually no hazard when they originate outside the body (Shapiro, 1981).

During the synthesis of radiolabeled compounds, the label is usually introduced as part of the molecular skeleton in a metabolically stable and, with tritium, nonexchangeable position. The *in vivo* stability of $^{14}$C labels is often reflected by the extent of $[^{14}C]$ carbon dioxide formation. The biologic stability of $^{3}$H labels can be estimated by the extent of tritiated water formation. The tritiated water concentration (dpm/ml) is urine samples collected during a designated time interval after dosing, assumedly after equilibrium is reached between urine and the body water pool, is determined. This value is extrapolated from the midpoint of the collection interval to zero time, based on the known half-life of tritiated water in the given species. The percentage of the radioactive dose that is transformed to tritiated water (% $^{3}$H$_2$O) can be calculated using the following equation:

$$\% \, ^{3}H_2O = \frac{^{3}H_2O \text{ concentration at zero time} \times \text{exchangeable body water volume}}{\text{radioactivity dose}}$$
$$\times \, 100\%$$

**TABLE 18.9. Properties of Primary Radioisotopes Employed in Pharmacokinetics**

| Property | $^{3}$H | $^{51}$Cr | $^{14}$C | $^{125}$I |
|---|---|---|---|---|
| Half-life (yr) | 12.3 | 27.8 (d) | 5730 | 13 (d) |
| Maximum beta energy (MeV) | 0.0186 | 0.752 | 0.156 | 2.150 |
| Average beta energy (MeV) | 0.006 | 0.049 | | |
| Range in air (mm) | 6 | 300 | | |
| Range in unit density material (mm) | 0.0052 | 0.29 | | |

Values for the exchangeable body water content as well as the half-life of tritiated water in some mammalian species that can be applied to the above equation were shown earlier in Table 18.3. If the molecule is likely to or is known to fragment into two major portions, it may be desirable to monitor both fragments by differential labeling ($^3$H and $^{14}$C).

The chemical and radiochemical purity of the labeled compound must be ascertained prior to use. In practice a value of 95% or greater is usually acceptable. The desired specific activity of the administered radioactive compound depends on the dose to be used as well as the species studied. Doses of $^{14}$C on the order of 5 μCi/kg for the dog and 20 μCi/kg for the rat have been found adequate in most studies, while doses of $^3$H are usually two to three times higher owing to lower counting efficiency of this isotope.

Liquid scintillation counting is the most popular technique for the detection and measurement of radioactivity. In order to count a liquid specimen such as plasma, urine, or digested blood or tissues directly in a liquid-scintillation spectrometer, an aliquot of the specimen is first mixed with a liquid scintillant. Aliquots of blood, feces, or tissue homogenates are air-dried on ash-free filter papers and are combusted in a sample oxidizer provided with an appropriate absorption medium and a liquid scintillant prior to counting. The liquid scintillant plays the role of an energy transducer, converting energy from nuclear decay into light. The light generates electrical signal pulses which are analyzed according to their timing and amplitude, and are subsequently recorded as a count rate, e.g., counts per minute (cpm). Based on the counting efficiency of the radionuclide used, the count rate is then converted to the rate of disintegration, disintegrations per minute (dpm), which is a representation of the amount of radioactivity present in the sample.

***Immunoassay Methods.*** Radioimmunoassay (RIA) allows measurement of biologically active materials which are not detectable by traditional cold chemistry techniques. RIAs can be used to measure molecules that cannot be radiolabeled to detectable levels *in vivo*. They also are used for molecules unable to fix complement when bound to antibodies, or they can be used to identify cross-reacting antigens that compete and bind with the antibody.

Competitive inhibition of radiolabeled hormone antibody binding by unlabeled hormone (either as a standard or an unknown mixture) is the principle of most RIAs. A standard curve for measuring antigen (hormone) binding to antibody is constructed by placing known amounts of radiolabeled antigen and the antibody into a set of test tubes. Varying amounts of unlabeled antigen are added to the test tubes. Antigen–antibody complexes are separated from the antigen and the amount of radioactivity from each sample is measured to detect how much unlabeled antigen is bound to the antibody. Smaller amounts of radiolabeled antigen–antibody complexes are present in the fractions containing higher amounts of unlabeled antigen. A standard curve must be constructed to correlate the percentage of radiolabeled antigen bound with the concentration of unlabeled antigen present.

Two methods are commonly employed in RIAs to separate antigen–antibody complexes. The first, the double-antibody technique, precipitates antigen–antibody complexes out of solution by utilizing a second antibody, which binds to the first antibody. The second most commonly used method is the dextran-coated activated charcoal technique. Addition of dextran-coated activated charcoal to the sample followed immediately by centrifugation absorbs free antigen and leaves antigen–antibody complexes in the supernatant fraction. This technique works best when the molecular weight of the antigen is 30 kilodaltons (kDa) or less. Also, sufficient carrier protein must be present to prevent adsorption of unbound antibody.

Once a standard curve has been constructed, the RIA can determine the concentration of hormone in a sample (usually plasma or urine). The values of hormone levels are usually accurate using the RIA, but certain factors (e.g., pH or ionic strength) can affect antigen binding to the antibody. Thus similar conditions must be used for the standard and the sample.

Problems of RIAs include lack of specificity. This problem is usually due to nonspecific cross-reactivity of the antibody. RIA represents an analytical approach of great sensitivity. Unlike assays that often require large amounts of tissue (or blood), the greater sensitivity of the RIAs or monoclonal antibody techniques can be achieved using small samples of biological fluids. Some of these RIA methodologies are more useful than others and to some extent depend on the degree of hormonal cross-reactions or, in the case of monoclonal antibody methods, their degree of sensitivity.

Enzyme-linked immunosorbent assay (ELISA) is comparable to the immuno-radiometric assay except that an enzyme tag is attached to the antibody instead of a radioactive label. ELISAs have the advantage of nonradioactive materials and produce an end product that can be assessed with a spectrophotometer. The molecule of interest is bound to the enzyme-labeled antibody, and the excess antibody is removed for immunoradiometric assays. After excess antibody has been removed or the second antibody containing the enzyme has been added (two-site assay), the substrate and cofactors necessary are added in order to visualize and record enzyme activity. The level of molecule of interest present is directly related to the level of enzymatic activity. The sensitivity of the ELISAs can be enhanced by increasing the incubation time for producing substrate.

Immunoradiometric assays (IRMAs) are like RIAs in that a radiolabeled substance is used in an antibody–antigen reaction, except that the radioactive label is attached to the antibody instead of the hormone. Furthermore, excess of antibody, rather than limited quantity, is present in the assay. All the unknown antigen becomes bound in an IRMA rather than just a portion, as in a RIA; IRMAs are more sensitive. In the one-site assay, the excess antibody that is not bound to the sample is removed by addition of a precipitating binder. In a two-site assay, a molecule with at least two antibody-binding sites is adsorbed onto a solid phase, to which one of the antibodies is attached. After binding to this antibody is completed, a second antibody labeled with $^{125}$I is added to the assay. This antibody reacts with the second antibody-binding site to form a "sandwich," composed of antibody-hormone-labeled antibody. The amount of hormone present is proportional to the amount of radioactivity measured in the assay.

With enzyme-multiplied immunoassay technique (EMIT) assays, enzyme tags are used instead of radiolabels. The antibody binding alters the enzyme characteristics, allowing for measurement of target molecules without separating the bound and free components (i.e., homogeneous assay). The enzyme is attached to the molecule being tested. This enzyme-labeled antigen is incubatcd with the sample and with antibody to the molecule. Binding of the antibody to the enzyme-linked molecule either physically blocks the active site of the enzyme or changes the protein conformation so that the enzyme is no longer active. After antibody binding occurs, the enzyme substrate and cofactor are added, and enzyme activity is measured. If the sample contains subject molecules, it will compete with enzyme-linked molecules for antibody binding, enzyme will not be blocked by antibody, and more enzyme activity will be measurable.

Most chemical entities can now be assessed using monoclonal antibody (MAb) techniques. It is possible to produce antisera containing a variety of polyclonal antibodies that recognize and bind many parts of the molecule. Polyclonal antisera can create some nonspecificity problems such as cross-reactivity and variation in binding affinity. Therefore it is oftentimes desirable to produce a group of antibodies that selectively bind to a specific region of the molecule (i.e., antigenic determinant). In the past, investigators produced antisera to antigenic determinants of the molecule by cleaving the molecule and immunizing an animal with the fragment of the hormone containing the antigenic determinant of interest. This approach solved some problems with cross-reactivity of antisera with other similar antigenic determinants, but problems were still associated with the heterogeneous collection of antibodies found in polyclonal antisera.

The production of MAbs offers investigators a homogenous collection of antibodies that could bind selectively to a specific antigenic determinant with the same affinity. In addition to protein isolation and diagnostic techniques, MAbs have contributed greatly to RIAs.

While MAbs offer a highly sensitive, specific method for detecting antigen, sometimes increasing MAb specificity compromises affinity of the antibody for the antigen. In addition, there is usually decreased complement fixation, and costs are usually high for preparing and maintaining hybridomas that produce MAbs (Table 18.10).

The monoclonal antibody techniques provide a means of producing a specific antibody for binding antigen. This technique is useful for studying protein structure relations (or alterations) and has been used for devising specific RIAs.

**TABLE 18.10. Advantages and Disadvantages of Monoclonal Antibodies Compared to Polyclonal Antisera**

| Advantages | Disadvantages |
| --- | --- |
| Sensitivity | Overly specific |
| Quantities available | Decreased affinity |
| Immunologically defined | Diminished complement fixation |
| Detection of neoantigens on cell membrane | Labor intensive; high cost |

### 18.4.2. Sampling Methods and Intervals

***Blood.*** Since blood (plasma and serum) is the most easily accessible body compartment, the blood concentration profile is most commonly used to describe the time course of drug disposition in the animal. With the development of sensitive analytical methods that require small volumes (100–200 µl) of blood, ADME data from individual rats can be obtained by serial sample collection. Numerous cannulation techniques have been utilized to facilitate repeated blood collection, but the animal preparation procedures are elaborate and tedious and are incompatible with prolonged sampling periods in studies involving a large number of animals. In contrast, noncannulation methods such as collection from the tail vein, orbital sinus, or jugular vein are most practical. Significant volumes of blood can be obtained from the intact rat by cardiac puncture, although this method can cause shock to the animal system and subsequent death.

Blood collection from the tail vein is a simple and rapid, nonsurgical method which does not require anesthesia. A relatively large number of serial samples can be obtained within a short period of time. However, this method is limited to relatively small sample volumes (< 250 µl per sample). Although larger volumes can be obtained by placing the rat in a warming chamber, this procedure could significantly influence the disposition of the test compound and therefore is not recommended for routine studies. Blood collected from the cut tail has been shown to provide valid concentration data for numerous compounds.

The rat is placed in a suitable restrainer with the tail hanging freely. The tail is immersed in a beaker of warm water (37–40°C) for 1 to 2 min to increase the blood flow. Using surgical scissors or a scalpel, the tail is completely transected approximately 5 mm above the tip. The tail is then gently "milked" by sliding the fingers down the tail from its base. It should be noted that excessive "milking" could cause damage to the blood capillaries or increase the white cell count in the blood. A heparinized micropipet of desired capacity (25–250 µl) is held at a 30 to 45° downward angle in contact with the cut end of the tail. This allows blood to fill the micropipet by capillary action. Application of gentle pressure with a gauze pad for approximately 15 s is sufficient to stop bleeding. A sufficient number of serial blood samples may be obtained to adequately describe the blood level profile of a compound.

If plasma is required, the blood may be centrifuged after sealing one end of the filled micropipet and placing it in a padded centrifuge tube. The volume of plasma is determined by measuring the length of plasma as a fraction of the length of the micropipet, multiplied by the total capacity of the pipet. The tube is then broken at the plasma/red blood cell interface and the sample is expelled using a small bulb. If serum is needed, the blood should be collected without using anticoagulants in the sampling tube.

Serial blood samples can also be collected from the orbital sinus, permitting rapid collection of larger (1–3 ml) samples.

***Excreta.*** Excretion samples commonly collected from the rat include urine, feces, bile, and expired air. With properly designed cages and techniques, the samples can be completely collected so that the mass balance is readily determined. These samples also serve to elucidate the biotransformation characteristics of the compound.

These samples can be easily collected through the use of suitable metabolism cages. Since rodents are coprophagic, the cage must be designed to prevent the animal from ingesting the feces as it is passed. Other main features of the cage should include a system to effectively separate urine from feces with minimal cross-contamination, a feed and water system that prevents spillage and subsequent contamination of collected samples, and collection containers that can be easily removed without disturbing the animal. Also, the cage should be designed so that it can be easily disassembled for cleaning or autoclaving.

Following dose administration, rats are placed in individual cages. The urine and feces that collect in containers are removed at predetermined intervals. The volume of urine and the weight of feces are measured. After the final collection, the cage is rinsed, normally with ethanol or water, to assure complete recovery of excreta. If the rats are also used for serial blood sampling, it is important that bleeding be performed inside the cage to avoid possible loss of urine or feces.

**Bile.** The bile is the pathway through which an absorbed compound is excreted in the feces. In order to collect this sample, surgical manipulation of the animal is necessary.

**Expired air.** For $^{14}$C-labeled chemicals, the tracer carbon may be incorporated *in vivo* into carbon dioxide, a possible metabolic product. Therefore, when the position of the radiolabel indicates the potential for biological instability, a pilot study to collect expired air and monitor its radioactivity content should be conducted prior to initiating a full-scale study. Expired air studies should also be performed in situations where the radiolabel has been postulated to be stable but analyses of urine and feces from the toxicokinetic study fail to yield complete recovery (mass balance) of the dose.

Following drug administration, the rat is placed in a special metabolism cage. Using a vacuum pump, a constant flow of room air (approx. 500 ml/min) is drawn through a drying column containing anhydrous calcium sulfate impregnated with a moisture indicator (cobalt chloride), and passed into a second column containing Ascarite$^{\text{(R)}}$ II, where it is rendered carbon dioxide free. The air is then drawn in through the top of the metabolism cage. Exhaled breath exiting the metabolism cage is passed through a carbon dioxide adsorption tower, where the expired $^{14}$CO$_2$ is trapped in a solution such as a mixture of 2-ethoxyethanol and 2-aminoethanol (2:1). The trapping solution is collected, replaced with fresh solution, and assayed at designated times postdose so that the total amount of radioactivity expired as labeled carbon dioxide can be determined.

**Milk.** The study of passage of a xenobiotic into milk serves to assess the potential risk to breast-fed infants in the absence of human data. The passage into milk can be estimated as the milk:plasma ratio of drug concentrations at each sampling time or that of the AUC values. Approximately 30 rats in their first lactation are used. The litter size is adjusted to about 10 within 1 to 2 days following parturition. The test compound is administered to the mothers 8 to 10 days after parturition. The rats are then divided into groups for milk and blood collection at designated times postdose. All sucklings are removed from the mother rats several hours before milking. Oxytocin, 1 IU per rat, is given intramuscularly 10 to 15 min before each collection of milk to stimulate milk ejection. The usual yield of milk is about 1 ml from each rat. Blood is obtained immediately after milking. In order to minimize the number of animals used, the sucklings can be returned to the mother rat which can then be milked again 8 to 12 hours later.

In all the fluid sampling techniques mentioned, the limitations of availability should be kept in mind. Table 18.11 presents a summary of such availability for the principle model species.

For topical exposures, determining absorption (into the skin and into the systemic circulation) requires a different set of techniques. For determining how much material is left, skin washing is required. There are two components to skin washing in the recovery of chemicals. The first component is the physical rubbing and removal from the skin surface. The second component is the surfactant action of soap and water. However, the addition of soap effects the partitioning. Some compounds may require multiple successive washing with soap and water applications for removal from skin.

Skin tape stripping can be used to determine the concentration of chemical in the stratum corneum at the end of a short application period (30 min) and by linear extrapolation predict the percutaneous absorption of that chemical for longer application periods. The chemical is applied to skin of animals or humans, and after a 30-minute skin contact application time, the stratum corneum is blotted and then removed by successive tape applications. The tape strippings are assayed for chemical content. There is a linear relationship between this stratum corneum reservoir content and percutaneous absorption. The major advantages of this method are (1) the elimination of urinary and fecal excretion to determine absorption and (2) the applicability to nonradiolabeled determination of percutaneous absorption, because the skin strippings contain adequate chemical concentrations for nonlabeled assay methodology.

Finally, a complete determination of the distribution and potential departing of a chemical and its metabolites requires some form of measurement or sampling of

**TABLE 18.11. Approximate Volumes of Pertinent Biological Fluids in Adult Laboratory Animals**

| Fluid | Rat | Mouse | Dog | Rabbit | Monkey |
|---|---|---|---|---|---|
| Blood (ml/kg) | 75 | 75 | 70 | 60 | 75 |
| Plasma (ml/kg) | 40 | 45 | 40 | 30 | 45 |
| Urine (ml/kg/day) | 60 | 50 | 30 | 60 | 75 |
| Bile (ml/kg/day) | 90 | 100 | 12 | 120 | 25 |

tissues or organs. Autoradiography provides a nonquantitative means of doing such, but quantitation requires actual collection and sampling of tissues. Table 18.6 provided guidance as to the relative percentage of total body mass that the organs constitute in the common model species.

***Sampling Interval.*** To be able to perform valid toxicokinetic analysis, it is not only necessary to properly collect samples of appropriate biological fluids, but also to collect a sufficient number of samples at the current intervals. Both of these variables are determined by the nature of the answers sought. Useful parameters in toxicokinetic studies are $C_{max}$, which is the peak plasma test compound concentration; $T_{max}$, which is the time at which the peak plasma test compound concentration occurs, $C_{min}$, which is the plasma test compound concentration immediately before the next dose is administered; AUC, which is the area under the plasma test compound concentration-time curve during a dosage interval, and $t_{\frac{1}{2}}$ which is the half-life for the decline of test compound concentrations in plasma. The samples required to obtain these parameters are shown in Table 18.12. $C_{min}$ requires one blood sample immediately before a dose is given and provides information on accumulation. If there is no accumulation in plasma, the test compound may not be detected in this sample.

Several $C_{min}$ samples are required at intervals during the toxicity study to check whether accumulation is occurring. CT is a blood sample taken at a chosen time after dosing and provides proof of absorption as required by the GLP regulations, but little else. $C_{max}$ requires several blood samples to be taken for its accurate definition as does $T_{max}$; these two parameters provide information on rate of absorption. AUC also requires several blood samples to be taken so that it can be calculated: it provides information on extent of absorption. The half-life, $t_{\frac{1}{2}}$ requires several samples to be taken during the terminal decline phase of the test compound concentration-time curve: this parameter provides information on various aspects such as any change in the kinetics of the test compound during repeated doses or at different dose levels. Depending on the other parameters obtained, the accumulation

**TABLE 18.12. Blood Samples Required so that Certain Toxicokinetic Parameters can be Obtained and Calculated**

| Parameter | Blood sample required | Information obtained |
| --- | --- | --- |
| $C_{min}$ $(C_{24})$ | 24 h | Accumulation |
| CT | $T$ h | Proof of absorption |
| $C_{max}$ ($C$ peak) | Several[a] | Rate of absorption |
| $T_{max}$ ($T$ peak) | Several[a] | Rate of absorption |
| AUC | Several[a] | Extent of absorption |
| $t_{\frac{1}{2}}$ | Several[a] | Various |
| Accumulation ratio | Several after first and repeated doses | Extent of accumulation |

[a] Several samples to define concentration-time profile.

ratio can be calculated from $C_{min}$, $C_{max}$ and/or AUC when these are available after the first dose and after several doses to steady-state.

Operational and metabolic considerations generally make urine sampling and assay of limited value for toxicokinetic purposes.

***Study Type.*** Metabolic and pharmacokinetic data from a rodent species and a nonrodent species (usually the dog) used for repeat dose safety assessments (14 days, 28 days, 90 days or six months) are recommended. If a dose dependency is observed in metabolic and pharmacokinetic or toxicity studies with one species, the same range of doses should be used in metabolic and pharmacokinetic studies with other species. If human metabolism and pharmacokinetic data also are available, this information should be used to help select test species for the full range of toxicity tests, and may help to justify using data from a particular species as a human surrogate in safety assessment and risk assessment.

Metabolism and pharmacokinetic studies have greater relevance when conducted in both sexes of young adult animals of the same species and strain used for other toxicity tests with the test substance. The number of animals used in metabolism and pharmacokinetic studies would be sufficient to reliably estimate population variability. This usually means a separate (but parallel) set of groups of animals in rodent studies. A single set of intravenous and oral dosing results from adult animals, when combined with some *in vitro* kinetic results, may provide an adequate data set for the design and interpretation of short-term, subchronic and chronic toxicity studies.

Studies in multiple species may clarify what appear to be contradictory findings in toxicity studies (i.e., equal mg/kg body weight doses having less effect in one species than in another). If disposition and metabolite profiles are found to be similar, then differences in responses among species could more reliably be attributed to factors other than differences in metabolism. Studies of the pharmacokinetics and metabolism of a substance in neonatal and adolescent animals provide information about any changes in metabolism associated with tissue differentiation and development. Animals with fetuses of known gestational age should be used for determining the disposition of the test substance in the fetus. Dosage is by (to the maximum extent possible) the intended clinical route.

An acute intravenous study can provide accurate rates of metabolism without interference from intestinal flora, plus rates of renal and biliary elimination, if urine and bile are collected. This route also avoids the variability in delivered dose associated with oral absorption and ensures that the maximum amount of radiolabel is excreted in the urine or bile for purposes of detection. Once IV data and parameters are available, they can be used with plasma concentrations from limited oral studies to compute intestinal absorption via the ratio of Areas Under the (plasma and/or urine) Curves or via simulations of absorption with gastrointestinal absorption models.

In single-dose pharmacokinetic studies of oral absorption, the primary concerns are with the extent of absorption and peak plasma or target tissue concentrations of the test substance. If the test vehicle affects gastric emptying, it may be necessary to use both fasted and nonfasted animals for pharmacokinetic studies.

Blood (RBCs, plasma, and serum), urine, and feces are the most commonly collected samples. In addition, a few representative organ and tissue samples should be taken, such as liver, kidney, fat and suspected target organs. Sampling times should depend on the substance being tested and the route of administration. In general, an equal number of blood samples should be taken in each phase of the concentration-versus-time curve. Intravenous (IV) studies usually require much shorter, and more frequent, sampling than is required for oral dosing. Time spacing of samples will depend on the rates of uptake and elimination. In a typical IV study, blood and tissue samples are taken in a "powers of 2" series, i.e., samples at 2, 4, 8, 16, and 30 (32) minutes, 1, 2, 4, 8, and 16 hours. Similar coverage could be obtained with only 7 time points by using a "powers of 3" series: 3, 9, and 30 (27) minutes; 1, 3, 9, and 24 (27) hours. Oral dosing studies usually extend to at least 72 hours. Such a sampling scheme would provide data coverage for evaluation of absorption, elimination, enterohepatic recirculation and excretion processes.

The number of animals used in metabolism and pharmacokinetic studies should be large enough to reliably estimate population variability. In the case of rats and mice, tissue and/or blood sample size is usually the limiting factor: analysis of the substance may require 1 ml or more blood, but it is difficult to obtain multiple blood samples of this size from one animal. As a consequence, a larger number of animals is required (3–4 per time point, 7–9 time points) when small rodents are used. Such an approach has the advantage of allowing limited sampling of critical tissues (e.g., liver, fat) at each time point, an option which is usually unavailable with large animals. The use of humans and large animals generally permits collection of multiple (serial) blood samples. For outcrossing populations like humans and large animals, individual differences in the rates of biotransformation are likely to be greater than those of inbred rodent populations; under these circumstances, more samples/sex/group may be needed to reliably estimate variability.

Individual metabolism cages are recommended for collecting urine and feces in oral dosing studies. Excreta should be collected for at least 5 elimination half-lives of the test substance. When urine concentrations will be used to determine elimination rates, sampling times should be less than one elimination half-life (taken directly from the bladder in IV studies); otherwise, samples should be taken at equal time intervals.

The results of the preliminary biotransformation/kinetic study, together with the current regulatory metabolism studies and the 28- and 90-day studies should allow the selection of a relatively small number of appropriate tissues and/or fluids for monitoring purposes. Satellite groups of animals will provide the material for analysis. Methods must be developed to analyze nonradioactive test chemical. Obviously it is important to monitor blood. It is accessible, convenient and, in certain circumstances, sequential sampling from the same animal may be important. The most useful aspect of blood is that the results can be compared with those obtained in humans (see below). It is important, however, not to be constrained by this aspect. The most relevant tissues and body fluids should also be analyzed. These are target organs (if known) and indicator organs, tissues or fluids, i.e. those in which the concentration of pesticide or metabolite is a measure of that in the whole animal.

In cases where distribution varies with dose (if shown in the preliminary study), a larger number of organs or tissues would be chosen for monitoring.

Whether the parent drug or metabolite (or both) is chosen for analysis depends on the preliminary study. In principle, analysis for the parent compound should always be carried out; however, there are situations (e.g., rapid metabolism) when this is quite futile and a major retained metabolite should be used. Covalently bound metabolites are addressed in a later section.

Four occasions may be adequate for monitoring.

1. One month (equilibrium between intake of chemical and elimination of metabolites should be established; the time relates to the 28-day preliminary study).
2. Three months (confirmation of results at one month; relates to the 90-day study).
3. One year (coincides with the interim kill).
4. Two years (effects of age; coincides with termination of study).

Consideration should be given to the analysis of moribund animals.

*In Vitro Studies.* *In vitro* measurements employing enzymes, subcellular organelles, isolated cells and perfused organs may be used to augment the dose response information available from less extensive metabolic and pharmacokinetic studies. Because *in vitro* systems generally are less complex than whole animals, elucidation of a test compound's metabolic pathways and the pathways' kinetic characteristics may be facilitated. Such systems can be used to measure binding, adduct and conjugate formation, transport across cell membranes, enzyme activity, enzyme substrate specificity, and other singular objectives. Biochemical measurements that can be made using *in vitro* systems include: intrinsic clearances of enzymes in an organ or tissue, kinetic constants for an enzyme, binding constants, and the affinity of the test compound and its metabolites for the target macromoecules. The activity of a hepatic drug-metabolizing enzyme *in vivo* may be approximated by kinetic constants that are calculated from *in vitro* studies; when a first-order approximation is used, the ratio of $V_{\max}$ to $K_{\mathrm{m}}$ is equal to the intrinsic clearance of the drug. *In vitro* measurements made using readily accessible tissues and body fluids from animals and humans may also be useful in elucidating mechanisms of toxicity.

*Analysis of Data.* Data from all metabolism and pharmacokinetic studies should be analyzed with the same pharmacokinetic model and results should be expressed in the same units. Concentration units are acceptable if the organ or sample size is reported, but percent of dose/organ is usually a more meaningful unit. In general, all samples should be analyzed for metabolites that cumulatively represent more than 1% of the dose.

A variety of rate constants and other parameters can be obtained from IV and oral dosing data sets, provided that good coverage of the distribution, elimination, and absorption (oral dose) phase is available. Typical parameters calculated to characterize the disposition of a test substance are: half-lives of elimination and absorption; area under the concentration-versus-time curve (AUC) for blood; total body, renal and metabolic clearances (Cl); volume of distribution ($V_d$); bioavailability ($F$); and mean residence and absorption times (MRT, MAT). Some of these parameters, such as half-lives and elimination rates, are easily computed from one another; the half-life is more easily visualized than the rate constant.

Computation of oral absorption ($k_a$) and elimination (E) rates is often complicated by the "flip-flop" of the absorption and elimination phases when they differ by less than a factor of 3. Because of these analysis problems, computation of absorption and elimination rates should not be attempted on the basis of oral dosing results alone.

Blood-tissue uptake rates ($k_{jl}$) can often be approximated from data at early ($t < 10$ minutes) time points in IV studies, provided the blood has been washed from the organ (e.g., liver) or the contribution from blood to the tissue residue is subtracted (fat). High accuracy is not usually required since these parameters can be optimized to fit the data when they are used in more complex models. Tissue-blood recycling rates ($k_{lj}$) and residence times can be computed from partition coefficients if estimates of uptake rates are available.

Tissue : blood partition coefficients ($R_{jl}$) should be determined when steady-state has been achieved. Estimates based on samples obtained during the elimination phase following a single dose of the test substance may lead to underestimates of this ratio in both eliminating and noneliminating tissues unless its half-life is very long. Correction of these values for elimination has been described by several authors (Yacobi et al., 1989; Shargel and Yu, 1999; Renwick, 2000).

It may be important to determine the degree of plasma protein and red blood cell binding of the test substance; calculation of blood clearance rates using plasma or serum concentrations of the substance that have not been adjusted for the degree of binding may under or over-estimate the true rate of clearance of the test substance from the blood. This is usually done through experiments *in vitro*.

Two classical methods used in the analysis of pharmacokinetic data are the fitting of sums of exponential functions (2- and 3-compartment mammillary models) to plasma and/or tissue data, and less frequently, the fitting of arbitrary polynomial functions to the data (noncompartmental analysis).

Noncompartmental analysis is limited in that it is not descriptive or predictive; concentrations must be interpolated from data. The appeal of noncompartmental analysis is that the shape of the blood concentration-versus-time curve is not assumed to be represented by an exponential function and, therefore, estimates of metabolic and pharmacokinetic parameters are not biased by this assumption. In order to minimize errors in parameter estimates that are introduced by interpolation, a large number of data points that adequately define the concentration-versus-tie curve are needed.

Analysis of data using simple mammillary, compartmental models allows the estimation of all of the basic parameters mentioned here, if data for individual tissues are analyzed with one or two compartment models, and combined with results from two to three compartment analyses of blood data. "Curve Stripping" analysis can be applied to such simple models through the use of common spreadsheet programs (i.e., LOTUS 1-2-3), as long as a linear regression function is provided in the program. Optimization of the coefficients and exponents estimated may require the use of more sophisticated software: a number of scientific data analysis packages such as RS/1 and SigmaPlot have the necessary capabilities. Specialized programs such as NONLIN, CONSAM, or SIMUSOLV will be needed when more complex models must be analyzed. Coefficients and exponents from mammillary models can be used to calculate other parameters; however, they should not be taken too literally, since mammillary models assume that all inputs are to a central pool (blood), which communicates without limitation into other compartments. This approach does not include details such as blood flow limitations, anatomical volumes or other physiological limits in the animal.

Physiologically based pharmacokinetic models (PB-PK) were developed to overcome the limitations of simple mammillary models. Physiologically based models describe the disposition of test substances via compartmental models which incorporate anatomical, biochemical, and physiological features of specific tissues in the whole animal. The types of information added include organ-specific blood flows, volumes, growth models and metabolism rates. Metabolic parameters often are obtained from *in vitro* studies (i.e., enzyme reaction rates in cultured hepatocytes, plasma protein binding, etc.), while other parameters are becoming available as standard parameters in the literature. Parameters from mammillary models can be used to compute the value of parameters used in physiological pharmacokinetic models, using tissue-specific blood flows, anatomical volumes, and other information (literature values). Estimation of parameters for a simple mammillary model is often the first data reduction step in creating a physiological model.

Because PB-PK models are based on physiological and anatomical measurements and all mammals are inherently similar, they provide a rational basis for relating data obtained from animals to humans. Estimates of predicted disposition patterns for test substances in humans may be obtained by adjusting biochemical parameters in models validated for animals; adjustments are based on experimental results of animal and human *in vitro* tests and by substituting appropriate human tissue sizes and blood flows. Development of these models requires special software capable of simultaneously solving multiple (often very complex) differential equations, some of which were mentioned in this chapter. Several detailed descriptions of data analysis have been reported.

*Use of Data from Metabolism and Pharmacokinetic Studies.* Information from metabolism and pharmacokinetic studies can be used in the design and analysis of data from other toxicity studies. Some examples are described below.

DESIGN OF TOXICITY STUDIES. The concentration-versus-time curve, peak and steady-state concentrations of the test substance in blood or plasma provide information on the distribution and persistence of the substance in the animal which may suggest essential elements in the design of the toxicity studies. For example, when metabolic and pharmacokinetic studies indicate that the test compound accumulates in the bone marrow, long-term toxicity tests should include evaluation of the test compound's effect on hematopoietic function and morphology. If a test compound is found to accumulate in milk, an investigator may need to plan to perform reproductive toxicity studies with *in utero* exposure and a nursing phase (cross-fostering study). In addition, information from metabolic and pharmaco-kinetic studies can be used to predict the amount of test compound that enters biological compartments (tissues, organs, etc.) that may not suffer a toxic insult but may serve as depots for indirect or secondary exposure.

### 18.4.3. Whole Body Autoradiography

Autoradiography is the production of an image in a photographic emulsion by the emission from a radioactive element. The term "autoradiography" is preferred to radioautography. Prefixes are added to words to further classify the concept. Therefore, the process is "auto-" radiography for a "self-" radiograph and not a "radio-" autograph or one's transmitted signature (Waddell, 1972).

Whole Body Autoradiography (WBA) has been used with increasing frequency as a means of identifying tissues that concentrates test substances. This technique allows a small number of animals (5–10) to be used for screening purposes with a minimal investment in manual labor. FDA encourages the use of WBA with IV dosing, as a means of screening and selecting tissues of greatest relevance for later oral dosing studies. Animals used for WBA should generally be sacrificed before primary consideration in selecting specific tissues.

The most comprehensive technique currently available for the initial survey of the distribution of a drug is that of whole body autoradiography. The species of animals used include mice, rats, hamsters, monkeys, pigs, dogs, and ferrets. The most widely used animal has been the mouse, which has the advantages of requiring less isotope and being easier to section.

The animals are anesthetized and then frozen by immersion at various times after administration of the labeled compound in hexane or acetone cooled with dry ice. Since the freezing in the interior of the animals occurs slowly, large ice crystals form within these tissues, hence, subcellular localization of compounds is not possible.

The selection of times for freezing an animal after injection of a drug must be based on the information available on the rate of elimination of the compound from the animal by metabolism and excretion. In general, a geometric increase in time intervals is most useful. In order to have time intervals for comparison, we routinely have employed freezing times which are approximately multiples of three, namely two minutes, 6.5 minutes, 20 minutes, one hour, three hours, nine hours, and 24 hours. In certain cases, rapid elimination of the drug by the kidneys must be circumvented by ligation of the renal pedicles to avoid apparent localization from failure of the agent to reach equilibrium.

The frozen animal is frozen into a block of carboxymethylcellulose ice on the microtome stage. Although the Jung, type K, microtome has been used, the Leitz, model 1300, sledge microtome is more suitable, for its smaller size allows it to be mounted in an ordinary commercial freezer instead of a walk-in freeze room. The microtome stage must be designed for mounting in the vice by the front end of the stage.

Sections from 5 μm to approximately 80 μm-thick are taken onto #800 Scotch tape (Minnesota Mining & Mfg. Co.). Before removal from the freezer, the sections must be allowed to dry thoroughly so that no ice remains that can melt and allow movement of the isotope. After drying, if covered to prevent condensation of moisture on the sections, the sections may be transferred from the freezer to room temperature.

X-ray films which produce the most satisfactory autoradiograms are Kodak industrial type AA and Gevaert Structurix D-7. Both are fine grain films which have been demonstrated not to produce chemical artifacts. Approximately six times faster, Kodak No Screen and Kodirex may be used for rapid screening and timing of autoradiograms. However, they occasionally produce artifacts and should not be relied on for interpretation. Some investigators have used photographic emulsions such as Ilford G-5, 10 μm-thick, preapplied to glass plates. The increased cost and likelihood of breakage, however, hardly justify the small improvement in resolution for whole-body sections.

Exposure of the photographic emulsion by the radioactivity of the tissue section should be at freezer temperatures to prevent autolysis of the tissue. After exposure of the X-ray film, sections with isotopes which have a long half-life may be placed against fresh X-ray film for additional sets of autoradiograms with either a longer or shorter exposure time. This procedure is useful for revealing relative concentrations of radioactivity for areas that have either very high or very low concentrations after the first exposure. When no further autoradiograms are needed, the section can be stained with histological dyes to verify localizations of radioactivity.

Compounds that fluoresce under ultraviolet light can be visualized in the tissue sections and their locations recorded with color film. Whole-body tissue sections can be used for histochemical localizations for comparison with the autoradiograms. Furthermore, the areas can be removed, extracted, and the extract chromotographed to identify the chemical nature of the radioactivity revealed by the autoradiogram.

Although the whole-body technique will allow localization of an increased concentration of an isotope in a tissue or occasionally a cell type, other techniques must be used for single cells and subcellular localization. A nuclear tract plate is prepared by dipping the plate in a 12% solution of glycerine in absolute ethyl alcohol and allowing it to drain for 10 minutes in a vertical position before approximating the section on tape. After the emulsion is exposed, soaking in xylene removes the tape but leaves the section attached to the nuclear tract plate. The Ilford G-5 nuclear tract plates with 10 μm emulsions are most satisfactory. The increased resolution gained by the finer grained Ilford K and L emulsions is warranted only for tissues that are well preserved and relatively free of ice crystal artifacts. Kodak NTB emulsions seem to produce more pressure artifacts than the Ilford plates.

Comparison of various techniques of autoradiography for diffusible compounds clearly demonstrates that no solutions can be used in processing the tissue. These investigators have dried thin sections of liver and uterus at temperatures below

−60°C. These freeze-dried sections were dry mounted on microscope slides which had been precoated with either Kodak NTB-3 or NTB-10 emulsion. Other techniques which thawed the frozen section, embedded the tissue in paraffin or dipped the section in liquid emulsion were demonstrated to translocate diffusible compounds. Many other similar attempts have been and are currently being made to localize diffusible compounds by autoradiography at the electron microscope level.

## 18.5. PHYSIOLOGICALLY BASED PHARMACOKINETIC (PBK) MODELING

Pharmacokinetic modeling is the process of developing mathematical explanations of absorption, distribution, metabolism, and excretion of chemicals in organisms. Two commonly used types of compartmental pharmacokinetic models are (a) data-based and (b) physiologically based. The data-based pharmacokinetic models correspond to mathematical descriptions of the temporal change in the blood and tissue level of a xenobiotic in the animal species of interest. This procedure considers the organism as a single homogeneous compartment or as a multi-compartmental system with elimination occurring in specific compartments of the model. The number, behavior, and volume of these hypothetical compartments are estimated by the type of equation chosen to describe the data, and not necessarily by the physiological characteristics of the model species in which the blood and tissue concentration data were acquired.

Whereas these data-based pharmacokinetic models can be used for interpolation, they should not be used for extrapolation outside the range of doses, dose routes, and species used in the study on which they were based. In order to use the data-based models to describe the pharmacokinetic behavior of a chemical administered at various doses by different routes, extensive animal experimentation would be required to generate similar blood-time course data under respective conditions. Even within the same species of animal, the time-dependent nature of critical biological determinants of the disposition (e.g., tissue glutathione depletion and resynthesis) cannot easily the included or evaluated with the data-based pharmaco-kinetic modeling approach. Further, due to the lack of actual anatomical, physio-logical, and biochemical realism, these data-based compartmental models cannot easily be used in interspecies extrapolation, particularly to predict pharmacokinetic behavior of chemicals in humans. These various extrapolations, which are essential for the conduct of dose-response assessment of chemicals, can be performed more confidently with a physiologically based pharmacokinetic modeling approach. This section presents the principles and methods of physiologically based pharmaco-kinetic modeling as applied to the study of toxicologically important chemicals.

PBPK modeling is the development of mathematical descriptions of the uptake and disposition of chemicals based on quantitative interrelationships among the critical biological determinants of these processes. These determinants include partition coefficients, rates of biochemical reactions and physiological characteristics of the animal species. The biological and mechanistic basis of the PBPK models enable them to be used, with limited animal experimentation, for extrapolation of the kinetic behavior of chemicals from high dose to low dose, from one exposure route to another, and from test animal species to people.

The development of PBPK models is performed in four interconnected steps: model representation, model parameterization, model stimulation, and model validation. Model representation involves the development of conceptual, functional, and computational descriptions of the relevant compartments of the animal as well as the exposure and metabolic pathways of the chemical. Model parameterization involves obtaining independent measures of the mechanistic determinants, such as physiological, physicochemical, and biochemical parameters, which are included in one or more of the PBPK model equations. Model simulation involves the prediction of the uptake and disposition of a chemical for defined exposure scenarios, using a numerical integration algorithm, simulation software, and a computer. Finally, the model validation step involves the comparison of the *a priori* predictions of the PBPK model with experimental data to refute, validate, or refine the model description, and the characterization of the sensitivity of tissue dose to changes in model parameter values. PBPK models after appropriate testing and validation can be used to conduct extrapolations of the pharmacokinetic behavior of chemicals from one exposure route or scenario to another, from high dose to low dose, and from one species to another.

The PBPK model development for a chemical is preceded by the definition of the problem, which in toxicology may often be related to the apparent complex nature of toxicity. Examples of such apparent complex toxic responses include nonlinearity in dose-response, sex and species differences in tissue response, differential response of tissues to chemical exposure, qualitatively and/or quantitatively difference responses for the same cumulative dose administered by different routes and scenarios, and so on. In these instances, PBPK modeling studies can be utilized to evaluate the pharmacokinetic basis of the apparent complex nature of toxicity induced by the chemical. One of the values of PBPK modeling, in fact, is that accurate description of target tissue dose often resolves behavior that appears complex at the administered dose level.

The principal application of PBPK models is in the prediction of the target tissue dose of the toxic parent chemical or its reactive metabolite. Use of the target tissue dose of the toxic moiety of a chemical in risk assessment calculations provides a better basis of relating to the observed toxic effects than the external or exposure concentration of the parent chemical. Because PBPK models facilitate the prediction of target tissue dose for various exposure scenarios, routes, doses, and species, they can help reduce the uncertainty associated with the conventional extrapolation approaches. Direct application of modeling includes

- High-dose–low-dose extrapolation;
- Route-route extrapolation;
- Exposure scenario extrapolation;
- Interspecies extrapolation.

## 18.6. POINTS TO CONSIDER

Stereoisomerism will influence metabolism and toxicity. For example, Lu et al. (1998) reported a comparison of $(S)$-$(-)$Ifosfamide and $(R)$-$(+)$-Ifsosfamide. They demonstrated that there were significant differences between the two stereoisomers with regard to pharmacokinetic behavior and major metabolite formation, as shown in Table 18.13.

In addition, treatment of animals with phenobarbital not only increased overall rates of metabolism and clearance, but also shifted the metabolite patterns. One of the more common methods used for determining an exposure to (or the amount of a metabolite produced) is to determine an area under the curve (AUC) for the metabolite. Further, one of the more common methods for representing a racemically preferred metabolite is to calculate the ratio of the $R$ to the $S$. For example, the 3-decholoro metabolite of ifosfamide was produced in higher amounts from the $R$ enantiomer while the 2-decholorometabolite was the major metabolite produced from the $R$ enantiomer in naive animals. Treatment with phenobarbital shifted the metabolism so that the 3-dechloro metabolite was no longer the major metabolite for the $S$ enantiomer.

Additionally, protein binding of a drug should be evaluated very early in development. Drugs with significant binding have a greater poleplia for adverse drug : drug interactions.

## 18.7. BIOLOGICALLY DERIVED MATERIALS

The progress and products of biotechnology have brought some new challenges to the assessment of pharmacokinetics and toxicokinetics. While the reasons for needing this data (demonstrating, exposure, displaying dose dependency, correlating any findings of toxicity to exposure and determining steady-state for systemic agent

**TABLE 18.13. Example of Stereoselective Differences in Metabolism (R) versus (S) Ifosfamide[a]**

| Parameter | Phenobarb | R | S | R/S |
|---|---|---|---|---|
| Term half-life | − | 34.3 | 41.8 | 0.820 |
| (min) | + | 19.8 | 19.41 | 1.02 |
| AUC | − | 4853 | 6259 | 0.820 |
| ($\mu$M*min) | + | 1479 | 1356 | 1.03 |
| 2-dehloro metabolite | − | 799 | 2794 | 0.287 |
| AUC | + | 229 | 1205 | 0.186 |
| 3-dehloro metabolite | − | 1380 | 996 | 1.41 |
| AUC | + | 192 | 1175 | 0.159 |

[a] Animals were pretreated with phenobarbital (80 mg/kg) for four days.
*Source:* Adapted from Lu et al., 1998.

levels) are certainly as compelling as with traditional drugs, there are a whole set of special problems involved.

These special concerns for biologically derived products are:

### Assay Sensitivity/Specificity

- Needs to be at 1 ng/ml or lower.
- Cross reactivity to native protein may confound results.
- If test article is the same as native protein, how do you tell the difference?
- Western blot can be used to demonstrate specificity.
- Antibody interference may occur with assay.

### Low Systemic Levels

- Rapid metabolism.
  Metabolites may be endogenous proteins or amino acids.
- Extensive metabolism.
  Metabolites may be incorporated into cell structures rapidly.
- Rapid distribution.
- Rapid hepatic clearance.
- Route of administration may bypass systemic circulation.
  *SC.*
  *ICV; IT.*

### Endogenous Protein

- May cross react and lead to false positive blood levels.
- Can radiolabel to tell difference between administered molecule and endogenous molecule.
  However, the label may lead to different distibution.
  What is the specific activity if diluted with unlabeled endogenous material?

### Sample Volume

- May need to be large to increase sensitivity.
- But also may need to be small because of competing assays.
  Immune factors (antibodies, globulins).
  Hormones.
  Disease state modifiers.
  In humans, concomitant medications.
- Available test material supply will be very limited in early development.

The upshot of these points is that it may not be practical to follow established guidelines for ADME evaluation. Binding proteins, immunoreactive metabolites and antibodies could interfere with the immunoassays used to measure the activity of biotechnologically derived pharmaceuticals. The link between immunoreactivity and pharmacological activity may be difficult to establish, making the data difficult to interpret. In radiolabelled distribution studies, if the label alters the physicochemical and biological properties of the test material, its pharmacokinetic behavior may change. These analytical difficulties may preclude accurate characterization of the distribution, metabolism and excretion of a protein.

AUC and $C_{max}$ are commonly measured to identify safety ratios for new chemical entities. Since the analytical methods used for biotechnologically derived pharmaceuticals may lack specificity, a clinical marker of biological activity or efficacy may sometimes be more appropriate than exposure data.

It is therefore essential that before pivotal (repeat dose) preclinical studies are initiated, bioanalytical assay development must be completed. This has to cover potential test species, normal and diseased humans. The assays must be validated in the sampling matrix of the toxicity test species, and one should also develop suitable assays for antibodies to the test article.

## REFERENCES


Bronaugh, R.L. (1998) Methods for *in vitro* percutaneous absorption. In: *Dermatotoxicology Methods* (Marzulli, F.N. and Maibach, H.I., Eds.), Taylor & Francis, Philadelphia.

Caldwell, W.S., Byrd, C.D., DeBethizz, J.D. and Brooks, P.A. (1994). Modern instrumental methods for studying mechanisms of toxicity. In: *Principles and Methods of Toxicology* (Hayes, A.W., Ed.), Raven Press, New York.

Connally, R. and Anderson, M. (1991). Biologically based pharmacokinetic models: Tools for toxicological research risk assessment. *Annu. Rev. Pharmacol. Toxicol.* 31: 503–523.

Draper, A., Madan, A., Smith, K. and Parkinson, A. (1998). Development of a non-high pressure liquid chromatography assay to determine testosterone hydroxylase (CYP3A) activity in human liver microsomes. *Drug Metab. Dispos.* 26: 299–304.

FDA (2000). *Redbook II*, pp. 138–148.

Gabrielsson, J. and Weiner, D. (1997). *Pharmacokinetic/Pharmacodynamic Data Analysis: Concepts and Applications.* Apotekarsociateten, Stockholm.

Gad, S.C. and Chengelis, C.P. (1997). *Acute Toxicology Testing*, 2nd ed. Academic Press, San Diego, CA.

Gad, S.C. and Chengelis, C.P. (Eds.). (1992). *Animal Models in Toxicology.* Marcel Dekker, New York.

Garner, C. and Matthews, H. (1998). The effect of chlorine substitution on the dermal absorption of polychlorinated biphenyls. *Toxicol. Appl. Pharmacol.* 149: 150–158.

Goldstein, A., Aronow, L. and Kalman, S. (1974). *Principles of Drug Action: The Basis of Pharmacology.* Wiley, New York.

Griffin, R., Godfrey, V., Kim, Y. and Burka, L. (1997). Sex-dependent differences in the disposition of 2,4-dichlorophenoxyacetic acid in Sprague-Dawley rats, B6C3F1 mice and Syrian hamsters. *Drug Metab. Dispos.* 25: 1065–1071.

Holland, J., Kao, M. and Whitaker, M.J. (1984). A multisample apparatus for kinetic evaluation of skin penetration *in vitro*: The influence and metabolic status of the skin. *Toxicol. Appl. Pharmacol.* 72: 272–280.

ICH (2000). Toxicokinetics. In: *International Conference on Harmonization: Safety.* Interpharm Press, Inc, Buffalo Grove, IL.

Keberle, G., Brindle, S.D. and Greengard, P. (1971). The route of absorption of intraperitoneally administered compounds. *J. Pharmacol. Exp. Ther.* 178: 562–566.

La Du, B., Mandel, H. and Way, E. (1972). *Fundamentals of Drug Metabolism and Drug Disposition.* Williams & Wilkins, Baltimore, MD.

Lu, H., Wang, J., Chan, K. and Young, D. (1998). Effects of phenobarbital of stereoselective metabolism of ifosfamide in rats. *Drug Metab. Dispos.* 26: 476–482.

Meyer, U.A. (1994). The molecular basis of genetic polymorphisms of drug metabolism. *J. Pharm. Pharmacol.* (suppl 1): 409–415.

Monostory, K., Jemnitz, K., Vereczkey, L. and Czira, G. (1997). Species differences in metabolism of panomifene, an analogue of tamoxifen. *Drug Metab. Dispos.* 25: 1370–1378.

Mugfor, C. and Kidderis, G. (1998). Sex-dependent metabolism of xenobiotics, *Drug Metab. Rev.*, pp. 441–498.

O'Reilly, W.J. (1972). Pharmacokinetics in drug metabolism and toxicology. *Can. J. Pharm. Sci.* 7: 66–77.

Parkinson, A. (1996). Biotransformation of xenobiotics. In *Cassarett & Doull's Toxicology: The Basic Science of Poisons.* 5th ed. (Klaassen, C., Ed.). McGraw-Hill, New York.

Pratt, W.B. and Taylor, P. (1990). *Principles of Drug Action: The Basis of Pharmacology,* 3rd ed. Wiley, New York.

Renwick, A.G. (2000). Toxicokinetics. In: *General and Applied Toxicology* (Ballantyne, B., Marrs, T. and Syversen, T., Eds.). Grove's Dictionaries, New York.

Smith, D. (1991). Species differences in metabolism and pharmacokinetics: are we close to an understanding? *Drug Metab. Rev.* 23: 355–373.

Shapiro, J. (1981). *Radiation Protection*, 2nd ed., Harvard University Press, Cambridge, MA, pp. 12–18.

Shargel, L. and Yu, A.B.C. (1999). *Applied Biopharmaceutics and Pharmacokinetics.* Appleton & Lange, New York.

Tse, F.L.S. and Jaffe, J.M. (1991). *Preclinical Drug Disposition.* Marcel Dekker, New York.

Vinegar, A. and Jepson, G. (1996). Cardiac sensitization thresholds of halon replacement chemicals in humans by physiologically based pharmacokinetic modeling. *Risk Analysis* 16: 571–579.

Waddell, W.J. (1972). Autoradiography in drug dispositions studies. In: *Fundamentals of Drug Metabolism and Drug Disposition* (La Du, B.N., Mandel, H.G. and Way, E.L., Eds.). Williams & Wilkens, New York, pp. 505–514.

Wang, Y.M. and Reuning, R. (1994). A comparison of two surgical techniques for the preparation of rats with chronic bile duct canulae for the investigation of enterohepatic circulation. *Lab. Anim. Sci.* 44: 479–485.

Yacobi, A., Skelly, J.P. and Batera, V.K. (1989). *Toxicokinetics and New Drug Development.* Pergamon Press, New York.

# 19

# SAFETY PHARMACOLOGY

## 19.1. INTRODUCTION

Safety pharmacology is the evaluation and study of the pharmacologic effects of a potential drug that is unrelated to the desired therapeutic effect, and therefore may present a hazard—particularly in individuals who already have one or more compromised or limited organ system functions. Unlike other nonclinical evaluations of the safety of a drug, these evaluations are usually conducted at doses close to the intended clinical dose.

General/safety pharmacology has been an emerging discipline within the pharmaceutical industry, in which unanticipated effects of new drug candidates on major organ function (i.e., secondary pharmacological effects) are critically assessed in a variety of animal models. A survey was conducted to obtain customer input on the role and strategies of this emerging discipline, which was overlooked in importance by all but a few (Zbinden, 1966, 1984) for many years. The Japanese clearly became the leaders in developing and requiring such information, while the United States was (and remains) in a position behind Japan and the EU both in having formal requirements and in implementing industrial programs. While major companies were aware and largely addressing the need by the mid-1990s (Murphy et al., 1994; Sullivan and Kinter, 1995), it wasn't until July of 2001 that FDA guidelines were published (FDA, 2001).

Most companies conduct evaluations of cardiovascular and CNS functions, fewer evaluate respiratory, gastrointestinal and renal functions; a few conduct a ligand-binding/activity panel as part of their pharmacological profiling. Resources to complete a company's standard safety pharmacology program are approximately 1–4 full-time persons per compound. One-third of companies use a maximum tolerated dose (MTD) for safety pharmacology studies, two-thirds use multiples of

737

pharmacological or therapeutic doses. Approximately half conduct safety pharmacology studies to Good Laboratory Practices (GLPs) and use the 1992 Japanese guidelines only as a guide or outline. Company clinicians are most often cited as the "primary customer" for whom safety pharmacology studies are done, followed by research and development scientists, and then regulatory authorities. These results suggest that most companies primarily conduct safety pharmacology for its contribution to risk assessment and critical care management.

It is recognized to be important that the tests employed detect bidirectional drug effects and that the tests performed be validated in both directions with appropriate reference (control) substances. This requirement is less appropriate for multiparameter procedures. Blind testing could be an advantage. Ethical considerations are important, but the ultimate ethical criterion is the assessment of risk for humans. Safety pharmacology studies should not be over-inclusive, but should be performed to the most exacting standards, including Good Laboratory Practice (GLP) compliance. Availability of safety pharmacology data is acknowledged to be important during the planning stage for phase I studies, but such is still less often the case than not. Partly this arises from the viewpoint that human tolerance (particularly in a well-designed and executed Phase I study in normal volunteers) is, in itself, an adequate assessment of safety pharmacology. This is, of course, backwards: such human tolerance is properly an extension (and expression) of the nonclinical safety pharmacology.

The other point of view in the past has been that properly executed repeated dose preclinical safety studies meeting the current design will (or could) fill these needs. Recognizing that undesired pharmacological activities of novel drugs or biologicals may limit development of a therapeutic agent prior to the characterization of any toxicological effects in rodent species, general pharmacology assays have traditionally been used to screen new agents for pharmacological effects on the central and peripheral nervous systems, the autonomic nervous system and smooth muscles, the respiratory and cardiovascular systems, the digestive system, and the physiological mechanisms of water and electrolyte balance. In large animal species, such as dogs and nonhuman primates, smaller numbers of animals per study limit their use for screening assays, but these species may play an important role in more detailed mechanistic studies. For drugs and biologicals that must be tested in nonhuman primates because of species-specific action of the test agent, functional pharmacology data are often collected during acute or subacute toxicity studies. This requires careful experimental design to minimize any impact that pharmacological effects or instrumentation may have on the assessment of toxicity. In addition, with many new therapies targeted at immunological diseases, the pharmacological effect of therapeutics on the immune system presents new challenges for pharmacology profiling. The applications of pharmacology assays by organ systems in both rodent and large animal species are discussed in this chapter as well as practical issues in assessing pharmacological endpoints in the context of toxicity studies (Martin et al., 1997; Folke, 2000; Hite, 1997).

In Europe, the numbers of registered drugs and drug expenditure are increasing rapidly. Within the European Union (EU) there are no longer any regulations requiring that new drugs have to be better than old ones. At the same time, pharmacoepidemiology studies in Europe and in the United States show that adverse drug reactions now may account for up to 10% of the admissions of patients to hospitals at a cost of hundreds of millions of U.S. dollars annually (Sjoquist, 2000). This represents a considerable increase compared to 20 years ago. A partial explanation is the many shortcomings of clinical trials and their relevance for health care. Adverse drug reactions are often poorly studied and documented in these studies and very seldom included in health economical analyses of the value of new drugs. Pharmacovigilance is product oriented—rather than utilization oriented and quite invisible in clinical medicine. This is regrettable, since up to 50% of adverse drug reactions (ADRs) are dose-dependent and thus preventable. Hopefully, the rapid progress in molecular and clinical pharmacogenetics will provide new tools for clinicians to choose and dose drugs according to the individual needs of patients. A good starting point for those not well versed in pharmacology and the range of potential mechanisms of action and of interaction can be found in Goodman and Gilman (Hardmon and Limbird, 1996).

## 19.2. REGULATORY REQUIREMENTS

While the ICH guidelines promulgated in November of 2000 (due to be implemented in Europe in June of 2001) are the announced international standards for regulation, the actual situation in different countries remains very mixed (Olejiniczak, 1999; Fujimori, 1999).

Japan continues to operate in conformance to its MHW draft, "Guidelines for Safety Pharmacology Studies". In 1999, this was revised. The basic principle of the revision is to harmonize the guideline with international concepts. The working group decided to change the title of "General Pharmacology" to "Safety Pharmacology," because the objective of this guideline is to assess the safety of a test substance in humans by examining the pharmacodynamic properties of the substance. The proposed guideline includes studies on vital functions as essential studies that should be performed prior to human exposure. Studies are also required to be conducted when unpredictable or unexpected observed effects are concerned. The working group recommends a case-by-case approach to select the necessary test items in consideration of the variable information available (Matsuzawa et al., 1997).

In the EU, the CPMP issued a draft "Note for Guidance on Safety Pharmacology Studies in Medicinal Product Development" in 1998, but it has not yet been finalized or put in force, and as of the middle of 2001, USFDA has remained mute on guidelines.

The actual requirements of the November 8, 2000 ICH guidelines are broadly outlined. They call for the conduct of studies in a core battery to assess effects on the cardiovascular (Table 19.1), respiratory (Table 19.2), central nervous system (Table 19.3) and secondary organ system (Table 19.4) effects. Follow-up studies for the care battery are also required on a case-by-case basis for the three main organ systems.

**TABLE 19.1. Cardiovascular System Safety Pharmacology Evaluations**

Core
 Hemodynamics (blood pressure, heart rate)
 Autonomic function (cardiovascular challenge)
 Electrophysiology (EKG in dog)

QT prolongation (non-core)
 An additional guideline, ICHS7B, is in preparation which will address the assessment of
  potential for QT prolongation. In the meantime, CPMP 986/96 indicates the following
  preclinical studies should be conducted prior to first administration to humans:
 Cardiac action potential *in vitro*
 ECG (QT measurements) in a cardiovascular study which would be covered in the core
  battery
 HERG channel interactions (HERG expressed in HEK 293 cells)

- *Central Nervous System.* Behavioral pharmacology, learning and memory,
  specific ligand binding, neurochemistry, visual, auditory and/or electrophysiology examinations, and so on.
- *Cardiovascular System.* Behavioral pharmacology, learning and memory,
  specific ligand binding, neurochemistry, visual, auditory and/or electrophysiology examinations, and so on.
- *Respiratory System.* Tidal volume, bronchial resistance, compliance, pulmonary arterial pressure, blood gases.

Conditions are also defined under which studies are not necessary.

 Locally applied agents (e.g., dermal or ocular) where systemic exposure or
  distribution to the vital organs is low;
 Cytotoxic agents for treatment of end-stage cancer patients;
 Biotechnologically-derived products that achieve highly specific receptor target-
  ing (refer to toxicology studies);
 New salts having similar pharmacokinetics and pharmacodynamics.

**TABLE 19.2. Respiratory System Safety Pharmacology Evaluation**

Respiratory functions
 Measurement of rate and relative tidal volume in conscious animals

Pulmonary function
 Measurement of rate, tidal volume and lung resistance and compliance in anaesthetized
  animals

**TABLE 19.3. Central Nervous System (CNS) Safety Pharmacology Evaluation**

Irwin test
  General assessment of effects on gross behavior and physiological state[a]
Locomotor activity
  Specific test for sedative, excitatory effects of compounds
Neuromuscular function
  Assessment of grip strength
Rotarod
  Test of motor coordination
Anaesthetic interactions
  Test for central interaction with barbiturates
Anti/proconvulsant activity
  Potentiation or inhibition of effects of pentylenetetrazole
Tail flick
  Tests for modulation of nociception (also hot plate, Randall Selitto, tail pinch)
Body temperature
  Measurement of effects on thermoregulation
Autonomic function
  Interaction with autonomic neurotransmitters *in vitro* or *in vivo*
Drug dependency
  Test for physical dependence, tolerance and substitution potential
Learning and memory
  Measurement of learning ability and cognitive function in rats

[a]Usually a functional observational battery (FOB) is integrated into a rodent (rat) repeat dose toxicity study to meet this requirement.


**TABLE 19.4. Secondary Organ System Safety Pharmacology Evaluation**

Renal system
  Renal function: Measurement of effects on urine excretion in saline loaded rats
  Renal dynamics: Measurement of renal blood flow, GFR and clearance

GI system
  GI function: Measurement of gastric emptying and intestinal transit
  Acid secretion: Measurement of gastric acid secretion (Shay rat)
  GI irritation: Assessment of potential irritancy to the gastric mucosa
  Emesis: nausea, vomiting

Immune system
  Passive cutaneous anaphylaxis (PCA)-Test for potential antigenicity of compounds

Other
  Blood coagulation
  —*In vitro* platelet aggregation
  *In vitro* hemolysis

## 19.3. STUDY DESIGNS AND PRINCIPLES

As a starting place, unlike older pharmacology studies, safety pharmacology studies are normally conducted as GLP studies. At the same time, unlike other safety assessment studies, these do not need to vastly exceed intended therapeutic doses so as to identify signs of toxicity. In this sense, they are closer to hazard tests.

General guidance for dose (or concentration) section for such studies:

- *In vivo Studies:*

  Designed to define the dose response curve of the adverse effects .

  Doses should include and exceed primary pharmacodynamic or therapeutic range.

  In absence of safety pharmacology parameters, the highest doses equal or exceed some adverse effects (toxic range).

- *In vitro Studies*

  Generally designed to establish an effect-concentration relationship (range of concentrations).

Considerations in the selection and design of specific studies are straightforward. The following factors should be considered (selection):

Effects related to the therapeutic class.

Adverse effects associated with members of the chemical or therapeutic class.

Ligand binding or enzyme data suggesting a potential for adverse effects.

Data from investigations that warrant further investigation.

A hierarchy of organ systems can be developed:

Importance with respect to life-supporting functions:
   Cardiovascular;
   Respiratory;
   Central nervous system.

Functions which can be transiently disrupted without causing irreversible harm. The absence of observed activity may represent either a true or false negative effect. If an assay is valid for the particular test article and fails to indicate activity, it is an appropriate indicator of future events (Green, 1997). However, if the assay is insensitive or incapable of response, the test represents a form of bias, albeit unconscious. Many biological products demonstrate a specificity of response that limits the utility of commonly employed safety studies. Specificity for many biologies arises from both their physicochemical properties and their similarity to endogenous substances that are regulated in a carefully controlled manner. To overcome the issue of lack of predictive value, various approaches may be used. For example, a multiple testing strategy of mutually reinforcing studies may be employed or safety studies may be adaptively fit to the biological circumstance.

A separate issue is how and when to consider isomers, metabolites and the actual finished product.

Generally, parent compound and its major metabolite(s) that achieve systemic exposure should be evaluated

It may be important to test active metabolites from humans.

Testing of individual isomers should also be considered.

Studies with the finished product only necessary if kinetics and dynamics are substantially altered in comparison to the active substance previously tested.

There are also special considerations as to how to statistically evaluate specific aspects of these studies. Specifically, analysis of time to event becomes very important (Anderson et al., 2000).

## 19.4. ORGAN SYSTEM SPECIFIC TESTS

### 19.4.1. Cardiovascular

The cardiovascular system is one of the primary vital functions that have to be examined during safety pharmacology studies. Cardiovascular system functioning is maintained by cardiac electrical activity and by pump-muscle function, which contribute to hemodynamic efficacy. The aim of cardiovascular safety pharmacology is to evaluate the effects of test substances on the most pertinent components of this system, in order to detect potentially undesirable effects before engaging in clinical trials (Lacroix and Provost, 2000). In the basic program, a detailed hemodynamic evaluation is carried out in the anaesthetized dog. It is completed by cardiac and/or cellular electrophysiology investigations in order to assess the arrhythmogenic risk. The basic program can be preceded by rapid and simple testing procedures, during the early drug discovery stage. It should be completed, if necessary, by specific supplementary studies, depending on the data obtained during the early clinical trials.

### 19.4.2. Hemodynamics, ECG, and Respiration in Anaesthetized Dogs or Primates

Anaesthetized studies conducted using data capture systems to record six lead ECG (I, II, III, $aV_1$, and $aV_f$), left ventricular pressure variables, arterial blood pressure and respiratory measurement of arterial blood flow in selected vascular beds, cardiac output and arterial blood gas measurement. ECG intervals are measured from the lead II ECG and Q-T interval can be corrected for heart rate using Bazett's, Friderecia's or Van De Water's formulas.

### 19.4.3. Cardiac Conduction Studies

In addition to the above hemodynamic measurements, intraventricular, intra-arterial and atrioventricular conduction times and velocities can be measured using epicardial electrodes in the anesthetized and thoracotomized dog.

### 19.4.4. Conscious Rodent, Dog, and Primate Telemetry Studies

Effects on blood pressure, heart rate, lead II ECG, core body temperature, and locomotor activity can be explored using DataSciences telemetry implanted devices in rats, guinea-pigs, dogs, or primates. Effects on behavior can be captured on video using CCTV for dog and primate studies. Repeated administration and interaction studies can be performed.

### 19.4.5. Six Lead ECG Measurement in the Conscious Dog

Conscious studies using devices for measurement of blood pressure and six chest lead ECG measurements (V2, V4, V6, V10, rV2 and rV4). ECG interval analysis is performed on the V2 lead (RR, PR, QT, QTc intervals, QRS duration). QT dispersion can also be measured. Locomotor activity can be monitored and behavior captured on video using CCTV.

In addition to validated systems for automatic measurement of ECG parameters, ECGs can be reviewed by veterinary cardiology services to detect any transparent abnormalities.

Colonies of telemetered animals can be set up and maintained for repeat use.

Respiration rate measurements can be taken from dogs in slings using a pneumograph system.

An animal specific correction of QT interval can also be derived for each dog or primate based on individual variability of QT interval with rate using the Framingham equation.

Recent concerns over the arrhythmogenic effects of a number of marketed compounds have resulted in the issue of the "Points to Consider" document, CPMP 986/96 by the EMA (European Medicines Agency) (available at http://www.eudra/org/humandocs/PDFs/SWP/098696en.pdf).

Studies to assess the effects of compound and any known metabolites on ECG and cardiac action potentials are recommended. Changes in action potential duration and other parameters measured are a functional consequence of effects on the ion channels which contribute to the action potential. This *in vitro* test is considered to provide a reliable risk assessment of the potential for a compound to prolong Q-T interval in humans.

### 19.4.6. Systems for Recording Cardiac Action Potentials

These include a range of currently available methodologies, some of which can be incorporated into existing study designs.

Isolated ventricular Purkinje fibers from dog or sheep.

Isolated right ventricular papillary muscle from guinea pig.

Continuous intracellular recording of action potentials and on-line analysis of resting membrane potential, maximum rate of depolarization, upstroke amplitude and action potential duration using Notocord HEM data acquisition system.

Assessment of use-dependent and inverse use-dependent actions by stimulation at normal, bradycardic and tachycardic frequencies.

### 19.4.7. Special Case (and Concern): Q-T Prolongation

Drugs that alter ventricular repolarization (generally recognized as drugs that "prolong the Q-T interval") have been associated with malignant ventricular arrhythmias (especially the distinctive polymorphic ventricular tachycardia called torsade de pointes) and death (Fenichel and Koerner, 1999). Many of the drugs now known to alter ventricular repolarization were developed as antiarrhythmics (e.g., dofetelide, sotalol), but others (e.g., cisapride, terfenadine) were developed without the expectation of any effect upon electrically excitable membranes.

The association between abnormalities of repolarization and life-threatening arrhythmias is stronger than some other associations between laboratory abnormalities and clinical events. For example, there are drugs (tacrine) and inborn errors of metabolism (Gilbert's syndrome) that cause wild excursions in liver-function tests, but with no adverse consequences. In contrast, although the severity of proarrhythmia at a given Q-T duration varies from drug to drug and from patient to patient, no drug is known to alter ventricular repolarization without inducing arrhythmias*, and each of the several congenital long-Q-T syndromes is associated with an elevated incidence of malignant arrythmias.

With any given repolarization-altering drug, the risk of malignant arrhythmia seems to increase with increasing Q-T interval, but there is no well-established threshold duration below which a prolonged Q-T interval is known to be harmless. The extent of Q-T prolongation seen with a given drug and patient may be nonlinearly related to patient factors (sex, electrolyte levels, and so on) and to serum levels of the drug and/or its metabolites. The actual incidence of malignant

---

*Some QT-prolonging drugs [e.g., amiodarone; see Hohnloser, S.H., Klingenheben, T. and Singh, B.N. (1994). Amiodarone-associated proarrhythmic effects, *Ann. Intern. Med.* 121(7): 529–535] are not reported to have caused many arrhythmic deaths, but this observation must be interpreted carefully. In a population with a high incidence of life-threatening arrhythmias, a drug with both proarrhythmic and antiarrhythmic effects might cause a net reduction in arrhythmias, and the arrhythmias that it had induced might not be attributed to it. In a population whose native arrhythmias were not life-threatening, the same drug might result in a net decrease in mortality.

arrhythmias, even in association with the drugs most known to induce them, is relatively low, so failure to observe malignant arrhythmias during clinical trials of ordinary size and duration does not provide substantial reassurance.

Abnormal repolarization and the associated arrhythmias are the end results of a causative chain that starts with alterations in the channels of ionic flux through cell membranes. Some cells (e.g., those of the Purkinje system or midmyocardium) seem especially susceptible to these changes. At a substrate level, the links on the chain are alterations in the time-course of the action potential, alteration in the propagation of action potentials within a given cell, and alterations in the propagation of action potentials from cell to cell within syncitia and from tissue to tissue within the heart. At a higher level of aggregation, one sees "afterdepolarizations" in the terminal portion of the action potential; spontaneous beats triggered by afterdepolarizations; propagation of these beats to other cells; and re-entrant excitation.

With these considerations in mind, the problem of altered repolarization should be integrated into drug development (Malik and Camm, 2001) by

*In vitro* screening of the drug and its metabolites for effects on ion channels (especially $I_{Kr}$).

*In vitro* screening of the drug and its metabolites for effects on action-potential duration.

Screening of the drug and its metabolites for altered repolarization in animal models.

Focused preclinical studies for proarrhythmia if altered repolarization is seen in preclinical screening or in patients.

Some specific techniques which can be employed include the following.

1. *Cloned Human Potassium Channels.* Assessment of effects on cloned HERG K channels stably expressed in a cell line by measurement of whole cell K current ($I_{Kr}$) using voltage clamp. Other cloned human ion channels (e.g., KvLQT1/minK-IKs currents) are also possible.

2. *Cardiac Action Potential In Vitro Purkinje Fibers.* Intracellular recording of action potentials from cardiac Purkinje fibers isolated from dog or sheep ventricle. Measurement of maximum rate of depolarization and action potential duration to detect sodium and potassium channel interactions, respectively, according to recommendations in EMA CPMP "Points to Consider" document, CPMP 986/96 (1998).

3. *Monophasic Action Potential in Anesthetized Guinea Pigs.* Epicardia monophasic action potential recording using suction/contact pressure electrodes are emplaced, allowing simultaneous measurement of ECG and heartrate.

4. *ECG by Telemetry in Conscious Guinea Pigs.* Lead II ECG recording using DataSciences telemetry device. Repeated administration and interaction studies can be performed.

5. *Hemodynamics and ECG in Anesthetized or Conscious Dogs or Primates:*

Conscious studies using DataSciences telemetry for blood pressure and lead II ECG or the ITS system for blood pressure and six chest lead ECG measurements (including QT dispersion).

Anaesthetized studies using $MI^2$ data capture system with additional measurement of blood flow in selected vascular beds, cardiac output, respiratory and left ventricular function.

### 19.4.8. Relevance of HERG to QT Prolongation

Compounds that are associated with ADRs of QT prolongation, arrhythmias such as torsades de pointes and sudden death, predominantly have a secondary pharmacological interaction with the rapidly activating delayed rectifier potassium channel $I_{Kr}$. The gene encoding this channel has been identified as HERG (human *ether-á-go-go related gene*). Testing of compounds for interactions with the HERG channel allows the identification of potential risk of QT prolongation in humans and can be used as a screen in development candidate selection.

***Expression and Recording Systems.*** HEK-293 cells have been transfected with cDNA for HERG-1 to produce a stable expression system. The cell line has been obtained under license for the laboratory of Craig January at the University of Wisconsin (Mohammad et al., 1997).

### 19.5. CENTRAL NERVOUS SYSTEM

There are four broad classes of approaches to assessing nervous system effects of drugs in animals.

### 19.5.1. Intact Animal Functional Testing

The front end of this tier approach is a screen, the functional observation battery (FOB) Gad (1982) or Irwin (1968) screen. This is the tool of choice for initial (and for most of the compounds covered by this volume, the only screen tests for) identification of potentially neurotoxic chemicals. The use of such screens, other behavioural test methods, or what are generally called clinical observations does, however, warrant one major caution or consideration. That is that short-term (within 24 hr of dosing or exposure) observations are insufficient on their own to differentiate between pharmacologic (reversible in the short term) and toxicological (irreversible) effects.

The most generally useful test or detector for a neurotoxicant is enhanced careful observation of animals during such traditional toxicology studies as acute and subchronic oral and reproductive and teratology studies. A formal means of ensuring such a set of observations is to use an observational screen as proposed by several researchers (Haggerty, 1991; Mattson et al., 1996). Such a screen, integrated into the normal course of other systemic toxicity studies, is the initial step in evaluating the potential for neurotoxicity of a compound and the one step I believe is essential for all new materials in terms of protecting against possible neurotoxicity.

There are many variations on the design and contact of such a screen. All have their origin in the work of neurologic and behavioural pharmacologists such as Smith (1961), Irwin (1962, 1964), and Campbell and Richter (1967). The approach presented here is based on the author's own methodology (6), which has been adopted as the starting point for such a screen by the U.S. Environmental Protection Agency (EPA), U.S. Food & Drug Administration (FDA), and the Organization for Economic Cooperation and Development (OECD).

The following set of observations/measures are performed on animals (rats and/or mice) that constitute the experimental and control groups in standard acute, subacute, subchronic, reproductive, developmental, and chronic toxicity studies. Technicians can be trained to screen animals after approximately 6 hr with reinforcement conducted over one week. The screen replaces clinical observations performed prior to dosing, and, in the case of an acute study at 1 hr, 24 hr, 4, 7, and 14 days after dosing/exposure (unless a vehicle such as propylene glycol, which masks neurological effects by its transitory character is used, in which case the 1 hr measurement is replaced by a 6 hr measurement). For a repeated dosage study, as appropriate, the screen can be performed at 1 hr, 1, 7, 14, 30 days, and once a month thereafter. A trained technician takes from 3 to 5 min to screen a single animal.

In preparation for the screen, a sufficient number of scoring sheets are filled in with the appropriate information. Then the cart employed as a mobile testing station is checked to ensure that all the necessary equipment (empty wire-bottom cage, blunt probe, penlight, 1/2 in. diameter steel rod, force transducer, ink pad, pad of blotting paper, ruler, and electronic probe thermometer) are on the cart and in forking order. Each animal is then evaluated by the following procedures.

### Locomotor Activity

The animal's movements (walking, jumping) while on the flat surface of the cart are evaluated quantitatively on a scale of 1 (hypoactive) to 5 (hyperactive), with 3 being the normal state. The data can be upgraded to interval data if one has and utilizes one of the electromagnetic activity-monitoring instruments.

### Righting Reflex

For rats and mice, the animal is either grasped by its tail and flipped in the air or held upside down and allowed to drop (2 ft above the cart surface) so that it turns head over heels. The normal animal should land squarely on its feet. If it lands on its side, score 1 point; if on its back; score 2 points. Repeat 4 times and record its total score. For a rabbit, when placed on its side on the cart, does the animal regain its feet without noticeable difficulty?

### Grip Strength

For rats and mice, the animal is held by the tail and allowed to grasp the crossbar of a strain gauge designed for the purpose. The tension on the tail is slowly increased until the animal loses its grip, and the resulting value recorded. This procedure is repeated twice for each animal.

## Body Temperature

The electronic probe thermometer (with a blunt probe) is used to take a rectal temperature, allowing equilibrium for 30 sec before the reading is recorded.

## Salilvation

Discharge of clear fluid from mouth, most frequently seen as beads of moisture on lips in mice and rats or as a fluid flow from the mouth in rabbits. Normal state is to see none, in which case the score sheet space should be left blank. If present, a plus sign should be recorded in the blank.

## Startle Response

With the animal on the cart, the metal cage is struck with the blunt probe. The normal animal should exhibit a marked but short-duration response, in which case the space on the scoring sheet should be left blank. If present, a plus sign should be entered.

## Respiration

While at rest on the cart, the animal's respiration cycle is observed and evaluated on a scale from 1 (reduced) to 5 (increased), with 3 being normal.

## Urination

When returning the animal to its case, examine the pan beneath the cage for signs of urination and evaluate on a scale of 1 (lacking) to 5 (polyuria).

## Mouth Breathing

Rats and mice are normally obligatory nose breathers. Note whether each animal is breathing through its mouth (if it is, place a check in the appropriate box).

## Convulsions

If clonic or tonic convulsions are observed, they should be graded for intensity (1, minor, 5, marked) and the type and intensity recorded.

## Pineal Response (Rabbits Only)

When a blunt probe is lightly touched to the inside of the ear, the normal animal should react by moving its ear and head reflexively. If this response is present (normal case), the space should be left blank. If absent, a minus sign should be entered in the blank.

### Piloerection

Determine whether the fur on the animal's back is raised or elevated. In the normal case (no piloerection), leave the space blank. If piloerection is present, a plus sign should be entered in the blank.

### Diarrhea

In examining the pen beneath an animal's cage, note if there are any signs of loose or liquid stools. Normal state is for there to be none, in which case a 1 should be recorded in a scale of 1 (none) to 5 (greatly increased).

### Pupil Size

Determine if pupils are constricted or dilated and grade them on a scale of 1–5, respectively.

### Pupil Response

The beam of light from the pen light is played across the eyes of the animal, and changes in pupil size are noted. In the normal animal, the pupil should constrict when the beam is on it and then dilate back to normal when the light is removed. Note if there is no response by recording a minus sign in the blank space).

### Lacrimation

The animal is observed for the secretion and discharge of tears. In rats and mice the tears contain a reddish pigment. No discharge is normal, and in this case the box should be left blank. If discharge is present, a plus sign should be entered.

### Impaired Gait

The occurrence of abnormal gait is evaluated. The most frequent impairments are waddling (W), hunched gait (H), or ataxia (A, the inability of all the muscles to act in unison). Record the extent of any impairment on a scale of 1 (slight) to 5 (marked).

### Stereotype

Each animal is evaluated for stereotypic behavior (isolated motor acts or partial sequences of more complex behavioural patterns from the repertoire of a species, occurring out of context and with an abnormally high frequency). These are graded on a scale of 0–5 (as per Sturgeon et al., 1979) if such signs are present.

### Toe Pinch (Rats and Mice Only)

The blunt probe is used to bring pressure to bear on one of the digits of the hind limb. This should evoke a response from the normal animal, graded on a scale from 1 (absent) to 5 (exaggerated).

### Tail Pinch

The procedure detailed above is utilized with the animal's tail instead of its hind limb, and is graded on the same scale.

### Wire Maneuver (Rats and Mice Only)

The animal is placed on the metal or wooden rod suspended parallel to the card 2 feet above it. Its ability to move along the rod is evaluated. If impaired, a score of from 1 (slightly impaired) to 5 (unable to stay on the rod) is recorded. The diameter of the rod relative to the animal is critical. Larger animals need thicker rods.

### Hind Leg Splay

The rat or mouse is then held 30 cm above a sand table placed on the cart, and dropped, and the distance between the prints of the two hind paws is measured.

### Positional Passivity

When placed in an awkward position (such as on the edge of the top of the wire-bottom cage) on the cart surface, does the animal immediately move into a more normal position? If not, a score should be recorded on a scale of 1 (slightly impaired) to 5 (cataleptic).

### Tremors

These are periods of continued fine movements, usually starting in the limbs (and perhaps limited to them). Absence of tremors is normal, in which case no score is recorded. If present, they are graded on a scale of 1 (slight and infrequent) to 5 (continuous and marked).

### Extensor Thrust.

The sole of either hind foot is pressed with a blunt object. A normal animal will push back against the blunt object. If reduced or absent, this response should be graded on a scale of 1 (reduced) to 5 (absent).

### Positive Geotropism

The animal is placed on the inclined (at an angle of $-30°$C) top surface of the wire cage with its head facing downward. It should turn 180° and face "uphill," in which case the space on the form should be left blank. If this occurs, a negative sign should be recorded in the blank.

### Limb Rotation

Take hold of a animal's hind limbs and move them through their normal place of rotation. In the normal state, they should rotate readily but there should be some resistance. The variations from normal are no resistance (1) to markedly increased resistance or rigidity (5), with 3 being normal.

There are a number of other tests which may be added to a behavioral screen to enhance its sensitivity. These methods tend to require more equipment and effort, so if several compounds are to be screened, their inclusion in a screen must be carefully considered. An example of such methods is the "narrowing bridge" technique. All these methods require some degree of training of animals prior to their actual use in test systems.

The narrowing bridge test measures the ability of a rat to perform a task requiring neuromuscular control and coordination. Any factor that renders the neuromuscular system of the rat less effective will be expected to result in the rat obtaining a higher score on this test. Therefore, the test cannot by itself discriminate between injuries to the brain (e.g., degenerative changes or tumors), spinal cord, muscle, or peripheral nerve. In addition, compounds that exert a pharmacological action on the central or peripheral nervous systems will be expected to alter the performance of rats on this test. However, a study of the manner in which the performance of the rat alters with time plus clinical examination will enable, in many cases, a distinction to be made between these different possibilities.

The main use of the test is in the study of peripheral neuropathy. It has been demonstrated that this test will detect acrylamide neuropathy 1 week before any clinical signs of neuropathy are present. It also claimed that this test is the most sensitive method for detecting hexane neuropathy.

The narrowing bridge consists of three 1.5 m wooden bridges, 23 cm above the ground arranged at right angles. The widths of the three bridges are 2.5, 2.0, and 1.8 cm, respectively. The rat is placed at the end of the 2.5 cm wide bridge and must traverse the three bridges to get to the home cage. The number of times the rat slips is counted. The score on each section of the bridge is calculated as follows:

| Bridge width | Score |
| --- | --- |
| 2.5 cm | number of slips $\times 3$ |
| 2.0 cm | number of slips $\times 2$ |
| 1.8 cm | number of slips $\times 1$ |

The total is calculated by adding the scores from the three sections of the bridge. The test is repeated 3 times and the measure of the performance of the rat in the test is the mean of the three total scores. Animals are trained to navigate the bridge system for 5 consecutive days prior to receiving any test compound.

### 19.5.2. Isolated Tissue Assays

The classic approach to screening for nervous system effect is a series of isolated tissue preparation bioassays, conducted with appropriate standards, to determine if the material acts pharmacologically directly on neural receptor sites or transmission properties. Though these bioassays are normally performed by a classical pharmacologist, a good technician can be trained to conduct them. The required equipment consists of a Mangus (or similar style) tissue bath (Turner, 1965; Offermeier and Ariens, 1966; Nodine and Seigler, 1964), a physiograph or kymograph, force transducer, glassware, a stimulator and bench spectrophotometer. The assays utilized in the screening battery are listed in Table 19.5, along with the original reference describing each preparation and assay. The assays are performed as per the original author's descriptions with only minor modifications, except that control standards (as listed in Table 19.5) are always used. Only those assays that are appropriate for the neurological/muscular alterations observed in the screen are utilized. Note that all these are intact organ preparations, not minced tissue preparations as others (Bondy, 1979) have recommended for biochemical assays.

The first modification in each assay is that, where available, both positive and negative standard controls (pharmacological agonists and antagonists, respectively) are employed. Before the preparation is utilized to assay the test material, the tissue preparation is exposed to the agonist to ensure that the preparation is functional and to provide a baseline dose-response curve against which the activity of the test material can be quantitatively compared. After the test material has been assayed (if a dose-response curve has been generated), one can determine whether the antagonist will selectively block the activity of the test material. If so, specific activity at that receptor can be considered as established. In this assay sequence, it must be kept in mind that a test material may act to either stimulate or depress activity, and therefore the roles of the standard agonists and antagonists may be reversed.

Commonly overlooked when performing these assays is the possibility of metabolism to an active form that can be assessed in this *in vitro* model. The test material should be tested in both original and "metabolized" forms. The metabolized form is prepared by incubating a 5% solution (in aerated Tyrodes) or other appropriate physiological salt solution with strips of suitably prepared test species liver for 30 min. A filtered supernatant is then collected from this incubation and tested for activity. Suitable metabolic blanks should also be tested.


### 19.5.3. Electrophysiology Methods

There are a number of electrophysiological techniques available which can be used to detect and/or assess neurotoxicity. These techniques can be divided into two broad general categories; those focused on central nervous system (CNS) function and those focused on peripheral nervous system function, (Seppalainer, 1975).

First, however, the function of the individual components of the nervous system, how they are connected together, and how they operate as a complete system should be very briefly overviewed.

Data collection and communication in the nervous system occurs by means of graded potentials, action potentials, and synaptic coupling of neurons. These electrical potentials may be recorded and analyzed at two different levels depending

**TABLE 19.5. Isolated Tissue Pharmacologic Assays**

| Assay system | Endpoint | Standards (agonist/antagonist | References |
| --- | --- | --- | --- |
| Rat ileum | General activity | None (side-spectrum assay for intrinsic activity) | Domer, 1971 |
| Guinea pig vas deferens | Muscarinic nicotinic or Muscarinic | Methacholine/atropine<br>Methacholine/hexamethonium | Leach, 1956 |
| Rat serosal strip | Nicotinic | Methacholine/hexamethonium | Khayyal, et. al., 1974 |
| Rat vas deferens | Alpha adrenergic | Norepinephrine/phenoxybenzamine | Rossum, 1965 |
| Rat uterus | Beta adrenergic | Epinephrine/propranol | Levy and Tozzi, 1963 |
| Rat uterus | Kinin receptors | Bradykinin/none | Gecse, et. al., 1976 |
| Guinea pig tracheal chain | Dopaminergic | Dopamine/none | Domer, 1971 |
| Rat serosal strips | Tryptaminergic | 5-Hydroxytryptamine (serotonin)/dibenzyline or lysergic acid dibromide | Lin and Yeoh, 1965 |
| Guinea pig tracheal chain | Histaminergic | Histamine/benadryl | Castillo and De Beer, 1947a, b |
| Guinea pig ileum (electrically stimulated) | Endorphin receptors | Methenkephaline/none | Cox, et al., 1975 |
| Red blood cell hemolysis | Membrane stabilization | Chloropromazine (not a receptor-mediated activity) | Seeman and Weinstein, 1966 |
| Frog rectus abdominis | Membrane depolarization | Decamethonium iodide (not a receptor-mediated activity) | Burns and Paton, 1951 |

on the electrical coupling arrangements: individual cells (that is, intracellular and extracellular) or multiple cell (e.g., EEG, evoked potentials (EPs), slow potentials). These potentials may be recorded in specific central or peripheral nervous system areas (e.g., visual cortex, hippocampus, sensory and motor nerves, muscle spindles) during various behavioral states or in *in vitro* preparations (e.g., nerve-muscle, retinal photoreceptor, brain slice).

***19.5.3.1. CNS Function: Electroencephalography.*** The electroencephalogram (EEG) is a dynamic measure reflecting the instantaneous integrated synaptic activity of the CNS, which most probably represents, in coded form, all ongoing processes under higher nervous control. Changes in frequency, amplitude, variability, and pattern of the EEG are thought to be directly related to underlying biochemical changes, which are believed to be directly related to defined aspects of behavior. Therefore, changes in the EEG should be reflected by alterations in behavior and vice versa.

The human EEG is easily recorded and readily quantified, is obtained noninvasively (scalp recording), samples several regions of the brain simultaneously, requires minimal cooperation from the subject, and is minimally influenced by prior testing. Therefore, it is a very useful and recommended clinical test in cases in which exposure to drugs produces symptoms of CNS involvement and in which long-term exposures to high concentrations are suspected of causing CNS damage.

Since the EEG recorded using scalp electrodes is an average of the multiple activity of many small areas of cortical surface beneath the electrodes, it is possible that in situations involving noncortical lesions, the EEG may not accurately reflect the organic brain damage present. Noncortical lesions following acute or long-term low-level exposures to toxicants are well documented in neurotoxicology (Norton, 1980). The drawback mentioned earlier can be partially overcome by utilizing activation or evocative techniques, such as hyperventilation, photic stimulation, or sleep, which can increase the amount of information gleaned from a standard EEG.

As a research tool, the utility of the EEG lies in the fact that it reflects instantaneous changes in the state of the CNS. The pattern can thus be used to monitor the sleep-wakefulness cycle activation or deactivation of the brainstem, and the state of anesthesia during an acute electrophysiological procedure. Another advantage of the EEG, which is shared by all CNS electrophysiological techniques, is that it can assess the differential effects of toxicants (or drugs) on various brain areas or structures. Finally, specific CNS regions (e.g., the hippocampus) have particular patterns of after-discharge following chemical or electrical stimulation which can be quantitatively examined and utilized as a tool in neurotoxicology.

The EEG does have some disadvantages, or, more correctly, some limitations. It cannot provide information about the effects of toxicants on the integrity of sensory receptors or of sensory or motor pathways. As a corollary, it cannot provide an assessment of the effects of toxicants on sensory system capacities. Finally, the EEG does not provide specific information at the cellular level and therefore lacks the rigor to provide detailed mechanisms of action.

Rats represent an excellent model for EEGs as they are cheap, resist infection during chronic electrode and cannulae implantation, and are relatively easy to train so that behavioral assessments can be made concurrently.

Depending on the time of drug exposure, the type of scientific information desired, and the necessity of behavioral correlations, a researcher can perform acute and/or chronic EEG experiments. Limitations of the former are that most drugs that produce general anesthesia modify the pattern of EEG activity and thus can complicate subtle effects of toxicants. However, this limitation can be partially avoided if the effect is robust enough. For sleep–wakefulness studies, it is also essential to monitor and record the electromyogram (EMG).

Excellent reviews of these electrophysiology approaches can be found in Fox et al. (1982) and Takeuchi and Koike (1985).

### 19.5.4. Neurochemical and Biochemical Assays

Though some very elegant methods are now available to study the biochemistry of the brain and nervous system, none has yet discovered any generalized marker chemicals which will serve as reliable indicators or early warnings of neurotoxic actions or potential actions. There are, however, some useful methods. Before looking at these, however, one should understand the basic problems involved.

Normal biochemical events surrounding the maintenance and functions of the nervous system centers around energy metabolism, biosynthesis of macromolecules, and neurotransmitter synthesis, storage, release, uptake, and degradation. Measurement of these events is complicated by the sequenced nature of the components of the nervous system and the transient and labile nature of the moieties involved. Use of measurements of alterations in these functions as indicators of neurotoxicity is further complicated by our lack of a complete understanding of the normal operation of these systems and by the multitude of day-to-day occurrences (such as diurnal cycle, diet, temperature, age, sex, and endocrine status) which are constantly modulating the baseline system. For detailed discussions of these difficulties, the reader is advised to see Damstra and Bondy (1980, 1982).

### 19.6. RESPIRATORY SYSTEM

The known effects of drugs, from a variety of pharmacologic/therapeutic classes, on the respiratory system and worldwide regulatory requirements support the need for conducting respiratory evaluations in safety pharmacology. The objective of studies is to evaluate the potential for drugs to cause secondary pharmacologic or toxicologic effects that influence respiratory function. Changes in respiratory function can result either from alterations in the pumping apparatus that controls the pattern of pulmonary ventilation or from changes in the mechanical properties of the lung that determine the transpulmonary pressures (work) required for lung inflation and deflation. Defects in the pumping apparatus are classified as hypo- or hyperventilation syndromes and are evaluated by examining ventilatory parameters in a conscious animal model. The ventilatory parameters include respiratory rate, tidal volume, minute volume, peak (or mean) inspiratory flow, peak (or mean) expiratory flow, and fractional inspiratory time. Defects in mechanical properties of the lung are classified as obstructive or restrictive disorders and can be evaluated in animal models by performing flow-volume and pressure-volume maneuvers, respectively. The parameters used to detect airway obstruction include peak expiratory flow, forced expiratory flow at 25 and 75% of forced vital capacity, and a timed forced expiratory volume, while the parameters used to detect lung restriction include total lung capacity, inspiratory capacity, functional residual capacity, and compliance. Measurement of dynamic lung resistance and compliance, obtained continuously during tidal breathing, is an alternative method for evaluating obstructive and restrictive disorders, respectively, and is used when the response to drug treatment is expected to be immediate (within minutes post-dose). The species used in safety pharmacology studies are the same as those used in toxicology studies since pharmacokinetic and toxicologic/pathologic data are available in these species. These data can be used to help select test measurement intervals and doses and to aid in the interpretation of functional change. The techniques and procedures for measuring respiratory function parameters are well established in guinea pigs, rats and dogs (Murphy, 1994).

## 19.7. SECONDARY ORGAN SYSTEMS

The kidneys are an important target for toxic effects of drug candidates. It is mandatory to select accurate, clinically relevant parameters in order to be in a position to detect putative nephrotoxic effects during the safety pharmacology program. The glomurelar filtration rate appears to be of major interest since it is associated with the definition of acute renal failure. Measurement of the renal blood flow, proteinuria, enzymuria, fractional excretion of sodium, and so on are also highly useful to detect any possible renal impact of a new compound. Although the rat is, by far, the most widely used animal species, there are no specific (clinically relevant) reasons to choose it. Various parameters may vary according to the species, sex, strain, age, and so on. Since in most cases acute renal failure occurs following administration of drugs in patients with pre-existing risk factors, it is suggested that sensitized animal models be validated and used (salt depletion, dehydration, coadministration of pharmacologic agents, etc.).

The potential effects of new drugs on the digestive system can be examined in a number of model systems of which intestinal motility in the mouse and/or gastric emptying in the rat are examples recommended for safety pharmacology evaluation. Intestinal motility, assessed by the transit of carmine dye in the mouse and gastric motility, assessed by stomach weight in the rat, were examined using a range of clinical drugs or potent pharmacological agents known to affect gastrointestinal function. Assessment of both models in the guinea pig was also evaluated. Activity was demonstrated with codeine, diazepam, atropine and CCK-8 (all of which inhibited gastric function). However, neither model gave consistent and reliable results with the remaining reference compounds, namely metoclopramide, bethanechol, cisapride, deoxycholate, carbachol and domperidone. This investigation questions the usefulness of simple models of gastrointestinal transport in the rodent as a means of detecting potential effects of a new drug on the digestive system. This finding should be of concern to the pharmaceutical industry as these simple models are routinely used as part of a regulatory safety pharmacology "package" of studies.

A number of classic assays have been designed to examine the effects of a test article on gastrointestinal function. Gastrointestinal transit rate is most often measured with a test employing a forced meal of an aqueous suspension of activated charcoal (Janssen and Jageneau, 1957). The test article is given via the appropriate route at a pre-set time prior to the charcoal meal. For example, a compound intended for use via intravenous injection would be injected intravenously in mice 30 min prior to delivering a charcoal meal by gavage. The distance traveled from the stomach by the black-colored charcoal meal to a specific anatomic location within the intestine is measured at a fixed time after this meal, usually 20 or 30 min later. In validating this procedure at Mason Laboratories, we tested the ability of a parasympatholytic agent, intravenous atropine sulfate, to inhibit gastrointestinal transit. In a dose-dependent fashion, 30 and 50 mg/kg atropine sulfate significantly decreased the distance traveled by the charcoal meal.

Another important safety assay of the gastrointestinal system is the influence of test article on the formation of ulcers (Shay et al., 1945). After overnight fasting, young rats are given the test article and euthanized 4 or 6 h later. The mucosal surface of the stomach and duodenum is scored for the presence of hyperemia, hemorrhage, and ulcers. The dose-dependent ulcerative properties of NSAIDs (non steroidal anti-inflammatory drugs) are clearly demonstrated in this assay, making it important in the development of other NSAIDs that are not as caustic to the gastrointestinal mucosa (Bramm et al., 1981; Cashin et al., 1977; Diadone et al., 1994; Darias et al., 1994).

Additional digestive system safety pharmacology tests include effects of test articles on gastric emptying rate and gastric secretion. Gastric emptying rate is measured in rats using a solution of phenol red (or Evans blue) delivered via oral gavage a pre-set time after administration of the test article (Megens et al., 1991). The dilution of phenol red after 30 min in the rat's stomach is determined colorimetrically at 558 nm in a spectrophotometer. This is compared to a group of control rats that are euthanized immediately after phenol red administration. The influence of test articles on gastric juice secretion is accomplished by ligating the pyloric sphincter under anesthesia in rats following a fasting period (Graf et al., 1982; Shay et al., 1945; Takasuna et al., 1992). Immediately after recovery from anesthesia, each rat is given a pre-set dose of the test article. The fluid content of the rat's stomach is recovered after a set period of time, usually 4 h. The volume and contents of the stomach are measured to determine the effect of the test article on gastric secretions. Electrolyte concentrations, pH, and protein content of gastric secretions can be measured in this assay (Takasuna et al., 1992).

### 19.7.1. Gastric Emptying Rate and Gastric pH Changes: A New Model

Sometimes new technologies for safety pharmacology can come from clinical settings. The Heidelberg pH Capsule (HC) was developed over 30 years ago at Heidelberg University in West Germany. H. G. Noller invented and first tested this device on over 10,000 adult patients over a three-year period. The HC is a pill-sized device containing an antimony-silver chloride electrode for measuring pH and a high-frequency transmitter operating at an average frequency of 1.9 MHz. The transmitter in the HC is activated by immersion in physiologic saline by a permeable membrane enclosing the battery compartment. Thus, when a patient swallows the HC, the fluid contents of the stomach activate the transmitter. Transmitted signals are picked up via a belt receiver and can be displayed and recorded. The profile of changes in pH over time correlate with the movement of the HC through the different regions of the gastrointestinal tract (Mojaverian et al., 1989). The pH of the fasted human stomach is very acidic, on average about pH 1. When the HC moves through the pyloric sphincter and into the duodenum, there is a rapid increase in pH of over 4 pH units. Thus, one can get a fairly precise measure of gastric emptying rate in humans with this noninvasive technique. Additional pH changes have been correlated with transition of the HC through the duodenum, jejunum, and the colon.

Mojaverian and colleagues have used the HC extensively to examine the influence of gender, posture, age, and content and frequency of food ingestion on the gastric emptying rate (or gastric residence time) in healthy volunteers (Mojaverian et al., 1989; Mojaverian et al., 1991). While developed for clinical use in people, the HC may be a useful tool for measuring important digestive system parameters in laboratory animals. The size of the HC, approximately the size of a No. 1 gelatin capsule (7 mm diameter, 20 mm long) prohibits its use in small animals (Mojaverian et al., 1989). It may be useful in studies with dogs and possibly in nonhuman primates. In particular, the HC could be used to measure gastric emptying rate in a totally noninvasive manner in dogs (Itoh et al., 1986). Dogs are readily trainable to accept pills and to wear a receiver belt and could be tested after administration of a test compound (Lui et al., 1986; Vashi and Meyer, 1988). This technique for measuring gastric emptying rate in dogs is also advantageous in that it is not a terminal procedure. The influence of test articles on the pH within different portions of the gastrointestinal system could also be measured with the HC (Youngberg et al., 1985). The major drawback for using the HC for safety pharmacology screening is the price of the capsules and the receiver system.

### 19.8. SUMMARY

The initiative to add mandated safety pharmacology studies to the drug development process is overdue in arriving. However, its actual implementation and the use of the resulting data in risk/benefit decision will take some time to be worked out. During the year 2001, many small companies were put in a difficult position when the requirement for testing prior to IND filing was imposed midway through the year. The exact requirements that FDA expects will be met are still open to discussion.


## REFERENCES


Anderson, H., Spliid, H., Larsen, S. and Dall, V. (2000). Statistical analysis of time to event data from preclinical safety pharmacology studies. *Tox. Methods* 10: 111–125.

Bondy, S.C. (1979). Rapid screening of neurotoxic agents by *in vivo* means. In: *Effects of Food and Drugs on the Development and Function of the Nervous System: Methods for Predicting Toxicity.* Gryder, R.M. and Frankos, V.H., (Eds.) Office of Health Affairs, FDA, Washington, D.C., pp. 133–143.

Bramm, E., Binderup, L. and Arrigoni-Martelli, E. (1981). An unusual profile of activity of a new basic anti–inflammatory drug, timegadine. *Agents Actions* 11: 402–409.

Burns, B.D. and Paton, W.D.M. (1951). Depolarization of the motor end–plate by decamethonium and acetylcholine. *J. Physiol. (London)* 115: 41–73.

Campbell, D. and Richter, W. (1967). Whole animal screening studies. *Act. Pharmacol.* 25:345–363.

Cashin, C. H., Dawson, W. and Kitchen, E.A. (1977). The pharmacology of benoxaprofen (2-[4-chlorophynl]-α-methyl-5-benzoxazole acetic acid), LRCL 3794, a new compound with anti–inflammatory activity apparently unrelated to inhibition of prostaglandin synthesis. *J. Pharm. Pharmacol.* 29: 330–336.

Castillo, J.C. and De Beer, E.J. (1947a). The guinea pig tracheal chain as an assay for histamine agonists. *Fed. Proc.* 6: 315.

Castillo, J.C. and De Beer, E.J. (1947b). The tracheal chain. *J. Pharmacol. Exp. Ther.* 90: 104.

CPMP (1998). Note for Guidance on Safety Pharmacology Studies in Medicinal Product Development.

Cox, B.M., Opheim, K.E., Teschemach, H. and Goldstein, A. (1975). A peptide–like substance from pituitary that acts like morphine 2. Purification and properties. *Life Sci.* 16: 1777–1782.

Damstra, T. and Bondy, S.C. (1980). The current status and future of biochemical assays for neurotoxicity. In: *Experimental and Clinical Neurotoxicology.* (Spencer, P.S. and Shaumberg, H.H.) Williams and Wilkins, Baltimore, pp. 820–833.

Damstra, T. and Bondy, S.C. (1982). Neurochemical approaches to the deletion of neurotoxicity. In *Nervous System Toxicology.* (Mitchell, C.L., Ed.) Raven Press, New York, pp. 349–373.

Darias, V., Abdallah, S.S., Tello, M.L., Delgado, L.D. and Vega, S. (1994). NSAI activity study of 4-phenyl-2-thioxo-benzo[4,5]thieno[2,3-*d*]pyrimidine derivatives. *Arch. Pharm. (Weinheim)* 327: 779–783.

Diadone, G. Maggio, B., Raff, D., Plescia, S., Bajardi, M.L., Caruso, A., Cutuli, V.M.C. and Amico-Roxas, M. (1994). Synthesis and pharmacological study of ethyl 1-methyl-5-[2-substituted-4-oxo-3(4*H*0-quinazolinyl]-1*H*)-pyrazole-4-acetates. *Eur. J. Med. Chem.* 29: 707–711.

Domer, F. R. (1971). *Animal Experiments in Pharmacological Analysis.* Charles C. Thomas, Springfield, IL, pp. 98, 115, 155, 164, 220.

FDA (2001) *Guidance for Industry: STA Safety Pharmacology Studies Rev Human Pharmaceuticals*, USHHS, Washington, D.C.

Fenichel, R.P. and Koerner, J. (1999). Development of drugs that alter ventricular repolarization. Internet–based draft.

Folke, S. (2000). Drug safety in relation to efficacy: the view of a clinical pharmacologist. *Pharmacol. Toxicol.* 86: 30–32.

Fox, D.A., Lowndes, H.E. and Bierkamper, G.G. (1982). Electrophysiological techniques in neurotoxicology. In: *Nervous System Toxicology.* (Mitchell, C.L., Ed.). Raven Press, New York, pp. 299–336.

Fujimori, K. (1999). The role of general pharmacological studies and pharmacokinetics in the evolution of drugs (1): The role of general/safety pharmacology studies in the development of pharmaceuticals: International harmonization guidelines. *Folia Pharmacologica Japonica* 13: 31–39.

Gad, S.C. (1982). A neuromuscular screen for use in industrial toxicology. *J. Toxicol. Environ. Health* 9: 691–704.

Gecse, A., Zsilinsky, E. and Szekeres, L. (1976). Bradykinin antagonism. In *Kinins; Pharmacodynamics and Biological Roles.* Sicuteri, F., Back, N. and Haberland, G., Eds.). Plenum Press, New York, pp. 5–13.

Green, M.D. (1997). Problems associated with the absence of activity in standard models of safety pharmacology used to assess biological products. *Int. J. Toxicol.* 16: 33–40.

Graf, E., Sieck, A., Wenzl, H. and Winkelmann, J. 1982. Animal experiments on the safety pharmacology of lofexidine. *Arzneim.-Forsch./Drug Res.* 32(II)(8a): 931–940.

Haggerty, G.C. (1991). Strategies for and experience with neurotoxicity testing of new pharmaceuticals. *J. Am. Coll. Toxicol.* 10: 677–687.

Hardman, J.C. and Limbird, L.E. (1996). *Goodman & Gilman's The Pharmacological Basis of Therapeutics*, 9th ed. McGraw-Hill, New York.

Hite, M. (1997). Safety pharmacology approaches. *Int. J. Toxicol.* 16: 23–31.

ICH (2000). Safety Pharmacology Studies for Human Pharmaceuticals, *97A*, ICH.

Irwin, S. (1962). Drug screening and evaluation procedures. *Science* 136: 123–128.

Irwin, S. (1964). Drug screening and evaluation of new compounds in animals. Animal and clinical pharmacologic techniques. In: *Drug Evaluation.* Nodine, J. and Sieger, P. (Eds.) Year Book Medical Publishers, Inc., Chicago, pp. 26–54.

Irwin, S. (1968). Comprehensive observational assessment: la. A systematic, quantitative procedure for assessing the behavioral and physiologic state of the mouse. *Psychopharmacologia (Berlin)* 13: 222–257.

Itoh, T., Higuchi, T., Gardner, C.R. and Caldwell, L. 1986. Effect of particle size and food on gastric residence time of nondisintegrating solids in beagle dogs. *J. Pharm. Pharmacol.* 38: 801–806.

Janssen, P.A.J. and Jageneau, A.H. (1957). A new series of potent analgesics: Dextro 2 : 2-diphenyl-3-methyl-4-morpholino-butyrylpyrrolidine and related amides. *J. Pharm. Pharmacol.* 9: 381–400.

Khayyal, M.T., Tolba, N.M., El–Hawary, M.B. and El-Wahed, S.A. (1974). A sensitive method for the bioassay of acetylcholine. *Eur. J. Pharmacol.* 25: 287–290.

Lacroix, P. and Provost, D. (2000). Basic safety pharmacology: the cardiovascular system. *Therapie* 55: 63–69.

Leach, G.D.H. (1956). Estimation of drug antagonisms in the isolated guinea pig vas deferens. *J. Pharm. Pharmacol.* 8: 501.

Levy, B. and Tozzi, S. (1963). The adrenergic receptive mechanism of the rat uterus. *J. Pharmacol. Exp. Ther.* 142: 178.

Lin, R.C.Y. and Yeoh, T.S. (1965). An improvement of Vane's stomach strip preparation for the assay of 5-hydroxy-tryptamine. *J. Pharm. Pharmacol.* 17: 524–525.

Lui, C.Y., Amidon, G.L., Berardi, R.R., Fleisher, D., Youngberg, C.A. and Dressman, J.B. (1986). Comparison of gastrointestinal pH in dogs and humans: implications on the use of the beagle dog as a model for oral absorption in humans. *J. Pharm. Sci.* 75: 271–274.

Malik, M. and Camm, A.J. (2001). Evaluation of Drug-induced QT interval prolongation: Implications for drug approval and labeling. *Drug Safety* 24: 323–351.

Martin, L.I., Horvath, C.J. and Wyand, M.S. (1997). Safety pharmacology screening: practical problems in drug development. *Int. J. Toxicol.* 16: 41–65.

Matsuzawa, T., Hashimoto, M, Nara, H., Yoshida, M., Tamura, S. and Igarashi, T. (1997). Current status of conducting function tests in repeated dose toxicity studies in Japan. *J. Toxicol. Sci.* 22: 374–382.

Mattson, J.L., Spencer, P.J. and Albee, R.R. (1996). A performance standard for clinical and functional observational battery examination of rats. *J. Am. Coll. Toxicol.* 15: 239.

Megens, A.A.H.P., Awouters, F.H.L. and Niemegeers, C.J.E. (1991). General pharmacology of the four gastrointestinal motility stimulants bethanechol, metoclopramide, trimebutine, and cisapride. *Arzneim.-Forsch./Drug Res.* 41(I)(6): 631–634.

Mohammad, A.H., Jabed, C.W. and Jones, R.W. (1997). Blockage of the HERG human cardiac K channel by gastrointestinal prokinetic agent cisapride. *Am. J. Physiol.* 273, H2534–H2538.

Mojaverian, P., Chan, K., Desai, A. and Vivian, J. (1989). Gastrointestinal transit of a solid indigestible capsule as measured by radiotelemetry and dual gamma scintigraphy. *Pharm. Res.* 6: 717–722.

Mojaverian, P., Reynolds, J.C., Ouyang, A., Wirth, F., Kellner, P.E. and Vlasses, P.H. (1991). Mechanism of gastric emptying of a nondisintegrating radiotelemetry capsule in man. *Pharm. Res.* 8: 97–100.

Murphy, D.J. (1994). Safety pharmacology of the respiratory system: Techniques and study design. *Drug Dev. Res.* 32: 237–246.

Nodine, J.H. and Sieger, P.E. (1964) *Animal and Clinical Pharmacologic Techniques in Drug Evaluation*, pp. 36–38, Year Book Medical Publishers, Inc., Chicago.

Norton, S. (1980). Toxic responses of the central nervous system. In *Toxicology: The Basic Science of Poisons*, 2nd ed. Doull, J., Klaassen, C.D. Amdur, M.O., (Eds.). Macmillan, New York.

Offermeier, J. and Ariens, E.J. (1966). Serotonin I. Receptors involved in its action *Arch. Int. Pharmacodyn. Ther.* 64: 92–215.

Olejiniczak, K. (1999). Development of a safety pharmacology guideline. *Human Exper. Toxicol.* 18: 502.

Rossum, J. M. van (1965). Different types of sympathomimetic $\beta$-receptors. *J. Pharm. Pharmacol.* 17: 202.

Seeman, P. and Weinstein, J. (1966). Erythrocyte membrane stabilization by tranquilizers and antihistamines. *Biochem. Pharmacol.* 15: 1737–1752.

Seppalainen, A.M. (1975). Applications of neurophysiological methods in occupational medicine: A review. *Scand J. Work Envirn. Health* 1: 1–14.

Shay, H., Komarox, S.A., Fels, S.S., Meranze, D., Gruenstein, M. and Siplet, H. (1945). A simple method for the uniform production of gastric ulceration in the rat. *Gastroenterology* 5: 43–61.

Smith, W.G. (1961). Pharmacological screening tests. In: *Progress in Medicinal Chemistry, vol. 1.* Ellis, G. and West, G. (Eds.). Butterworth, Washington, D.C. pp. 1–33.

Sjouist, F. (2000). Drug-related hospital admissions. *Ann. Pharmacol.* 34: 832–839.

Sturgeon, R.D., Fessler, R.G. and Meltzter, H.Y. (1979). Behavioral rating scales for assessing phencylidine induced locomotor activity, stereotyped behavior and ataxia in rats. *Eur. J. Pharmacol.* 59: 169–179.

Sullivan, A.T. and Kinter, L.B. (1995). Status of safety pharmacology in the pharmaceutical industry 1995. *Drug Dev. Res.* 35: 166–172.

Takasuna, K., Kasai, Y., Usui, C., Takahashi, M., Hirohashi, M., Tamura, K. and Takayama, S. (1992). General pharmacology of the new quinolone anti–bacterial agent levofloxacin. *Arzneim.-Forsch./Drug Res.* 42(I)(3a): 408–418.

Takeuchi, Y. and Koike, Y. (1985). Electrophysiological methods for the *in vivo* assessment of neurotoxicology. In *Neurotoxicology*. Edited by (Blum, K. and Manzo, L., (Eds.) Marcel Dekker, New York, pp. 613–629.

Turner, R.A. (1965). *Screening Methods in Pharmacology,* Vols. I and II. Academic Press, New York, pp. 42–47, 60–68, 27–128.

Vashi, V.I. and Meyer, M.C. (1988). Effect of pH on the *in vitro* dissolution and *in vivo* absorption of controlled–release theophylline in dogs. *J. Pharm. Sci.* 77: 760–764.

Youngberg, C.A., Wlodyga, J., Schmaltz, S. and Dressman, J.B. (1985). Radio–telemetric determination of gastrointestinal pH in four healthy beagles. *Amer. J. Vet. Res.* 46: 1516–1521.

Zbinden, G. (1984). Neglect of function and obsession with structure in toxicity testing. In Proc. *Ninth Int. Cong. Pharmacol.,* Vol. 1. Macmillan, New York, 43–49.

Zbinden, G. (1966). The significance of pharmacologic screening tests in the preclinical safety evaluation of new drugs. *J. New Drugs* 6: 1–7.

# 20

# EVALUATION OF HUMAN TOLERANCE AND SAFETY IN CLINICAL STUDIES: PHASE I AND BEYOND

## 20.1. THE PHARMACEUTICAL DEVELOPMENT PROCESS AND SAFETY

As explained at the beginning of this volume, the pharmaceutical development process is a long (13–16 years from drug inception to market approval) and costly ($250 million to $500 million, depending on how one allocates costs) process, even when successful. It is shaped by medical needs, regulatory requirements, economics, our understanding of sciences and diseases, and limitations of technology. All of these interact to shape a process which serves to iteratively reduce risks (to both economic and human safety), with the probability of failure being reduced in a stepwise fashion (Matoren, 1984; PhRMA, 2000). Figure 20.1 briefly summarizes this process.

For our purposes (that is, for a safety assessment perspective), the purpose of all nonclinical (animal and *in vitro*) testing is to reduce the risks and probability of adverse events in humans. But between initial nonclinical testing (and concurrent with additional animal testing) and a drug's reaching the marketplace, the potential for having adverse effects in the general patient population it is intended for is further guarded against by a scheme of increasingly more powerful human (or "clinical") trials (Piantadosi, 1997; Nylen, 2000). How safety is evaluated in these is the subject of this chapter. The most common "unexpected" (from nonclinical trial results) safety findings in initial trials involve the skin (dermatitis of one form or another) and liver (Kaplowilz, 2001).

764

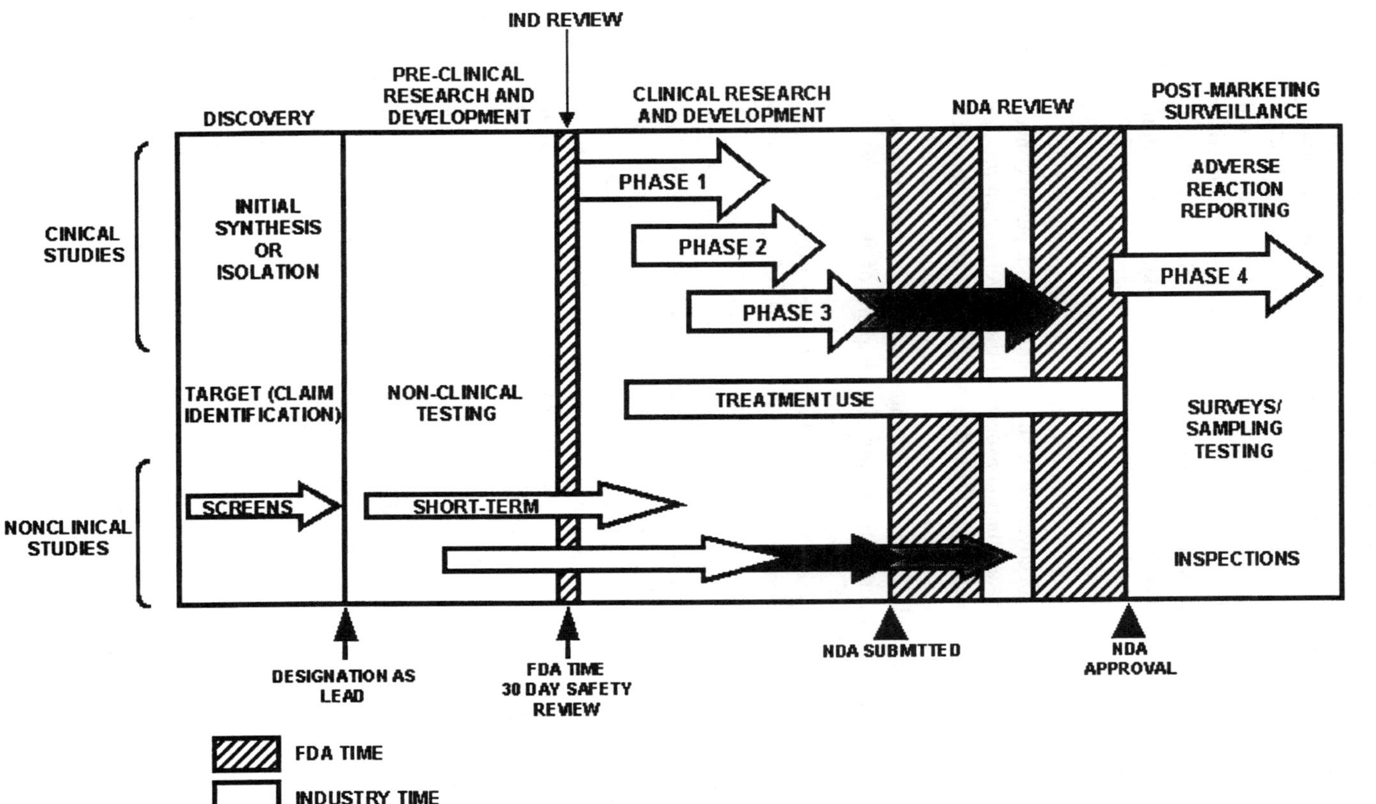


**FIGURE 20.1.** The pharmaceutical development process, viewed as four stages (discovery, preclinical development, clinical development, and NDA review) as well as the important post-market surveillance phase.

Except for those cases where there is substantial potential to save or extend lives (such as anticancer and anti-AIDS drugs) or where the intended target diseases are chronic and severe (Parkinson's or MS) or the routes of administration are invasive (interathecal), the initial evaluations in humans are performed in "normal," healthy volunteers with the primary objective being limited to defining the limits of tolerance (safety) of the potential drug and its pharmacokinetic characteristics. These trials may also seek to detect limited (usually surrogate, that is, indirect) indicators of efficacy, but are severely limited in doing so (Biomarker Definitions Working Group, 2001). Later trials look at the drug's actions on carefully defined groups of patients.

With the number of drugs withdrawn from the marketplace since 1990* (or, perhaps, the degree of media coverage of such withdrawals), public concern with the workings of the drug safety evaluation aspects of the development process has risen sharply (Ganter, 1999; Wechsler, 2001). It is currently estimated that in the United States, adverse drug reactions (ADRs) rank between the fourth to sixth leading cause of death (Eikelblom et al., 2001). While improvements in the nonclinical of drug safety assessment (as covered in the first 19 chapters of this book) are possible and even likely, clearly the clinical aspects (the subject of this chapter) are likely to be where most improvement is likely. This will come from both better selection of subjects for inclusion in trials and a better understanding of individual or subpopulation differences in human responses to drugs.

While there is much press about the concern that the "increased pace of drug approval" has caused the release onto the market of less safe drugs (Willman, 2000), the causes are more mundane and of much longer standing. An important reason for the high incidence of serious and fatal ADRs is that the existing drug development paradigms do not generate adequate information on the mechanistic sources of marked variability in pharmacokinetics and pharmacodynamics of new therapeutic candidates, precluding treatments from being tailored for individual patients (Ozdemir et al., 2001).

Pharmacogenetics is the study of the hereditary basis of person-to-person variations in drug response. The focus of pharmacogenetic investigations has traditionally been unusual and extreme drug responses resulting from a single gene effect. The Human Genome Project and recent advancements in molecular genetics now present an unprecedented opportunity to study all genes in the human genome, including genes for drug metabolism, drug targets, and postreceptor second messenger mechanisms, in relation to variability in drug safety and efficacy. In addition to sequence variations in the genome, high throughput and genome-wide transcript profiling for differentially regulated mRNA species before and during drug treatment will serve as important tools to uncover novel mechanisms of drug action. Pharmacogenetic-guided drug discovery and development represent a departure for the conventional approach which markets drugs for broad patient populations, rather than smaller groups of patients in whom drugs may work more optimally.

*See Table 1.1

Pharmacogenetics provides a rational framework to minimize the uncertainty in outcome of drug therapy and clinical trials and thereby should significantly reduce the risk of drug toxicity. The reader is referred to the Internet sources in Table 20.1 for more details on pharmacogenetics and drug development. Potential improvements in patient inclusion criteria will be addressed later in this chapter.

### 20.1.1. Pharmacokinetics

Current costs and time pressures for developing a new therapeutic motivate companies to make the best possible decision as to whether to continue or abandon the development of a new drug based on a likelihood matrix for three factors: does it work (efficacy), is it acceptably tolerated at therapeutic doses (safety) and is it possible to deliver those therapeutic doses to the target sites/organs economically via the desired route (bioavailability). These likelihoods change most rapidly in early phase development and most compounds abandoned during clinical development are abandoned in this phase, with the most common reason begin unsuitable pharmacokinetics (is it absorbed and does it stay at therapeutic levels for an optimal or near optimal period? Rolan, 1997). Hence the assessment of pharmacokinetics in early phase drug development is strategically important. Some of the drug development issues which are likely to be answered at least in part by a thoughtful interpretation of pharmacokinetic data include the following.

1. Is the compound adequately absorbed to be likely to have a therapeutic effect?
2. Is the compound absorbed with a speed consistent with the desired clinical response?
3. Does the compound stay in the body long enough to be consistent with the desired duration of action?
4. Is the within- or between-subject variability acceptable given the likely therapeutic index of the compound?
5. Is there evidence of a formulation problem?
6. Is there a dose range which produces plasma (or tissue) concentrations which are likely to be associated with a desired clinical response, or which gives rise to safety concerns?
7. Is there a relationship between plasma concentrations and a relevant measure of drug effect?
8. Are metabolites produced which may confound the therapeutic response or safety profile?
9. From the absorption, metabolism, and excretion profile, are there subsets of the target population which may behave differently from expected?
10. Considering the above issues, what is a suitable dosing regimen for clinical efficacy trials?

**TABLE 20.1. Educational Sources on Pharmacogenetics and Drug Development Available on the World Wide Web**

| Source | Focus | Web Address |
| --- | --- | --- |
| Affymetrix | DNA microarray technology | www.affymetrix.com |
| Celera Genomics | Human genome sequencing and variation | www.celera.com |
| Center for Drug Development Science | Drug development | www.dml.georgetown.edu/depts/pharmacology/cdds/index.html |
| Center for Ecogenetics and Environmental Health | Gene-environment interactions | depts.washington.edu/ceeh |
| Cold Spring Harbor Laboratory | Genetics education | www.cshl.org |
| Food and Drug Administration | Drug development and regulation | www.fda.gov |
| Genaissance Pharmaceuticals | Human genetic variation | www.genaissance.com |
| Genset Corporation | Genomics and drug development | www.genxy.com/index/html |
| Human Genic Bi-allelic Sequences Database | SNPs[a] | http://hgbase.cgr.ki.se |
| Human Genome Project | Human genetic variation | www.ornl.gov/TechResources/Human_Genome/home.html |
| Karolinska Institute | Genetics of drug metabolism | www.imm.ki.se/CYPalleles |
| National Institutes of Health | Glossary of genetic terms | www.nhgri.nih.gov/DIR/VIP/Glossary |
| Nature Genetics | Genomics | http://www.nature.com/genomics |
| Orchid Biocomputer | SNPs[a] | www.snps.com |
| Pharsight Corporation | Drug development | www.pharsight.com |
| SNP Consortium | Human genetic variation | Snp.cshl.org |
| Stanford University | Genome resources | www-genome.stanford.edu/index.html |
| Whitehead Institute | Genome resources | www-genome.wi.mit.edu |

[a]SNPs = single-nucleotide polymorphisms.

As most drugs are preferably given orally, absorption which is complete, consistent and predictable is desirable. Although it may be possible from solubility, lipophilicity, pKa, molecular size, and animal data to make some prediction about likely absorption, only a study in humans will give quantitative data as the mechanisms of drug absorption are complex and still incompletely understood (Washington et al., 2001). It may be helpful here to distinguish between the terms "absorption" and "bioavailability."

"Absorption" refers to the fraction of the administered dose which is taken into the body. If a drug is taken up into intestinal cells but then extensively metabolized, it is still regarded as having been absorbed. However, for drug to be "bioavailable," unchanged drug must reach the systemic circulation. Hence a drug with a very high first-pass metabolism might be well absorbed but poorly bioavailable. Although in therapeutic terms poor absorption and poor bioavailability pose similar problems, it is important to distinguish between them, because there are likely to be different possible solutions. Poor absorption might be approached by reformulation, change in the route of administration, or the development of a prodrug; extensive presystemic metabolism might only be avoided by change in the route of administration or chemical modification. Poor absorption is still frequently encountered in modern drug development, because the rational drug discovery process often puts more emphasis on potency and selectivity (because these programs are run by biochemists and pharmacologists) than factors likely to be associated with good absorption. This can result in lead compounds that perform very well *in vitro* but which may present major bioavailability and/or formulation problems (see discussion of this by Rolan et al., 1994).

Quantitative assessment of the extent of absorption (absolute bioavailability) is most rigorously obtained by comparison of the areas under the plasma concentration-time curves (after adjusting for dose) following IV and oral administration. However, even after oral administration alone some idea of absorption or bioavailability can be obtained in the following ways:

1. If a drug is not substantially metabolized, urinary excretion of unchanged drug may be a useful measure of absorption and bioavailability.

2. If a drug is substantially metabolized but it is reasonable to assume that metabolites are not produced in the gut lumen, urinary recovery of drug and metabolites might be a useful measure of absorption.

3. If the "apparent" plasma clearance (dose/area under the plasma concentration-time curve, equivalent to true clearance/fraction of dose absorbed) gives an implausibly high value of clearance (e.g., greater than hepatic and renal plasma flow), it is likely the bioavailability is low. However, this could be due to presystemic metabolism in addition to low absorption.

4. If there is a very large within- or between-subject variability in "apparent" clearance this might indicate variable absorption or bioavailability, which in turn is often seen when absorption or bioavailability is low.

Determining whether absorption is related to the formulation or to an intrinsic property of the molecule can be obtained by comparing absorption from a solid formulation and an oral solution, ideally with an IV solution as a reference.

Some idea of the rate of absorption can be obtained from examination of the plasma concentration-time profile. It should be remembered, however, that the time to maximum plasma concentration ($t_{max}$) is not when absorption is complete but when the rates of drug absorption and elimination are equal. Thus two drugs with the same absorption rate will differ in $t_{max}$ if elimination rates differ. Assessment of the rate of absorption can also be confounded by complex or slow drug distribution. For example, the calcium-channel blocker amlodipine has a much later $t_{max}$ than other similar drugs. This is not due to slow absorption but to partitioning in the liver membrane with slow redistribution. A quantitative assessment of the rate of absorption can be obtained by deconvolution of plasma profiles following IV and oral administration.

***Relating the Time-Course of Plasma Concentrations to the Time-Course of Effect.*** A critical decision to be made after the first human study is whether the compound's speed of onset and duration of action are likely to be consistent with the desired clinical response. Speed of onset is clearly of interest for treatments which are taken intermittently for symptoms relief, for example, acute treatments for migraine, analgesics, or antihistamines for hay fever. Duration of action phase I is particularly important when the therapeutic effect needs to be sustained continuously, such as for anticonvulsants. The first information on the probable time course of action often comes from the plasma pharmacokinetic profile. However, it has become increasingly evident that the kinetic profile alone may be misleading, with the concentration-time and the effect-time curves being substantially different. Some reasons for this, with examples, include

1. The effect may be delayed with respect to plasma concentration because of slow uptake into the target tissue from the plasma. A well-known example is digoxin, where there is a delay of several hours between peak plasma concentration and peak effect.

2. The effect may wane faster than the plasma elimination curve due to tolerance, for example, benzodiazepines and nitrates.

3. The effect may persist despite apparent elimination from plasma. This can occur with an irreversible effect of the drug (e.g., acetylation of platelet cyclo-oxygenase by aspirin). Another reason is very tight binding of the drug near the receptor (e.g., salmeterol) or concentration and trapping in the target tissue (moeprazole).

4. The formation of active metabolites may also contribute to a delay in onset and/or prolongation of action.

Some of these mechanisms may become apparent during animal pharmacology studies, but the clinical pharmacologist must always be aware of the possible discrepancy between concentration and effect-time curves. Clearly, if a relevant drug effect can also be measured in early human studies, establishing a relationship between plasma concentration and effect may be possible. If the desired clinical effect can be measured directly (e.g., blood pressure for an antihypertensive drug), the pharmacokinetic profile may not contribute greatly to the assessment of time course of action, but these circumstances are the exception rather than the rule. Because of the many causes of discrepancies between the time course of drug concentrations and effect, and often the difficulty in measuring the clinical effects directly, a potentially useful approach comes from the use of surrogate markers of drug effect (discussed elsewhere in this book) combined with pharmacokinetic-pharmacodynamic modeling to explore the relationships between dose, plasma concentrations, and effects.

## 20.1.2. Safety of Clinical Trial Subjects

While there continues to be increased interest in and concern about the safety of marketed ("approved") drugs [Ioannidis and Lau (2001), for example, have published a study showing that adverse safety findings is frequently low compared to actual numbers], as of this writing the public's confidence in the safety of participants in trials is at a low level (Shalala, 2000). Certainly, the FIAU tragedy (Meinert, 1996) and the case of the death of a healthy volunteer in a Johns Hopkins trial brought this issue to the forefront of the public mind. Amid estimates of as many as 5,000 subject deaths per year in federally funded clinical trials (out of seven million individuals enrolled in such trials) (Shamoo, 2000; Wilson, 1998; Davis, 1998; Association of American Universities, 2000; Henney, 2000), the current guidelines and procedures should be clearly understood and carefully adhered to, but are likely to be changed. As a starting place, Table 20.2 presents a glossary of key terms employed in this discussion.

There are international regulations which govern (on a country-by-country basis) the conduct of clinical trials, with many national governments expecting researchers to follow specific guidelines, such as given in the International Conference on Harmonization (ICH, 1997) *Guideline for Good Clinical Practice*. Regulations and guidelines are generally based on the principles of the Nuremberg Convention. The Nuremberg Code was written in 1946 in an effort to prevent recurrence of the human experimentation atrocities of World War II. This document states that all research in humans should be done with the well-being of the subject of primary concern (Schmidt, 2001).

The 1964 Declaration of Helsinki includes significant detail about clinical trial practices and the rights of potential subjects to be informed about risks, benefits, and alternative therapies (World Medical Association, 2001). It has been amended several times, most recently in 2000, when the use of placebos in trials employing patients was pronounced to be unethical (Mackintosh, 2001). Together, several parts of the U.S. *Code of Federal Regulations* (21 CFR 50, 21 CFR 54, 21 CFR 56, 21 CFR 312) constitute the Good Clinical Practice (GCP) regulations for studies conducted in the United States. The regulations detail the responsibilities of

**TABLE 20.2. Key Terms**

Adverse event (or Adverse experience): Any untoward medical occurrence in a patient or clinical investigation subject administered a pharmaceutical product and which does not necessarily have to have a causal relationship with this treatment.

Adverse drug reaction (ADR): In the preapproval clinical experience with a new medicinal product or its new usages, particularly as the therapeutic dose(s) may not be established "all noxious and unintended responses to a medicinal product related to any dose should be considered adverse drug reactions."

IND: Investigational New Drug application, filed with FDA after preclinical testing is complete asking for permission to proceed with human tests.

Efficacy pharmacology: Evaluation of a drug's characteristics, effects, and uses with regard to the target illness, and its interactions with living organisms.

Healthy volunteer: A healthy person who agrees to participate in a clinical trial for reasons other than medical and receives no direct health benefit from participating.

Human subject: An individual who is or becomes a participant in research, either as a recipient of the test article or as a control. A subject may be either a healthy human or a patient. [21 CFR (*Code of Federal Regulations*) 50.3].

Nonclinical studies: Studies in living systems (animals or cells) other than humans.

Phase I: Initial safety trials on a new medicine in which investigators attempt to establish the dose range tolerance for single and multiple doses in about 20–80 healthy volunteers.

Phase II: Pilot clinical trials to evaluate efficacy, safety, and therapeutic dose ranges in selected populations of about 100–300 subjects who have the disease or condition to be treated, diagnosed, or prevented.

Phase III: Multicenter studies in populations of perhaps 100–3000 subjects (or more) for whom the medicine is eventually intended.

Phase IV: Postmarketing trials to provide additional details about the product's safety, efficacy, and additional uses.

Preclinical studies: Animal studies that support Phase I safety and tolerance studies and must comply with Good Laboratory Practice (GLP). Other preclinical studies are done in discovery research laboratories to support drug efficiency claims.

Serious adverse event: A serious adverse event (experience) or reaction is any untoward medical occurrence that at any dose:
    Results in death.
    Is life-threatening.
    Requires inpatient hospitalization or prolongation of existing hospitalization.
    Results in persistent or significant disability/incapacity.
    Is a congenital anomaly or birth defect.

Subject/trial subject: An individual who participates in a clinical trial, either as recipient of the investigational product(s) or as a control. (ICH) See also healthy volunteers, human subject. (ICH 1.57)

Unexpected adverse drug reaction: An adverse reaction, the nature or severity of which is not consistent with the applicable product information (e.g., investigator's brochure for an unapproved investigational medicinal product).

sponsors, investigators, and IRBs (institutional review boards), and also outline monitoring practices to ensure regulatory and study design compliance and subject safety. Similarly, the ICH guidelines on GCP provides detailed instructions for investigators, institutions, sponsors, and IRBs.

As with preclinical matters, during the 1990s, the International Conference on Harmonization brought together regulatory agencies and industry representatives from the United States, Europe and Japan, and observers from all over the world to agree to a single set of technical requirements for the registration of pharmaceuticals for human use. This process is now almost complete. The ICH Guideline for Good Clinical Practice has been adopted by the three lead regions and by many other countries (ICH, 1997). As developing nations begin establishing practices for the testing and registration of new molecular entities, many are using ICH guidelines as standards.

Thus, during the past 50 years, the conduct of clinical drug research has improved because of regulations, guidelines, and policies put in place to protect subjects. Individual pharmaceutical companies have used these guidelines and regulations as the basis for their standard operating procedures (SOPs), technical operations policies, and training programs to direct work processes and staff in their research. Most companies have created quality assurance (QA) units to oversee their researchers' adherence to agency guidelines and regulations and to their own company policies and practices.

In the United States, no clinical drug research can begin without prior FDA review of the Investigational New Drug application, which includes the human testing protocol and associated preclinical testing results. While formal FDA approval of such an application is not legally a requirement, assent before preceding is a prudent goal. Regulators in some countries require only notification of intent to initiate first-in-human studies. Before moving on to Phase II or Phase III studies, pharmaceutical companies and other sponsors must submit the information gathered to date for agency reviews.

For new chemical entities (NCEs), new indications or new formulations companies must file an investigational new drug application (IND), which must be approved by the FDA before a drug can be used in humans. The requirements for ADR reporting for investigational new drugs are thus known as the IND regulations. Before a new product can be marketed, companies must file a new drug application (NDA) and have it approved by the FDA. The requirements for ADR reporting after marketing are thus known as the NDA regulations. Both sets of regulations can apply to a drug at the same time; for instance the NDA regulations apply to any marketed forms, but the IND regulations apply to a new indication or formulation. At the time of writing, the current regulations are in Title 21 of the *Code of Federal Regulations* (21 CFR) as follows.

- 21 CFR 312.32 Safety reports for investigational products subject to an IND application (published 1987).
- 21 CFR 314.80 Post-marketing reporting of ADEs (NDA) (published 1985).

- 21 CFR 600.80 Post-marketing reporting of adverse experiences for licensed biological products (includes vaccines) (published 1994).

See also CFR Web site, http://www.access.gpo.gov/nara/cfr/index.html. An August 1997 guideline, *Post-Marketing Adverse Experience Reporting for Human Drug and Licensed Biological Products: Clarification of What to Report*, defined the minimum data relevant for a safety report as

- An identifiable patient;
- An identifiable reporter;
- A suspect drug or biological product;
- An adverse event or fatal outcome.

If any of these items remain unknown after being actively sought, a report should not be submitted to the FDA. The guideline also clarifies that adverse experiences derived during planned contacts and active solicitation of information from patients (e.g., company sponsored patients' support programs, disease management programs) should be handled as safety information from a post-marketing study (i.e., for expedited reporting, events must be serious, unexpected, and with a reasonable possibility that the drug caused the event).

See also Center for Drug Evaluation and Research (CDER) guidance page: http://www.fda.gov/cder/guidance/index.htm.

These regulations and the guidelines have recently been extensively indexed in two publications in the *Drug Information Journal*—Curran and Engle (1977) and Curran and Sills (1990).

In the *Federal Register* of 27 October 1994, the FDA published a proposed rule to amend the regulations to provide consistency with certain standardized definitions, procedures and formats developed by the ICH and CIOMS. The FDA received many comments on these proposals and finally published detailed amended expedited safety reporting regulations, implementing ICH 2 October 1997 (*Federal Register*, 7 October 1997, Volume 62, Number 194, pp. 52237–52253). A revision of the associated guideline has also been proposed by the FDA, but was not available at the time of writing.

These new regulations for expedited reporting were effective 180 days later on 6 April 1998, but companies could comply with the provisions of this final rule before its effective date. Key points from the new regulations are described below. The amendments to the periodic post-marketing safety reporting regulations were delayed awaiting further consideration of the ICH E2C guideline.

***IND Regulations.*** In 1994 the FDA proposed to amend requirements for clinical study design, conduct, and annual sponsor reporting in the IND regulations as a result of events with fialuridine. In the light of comments received, the FDA withdrew the proposed amendments and proposed developing a guidance document with recommendations on study design and monitoring of investigational drugs used to treat serious and potentially fatal illnesses, with particular attention to detection of adverse events similar to those caused by underlying disease.

***Increased Frequency Reports.*** The requirement for increased frequency reports for serious expected ADRs with marketed products is revoked. This was also published in the *Federal Register* of 25 June 1997 (Volume 62, Number 122, pp. 34166–34168). The rationale for this was that despite receiving many such reports, only a small number of drug safety problems were identified.

***Reporting Forms.*** FDA form 3500/3500A (see Figure 20.1) is the standard form for notifying expedited reports and can also be used by companies to submit IND safety reports. Foreign cases may be reported on the CIOMS I form.

***Definitions.*** The definition of "serious" has been revised to make it consistent with ICH E2A and is the same for INDs and NDAs (see Table 21.2).

The definition of "unexpected" for IND reporting is

Any adverse drug experience, the specificity or severity of which is not consistent with the current investigator brochure; or if an investigator brochure is not required or available, the specificity or severity of which is not consistent with the risk information described in the general investigational plan or elsewhere in the current application, as amended. For example, under this definition, hepatic necrosis would be unexpected (by virtue of greater severity) if the investigator brochure only referred to elevated hepatic enzymes or hepatitis. Similarly, cerebral thromboembolism and cerebral vasculitis would be unexpected (by virtue of greater specificity) if the investigator brochure only listed cerebral vascular accidents. "Unexpected," as used in this definition, refers to an adverse drug experience that has not been previously observed (e.g., included in the investigator brochure) rather than from the perspective of such experience not being anticipated from the pharmacological properties of the pharmaceutical product.

***Time Frames.*** The time period for submitting written IND safety reports has been revised from ten working days to 15 calendar days. For telephone reports (fatal and life-threatening unexpected reactions), it has been revised from three working days to seven calendar days. Such reports can also be made by fax. Telephone reporting was previously restricted to clinical studies conducted under the IND, but under the new rule, telephone reporting within seven calendar days applies to any unexpected fatal or life-threatening reaction from any source.

The time period for submitting NDA alert reports (serious and unexpected) has been revised from 15 working days to 15 calendar days.

Wherever human drug research in conducted, national regulations call for an independent ethical review of the study plan. In countries where a guideline on Good Clinical Practices (GCP) is used, ethics review bodies are made up of medical professionals from the institution, nonmedical personnel, and community members. Sponsor companies and involved investigators have no voting representation on these review boards, nor may they be present during the voting on the research approval. The investigator conducting the study may, however, present the protocol and answer questions at the IRB review meeting. The company sponsoring the trial is not allowed to participate in IRB meetings as a matter of routine, although a representative might be invited to explain or clarify the protocol to the ethics review body.

***Informed Consent.*** This must be obtained from study participants in writing before any study-related activities are performed. Regulations clearly describe the required elements of the consent document and the consent process to be followed. A good informed consent process can help ensure that potential subjects understand the nature of the studies they will enter, the type of treatments they will undergo, alternative therapies currently available, and any particular hazards they might experience. They must be informed that they can withdraw from the study at any time without penalty. Subjects are to be asked for their consent to release information from their medical records and told that the medical information may be inspected by sponsor company and regulatory agency representatives. They are to be informed that the results of the trials may be used publicly, but anonymously.

***Drug Supplies.*** These must be accounted for throughout the trial and reconciled at the end of the trial. These practices are designed to prevent the misuse or inappropriate redistribution of the investigational drug and to help ensure compliance with the protocol.

***Adverse Events.*** Unexpected drug reactions, and drug side effects experienced and reported by subjects or observed by clinical investigators are all to be recorded and promptly reported to sponsor companies. It is clear, however, that there are differences in reporting standards between companies and between countries (Hayachi and Walker, 1996). There is also, however, a marked difference in reporting standards and rates in U.S. clinical trials between different medical areas (Ioannides and Lau, 2001). The investigators involved with subject care and the pharmaceutical company sponsor are then to analyze each event for "causality" and "relatedness" to administration of the drug: Did this reaction occur because of the drug or because of something else such as the progression of the disease symptoms, other medications being taken, or unrelated causes? Such safety information is then to be forwarded to the appropriate IRB or ethics committee and regulatory agencies. The sponsor company is to send periodic updates to investigators, alerting them to new serious or unexpected drug reactions.

Company physicians are expected to continuously analyze the adverse drug event data coming in from worldwide trials for trends and patterns that could foretell a drug safety problem. Drug companies frequently set up data and safety monitoring boards (DSMBs), composed of noncompany medical experts and statisticians who impartially evaluate safety as the study progresses and are responsible for alerting the sponsor to unanticipated problems. Regulatory agencies also watch for trends, because they are often in the best position to see safety trends across classes of drugs from any different companies.

Sponsor companies use quality assurance units independent of the clinical research group to audit medical operations. Their role is to ensure that regulatory standards and company policies and procedures for clinical research are being followed in all countries where research is being conducted.

***Regulatory Agencies.*** Their duties are to oversee sponsor organizations, clinical trial processes, and clinical trial sites to verify that sponsors are conducting trials appropriately. Existing FDA regulations conform to ICH guidelines. When deficiencies are noted, agency inspectorates can restrict and penalize the offending academic institutional review board, investigator, and/or the sponsor company. Investigator sites (including, in extreme cases, entire universities) can be prohibited from conducting clinical research. Company studies can be rejected by regulatory agencies.

***Continuous Safety Monitoring.*** Medical staff members at the clinical trial site and at the sponsor company are expected to be continuously alert to adverse drug reactions or unexpected and serious medical problems that might be attributed to the new medication begin tested. The investigator and the site staff examine subjects and take vital sign measurements on the schedule designated by the protocol, the guide for study conduct. Each drug, as shown in its preclinical studies, has unique characteristics, and the potential for adverse events or side effects that investigators need to watch for during the clinical trial. Because of this, safeguard activities are built into the protocol, such as the time intervals between subject visits, how often subjects are to be questioned and examined, the specific medical tests to be run at various time points, and the special diagnostic tests or interviews to be conducted. Staff members at the clinical site must record the medical information from these tests and from interviews and medical histories. Site staff must also transfer information from the medical source documents to the case report forms (CRFs) specific to the study. The CRFs contain key information required for the protocol. Clinical research associates and physicians are required to review the information regularly and to immediately report anything alarming to the IRB and regulatory agencies for further evaluation.

***Sponsor Pharmacovigilance.*** Dedicated departments in pharmaceutical companies, often called pharmacovigilance groups, receive, review, analyze, follow up on, and appropriately distribute safety-related information from new drug trials. These groups sometimes staff hot lines and question and answer services to provide up-to-date answers to drug-related questions. Safety information is to be reported to regulatory agencies at specified intervals and at milestone time points throughout all phases of drug development. The post-approval aspects of this effort are the core of the subject of Chapter 22.

***Sponsor Monitoring.*** Another important oversight process to ensure quality, compliance, and subject safety, monitors may be employees of the sponsor's medical staff or a contract research organization, or may be independent contractors. In each case, they represent the sponsor, and visit investigator sites regularly, perhaps every four to eight weeks. They examine subject records in detail and verify that the correct information was transferred to the clinical trial case report forms, a process called source data verification. During their site visits, monitors also examine administrative and regulatory documents, including drug supply and dosing records, adverse events documentation and reporting, the informed consent process and forms, and case report forms.

Ensuring subject safety must be of the foremost concern during the entire drug development process, especially in clinical trials. The gradual dosing of a drug candidate in healthy human volunteer subjects is performed under tightly controlled conditions and under the direction and scrutiny of physicians trained in clinical pharmacology. A drug candidate's progress toward broader testing in a population of individuals with the disease or condition to be treated also moves prudently and in well-defined steps.

### 20.1.3.  Limitations on/of Clinical Trials

Before looking more closely at the definition, structure and designs of trials, one should understand their limitations. These are regulatory, economic, legal and due to custom.

First, the most recent (October, 2000) revision of the Declaration of Helsinki (World Medical Association, 2000) calls for discontinuing the use of placebo controlled trials in patients. While this is not currently binding on U.S. trials (FDA has specifically said that they will not mirror this as a requirement), and is intended to protect the health of participating patient subjects by precluding having some denied existing efficacious treatments (which would be the effect in most—but not all—cases), it will also likely cause the numbers of subjects required in a trial to increase. This will further stretch the economic aspects of limitations on the power of trials to assess potential drug safety in what will be the intended patient population. Trials are already very expensive; each additional subject enrolled costs $15,000 or more in a Phase II or III trial.

The legal (or rather, litigation) limitations are that any adverse event in a trial (or resulting from it) exposes a sponsor to potential litigation. Accordingly, trials are designed to exclude not only those individuals who are not in the precisely designed subject disease population, but also those who represent potential additional risk subpopulations (the elderly, the young, those currently taking other drugs, minorities and women who are or may become pregnant) or who are likely to eventually use the drug when it enters the marketplace.

Custom (continuing to do things as they have previously been done) also limits the power of trials to identify safety issues. While there are now regulatory inducements to include more women, the young, and ethnic minorities in trials, the first two groups still are not proportionately incorporated because of both the perceived risks of adverse events that they represent and because historically they have not been. Ethnic minorities, particularly African Americans, present a different problem in that there is a historically based resistance to participation in such trials.

## 20.2. THE CLINICAL TRIALS PROCESS

While the numbers of animals involved in research is tracked closely and is well known, such is not the case for human subjects involved in clinical trials. We simply do not know how many are involved in such trials in the United States, much less worldwide. Though the NIH does track closely how many dollars and individuals are involved in research it funds ($12.7 billion and seven million subjects in 1997), the same is not true for privately funded research (where the numbers are greater). And while there is now a Web site where one can examine the numbers and types of efficacy trials open, the same is not true for Phase I tolerance and pharmacokinetic trials, where most potential drugs cease development.

Clinical drug development is often described as consisting of four distinct phases (Phases I–IV). It is important to recognize that the phase of development provides an inadequate basis for classification of clinical trials because one type of trial may occur in several phases (see Figure 20.2). Table 20.3 presents a preferable (objective-based) classification of trial types. It is important to appreciate that the phase label is a description, not a set of requirements. It is also important to realize that these temporal phases do not imply a fixed order of studies since for some drugs in a development plan the typical sequence will not be appropriate or necessary. For example, although human pharmacology studies are typically conducted during Phase I, many such studies are conducted at each of the other three stages, but nonetheless sometimes labeled as Phase I studies. Figure 20.2 demonstrates this close but variable correlation between the two classification systems. The distribution of the points of the graph shows that the types of study are not synonymous with the phases of development.

Drug development is ideally a logical, step-wise procedure in which information from small early studies is used to support and plan later larger, more definitive studies. To develop new drugs efficiently, it is essential to identify characteristics of the investigational drugs in the early stages of development and to plan an appropriate development based on this profile.

Initial trials provide an early evaluation of short-term safety and tolerability and can provide pharmacodynamic and pharmacokinetic information needed to choose a suitable dosage range and administration schedule for initial exploratory therapeutic trials. Later confirmatory studies are generally larger and longer and include a more diverse patient population. Dose-response information should be obtained at all stages of development, from early tolerance studies, to studies of short-term pharmacodynamic effect, to large efficacy studies. Throughout development, new data may suggest the need for additional studies that may commonly be part of an earlier phase. For example, blood level data in a late trial may suggest a need for a drug–drug interaction study, or adverse effects may suggest the need for further dose finding and/or additional nonclinical studies. In addition, to support a new marketing application approval for the same drug, for instance, for a new indication, pharmacokinetic or therapeutic exploratory studies are considered to be in Phase I or Phase II of development.

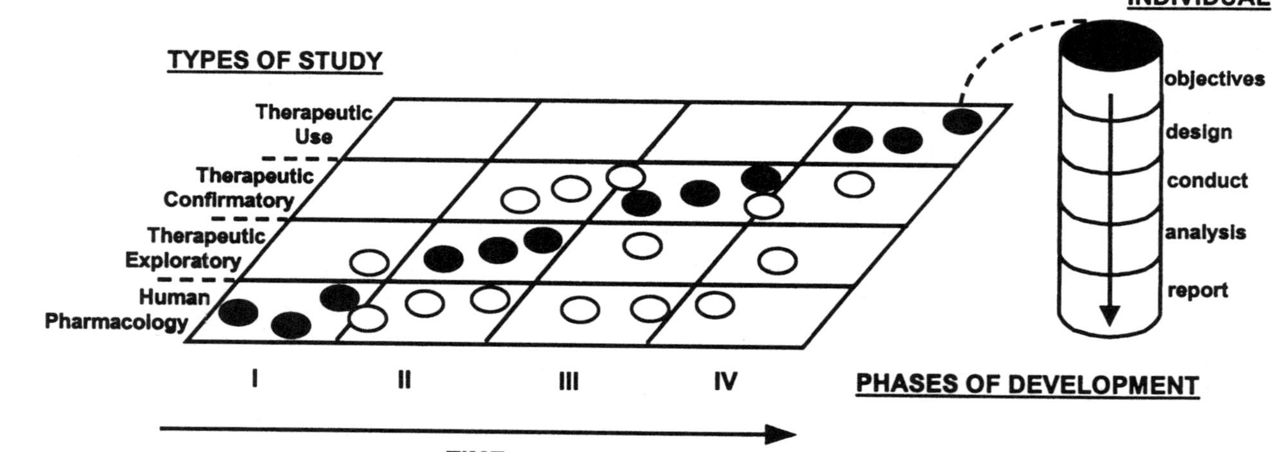



**FIGURE 20.2.** This matrix illustrates the relationship between the phases of development and types of study by objective that may be conducted during each clinical development of a new medicinal product. The shaded circles show the types of the study most usually conducted in a certain phase of development; the open circles show certain types of study that may be conducted in that phase of development but are less usual. Each circle represents an individual study. To illustrate the development of a single study, one circle is joined by a dotted line to an inset column that depicts the elements and sequence of an individual study.

**TABLE 20.3. An Approach to Classifying Clinical Studies According to Objective**

| Type of Study | Objective of Study | Study Examples |
| --- | --- | --- |
| Human pharmacology (Phase I) | Assess tolerance | Dose-tolerance studies |
| | Define/describe pharmacokinetics and pharmacodynamics | Single and multiple dose PK and/or PD studies |
| | Explore drug metabolism and drug interactions | Drug interaction studies |
| | Estimate activity | |
| Therapeutic exploratory (Phase Ib/II) | Explore use for the targeted indication | Earliest trials of relatively short duration in well-defined narrow patient populations, using surrogate or pharmacological endpoints or clinical measures |
| | Estimate dosage for subsequent studies | |
| | Provide basis for confirmatory study design, endpoints, methodologies | Dose-response exploration studies |
| Therapeutic confirmatory (Phase III) | Demonstrate/confirm efficacy | Adequate and well controlled studies to establish efficacy |
| | Establish safety profile | Randomized parallel dose-response studies |
| | Provide an adequate basis for assessing the benefit/risk relationship to support licensing | Clinical safety studies |
| | Establish dose-response relationship | Studies of mortality/morbidity outcomes |
| | | Large simple trials |
| | | Comparative studies |
| | | Comparative effectiveness studies |
| Therapeutic use (Phase III/IV) | Refine understanding of benefit/risk relationship in general or special populations and/or environment | Studies of mortality/morbidity outcomes |
| | Identify less common adverse reactions | Studies of additional endpoints |
| | Refine dosing recommendation | Large simple trials |
| | | Pharmacoeconomic studies |

*Phase I* starts with the first-in-man administration of an investigational new drug. Although human pharmacology studies are typically identified with Phase I, they may also be indicated at other points in the development sequence. Studies in this phase of development usually have nontherapeutic objectives and may be conducted in healthy volunteer subjects or certain types of patients, for example, patients with mild hypertension. Drugs with significant potential toxicity, (cytotoxic drugs) or risks due to route of administration (such as intrathecal) are usually studied in patients. Studies in this phase can be open, baseline controlled or may use randomization and blinding to improve the validity of observations.

Studies conducted in Phase I typically may involve one or a combination of the following:

1. *Estimation of Initial Safety and Tolerability.* The initial and subsequent administration of an investigational new drug into humans is usually intended to determine the tolerability of the does range expected to be needed for later clinical studies and to determine the nature of adverse reactions that can be expected. These studies typically include both single and multiple dose administration.

2. *Pharmacokinetics.* Characterization of a drug's absorption, distribution, metabolism, and excretion continues throughout the development plan. Such preliminary characterization is an important goal of Phase I. Pharmacokinetics may be assessed via separate studies or as a part of efficacy, safety and tolerance studies. Pharmacokinetic studies are particularly important to assess the clearance of the drug and to anticipate possible accumulation of parent drug or metabolites and potential drug–drug interactions. Some pharmacokinetic studies are commonly conducted in later phases to answer more specialized questions. For many orally administered drugs, especially modified release products, the study of food effects on bioavailability is important. Obtaining pharmacokinetics information in sub-populations such as patients with impaired elimination (renal or hepatic failure), the elderly, children, women and ethnic subgroups should be considered. Drug–drug interaction studies are important for many drugs and are generally performed in phases beyond Phase I. But studies in animals and *in vitro* studies of metabolism and potential interactions may lead to doing such studies earlier.

3. *Assessment of Pharmacodynamics.* Depending on the drug and the endpoints studied, pharmacodynamic studies and studies relating drug blood levels to response (PK/PD studies) may be conducted in healthy volunteer subjects or in patients with the target disease. In patients, if there is an appropriate measure, pharmacodynamic data can provide early estimates of activity and potential efficacy and may guide the dosage and dose regimen in later studies.

4. *Early Measurement of Drug Activity.* Preliminary studies of activity or potential therapeutic benefit may be conducted in Phase I as a secondary objective. Such studies are generally performed in later phases but may be appropriate when drug activity is readily measurable with a short duration of drug exposure in patients at this early stage. Frequently such evaluations are done in what are called Phase Ib studies.

*Phase II* is usually considered to start with the initiation of studies in which the primary objective is to explore therapeutic efficacy in patients.

Initial therapeutic exploratory studies may use a variety of study designs, including concurrent controls and comparison with baseline status. Subsequent trials are usually randomized and concurrently controlled to evaluate the efficacy of the drug and its safety for a particular therapeutic indication. Studies in Phase II are typically conducted in a group of patients who are selected by relatively narrow criteria, leading to a relatively homogeneous population, and are closely monitored.

An important goal for this phase is to determine dose levels and regimen for Phase III trials. Early studies in this phase often utilize dose escalation designs to give an early estimate of dose response, and later studies may confirm the dose-response relationship for the indication in question by using recognized parallel dose-response designs (could also be deferred to Phase III). Confirmatory dose response studies may be conducted in Phase II or deferred until Phase III. Doses used in Phase II are usually but not always less than the highest doses used in Phase I.

Additional objectives of clinical trials conducted in Phase II may include evaluation of potential study endpoints, therapeutic regimens (including concomitant medications) and target populations (e.g., mild versus severe disease) for further study in Phase II or III. These objectives may be served by exploratory analyses, examining subsets of data and by including multiple endpoints in trials.

*Phase III* usually is considered to begin with the initiation of studies in which the primary objective is to demonstrate, or confirm, therapeutic benefit.

Studies in Phase III are designed to confirm the preliminary evidence accumulated in Phase II that a drug is safe and effective for use in the intended indication and recipient population. These studies are intended to provide an adequate basis for marketing approval. Studies in Phase III may also further explore the dose-response relationship, or explore the drug's use in wider populations, in different stages of disease, or in combination with another drug. For drugs intended to be administered for long periods, trials involving extended exposure to the drug are ordinarily conducted in Phase III, although they may be started in Phase III. ICH E1 and ICH E7 describe the overall clinical safety database considerations for chronically administered drugs and drugs used in the elderly. These studies carried out in Phase III complete the information needed to support adequate instructions for use of the drug (official product information).

*Phase IV* begins after drug approval. Once rare, there are now commonly required therapeutic use studies that go beyond the prior demonstration of the drug's safety, efficacy and dose definition.

Studies in Phase IV are all studies (other than routine surveillance) performed after drug approval and related to the approved indication. They are studies that were not considered necessary for approval but are often important for optimizing the drug's use. They may be of any type but should have valid scientific objectives. Commonly conducted studies include additional drug–drug interaction, dose-response or safety studies, and studies designed to support use under the approved indication, for instance, mortality/morbidity studies, epidemiological studies.

***Development of an Application Unrelated to Original Approved Use.*** After initial approval, drug development may continue with studies of new or modified indications, new dosage regimens, new routes of administration or additional patient populations. If a new dose, formulation, or combination is studied, additional human pharmacology studies may be indicated, necessitating a new development plan.

The need for some studies may be obviated by the availability of data from the original development plan or from therapeutic use.

### 20.2.1. Special Considerations

A number of special circumstances and populations require consideration on their own when they are part of the development plan.

***Studies of Drug Metabolites.*** Major active metabolite(s) should be identified and deserve detailed pharacokinetic study. Timing of the metabolic assessment studies within the development plan depends on the characteristics of the individual drug.

***Drug–Drug Interactions.*** If a potential for drug–drug interaction is suggested by metabolic profile, by the results of nonclinical studies, or by information on similar drugs, studies on drug interaction during clinical development are highly recommended. For drugs that are frequently coadministered it is usually important that drug–drug interaction studies be performed in nonclinical and, if appropriate, in human studies. This is particularly true for drugs that are known to alter the absorption or metabolism of other drugs, or whose metabolisms or excretion can be altered by effects by other drugs.

***Special Populations.*** Some groups in the general population may require special study because they have unique risk/benefit considerations that need to be taken into account during drug development or because they can be anticipated to need modification of use of the dose or schedule of a drug compared to general adult use. Pharmacokinetic studies in patients with renal and hepatic dysfunction are important to assess the impact of potentially altered drug metabolism or excretion. Specific ICH and FDA documents address such issues for geriatric patients and patients from different ethnic groups. The need for nonclinical safety studies to support human clinical trials in special populations is addressed in the ICH M3 document.

A key issuc is thus when to perform kinetic studies in special patients groups (elderly, patients with renal or hepatic disease) and how. As the elderly are the majority users of many medicines, the subject of evaluating new drugs in the elderly is a major issue which is discussed in detail elsewhere. Unless a medication is unlikely to be used in the elderly some data will be required by regulators for registration. However, an important issue in early phase development is whether to perform a separate elderly volunteer kinetic and tolerability study before elderly patients are included in later phase clinical trials. The major argument for doing so includes the possible reluctance of clinical investigators to enroll elderly patients without such data being available because of safety concerns; however, the utility of such studies has been questioned. The subjects in elderly volunteer studies are usually in much better health than the general population they are intended to represent. Also, the elderly may differ from the young not so much in terms of mean kinetic parameters but the variability in the elderly may be much greater. The relatively small sample size (typically 12–18) may not allow a good estimation of the variability within the elderly population. For these reasons the FDA have recommended that information about the kinetics of a drug in the elderly should come from a larger group representative of the target population and this can be done in the efficacy clinical trials. Although these data are useful, it is not always an acceptable substitute for a specific elderly volunteer pharmacokinetic study because the information is only available after many patients have been exposed rather than before and clinical investigators may be reluctant to enroll patients without such data in advance. In practice, for a drug likely to be given to the elderly, an elderly volunteer study should be performed soon after a young healthy volunteer study to expand the potential population for efficacy studies as much as possible. If elderly patients are then included in the main efficacy–safety studies, the population approach can then be used to explore the pharmacokinetic variability in this subset of the population and whether this is associated with an altered clinical outcome.

A similar rationale can be used to decide whether special kinetic (and possibly, dynamic) studies should be performed in patients with renal or hepatic disease. For example, if the compound is largely metabolized to inactive metabolites, renal function can reasonable be expected not to have a major effect on kinetics. However, regulators usually will want some information as some expectations do exist to the above assumption. An example is the "futile cycle" involving some NSAIDS, where prolonged residence of inactive acyl glucuronide metabolites in the plasma in patients with renal disease allows breakdown back to the parent molecule, resulting in accumulation (Sallustio et al., 1989). As outlined above, a population approach could be used to screen for an effect of disease on drug kinetics, but some investigators may need reassurance before enrolling patients in trials. A small study in patients with advanced renal disease may be able to provide this reassurance. Liver disease can be handled similarly for drugs which are primarily eliminated renally.

The safety of marketed drugs could be significantly improved if the subject groups involved in Phase II and III trials better reflected the patient populations that will use drugs. By excluding "representatives" for what will clearly be subpopulations utilizing a drug (those using other drugs or with other diseases), many clear safety questions go unasked. The same is, to some degree, true about preclinical animal studies where only healthy young animals are employed rather than (perhaps) some disease model groups which might serve as better predictors of patient safety concerns.

### 20.2.2. Institutional Review Boards (IRBs) in the Clinical Trial Process

Clinical drug trials represent research with human subjects (Cato, 1988). All research involving human subjects that is supported by the federal government or the results of which are to be used in applications for drug or device approval must be conducted in accordance with regulations promulgated by the Department of Health and Human Services (HHS) (45 CFR 46) and the Food and Drug Administration (21 CFR 56). The regulations of both the HHS and the FDA require that an IRB "…shall review and have authority to approve, required modifications in (to secure approval), or disapprove all research activities covered by [the] regulations" (45 CFR 46, 21 CFR 56).

The review of clinical drug trials by IRBs raises a number of interesting and difficult issues. These relate to the origin and sponsor of the proposed trial, the nature of the institution the IRB serves, and the manner in which the norms for determining ethical conduct in clinical trials can be applied to specific trials.

Here the ethical principles underlying research involving human subjects, the legal authority for IRBs, and the regulatory requirements affecting the operations of IRBs are reviewed. We will then discuss the role of IRBs in reviewing clinical trials by examining how IRBs can assess the scientific design of trials, the competency of the investigator, the manner of selecting subjects for the trial, the balance of risks and benefits, informed consent, and provisions for compensating for research-related injuries.

***Legal Authority for IRBs.***   The legal authority for IRBs derives from two parallel sets of federal regulations. One set of regulations was promulgated by the Department of Health and Human Services and implements the 1974 amendments to the Public Health Services Act (National Research Act, 1974). These regulations are codified in Title 45 of the *Code of Federal Regulations* (CFR), Part 46. The second set of regulations was promulgated by the FDA under the Federal Food, Drug and Cosmetic Act. These regulations are codified in Title 21 of the CFR; regulations pertaining to IRBs are in Part 50 and those pertaining to informed consent are in Part 56.

The FDA has the legal authority to regulate clinical investigations in the United States when the investigational products move across state or national boundaries. Under the FDA regulations, review and approval by an IRB is required for any experiment that involves a test article and one or more human subjects, either patients or healthy persons, and that is subject to the requirements for prior submission to the FDA (21 CFR 50.3). Such review is also required for any experiment the results of which are intended to be submitted later to, or held for inspection by the FDA.

The regulations of the FDA are identical or similar to those of the ICH and HHS in nearly all essential respects. Such differences as do exist reflect the different statutory authority under which the separate sets of regulations were promulgated and the difference in mission between the FDA and the National Institutes of Health (NIH), the agency within HHS charged with overseeing the implementation and enforcement of the HHS regulations. The difference in mission between the FDA and the NIH is reflected in the FDA's approach to compliance with its regulations utilizing its traditional tools of inspections and audits.

The FDA regulations specify requirements for IRB membership, function, and operation, and the criteria according to which approval may be given for conducting research. Since these requirements are similar, a single committee should be established to undertake the activities required by both sets of regulations. Additionally, the FDA regulations allow a wide variety of ways in which private practitioners not affiliated with an institution can obtain necessary IRB review of their clinical research activities. The basic ethical tenets governing the actions of an IRB should include (Sharp, 2001).

1. Risks to subjects are minimized: (i) by using procedures which are consistent with sound research design and which do not unnecessarily expose subjects to risk; and (ii) whenever appropriate, by using procedures already being performed on the subjects for diagnostic or treatment purposes.
2. Risks to subjects are reasonable in relation to anticipated benefits, if any, to subjects, and the importance of the knowledge that may reasonably be expected to result.
3. Selection of subjects is equitable.
4. Informed consent will be sought from each prospective subject or the subject's legally authorized representative.
5. Informed consent will be appropriately documented.

Additional requirements are that adequate provisions exist for monitoring the data collected, adequate provisions exist to protect the privacy of subjects and maintain the confidentiality of the data, and that appropriate safeguards be included to protect the rights and welfare of subjects who are "…vulnerable to coercion or undue influence…or persons who are economically or educationally disadvantage…" (45 CFR 46.1).

Before a trial initiates, formal review by an institutional IRB that agrees to assume this additional function or by IRBs formed by a local or state health agency, a medical school, a medical society, a state licensing board, or a nonprofit or for-profit independent group is required. All IRBs, regardless of sponsorship, that are assuming responsibilities for reviewing and approving clinical research protocols subject to FDA authority must comply with the IRB regulations set out by the FDA.

***Duties of IRBs.*** IRBs are required to review and have the authority to approve, require modifications in, or disapprove all research activities covered by the regulations [45 CFR 46.109(b)]. They must require that information given to subjects as part of informed consent is in accordance with the general requirements for informed consent that are set out in the regulations. Additionally, they may require that other information be given to subjects when they judge that such information would further protect the rights and welfare of the subjects [45 CFR 46.109(c)].

IRBs must require documentation of informed consent in all studies except those specified in the regulations in which documentation may be waived. Clinical drug trials are not among the classes of studies in which documentation of informed consent may be waived.

IRBs must provide written notification to investigators and institutions of their decisions to approve, require modifications in, or disapprove proposed research activities. Decisions to disapprove a proposed research proposal must be accompanied by a statement of reasons for the decision and provide the investigator an opportunity to respond in person or in writing.

IRBs must conduct continuing reviews of research they approve at least once each year. More frequent reviews may be required if the risk of a particular research project so warrants. IRBs have the authority to suspend or terminate approval of research that is not being conducted in accordance with their requirements or that has been associated with unexpected serious harm to subjects. Such action must be accompanied by a statement of reasons for it and be communicated to the investigator, appropriate institutional officials, and the Secretary of HHS.

The regulations require that IRBs must follow the written procedures that are set out in the assurances they have filed with HHS, review proposed research at convened meetings at which a majority of the IRB members are present, vote approval by a majority of members present at the meeting, and be responsible for reporting to the appropriate institutional official and the Secretary of HHS "...any serious or continuing noncompliance by investigators with the requirements and determination of the IRB."

Institutions that are cooperating in multi-institutional studies, such as clinical drug trials, must each review and approve the proposed studies. Such institutions may, however, use joint review, rely on the review of another qualified IRB, or utilize similar arrangements to avoid duplication of efforts (Cato, 1988).

***Informed Consent.*** Assuring that adequate provisions exist for securing informed consent is a central duty of IRBs, and that which is seemingly the most visualized when it fails (Office of the Inspector General, 2000a, b). The requirements for informed consent are specified in international guidelines and the federal regulations. These require that investigators "shall seek such consent only under circumstances that provide the prospective subject...sufficient opportunity to consider whether or not to participate and that minimize the possibility of coercion or undue influence. The information that is given to the subject...shall be in language that is understandable to [him]" (45 CFR 46.116). The regulations further stipulate that "No informed consent, whether oral or written, may include any exculpatory language through which the subject...is made to waive or appear to waive any of the subject's legal rights, or releases or appears to be release the investigator, the sponsor, the institution or its agents from liability from negligence."

The federal regulations specify the information that shall be provided to each subject.

1. A statement that the study involves research, an explanation of the purposes of the research and the expected duration of the subject's participation, a description of the procedures to be followed, and identification of any procedures which are experimental.

2. A description of any reasonably foreseeable risks or discomforts to the subjects.

3. A description of any benefits to the subject or to others which may reasonably be expected from research.

4. A disclosure of appropriate alternative procedures or courses of treatment, if any, that might be advantageous to the subject.

5. A statement describing the extent, if any, to which confidentiality of records identifying the subject will be maintained.

6. For research involving more than minimal risk, an explanation as to whether any compensation and an explanation as to whether medical treatments are available if injury occurs and, if so, what they consist of, or where further information may be obtained.

7. An explanation of whom to contact for answers to pertinent questions about the research and research subject's rights, and whom to contact in the event of a research-related injury to the subject.

8. A statement that participation is voluntary, refusal to participate will involve no penalty or loss of benefits to which the subject is otherwise entitled, and the subject may discontinue participation at any time without penalty or loss of benefits to which the subject is otherwise entitled.

In addition to these basic elements of informed consent, IRBs shall also require that information shall be provided, where indicated, to the effect that (1) the particular treatment or procedure being tested may involve risks to the subject that are currently unforeseeable; (2) foreseeable circumstances may exist under which continued participation by the subject may be terminated by the investigator without regard to the subject's consent; (3) additional costs to the subject may results from participation in the research; (4) the consequences of a decision to withdraw; and (5) significant findings that may influence a subject's continued participation will be related to the subject.

In addition to the elements enumerated in the federal regulations, IRBs must consider whether consent forms should include the fact of randomization in the case of prospective randomized clinical trials.

Those who feel that the fact of randomization need not be disclosed to prospective subjects argue that since the alternative treatments to be tested are not known to produce significantly different results and since the physician would have to make an arbitrary selection of one treatment or the other for a particular patient, notification that selection of treatment is by computer rather than by the patient's own physician does not provide additional protection for the subjects and is unnecessary. The response to this contention is that a subject's ability to exercise full autonomy over what will be done with his or her own body is best served by notifying the subject as to how the treatment will be selected and by whom, even if the selection process is equally arbitrary whatever process is used.

The weight of the arguments favors the notion that for consent to be fully informed, subjects must be notified that their treatments will be allocated in a random manner, that is, selected by a process other than the judgment of their own physician. The meaning of the concept of randomization and the fact that it will be the manner by which treatment is selected is therefore considered to be an important and integral part of informed consent for participation in randomized clinical trials.

Implicit in the elements that comprise informed consent for subjects participating in clinical trials is that subjects will be notified of the nature of their disease. Current bioethical thinking views this to be essential in order for patients/subjects to give legally effective informed consent. The current practice in the United States is that informed consent to participate in clinical trials requires that patients be notified of their diagnosis. Accordingly, a statement regarding the diagnosis is required in consent forms for participation in clinical trials that are sponsored by national cooperative groups. The Tuskegee study on syphillis is an excellent example of the results of not informing patients (Jones, 1993). It is of interest that other Western countries do not feel that it is necessary or even appropriate to inform patients of their diagnosis as part of the consent process.

Increased incidents in clinical trials have lead to a recognition of the weaknesses of informed consent procedures. Actually, the FDA has reported that such deficiencies are the poorest area of GCP compliance for more than 12 years (*FDA Reports*, 2000, Office of Inspector General, 2000a, b).

## 20.3. DRUG FORMULATIONS AND EXIPIENTS

It should never be lost sight of that one of the major reasons for the 1938 FD&C Act was a public health disaster caused by a drug formulation mistake. In the 1930s, the Massengill Company's use of diethylene glycol in elixir of sulfanilamide led to 105 deaths. This same disaster was, by the way, repeated in Haiti in 1995 and 1996 (O'Brien et al., 1998). Such considerations are also overlooked in clinical safety evaluations, though the history of their directly and indirectly causing problems, even to the current day, is extensive (Winek, 2000).

Preclinical animal studies are usually performed with simple formulations which are appropriate for the route investigated in the (nonhuman) species involved. While similar simple formulations or approaches (such as capsules) are also employed for first-in-man studies, as development proceeds, efforts are made to develop formulations which optimize bioavailability. This may lead to effects not seen in earlier animal (or, indeed, human) studies, a factor that should be kept in mind in both study design and interpretation.

It is essential that formulations used in clinical trials should be well characterized, including information on bioavailability wherever feasible. The formulation should be appropriate for the stage of drug development. Ideally, the supply of a formulation will be adequate to allow testing in a series of studies that examine a range of doses. During drug development, different formulations of a drug may be tested. Links between formulations, established by bioequivalence studies or other means are important in interpreting clinical study results across the development program.

Safety limitations on formulations usually arise from local tissue tolerance concerns at the site of administration for drugs other than oral.

## 20.4. PHASE I DESIGNS

Phase I clinical trials are the first studies in which a new drug is administered to human subjects. The primary purpose of Phase I studies of new drugs is to establish a safe dose and schedule of administration (O'Grady and Linet, 1990). Other purposes are to determine the types of side effects and toxicity and organ systems involved, to assess evidence for efficacy, and to investigate basic clinical pharmacology of the drug. Not all of these goals can be met completely in any Phase I trial, in part because the number of patients treated is small. However, well-conducted Phase I studies can achieve substantial progress toward each of these goals. Phase I trials are not synonymous with dose-response studies, but they have many characteristics in common.

The initial phase of clinical testing has the following objectives.

1. Establish a dose–response pharmacodynamic profile by using initial doses projected to be therapeutic in humans. The dose required is predicted on the basis of blood levels found in animal screens.

2. Determine the pharmacokinetic profile for initial titration and maintenance of steady state for chronically administered drugs.

3. Design a safe dosage regimen for efficacy testing in adults, pediatric, or elderly.

4. Estimate efficacy information necessary to make sample size determinations for Phase II studies and establish adequate duration of treatment.

5. Determine the drug interaction potential when concurrent medications are administered, as well as food interaction, assess the enzyme induction potential, and assess the need for therapeutic drug monitoring during efficacy testing.

6. Establish the requirements for the final formulation.

The initial strategy for Phase I is to conduct a single-dose safety study in normal volunteers. The first trial demands close 24-hour supervision in a clinical setting. Ethical considerations may, however, demand that only patients be used, for example, when evaluating an anticancer agent with predictable toxicity. A repeat dose tolerance and pharmacokinetic study in normal or patient volunteers is then conducted for chronically administered drugs. These studies will provide the necessary safety information to support efficacy testing.

Sometimes investigators say that Phase I studies are not "clinical trials" because there is no treatment comparison being made (except that frequently a placebo is employed). Such treatment comparisons are not a prerequisite for experiments. Because Phase I trials rely on investigator controlled treatment administration and subsequent structured observations, they are clinical trials.

In the development of cytotoxic drugs in oncology, dose-finding usually means establishing a "maximum tolerated dose" (MTD). This is the dose associated with serious but reversible side effects in a sizable proportion of patients and the one that offers the best chance for a favorable therapeutic ratio. Side effects from cytotoxic drugs tend to be serious and are referred as toxicities. Investigators are interested not only in the organ systems involved, but also in the duration, reversibility, and probability of specific toxicities. In this setting, evidence of efficacy is usually weak or nonexistent, because many patients receive what turn out to be subtherapeutic doses of the drug.

For all Phase I studies, learning about basic pharmacokinetics (clinical pharmacology) is important and includes measuring drug uptake, metabolism, distribution, and elimination. This information is vital to the future development and use of the drug, and is helpful in determining the relationship between blood levels and side effects, if any. These goals indicate that the major areas of concern in designing Phase I trials will be selection of patients, choosing a starting dose, rules for escalating dose, and methods for determining the MTD or safe dose.

If basic pharmacology were the only goal of a Phase I study, the patients might be selected from any underlying disease and without regard to functioning of specific organ systems. However, Phase I studies are usually targeted for patients with the specific condition under investigation. For example, in Phase I cancer trials, patients are selected from those with a disease type targeted by the new drug. Because the potential risks and benefits of the drug are unknown, patients often are those with relatively advanced disease. It is usually helpful to enroll patients with a normal cardiac, hepatic, and renal function. Because bone marrow suppression is a common side effect of cytotoxic drugs, it is usually helpful to have normal hematologic function as well when testing new drugs in cancer patients. In settings other than cancer, the first patients to receive a particular drug might have less extensive disease or even be healthy volunteers.

### 20.4.1. First Administration: Single Dose

First-time administration of single doses of new drugs are undertaken using a wide range of study design, but essentially there are several basic designs available which are modified to meet the needs of a given study. Fundamental to all designs is that in the interests of safety, successive subjects are exposed to increasing doses of the drug. The fact that doses are titrated upward either in the same subject or groups of subjects and not randomized to remove the potential for bias can be argued as a design weakness, but there is no alternative. Nevertheless, an ordered dose response can be taken as reasonable evidence of a drug-related effect. In addition, the use of placebo, which enables studies to be conducted on either a single- or a double-blind basis, will help to minimize bias. For this reason, placebo control is an integral part of a Phase I study. Unwanted feelings or sensations are common occurrences in everyday life; hence it is to be expected that adverse events will be encountered during Phase I studies. Adverse events may be drug-related, study-related, or result from something which has nothing to do with the drug or the study. They may act singly or in combination. For example, headache, which is one of the commonest if not the commonest symptom reported by volunteers taking part in Phase I studies, can result from any one of the following: fasting, caffeine withdrawal, feeling anxious about the study, an impending attack of influenza, or a combination of all four factors. Thus without placebo control it becomes difficult to differentiate between headache which is drug-related, and headache which is nondrug-related. But a placebo is not only of value in helping to distinguish between drug- and nondrug-related subjective effects, it also plays a role in the interpretation of results from laboratory and other safety tests and pharmacological tests which may be influenced by diverse factors such as diet, physical activity, mental state, circadian or other biological rhythms, and asymptomatic illnesses, such as subclinical viral infections.

The different designs available for a first-time-in-humans study all have their own advantages and disadvantages (Fleiss, 1986; Spilker, 1991). At the end of the day it is up to the investigator to weigh the pros and cons of each and then to choose the design which best meets the aims of the study. In an attempt to examine their strengths and weaknesses, let us consider some designs open to an investigator who wishes to undertake a single rising dose safety and tolerability study with a new drug. A typical protocol might require

- Placebo control;
- The dose be increased from X (first dose) to 64 X (top dose);
- Two-fold increases in successive doses (within or between subjects);
- A seven-day within subject washout period;
- A minimum of four subjects to receive each dose level.

Some design options are shown in Tables 20.4 through 20.8, while the implications for going with one or other in terms of subject numbers, number of clinic visits, highest first dose given to a subject, biggest increment in dose, and time to complete the study are given in Table 20.9.

Design types A and B require more than threefold the number of volunteers needed for the other designs, but also gives the clearest picture of the pharmacokinetics and tolerance of a single dose. This requirement is compounded by the fact

**TABLE 20.4. Phase I Study: Type A**

| Group | Placebo | $X^a$ | 2X | 4X | 8X | 16X | 32X | 64X |
|---|---|---|---|---|---|---|---|---|
| | | Number of Subjects Who Received Each Treatment | | | | | | |
| 1 | 2 | 3 | | | | | | |
| 2 | 2 | | 3 | | | | | |
| 3 | 2 | | | 3 | | | | |
| 4 | 2 | | | | 3 | | | |
| 5 | 2 | | | | | 3 | | |
| 6 | 2 | | | | | | 3 | |
| 7 | 2 | | | | | | | 3 |

[a]First dose.

**TABLE 20.5. Phase I Study: Type B**

| Group | Placebo | $X^a$ | 2X | 4X | 8X | 16X | 32X | 64X |
|---|---|---|---|---|---|---|---|---|
| | | Number of Subjects Who Received Each Treatment | | | | | | |
| 1 | 2 | 3 | 1 | | | | | |
| 2 | 2 | | 2 | 1 | | | | |
| 3 | 2 | | | 2 | 1 | | | |
| 4 | 2 | | | | 2 | 1 | | |
| 5 | 2 | | | | | 2 | 1 | |
| 6 | 2 | | | | | | 2 | 1 |
| 7 | 2 | | | | | | | 2 |

[a]First dose.

**TABLE 20.6. Phase I Study: Type C**

| No. Visits[a] | Volunteer No. | Treatment | | | |
|---|---|---|---|---|---|
| 2 | 1–4 | $X^b$ | 2X | 4X | (P)[c] |
| 2 | 5–8 | 4X | 8X | 16X | (P) |
| 2 | 9–12 | 16X | 32X | 64X | (P) |

[a]Volunteers receive three doses of drug on one visit and placebo on the other visit.
[b]First dose.
[c]Randomized placebo.

that one-third of the volunteers will receive placebo. The number of volunteers on placebo in each group is open to the investigator's choice, but a balanced (even number of each) design again is easiest to interpret. Whichever way, types A and B require large numbers of subjects, which could present problems when recruiting suitable subjects. The situation is made more difficult when numbers on the volunteer panel are limited (which often is the case) and when one is attempting to recruit the best available volunteers who also satisfy the inclusion–exclusion criteria for a first-time-in-humans study. It can also be argued that if the drug under test proved to be toxic, then more subjects would be exposed to its harmful effects. On the other hand, if the drug turns out to be well-tolerated it can be argued equally

**TABLE 20.7. Phase I Study: Type D**

| No. Visits[a] | Volunteer No. | Treatment | | | |
|---|---|---|---|---|---|
| 4 | 1–4 | $X^b$ | 2X | 4X | (P)[c] |
| 4 | 5–8 | 4X | 8X | 16X | (P) |
| 4 | 9–12 | 16X | 32X | 64X | (P) |

[a]Volunteers receive three doses of drug on one visit and placebo on the other visit.
[b]First visit.
[c]Randomized placebo.

**TABLE 20.8. Phase I Study: Type E**

| Visit | Volunteer No. | | Volunteer No. | | Volunteer No. | |
|---|---|---|---|---|---|---|
| 1 | 1 | P[b] | 5 | X[a] | 9 | 2X |
|   | 2 | X[a] | 6 | P[b] | 10 | 2X |
|   | 3 | X[a] | 7 | 2X | 11 | P[b] |
|   | 4 | X[a] | 8 | 2X | 12 | 4X |
| 2 | 1 | 4X | 5 | P[b] | 9 | 4X |
|   | 2 | 4X | 6 | 4X | 10 | P[b] |
|   | 3 | 4X | 7 | 4X | 11 | 8X |
|   | 4 | P[b] | 8 | 4X | 12 | 8X |
| 3 | 1 | 8X | 5 | 16X | 9 | P[b] |
|   | 2 | 8X | 6 | 16X | 10 | 16X |
|   | 3 | P[b] | 7 | 16X | 11 | 16X |
|   | 4 | 16X | 8 | P[b] | 12 | 16X |
| 4 | 1 | 16X | 5 | 32X | 9 | 64X |
|   | 2 | P[b] | 6 | 32X | 10 | 64X |
|   | 3 | 32X | 7 | P[b] | 11 | 64X |
|   | 4 | 32X | 8 | 64X | 12 | P[b] |

[a]First dose.
[b]Placebo.

well that exposing a larger number of subjects is a better basis on which to proceed to the next study.

Types A and B, however, have two clear advantages over the other designs. First, as only one visit to the clinic is required, this will encourage the volunteer to take part in and complete the study. Second, they are ideal designs for drugs with long (or unclear) pharmacological, clinical or chemical half-lives when a seven-day washout period is an inadequate time for the drug effects to disappear or for it to be cleared form the body.

In the interests of safety, the lower the dose the volunteer is given on the first exposure to the drug the better. However, as it is impractical to start everyone off with dose X, the next best thing one can do is to keep the first dose given to a volunteer in each group as low as possible within the confines of the design of the study. In this respect, type E works best and types A and B do badly.

**TABLE 20.9. Comparisons of Study Types**

| | A | B | C | D | E |
|---|---|---|---|---|---|
| No. of volunteers | 12 | 12 | 12 | 42 | 42 |
| No. of clinic visits | 4 | 4 | 2 | 1 | 1 |
| Highest first dose to a subject | 16X | 8X | 16X | 64X | 64X |
| Largest within subject increment in dose | X2 | X2 | X16 | X2 | — | — |
| Time to do study | 9 weeks | 4 weeks | 3 weeks | 3–6 weeks[a] | 3–6 weeks[a] |

[a]Dependent upon whether dosing takes place once or twice weekly.

With types D and C, twofold increments in dose are uniformly made throughout the whole dose range. This is in contrast to type E, in which the size of dosage increments over the dose range within subjects varies between 2- and 16-fold. Thus type E might be an unwise choice for a drug anticipated to have a narrow therapeutic index or a steep dose response.

Assuming the study goes according to plan (which is often not the case in first-administration studies) and depending upon the study design used, it will take between three and nine weeks to complete. However, although type C (in which the dose is increased stepwise on the same study day) offers the advantage of speed, the fact that it can only really be used for drugs given by the intravenous route and for drugs with rapid onsets and offsets of action limits its usefulness in practice.

### 20.4.2. First Administration in Humans: Repeat Dose

In clinical practice, drugs are often prescribed for illnesses which require regular treatment for days, weeks, months, or years. For drugs used in this way (or for which off label use is likely to be this way), testing on a repeat dose basis in volunteers is required to evaluate safety and tolerability before treating patients. As with first-time single-dose studies, first-time repeat dose studies can be undertaken using different designs but with the emphasis again on safety and tolerability. The cornerstone design is a randomized, rising dose, placebo-controlled group comparative evaluation. Whichever design is used, the investigator has to decide upon an appropriate dosing schedule. The choice of a unit dose and dosing interval depends primarily upon the results from the single-dose study. To illustrate this point, if one assumes that the top dose (i.e., 64 X) given in the previously described single-dose study proved to be well-tolerated, then one might opt for the dosing schedule given in Table 20.10. Of course, the frequency of dosing will depend upon the pharmacodynamic and/or pharmacokinetic profile of the drug. Ideally, dosing should be continued until steady-state plasma concentrations of drug have been achieved, but this may not be practical for drugs with long half-lives. More often than not volunteers are dosed for 7 to 10 days, but in certain circumstances if toxicological clearance is available and there is a definite need to do so, volunteers may be dosed for four weeks. Even if the intent is to dose more than once daily (as in Table 20.10 where twice-daily [b.i.d.] dosing is required), giving single doses on the mornings of day 1 and the last day of dosing (i.e., day 7) offers certain advantages. For example,

**TABLE 20.10. Design and Dosing Schedule for a First Repeat-Dose Phase I Study**

| Group | Day 1 | Day 2–6 | Day 7 |
|---|---|---|---|
| 1 | 8X | 8X b.i.d.[a] | 8X |
| 2 | 16X | 16X b.i.d. | 16X |
| 3 | 32X | 32X b.i.d. | 32X |

[a]b.i.d. = twice daily.

it allows for a longer period to assess tolerability before the second dose of drug is given to a volunteer who more than likely will not have been exposed to the drug previously. It also enables comparisons to be made between drug plasma concentration time profiles over 24 h and the elimination kinetics of the drug at the start and end of dosing.

In the interests of safety, doses are increased between groups sequentially and as a rule dosing is completed in the previous group before dosing is started in the next group. However, if groups are to be dosed for more than 7 to 10 days or a large number of increments in dose is planned, particularly if more than one dosing frequency is under test, the investigator might choose to overlap dosing between one group and the next thus enabling the study to be completed in a reasonable time frame. Within each group, volunteers are randomly allocated to receive drug or placebo. The size of the groups usually varies between 6 and 12 with the numbers of subjects receiving drug and placebo in a group being subject to investigator preference.

***Number of Subjects.*** In a Phase I trial, a sufficient number of subjects must be included in a study if valid conclusions are to be drawn from the results. Studies in healthy volunteers and patients are inherently flawed when it comes to assessing safety and tolerability because of the small numbers of subjects involved, and only the most guarded of conclusions are possible. It is easier to draw valid conclusions in respect to drug action involving pharmacodynamic, surrogate, or clinical endpoints because one is able to specify beforehand the magnitude of the difference which constitutes a useful drug effect, and thus calculate the numbers of studies, except that regulatory authorities rather than the investigator specify the criteria which have to be met to enable different formulations to be judged bioequivalent.

### 20.4.3. Route of Administration

Just as new drugs must be tested in animals by the route to be used in humans, so must they be tested in volunteers using the intended route for patients. But there are clear benefits in testing all drugs when going into humans for the first time using intravenous infusions, even if systemic exposure in patients will be achieved by another route. These benefits relate primarily to the fact that intravenous infusion allows for precise control of drug administration.

In the event of a serious or otherwise distressing adverse event during the infusion, drug delivery can be halted.

As the drug is delivered directly into the bloodstream, this ensures 100% exposure and overcomes problems relating to bioavailability which may occur with other routes, but in particular dosing by the oral route when the drug may be destroyed in the GI tract or metabolized presystemically in the gut wall or in the liver.

Delivery of the full dose into the bloodstream, coupled with a uniform delivery rate, results in less variability in plasma or tissue concentrations of drug than is possible using oral dosing, where not only the extent but also the rate of absorption from the GI tract can vary considerably between subjects. Less intersubject variability in plasma concentrations of drug in turn enables the study to be done using smaller numbers of subjects, and also offers advantages for drugs it is anticipated might have narrow therapeutic ratios.

Intravenous dosing allows the true disposition kinetics of the drug to be evaluated and makes the assessment of PK/PD relationships easier to perform.

Pharmacokinetic scaling between species, that is, animals to humans, is made simpler as fewer assumptions need to be made about extent and rate of exposure in humans. This in turn helps in further dose selection for human studies.

Blinding of studies is made easier when intravenous dosing is used; that is, there is no need to produce matching placebos while intravenous dosing overcomes any problems relating to taste, which can make it difficult in blind studies involving oral dosing.

The primary disadvantage of using intravenous dosing for first-time-in-humans studies is that additional resources will be needed to be spent in toxicology, establishing dosage form stability, and for mutation development on a drug which might fail at the first hurdle in humans, as indeed many do. For this reason investigators often prefer to administer drugs for the first time in healthy volunteers using the route to be used in patients and dose intravenously to establish the drug's pharmacokinetic profile only when they feel reasonably certain that it is likely to be a candidate for further development.

## 20.5. CLINICAL TRIAL SAFETY INDICATORS

One major purpose of preclinical (animal) toxicity studies of a potential new drug is to identify the toxic effects which most commonly occur at doses nearest to those to be used in humans. These observations serve to help ensure that care is taken to detect any such effects in humans. Additionally, a broad range of other indicators of adverse drug action may be identified to ensure that their occurrence is looked for. These are also commonly called safety parameters.

Because of the relatively small numbers of volunteers and patients involved, only the most common of drug-related adverse events are likely to be detected during early studies (O'Grady and Joubert, 1997). For example, to have a 95% chance of picking up three subjects who have experienced an adverse reaction (with no background incidence) which occurs in 1 in every 100 subjects treated with the drug, it would need to be given to 650 subjects. Matters are made worse when the adverse event in question also occurs in the general population, which is usually the case with the kind of symptoms reported by volunteers and patients taking part in drug studies. No matter how good the study design, nothing can compensate for this problem of inadequate numbers. In this respect all of the study designs described earlier are more or less equally adequate or inadequate as the case may be.

Monitoring for drug-related adverse events employs the same or similar methods in both volunteers and patients. In both cases assessments of tolerability and safety are based upon symptom reports, routine laboratory safety screens, EKG monitoring, and on occasion, special tests designed to detect unwanted effects associated with a particular class of drug. The chances of obtaining reliable information on a drug's safety profile are enhance by detailed and careful monitoring. Symptoms may be reported spontaneously or elicited in reply to standard questions. Open questions such as "How are you feeling?" are to be preferred to leading questions on the basis that they result in fewer reports of adverse events. If leading questions are used, they need to be carefully worded. A certain amount of basic information is required on all adverse events, that is, type, severity, time of onset in relation to time of dosing, duration, and causality. Attributing the cause of an unwanted effect to the drug or some other factor can be difficult, particularly when little is known about the drug, as is often the case at the state of initial studies in volunteers or patients. Rechallenge with the drug ideally using the same dose or, if need be (because the event caused a degree of discomfort), a reduced dose is probably the single best way of proving or disproving a causal relationship. But the rechallenge procedure must be designed using placebo as comparator under double-blind conditions. Obviously, rechallenges can be done only if the adverse event was reversible, did not cause excessive discomfort, and most important, was not life threatening. The question of assessing attributions or causality is considered in detail later in this chapter (Section 20.6).

### 20.5.1. Overall Approach to Assessing Safety

***Choosing Safety Parameters.*** Choosing the appropriate safety parameters for a clinical trial depends on a number of factors. A selected list of examinations and tests commonly used to assess the safety of medicines is given in Table 20.11. The majority of these tests will not be conducted in most drug trials. An assessment of the quantity and quality of prior experience and previous data obtained with the therapeutic is essential to enable one to decide which specific safety tests to incorporate in a medicine trials. The choice of safety parameters requires both data in areas where there are indications of potential (or actual) safety problems to monitor and also additional experience and data with a new drug. Until a sufficient body of safety data has accumulated, more laboratory parameters of safety are generally included than will be needed at a later date. The nature of the clinical trials and efficacy tests used may dictate that certain safety parameters should or should not be included (e.g., in testing a new anticancer medicine, it may be necessary to perform a bone marrow biopsy and smear to confirm the lack of toxicity, and in assessing an agent in anesthetized patients, the appropriate tests to ensure the patient's safety while under anesthesia must be performed). If, on the basis of preclinical pharmacological or toxicological data, any toxicity is either anticipated or considered possible, then an attempt should be made to evaluate patients for those possible problems. The anticipated use(s) of a therapeutic will also influence which

**TABLE 20.11. Selected List of Examinations and Tests Used to Evaluate Safety**

A. Clinical Examinations
1. Physical
2. Vital signs (usually considered as part of the physical examination)
3. Height and weight (state of dress is usually specified, e.g., socks)
4. Neurological or other specialized clinical examinations

B. Clinical Laboratory examinations
1. Hematology (see Table 20.12)
2. Clinical chemistry (see Table 20.13)
3. Urinalysis (see Table 20.12)
4. Virology (viral cultures or viral serology)
5. Immunology or immunochemistry (e.g., immunoglobins, complement)
6. Serology
7. Microbiology (including bacteriology and mycology)
8. Parasitology (e.g., stool for ova and protozoa)
9. Pulmonary function tests (e.g., arterial blood gas)
10. Other biological tests (e.g., endocrine, toxicology screen)
11. Stool for occult blood (specify hemoccult or guaiac method)
12. Skin tests for immunologic competence
13. Medicine screen (usually in urine) for detection of illegal or nonprotocol-approved medicines
14. Bone marrow examination
15. Gonadal function (e.g., sperm count, sperm motility)
16. Genetics studies (e.g., evaluate chromosomal integrity)
17. Stool analysis using *in vivo* dialysis

C. Probe for adverse reactions

D. Psychological and psychiatric tests and examinations
1. Psychometric and performance examinations
2. Behavioral rating scales
3. Dependence liability

E. Examinations requiring specialized equipment (selected examples)
1. Audiometry
2. Electrocardiogram (EKG)
3. Electroencephalogram (EEG)
4. Electromyography (EMG)
5. Stress test
6. Endoscopy
7. Computed tomography (CT) scans
8. Ophthalmological examination
9. Ultrasound
10. X-rays
11. Others

safety parameters are chosen for evaluation (e.g., ophthalmological tests would be included for drugs intended for ocular use).

***Measuring Safety Parameters.*** After specific safety parameters are chosen, it is necessary to determine how thorough an evaluation of each parameter should be conducted. It is also possible that different types of examinations would be suitable at different points of a clinical trial. For example, a physical examination may be specified to include more or fewer measurements or facets, and a complete examination may not be necessary or even suitable during some periods of clinical trial.

Vital signs may be measured with the patient in a supine, seated, and/or erect position. Both supine and erect positions are usually used if orthostatic changes are being evaluated. The need for such data will depend on the situation, but the position of the patients for this examination, as well as the period of time desired for stabilization, should be noted in the protocol.

***Parameters that Measure Either Safety or Efficacy.*** Certain parameters may, of course, be either safety or efficacy parameters, or both. The electroencephalogram (EEG) is an example. Blood pressure is another. It is thus important to establish clearly in the protocol whether each parameter is being incorporated in the protocol for safety or efficacy evaluations. Almost any safety parameter can be used for measuring efficacy.

***Appropriateness of Each Parameter for the Clinical Trial and Patient.*** There are four categories of appropriateness of safety tests used in clinical trials.

1. Appropriate for patients, but not necessary for the clinical trial. All of these tests should be included in the clinical trial. They indirectly benefit the trial because they may be monitored for progress or trends or they may simply ensure that patients are receiving appropriate care.

2. Appropriate for the clinical trial, but not necessary for the patients. These tests should be included in the clinical trial if they do not place the patient at unacceptable risk or discomfort. If any tests are deemed unethical in the context of the trials and the patients enrolled, then they should be excluded.

3. Appropriate for both patients and the clinical trial. All of these tests should be included in the clinical trial.

4. Appropriate for neither patients or the clinical trial. All of these tests should be identified and excluded from the clinical trial.

### 20.5.2. Precautions

Clinical laboratory parameters must be specified individually in the protocol. Abbreviations such as "SMA-6" or "SMA-12" are not acceptable, as different laboratories include different tests in their "SMA-6" (or "SMA-12") battery, and using these abbreviations without an explanation can adversely affect the clarity of the protocol and possibly lead to the collection of data on divergent parameters at different sites. Other precautions to consider prior to initiating a clinical trial are to decide if (1) severely abnormal results should be routinely confirmed; (2) samples should be divided and sent to two separate laboratories when specified abnormalities are determined; (3) additional tests should be routinely requested if specified abnormalities are observed; (4) medical consultants should examine patients whenever severe abnormalities are observed; and (5) aliquots of known concentrations of standard drugs should be sent to laboratories for confirmatory measurements and interlaboratory evaluation.

***Summary of Tests.*** Common dermatological tests are shown in Table 20.15 and ophthalmological tests in Table 20.14. Note that any of these tests could be utilized as measures of efficacy if they addressed the clincial trial objectives. Selected pointers are given in Table 20.13. Specific tests that may be used in hematology, clinical chemistry, and urinalysis are shown in Table 20.12, adult and pediatric behavioral rating scales in Tables 20.16 and 20.17, and psychometric and performance tests in Table 20.18.

***Choosing Laboratory Tests.*** There is no standardized series of laboratory parameters that are evaluated in all clinical trials, nor is there a single standard for drugs in Phases I, II, or III. There are, however, broad general guidelines for laboratory tests that reperformed at each stage of clinical development.

***Tests in Phase I.*** In Phase I clinical trials, there is the greatest need to obtain a wide variety of laboratory evaluations as part of developing the safety profile on a new medicine. This entails an evaluation of the basic hematology, clinical chemistry, and urinalysis parameters (Table 20.12). There will never be 100% agreement among investigators and/or clinical scientists as to which specific tests constitute a "basic" workup.

***Tests in Later Phases.*** The total number of normal laboratory values that is sufficient to collect on a new drug to demonstrate safety is impossible to specify. Numerous factors must be considered, such as the toxicological profile on other safety parameters and the expected use of the drug in patients. It is important to determine if a therapeutic agent is to be used topically or parenterally, whether it is to be used in generally healthy patients or in seriously ill patients, whether it is a "me-too" drug or a totally novel drug chemically, and whether it will be life-saving or provide a minimal therapeutic effect. The number of laboratory tests performed usually decreases as an investigational drug moves closer to the market, but one or more tests may be added to the list in Table 20.12 and studied in great detail.

***Tests in Medical Practice.*** The ordering of laboratory tests in medical practice (as opposed to Phase I clinical trials) is extremely inefficient and often irrational. This suggests the need in some clinical situations to develop logical protocols and

**TABLE 20.12. Hematology, Clinical Chemistry, and Urinalysis Parameters Usually Evaluated During the Development of a New Therapeutic Agent**

A. Hematology
   1. Red blood cell (RBC) count
   2. Hemoglobin
   3. Hematocrit
   4. White blood cell (WBC) count and differential
   5. Platelet estimate or platelet count
   6. Red blood cell indices (MCV, MCH, MCHC)[a]
   7. Prothrombin (PT), partial thromboplastin time (PTT)
   8. Reticulocytes
   9. Fibrinogen
  10. Any additional tests suggested by previous data

B. Clinical Chemistry
   1. Albumin
   2. Albumin/globulin ratio
   3. Alkaline phosphatase (and/or its isoenzymes)
   4. Amylase
   5. Bilirubin, total and direct
   6. Bicarbonate (carbon dioxide)
   7. BUN/creatinine ratio
   8. Calcium
   9. Chloride
  10. Cholesterol (and/or a lipid panel)
  11. Creatinine
  12. Creatine phosphokinase (CPK)
  13. $\gamma$-Glutamyl transferase (GGT)
  14. Globulin
  15. Glucose, nonfasting or fasting
  16. Glucose-6-phosphate dehydrogenase (G6PD)
  17. Glutamate oxalacetic transaminase (SGOT), now frequently referred to as aspartate aminotransferase (AST)
  18. Glutamate pyruvate transaminase (SGPT), now frequently referred to as alanine aminotransferase (ALT)
  19. Iron (and/or other related parameters such as ferritin, total iron binding capacity)
  20. Lactic acid dehydrogenase, total (LDH, and/or its isoenzymes)
  21. Inorganic phosphorus
  22. Potassium
  23. Sodium
  24. Total iron binding capacity
  25. Total protein
  26. Triglycerides
  27. Urea nitrogen (BUN)
  28. Uric acid

C. Hormones and/or other chemical substances in blood

D. Urinalysis[b]
   1. Appearance and color
   2. Specific gravity

*(continued)*

**TABLE 20.12.** (*continued*)

3. Acetone
4. Protein
5. Glucose
6. PH
7. Bile
8. Irobilinogen
9. Occult blood
10. Microscopic evaluation of sediment
    a. Red blood cells (Number per high-power field)
    b. White blood cells (number per high-power field)
    c. Casts (describe and give number per high- or low-power field)
    d. Crystals (describe and given number per high-power field)
    e. Bacteria (generally rated as few, many or loaded)
    f. Epithelial cells (number per low-power field)

E. Other urine tests sometimes evaluated
    1. Creatinine (actual values are preferable to estimated values)
    2. Electrolytes (usually sodium, potassium and chloride)
    3. Protein
    4. Specific hormones or chemicals
    5. 24-hour collections for specific evaluations

[a]MCH, mean corpuscular hemoglobin = hemoglobin divided by RBC count; MCHC, mean corpuscular hemoglobin concentration = hemoglobin divided by hematocrit; MCV, mean corpuscular volume = hematocrit divided by RCB count.

[b]Sample codes used to quantify several parameters in the urinalysis are the following. Protein, glucose, ketones, bilirubin: 0, none or negative; 0.5, trace or positive (qualitative); 1, + or 1+ ; 2, ++ or 2+ ; 3, +++ or 3+ ; 4, ++++ or 4+ . Epithelial cells, crystal, WBC, RBC, casts: 0, none or negative; 0.5, rare, occasional, few present, trace (1–5); 1, several, mild (6–10); 2, moderate (11–25); 3, many, much (26–50); 4, loaded, severe (>50). Bacteria: 0, none or negative; 0.5, rare, trace, occasional, few several (1–10); 1, mild (11–50); 2, moderate (51–75); 3, many, numerous (76–100); 4, loaded, severe (>100).

**TABLE 20.13. Selected Considerations Pertaining to Laboratory Data**

1. Ask the laboratory to maintain assayed samples that are of particular importance; if questions arise as to the accuracy of results it might be possible to retest the original samples.
2. If laboratory problems are anticipated, divide the initial (and subsequent) samples and send them to two different laboratories, or to the same laboratory at two different times.
3. If laboratory samples for a complete blood count are going to remain unexamined for a long period of time (e.g., sample obtained on Sunday), prepare a fresh smear so that a comparison may be made with one made 24 or more hours later, because abnormalities may occur when a sample lies around even when it is kept at an appropriate temperature.

algorithms for physicians to follow in ordering tests, particularly when the technology is changing (e.g., hepatitis), in therapeutic areas in which an excessive number of tests are often ordered (e.g., thyroid tests) or when hospitals have developed their own approaches to diagnosis (e.g., use of cardiac isoenzymes in diagnosing a myocardial infarction).

***Less Commonly Used Methods.*** Evaluations of virtually any biological fluid, tissue or sense (taste, smell, hearing, sight, and touch) can be conducted to ascertain the safety of a drug (several have been reported to affect taste in some patients, and there are many other examples involving medicine-induced effects on one of the other senses). The choice of tests will depend on experience with the medicine and suspicions about possible problems. Drugs should also be reviewed for teratogenic potential, drug dependence, liability, and carcinogenicity.

***Identifying the Most Important Laboratory Analytes to Monitor in a Clinical Trial.*** A choice often must be made among the numerous laboratory analytes that could be measured in a clinical trial. This choice is based on (1) past experience with the treatment(s) being evaluated, (2) therapeutic claim, (3) cost of the tests, (4) convenience of obtaining samples, (5) resources available, (6) state-of-the-art concept of the data's importance, and (7) the ability of data obtained to convince both regulators and medical practitioners. To arrive at a decision given these and other previously discussed factors may be difficult.

***Uses of Specific Laboratory Tests to Discover, Confirm, and/or Exclude a Disease.*** Some tests can confirm the diagnosis of a disease (e.g., tissue histology from a bronchoscopic biopsy to confirm lung cancer), but cannot be used to exclude the disease or discover the disease in routine screening. Other tests can be used both to confirm and to exclude the diagnosis of a disease (e.g., glucose tolerance test for diabetes mellitus), but are too inconvenient to be used to discover the disease in routine screening. The uses of each laboratory test to discover, confirm, or exclude a disease should be considered before a test is simply added to a clinical trial protocol. This ensures that the test is appropriate in the context of the planned clinical trial.

***Hematology.*** A basis hematology evaluation usually includes determination of hemoglobin, hematocrit, red blood cell (RBC) count, white blood cell (WBC) count, RBC indices [mean corpuscular hemoglobin (MCH), mean corpuscular hemoglobin concentration (MCHC), and mean corpuscular volume (MCV)], and a platelet count. The white blood cell differential count is usually not required as part of a basic hematological workup unless a specific parameter of the differential count is being evaluated. Nonetheless, a white blood cell differential count is often obtained in Phase I and generally provides useful (though often negative) information. Other hematological parameters (some of which are indicated in Table 20.12) are not usually obtained unless there is a specific reason to do so.

### 20.5.3. Clinical Chemistry

A measurement of renal function (creatinine and/or BUN) is an "essential" test for most clinical studies, as is the inclusion of an panel of liver function tests (SGOT, SGPT, LDH, CPK, GGT, and/or alkaline phosphatase). The specific tests chosen to be included in a study are somewhat dependent on both the investigator's and/or clinical scientist's experiences and the characteristics of the drug. Other important parameters to measure include serum electrolytes and at least some of the tests listed in Table 20.12.

***Drug Levels in Plasma.*** Drug levels may also be measured in a clinical trial. Such levels are usually part of a pharmacokinetic analysis but also provide important safety data. This information would be particularly relevant in cases of suspected or actual drug overdosage, drug interactions, to correlate medicine levels with toxic events, or in other situations. It must be clarified whether free levels of the drug and/or the protein bound will be measured by the laboratory.

***Total Blood That May Be Taken from Patients.*** The total amount of blood that may be taken from a subject in most therapeutic trials should be limited to one unit (about 460 ml) per 8-week period.

### 20.5.4. Urinalysis

Most clinical laboratories have established a standard battery of tests that includes most or all of the basic parameters listed in Table 20.12. If a dipstick is used to test the urine for several parameters, it is useful to use one that measures occult blood, even if a microscopic examination will count the number of red blood cells per high-power field. The means of obtaining the specimen should be indicated (i.e., normal voiding sample, clean catch, midstream, catheterization, suprapubic tap, or cytoscopy), especially in clinical trials in which an antidiuretic or antibiotic (or other relevant drug) is being tested.

It is usually unnecessary to obtain a microscopic examination on all urinalyses unless there are reasons to believe that important information and data may be lost. This is particularly true after it has been demonstrated that the test treatment does not affect the parameters measured in the microscopic evaluation of urine.

### 20.5.5. Urine Screens

A urine screen can be used to confirm generally that patients being screened or entering the baseline period of the clinical trial are not using agents (legal or otherwise) contraindicated in the protocol. It can also be used on a scheduled or random basis during the study to confirm that patients are not using such agents. The urine screen is limited in that it is unable to detect positive compliance with the protocol and only measures certain aspects of compliance failure. If urine tests will be conducted at unannounced times in the clinical trial, then this point must be mentioned in the informed consent.

The number of agents tested in the urine screen is generally determined individually for each clinical trial, since there is a wide variety of possible drugs that may be measured. The choice of drugs to screen will be based on their relative importance for the trial plus the cost and reliability of the methodology. Results of urine screens are usually best viewed in qualitative (i.e., present or absent) rather than quantitative terms. The identification of specific drugs in a patient's urine may help in explaining unusual adverse reactions, laboratory abnormalities, or other events. Urine screens may detect the presence of the therapeutic under study. If the urine screen is able to detect the presence of the study drug, and this is reported as an unknown drug that is present or as a false positive for another drug, then it could essentially unblind a double-blind clinical trial. To prevent this situation from occurring, data from urine screens may be reported to a nonblinded monitor rather than to the investigator. If a sample of the study drug is put in urine at a physiological concentration and sent to the laboratory, the possibility of cross-reactivity with known agents may be assessed prior to initiation of the trial.

***Type of Container to Be Used.*** The specific type of contained used to collect blood or urine samples is sometimes indicated in a protocol, especially if a special anticoagulant or additive is required or if other specific conditions of sample collection and handling are required. It is generally not necessary to provide this information for commonly requested laboratory tests.

***Use of International System Units.*** Although the international system of laboratory analyte units is almost universally agreed upon, many people in the United States resist using it. Typically, these are physicians (and others) who desire to retain the system with which they were trained, which makes mores sense to them.

### 20.5.6. Identifying New Diagnostic Laboratory Tests

Numerous laboratory tests are periodically performed as aids in the diagnosis of disease states. The standards that must be met before a new test is accepted are extremely high, particularly in terms of calculated rates of false-positive and false-negative results. It is proposed that a five-step process leading up to acceptance of a new diagnostic test.

### 20.5.7. Ophthalmological Examination

Various parts of the ophthalmological examination are shown in Table 20.14. The most important common ophthalmological test to evaluate patients for the occurrence of chronic drug-induced toxicity is slit-lamp examination. Specific types of drugs with known potential for ocular toxicity may require that special attention be directed to other evaluations shown in Table 20.14. Most drugs that are to be taken

**TABLE 20.14. Procedures and Tests Performed in Ophthalmological Examination**

1.  Ophthalmological history (attention is paid to patient family history plus patient's diseases and drug reactions
2.  Visual acuity corrected (i.e., with glasses present)
3.  External ocular examination (i.e., check for inflammation, ptosis, nystagmus, tearing, proptosis and other abnormalities)
4.  Extraocular muscle testing
5.  Pupil size and evaluation (in darkened room with controlled illumination)
6.  Slit-lamp biomicroscopy (with dilated pupils)
7.  Tonometry (occular pressure)
8.  Ophthalmoscopy with fundus photographs
9.  Visual field testing and color vision testing
10. Goniscopy[a]
11. Lacrimation[a] (Schirmer test)

[a]These tests are of minimal value in determining ocular toxicity and are not recommended for routine use in ophthalmological examination to detect drug toxicities.

systemically require at least some evaluation of ocular safety prior to approval for marketing.

### 20.5.8. Dermatological Examinations

A few selected safety measurements and tests for specialized dermatological examination are listed in Table 20.15.

In evaluating the safety of drugs using laboratory or other tests, it is important to develop data that helps establish the nature and magnitude of any issue or problem (real or potential) that arises with abnormal laboratory data. Data obtained must also measure the strength of the association between the drug and the event noted or of the serial trends that are observed. While this information is being collected, the definitive courses of action in dealing with the issue or problem can be developed and evaluated. These countermeasures may take the form of (1) periodic monitoring [i.e., prothrombin (PT) or partial thromboplastin time (PTT) times for patients receiving anticoagulants], (2) cessation of medicine treatment, (3) decreasing the dose or changing the dose schedule, (4) initiating countertreatment, (5) specific

**TABLE 20.15. Selected Examples of Safety Measurements and Tests for a Specialized Dermatological Examination**

1.  Biopsy
2.  Erythema at site of lesion
3.  Absorption of medications systemically (e.g., blood levels)
4.  Signs and symptoms of absorption
5.  Interactions with standard treatment (e.g., ultraviolet light)

antidotes may be used to counter or reverse medicine effects, (6) increasing surveillance of the patient, or (7) various other alternatives.

### 20.5.9. Deaths in Clinical Trials

Certain ADRs may be sufficiently alarming as to require very rapid notification to regulators in countries where the medicinal product or indication, formulation or population for the medicinal product are still not approved for marketing because such reports may lead to consideration of suspension of, or other limitations to, a clinical investigations program. Fatal or life-threatening, unexpected ADRs occurring in clinical investigations qualify for very rapid reporting. Regulatory agencies should be notified (e.g., by telephone, facsimile transmission or in writing) as soon as possible, but no later than seven calendar days after first knowledge by the sponsor that a case qualifies, followed by a report that is as complete as possible within eight additional calendar days. This report must include an assessment of the importance and implication of the findings, including relevant previous experience with the same or similar medicinal products.

Determining the cause of deaths in clinical trials is extremely important, but this goal is often difficult or impossible to achieve. Investigators should be prepared to present reasons to family members to convince them of the importance of conducting an autopsy. Such an autopsy should include examination of the brain, whenever possible.

Any history of drug or alcohol abuse by a patient should trigger a request for appropriate blood and urine tests. Blood samples should always be taken to assess the levels of study drugs and any concomitant agents used. The drug containers should always be analyzed to confirm their contents. This usually entails sending these drugs to their manufacturer.

The circumstances surrounding the patient's death should be as well documented as possible, including a description of all possible influences of the clinical trial procedures on the death, even influences that are clearly independent of the medicine(s) being tested. Even procedures in a clinical trial apparently unrelated to a patient's death may have contributed to the death in some way. For example, these procedures could include (1) the requirement for excessive physical exertion, (2) prolonged periods of psychologically difficult testing that lead to extreme fatigue, or (3) giving patients many (e.g., 30) large capsules to ingest per day that lead to choking or aspiration.

Evaluation of the data surrounding the death by physicians who are unassociated with the clinical trial lends additional credibility to the report and conclusions. Physician biases probably will strongly influence their decision regarding the association of a patient's death with the clinical trial, and this factor must be considered in interpreting their report. This is particularly true for developing survival curves in cancer or other often fatal diseases, when deaths unrelated to the disease or to the treatment are excluded from the analysis.

### 20.5.10. Behavioral Rating Scales, Performance, Personality, and Disability Tests

A number of behavioral ratings scales and psychometric and performance tests, listed in Tables 20.16 to 20.18, are briefly summarized below, since many of these scales and tests may be used to evaluate safety as well as efficacy. The following comments on the tests provide only a few highlights; readers who are interested in more details are advised to obtain additional information before choosing the tests that appear most relevant to be included in their particular protocol.

These scales may be used either as part of a clinical trial or as major endpoints in an efficacy trial. Here they are described as a means of obtaining ancillary data on psychological factors in a clinical trial. If these scales are used to demonstrate efficacy, it is mandatory to include only those scales known to be valid.

Unless otherwise noted, all of the adult and children's behavioral scales are given once pretreatment and at least once post-treatment (depending on the trial design, subject drug pharmacokinetics, and length of the trials). Investigators may schedule additional evaluations with these tests, but this is usually not done at less than weekly or biweekly intervals. Many tests provide data on both a total score and

**TABLE 20.16. Adult Behavioral Rating Scales**[a]

| | Scale Rated by | | |
|---|---|---|---|
| Scale | Professional | | Subject |
| 1. Anxiety Status Inventory (ASI) | X | | |
| 2. Beck Depression Inventory (Beck) | | | X |
| 3. Brief Psychiatric Rating Scale (BPRS) | X | | |
| 4. Carroll Depression Scale | | | X |
| 5. Clinical Global Impression (CGI) | X | or | X |
| 6. Clyde Mood Scale | X | | |
| 7. Covi Anxiety Scale | X | | |
| 8. Crichton Geriatric Rating Scale | X | | |
| 9. Depression Status Inventory | X | | |
| 10. Hamilton Anxiety Scale (HAMA) | X | | |
| 11. Hamilton Depression Scale (HAMD) | X | | |
| 12. Hopkin Symptom Checklist (HSCL) | | | X |
| 13. Inpatient Multidimensional Psychiatric Scale (IMPS) | X | | |
| 14. Nurses Observation Scale for Inpatient Evaluation (NOSIE) | X | | |
| 15. Plutchik Geriatric Rating Scale (PLUT) | X | | |
| 16. Profile of Mood States (POMS) | | | X |
| 17. Sandoz Clinical Assessment—Geriatric | X | | |
| 18. Self-Report Symptom Inventory (SCL-90) | | | X |
| 19. Wittenborn Psychiatric Rating Scale (WITT) | X | | |
| 20. Zung Self-Rating Anxiety Scale (SAS) | | | X |
| 21. Zung Self-Rating Depression Scale (SDS) | | | X |

[a]Standard abbreviations are used (See *ECDEU Assessment Manual for Psychopharmacology*, Guy, 1976). Additional tests are described in *Mental Measurements Yearbook* (Buros, 1978).

**TABLE 20.17. Pediatric Behavioral Rating and Diagnostic Scales**

1. Children's Behavior Inventory (CBI)
2. Children's Diagnostic Classification (CDC)
3. Children's Diagnostic Scale (CDS)
4. Children's Psychiatric Rating Scale (CPRS)
5. Clinical Global Impression (CGI)
6. Conners Parent Questionnaire (PO)
7. Conners Parent-Teacher Questionnaire (PTO)
8. Conners Teacher Questionnaire (TO)
9. Devereux Child Behavior Rating Scale
10. Devereux Elementary School Behavior Rating Scale
11. Dosage Record and Treatment Emergent Symptoms (DOTES)
12. Stereotyped Behavior in Retarded

subtest (factor) scores. The times given to complete tests are subject to significant variation depending on the anxiety and characteristics of the patient and/or the experience of the professional. The times listed do not include either scoring or preliminary and/or necessary observations of the patient.

## 20.5.11. Adult Behavioral Rating Scales

*Anxiety Status Inventory.* The Anxiety Status Inventory (ASI) scale is the professional-rated version of the Zung Self-Rating Anxiety Scale (SAS). Both tests (ASI

**TABLE 21.18. Psychometric and Performance Tests[a]**

| Test | For Use in | |
| --- | --- | --- |
| | Adults | Children |
| 1. Bender-Gestalt Test | X | X |
| 2. Conceptual Clustering Memory Test | X | X |
| 3. Digital Symbol Substitution Test | X | X |
| 4. Embedded Figures Test | X | X |
| 5. Frostig Development Test of Visual Perception | | X |
| 6. Goodenough-Harris Figure-Drawing Test (GOOD) | | X |
| 7. Peabody Picture Vocabulary Test | | X |
| 8. Porteus Mazes | X | X |
| 9. Reaction Time | X | X |
| 10. Vigilance Tests | X | X |
| 11. Wechsler Adult Intelligence Scale (WAIS) | X | |
| 12. Wechsler Intelligence Scale for Children (WISC) | | X |
| 13. Wechsler Memory Scale (WMEN) | X | X |
| 14. Wide Range Achievement Test (WRAT) | | X |

[a] Additional tests are described in *Mental Measurements Yearbook* (Buros, 1978).

and SAS) contain 20 items, each with a four-point scale, and are designed for use in adults diagnosed as having anxiety neurosis. Both assess anxiety as a clinical disorder rather than a "feeling state." The tests rate either the present time or the average status of the patient during the week preceding the evaluation. The ASI takes up to 15 to 20 minutes to complete and gives two scores: state anxiety and trait anxiety.

***Beck Depression Inventory.*** The Beck Depression Inventory (Beck) test may be used to measure the depth of depression as a rapid screen for depressed patients. It is a self-rating scale of 21 items (13 in a shortened form), with each item rated on a four-point scale. It measures the immediate present and has been used in anti-depressant medicine trials. The original 21-item scale can be completed in about 10 minutes and the test is able to discriminate between anxiety and depression. No subtests are present in the Beck.

***Brief Psychiatric Rating Scale.*** The Brief Psychiatric Rating Scale (BPRS) is used primarily in adult inpatients to evaluate treatment response in medicine trials and in nonmedicine clinical treatment, but it is also used in some outpatient trials. Abbreviated instructions are printed on the form. Ratings are based on observations of patients. Originally developed for psychopharmacologic research, this test contains 18 symptoms, each rated on a seven-point severity scale. It requires approximately 20 minutes to complete and rates the period of time since the last test. If the test is being used for the first time, it rates the previous week. Five separate subscales are obtained: anxiety-depression, anergia, thought disturbance, activation, and hostility-suspiciousness.

***Carroll Rating Scale for Depression.*** The Carroll Rating Scale for depression (52-item self-rating scale) is scored with "yes" or "no" answers by patients. It was designed to match closely the information content and specific items included in the Hamilton rating scale. It has been validated by comparisons with both the Hamilton Depression Scale (HAMD) and Beck and requires approximately 20 minutes to complete. Seventeen components of depression are measured.

***Clinical Global Impressions.*** Although the ECDEU *Assessment Manual for Psychopharmacology* (Guy, 1976) provides a formal test for the Clinical Global Impression (CGI) Scale, numerous investigators have modified the three major questions as well as the scales used in order to fit this test to their own clinical trials. The three questions, which may be applied in almost all Phase II and Phase III clinical trials, are

1. *Severity of illness.* "Considering your total clinical experience with this particular population, how mentally ill [the investigator may substitute a more appropriate term if this is not applicable] is the patient at this time?
2. *Global improvement.* Rate total improvement, whether or not in your judgment it is due entirely to medicine treatment.

3. *Efficacy Index.* Rate this item on the basis of medicine effect only. [This utilizes a rating of both efficacy and adverse reactions and divides the efficacy score by the adverse reaction score to form a ratio (efficacy index).]

Severity of illness is the only one of these three rated pretreatment. All three questions may be rated posttreatment, and additional ratings are possible during a clinical trial. The CGI measure, which is widely used in all types of medicine trials, is generally well accepted.

A scale of two to nine gradations is usually used for questions (1) and (2), although five or so gradations are probably most common. A typical five-point scale for question (2) would be that the patient is rated as 1 (much worse), 2 (minimally worse), 3 (unchanged), 4 (minimally improved), or 5 (markedly improved).

***Clyde Mood Scale.*** The Clyde Mood Scale test may be used as either a self-rated or observer-rated scale. It contains 48 items to measure mood and has been shown to be sensitive to medicine effects. The test takes 5 to 15 minutes to complete and measures the immediate present in a patient or normal individual. The test gives six scores: friendly, aggressive, clear-thinking, sleepy, unhappy, and dizzy.

***Covi Anxiety Scale.*** The Covi Anxiety Scale is a global observer's rating scale of patient anxiety. There are three items that are each rated on a 0–5 scale. The test is simple to use and requires only a few minutes to complete.

***Crichton Geriatric Rating Scale.*** The Crichton Geriatric Rating Scale test measures the level of behavioral function in elderly psychiatric patients using a five-point scale on 11 items. It rates either the present or the period within the last week and takes 5 to 10 minutes to complete.

***Depression Status Inventory.*** The Depression Status Inventory (DSI) scale is the professional's version of the Zung Self-Rating Depression Scale (SDS). Each of the two scales (DSI and SDS) consists of the same 20 items rated on a four-point scale and is applied to adults with depressive symptomatology. The DSI is completed by the professional, and the SDS is completed by the patient. Both tests take about 5 to 10 minutes to complete. The DSI rates either the present situation or the last week prior to the test, and a total score is obtained.

***Hamilton Anxiety Scale.*** The Hamilton Anxiety (HAMA) scale was designed to be used in adult patients who already have a diagnosis of anxiety neurosis rather than for making a diagnosis of anxiety in patients who have other problems. The test contains 14 items, each with a five-point scale, and is completed by a physician or psychologist. The test emphasizes the patient's subjective state. The two subscales determined are somatic anxiety and psychic anxiety.

***Hamilton Depression Scale.*** The HAMD is one of the most widely used tests to evaluate the severity of depressive illness quantitatively in adults. The most widely used form of this test contains 21 items covering a broad range of symptomatology, with a three- to five-point scale for most items. The minimum time required to complete this test is usually 10 to 20 minutes, and it requires a skilled interviewer. Either the present time or the period within the last week is rated. Six subscales are obtained in the HAMD: anxiety/somatization, weight, cognitive disturbance, diurnal variation, retardation, and sleep disturbance.

***Hopkins Symptom Checklist.*** The Hopkins Symptom Checklist (HSCL) is a scale that has been used to measure the presence and intensity of various symptoms in outpatient neurotic patients. It is a 58-item self-rating scale and has generally been replaced by the Self-Report Symptom Inventory (SCL-90). It measures the symptoms during the past week and requires approximately 20 minutes to complete. There are five subtests: somatization, obsessive-compulsive, interpersonal sensitivity, depression, and anxiety.

***Inpatient Multidimensional Psychiatric Scale.*** The Inpatient Multidimensional Psychiatric Scale (IMPS) is used to measure psychotic syndromes in hospitalized adults capable of being interviewed. The 89 items are rated on the basis of a psychiatric interview. This test has been well validated and requires 10 to 15 minutes following a 35- to 45-minute interview. There are ten scores: excitement, hostile belligerence, paranoid projection, grandiose expansiveness, perceptual distortions, anxious intropunitiveness, retardation and apathy, disorientation, motor disturbances, and conceptual disorganization.

***Nurses Observation Scale for Inpatient Evaluation.*** The Nurses Observation Scale for Inpatient Evaluation (NOSIE) (30-item test) is used by nursing personnel to rate a patient's behavior on the ward, with a five-point scale for each item. This test is widely used and is well accepted for adult inpatients. The test, which rates the most recent three days, is relatively easy to use and requires three to five minutes to complete.

***Plutchik Geriatric Rating Scale.*** The Plutchik Geriatric Rating Scale (PLUT) (31-item test) is designed to measure the degree of geriatric functioning in terms of both physical and social aspects. The three-point scale for each item is completed on the basis of direct observation of the patient's behavior and takes 5 to 10 minutes to complete. The subscales measure overall dysfunction, aggressive behavior, sleep disturbance, social isolation, sensory impairment, work and activities, and motor impairment.

***Profile of Mood States.*** Profile of Mood States (POMS) self-rating scale is used in both normals and psychiatric outpatients to evaluate feelings, affect, and mood. It has been widely used in medicine trials. The 65 adjectives included in this test may be used to rate the present and/or previous week. This test requires from 5 to 10 minutes to complete and provides scores for six subtests: tension-anxiety, depression-dejection, anxiety-hostility, vigor, fatigue, and confusion.

***Sandoz Clinical Assessment-Geriatric.*** The Sandoz Clinical Assessment-Geriatric (SCAG) test measures 18 individual symptoms plus a global rating using a seven-point scale similar to those used in the Brief Psychiatric Rating Scale. It measures the present period or that within the last week, requires about 10 to 15 minutes to complete, and does not contain subtests.

***Self-Report Symptom Inventory.*** Each of the 90 items in the SCL-90 uses a five-point scale of distress. It was designed as a general measure of symptomatology for use by adult psychiatric outpatients in either a research or clinical setting. It rates either the present or previous week. It requires about 15 minutes for the patient to complete this form and about 5 minutes for a technician to verify identifying information. This test is sensitive to drug effects and may be used with inpatients. Nine subscales are measured: somatization, obsessive-compulsive, interpersonal sensitivity, depression, anxiety, anger-hostility, phobic anxiety, paranoid ideation, and psychoticism.

***Wittenborn Psychiatric Rating Scale.*** The ECDEU version [Wittenborn Psychiatric Rating Scale (WITT)] is a 17-item test shortened from the original 72-item test. All but one item use a four-point scale, and the test takes 5 to 10 minutes to complete. It is used for both in- and outpatients and rates either the present or previous week. This test is not intended to make diagnoses but to reflect changes within one patient and to provide a basis for comparing different patients. This test provides descriptive, as opposed to etiological or prognostic, information on patients and includes the following subscales: anxiety, somatic-hysterical, obsessive-compulsive-phobic, depressive retardation, excitement, and paranoia.

***Zung Self-Rating Anxiety Scale.*** The SAS test requires approximately 5 to 10 minutes to complete.

***Zung Self-Rating Depression Scale.*** The SDS test requires approximately 5 to 10 minutes to complete.

### 20.5.12. Pediatric Behavioral Rating and Diagnostic Scales

Many of the behavioral rating scales described for adults are not suitable for use in the pediatric population. Special tests have been designed, and a number of pediatric behavioral rating scales are presented in Table 20.17. General comments on these tests are presented below. A further description of rating scales used in pediatric medicine trials is given in the *ECDEU Assessment Manual For Psychopharmacology* by Guy (1976). His article is a practical guide to identifying appropriate scales for a particular situation. Conners discusses the two broad approaches of many pediatric rating scales as either "rating current behaviors, symptoms or states;

or. . .describing basic traits, dispositions, and personality characteristics." The choice of one of these two approaches depends in part on the purpose of using a scale in a medicine trial. Three general purposes have been suggested for using a behavioral test: prediction, measurement of change, and classification. The choice of one of these three purposes usually implies that one of the two specific approaches implicit in the pediatric behavioral scales will be more appropriate.

1. To be able to predict something about a patient, choose a scale that rates basic traits.
2. To measure change in a patient, choose a scale that rates current symptoms.
3. To assess a patient's classification, choose a scale that rates either basic traits or current symptoms, depending on the purpose of the classification.

The type of patient population and the desired format of the test to be used in a clinical trial also influence the particular scale(s) chosen.

An evaluation system that can be used in a wide variety of pediatric inpatients is the Children's Behavior Inventory.

***Children's Behavior Inventory.*** The Children's Behavior Inventory (CBI) is a 139-item, two-point (yes–no) scale to record maladaptive behavior in children aged 1 to 15 years. Relatively little training is needed to administer this test. It is easily used by nurses, teachers, graduate students, psychologists, and others. This test usually requires at least two hours of observation of the child, but better reliability is achieved if behavior is observed over an eight-hour period. Nine subtest scores are provided: anger-hostility, conceptual dysfunctioning, fear and worry, incongruous behavior, incongruous ideation, lethargy-dejection, perceptual dysfunctioning, physical complaints, and self-deprecation.

***Children's Diagnostic Classification.*** Children's Diagnostic Classification (CDC) test may be used instead of the Children's Psychiatric Rating Scale (CPRS) to arrive at a diagnosis. This differs from the CPRS in that it is highly directed and leads the observer to a diagnosis. It rates the current status of the child and may be used at pretreatment and/or the termination of the clinical trial.

***Children's Diagnostic Scale.*** The Children's Diagnostic Scale (CDS) is used in children up to 15 years of age to assist in the diagnosis and classification of the child's condition. It contains 13 items, eight of which have a seven-point scale. The others are specific diagnostic questions. It measures current status only and is mainly used at the start of a study, although it may be used at the termination of the study as well.

***Children's Psychiatric Rating Scale.*** The CPRS is a comprehensive scale to assess a wide range of psychopathologies in children up to age 15. It contains 63 items, with a seven-point scale derived from the Brief Psychiatric Rating Scale (BPRS). This test rates 28 items by direct observation of the child, based on behavior expressed during the interview, and rates other items based on the child's reports of events that occurred either over the preceding week or that occurred during the interview. Scores of 15 separate clusters of the rated items are provided as well as the overall score.

***Clinical Global Impression.*** See adult behavioral rating scale description of the CGI.

***Conners Parent Questionnaire.*** Conners Parent Questionnaire (PQ) is a 94-item checklist of symptoms that evaluates common behavior disorders using a four-point scale in children up to 15 years of age and takes 15 to 20 minutes to complete. It is used once pretreatment and may be repeated but is often replaced after the first use by the 11-item Conners Parent-Teacher Questionnaire (PTQ). There are eight subscales: conduct problem, anxiety, impulsive-hyperactive, learning problem, psychosomatic, perfectionism, antisocial, and muscular tension.

***Conners Parent–Teacher Questionnaire.*** See descriptions above for Conners Parent Questionnaire and below for the Conners Teacher Questionnaire (TQ). The PTQ is used in conjunction with either the PQ to TQ and yields a total score only (i.e., no subscales are given). The PTQ takes about five minutes to complete and is not used pretreatment.

***Conners Teacher Questionnaire.*** The TQ form was designed to obtain teacher evaluations of children up to age 15 in terms of their interactions with peers and their ability to cope with the school environment and requirements. There are 41 items, and the first 39 have a four-point scale. Question 40 deals with the teacher's evaluation of the child's severity of illness, and question 41 deals with global improvement in four different areas. This test is used once at pretreatment and as needed afterwards. It takes about 15 minutes to complete and covers either the present or any interval period up to one month. A shorter 11-item PTQ is often used after the initial use of the 41-item TQ. The five subscales included are conduct, inattentive-passive, tension-anxiety, hyperactivity, and social ability.

***Devereux Child Behavior Rating Scale.*** The Devereux Child Behavior Rating Scale contains 97 items and is similar to the Devereux Teacher Scale. It is used for emotionally disturbed and mentally retarded children aged 8 to 12 years. Besides being easy to use, this scale is well researched and discussed in the literature. It requires 10 to 20 minutes to complete by clinicians, child care workers, parents, or others and gives 17 scores. There is a Devereux Adolescent Behavior Rating Scale for children from ages 13 to 18.

***Devereux Elementary School Behavior Rating Scale.*** The Devereux Elementary School Behavior Rating Scale is a widely used test incorporating 47 items that have a high test-retest reliability. It uses a checklist format and is easy to use (requires 10 min). There are 11 factor scores and three item scores.

### 20.5.13. Psychometric and Performance Tests

The psychometric and performance tests presented in Table 20.18 may be grouped as being applicable for use in either children or adults. In children, the tests measure intellect (GOOD, Porteus Mazes, WISC, Peabody), achievement (WRAT), and motor performance (vigilance tests, reaction time). There are other tests that may be used to measure learning, although many of these tests utilize equipment and are not described. All of these tests (unless otherwise noted) are given once pretreatment, at least once posttreatment, and at additional times if desired by the investigator. The contribution of learning in the scores obtained at second and third testings is usually unknown. The methods used to motivate patients to perform to the best of their ability in all tests must be standardized and reported.

***Bender–Gestalt Test.***  The Bender–Gestalt is a nonverbal performance test in which the individual copies a design shown on a card. It is often used to identify a problem of visual perception and/or motor performance or minimal brain dysfunction in children.

The scoring used for children (age 4 or 5–11 years) differs from that used for adults (age 15–adult). This test measures perceptual maturity, possible neurological impairment, and emotional adjustment in children. It measures maturation, intelligence, psychological disturbance, and cortical impairment in adults. The test requires 10 minutes to complete. Scores may fluctuate from test to test and thus must be interpreted carefully.

***Conceptual Clustering Memory Test.***  For the Conceptual Clustering Memory Test, patients are given a list of 24 specific words from a number of different categories such as birds, cars, or types of drinks. The words are presented one at a time over two minutes, after which patients are asked to recall as many of the specific words as possible. The test measures the total recall as well as the degree to which words of a specific category (e.g., animals) are recalled from the cluster of words given in that category (e.g., dog, cat, cow).

***Digital Symbol Substitution Test.***  A subtest of the Wechsler Adult Intelligence Scale (WAIS), the Digital Symbol Substitution test measures sensory-motor integration and learning relationships of symbols. It has been used in many psychopharmacological studies. Subjects are given different forms of this test at each session. The test requires the patient to match as many of 100 symbols to their respective numerals, found in a code key, as possible within 60 seconds.

***Embedded Figures Test.***  For the Embedded Figures Test, patients are shown a complex design and must identify as quickly as possible a simple figure that is "embedded" within the design. Twenty-four embedded figures are included, and a maximum of three minutes is allowed for each one.

***Frostig Developmental Test of Visual Perception.*** The Frostig Developmental Test of Visual Perception (FROST) measures the development of perceptual skills in children from four to eight years of age or in older children with learning difficulties. It may be administered individually (requires 30–45 minutes) or to groups (requires 40–60 minutes).

***Goodenough–Harris Figure-Drawing Test.*** The Goodenough–Harris Figure-Drawing Test is a brief (10–15 minute) easy to use test for children 4 to 15 years of age to measure intellectual maturity.

***Peabody Picture Vocabulary Test.*** The Peabody Picture Vocabulary Test is a rapid 10–15-minute intelligence test for children aged 2.5 to 18 years that is useful when there is inadequate time to give the WISC.

***Porteus Mazes.*** The Porteus Mazes is a nonverbal test that has been shown to be sensitive to medicine effects in both children (over three years) and adults. The test has three series of mazes to prevent score improvement on retesting with the same test. It requires about 25 minutes and provides both a qualitative and quantitative score.

***Reaction Time.*** There are many different tests used to measure reaction time. These tests measure the period of time between the presentation of a stimulus to a patient and the onset of the resulting response. The signal is usually a visual or auditory stimulus, and the onset of a motor reaction, such as the lifting of a finger, arm, or leg or the pressing of a buzzer, is used to measure the speed of response.

In simple reaction times, a stimulus is presented that always requires the same response, even if the nature of the stimulus changes. A complex reaction time requires the patient to respond to some stimuli but not to others.

***Vigilance Tests.*** Numerous tests have been designed to measure vigilance. In these tests, patients are requested to respond in some manner to certain stimuli or occurrences but not to others. The stimuli may be controlled to present minimally perceived signals that require vigilance on the part of the patient.

***Wechsler Adult Intelligence Scale.*** The WAIS consists of 11 subtests: six verbal tests and five performance tests. This provides an age-related IQ in adults from 16 to 75 years of age; that is, the test measures intelligence of persons in relation to their age group and not to the entire population. It may be used either as an initial assessment or as a tool to measure change. The test, which takes 40 to 60 minutes to complete, provides 13 scores in verbal and performance categories plus a total score.

***Wechsler Intelligence Scale for Children.*** The Wechsler Intelligence Scale for Children (WISC) was extensively revised in 1974 and became the WISC-R, which requires 40 to 60 minutes to complete. This widely used scale in children from 6 to 16 years of age may be used for either screening or baseline data or as a measure of change. There is a "preschool and primary scale of intelligence" version that may be used in children from 4 to $6\frac{1}{2}$ years of age (requires 50–75 minutes). The WISC-R has six verbal and six performance subtests.

***Wechsler Memory Scale.*** The Wechsler Memory (WMEM) Scale is a brief test that is used to measure memory deficits. There are two forms of the test, and they are generally alternated to avoid a training effect in children taking the test on two or more occasions.

***Wide Range Achievement Test.*** The Wide Range Achievement Test (WRAT) is used in children from age five years to adults in college. It assesses basic skills in reading, spelling, and mathematics. It is simple, easy to administer, and requires 20 to 30 minutes to complete.

### 20.5.14. Personality Tests

In addition to the above behavioral and performance tests, there are a number of well-known tests of personality that may provide useful information in select clinical studies. The most well known of these tests is the Minnesota Multiphasic Personality Inventory (MMPI). This test consists of 550 affirmative statements to which a true or false response is given and requires about one hour to complete. It is given to adults over the age of 16 and is scored for ten scales: depression, hysteria, hypochondriasis, psychopathic deviate, masculinity-femininity, paranoia, hypomania, schizophrenia, psychasthenia, and social introversion.

### 20.6. ASSESSMENT OF UNWANTED DRUG EFFECTS

As presented in Section 20.5, a number of factors in clinical trial design make the identification and evaluation of adverse effects a challenge. Actions in addressing these challenges include the following.

***Separation of Adverse Reactions from Placebo Reactions.*** Since adverse non-drug symptoms are common (Reidenberg and Lowenthal, 1968) and are not easily separated from drug-induced symptoms, both must be collected for analysis if a complete profile of adverse reactions is to be made. However, this technique can only be used in controlled studies, ideally with placebo, as well as with other standard drugs. The temptation to subtract the number of the particular AR in the placebo group from the number in the active drug group as follows:

Drug group − placebo group = number of adverse reactions to drugs

should be resisted because:

- The difference may not be statistically significant and may have arisen by chance.

- Although the total number of events may be statistically different in the two treatment groups, it is also necessary to establish whether the numbers of patients afflicted with the AE are different and vice versa.
- Having established that there is a significant difference between the two treatment groups for the number of events and the number of patients afflicted, the severity of the ADRs in the two groups should be compared.

A further problem is that due to classification, some terms may include more than one type of abnormality (e.g., the incidence of "blurred vision" may be equal in both groups, but there may be several cases of tunnel vision with the trial drug but because there is no code for tunnel vision it is coded under a more general term). Another problem is that the symptoms forming a syndrome are often coded separately and individually there may be no difference between two drugs, but when the cases are examined there may be a combination of symptoms with one drug that warrant being called a syndrome. It is therefore essential to read the individual original description of the AEs before making a judgement. This area has been explored more fully by Bernstein and he has added bias to the equation:

$$\text{Attributable AEs} = \text{drug group AEs} - \text{placebo group AEs} + / - \text{bias}$$

Bias is equal to the base line (B) frequency and severity of the AE multiplied by pharmacological clinical activity of the drug (AD) minus the pharmacological clinical activity of the placebo (AP):

$$\text{Bias} = B\,(AD - AP)$$

The argument is that the disease or a symptom or sign of the disease and the drug ADR may interact as follows:

1. *Compliance.* Early improvement may cause the patient to stop the drug and the improvement of the ADR may be inappropriately assigned to tachyphylaxis of the ADR; failure of the disease to improve may persuade the patient to add a rescue drug or increase the dose of the study drug or even stop the drug; impaired mental or cognitive function due to the disease may affect compliance.

2. The disease may alter the absorption, distribution, metabolism, or elimination of the drug (e.g., alteration of the blood–brain barrier by the disease may allow the drug to affect the brain).

3. Observational bias of convalescence (e.g., severe pain causing insomnia may require morphine causing compensatory hypersomnia in excess of that caused by morphine alone).

4. Observational bias by halo effects. Perception of an ADR may be swamped by the symptoms of the disease, thus as the disease symptoms resolve the ADR becomes apparent.

5. Unblinding. If the patient or physician are unblinded due to rapid improvement of the disease or an ADR they may be led to expect ADRs with the active treatment.

6. Pharmacological clinical activity bias. An AE that is already present due to the disease may be increased if it is also an ADR of the drug or vice versa. For example, the diarrhea of gastroenteritis may be alleviated by codein-containing preparations given to relieve pain while the inertia of a severely depressed patient may be sufficiently resolved by an antidepressant to enable the patient to commit suicide.

Adverse drug reactions that are similar to common nondrug AEs are rarely described or investigated sufficiently for a causal relationship for each individual event to be established. If they cannot be distinguished qualitatively, the correct quantitative procedure is to compare them using nonparametric statistics, giving the confidence limits for the incidences of ADRs. Small studies ($n < 30$) have little chance of separating ADRs from placebo or nondrug events unless they are very common and specific to the drug. The situation is worsened by the fact that members of a placebo group have a tendency to "catch" AEs from the active drug group, therefore changing a relatively specific ADR to a nonspecific event.

### 20.6.1. Base Case Causality of Single-Event Adverse Drug Reactions

The analysis and evaluation of adverse drug reactions (ADRs) is a major problem in both the development of new drugs and in the postmarketing surveillance period. Just as there are standards and requirements established as guidelines in the chemical, pharmacological, and toxicological phases preceding the marketing of a new drug, there are also guidelines for causality assessment of individual human cases in both pre- and postapproval for new drugs.

The most common problem of assessment is the single-event ADR case. Presented here is an approach to such single-event ADR cases. This methodology, relating to the use of therapeutic, diagnostic, and prophylactic-type drugs in a clinical setting, should permit the diagnostician to make one of three responses after an assessment of an ADR case: an assured *yes*, a firm *no*, or a reasoned admission of *uncertainty*. The clinicopathological picture presented by the ADR case is often not readily distinguishable from nondrug-induced diseases. The clinical and morphologic findings of ADRs have the same limited number of final common paths that characterize these other (nondrug) human illnesses.

There are three major requirements for establishing the occurrence of an ADR:

1. The possibility and likelihood of a causal relationship between the drug and the ADR must be confirmed by establishing its eligibility.
2. Linkage of the drug with the clinicopathological findings made.
3. The degree of certainty of this drug linkage should be determined.

As an initial background for developing this algorithm or methodology, Figure 20.3 is offered for consideration and orientation. This figure has the basic elements of a "time flow chart," which has considerable utility in evaluating ADR cases.

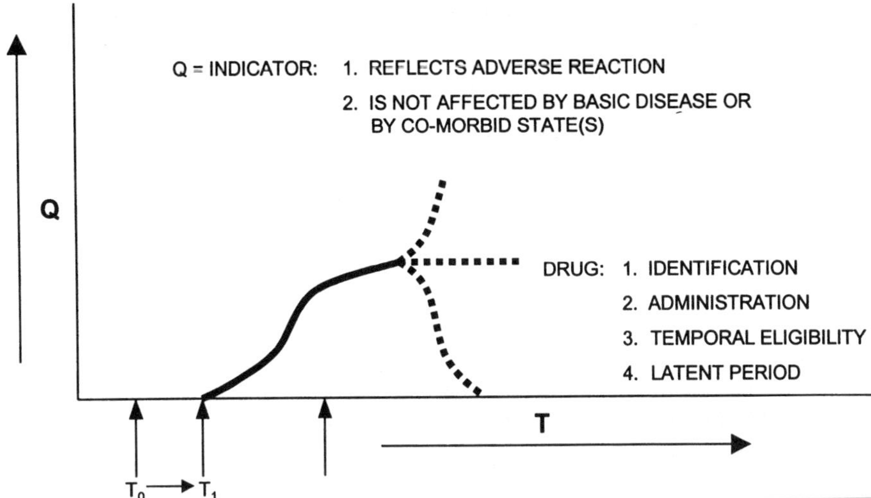



**FIGURE 20.3.** An adverse drug reaction (the curve Q) is plotted against time (the abscissa $T$). Dashed lines show the three courses an ADR can take: increasing severity to death; leveling off to chronicity; or return to the abscissa, indicating recovery. Four criteria that must be met before the drug is eligible to be an empiric correlate of Q (the adverse drug reaction) are listed.

In this graphical representation of an ADR, the ordinate (Q) represents any of the findings of an ADR. *Specifically,* Q may be a symptom (pain, nausea, etc.), a sign, a clinical laboratory result, a radiological finding, a morphological finding, or any combination of these. Synonyms for Q include marker, disease marker, signal, indicator, parameter, detector, response, and effect.

The abscissa is the time element ($T$), related to both the time of drug administration and to the dating of disease marker data. Both are usually plotted on the same time flow chart in a particular case.

This graphical representation of an ADR case will be used frequently in the assessment of eligibility and linkage determinations of ADRs. The four eligibility criteria are also listed in Figure 20.3.

***Administration of the Drug.*** As it is with accurate identification of a drug, so it is that its "administration" must at times be held in question. Subject compliance with the study protocol is not a rare problem in clinical trials. Complete noncompliance sometimes occurs.

***Temporal Eligibility.*** The time factor in assessment of ADRs is a very important one and in some cases is of critical diagnostic importance. This is true not only in establishing "eligibility" of the drug, but also in linking the drug to the reaction. On the other hand, the time element may be equally important in denying eligibility and also make linkage of the drug with the clinicopathological picture a most unlikely possibility.

It is quite apparent that a drug cannot be responsible for an ADR if the latter is already in progress before the drug is first administered. This dyssynchronicity is sometimes seen in both trials and later in the marketplace.

***Latent Period.*** Latent period refers to the time interval between the initial administration of the drug and the onset of the ADR (in Figure 20.3, it is the interval $T_0$ to $T_1$). The latent period is not rigidly fixed or exactly predictable, but it tends to fall within certain limits.

Characteristically, strychnine deaths occur in seconds to minutes. Most anaphylactic deaths occur within 20–30 minutes after contact with the lethal antigen, while jaundice associated with most drugs has its onset within three days to three weeks after the beginning of therapy. The fatal pancytopenia following chloramphenicol appears in one to three months, while hepatic angiosarcoma related to aflotoxin has a latent period of one to several decades. The ultimate in length of latency is one to several generations from a drug-induced mutational germ cell change to its manifestation in a conceptus.

Consideration of the latent period in an ADR is of use in an ADR assessment in one of two ways: the latent period may be too long, or it may be too short.

In summary, identification, administration, temporal eligibility, and latent period are the four criteria for establishing the eligibility of a drug to have caused an ADR. Emphasis should be placed on obtaining sufficiently detailed time-related data on drug administration and on the appearance of ADR markers. These data are a *sine qua non* in the assessment of drug eligibility.

***Linking the Drug with the Clinicopathological Findings.*** The second major task in analyzing an ADR case is to establish a connection or linkage between the drug and the clinicopathological findings (making empiric correlates of the drug and these findings).

Figure 20.4 is a time flow chart representing an ADR that itemizes six ways of making this linkage.

***Exclusion.*** Exclusion consists of selecting one drug from a group of drug candidates by the use of the time flow chart.

The exclusion method also includes instances in which drug candidates are themselves excluded from causation status because a nondrug etiology is clearly demonstrable (environmental or occupational factors, radiation injury, the underlying disease of the patient, or a comorbid state) that can reasonably account for the clinicopathology findings.

***Dechallenge.*** The principle involved in the dechallenge method of linkage is that if there is a reversible effect present, then removing the cause will eliminate the effect.

***Rechallenge.*** The principle involved in the rechallenge method of linkage of a therapeutic to an ADR is implied in the phrase *post hoc ergo propter hoc* (after this therefore because of this).

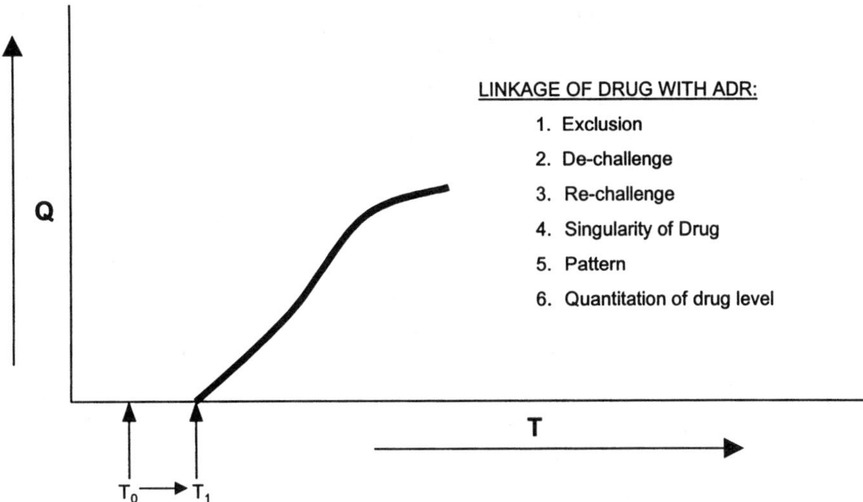


**FIGURE 20.4.** The six methods of linking a drug with an adverse drug reaction.

As applied, if a drug has been incriminated with a reaction, and the ADR disappeared when the drug was discontinued, a rechallenge with this drug followed by a return of the ADR would increase the probability that the drug and the ADR were empiric correlates. While intentional challenge is not often done, such a rechallenge may occur inadvertently.

***Singularity of the Drug.*** The principle involved in the singularity method of linking a drug with an ADR is based on two assumptions: Only one drug was administered, and there was no basic disease or co-morbid state that could be related to the ADR marker being used in the assessment.

***Pattern.*** The pattern method of linking a drug with an ADR shifts the focus of attention to the clinicopathological findings in an ADR, and away from the identification of the causative drug. This shift of emphasis is necessary when detailed time-related drug and disease marker data are unavailable to the evaluator of the case. The site-process profile may then be used as a guideline for searching past experience and the literature for cases that have matching features. Matching features found in the literature may include associations with certain drugs or chemicals, which serves as a guideline for a focused examination of the patient's history for the causative agent.

This "pattern" method may also be used in excluding drugs. If the drugs or chemicals suggested by the morphologic findings are not identified or disclosed by historical or toxicological efforts, then the morphologic changes appear to remain non drug or non-chemical related.

***Quantitation of Drug Level.*** Assessing an ADR case by quantitation of drug level brings our focus back to the search for and the identification of the causative agent by quantitative and objective data based on laboratory analysis of body fluids and/or viscera (Ozdemir et al., 2001). This method is applicable and strongest in the case of higher dose level. The feasibility of this approach is based on the availability of dependable information on lethal levels from past experience or preclinical work. Without this comparison information, there is no judgmental significance to toxicological levels in the case at hand.

Quantitated levels of drugs have limitations in diagnostic value. In adverse reactions in the hypersensitivity, idiosyncratic, and pharmacogenetic categories, drugs have been administered in therapeutic (not toxic) amounts, and blood and other body fluids and tissue levels have been found to lie within therapeutic ranges. Such analyses will confirm any prior administration of the drugs, but the problem of the etiological differential diagnosis will still remain.

In addition to quantitative approach, qualitative identification can be of value in appropriate instances. In some cases of ADRs, more than one of the six methods of drug linkage that are listed in Figure 20.4 may be used in causation analysis. In fact, multiple methods in the same case strengthens either the confirmation of the rejection of an ADR and its etiology.

***Difficulties in Assessing ADRs.*** Requirements for establishing eligibility and methods of linking a drug with an illness have been presented in the preceding discussion. This algorithm should constitute a blueprint for solving many if not most of the ADR problems in this area of medical diagnostics.

However, in the hands-on practice of the assessment of ADR cases, there are at least four major difficulties that stand in the way of such high diagnostic expectations. These four obstacles include the following:

1. *Incomplete Information.* Incomplete information is not unique to ADR evaluation but is common to all areas of medical practice. The lack of sufficiently detailed, time-related data on drug administration and disease markers may make it impossible to render a reasoned judgment on many ADR cases, leaving them in their original and unsatisfactory anecdotal status.

Denial to the evaluation of access to these required facts makes it impossible to make judgments on latent period and temporal eligibility; time flow charts cannot be utilized in exclusion, dechallenge, and rechallenge techniques. The diagnostic data base should also include information on any other drugs being administered or taken, concurrent comorbid states, and the existence of any preexisting occupational and environmental hazards.

2. *Polypharmacy.* In recent times, polypharmacy is the rule rather than the exception. Patients with complicated and prolonged illnesses may have 20–30 medications in their medical background. Cases of this sort may be of such complexity that even with ideally complete drug and disease marker information, diagnostic success may be elusive.

3. *Lack of Objective Means of Linking the Drug to the ADR.* Tests and

procedures that specifically and causally connect a drug to an illness are lacking. Our high-tech laboratory instrumentation is capable of identifying and quantifying extremely low levels of drugs and chemicals, but this type of information falls short of establishing causation.

4. *The Limited number of Toxicologic Responses in Human Disease.* There are a limited number of generic morphological reaction patterns that diseases fit into (inflammatory, congenital, neoplastic, degenerative, infiltrative, vascular, functional). In parallel, there are also a rather limited number of clinical symptoms and signs (pain, nausea, fever, lumps, etc.) that come to the attention of the practicing physician. There are a multitude of causes and a multitude of clinical conditions that funnel into these clinicopathological "final common paths." The algorithm previously described is an attempt to move from the generic to the specific in analyzing ADR causation.

Of the above four difficulties, only the first (incomplete information) is subject to at least some degree of improvement.

***Degree of Certainty.*** The third major task in analyzing and assessing ADRs is determining the degree of certainty one has as to the causal relationship between the drug and the clinicopathological findings. Interposed between the definitive causative and negative categories are three shades of certainty (probable, possible, and coincidental) that titrate between these two extremes. These degrees of certainty are defined as follows:

1. *Causative.* Cases in this class are those in which there is no doubt that a drug has caused the reaction. This category is essentially limited to drug overdose cases or those cases in which the causative agent can be objectively identified (asbestos bodies; granuloma encapsulated silica, etc.). Parenthetically, the overdose cases with drug levels in lethal ranges should have important negative findings: no anatomical cause of death at autopsy.

2. *Probable.* This term is equivalent to the phrase "consistent with," and cases in this category of certainty fall short of the "causative" designation because they lack an objective and quantitative laboratory finding that is the *sine qua non* of the causative category. Cases placed in this category have the following characteristics:

(a) The criteria of temporal eligibility and appropriateness of latent period have been met.

(b) The clinicopathological features are consonant with previous experience and literature precedent for the drug in question.

(c) Other causes (the basic disease, co-morbid states, and other modalities of therapy) have been eliminated from consideration.

(d) One or several means of linkage of the drug to the ADR have been utilized: exclusion, dechallenge, rechallenge, singularity of the drug, and pattern.

3. *Possible.* Cases are put in this category when the relationship between the drug and the clinicopathological findings can be neither confirmed nor denied. There are three subdivisions in this category.

(a) Cases with potential causes other than the drug in question. The clinicopathological picture could have been produced by the basic disease, a comorbid state, or by some other modality of therapy.

(b) Cases in which some of the criteria for eligibility and linkage have been met, but some have not because of lack of adequate information. Such a case could be put in this category temporarily while more information is awaited or placed here permanently if it were evident that further data would not be forthcoming.

(c) Cases that have met all the criteria of eligibility and linkage but for which there is no known precedent literature. Such a case might be a new and emergent ADR. It could be placed in the "possible" group, awaiting the appearance of similar cases for cluster studies at a later time.

4. *Coincidental.* Cases in this category include those that were indeed exposed to the drug in question but in which assessment of the case clearly reveals only an anecdotal association.

5. *Negative.* This category applies to those cases in which the alleged drug was not or could not have been in the patient's system at the time of the ADR. This circumstance could be related either to noncompliance, mislabeling of the drug, or historical misinformation.


## 20.7. CONCLUSION

The roles of the toxicologist in clinical trials are to:

1. Prospectively and retrospectively evaluate, explain and extrapolate from the relationships between nonclinical trial findings and adverse clinical trial events.
2. Provide mechanistic insight into the causes, treatment and avoidance (of further) undesired effects in a clinical trial.
3. Guide selection and refinement of subject profiles for clinical trials.

The ultimate expression of a toxicologist's preclinical labours which serves to address these moles are the safety sections of the investigations brochure (IB) and section 8 of the IND. Here are the last chances to guide a potential drug into safe development in humans.


## REFERENCES

Association of American Universities (2000). Task Force on Research Accountability: Report on University Protection of Human Beings Who are the Subjects of Research. Washington, D.C., June 28, 2000. www.aau.edu/HumSUbRpt06.28.00pdf

Biomarkers Definitions Working Group (2001). Biomarkers and surrogate endpoints: Preferred definitions and conceptual frameworks. *Clin. Pharmacol. Ther.* 69: 89–95.

Buros, O.K. (1978). *The Eight Mental Measurements Yearbook*. Gryphon Press, Highland Park, NJ.

Cato, A.E. (1988). *Clinical Drug Trials and Tribulations*. Marcel Dekker, New York.

CFR, Title 21, Parts 50, 54, 56, 312, 314. U.S. Government Printing Office, Washington, D.C. www.access.gpo.gov/nara/cfr/

Davis, R. (1998). Holes are growing in medical testing safety nets. *USA Today*, June 8, 1998, 19A–20A.

Eikelboom, J.W., Mehta, S.R., Pogue, J. and Yusuf, S. (2001). Safety Outcomes in Meta-analyses of Phase II versus Phase III Randomized Trials. *JAMA* 285: 444–450.

F-D-C Reports, Inc. (2000). FDA May Request "Intermediate" Enforcement Authority for Clinical Trials. *The Pink Sheet*, 62 (19): 16–17.

Fleiss, J.L. (1986). *The Design and Analysis of Clinical Experiments*. J Wiley, New York.

Gad, S.C. (1998). *Statistics and Experimental Design for Toxicologists*. CRC Press, Boca Raton, FL.

Ganter, J. (1999). Responding to industry critics: If the industry doesn't address concerns raised by the consumer press, who will? *Appl. Clinical Trials* 10, November, 1999.

Guy, W. (1976). *ECDEU Assessment Manual for Psychopharmacology*. U.S. DHEW Pub. No. (ADM) 76-338. U.S. Government Printing Office, Washington, D.C.

Hayachi, K. and Walker, A.M. (1996). Japanese and American reports of randomized trials: Difference in the reporting of adverse effects. *Controlled Clinical Trials* 17: 99–110

Henney, J.E. (2000). Remarks presented at the Association of American Medical Colleges Council on Teaching Hospitals Spring meeting, May 11, 2000. www.fda.gov/oc/speeches/2000/aamc511.html

ICH (1997). *General Considerations for Clinical Trials*, FDA, Washington, D.C.

Ioannides, J.P.A. and Lau, J. (2001). Completeness of safety reporting in randomized trials: An evaluation of 7 medical areas. *JAMA* 24: 437–443.

Jones, J.H. (1993). *Bad Blood: Tuskegee Syphilis Experiment*. Free Press, Berkeley.

Kaplowilz, N. (2001). Drug induced liver disorders: Implications for drug development and regulation. *Drug Information Journal*, 35: 347–400.

Mackintosh, D.R. (2001). Bye-Bye Placebos. *Appl. Clinical Trials*, April, 2001, pp. 47–49.

Matoren, G.M. (1984). *The Clinical Research Process in the Pharmaceutical Industry*. Marcel Dekker, New York.

Meinert, C.L. (1996). An open letter to the FDA regarding changes in reporting procedures for drugs and biologics proposed in the wake of the FIAU tragedy. *Controlled Clinical Trials* 17: 273–284.

Nylen, R.A. (2000). *The Ultimate Step-By-Step Guide to Conducting Pharmaceutical Clinical Trials in the USA*. RAN Institute, Tampa, FL.

O'Brien, K.L., Selaniko, J.D. and Heedivert, C. (1998). Epidemic of pediatric deaths from acute renal failure caused by diethylene glycol poisoning. *JAMA* 279: 1175–1180.

O'Grady, J. and Joubert, P.H. (1997). *Phase I/II Clinical Drug Trials*. CRC Press, New York.

O'Grady, J. and Linet, O.I. (1990). *Early Phase Drug Evaluations in Man*. CRC Press, New York.

Office of Inspector General (2000a). Protecting Human Research Subjects: Status of Recommendations, OEI-01-97-00197. Department of Health and Human Services, Washington, D.C., June 2000. www.dhhs.gov/progorg/oei/reports/a447.pdf

Office of Inspector General (2000b). Recruiting Human Subjects: Pressures in Industry-Sponsored Clinical Research, OEI-01-97-00195. Department of Health and Human Services, Washington, D.C., June 2000. www.hhs.gov/oig/oei/reports/a459.pdf

Ozdemir, V., Shear, N.H. and Kalow, W. (2001). What will be the role of pharmacokinetics in evaluating drug safety and minimizing adverse effects? *Drug Safety* 24: 75–85.

Pharmaceutical Research and Manufacturers Association (PhRMA) (2000). www.phrma.org/publications/publications/brochure/questions/whycostmuch.phtml.

Piantadosi, S. (1997). *Clinical Trials: A Methodologic Perspective.* J Wiley, New York.

Reidenberg, M.M. and Lowenthal, D.T. (1968). Adverse non-drug reactions, *N. Engl. J. Med.* 279: 678–679.

Rolan, P.E. (1997). The assessment of pharmacokinetics in early phase drug evaluations. *Handbook of Phase I/II Clinical Drug Trials,* (Grady, J.C. and Joubert, P.H., Eds.). CRC Press, Boca Raton, FL, pp. 169–175.

Rolan, P.E., Mercer, A.J., Weatherly, B.C., Holdich, T., Meire, H., Peck, R.W., Ridout, G. and Posner, J. (1994). Examination of some factors responsible for a food-induced increase in absorption of atovaquone. *Br. J. Clin. Pharmacol.* 37: 13–20.

Sallustio, B.C., Purdie, Y.J., Birkett, D.J. and Meffin, P.J. (1989). Effect of renal dysfunction on the individual components of the acyl-glucuronide futile cycle. *J. Pharmacol. Exp. Ther.* 25: 288–294.

Schmidt, M.J. (2001). Human safety in clinical research. *Appl. Clinical Trials* July, 2001, pp. 40–50.

Shalala, D. (2000). Protecting research subject—What must be done. *N. Engl. J. Med.,* 343 (11), pp. 808–810.

Shamoo, A.E. (2000). Future challenges to human subject protection. *Scientist,* 14 (13) 35, June 26, 2000. www.the-scientist.com/yr2000/jun/opin_000626.html

Sharp, S.M. (2001). The ethical foundations of clinical trials. *Appl. Clinical Trials* April, 2001, pp. 48–54.

Spilker, B. (1991). *Guide to Clinical Trials.* Raven Press, New York.

Washington, N., Washington, C., and Wislons, C.G. (2001). *Physiological Pharmaceutics.* Taylor & Francis, London.

Wechsler, J. (2001). Clinical trial safety and oversight top policy agenda. *Appl. Clinical Trials,* January 2001, pp. 18–21. www.actmagazine.com/articles/act/act0101_jill.pdf

Willman, D. (2000). Quickened pace of drug approvals by FDA taking toll. *San Jose Mercury News,* Dec. 28, 2000.

Wilson, D. (1998). A cautionary tale for human "guinea pigs." *News and Observer* May 8, 1998, p. 4E.

Winek, C.L. (2000). History of excipient safety and toxicity. *Excipient Toxicity and Safety,* (Werner, M.L., and Kotkoskie, L.A., Eds.). Marcel Dekker, New York, pp. 59–72.

World Medical Association (2000). Declaration of Helsinki: Ethical Principles for Medical Research Involving Human Subjects. Adopted by the 18th WMA General Assembly, Helsinki, Finland, June 1964; Amended by the 29th WMA, 1975; 35th WMA, 1983; 41st WMA, 1989; 48th WMA, Somerset West, Republic of South Africa, October 1996; and 52nd WMA, Edinburgh, Scotland, October 2000. www.wma.net/e/policy/17-c_e.html

# 21

# POSTMARKETING SAFETY EVALUATION: MONITORING, ASSESSING, AND REPORTING OF ADVERSE DRUG RESPONSES (ADRs)

## 21.1. INTRODUCTION

Once a new drug is approved it proceeds to market. While this represents the end of a long road, it is also the start of yet another. While careful work during development (both in animals and humans) serves to greatly reduce the potential safety issues around a new drug, it cannot totally eliminate them. One needs only to look at Table 21.1 to appreciate the history of market withdrawals due to safety issues in the modern era (1961–2001), or return to Table 1.1 to verify that the problem is still present and comparable to the past.

Tracking and continuing to evaluate the safety of a therapeutic agent once it is on the market is a complex task. Manufacturers are legally required to collect, analyze and report such data both nationally [by the Food and Drug Administration (FDA) in the United States and by equivalent organizations in other countries, but here the emphasis will be on the U.S. situation] and internationally (by WHO). There are regulatory reporting systems (that is, where the reports go directly to government agencies) and organizational reporting systems (organized around method of distribution, such as hospital pharmacies (ASHP, 1995; Hunziker et al., 1977) or by product type, such as radiopharmaceuticals). Poison control centers also monitor adverse drug reaction cases and rates (Chyka and McEommon, 2000; Chyka, 1999). The regulatory systems for such pharmacosurveillance in the United States are MedWatch (for human drugs), VAERS (for human vaccines) (Niu et al., 1998, 1999; Varrincchio, 1998) and the FDA-CVM system (for veterinary drugs) (Bukowski and

**TABLE 21.1. Therapeutic Products Withdrawn from the Marketplace Due to Safety Reasons in U.K. and/or USA 1961–1995**

| Drug (INN) | Trade Name | Therapeutic Class | Reason(s) for Withdrawal/Suspension of Product License | Launch Date | Countries | License Suspension or Market Withdrawal | Years on Market |
|---|---|---|---|---|---|---|---|
| Acetylsalicylic acid (pediatric) | Aspirin | Analgesic | Reye's Syndrome | 1899 | U.K. | 1986 | 87 |
| Alclofenac | Prinalgin | Non-steroidal anti-inflammatory drug (NSAID) | Skin and renal reactions Mutagenic metabolite | 1972 | U.K. | 1979 | 8 |
| Alphoxalone | Althesin | Anaesthetic | Allergic-type reaction | 1972 | U.K. | 1984 | 12 |
| Aminoglutethimide | Elipten | Anticonvulsant | Endocrinological | 1960 | U.S. | 1966 | 6 |
| | | | Reintroduced: Cushing's Syndrome | 1978 | U.S. | | |
| Aminopyrine | | Analgesic | Hematological | 1900 | U.S. | 1970 | 70 |
| | | | | 1900 | U.K. | 1975 | 75 |
| Astemizole | Hismanal | Antihistamine | Drug–drug interaction | 1988 | U.S. | 1999 | 11 |
| Azaribine | Triazure | Antipsoriatic | Neuropsychiatric coagulation disorders | 1975 | U.S. | 1976 | 1 |
| Benoxaprofen | Opren | NSAID | Cholestatic jaundice | 1980 | U.K. | 1982 | 2 |
| | | | Photosensitivity | 1982 | U.S. | 1982 | <1 |
| Benziodarone | Amplivix | Uricosuric Coronary dilator | Hepatic | 1962 | U.K. | 1964 | 2 |
| Bithionol | Actamer | Anthelminthic | Dermatological | ? | U.S. | 1967 | ? |
| Bronfemic sodium | Duract | NSAID | Liver damage | 1996 | U.S. | 1998 | 3 |
| Cerivastatin sodium | Baycol | Cholesterol lowerers | Muscle weakening | 1999 | U.S. | 2001 | 2 |
| Chlormadinone | Normenon | Hormone | Animal carcinogenicity | 1965 | U.S. | 1970 | 5 |
| | | | | 1996 | U.K. | 1970 | 4 |

| | | | | | | | |
|---|---|---|---|---|---|---|---|
| Cisapride | Propulsid | Heartburn | Cardiovascular irregularities | 1993 | U.S. | 2000 | |
| Clioquinol | Enterovioform | Antidiarrheal | Neuropsychiatric | 1930 | U.K. | 1981 | 51 |
| | | | | 1930 | U.S. | 1973 | 43 |
| Centoxin | HA-1A | Hu-anti-lipid A IgM monoclonal | Gram negative septicemia | 1990 | U.K. | 1992 | 2 |
| Danthron | Dorbanex | Laxative | Animal carcinogenicity | 1959 | U.S. | 1987 | 28 |
| | | | Reintroduced with restrictions | 1964 | U.K. | 1987 | 23 |
| Desensitizing vaccines | Various | Vaccine | Allergic-type reactions | ? | U.K. | 1989 | |
| Diamthazole | Asterol | Antifungal | Neuropsychiatric | ? | U.S. | 1970 | 17 |
| Dihydrostreptomycin | | Antibiotic | Neuropsychiatric | ? | U.S. | 1970 | ? |
| Dinoprostone | Propess | Hormone | Uterine hypertonus and fetal distress | 1989 | U.K. | 1990 | <1 |
| Dipyrone | | Analgesic | Hematological | 1930 | U.S. | 1977 | 47 |
| | | | | 1930 | U.K. | 1977 | 47 |
| Dithiazanine | | Anthelmintic | Metabolic Cardiovascular | ? | U.S. | 1964 | |
| Domperidone (injection) | Motilium | Antiemetic | Cardiovascular risk of overdose | 1984 | U.K. | 1986 | 2 |
| Doxylamine | Bendectin | Antihistamine | Fear of teratogenicity: dysmorphogenicity? | 1956 | U.S. | 1983 | 27 |
| Dicyclomine | Debendox | | | 1957 | U.K. | 1983 | 26 |
| Encainide | Enkaid | Antiarrhythmic | Cardiovascular | 1987 | U.S. | 1991 | 4 |
| Factor VIII | Factorate | Coagulation factor | Excess mortality risk Manufacture problem Risk of AIDS transmission | 1972 | U.K. | 1986 | 14 |

(continued)

**TABLE 21.1.** (*continued*)

| Drug (INN) | Trade Name | Therapeutic Class | Reason(s) for Withdrawal/Suspension of Product License | Launch Date | Countries | License Suspension or Market Withdrawal | Years on Market |
|---|---|---|---|---|---|---|---|
| Fenclofenac | Flenac | NSAID | Multiple: especially skin reactions | 1978 | U.K. | 1984 | 6 |
| Feprazone | Methrazone | NSAID | Multiple | 1976 | U.K. | 1984 | 8 |
|  |  |  |  |  |  | 1984 | 8 |
| Flosequinan | Manoplax | Heart failure | Increased mortality Lack of long-term efficacy | 1992 | U.K. | 1993 1993 | 9 months |
| Grepafloxacin | Raxar | Quinolone antibiotic | Q-T interval prolongation | 1997 | U.S. | 1999 | 23 months |
| Growth Hormone (natural) | Crescormon | Hormone | Manufacture problem | 1970 | U.K. | 1985 | 15 |
|  |  |  | Creutzfeldt–Jakob disease transmission | 1970 | U.S. | 1985 |  |
| Guanethidine | Ganda (high dose) | Anti-glaucoma eye drops | Ophthalmological | 1977 | U.K. | 1986 | 9 |
| Ibufenac | Dytransin | NSAID | Hepatic | 1966 | U.K. | 1968 | 2 |
| Indomethacin-R | Osmosin form | NSAID | Multiple gastrointestinal: 36 fatal small intestine perforations | 1982 | U.K. | 1983 | 9 months |
| Indoprofen | Flosint | NSAID | Gastrointestinal carcinogenicity | 1982 | U.K. | 1983 1984 | 1 ?2 |
| Iodinated casein strophantin | Coratose | Anorexiant | Metabolic | ? | ? | 1964 | ? |

| — | Lotanex | Irritable bowel syndrome | Ischemic colitis | 2000 | U.S. | 2000 | 9 months |
| Mebanazine | Actomol | Antidepressant | Hepatic drug interactions | 1963 | U.K. | 1975 | 12 |
| Megestrol acetate | Volidan 21 | Hormone | Carcinogenicity | 1963 | U.K. | 1970 1969 1975 | 7 |
| Methandrostenolone | Dianabol | Hormone | Endocrinological | 1960 | U.S. | 1982 | 12 |
| Methapyrilene | | H1 antihistamine | Carcinogenicity | 1947 | U.S. | 1979 | 31 |
| | | | | 1950 | U.K. | 1979 | 29 |
| Metipranolol | Glauline | Antiglaucoma eye drops | Ophthalmological: uveitis (high dose) | ? | U.K. | 1990 | ? |
| | | | Low-dose preparation | | | 1991 | |
| Metofoline | Versidyne | Analgesic | Experimental toxicity | ? | | 1965 | ? |
| Midefradil | Posicor | Calcium channel blocker | Lethal drug interadion (Inhibited liver enzymes) | 1996 | U.S. | 1998 | 3 |
| Mumps vaccine Urabe AM9 strain | Pariorix | Vaccine | Neuropsychiatric | 1988 | U.K. | 1992 | 4 |
| | | | Meningitis | 1988 | U.S. | 1992 | 4 |
| Neomycin (injection) | | Antibiotic | Misuse | ? | U.S. | 1989 | ? |
| | | | Irrigation of open wounds | | | | |
| Nialamide | Niamid | Antidepressant (MAOI) | Hepatic | 1959 | U.K. | 1978 | 19 |
| | | | Drug interactions | 1959 | U.S. | 1974 | 15 |
| Normifensin | Merital | Antidepressant | Hemolytic anemia | 1977 | U.K. | 1986 | 9 |
| | | | Hepatotoxicity-fetal hepatitis | | | | |
| Oxphenbutazone | Tanderil | NSAID | Hematological | 1960 | U.S. | 1985 | 25 |
| | | | Multiple | 1962 | U.K. | 1984 | 22 |
| Oxyphenisatin | Veripaque | Laxative | Hepatic | 1955 | U.K. | 1978 | 23 |
| | | | | 1957 | U.S. | 1972 | 15 |

(continued)

**TABLE 21.1.** (*continued*)

| Drug (INN) | Trade Name | Therapeutic Class | Reason(s) for Withdrawal/Suspension of Product License | Launch Date | Countries | License Suspension or Market Withdrawal | Years on Market |
|---|---|---|---|---|---|---|---|
| Perhexiline maleate | Pexid | | Hepatic damage<br>Peripheral neuropathy | 1975 | U.K. | 1985 | 10 |
| Phenacetin | — | Analgesic | Renal carcinogenicity | <1900<br>1900 | U.K.<br>U.S. | 1980<br>1983 | 80<br>83 |
| Phen-fen | Fenfuramine/dexafluramine | Diet aid | Heart valve abnormality | 1973 | U.S. | 1997 | 24 |
| Phenformin | Insoral<br>Dibotin | Antidiabetic | Metabolic | 1959<br>1959 | U.K.<br>U.S. | 1982<br>1977 | 23<br>18 |
| Phenoxypropazine | Drazine | Antidepressant (MAOI) | Hepatic | 1961 | U.K. | 1966 | 5 |
| Phenylpropanolamine | PPA | CTC ingredient | Drug interactions<br>Hemorrhagic stroke | 1936 | U.S. | 2001 | 65 |
| Pituitary chorionic hormone | | Hormone | Hypersensitivity | ? | U.K. | 1972 | ? |
| Polidexide | Secholex | Antihyperlipidemic | Experimental toxicity<br>Toxic impurities | 1974 | U.K. | 1975 | 1 |
| Practolol | Eraldin | Beta blocker | Oculomucocutaneous syndrome<br>Deafness<br>Sclerosing peritonitis | 1970 | U.K. | 1989 | 16 |
| Prenylamine | Segontin<br>Synadrin | Antianginal | Cardiovascular | 1973 | U.K. | 1989 | 16 |
| Pronethalol | Alderlin | Beta blocker | Animal carcinogenicity | 1963 | U.K. | 1965 | 2 |

| Remoxipride | Roxiam | Antipsychotic | Hematological–aplastic anemia | 1991 | U.K. | 1994 | 3 |
| Rotashield | — | Rotavirus vaccine | Bowel obstruction | 1998 | U.S. | 1999 | 1 |
| Somatropin | Crescormone | Natural growth hormone | Creutzfeldt–Jakob disease | 1973 | U.K. | 1985 | 12 |
| Sulfamethoxy-pyridazine | Lederkyn | Antiinfective | Hematological Dermatological | ? | U.K. | 1986 | ? |
| Supofren | Suprol | NSAID | Renal | 1986 | U.S. | 1987 1987 | 1 |
| Temafloxacin | Omniflox Teflox | Antiinfective | Hepatic dysfunction Hemolytic anemia Nephrological Anaphylaxis Metabolic | 1991 1992 | U.K. U.S. | 1992 1992 | 1 4 months |
| Terolidine | Micturin | Urinary incontinence | Cardiac arrhythmia | 1986 | U.K. | 1991 | 5 |
| Tetracycline (pediatric form) | Achromycin V | Antibiotic | Teeth discoloration | 1952 | U.S. | 1979 | 27 |
| Thalidomide | Contergan Distaval | Sedative Orphan Drug Inds | Teratogenicity Phocomelia | 1956 | U.K. | 1961 | 5 |
| Thenalidine | | H1 antihistamine | Hematological | | | 1961 | ? |
| Ticrynafen | Selacryn Diflurex | Diuretic | Hepatic | 1979 | U.S. | 1980 | 1 |
| Triazolam | Halcion | Hypnotic | Neuropsychiatric: memory loss, depression | 1979 | U.K. | 1991 | 12 |
| | | | | 1983 | U.S. | NW | |
| Triparanol | MER-29 | Antihyperlipidemic | Ophthalmological | 1959 | U.S. | 1962 | 3 |
| Troglitazone | Renzulin | Type II diabetes | Liver damage | 1996 | U.S. | 2000 | 5 |

(continued)

**TABLE 21.1.** (*continued*)

| Drug (INN) | Trade Name | Therapeutic Class | Reason(s) for Withdrawal/Suspension of Product License | Launch Date | Countries | License Suspension or Market Withdrawal | Years on Market |
|---|---|---|---|---|---|---|---|
| Trovafloxacin | Trovan | Antibiotic | Liver/kidney damage | 1992 | U.S. | 1999 (use severely restricted) | 7 |
| Tryptophan | Pacitron Optimax | Low protein diet reintroduced with OPTICs monitor | Eosinophilic myalgia syndrome | 1974 | U.S. | 1989 1990 | 15 |
| Vitamin E | E-Ferol | Vitamin | Hematological Hepatic Renal | 1983 | U.S. | 1984 | 1 |
| Zomepirac | Zomax | NSAID | Allergic-type reactions: fatal anaphylaxis | 1980 1981 | U.S. U.K. | 1983 1983 | 3 2 |
| Zimeldine | Zelmid | Antidepressant | Hepatotoxicity Neurological–peripheral neuropathy, Guillain–Barré syndrome | 1982 | U.K. | 1983 | 1 |

Wartenberg, 1996; Keller et al., 1998). One key difference of the U.S. systems from those in other countries is that they are voluntary (largely a reflection of the primarily private, that is, not national government, health care system in America).

There is no compulsion for physicians, hospitals or individuals to report adverse events to either the manufacturer or the government (though the marketing companies for a therapeutic are required to periodically send summaries of all reports of adverse events that they know of to the federal government). It is widely held that it is this voluntary (or "spontaneous") aspect which limits the effectiveness of the U.S. systems (Piazza-Hepp and Kennedy, 1995; Sharpe, 1988; White and Love, 1998; Goldman, 1998; Kennedy and Goldman, 1997; Brewer and Colditz, 1999). Studies have identified factors which influence (and limit) physician use of such systems (LaCalamita, 1995; Figueras et al., 1999), and newly marketed drugs are subject to a higher rate of underreporting of ADRs than are established drugs (Martin et al., 1998). It should be kept in mind that what we are considering here are adverse effects caused by the use of a drug as intended, and not by a medication error. Medication errors are at least as serious a problem (and complex an issue) as ADRs (Antonow et al., 2000), but are beyond the scope of this volume. Both companies and the regulatory agencies must collect reports of adverse events, evaluate them, and then decide on a correct course of action (ranging from doing nothing through improving labeling, then on to restricting access and/or requiring ongoing or increased medical surveillance of patients, to withdrawing the drug from the market).

## 21.2. CAUSES OF SAFETY WITHDRAWALS

It would be comforting to be able to state that the causes of postmarketing withdrawals from drugs were substantially different from those of failure of drugs in clinical trials. While the last few years (refer back to Table 1.1) are seemingly somewhat different from those in the past, the historic causes for the modern era (the last 40 years) are lead off by hepatic toxicity, also the primary cause for safety failure in early clinical trials.

Fung et al. (2001) have done an extensive assembly and analysis of safety withdrawal data through 1999, and Ajayi et al. (2000) have also analyzed factors increasing the likelihood of safety problems. Table 21.2 presents this author's extension of their work to the time of this writing (late in the third quarter of 2001), which changes the results but little. It should be noted that the rank orders of these two lists is different than the rank orders based on numbers of adverse events (see Holland and DeGruz, 1997). Adverse events can have a wide range of causes which may not even be due to unanticipated effects of a drug, but due to a medication error or something as mundane as the discrepancies between doses recommended in *The Physician's Desk Reference* and those recommended or reported in the medical literature (Cohen, 2001).

Failure to identify these largely predictable causes of failures in new therapeutic entities largely reflects both a continuing lack of recognition of the actual patient

**TABLE 21.2. Characteristics of Drug Safety Withdrawals (1960–August 2001)**

|  | Drugs | % of Total |
|---|---|---|
| A. Most Common Classes |  |  |
| NSAIDs | 16 | 13 |
| Nonnarcotic analgesics | 10 | 8 |
| Antidepressants | 9 | 7 |
| Vasodilators | 7 | 6 |
| Anorexiants | 5 | 4 |
| CNS stimulants | 5 | 4 |
| Barbiturates | 5 | 4 |
| Anesthetics | 4 | 3 |
| Antihistamines | 4 | 3 |
| Antibiotics | 3 | 2 |
| B. Most Common Causes of Withdrawal |  |  |
| Hepatic toxicity |  | 26 |
| Hematologic toxicity (bone marrow suppression) |  | 10 |
| Cardiovascular toxicity |  | 6 |
| Carcinogenicity |  | 6 |
| Renal toxicity |  | 5 |
| Drug interactions |  | 4 |
| Neurotoxicity |  | 4 |
| Behavioral effects |  | 4 |
| Abuse potential |  | 4 |

populations utilizing drugs with their existing pathophysiological characteristics (Table 21.3) and the limitations of the currently employed clinical trial scheme (Table 21.4). While such efforts as mandatory assessment of safety pharmacology features will serve to improve the situation, for the foreseeable future it remains vital to ensure that our pharmacovigilance systems identify problems as soon as possible.

**TABLE 21.3. Factors that Increase Patient Risk for Adverse Drug Interactions**

| Factor | Group/Disorder |
|---|---|
| Age | Neonates, elderly |
| Gender | Women |
| Genetic phenotype | Slow metabolizers |
| Chronic disease | Moderate/severe renal or hepatic impairment, CHF, cirrhosis |
| Acute illness | Pneumonia, influenza |
| Metabolic disturbances | Hypothyroidism, hypoxia |
| Multiple drug use | Elderly, HIV patients |
| Multiple prescribing physicians | Elderly |
| Use of drugs with a low therapeutic index |  |
| Use of drugs that are enzyme inhibitors or inducers |  |

**TABLE 21.4. Limitations of the FDA's Current Clinical Trials**

| | |
|---|---|
| 1. Too few | Prior to approval, most drugs are administered to 2,000 to 3,000 patients. (To obtain an 80% probability of detecting an adverse drug event that occurs in one out of every 10,000 recipients, 16,000 patients must receive the drug). |
| 2. Too simple | Premarketing trials often exclude patients with complicated medical histories or medication regimens. It is easier to demonstrate efficacy without including these complex patients. |
| 3. Too median | Most premarketing trials exclude patient populations such as pediatric, geriatric, lactating, and pregnant patients. |
| 4. Too narrow | Premarketing trials are generally intended to investigate a drug for a single indication. After release to the market, the drug may be used to treat other conditions in different populations with varying medical histories. |
| 5. Too brief | Adverse drug events that occur only with chronic use will not be detected in the relatively short clinical trial. |

*Source:* Rogers, 1987.

## 21.3. REGULATORY REQUIREMENTS

Regulations and guidelines concerning pharmacovigilance have been in a continuous state of change and development in recent years. A discussion of these should start with the understanding of the individual incident, or "case".

A "case" is a basic unit of drug safety surveillance. It is used to assure, to the greatest extent possible, the safety of approved drug products that are still in use. The basic unit of all postmarketing safety submissions is the adverse drug experience "case", which is an individual adverse drug experience.

FDA has explicit requirements for reporting of adverse event cases for drugs. A postmarketing adverse drug experience source can be categorized into the several sample categories: clinical trial, nonclinical trial and regulatory authority, nonclinical trial and literature, nonclinical trial and all other. This chapter only deals with spontaneous experiences: nonclinical trial adverse drug experiences reported to the industry any time after a marketed drug product achieves marketing approval from FDA (Adams et al., 1997).

When one looks at a typical case folder, he notices that certain types of information are on or in the folder.

- The outside of a folder is identified by a (alpha) numeric code;
- There is an "initial" report;
- There is either at least one letter requesting additional information regarding the initial report or documentation reflecting the failed attempts to obtain additional information;
- There is at least one "follow-up" report;

- The spontaneous report event is categorized as serious or nonserious, expected or unexpected;
- The source is either literature, regulatory authority or spontaneous;
- There is at least one MedWatch form or CIOMS I form for each report.

Everything in a given case folder is present because of an FDA regulation requirement or a related company-written standard operating procedure.

The number on the outside of the case is required to be numeric or alphanumeric, not the name of the patient. Patient names are not permitted to be publicly disclosed in the context of a MedWatch report according to 21 CFR 21.63(f). The initial report is the first reported information received by the company about an individual's adverse drug experience. There must be a "prompt" attempt to obtain follow-up information about each initial report. The attempt(s) are made according to the company's written procedures. If the written safety procedures are not followed, the safety reports are not appropriately submitted, or the safety records are not appropriately kept, FDA has the authority under Section 80 of Part 315 to withdraw the market NDA. The follow-up report is the format for submitting additional information about an experience. Each case regards only one individual unless the experience is both temporally and clinically unrelated to a second event experienced by the same person taking the same drug product.

Table 21.5 summarizes FDA reporting requirements for spontaneous reports in terms of how the case event is first submitted to the agency. The definitions of serious, unexpected, and so forth, are in 21 CFR 314.80(a) (CFR, 1994).

### 21.3.1. The 15-Day Report versus the U.S. Periodic Report

Postmarketing adverse drug experiences are reported to a drug company by the public via regulatory authorities, literature, attorneys, consumers, and health

**TABLE 21.5. How a Spontaneous Drug Case is First Submitted to the Food and Drug Administration**

| Case Source/Case Type | Report Submitted |
| --- | --- |
| Foreign literature/NOT both serious and unexpected | NOT 15-day, NOT Periodic |
| Foreign literature/serious and unexpected | 15-day |
| U.S. Consumer/NOT both serious and unexpected | Periodic |
| U.S. consumer/serious, unexpected | 15-day |
| Foreign consumer/NOT both serious and unexpected | NOT 15-day, NOT Periodic |
| Foreign consumer/serious, unexpected | 15-day |
| FDA, initial/serious and unexpected | 15-day |
| FDA, initial/serious and unexpected | Periodic, NOT 15-day |
| International regulatory authority/serious and unexpected | 15-day |
| International regulatory authority/NOT serious and unexpected | NOT 15-day, NOT Periodic |

professionals. Sometimes a company receives a report of an adverse experience someone had after taking its drug product not from the public, but from FDA because instead of submitting the report to the company, the report was submitted directly to the agency. When FDA sends the applicant an initial MedWatch report, the information does not have to be resubmitted to the agency in an initial 15-day report if the information is serious and unexpected. This is because FDA already has knowledge of the report. However, the MedWatch report and its information are incorporated into the next periodic report of the product. FDA's MedWatch report obtained from a non-FDA source, would be submitted as a follow-up, expedited 15-day report (and should reference the source of the initial report).

If an initial 15-day report was submitted, and the first follow-up information reflects that the event is no longer classified as a 15-day report (never was serious and unexpected), the first follow-up report describes the change in the report classification but is a (first) follow-up 15-day report. Subsequent additional information is not submitted in the form of a 15-day report.

A periodic report contains certain information, such as the event terms submitted during the period, the dates that events of the period were submitted, an event term count by body system, and labeling changes made due to the period's adverse experiences. In addition to (and prior to) being incorporated into a periodic report, 15-day reports are submitted within 15 calendar days of the date the applicant received the data. All 15-day reports contain serious, unexpected events. Non-15-day reports are submitted periodically in FDA periodic reports.

If on a given day a serious, unexpected domestic report is received, it is submitted first on an FDA Form 3500A, within 15 calendar days of receipt, via the 15-day report and subsequently is incorporated (not in the form of an FDA Form 3500A) into a periodic report. If a report is received that is domestic but not both serious and unexpected, it is not submitted in a 15-day report but rather in the U.S. periodic report. A U.S. periodic report is submitted quarterly for the first three years after the date the product was approved by FDA for marketing (21 CFR 314.80). However, the March 2001 FDA guidance allows an applicant to request a 21 CFR 314.90 waiver of the U.S. periodic report reporting period and base the report not on the date of FDA marketing approval but instead on the international birth date (the first date the product was approved in the international community). The request for such a waiver should be submitted to Director; Office of Postmarketing Drug Risk Assessment; CDER; FDA; 5600 Fishers Lane; HFD-400, Rockville, MD 20857. The request should include the product's name, the date of FDA marketing approval, and the product's approved application number. In addition, an applicant may request a 21 CFR 314.90 waiver of the 21 CFR 314.80©(2)(ii) format of the periodic report submitted. If the waiver is granted, the ICH E2C Periodic Safety Update Report format may be used provided the content of the section 80©(2)(ii) information that is not in the body of the ICH E2C periodic report is found in appendices, that is, certain reports from consumers that are not in the body of the ICH E2C periodic report submission. 21 CFR 314.90 states, among other things, that the applicant may request FDA to waive any of the postmarketing requirements under 21 CFR 314.80.

ICH E2C and FDA March 2001 draft guidance *Postmarketing Safety Reporting for Human Drug and Biological Products Including Vaccines* are available at www.fda.gov/cder/guidance/index.htm; "case" requirements are accessible in 21 CFR 314.80.

The major change over the past few years has been a significant attempt to harmonize regulations under the aegis of the International Conference of Harmonization (ICH), and this is covered in some depth in the following. The latest response to the ICH in its three participating regions (Europe, U.S., and Japan) is also described together with an update on the current U.K. regulations. The ICH potentially offers real advantages to the pharmaceutical industry, but the process takes time and countries have adopted and implemented the guidance in slightly different ways and at different times. National regulations and guidelines are therefore bound to change in the near future as each country embraces the ICH.

The ICH of Technical Requirements for Registration of Pharmaceuticals for Human Use has brought together as equal partners the regulatory authorities of Europe, Japan and the U.S. and experts from the pharmaceutical industry in these regions to discuss scientific and technical aspects of product registration. The World Health Organization (WHO), European Free Trade Area (EFTA) and Canada are observers, and the International Federation of Pharmaceutical Manufacturers Association (IFPMA) ensures contact with the research-based industry outside the ICH regions.

The aim of the ICH is to achieve greater harmonization in the interpretation and application of technical guidelines and requirements for product registration and reduce or eliminate duplicate testing. This should result in better use of resources and eliminate unnecessary delay in the global development and availability of new medicines while maintaining safety guards on quality, safety and efficacy.

There are four broad topic areas within the ICH.

S    Safety (animal toxicology and pharmacology);
Q    Quality (pharmaceutical and analytical);
E    Efficacy (clinical);
M    Multidisciplinary topics.


Timely, complete reporting of adverse drug reactions (ADRs ) and medical device problems is essential to an effective national system of postmarketing surveillance. Pharmaceutical manufacturers are required by federal regulations to report all ADRs of which they are aware to FDA. However, many health care professionals do not think to report adverse events either to the manufacturers or to the agency. To encourage and facilitate the reporting of serious adverse events, FDA launched the MedWatch reporting program in June 1993. The MedWatch reporting form is used by health care professionals to voluntarily report ADRs and other problems with all FDA-regulated products used in medical therapy (drugs, biologics, medical devices, and special nutritional agents). The reporting of ADRs associated with vaccine products is the only exception, since reporting of those ADRs is mandatory. The form used for vaccines is the joint FDA/Centers for Disease Control and Prevention

Vaccine Adverse Event Reporting System (VAERS) form. For drugs and therapeutic biologics, the MedWatch (3500A) form replaces the 1639 reporting form.

FDA does not want reports on every adverse event observed; that would not be practical for reporters or FDA because of the sheer volume of adverse-event reports already being sent to the agency each year (about 130,000 in 1994). While 80–85% of these reports are submitted by the manufacturer, 10–15% are received by MedWatch directly from physicians, pharmacists, other health care professionals, and consumers. MedWatch encourages reporters to be selective by limiting their reports to events for which the outcome was serious (Table 20.2). This enables FDA to focus on those events with potentially the largest public health impact. Reporters are encouraged to fill out the reporting form as completely and accurately as possible.

From 1978 through 1990, the Centers for Disease Control and Prevention (CDC) and the Food and Drug Administration divided the responsibility for postmarketing surveillance of vaccines in the United States. FDA received reports of adverse events after vaccines were administered in the private sector; events occurring after the administration of vaccines purchased with public funds were reported to the Monitoring System for Adverse Events Following Immunization.

The monitoring system was a stimulated passive surveillance system. In other words, when vaccines purchased with federal funds were administered in the public sector, "Important Information" forms were given to recipients or their parents or guardians instructing them to report any illnesses requiring medical attention that occurred within four weeks of vaccination. System coordinators at each immunization project or grantee site and the state health department completed standardized forms that were reviewed for consistency and completeness and then forwarded to the CDC for data entry and analysis.

In response to the National Childhood Vaccine Injury Act of 1988, which required health workers to report vaccine adverse events, the CDC and the FDA collaborated in 1990 to implement the Vaccine Adverse Event Reporting System (VAERS) to monitor the safety of vaccines in both sectors. Health care professionals and parent or other caretakers are encouraged to report all clinically significant vaccine adverse events. Narrative diagnostic reports are reviewed and assigned standard codes using Coding Symbols for a Thesaurus of Adverse Reaction Terms. The source of the vaccines (public versus private provider) is recorded on the form.

The WHO system, created in response to the thalidomide disaster, seeks to capture worldwide adverse events and identifies problems (WHO, 1975; Olsson, 1998). It is proposed that all such gathered reports should first be analyzed for mortality effects and trends (Rose and Elnis, 2000) as such would identify the most critical trends and be easiest to evaluate.

## 21.4. MANAGEMENT OF ADR AND ADE DATA

In monitoring the safety of products, pharmaceutical companies need to comply with worldwide regulations as well as the primary requirement of helping doctors to prescribe safely. It is not intended to provide a comprehensive review in this chapter, but to provide an insight into the methods of managing ADR data.

### 21.4.1. Sources of Data

There can be an enormous variation in the nature and quality of data depending upon the source, and this must be considered when the data is processed, computerized and analyzed. Safety data may come from any of the sources mentioned in the following.

*Clinical Trials.* In Phase I studies, good documentation and additional investigations should be standard practice. Serious reactions are pretty unusual in these studies, which will detect only very common ADRs, in particular those that are pharmacologically mediated (e.g., bradycardia with beta adrenergic receptor antagonists).

Good documentation and follow-up should be possible in Phase II studies, but rare reactions will not be identified due to the small numbers of patients involved. The larger numbers in Phase III trials can pose problems, but these can be minimized by careful choice of investigators, good case report form design and procedures for follow-up. Phase IV studies are designed to test the efficacy and safety of the drug in clinical practice and often share the same constraints in patient numbers as premarketing trials.

*Postmarketing Surveillance Studies.* Any surveillance of safety of a drug after marketing is postmarketing surveillance (PMS) (now often referred to as a postauthorization safety study). In practice the distinction between Phase IV studies and PMS is blurred (e.g., German drug experience studies).

*Spontaneous Reports.* Spontaneous reports are the most effective means of identifying rare, serious adverse reactions (usually idiosyncratic or type B) after marketing despite the under-reporting that exists. Spontaneous reports are an unsolicited communication to a company, regulatory authority or other organization that describes an AE in a patient given one or more medical products. These reports do not originate from a study or from any organized data collection scheme. Unless indicated otherwise by the reporter, all spontaneous AEs are assumed to be possible ADRs. The quality and completeness of spontaneous reports is often inadequate. Pharmaceutical companies or regulatory authorities can only achieve good case documentation through effective data collection, detailed follow-up and the use of field workers for complex cases. The quality of spontaneous reports also varies from country to country. Some countries do not have a regulatory reporting form for ADRs. There are differences among countries in publicity of drug safety issues and drug regulations differ regarding the format, content and submission timeframes for ADR reporting.

Reports received by companies via regulatory authorities are often edited and poorly documented, but they cannot be ignored and should be handled alongside reports received directly. The FDA implemented the Medical Products Reporting Program (MedWatch) in 1993, which encourages health care providers to regard reporting as a fundamental professional and public health responsibility and submit serious AE reports directly to FDA on the FDA3500A form. FDA forwards these reports to the manufacturer, who is obliged to follow up with those reporting such events, and submit any relevant information obtained to FDA and other regulatory agencies worldwide as required. It is currently proposed that regulatory agencies (FDA) should take a more direct hand in these activities (Snidermann, 2000).

***Literature.*** The publication of case reports in medical and scientific journals is an important primary source of information on ADRs. Many ADRs are noted in medical and scientific journals before they become well known. For example, the association of thalidomide with birth defects was first noted in a letter to the *Lancet* in 1961. The quality of ADR reports in the published literature can be variable and has been the subject of much criticism and correspondence, though guidelines have been promulgated for these (Jones, 1982).

Despite the anecdotal nature and sometimes poor documentation, publication of case reports in journals remains one of the most useful primary sources of information on ADRs. ADR reports in the literature can be identified in several different ways. Prepublication manuscripts describing a spontaneous case report or an event from a clinical trial are sometimes provided by authors to the manufacturer of the drug and the regulatory authority in that country. Pharmaceutical companies are required to be aware of the literature as to the safety of their approved therapeutic products, and are assumed (by law) to be cognizant of such.

*Searching for ADRs in the Literature.* With the increasing number of scientific and biomedical journals there are more sources of ADR data on many drugs. Conversely, for some drugs, particularly those recently marketed, there is a scarcity of clinical publications and frequently there is an inadequate account of the adverse reaction profile. Searching for ADRs in the literature may be assisted by online databases such as MEDLINE (Index Medicus), EMBASE (Excerpta Medica) and secondary sources such as SEDBASE (Meyler's side effects of drugs) and ADIS online services such as REACTIONS. Many journals contain relevant information, but some specific ADR-related journals may assist in the search for information. Increasingly, the use of high-capacity storage systems such as compact disks (CD-ROM) has led to stand-alone systems for storage and search of the literature other than online systems. Integrated dictionaries have allowed the development of user-friendly information; however, due to the anecdotal nature of these reports, pharmaceutical companies should have a clear policy on how to handle them.

### 21.4.2. Information Required for Reports

In order to draw a conclusion about the possible relationship between a drug and an AE certain minimal information elements are required. Points considered essential for literature reports have been proposed (Jones, 1982) and some journals issue guidelines or checklists for potential authors. These can be adapted as a potential checklist for information that should be included in any ADR report as follows:

*Patient Demography.* Age, sex, body weight, height, race, pregnancy.

*Medical History.* Previous medical history and concurrent conditions, known allergies (including ADRs with similar drugs), previous experience with drug.

*Timing.* Duration of treatment with the suspect drug before AE.

*Concurrent Medications.* Details of other drugs including formulation, dose and duration.

*Dechallenge.* Action taken with the suspect drug (stopped, continued, dose reduction).

*Outcome.* Outcomes of the AEs.

*Alternative Causes.* What other factors could have accounted for the AE (diet, occupations exposure) and which were excluded?

*Rechallenge.* Was the patient rechallenged, and if so, what was the result?

*Relevant Additional Data.* Blood levels, laboratory data, biopsy data and where relevant, postmortem findings.

***Adverse Drug Reaction Forms and Form Design.*** Many forms are used by different organizations to collect ADR information. Most regulatory authorities have their own form (see Figure 21.1, the Food and Drug Administration 3500a). Although the content of these forms is similar, little attempt has been made to standardize the design other than by the Council for International Organization of Medical Sciences (CIOMS).

In order to design the best form for their needs, users must first define what data they wish to collect and which factors are of the greatest importance. In addition, all the usual factors in form design need to be considered (e.g., size, layout, color, print type, spacing, flow of questions, boxes, language, and instructions). A pilot to test the form should be carried out before formal introduction and use.

Consideration should be given to what happens to the form once it is returned. Form design will be affected depending upon whether it is intended to serve as a direct entry document (i.e., the data elements closely match the data entry screens), or whether a transcription document will be used.

The key factor in ADR form design is the compatibility with other forms required for output, most importantly regulatory authority forms. The FDA, for example, required ADR reports to be submitted on an FDA3500A (Figure 21.1). If the pharmaceutical company does not wish to collect data on an FDA3500A but must submit reports to the FDA, it will need to design a form that collects the same information. Adverse event report forms generally collect the basic data elements listed on page 850.

**Food and Drug Administration (FDA) 3500A**

# MED**W**ATCH

THE FDA MEDICAL PRODUCTS REPORTING PROGRAM

Approved by FDA on 3/27

Mfr report #

UF/Dist report #

FDA Use Only

---

**1. Patient identifier** — in confidence

**2. Age at time of event:** or________ **Date of birth:**

**3. Sex** ☐ female ☐ male

**4. Weight** ________lbs or ________kgs

**1. ☐ Adverse event and/or ☐ Product problem** (e.g., defects/malfunctions)

**2. Outcomes attributed to adverse event** (check all that apply)

death____________ (mo/day/yr)

☐ life threatening

☐ hospitalization – initial or prolonged

☐ disability

☐ congenital anomaly

☐ required interventio0n to prevent permanent impairment/damage

☐ other:____________

**3. Date of event** (mo/day/yr)

**4. Date of this report** (mo/day/yr)

**5. Describe event or problem**

**6. Relevant tests/laboratory data,** including dates

**7. Other relevant history, including preexisting medical conditions** (e.g. allergies, race, pregnancy, smoking and alcohol use, hepatic/renal dysfunction, etc.)

---

**1. Name** (give labeled strength & mfr/labeler, if known)

#1____________

#2

**2. Dose, frequency & route used**

#1____________

#2

**3. Therapy date** (if unknown, give duration) from/to (or best estimate)

#1____________

#2

**4. Diagnosis for use** (indication)

#1____________

#2

**5. Event abated after use stopped or dose reduced**

#1 ☐ yes ☐ no ☐ doesn't apply

#2 ☐ yes ☐ no ☐ doesn't apply

**6. Lot #** (if known)

#1________

#2

**7. Ex. date** (if known)

#1________

#2

**8. Event reappeared after reintroduction**

#1 ☐ yes ☐ no ☐ doesn't apply

#2 ☐ yes ☐ no ☐ doesn't apply

**9. NDC #** - for product problems only (if known)

#1    #2

**10. Concomitant medical products** and therapy dates (exclude treatment of event)

NI

**1. Contact office – name/address** (& mfring site for devices)

**2. Phone number**

**3. Report Source** (check all that apply)
☐ foreign
☐ study
☐ literature
☐ consumer
☐ health professional
☐ user facility
☐ company representative
☐ distributor
☐ other:

**4. Date received by manufacturer** (mo/day/yr)

**6. If IND, protocol #**

**5.** (A)NDA#________  IND#________  PLA#________

pre-1938 ☐ yes
OTC product ☐ yes

**7. Type of report** (check all that apply)
☐ 5-day    ☐ 15-day
☐ 10-day   ☐ periodic
☐ initial  ☐ follow-up

**9. Mfr. report number**

**8. Adverse event term(s)**

**1. Name, address & phone #**

**2. Health professional?** ☐ yes ☐ no

**3. Occupation**

**4. Initial reported also sent report to FDA** ☐ yes ☐ no ☐ unk

---

**FDA**

Domain Facsimile of FDA Form 3500A

Submission of a report does not constitute an admission that medical personnel, user facility, distributor, manufacturer or product caused or contributed to the event

**FIGURE 21.1.** The FDA Form 3500A (as MEDWATCH form) is used to make initial reports of each and every serious drug-related event. Its use by physicians and hospitals is voluntary, however.

- Patient demography.
- Relevant medical history and allergies.
- Suspect and concurrent drugs, route, indication.
- AE(s).
- Treatment and management of AE.
- Dechallenge, rechallenge, outcome.
- Relevant laboratory data.
- Reporter's opinion of causality.
- Report source of information.

The form can be printed as a folding postage prepaid envelope for domestic use to encourage a reply. The pharmaceutical company must be able to demonstrate due diligence in seeking relevant follow-up information on each AE report.

Within the next two years, several key regulatory authorities including the MCA (Medicines Control Agency) and FDA will require electronic data submission by companies for both expedited and nonexpedited case reports. The compatibility between the company's and the regulatory authority's databases with regard to content and format of the key data elements for transmission is a critical factor to success of these initiatives. The adoption of internationally sanctioned standards such as a dictionary of medical terms, various code lists (e.g., countries, routes, units), file formats, and periodic safety update reports are essential to enable efficient and accurate transmission. The International Conference on Harmonization (ICH) guideline (ICH E2B) defines data elements for transmission of individual case safety reports. The guidelines aim to standardize the data elements for all individual case safety reports regardless of source and destination and covers reports for both preapproval and postapproval periods. It also defines the minimum information for a report and the requirements for proper processing of the report. The medium for electronic submissions will be Electronic Data Interchange (EDI)-encrypted transmissions over the Internet.

***Computerization of Drug Safety Data: Data Collection and Input.*** "Rubbish in, rubbish out" applies to safety data as to any other computerized data. The enforced control of terms at entry can be linked to checking of data, which should form part of the quality control procedures. Such controls should be driven by the business so that clinical trial data, free from all errors and needed for statistical analysis, will probably involve double data entry whereas single data entry is generally considered adequate for AE databases used for signal generation and regulatory reporting.

Data are still generally typed into a database rather than electronically loaded from other systems. The first step of any data entry process should involve a check for duplicate cases. The need for decision making at the data entry stage will depend upon the type of database design. In all cases, there should be clear rules on how data should be entered into each field to ensure consistency and aid subsequent searching and outputting. This is particularly important when there are multiple users distributed over a number of international sites. Use of electronically available field specific lists of value and well-defined coding conventions will help with this.

In the future, data will increasingly be captured electronically. Image processing and developments in optical character recognition are already proving useful. Electronic data capture (using fax or pen-based methods) is used to collect data in some clinical trials.

With the increase in licensing agreements between pharmaceutical companies, safety data frequently needs to be exchanged between one or more parties. If the case volume is sufficient, it is worth considering electronic data exchange between the databases involved. In addition to preventing rekeying of data, this minimizes discrepancies between the data sets. With the adoption of proposed ICH standards in the future, this will become a much simpler process.

*Medical and Drug Terminology.* Medical and drug terminology is at the heart of the ADR systems. Accurate and consistent input of terms is critical for retrieval and analysis of ADR information. An integrated dictionary allows the capture of original text, which is autoencoded against the dictionary to retrieve the correct code for that piece of text. Coded information allows easy retrieval and analysis. The dictionary structure should allow different ways of grouping and analyzing data encompassing body systems at the highest level so that the specific reporter's wording should meet the following needs:

- Acceptable to all users of the system.
- New terms can be easily added.
- Specificity of the reported term preserved.
- Hierarchical structure to group terms at various levels of specificity.
- Logical groupings so similar terms are not scattered.
- A default grouping for each term.
- Unambiguous to enable autoencoding on input.

**Dictionaries.** This section compares commonly used dictionaries in monitoring drug safety. As electronic exchange of ADR data between industry and regulatory authorities in different countries increases, so dose the need for standardization of terminology (Benichou et al., 1991). MedDRA (Medical Dictionary for Drug Regulatory Affairs) has completed development with version 4.0 just being available, and is discussed later in this chapter. Table 21.4 presents a summary of its structure. (Brown et al., 1999; Gruchalla, 1995).

*Medical Term Coding Dictionaries.* It is logical to deal with AEs, indications, diseases, surgeries and procedures using one system for the following reasons:

- ADRs frequently mimic spontaneously occurring diseases, hence the same diagnosis or symptom could appear as an AE or disease.
- In the identification of new ADRs, it is important not to separate a possible side effect from a disease.
- Separate classifications can lead to confusion and add a layer of complexity when developing ADR systems.

Meaningful codes may or may not be needed for modern dictionaries. For example, the new Adverse Drug Reactions On-Line Information Tracking (ADROIT) dictionaries do not use meaningful codes, but rely on linkage of related terms and effective text processing. Where codes are considered necessary, they should be as short as possible (Westland, 1991). Whenever a system is used for AEs from the literature, spontaneous reports, clinical trials or a combination of these, the needs of the users of the system will influence the selection of the dictionary.

***MedDRA (Medical Dictionary for Regulatory Activities).*** MedDRA is a medical dictionary encompassing terms relevant to pre- and post-marketing phases of the regulatory process. It was developed by the MCA to support its information systems and has subsequently been further developed by the Medical Terminology Working Group. The objective is to harmonize standards for electronic submissions among regulatory authorities, between authorities and industry within and across regions. The aims of the dictionary are

- To address pre- and postmarketing AE reporting.
- To cover multiple medical product areas.
- To be available in multiple languages.
- To be available in multiple formats and platforms.
- To be well maintained.

The guiding principles are

To build from existing terminologies to maximize compatibility.
To focus on the international community need rather than optimizing on individual countries.
To ensure worldwide use through collaboration and participation in development.
To ensure mechanisms and structures are in place for translation into many languages.
To ensure long-term maintenance.

The scope of MedDRA is:

- Disease.
- Diagnoses.

There is a dual classification for some terms (e.g., 573.1 "Hepatitis in viral diseases classified elsewhere"), but this is not extensive. The dictionaries are very comprehensive with the exception of symptoms, which tend to be scattered. They have been widely used in coding patient histories and hospital charts.

ICD-9 CM is a clinical modification of ICD-9 and offers some advantages, particularly the inclusion of synonyms, but is constrained by systems that have used the older versions of ICD-9. ICD-10 is more comprehensive than any ICD revision to date (see Web sites). It extends well beyond the traditional causes of death and causes of hospitalization. The content has been expanded to include symptoms, signs, abnormal findings, factors related to lifestyle and other factors causing contact with health services.

- Signs and symptoms;
- Therapeutic indications;
- Investigation names and qualitative results;
- Medical and surgical procedures;
- Medical, social and family history;
- Terms from COSTART, WHO-ART, ICD-9, HARTS, J-Art.

The current structure of MedDRA is defined in Table 21.6. There will be a central maintenance organization responsible for development, user support, implementation and communication as well as an international user group. A management board will oversee the activities of the central maintenance organization with direction provided by the ICH Steering Committee. A standard medical dictionary will facilitate electronic data exchange between industry and regulatory authorities worldwide, as recommended by the ICH.

*FDA.* Under the March 2001 draft guidance *Postmarketing Safety Reporting for Human Drug and Biological Products Including Vaccines* (FDA, 2001), FDA will accept SAEs coded with either MedDRA, COSTART or WHO ART. MedDRA has been implemented for SAE coding in FDA's Adverse Event Reporting System (AERS) program. While FDA encourages companies to use MedDRA, the deadline for full MedDRA implementation is still pending.

*European Union (EU).* The European Agency for the Evaluation of Medical Products (EMEA) established January 2002 as the deadline for all electronically filed single case reports to be coded in MedDRA. All ADR drug reporting must be coded in MedDRA by January 2003.

*Japan.* MedDRA/J, the Japanese version of MedDRA, officially was issued on 28 December 1999 and the Ministry of Health highly recommended its use for ADR reporting beginning at the end of March 2000. However, J-ART terms are still applicable and upon submission to the ministry are begin converted to MedDRA/J terms. No firm deadline for full implementation has been issued.

MedDRA is available in English and Japanese only. The Maintenance and Support Services Organization (MSSO) is working on translations in French, Portuguese, German, Greek and Spanish. With their annual dues, subscribers can get MedDRA in English and one other European language (when available). Japanese or additional European languages will need to be purchased separately. The German and Portuguese translations were recently submitted to MSSO for review.

The most current version of MedDRA, 4.0, was released in July 2001. The cost of the dictionary depends on the type of organization and annual revenue. An annual

**TABLE 21.6. MedDRA Structure**

| Level of Hierarchy | Approximate Number of Terms | Definition | Example |
| --- | --- | --- | --- |
| System organ class | 26 | Broadest collection of concepts for retrieval; grouped by anatomy or physiology | Cardiac disorders |
| High-level group term | 334 | Broad concepts for linking clinically related terms; can be linked to one or more SOCs | Cardiac rhythm disorders |
| High-level term | 1663 | Groups of preferred terms related by anatomy, pathology, physiology, etiology, or function; can be linked to one or more high-level groups terms or SOCs | Tachyarrhythmia |
| Preferred term | 11,193 | International level of information exchange; single, unambiguous clinical concept | Ventricular tachycardia |
| Lowest-level term | 46,258 | Synonyms and quasi-synonyms; help define scope of preferred terms | Praoxysmal ventricular tachycardia |

subscription provides a company with all versions of MedDRA released during the year. All regulators are provided MedDRA free of charge. Otherwise, costs are as follows:

| | |
|---|---|
| Basic Service[a] | $3,000/year |
| System developer (no change requests) | $5,000/year |
| | |
| Core Service[b] | |
|     Under $10 million in annual revenue | $7,000/year |
|     $10–500 million in annual revenue | $12,000/year |
|     $500 million to $1 billion in annual revenue | $23,000/year |
|     $1–5 billion in annual revenue | $62,000/year |
|     More than $5 billion in annual revenue | $82,000/year |

[a]Basic service is reserved for nonprofit medical libraries, educational institutions and direct patient care providers. No change requests are available for this service.

[b]Core service subscribers have the ability to send in proposed changes to MSSO. AN individual core subscriber can send in up to 100 proposed changes a month. Any changes beyond that will be charged $325 per change. Collectively, no more than 9,000 change requests from all core subscribers can be received per year. Anything beyond that will be charged $325 per request and distributed among all core subscribers. A change must be medically valid and internally acceptable.

***Periodic Reports.*** Many regulatory authorities require detailed summary reports on groups of cases on a regular basis. The FDA requires annual progress reports for investigational compounds and periodic reports for marketed drugs either quarterly or annually depending upon the length of time the product has been on the U.S. market. CIOMS II guidelines recommend submission of line listings of serious, unlabelled spontaneous cases in conjunction with a summary of the drug safety profile on a six-monthly basis. These reports are well defined in format, content and submission time frame. Most major pharmaceutical companies produce them electronically.

The regulatory requirements, particularly regarding frequency of submission and content, differ in the three regions (Europe, Japan, and the United States). In order to avoid duplication of effort and to ensure that important data are submitted with consistency to regulatory authorities worldwide, the ICH3 Topic E2C Guideline on the Format and Content for Comprehensive Periodic Safety Update Reports (PSUR) 1996) of marketed medicine products ahs been developed. The general principles of this guideline include

One report is submitted for one active substance. All dosage forms as well as indications for a given active substance should be covered in one PSUR.

The focus is on ADRs, which include all spontaneous reports and all drug-related clinical trial and literature reports.

An international birthdate and frequency of review and reporting is defined. The international birthdate is the date of the first marketing authorization for the product granted to any company in any country in the world. Preparation of

PSURs should be based on data sets of six months or multiples thereof. The PSUR should be submitted within 60 days of the data lock point.

The reference safety information is the company core data sheet to determine whether an ADR is listed or unlisted.

ADR data are presented in line listings and/or summary tabulations.


## 21.5.  CAUSALITY ASSESSMENT

Decisions have to be made by pharmaceutical companies and regulatory authorities about whether a drug can cause a particular adverse event (AE) so that an appropriate action can be taken. What does "can cause" mean? Does it imply certainty? In many cases to wait for "certainty" before taking action would entail many patients suffering unnecessarily. The degree of certainty or "probability" required will vary according to the situation.

There are, nearly always, many factors other than the administration of a drug, that can cause an AE and will determine whether the AE will occur in a particular patient. The drug may be "the last straw that broke the camel's back". If an AE would not have occurred as and when it did but for the drug then the drug "caused" the AE (Hutchinson, 1992). So with an adverse drug interaction both drugs "caused" the AE. Using this definition the drug may only be a minor factor.

Certainty is rarely obtainable; perhaps an AE with a positive rechallenge where there is objective evidence and an absence of confounders in an individual case would be considered as certainty due to the drug. In the majority of cases action is needed before there is absolute certainty that a drug can cause an AE. This lack of certainty in individual cases has been described suing rather vague terms such as "almost certain", "probably", "possible", "unlikely", etc. These terms have also been defined, but each author has a slightly different definition (Venulet et al., 1982; Stephens et al., 1998).

Again, in epidemiological studies or clinical trials there is nearly always a degree of uncertainty due to bias, chance and confounders. In these studies uncertainty is measured in terms of $p$-values, odd ratios, and relative risks, and so on.

The differential diagnosis of AEs associated with a drug or drug(s) is an everyday part of a practicing clinician's life (Rogers, 1987). However, the term "causality assessment" is reserved for a similar process performed at one or more stages removed from the patient and with some important differences. Clinicians do not necessarily need to find out whether a drug caused an AE in order to satisfy themselves and their patients. They will be more interested in resolving the event as quickly as possible. If there is a possibility that the event might be an ADR, it may be resolved by either reducing the dose or stopping the drug or by treating the ADR while waiting for tolerance to develop, or it may resolve if any of the underlying factors are altered. The resolution of the AE might be because the event has been caused by the drug or it may have been a transient natural occurrence; either way the patient and doctor will welcome its disappearance. If, however, the doctor is interested in knowing whether it was an ADR, further investigations can be undertaken, as long as the patient is willing, until it is established or refuted.

When causality assessment is undertaken by a regulatory authority or a scientist or physician in industry, it is unlikely that the full details known to the clinic treating the patient will be reported, even after further inquiry is made. The only way to obtain all available data is usually by visiting the physician and, with permission, reading the notes and discussing the case with him or her.

### 21.5.1. Aims of Causality Assessment

Of the many similar events on an AE database, only a few have sufficient and relevant data to enable the assessor to decide that the AE was more likely caused by the drug than by any other cause or vice versa. A preliminary assessment (sometimes referred to as a "triage") can be made by placing the event into a category (e.g., probably, possible or unlikely, or using the EEC classification of A, B, or O) (Mezboom and Rozer, 1992). This will enable the company to extract the probably cases at regular intervals in order to consider whether there is a "signal". The possible and unlikely cases will probably not contribute much to this signal.

This preliminary assessment will need to be updated as and when further information becomes available. It should favor sensitivity over specificity so that a borderline possible–probable case is classified as "probable" rather than "possible" to make certain that the case is not lost when at a later stage the probable cases are picked out as a signal. A full assessment when all the information is available can then rectify any misclassifications.

### 21.6. COURSES OF CORRECTIVE ACTION

Identification of a safety issue with a marketed drug does not necessarily (or even usually) lead to the withdrawal of that therapeutic agent from the market. As noted at the beginning of this chapter, there are a range of possible actions.

- Change in dosage or dose form (reformation).
- Change in labeling (warnings).
- Restriction of situation of use (from open prescription to either clinician administration or hospital use only).
- Monitoring of patients during use.
- Restriction on use (that is, of patients allowed to use).
- Withdrawal from the market (usually a permanent step, but not always).

Which action(s) are taken depends on severity and incidence rates of the adverse response, technical details, the existence of alternative therapies, and the benefit of the use of the drug.

## 21.7. LEGAL CONSEQUENCES OF SAFETY WITHDRAWAL

Although in the context of personal injury claims an HMO and other parties (e.g., doctors, hospital) may all be the target of proceedings, it is usually the pharmaceutical company, perceived as having "deep pockets", that is the prime target for claimants. Claims for negligence based upon a failure to act with reasonable care (e.g., to obtain or act upon pharmacovigilance data) and/or the supply of a product that is "defective" in legal terms (e.g., because its labeling was not amended, pursuant to the receipt and review of pharmacovigilance data so as to give adequate warnings and precautions) are always possible.

Tables 21.7 and 21. 8 set out in very simple terms the necessary "ingredients" for establishing product liability, either in negligence or under statute: so-called strict liability.

All of the elements of each of these legal wrongs must be present in a given situation for liability to be established. In negligence therefore, where the claim is made against the person alleged to owe the duty of care (in the context of this chapter, this will be the company putting the product on the market), proof of causation, without a lack of reasonable care having occurred, will not afford the claimant a remedy. However, the chief distinction between negligent liability and so-called strict liability is that in the case of the latter, fault is not required to be

**TABLE 21.7. Criteria for Negligence: D + L + F + C = N**

| | |
|---|---|
| D: Duty of care | Owed to the claimant; easy to establish in the case of the supplier or manufacturer *vis á vis* the patient who uses the product |
| L: Lack of reasonable care | Evidenced by a failure to conduct operations according to accepted standards applicable at the time; that is, a breach of regulatory requirements, or possibly failure to take account of or apply (industry) guidelines |
| F: Foreseeable injury | Of the type likely to occur following failure (e.g., side effect of the drug) |
| C: Causation | The lack of reasonable care must have caused or contributed to the injury; if a label would not have been read by the patient in any event, an omission from it might not have caused injury |

**TABLE 21.8. Criteria for Strict Liability: D + D + C = SL**

| | |
|---|---|
| D: Defect | Widely defined; product design defect, manufacturing error (so that the product is less safe than persons generally would be entitled to expect), deficiency in "presentation" |
| D: Damage | To person or property flowing from the defect |
| C: Causation | See Table 21.7 |

shown. To establish strict liability, the claimant must establish against the "producer" (manufacturer or importer) that the product was "defective" (for the purpose of the law, this could refer to shortcomings in its presentation, design or manufacture) and that it caused the injury suffered.

It would not be at all unusual for claimants in personal injury actions to look for a regulatory compliance failure on the part of a company defendant. The demonstration of a regulatory breach will significantly assist the plaintiff in establishing lack of reasonable care (i.e., conduct falling below acceptable standards). In fact, whether the failure is alleged to be directly relevant to the injury or not, it can be used to demonstrate a general lack of care in the operation of corporate systems with prejudicial effect. Failure to warn is a common element of many pharmaceutical product liability cases, where the pleadings (of negligence and strict liability) might be expected to assert that had the labeling accurately dealt with contraindications, precautions and/or warnings, the patient would have avoided the injury allegedly suffered, either because the product would not have been used or administered at all, or the patient would have been monitored, advised (by the treating doctor), or managed differently so as to avert injury.

In a case where pharmacovigilance omissions are identified that can be said to lead to no or an insufficient response being adopted by the manufacturer (especially where the regulatory authorities have taken some form of action or simply criticized a company), the plaintiff is a significant way towards establishing a case for lack of reasonable care in negligence, or that the product was defective in strict liability terms, because it was not presented accurately and was therefore less safe than persons were entitled to expect, given the content of the labeling.

## REFERENCES


Adams, D.G., Cooper, R.M., and Kahan, J.S. (1997). *Fundamentals of Law and Regulation*, Vol. II. FDLI, Washington, D.C.

Ajayi, F.O., Sun, H. and Perry, J. (2000). Adverse drug reactions: A review of relevant factors. *J. Clin. Pharmacol.* 40: 1093–1101.

American Society of Hospital Pharmacy (1995). ASHP Guidelines on adverse drug reaction monitoring and reporting. *Am. J. Health Systems Pharm.* 52: 417–419.

Antonow, J.A., Smith, A.B. and Silver, M.P. (2000). Medication error reporting: A survey of nursing staff. *J. Nursing Care Quality* 15: 42–48.

Benichou, C., Danan, G. and Solal–Celignz, P. (1991). Standardization of international databases: Definitions of drug-induced blood cytopenias. *Int. J. Clin. Pharmacol. Toxicol.* 29: 75–81.

Brewer, T. and Colditz, G.A. (1999). Postmarketing surveillance and adverse drug reactions: Current perspectives and future needs. *JAMA* 281: 824–829.

Brown, E.G., Wood, L., and Wood, S. (1999). The Medical Dictionary for Regulatory Activities (MedDRA). *Drug Safety* 20: 109–117.

Bukowski, J.A. and Wartenberg, D. (1996). Comparison of adverse drug reaction reporting in veterinary and human medicine. *JAVMA* 209: 40–45.

CFR (1994). Postmarketing reporting of adverse drug experiences. CFR 314.80.

Chyka, P.A. (1999). Role of poison centers in adverse drug reaction monitoring. *Vet. Sc. Human Toxicol.* 41: 400–402.

Chyka, P.A. and McEommon, S.W. (2000). Reporting of adverse drug reactions by poison control centers in the United States. *Drug Safety* 23: 87–93.

Cohen, J.S. (2001). Dose discrepancies between the *Physicians Desk Reference* and the medical literature and their possible roles in the high incidence of dose-related adverse drug events. *Archives of Internal Medicine* 161: 957–964.

FDA (2001). *Postmarketing Safety Reporting for Human Drug and Biological Products Including Vaccines.* Draft Guidance, March, 2001.

Figueras, A., Tato, F., Fontainas, J. and Gestal-Otero, J.J. (1999). Influence of physician's attitudes on reporting adverse drug events: A case-control study. *Medical Care* 37: 809–814.

Fung, M., Thorton, A., Mazbeck, K., Wu, J.H., Hornbuckle, K., and Muniz, E. (2001). Evaluation of the characteristics of safety withdrawal of premarketing prescription drugs from worldwide pharmaceutical markets—1960 to 1999. *Drug Information J.* 35: 293–317.

Goldman, S.A. (1998). Limitations and strengths of spontaneous reports data. *Clin. Ther.* 201: Supplement C, CAO-58.

Gruchalla, R.S. (1995). A one-year perspective on MedWatch: The Food and Drug Administration's new medical products reporting program. *J. Allergy Clinical Immunology* 95: 1153–1157.

Holland, E.G. and DeGruz, F.V. (1997). Drug-induced disorders. *American Family Physician* 56: 1781–1788.

Hunziker, T., Kunyi, U.P., Braunschweig, S., Zehnder, D. and Hoigne, R. (1977). Comprehensive hospital drug monitoring (CHDM): adverse skin reactions, a 20-year survey. *Allergy,* 52: 388–393.

Hutchinson, T.A. (1992). Causality assessments of suspected adverse drug reactions. In *Detection of New Adverse Drug Reactions* (Stephens, M.B.D., Ed.). Macmillan, Press, London.

Jones, J.K. (1982). Criteria for journal reports of suspected adverse drug reactions. *Clin. Pharm.* 1: 554–555.

Keller, W.C., Bataller, N. and Oeller, D.S. (1998). Processing and evaluation of adverse drug experience reports at the Food and Drug Administration Center for Veterinary Medicine. *JAVMA* 213: 208–211.

Kennedy, D.L. and Goldman, S.A. (1997). Monitoring for Adverse Drug Events. *American Family Physician* 56: 1748–1788.

LaCalamita, S. (1995). Top 10 reasons for not reporting adverse drug reactions. *Hospital Pharmacy,* 30: 245–246.

Martin, R.M., Kapoor, K.V., Wilton, L.V. and Mann, R.O. (1998). Underreporting of suspected adverse drug reactions to newly marketed ("black triangle") drugs in general practice: Observational study. *Br. J. Med.* 317: 119–120.

Mezboom, R.H.B. and Rozer, R.J. (1992). Causality classification at pharmacovigilance centers in the European Community. *Pharmacoepidemiol Drug Safety* 1: 87–97.

Niu, M.T., Rhodes, P., Saline, M., Livelz, T., Davis, D.M., Black, S., Shinefield, H., Chen, R.T., Ellenberg, S.S. and the VAERS and VSD Working Groups (1998). Comparative safety of two recombinant hepatitis B vaccines in children: Data from the Vaccine Adverse Event Reporting System (VAERS) and Vaccine Safety Data links (VSD). *J. Clin. Epidemiol.* 51: 503–510.

Niu, M.T., Saline, M.E. and Ellenberg, S.S. (1999). Neonatal deaths after hepatitis B vaccine: The vaccine adverse event reporting system, 1991–1998. *Arch. Pediatr. Adolesc. Med.* 153: 1279–1282.

Olsson, S. (1998). The role of the WHO Programme on International Drug Monitoring in coordinating worldwide drug safety efforts. *Drug Safety* 19: 1–10.

Piazza-Hepp, T.D. and Kennedy, D. L. (1995). Reporting of adverse events to MedWatch. *AJHSP* 52: 1436–1439.

Rogers, A.S. (1987). Adverse drug events: identification and attribution. *Drug Intell. Clin. Pharm.* 21: 915–920.

Rose, J.C. and Elnis, A.S. (2000). A mortality index for postmarketing surveillance of new medications. *Am. J. Emergency Med.* 18(2): 176–179.

Sharpe, R. (1998). MedWatch system comes under fire. *Wall Street Journal*, June 24, 1988, p. B5.

Snidermann, O.A. (2000). The need for greater involvement of regulatory agencies in assessing adverse drug reactions. *CMAJ* 162: 209–210.

Stephens, M.D.B., Talbot, J.C.C. and Routledge, P.A. (1998). *Detection of New Adverse Drug Reactions*, 4th ed. Grove Dictionaries, New York.

Varrincchio, F. (1998). The vaccine adverse event reporting system. *Clin. Toxicology* 36: 765–768.

Venulet, J., Blattner, R., Von Bülow, J., and Bernecker, G.C. (1982). How good are articles on ADR? *Br. Med. J.* 284: 252–254.

Westland, M.M. (1991). Coding: The mortar in the bricks of data analysis. *Drug Inform. J.* 25: 197–200.

White, G.G. and Love, L. (1998). The MedWatch Program. *Clinical Toxicology* 36: 145–149.

WHO (1975). *Requirements for Adverse Drug Reaction Reporting*. WHO, Geneva.

# 22

# STATISTICS IN PHARMACEUTICAL SAFETY ASSESSMENT

## 22.1. INTRODUCTION

This chapter has been written for the practicing toxicologists, as a practical guide to the common statistical problems encountered in drug safety assessment and the methodologies that are available to solve them. The chapter has been enriched by the inclusion of discussions of why a particular procedure or interpretation is recommended, by the clear enumeration of the assumptions that are necessary for a procedure to be valid, and by discussion of problems drawn from the actual practice of toxicology and toxicologic pathology.

Studies continue to be designed and executed to generate increased amounts of data. The resulting problems of data analysis have then become more complex and toxicology has drawn more deeply from the well of available statistical techniques. Statistics has also been a very active and growing discipline during the last thirty-five years, to some extent, at least, because of the parallel growth of toxicology. These simultaneous changes have led to an increasing complexity of data and, unfortunately, to the introduction of numerous confounding factors which severely limit the utility of the resulting data in all too many cases.

A major difficulty is that there is a very real necessity to understand the biological realities and implications of a problem, as well as to understand the peculiarities of toxicological data before procedures are selected and employed for analysis. These characteristics include the following.

862

1. The need to work with a relatively small sample set of data collected from the members of a population (laboratory animals) that is not actually our population of interest (that is, humans or a target animal population).

2. Dealing frequently with data resulting from a sample that was censored on a basis other than by the investigator's as design. By censoring, of course, we mean that not all data points were collected as might be desired. This censoring could be the result of either a biological factor (the test animal being dead or too debilitated to manipulate) or a logistic factor (equipment being inoperative or a tissue being missed in necropsy).

3. The conditions under which our experiments are conducted are extremely varied. In pharmacology (the closest cousin to at least classical toxicology), the possible conditions of interaction of a chemical or physical agent with a person are limited to a small range of doses via a single route over a short course of treatment to a defined patient population. In toxicology however, all these variables (dose, route, time span and subject population) are determined by the investigator.

4. The time frames available to solve our problems are limited by practical and economic factors. This frequently means that there is no time to repeat a critical study if the first attempt fails. So a true iterative approach is not possible.

The training of most pathologists in statistics remains limited to a single introductory course which concentrates on some theoretical basics. As a result, the armertarium of statistical techniques of most toxicologists is limited and the tools that are usually present ($t$-tests, chi-square, analysis of variance, and linear regression) are neither fully developed nor well understood. It is hoped that this chapter will help change this situation.

As a point of departure toward this objective, it is essential that any analysis of study results be interpreted by a professional who firmly understands three concepts: the difference between biological significance and statistical significance, the nature and value of different types of data, and causality.

For the first concept, we should consider the four possible combinations of these two different types of significance, for which we find the relationship

|  |  | Statistical Significance | |
|---|---|---|---|
|  |  | No | Yes |
| Biological | No | Case I | Case II |
| Significance | Yes | Case III | Case IV |

Cases I and IV give us no problems, for the answers are the same statistically and biologically. But Cases II and III present problems. In Case II (the "false positive"), we have a circumstance where there is a statistical significance in the measured difference between treated and control groups, but there is no true biological significance to the finding. This is not an uncommon happening, for example, in the case of clinical chemistry parameters. This is called a type I error by statisticians, and the probability of this happening is called the (alpha) level. In Case III (the "false negative"), we have no statistical significance, but the differences between groups are biologically–toxicologically significant. This is called a type II error by statisticians, and the probability of such an error happening by random chance is called the $\beta$ (beta) level. An example of this second situation is when we see a few of a very rare tumor type in treated animals. In both of these latter cases, numerical analysis, no matter how well done, is no substitute for professional judgment. Along with this, however, one must have a feeling for the different types of data and for the value or relative merit of each. Note that the two error types interact, and in determining sample size we need to specify both $\alpha$ and $\beta$ levels (Diem and Lentner, 1975). Table 22.1 demonstrates this interaction in the case of tumor or specific lesion incidence.

The reasons that biological and statistical significance are not identical are multiple, but a central one is certainly causality. Through our consideration of statistics, we should keep in mind that just because a treatment and a change in an observed organism are seemingly or actually associated with each other does not "prove" that the former caused the latter. Though this fact is now widely appreciated for correlation (for example, the fact that the number of storks' nests found each year in England is correlated with the number of human births that year does not mean that storks bring babies), it is just as true in the general case of significance. Timely establishment and proof that treatment causes an effect requires an understanding of the underlying mechanism and proof of its validity. At the same time, it is important that we realize that not finding a good correlation or suitable significance associated with a treatment and an effect likewise does not prove that the two are not associated, that a treatment does not cause an effect. At best, it gives us a certain level of confidence that under the conditions of the current test, these items are not associated.

These points will be discussed in greater detail in the "Assumptions" section for each method, along with other common pitfalls, and shortcomings associated with

**TABLE 22.1. Sample Size Required to Obtain a Specified Sensitivity at $p < 0.05$**

| Background Tumor Incidence | $P$[a] | \multicolumn{10}{c}{Treatment Group Incidence} |
|---|---|---|---|---|---|---|---|---|---|---|---|
| | | 0.95 | 0.90 | 0.80 | 0.70 | 0.60 | 0.50 | 0.40 | 0.30 | 0.20 | 0.10 |
| 0.30 | 0.90 | 10 | 12 | 18 | 31 | 46 | 102 | 389 | | | |
| | 0.50 | 6 | 6 | 9 | 12 | 22 | 32 | 123 | | | |
| 0.20 | 0.90 | 8 | 10 | 12 | 18 | 30 | 42 | 88 | 320 | | |
| | 0.50 | 5 | 5 | 6 | 9 | 12 | 19 | 28 | 101 | | |
| 0.10 | 0.90 | 6 | 8 | 10 | 12 | 17 | 25 | 33 | 65 | 214 | |
| | 0.50 | 3 | 3 | 5 | 6 | 9 | 11 | 17 | 31 | 68 | |
| 0.05 | 0.90 | 5 | 6 | 8 | 10 | 13 | 18 | 25 | 35 | 76 | 464 |
| | 0.50 | 3 | 3 | 5 | 6 | 7 | 9 | 12 | 19 | 24 | 147 |
| 0.01 | 0.90 | 5 | 5 | 7 | 8 | 10 | 13 | 19 | 27 | 46 | 114 |
| | 0.50 | 3 | 3 | 5 | 5 | 6 | 8 | 10 | 13 | 25 | 56 |

[a]$P$ = power for each comparison of treatment group with background tumor incidence.

the method. To help in better understanding the chapters to come, terms frequently used in discussion throughout this book are presented in Table 22.2.

Each measurement we make, each individual piece of experimental information we gather, is called a datum. However we gather and analyze multiple pieces at one time, the resulting collection is called data.

Data are collected on the basis of their association with a treatment (intended or otherwise) as an effect (a property) that is measured in the experimental subjects of a study, such as body weights. These identifiers (that is, treatment and effect) are termed variables. Our treatment variables (those that the researcher or nature control,

**TABLE 22.2. Some Frequently Used Terms and Their General Meanings**

| Term | Meaning |
| --- | --- |
| 95 percent confidence interval | A range of values (above, below or above and below) the sample (mean, median, mode, etc.) has a 95 percent chance of containing the true value of the population (mean, median, mode). Also called the fiducial limit equivalent to the $p < 0.05$ |
| Bias | Systemic error as opposed to a sampling error. For example, selection bias may occur when each member of the population does not have an equal chance of being selected for the sample |
| Degrees of freedom | The number of independent deviations, usually abbreviated $df$ |
| Independent variables | Also known as predictors or explanatory variables |
| $P$-value | Another name for significance level; usually 0.005 |
| Power | The effect of the experimental conditions on the dependent variable relative to sampling fluctuation. When the effect is maximized, the experiment is more powerful. Power can also be defined as the probability that there will not be a Type II error $(1-\beta)$. Conventionally, power should be at least 0.07 |
| Random | Each individual member of the population has the same chance of being selected for the sample |
| Robust | Having inferences or conclusions little effected by departure from assumptions |
| Sensitivity | The number of subjects experiencing each experimental condition divided by the variance of scores in the sample |
| Significance level | The probability that a difference has been erroneously declared to be significant, typically 0.005 and 0.001 corresponding to 5 percent and 1 percent chance of error |
| Type I Error (false positives) | Concluding that there is an effect when there really is not an effect. Its probability is the alpha level |
| Type II Error (false negatives) | Concluding there is no effect when there really is an effect. Its probability is the beta level |

*Source:* Marriott (1991).

and that can be directly controlled) are termed independent, while our effect variables (such as weight, life span, and number of neoplasms) are termed dependent variables; their outcome is believed to be dependent on the "treatment" being studied.

All the possible measures of a given set of variables in all the possible subjects that exist is termed the population for those variables. Such a population of variables cannot be truly measured; for example, one would have to obtain, treat and measure the weights of all the Fischer-344 rats that were, are, or ever will be. Instead, we deal with a representative group, a sample. If our sample of data is appropriately collected and of sufficient size, it serves to provide good estimates of the characteristics of the parent population from which it was drawn.

### 22.1.1. Bias and Chance

Any toxicological study aims to determine whether a treatment elicits a response. An observed difference in response between a treated and control group need not necessarily be a result of treatment. There are, in principle, two other possible explanations: *bias*, or systematic differences other than treatment between the groups, and *chance*, or random differences. A major objective of both experimental design and analysis is to try to avoid bias. Wherever possible, treated and control groups to be compared should be alike in respect of all other factors. Where differences remain, these should be corrected for in the statistical analysis. Chance cannot be wholly excluded, since identically treated animals will not respond identically. While even the most extreme difference might in theory be due to chance, a proper statistical analysis will allow the experimenter to assess this possibility. The smaller the probability of a "false positive", the more confident the experimenter can be that the effect is real. Good experimental design improves the chance of picking up a true effect with confidence by maximizing the ratio between "signal" and "noise".

### 22.1.2. Hypothesis Testing and Probability ($p$) Values

A relationship of treatment to some toxicological endpoint is often stated to be "statistically significant ($p < 0.05$)". What does this really mean? A number of points have to be made. *First*, statistical significance need not necessarily imply biological importance, if the endpoint under study is not relevant to the animal's wellbeing. *Second*, the statement will usually be based only on the data from the study in question and will not take into account prior knowledge. In some situations, for example, when one or two of a very rare tumor type are seen in treated animals, statistical significance may not be achieved but the finding may be biologically extremely important, especially if a similar treatment was previously found to elicit a similar response. *Third*, the $p$ value does not describe the probability that a true effect of treatment exists. Rather, it describes the probability of the observed response, or one more extreme, occurring on the assumption that treatment actually had no effect whatsoever. A $p$ value that is not significant is consistent with a treatment having a small effect, not detected with sufficient certainty in this study. *Fourth*, there are two types of $p$ value. A "one-tailed" (or one-sided) $p$ value is the probability of getting by chance a treatment effect in a specified direction as great as or greater than that observed. A "two-tailed" $p$ value is the probability of getting, by chance alone, a treatment difference in either direction which is as great as or greater than that observed. By convention $p$ values are assumed to be two-tailed unless the contrary is stated. Where, which is unusual, one can rule out in advance the possibility of a treatment effect except in one direction, a one-tailed $p$ value should be used. Often, however, two-tailed tests are to be preferred, and it is certainly not recommended to use one-tailed tests and *not* report large differences in the other direction. In any event, it is important to make it absolutely clear whether one- or two-tailed tests have been used.

It is a great mistake, when presenting results of statistical analyses, to mark, as do some laboratories, results simply as significant or not significant at one defined probability level (usually $p < 0.05$). This poor practice does not allow the reader any real chance to judge whether or not the effect is a true one. Some statisticians present the actual $p$ value for every comparison made. While this gives precise information, it can make it difficult to assimilate results from many variables. One practice I recommend is to mark $p$ values routinely using plus signs to indicate positive differences (and minus signs to indicate negative differences): $+++p, 0.001$, $++0.001 \leq p < 0.01, +0.01p < 0.05, (+\_0.05 \leq p < 0.1$. This highlights significant results more clearly and also allows the reader to judge the whole range from "virtually certain treatment effect" to "some suspicion". Note that using two-tailed tests, bracketed plus signs indicate findings that would be significant at the conventional $p < 0.05$ level using one-tailed tests but are not significant at this level using two-tailed tests. This "fiducal limit" ($p < 0.05$) implies a false positive incidence of 1 in 20, and though now imbedded in regulation, practice, and convention, was somewhat an arbitrary choice to begin with. In interpreting $p$ values it is important to realize they are only an aid to judgment to be used in conjunction with other available information. One might validly consider a $p < 0.01$ increase as chance when it was unexpected, occurred only at a low dose level with no such effect seen at higher doses, and was evident in only one subset of the data. In contrast, a $p < 0.05$ increase might be convincing if it occurred in the top dose and was for an endpoint one might have expected to be increased from known properties of the chemical or closely related chemicals.

### 22.1.3. Multiple Comparisons

When a $p$ value is stated to be $<0.05$, this implies that, for that particular test, the difference could have occurred by chance less than 1 time in 20. Toxicological studies frequently involve making treatment-control comparisons for large numbers of variables and, in some situations, also for various subsets of animals. Some statisticians worry that the larger the number of tests the greater is the chance of picking up statistically significant findings that do not represent true treatment effects. For this reason, an alternative "multiple comparisons" procedure has been proposed in which, if the treatment was totally without effect, then 19 times out of

20 *all* the tests should show nonsignificance when testing at the 95% confidence level. Automatic use of this approach cannot be recommended. Not only does it make it much more difficult to pick up any real effects, but also there is something inherently unsatisfactory about a situation where the relationship between a treatment and a particular response depends arbitrarily on which other responses happened to be investigated at the same time. It is accepted that in any study involving multiple endpoints there will inevitably be a gray area between those showing highly significant effects and those showing no significant effects, where there is a problem distinguishing chance and true effects. However, changing the methodology so that the gray areas all come up as nonsignificant can hardly be the answer.

### 22.1.4. Estimating the Size of the Effect

It should be clearly understood that a $p$ value does not give direct information about the size of any effect that has occurred. A compound may elicit an increase in response by a given amount, but whether a study finds this increase to be statistically significant will depend on the size of the study and the variability of the data. In a small study, a large and important effect may be missed, especially if the endpoint is imprecisely measured. In a large study, on the other hand, a small and unimportant effect may emerge as statistically signficant.

Hypothesis testing tells us whether an observed increase can or cannot be reasonably attributed to chance, but not how large it is. Although much statistical theory relates to hypothesis testing, current trends in medical statistics are towards confidence interval estimation with differences between test and control groups expressed in the form of a best estimate, coupled with the 95% confidence interval (CI). Thus, if one states that treatment increases response by an estimated 10 units (95% CI 3–17 units), this would imply that there is a 95% chance that the indicated interval includes the true difference. If the lower 95% confidence limit exceeds zero, this implies that the increase is statistically significant at $p < 0.05$ using a two-tailed test. One can also calculate, for example, 99% or 99.9% confidence limits, corresponding to testing for significance at $p < 0.01$ or $p < 0.001$.

In screening studies of standard design, the tendency has been to concentrate mainly on hypothesis testing. However, presentation of the results in the form of estimates with confidence intervals can be a useful adjunct for some analyses and is very important in studies aimed specifically at quantifying the size of an effect.

Two terms refer to the quality and reproducibility of our measurements of variables. The first, accuracy, is an expression of the closeness of a measured or computed value to its actual or "true" value in nature. The second, precision, reflects the closeness or reproducibility of a series of repeated measurements of the same quantity.

If we arrange all of our measurements of a particular variable in order as a point on an axis marked as to the values of that variable, and if our sample were large enough, the pattern of distribution of the data in the sample would begin to become apparent. This pattern is a representation of the frequency distribution of a given population of data; that is, of the incidence of different measurements, their central tendency, and dispersion. The most common frequency distribution, one we will talk about throughout this chapter, is the normal (or Gaussian) distribution. The normal distribution is such that two-thirds of all values are within one standard deviation of the mean (or average value for the entire population) and 95% are within 1.96 standard deviations of the mean. Symbols used are $\mu$ for the mean and $\sigma$ for the standard deviation. Other common frequency distributions, such as the binomial, Poisson and chi square, are sometimes encountered.

In all areas of biological research, optimal design and appropriate interpretation of experiments require that the researcher understand both the biological and technological underpinnings of the system being studied and of the data being generated. From the point of view of the statistician, it is vitally important that the experimenter both know and be able to communicate the nature of the data, and understand its limitations. One classification of data types is presented in Table 22.3.

The nature of the data collected is determined by three considerations. These are the biological source of the data (the system being studied), the instrumentational and techniques being used to make measurements, and the design of the experiment. The researcher has some degree of control over each of these, the least over the biological system (he or she normally has a choice of only one of several models to study) and the most over the design of the experiment or study. Such choices, in fact, dictate the type of data generated by a study.

Statistical methods are based on specific assumptions. Parametric statistics, those most familiar to the majority of scientists, have more stringent underlying assumptions than do nonparametric statistics. Among the underlying assumptions for many parametric statistical methods (such as the analysis of variance) is that the data are continuous. The nature of the data associated with a variable (as described previously) imparts a "value" to that data, the value being the power of the statistical tests which can be employed.

**TABLE 22.3. Types of Variables (Data) and Examples of Each Type**

| Classified by | | Type | Example |
| --- | --- | --- | --- |
| Scale | Continuous | Scalar | Body weight |
| | | Ranked | Severity of a lesion |
| | Discontinuous | Scalar | Weeks until the first observation of a tumor in a carcinogenicity study |
| | | Ranked | Clinical observations in animals |
| | | Attribute | Eye colors in fruit flies |
| | | Quantal | Dead/alive or present/absent |
| Frequency distribution | | Normal | Body weights |
| | | Bimodal | Some clinical chemistry parameters |
| | | Others | Measures of time-to-incapacitation |

Continuous variables are those that can at least theoretically assume any of an infinite number of values between any two fixed points (such as measurements of body weight between 2.0 and 3.0 kilograms). Discontinuous variables, meanwhile, are those which can have only certain fixed values, with no possible intermediate values (such as counts of five and six dead animals, respectively).

Limitations on our ability to measure constrain the extent to which the real-world situation approaches the theoretical, but many of the variables studied in toxicology are in fact continuous. Examples of these are lengths, weights, concentrations, temperatures, periods of time, and percentages. For these continuous variables, we may describe the character of a sample with measures of central tendency and dispersion that we are most familiar with: the mean, denoted by the symbol $\bar{x}$ and also called the arithmetic average, and the standard deviation SD, denoted by the symbol $\sigma$ and calculated as being equal to

$$\sqrt{\frac{\sum X^2 - \dfrac{(\sum X)^2}{N}}{N-1}}$$

where $X$ is the individual datum and $N$ is the total number of data in the group.

Contrasted with these continuous data, however, we have discontinuous (or discrete) data, which can only assume certain fixed numerical values. In these cases our choice of statistical tools or tests is, as we will find later, more limited.

## 22.1.5. Functions of Statistics

Statistical methods may serve to do any combination of three possible tasks. The one we are most familiar with is hypothesis testing, that is, determining if two (or more) groups of data differ from each other at a predetermined level of confidence. A second function is the construction and use of models which may be used to predict future outcomes of chemical–biological interactions. This is most commonly seen in linear regression or in the derivation of some form of correlation coefficient. Model fitting allows us to relate one variable (typically a treatment or "independent" variable) to another. The third function, reduction of dimensionality, continues to be less commonly utilized than the first two. This final category includes methods for reducing the number of variables in a system while only minimally reducing the amount of information, therefore making a problem easier to visualize and to understand. Examples of such techniques are factor analysis and cluster analysis. A subset of this last function, discussed later under "descriptive statistics", is the reduction of raw data to single expressions of central tendency and variability (such as the mean and standard deviation).

There is also a special subset of statistical techniques that is part of both the second and third functions of statistics. This is data transformation, which includes such things as the conversion of numbers to log or probit values.

### 22.1.6.  Descriptive Statistics

Descriptive statistics are used to summarize the general nature of a data set. As such, the parameters describing any single group of data have two components. One of these describes the location of the data, while the other gives a measure of the dispersion of the data in and about this location. Often overlooked is the fact that the choice of which parameters are used to give these pieces of information implies a particular type of distribution for the data.

Most commonly, location is described by giving the (arithmetic) mean and dispersion by giving the standard deviation (SD) or the standard error of the mean (SEM). The calculation of the first two of these has already been described. If we again denote the total number of data in a group as $N$, then the SEM would be calculated as

$$\mathrm{SEM} = \frac{\mathrm{SD}}{\sqrt{N}}$$

The use of the mean with either the SD or SEM implies, however, that we have reason to believe that the sample of data being summarized are from a population that is at least approximately normally distributed. If this is not the case, then we should rather use a set of statistical descriptions which do not require a normal distribution. These are the median, for location, and the semiquartile distance, for a measure of dispersion. These somewhat less familiar parameters are characterized as follows.

***Median.*** When all the numbers in a group are arranged in a ranked order (that is, from smallest to largest), the median is the middle value. If there is an odd number of values in a group, then the middle value is obvious (in the case of 13 values, for example, the seventh largest is the median). When the number of values in the sample is even, the median is calculated as the midpoint between the $(N/2)$th and the $([N/2] + 1)$th number. For example, in the series of numbers 7, 12, 13, 19 the median value would be the midpoint between 12 and 13, which is 12.5.

The standard deviation (SD) and the standard error of the mean (SEM) are related to each other but yet are quite different.

The SEM is quite a bit smaller than the SD, making it very attractive to use in reporting data. This size difference is because the SEM actually is an estimate of the error (or variability) involved in measuring the means of samples, and not an estimate of the error (or variability) involved in measuring the data from which means are calculated. This is implied by the *Central Limit Theorem*, which tells us three major things.

The distribution of sample means will be approximately normal regardless of the distribution of values in the original population from which the samples were drawn.

The mean value of the collection.

The standard deviation of the collection of all possible means of samples of a given size, called the standard error of the mean, depends on both the standard deviation of the original population and the size of the sample.

The SEM should be used only when the uncertainty of the estimate of the mean is of concern, which is almost never the case in toxicology. Rather, we are concerned with an estimate of the variability of the population for which the standard deviation is appropriate.

***Semiquartile Distance.***   When all the data in a group are ranked, a quartile of the data contains one ordered quarter of the values. Typically, we are most interested in the borders of the middle two quartiles $Q_1$ and $Q_3$, which together represent the semiquartile distance and which contain the median as their center. Given that there are $N$ values in an ordered group of data, the upper limit of the $j$th quartile $(Q_j)$ may be computed as being equal to the $[(jN - 1)/4$th] value. Once we have used this formula to calculate the upper limits of $Q_1$ and $Q_3$, we can then compute the semiquartile distance (which is also called the quartile deviation, and as such is abbreviated as QD) with the formula $QD = (Q_3 - Q_1)/2$.

For example, for the fifteen-value data set 1, 2, 3, 4, 4, 5, 5, 5, 6, 6, 6, 7, 7, 8, 9, we can calculate the upper limits of $Q_1$ and $Q_3$ as

$$Q_1 = \frac{1(15 + 1)}{4} = \frac{16}{4} = 4$$

$$Q_3 = \frac{3(15 = 1)}{4} = \frac{48}{4} = 12$$

The fourth and twelfth values in this data set are 4 and 7, respectively. The semiquartile distance can then be calculated as

$$QD = \frac{7 - 4}{2} = 1.5$$

There are times when it is desired to describe the relative variability of one or more sets of data. The most common way of doing this is to compute the coefficient of variation (CV), which is calculated simply as the ratio of the standard deviation to the mean, or

$$CV = \frac{SD}{\overline{X}}$$

A CV of 0.2 or 20% thus means that the standard deviation is 20% of the mean. In toxicology the CV is frequently between 20 and 50% and may at times exceed 100%.

## 22.2. EXPERIMENTAL DESIGN

Toxicological experiments generally have a two-fold purpose. The first question is whether or not an agent results in an effect on a biological system. The second question, never far behind, is how much of an effect is present. It has become increasingly desirable that the results and conclusions of studies aimed at assessing the effects of environmental agents be as clear and unequivocal as possible. It is essential that every experiment and study yield as much information as possible, and that the results of each study have the greatest possible chance of answering the questions it was conducted to address. The statistical aspects of such efforts, so far as they are aimed at structuring experiments to maximize the possibilities of success, are called experimental design.

The four basic statistical principles of experimental design are replication, randomization, concurrent ("local") control and balance. In abbreviated form, these may be summarized as follows.

1. *Replication.* Any treatment must be applied to more than one experimental unit (animal, plate of cells, litter of offspring, etc.). This provides more accuracy in the measurement of a response than can be obtained from a single observation, since underlying experimental errors tend to cancel each other out. It also supplies an estimate of the experimental error derived from the variability among each of the measurements taken (or "replicates"). In practice, this means that an experiment should have enough experimental units in each treatment group (that is, a large enough $N$) so that reasonably sensitive statistical analysis of data can be performed. The estimation of sample size is addressed in detail later in this chapter.

2. *Randomization.* This is practiced to ensure that every treatment shall have its fair share of extreme high and extreme low values. It also serves to allow the toxicologist to proceed as if the assumption of "independence" is valid. This is, there is no avoidable (known) systematic bias in how one obtains data.

3. *Concurrent Control.* Comparisons between treatments should be made to the maximum extent possible between experimental units from the same closely defined population. Therefore, animals used as a control group should come from the same source, lot, age, and so on as test group animals. Except for the treatment being evaluated, test and control animals should be maintained and handled in exactly the same manner.

4. *Balance.* If the effect of several different factors is being evaluated simultaneously, the experiment should be laid out in such a way that the contributions of the different factors can be separately distinguished and estimated. There are several ways of accomplishing this using one of several different forms of design, as will be discussed later.

There are ten facets of any study which may affect its ability to detect an effect of a treatment. The first six concern minimizing the role of chance and the last four relate to avoidance of bias.

### 22.2.1. Choice of Species and Strain

Ideally, the responses of interest should be rare in untreated control animals but should be reasonably readily evoked by appropriate treatments. Some species or specific strains, perhaps because of inappropriate diets (Roe, 1989), have high background tumor incidences which make increases both difficult to detect and difficult to interpret when detected.

### 22.2.2. Sampling

Sampling—the selection of which individual data points will be collected, whether in the form of selecting which animals to collect blood from or to remove a portion of a diet mix from for analysis—is an essential step upon which all other efforts towards a good experiment or study are based.

There are three assumptions about sampling which are common to most of the statistical analysis techniques that are used in toxicology. These are that the sample is collected without bias, that each member of a sample is collected independently of the others and that members of a sample are collected with replacements. Precluding bias, both intentional and unintentional, means that at the time of selection of a sample to measure, each portion of the population from which that selection is to be made has an equal chance of being selected. Ways of precluding bias are discussed in detail in the section on experimental design.

Independence means that the selection of any portion of the sample is not affected by and does not affect the selection or measurement of any other portion.

Finally, sampling with replacement means that in theory, after each portion is selected and measured, it is returned to the total sample pool and thus has the opportunity to be selected again. This is a corollary of the assumption of independence. Violation of this assumption (which is almost always the case in toxicology and all the life sciences) does not have serious consequences if the total pool from which samples are sufficiently large (say 20 or greater) so that the chance of reselecting that portion is small anyway.

There are four major types of sampling methods: random, stratified, systematic, and cluster. Random is by far the most commonly employed method in toxicology. It stresses the fulfillment of the assumption of avoiding bias. When the entire pool of possibilities is mixed or randomized (procedures for randomization are presented in a later section), then the members of the group are selected in the order that are drawn from the pool.

Stratified sampling is performed by first dividing the entire pool into subsets or strata, then doing randomized sampling from each strata. This method is employed when the total pool contains subsets that are distinctly different but in which each subset contains similar members. An example is a large batch of a powdered pesticide in which it is desired to determine the nature of the particle size distribution. Larger pieces or particles are on the top, while progressively smaller particles have settled lower in the container and at the very bottom, the material has been packed and compressed into aggregates. To determine a timely representative answer, proportionally sized subsets from each layer or strata should be selected, mixed and randomly sampled. This method is used more commonly in diet studies.

In systematic sampling, a sample is taken at set intervals (such as every fifth container of reagent or taking a sample of water from a fixed sample point in a flowing stream every hour). This is most commonly employed in quality assurance or (in the clinical chemistry lab) in quality control.

In cluster sampling, the pool is already divided into numerous separate groups (such as bottles of tablets), and we select small sets of groups (such as several bottles of tablets) then select a few members from each set. What one gets then is a cluster of measures. Again, this is a method most commonly used in quality control or in environmental studies when the effort and expense of physically collecting a small group of units is significant.

In classical toxicology studies sampling arises in a practical sense in a limited number of situations. The most common of these are

1. Selecting a subset of animals or test systems from a study to make some measurement (which either destroys or stresses the measured system, or is expensive) at an interval during a study. This may include such cases as doing interim necropsies in a chronic study or collecting and analyzing blood samples from some animals during a subchronic study.

2. Analyzing inhalation chamber atmospheres to characterize aerosol distributions with a new generation system.

3. Analyzing diet in which test material has been incorporated.

4. Performing quality control on an analytical chemistry operation by having duplicate analyses performed on some materials.

5. Selecting data to audit for quality assurance purposes.

### 22.2.3. Dose Levels

This is a very important and controversial area. In screening studies aimed at hazard identification it is normal, in order to avoid requiring huge numbers of animals, to test at dose levels higher than those to which man will be exposed, but not so high that marked toxicity occurs. A range of doses is usually tested to guard against the possibility of a inappropriate selection of an appropriate high dose, and that the metabolic pathways at the high doses differ markedly from those at lower doses and, perhaps, to ensure no large effects occur at dose levels in the range to be used by humans. In studies aimed more at risk estimation, more and lower doses may be tested to obtain fuller information on the shape of the dose-response curve.

### 22.2.4. Number of Animals

This is obviously an important determinant of the precision of the findings. The calculation of the appropriate number depends on: (1) the critical difference, that is, the size of the effect it is desired to detect; (2) the false positive rate, that is, the probability of an effect being detected when none exists (equivalent to the "$\alpha$ level" or "Type I error"), (3) the false-negative rate, that is, the probability of no effect being detected when one of exactly the critical size exists (equivalent to the "$\beta$ level" or "type II error"); and (4) some measure of the variability in the material.

Tables relating numbers of animals required to obtain values of critical size, $\alpha$ and $\beta$ are given in Kraemer and Thiemann (1987) and Gad (1998) and software is also available for this purpose. As a rule of thumb, to reduce the critical difference by a factor of $n$ for a given $\alpha$ and $\beta$, the number of animals required will have to increased by a factor of $n^2$.

### 22.2.5. Duration of the Study

It is obviously important not to terminate the study too early for fatal conditions, which are normally strongly age-related. Less obviously, going on for too long in a study can be a mistake, partly because the last few weeks or months may produce relatively few extra data at a disporportionate cost, and partly because diseases of extreme old age may obscure the detection of tumors and other conditions of more interest. For nonfatal conditions, the ideal is to sacrifice the animals when the average prevalence is around 50%.

### 22.2.6. Stratification

To detect a treatment difference with accuracy, it is important that the groups being compared are as homogeneous as possible with respect to other known causes of the response. In particular, suppose that there is another known important cause of the response for which the animals vary, so that the animals are a mixture of hyper- and hyporesponders from this cause. If the treated group has a higher proportion of hyperresponders it will tend to have a higher response even if treatment has no effect. Even if the proportion of hyperresponders is the same as in the controls, it will be more difficult to detect an effect of treatment because of the increased between-animal variability.

Given that this other factor is known, it will be sensible to take it into account in both the design and analysis of the study. In the design, it can be used as a "blocking factor" so that animals at each level are allocated equally (or in the correct proportion) to control and treated groups. In the analysis, the factor should be treated as a stratifying variable, with separate treatment-control comparisons made at each level, and the comparisons combined for an overall test of difference. This is discussed later, where we refer to the factorial design as one example of the more complex designs that can be used to investigate the separate effect of multiple treatments.

### 22.2.7. Randomization

Random allocation of animals to treatment groups is a prerequisite of good experimental design. If not carried out, one can never be sure whether treatment-control differences are due to treatment or to "confounding" by other relevant factors. The ability to randomize easily is a major advantage animal experiments have over epidemiology.

While randomization eliminates bias (as least in expectation), simple randomization of all animals may not be the optimal technique for producing a sensitive test. If there is another major source of variation (e.g., sex or batch of animals), it will be better to carry out stratified randomization (i.e., carry out separate randomizations within each level of the stratifying variable).

The need for randomization applies not only to the allocation of the animals to the treatment, but also to anything that can materially affect the recorded response. The same random number that is used to apply animals to treatment group can be used to determine cage position, order of weighing, order of bleeding for clinical chemistry, order of sacrifice at terminations and so on.

### 22.2.8. Adequacy of Control Group

While historical control data can, on occasion, be useful, a properly designed study demands that a relevant concurrent control group be included with which results for the test group can be compared. The principle that like should be compared with like, apart from treatment, demands that control animals should be randomized from the same source as treatment animals. Careful consideration should also be given to the appropriateness of the control group. Thus, in an experiment involving treatment of a compound in a solvent, it would often be inappropriate to include only an untreated control group, as any differences observed could only be attributed to the treatment-solvent combination. To determine the specific effects of the compound, a comparison group given the solvent only, by the same route of administration, would be required.

It is not always generally realized that the position of the animal in the room in which it is kept may affect the animal's response. An example is the strong relationship between incidence of retinal atrophy in albino rats and closeness to the lighting source. Systematic differences in cage position should be avoided, preferably via randomization.

We have now become accustomed to developing exhaustively detailed protocols for an experiment or study prior to its conduct. *A priori* selection of statistical methodology (as opposed to the *post hoc* approach) is as significant a portion of the process of protocol development and experimental design as any other and can measurably enhance the value of the experiment or study. Prior selection of statistical methodologies is essential for proper design of other portions of a protocol such as the number of animals per group or the sampling intervals for body weight. Implied in such a selection is the notion that the toxicologist has both an indepth knowledge of the area of investigation and an understanding of the general principles of experimental design, for the analysis of any set of data is dictated to a large extent by the manner in which the data are obtained.

A second concept and its understanding are essential to the design of experiments in toxicology, that of censoring. Censoring is the exclusion of measurements from certain experimental units, or indeed of the experimental units themselves, from consideration in data analysis or inclusion in the experiment at all. Censoring may occur either prior to initiation of an experiment (where, in modern toxicology, this is almost always a planned procedure), during the course of an experiment (when they are almost universally unplanned, resulting from such as the as the death of animals on test), or after the conclusion of an experiment (when usually data are excluded because of being identified as some form of outlier).

In practice, *a priori* censoring in toxicology studies occurs in the assignment of experimental units (such as animals) to test groups. The most familiar example is in the common practice of assignment of test animals to acute, subacture, subchronic and chronic studies, where the results of otherwise random assignments are evaluated for body weights of the assigned members. If the mean weights are found not be comparable by some pre-established criterion (such as a 90% probability of difference by analysis of variance) then members are reassigned (censored) to achieve comparability in terms of starting body weights. Such a procedure of animal assignment to groups is known as a *censored randomization*.

The first precise or calculable aspect of experimental design encountered is determining sufficient test and control group sizes to allow one to have an adequate level of confidence in the results of a study (that is, in the ability of the study design with the statistical tests used to detect a true difference, or effect, when it is present). The statistical test contributes a level of power to such a detection. Remember that the power of a statistical test is the probability that a test results in rejection of a hypothesis, $H_0$ say, when some other hypothesis, $H$, say, is valid. This is termed the power of the test "with respect to the (alternative) hypothesis $H$."

If there is a set of possible alternative hypotheses, the power, regarded as a function of $H$, is termed the *power function* of the test. When the alternatives are indexed by a single parameter $\theta$, simple graphical presentation is possible. If the parameter is a vector $\theta$, one can visualize a *power surface*.

If the power function is denoted by $\beta(\theta)$ and $H_0$ specifies $\theta = \theta_0$, then the value of $\beta$ (II), the probability of rejecting $H_0$ when it is in fact valid, is the significance level. A test's power is greatest when the probability of a type II error is the least. Specified powers can be calculated for tests in any specific or general situation.

Some general rules to keep in mind are

- The more stringent the significance level, the greater the necessary sample size. More subjects are needed for a one percent level test than for a five percent level test.

- Two-tailed tests require larger sample sizes than one-tailed tests. Assessing two directions at the same time requires a greater investment.

- The smaller the critical effect size, the larger the necessary sample size. Subtle effects require greater efforts.

- Any difference can be significant if the sample size is large enough.

- The larger the power required, the larger the necessary sample seize. Greater protection from failure requires greater effort. The smaller the sample size, the smaller the power, that is, the greater the chance of failure.

- The requirements and means of calculating necessary sample size depends on the desired (or practical) comparative sizes of test and control groups.

This number ($N$) can be calculated, for example, for equal sized test and control groups, using the formula

$$N = \frac{(t_1 + t_2)^2}{d^2} S$$

where $t_1$ is the one-tailed $t$ value with $N - 1$ degrees of freedom corresponding to the desired level of confidence, $t_2$ is the one-tailed $t$ value with $N - 1$ degrees of freedom corresponding to the probability that the sample size will be adequate to achieve the desired precision, $S$ is the sample standard deviation, derived typically from historical data and calculated as

$$S = \sqrt{\frac{1}{N - 1} \sum (V_1 - V_2)^2}$$

There are a number of aspects of experimental design which are specific to the practice of toxicology. Before we look at a suggestion for step-by-step development of experimental designs, these aspects should first be considered.

1. Frequently, the data gathered from specific measurements of animal characteristics are such that there is wide variability in the data. Often, such wide variability is not present in a control or low-dose group, but in an intermediate dosage group variance inflation may occur. That is, there may be a large standard deviation associated with the measurements from this intermediate group. In the face of such a set of data, the conclusion that there is no biological effect based on a finding of no statistically significance effect might well be erroneous.

2. In designing experiments, one should keep in mind that potential effect of involuntary censoring on sample size. In other words, though a study might start with five dogs per group, this provides no margin should any die before the study is ended and blood samples are collected and analyzed. Just enough experimental units per group frequently leaves too few at the end to allow meaningful statistical analysis, and allowances should be made accordingly in establishing group sizes.

3. It is certainly possible to pool the data from several identical toxicological studies. One approach to this is meta-analysis, considered in detail later in this chapter. For example, after first having performed an acute inhalation study where only three treatment group animals survived to the point at which a critical measure (such as analysis of blood samples) was performed, we would not have enough data to perform a meaningful statistical analysis. We could then repeat the protocol with new control and treatment group animals from the same source. At the end, after assuring ourselves that the two sets of data are comparable, we could combine (or pool) the data from survivors of the second study with those from the first. The costs

of this approach, however, would then be both a greater degree of effort expended (than if we had performed a single study with larger groups) and increased variability in the pooled samples (decreasing the power of our statistical methods).

4. Another frequently overlooked design option in toxicology is the use of an unbalanced design, that is, of different group sizes for different levels of treatment.

There is no requirement that each group in a study (control, low dose, intermediate dose and high dose) have an equal number of experimental units assigned to it. Indeed, there are frequently good reasons to assign more experimental units to one group than to others, and, as we shall see later all the major statistical methodologies have provisions to adjust for such inequalities, within certain limits. The two most common uses of the unbalanced design have larger groups assigned to either the highest dose, to compensate for losses due to possible deaths during the study, or to the lowest dose to give more sensitivity in detecting effects at levels close to an effect threshold or more confidence to the assertion that no effect exists.

5. We are frequently confronted with the situation where an undesired variable is influencing our experimental results in a nonrandom fashion. Such a variable is called a confounding variable; its presence, as discussed earlier, makes the clear attribution and analysis of effects at best difficult, and at worst impossible. Sometimes such confounding variables are the result of conscious design or management decisions, such as the use of different instruments, personnel, facilities, or procedures for different test groups within the same study. Occasionally, however, such confounding variables are the result of unintentional factors or actions, in which there is, as it is called, a lurking variable. Examples of such variables are almost always the result of standard operating procedures being violated: water not being connected to a rack of animals over a weekend, a set of racks not being cleaned as frequently as others, or a contaminated batch of feed being used.

6. Finally, some thought must be given to the clear definition of what is meant by experimental unit and concurrent control.

The experimental unit in toxicology encompasses a wide variety of possibilities. It may be cells, plates of microorganisms, individual animals, litters of animals, and so on. The importance of clearly defining the experimental unit is that the number of such units per group is the $N$ which is used in statistical calculations or analyses and critically affects such calculations. The experimental unit is the unit which receives treatments and yields a response which is measured and becomes a datum.

A true concurrent control is one that is identical in every manner with the treatment groups except for the treatment being evaluated. This means that all manipulations, including gavaging with equivalent volumes of vehicle or exposing to equivalent rates of air exchanges in an inhalation chamber, should be duplicated in control groups just as they occur in treatment groups.

The goal of the four principles of experimental design is statistical efficiency and the economizing of resources.The single most important initial step in achieving such an outcome is to clearly define the objective of the study: get a clear statement of what questions are being asked.

For the reader who would like to further explore experimental design, there are a number of more detailed texts available which include more extensive treatments of the statistical aspects of experimental design (Cochran and Cox, 1975; Diamond, 1981; Federer, 1955; Hicks, 1982; Kraemer and Thiemann, 1987 and Myers, 1972).

There are four basic experimental design types used in toxicology. These are the randomized block, latin square, factorial design, and nested design. Other designs that are used are really combinations of these basic designs, and are very rarely employed in toxicology. Before examining these four basic types, however, we must first examine the basic concept of blocking.

Blocking is, simply put, the arrangement or sorting of the members of a population (such as all of an available group of test animals) into groups based on certain characteristics which may (but are not sure to) alter an experimental outcome. Such characteristics, which may cause a treatment to give a differential effect, include genetic background, age, sex, overall activity levels and so on. The process of blocking then acts (or attempts to act), so that each experimental group (or block) is assigned its fair share of the members of each of these subgroups.

We should now recall that randomization is aimed at spreading out the effect of undetectable or unsuspected characteristics in a population of animals or some portion of this population. The merging of the two concepts or randomization and blocking leads to the first basic experimental design, the randomized block. This type of design requires that each treatment group have at least one member of each recognized group (such as age), the exact members of each block being assigned in an unbiased (or random) fashion.

The second type of experimental design assumes that we can characterize treatments (whether intended or otherwise) as belonging clearly to separate sets. In the simplest case, these categories are arranged into two sets which may be thought of as rows (for, say, source litter of test animal, with the first litter as row 1, the next as row 2, etc.) and the secondary set of categories as columns (for, say, ages of test animals, with 6 to 8 weeks as column 1, 8 to 10 weeks as column 2 and so on). Experimental units are then assigned so that each major treatment (control, low dose, intermediate dose, etc.) appears once and only once in each row and each column. If we denote our test groups as A (control), B (low), C (intermediate) and D (high), such as assignment would appear as shown in the table.

|  | Age | | | |
| --- | --- | --- | --- | --- |
| Source Litter | 6–8 weeks | 8–10 weeks | 10–12 weeks | 12–14 weeks |
| 1: | A | B | C | D |
| 2: | B | C | D | A |
| 3: | C | D | A | B |
| 4: | D | A | B | C |

The third type of experimental design is the factorial design, in which there are two or more clearly understood treatments, such as exposure level to test chemical, animal age, or temperature. The classical approach to this situation (and to that described under the latin square) is to hold all but one of the treatments constant; and at any one time to vary just that one factor. Instead, in the factorial design all levels of a given factor are combined with all levels of every other factor in the experiment. When a change in one factor produces a different change in the response variable at one level of a factor than at other levels of this factor, there is an interaction between these two factors which can then be analyzed as an interaction effect.

The last of the major varieties of experimental design are the nested designs, where the levels of one factor are nested within (or are subsamples of) another factor. That is, each subfactor is evaluated only within the limits of its single larger factor.

## 22.3.  DATA RECORDING

Two distinct sources of systematic bias may occur in data recording. One is that awareness of treatment may, consciously or subconsciously, affect the values recorded by the measurer. This can be avoided by organizing data recording so that observations are made blind. The second is that there is a systematic shift in the standard of measurement with time, coupled with a tendency for different groups to be measured at different time points. This is particularly important when a pathologist grades a lesion for severity and when the control and high-dose animals are read before the intermediate-dose animals. In some situations it may be necessary to reread all the slides blind and in random order to be sure that diagnostic drift is avoided (Gad and Taulbee, 1996).

Valid analysis cannot be conducted unless one can distinguish animals which were examined and did not have the relevant response and animals which were not examined. It can also be important clearly to identify why data are missing. Table 22.4 identifies some basic rules for effective design of data collection forms.

## 22.4.  GENERALIZED METHODOLOGY SELECTION

One approach for the selection of appropriate techniques to employ in a particular situation is to use a decision-tree method. Figure 22.1 is a decision tree that leads to the choice of one of three other trees to assist in technique selection, with each of the subsequent trees addressing one of the three functions of statistics that was defined earlier in this chapter. Figure 22.2 is for the selection of hypothesis-testing procedures, Figure 22.3 for modeling procedures, and Figure 22.4 for reduction of dimensionality procedures. For the vast majority of situations, these trees will guide the user into the choice of the proper technique. The tests and terms in these trees will be explained subsequently.

**TABLE 22.4. Rules for Form Design and Preparation**

---

Forms should be used when some form of repetitive data must be collected. They may be either paper or electronic.

If only a few (two or three) pieces of data are to be collected, they should be entered into a notebook and not onto a form. This assumes that the few pieces are not a daily event, with the aggregate total of weeks/months/years ending up as lots of data to be pooled for analysis.

Forms should be self-contained, but should not try to repeat the content of the SOPs or method descriptions.

Column headings on forms should always specify the units of measurement and other details of entries to be made. The form should be arranged so that sequential entries proceed down a page, not across. Each column should be clearly labeled with a heading that identifies what is to be entered in the column. Any fixed part of entries (such at °C) should be in the column header.

Columns should be arranged from left to right so that there is a logical sequential order to the contents of an entry as it is made. An example would be date/time/animal number/ body weight/name of the recorder. The last item for each entry should be the name or unique initials of the individual who made the data entry.

Standard conditions that apply to all the data elements to be recorded on a form or the columns of the form should be listed as footnotes at the bottom of the form.

Entries of data on the form should not use more digits than are appropriate for the precision of the data being recorded.

Each form should be clearly titled to indicate its purpose and use. If multiple types of forms are being used, each should have a unique title or number.

Before designing the form, carefully consider the purpose for which it is intended. What data will be collected, how often, with what instrument, and by whom? Each of these considerations should be reflected in some manner on the form.

Those things which are common/standard for all entries on the form should be stated as such once. These could include such things as instrument used, scale of measurement (°C, F, or K), or the location where the recording is made.

---

## 22.5. STATISTICAL ANALYSIS: GENERAL CONSIDERATIONS

### 22.5.1. Variables to be Analyzed

Although some pathologists still regard their discipline as providing qualitative rather than quantitative data, it is abundantly clear that pathology, when applied to routine screening of animal toxicity and carcinogenicity studies, has to be quantitative to at least some degree so that statistical inferences and statements can be made about possible treatment effects. Inevitably, there will be some descriptive text which will not be appropriate for statistical analysis. However, the main objective of the pathologist should be to provide information on the presence or absence (with severity grade or size where appropriate) of a list of conditions, consistently recorded from animal to animal and classified by well-defined criteria, which can be validly used in a statistical assessment.

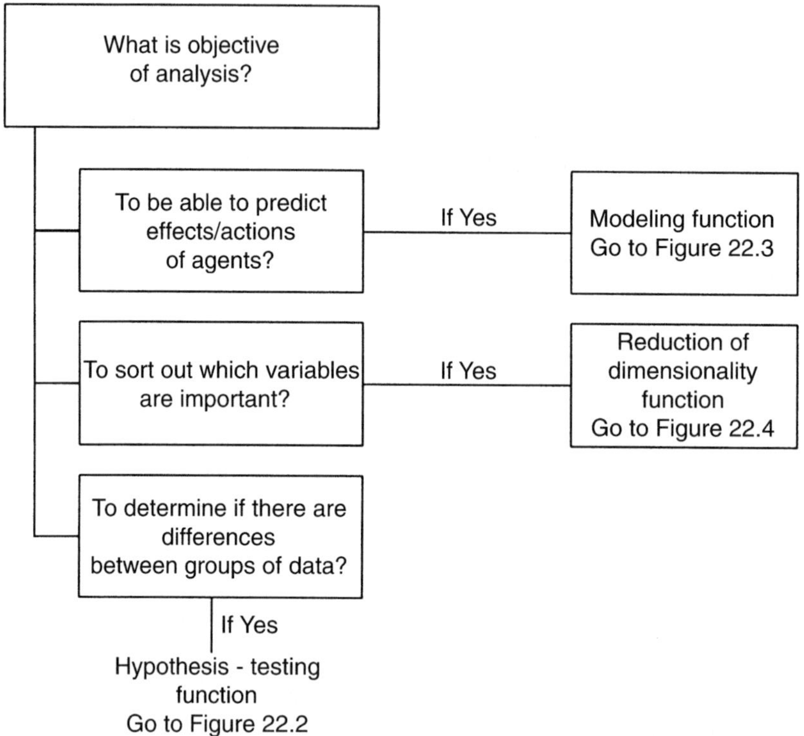



**FIGURE 22.1.** Overall decision tree for selecting statistical procedures.

Given that statistical analysis is worth doing and data are available that would be analyzed, should one then analyze all the endpoints recorded? Some arguments none of which really holds water, have been put forward against analyzing all the endpoints studies.

One argument is that some endpoints are not of interest. Perhaps the study is essentially a carcinogenicity study, so that nonneoplastic endpoints are not considered to be "background pathology" and almost *per se* unrelated to treatment. However, if the pathologist has gone to the trouble of recording the data, then surely, in general, they ought to be analyzed. The costs of the statistical analysis are much less than those of doing the study and the pathology. While one might justify failure to analyze nonneoplastic data where tumor analysis has already shown that the compound is clearly carcinogenic and no longer of market potential, the general rule ought to be to analyze everything that has been specifically investigated.

Another argument put forward against doing multiple analyses is that it may yield many chance significant $p$ values that have to be considered and evaluated for biological significance in the context of the entire set of available data. The whole context of dose response, as summarized in Table 22.5, must be kept in mind. A detailed look at the data can only aid interpretation, provided that one is not

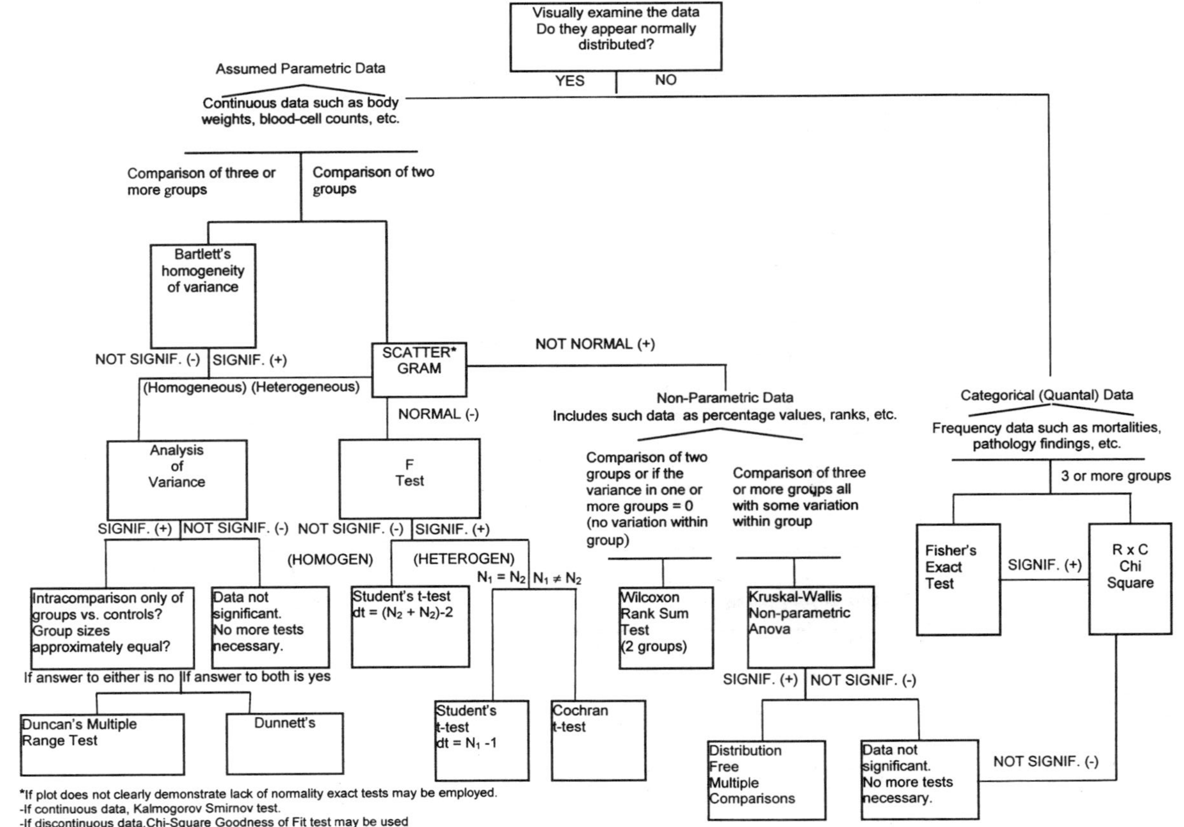


**FIGURE 22.2.** Decision tree for selecting hypothesis-testing procedures.

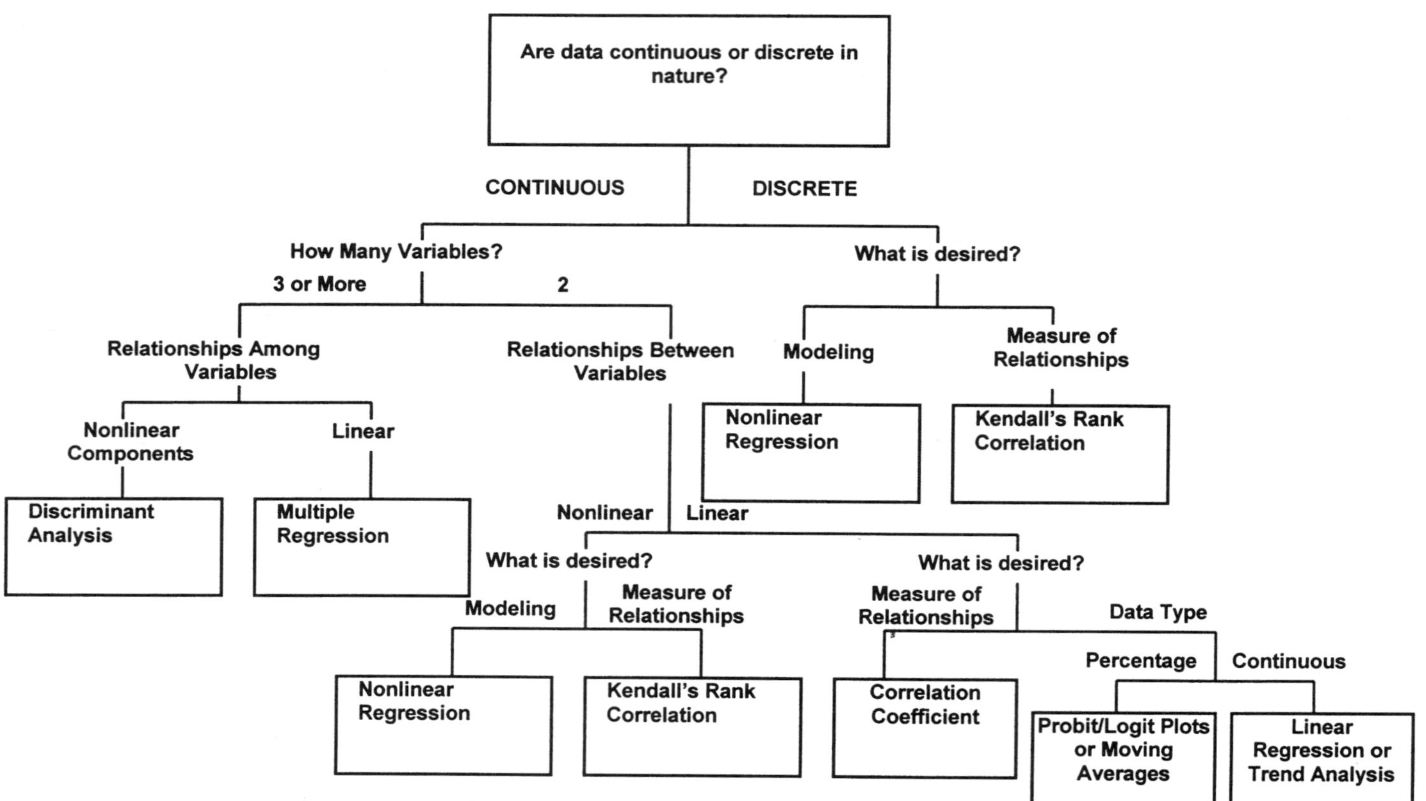


**FIGURE 22.3.** Decision tree for selecting modeling procedures.

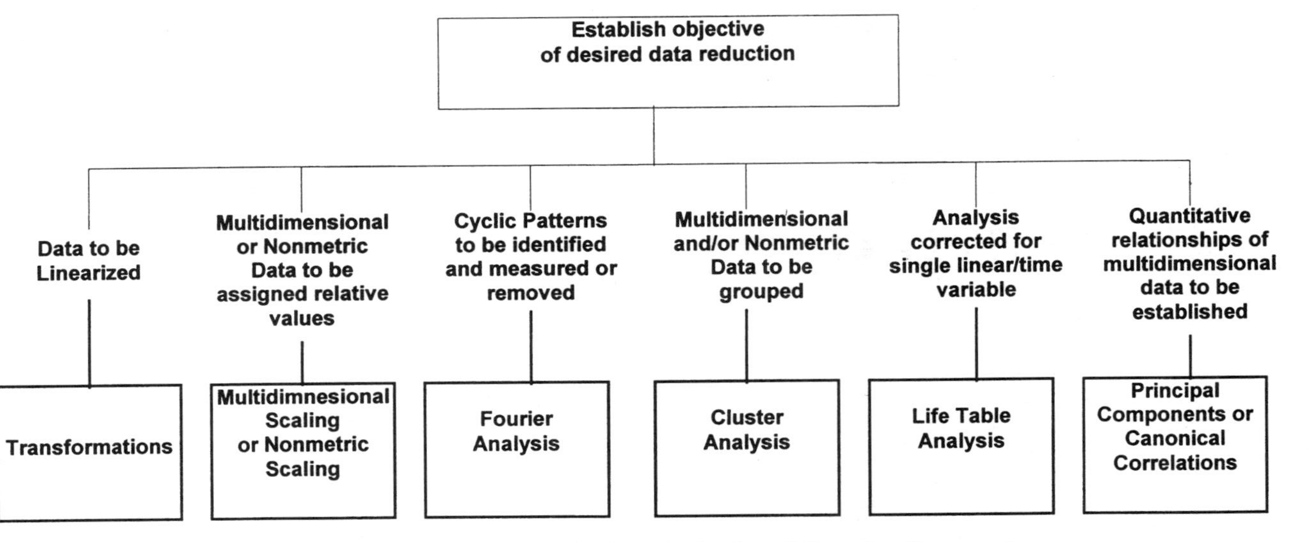


**FIGURE 22.4.** Decision tree for selection of reduction of dimensionality procedures.

887

**TABLE 22.5. The Three Dimensions of Dose Response**

As dose increases:
Incidence of responders in an exposed population increases
Severity of response in effected individuals increases
Time to occurrence of response or of progressive stage of response decreases

hidebound by the false argument that statistical significance necessarily equates with biological importance and definitely indicates a true effect of treatment.

Finally, some endpoints occur only very rarely. One must then be clear what "very rarely" is. For a typical study with a control and three dose groups of equal size, one would get a significant trend statistics if all three cases occurred at the top dose level or in the control group (two-tailed $p \approx 0.03$), so a total of three cases will normally be enough for statistical analysis. Endpoints occurring once or twice only are not worth analyzing formally, although, if only seen in the top dose group, they may be worth noting in the report. This is especially true if they are lesions that are rarely reported.

## 22.5.2. Combination of Pathological Conditions

There are four main situations where one might consider combining pathological conditions in a statistical analysis.

The first is when essentially the same pathological condition has been recorded under two or more different names or even under the same name in different places. Here failure to combine these conditions in the analysis may severely limit the chances of detecting a true treatment effect. It should be noted, however, that grouping together conditions which are actually different may also result in the masking of a true treatment effect, particularly if the treatment has a very specific effect.

The second is when separately recorded pathological conditions form successive steps on the pathway of the same process. The most important example of this is for the incidence of related types of malignant tumor, benign tumor, and focal hyperplasia. It will normally be appropriate to carry out analyses of (1) incidence of malignant tumor, (2) incidence of benign or malignant tumor and, where appropriate, (3) incidence of focal hyperplasia, benign or malignant tumor. It will not normally be appropriate to carry out analyses of benign tumor incidence only or of the incidence of hyperplasia only.

The third situation for combining is when the same pathological condition appears in different organs as a result of the same underlying process. Examples of this are the multicentric tumors (such as myeloid leukaemia, reticulum cell sarcoma and lymphosarcoma) or certain non-neoplastic conditions (such as arteritis/peri-arteritis and amyloid degeneration). Here analysis will normally be carried out only of incidence at any site, although in some situations site-specific analyses might be worth carrying out.

The final situation where an analysis of combined pathological conditions is normal is for analyses of overall incidence of malignant tumor at any site, of benign or malignant tumor at any site or of multiple tumor incidence. While analyses of tumor incidence at specific sites are normally more meaningful, since treatments often affect only a few specific sites, these additional analyses are usually required to guard against the possibility that treatment had some weak but general tumor-enhancing effect not otherwise evident.

In some situations, one might also envisage analyses of other combinations of specific tumors, such as tumors at related sites (e.g., endocrine organs if the compound had a hormonal effect) or of similar histological type.

### 22.5.3. Taking Severity into Account

The same line or argument that suggests that if the pathologist records data they should be analyzed, also suggests that if the pathologist chooses to grade a condition for severity, the grade should be taken into account in the analysis. There are two ways to carry out analysis when the grade has to be taken into account. In one, analyses are carried out not only of whether or not the animal has a condition, but also of whether or not the condition is at least grade 2, at least grade 3, and so on. In the other approach, nonparametric (rank) methods are used. The latter approach is more powerful, as it uses all the information in one analysis, although the output may not be so easily understood by those without some statistical training.

Note that the analyses based on grade can be carried out only if grading has been consistently applied throughout. If a condition has been scored only as present or absent for some animals, but has been graded for others, it is not possible to carry out graded analyses unless the pathologist is willing to go back and grade the specific animals showing the condition.

### 22.5.4. Using Simple Methods That Avoid Complex Assumptions

Different methods for statistical analysis can vary considerably in their complexity and in the number of assumptions they make. Although the use of statistical models has its place, more so for effect estimation than for hypothesis testing, and more so in studies of complex design than in those of simple design, there are advantages in using, wherever possible, statistical methods that are simple, robust, and make as few assumptions as possible. There are three reasons for this. First, such methods are more generally understandable to the toxicologist. Second, there are hardly ever extensive enough data in practice to validate any given formal model fully. Third, even if a particular model were known to be appropriate, the loss of efficiency in using appropriate simpler methods is often only very small.

The methods we advocate for routine use for the analysis of tumor incidence tend, therefore, not to be based on the use of formal parametric statistical models. For example, when studying the relationship of treatment to incidence of a pathological condition and wishing to adjust for other factors (in particular, age at death) that might otherwise bias the comparison, methods involving "stratification" are recommended, rather than a multiple regression approach or time-to-tumor models. Analysis of variance (ANOVA) methods can be useful in the case of continuously distributed data for estimating treatment effects. However, they involve underlying assumptions (normally distributed variables, variability equal in each group). If these assumptions are violated, nonparametric methods based on the rank of observations, rather than their actual value, may be preferable for hypothesis testing.

### 22.5.5. Using All the Data

Often information is available about the relationship between treatment and a condition of interest for groups of animals differing systematically in respect of some other factor. Obvious examples are males and females, differing times of sacrifice, and differing secondary treatments. While it will be necessary, in general, to look at the relationsip within levels of this other factor, it will also be advisable to try to come to some assessment of the relationsip over all levels of the other factor, and where a combined inference is not sensible, but in far more situations this is not the case, and using all the data in one analysis allows a more powerful test of the relationsip under study. Some scientists consider that conclusions for males and females should always be drawn separately, but there are strong statistical arguments for a joint analysis.

### 22.5.6. Combining, Pooling, and Stratification

Suppose, in a hypothetical study of a toxic agent which induces tumors that do not shorten the lives of tumor-bearing animals, the data regarding the number of animals with tumor out of number examined are as follows:

|  | Control | Exposed | Combined |
|---|---|---|---|
| Early deaths | 1/20 (5%) | 18/90 (20%) | 19/110 (17%) |
| Late deaths | 24/80 (30%) | 7/10 (70%) | 31/90 (34%) |
| Total | 25/100 (25%) | 25/100 (25%) | 50/200 (25%) |

It can be seen that if the time of death is ignored and the *pooled* data are studied, the incidence of tumors is the same in each group, resulting in the *false* conclusion that treatment had no effect. Looking within each time of death, however, an increased incidence in the exposed group can be seen. An appropriate statistical method would *combine* a measure of difference between the groups based on the early deaths and a measure of difference based on the late deaths, and conclude *correctly* that incidence, after adjustment for time of death, is greater in the exposed groups.

In this example, time of death is the stratifying variable, with two strata: early deaths and late deaths. The essence of the methodology is to make comparisons only within strata (so that one is always comparing like with like except in respect of treatment) and then to combine the differences over strata. Stratification can be used to adjust for any variable, or indeed combinations of variables.

Some studies are of factorial design, in which combinations of treatments are tested. The simplest such design is one in which four equal sized groups of animals receive (1) no treatment, (2) treatment A only, (3) treatment B only and (4) treatments A and B. If one is prepared to assume that any effects of the two treatments are independent, one can use stratification to enable more powerful tests to be conducted of the possible individual treatment effects. Thus, to test for effects of treatment A for example, one conducts comparisons in two strata, the first consisting of groups 1 and 2 not given treatment B and the second consisting of groups 3 and 4 given treatment B. Combination of results from the two strata is based on twice as many animals, and is therefore markedly more likely to detect possible effects of treatment A than is a simple comparison of groups 1 and 2. There is also the possibility of identifying interactions, such as synergism and antagonism, between the two treatments.

In some routine long-term screening studies, the study design involved five groups of (usually) 50 animals of each sex, three of which are treated with successive doses of a compound and two of which are untreated controls. Assuming that there is no systematic difference between the control groups (e.g., the second control group in a different room or from a different batch of animals), it will be normal to carry out the main analyses with the control groups treated as a single group of 100 animals. It will usually be a sensible preliminary precaution to carry out additional analyses comparing incidences in the two control groups.

### 22.5.7. Trend Analysis, Low-Dose Extrapolation, and NOEL Estimation

While comparisons of individual treated groups with the control group are important, a more powerful test of a possible effect of treatment will be to carry out a test for a dose-related trend. This is because most true effects of treatment tend to result in a response which increases (or decreases) with increasing dose, and because trend tests take into account all the data in a single analysis. In interpreting the results of trend tests, it should be noted that a significant trend does not necessarily imply an increased risk at lower doses. Nor, conversely, does a lack of increase at lower doses necessarily indicate evidence of a threshold (i.e., a dose below which no increase occurs).

Note that the testing for trend is seen as a more sensitive way of picking up a possible treatment effect than simple pairwise comparisons of treated and control groups. Attempting to estimate the magnitude of effects at low doses, typically below the lowest positive dose tested in the study, is a much more complex procedure, and is heavily dependent on the assumed functional form of the dose-response relationship.

Deterministic trend models are based on the assumption that the trend of a time series can be approximated closely by simple mathematical functions of time over the entire span of the series. The most common representation of a deterministic trend is by means of polynomials or of transcendental functions. The time series from which the trend is to be identified is assumed to be generated by a nonstationary process where the nonstationarity results from a deterministic trend. A classical model is the regression or error model (Anderson, 1971) where the observed series is treated as the sum of a systematic part or trend and a random part or irregular. This model can be written as

$$Z_t = Y_t + U_t'$$

where $U_t$ is a purely random process; that is, $U_t \sim$ i.i.d. $(O, 2/u)$ (independent and identically distributed with expected value 0 and variance $\sigma(2/u)$).

Trend tests are generally described as "$k$-sample tests of the null hypothesis of identical distribution against an alternative of linear order," i.e., if sample I has distribution function $F_i$, $i = 1$ then the null hypothesis

$$H : F_1 = F_2 = \cdots = F_k$$

is tested against the alternative

$$H1 : F_1 \geq F_2 \geq \cdots = F_k$$

(or its reverse), there at least one of the inequalities is strict. These tests can be thought of as special cases of tests of regression or correlation in which association is sought between the observations and its ordered sample index. They are also related to analysis of variance except that the tests are tailored to be powerful against the subset of alternatives $H_1$, instead of the more general set $\{F_1 \neq F_j, \text{ some } i \neq j\}$.

Different tests arise from requiring power against specific elements or subsets of this rather extensive set of alternatives.

The most popular trend test in toxicology is currently that presented by Tarone in 1975 because it is that used by the National Cancer Institute in the analysis of carcinogenicity data. A simple, but efficient alternative is the Cox and Stuart test (Cox and Stuart, 1955) which is a modification of the sign test. For each point at which we have a measure (such as the indidence of animals observed with tumors) we form a pair of observations, one from each of the groups we wish to compare. In a traditional NCI bioassay this would mean pairing control with low dose and low dose with high dose (to explore a dose-related trend) or each time period observation in a dose group (except the first) with its predecessor (to evaluate a time-related trend). When the second observation in a pair exceeds the earlier observation, we record a plus sign for that pair. When the first observation is greater than the second, we record a minus sign for that pair. A preponderance of plus signs suggests a downward trend while an excess of minus signs suggests an upward trend. A formal test at a preselected confidence level can then be performed.

More formally put, after having defined what trend we want to test for, we first match pairs as $(X_1\text{-}X_{1+c}), (X_2, X_{2+c}), \ldots, (X_{n'-c}, X_{n'})$ where $c = (n')/2$ when $n'$ is even and $c = (n' + 1)/2$ when $n'$ is odd (where $n'$ is the number of observations in a set). The hypothesis is then tested by comparing the resulting number of excess positive or negative signs against a sign test table such as are found in Beyer.

We can, of course, combine a number of observations to allow ourselves to actively test for a set of trends, such as the existence of a trend of increasing difference between two groups of animals over a period of time. This is demonstrated in Example 22.1. In a chronic feeding study in rats, we tested the hypothesis that, in the second year of the study, there was a dose responsive increase in tumor incidence associated with the test compound. We utilize a Cox–Stuart test for trend to address this question. All groups start the second year with an equal number of animals.

### 22.5.8. Assumptions and Limitations

Trend tests seek to evaluate whether there is a monotonic tendency in response to a change in treatment. That is, the dose response direction is absolute: as dose goes up, the incidence of tumors increases. Thus the test loses power rapidly in response to the occurrences of "reversals", for example, a low-dose group with a decreased tumor incidence. There are methods (Dykstra and Robertson, 1983) which "smooth the bumps" of reversals in long data series. In toxicology, however, most data series are short (that is, there are only a few dose levels).

Tarone's trend test is most powerful at detecting dose-related trends when tumor onset hazard functions are proportional to each other. For more power against other dose related group differences, weighted versions of the statistic are also available (Breslow, 1984; Crowley and Breslow, 1984).

In 1985, the United States *Federal Register* recommended that the analysis of tumor incidence data be carried out with a Cochran–Armitage (Armitage, 1955; Cochran, 1954) trend test. The test statistic of the Cochran–Armitage test is defined as this term:

$$T_{CA} = \sqrt{\frac{N}{(N-r)r}, \frac{\sum_{i=0}^{k}\left(R_1 - \frac{n_1}{N}r\right)d_1}{\sqrt{\sum_{i=0}^{k}\frac{n_i}{N}d_i^2 - \left(\sum_{i=0}^{k}\frac{n_i}{N}d_1\right)^2}}}$$

with dose scores $d_i$. Armitage's test statistic is the square of this term ($T_{CA}^2$). As one-sided tests are carried out for an increase of tumor rates, the square is not considered. Instead, the above-mentioned test statistic which is presented by Portier and Hoel (1984) is used. This test statistic is asymptotically standard normal distributed. The Cochran–Armitage test is asymptotically efficient for all monotone alternatives (Tarone, 1975), but this result only holds asymptotically. And tumors are rare events, so the binominal proportions are small. In this situation approximations may become unreliable.

**EXAMPLE 22.1. Use of a Trend Text to Assess Tumorigenic Dose Response**

| | Control | | | | | Low Doses[a] | | |
|---|---|---|---|---|---|---|---|---|
| Month of Study | Total X Animals with Tumors | Change $[X_{A-B}]$ | Total Y Animals with Tumors | Change $[Y_{A-B}]$ | Compared to Control (Y-X) | Total Z Animals with Tumors | Change $[Z_{A-B}]$ | Compared to Control (Z-X) |
| 12(A) | 1 | NA | 0 | NA | NA | 5 | NA | NA |
| 13(B) | 1 | 0 | 0 | 0 | 0 | 7 | 2 | (+)2 |
| 14(C) | 3 | 2 | 1 | 1 | (−)1 | 11 | 4 | (+)2 |
| 15(D) | 3 | 0 | 1 | 0 | 0 | 11 | 0 | 0 |
| 16(E) | 4 | 1 | 1 | 0 | (−)1 | 13 | 2 | (+)1 |
| 17(F) | 5 | 1 | 3 | 2 | (+)1 | 14 | 1 | 0 |
| 18(G) | 5 | 0 | 3 | 0 | 0 | 15 | 1 | (+)1 |
| 19(H) | 5 | 0 | 5 | 2 | (+)2 | 18 | 3 | (+)3 |
| 20(I) | 6 | 1 | 6 | 1 | 0 | 19 | 1 | 0 |
| 21(J) | 8 | 2 | 7 | 1 | (−)1 | 22 | 3 | (+)1 |
| 22(K) | 12 | 4 | 9 | 2 | (−)2 | 26 | 4 | 0 |
| 23(L) | 14 | 2 | 12 | 3 | (+)1 | 28 | 2 | 0 |
| 24(M) | 18 | 4 | 17 | 5 | (+)1 | 31 | 3 | (−)1 |
| | | | Sum of signs | | 4 +<br>4 − | | Sum of signs | 6 +<br>1 − |
| | | | Y-X | | = 0<br>(No trend) | | Z-X | = 5 |

[a]Reference to a sign table is not necessary for the low-dose comparison (where there is no trend) but clearly shows the high dose to be significant at the $p \leq 0.5$ level.

Therefore, exact tests are considered that can be performed using two different approaches: conditional and unconditional. In the first case, the total number of tumors $r$ is regarded as fixed. As a result the null distribution of the test statistic is independent of the common probability $p$. The exact conditional null distribution is a multivariate hypergeometric distribution.

The unconditional model treats the sum of all tumors as a random variable. Then the exact unconditional null distribution is a multivariate binomial distribution. The distribution depends on the unknown probability.

Such low-dose extrapolation is typically only conducted for tumors believed to be caused by a genotoxic effect, which some, but by no means all, scientists believe have no threshold. For other types of tumors and for many nonneoplastic endpoints a threshold cannot be estimated directly from data at a limited number of dose levels; a no observed effect level (NOEL) can be estimated by finding the highest dose level at which there is no significant increase in effects.

A useful technique for determining if there is an effect of treatment on any toxicological parameter is the NOSTASOT method (Tukey et al., 1985; Antonello et al., 1993). This test is based on the principle that a possible toxicological effect of interest occurs with a normal dose response; that is, there is an increasing effect with increasing dosage. The data to be analyzed should be examined first to confirm that this principle is not violated. In this method, regression analysis is used to determine if there is an increased or decreased response in a parameter with increasing dosage. This method can be visualized as a plot of response versus dosage in which the analysis determines if the slope of the plotted line deviates significantly from zero.

This method can be used for essentially all parameters. Three analyses are performed, each with different spacing between dosage levels. The spacing in the first analysis is based on the arithmetic values of the dosage levels. The spacing in the second, referred to as the ordinal scaling, has equal spacing between dosage levels; that is, the control through high-dosage levels are assigned values of 0, 1, 2, and 3. In the third analysis, the log of the dosage level is used. Since the log of zero is impractical, the control group is assigned a value based on the spacing between the low- and middle-dosage levels according to a formula that assigns a log scale value to the control such that the ratio of the difference between the control and low-dose groups and the difference between the low- and middle-dose groups is equal both in absolute values and in log scale values. This places the control group at a reasonable distance from the low-dosage group. The lowest $p$ value among the three analyses— arithmetic, ordinal, and logarithmic—is taken as the $p$ value of the overall analysis based on the assumption that, if there is a dosage-related effect, the method of analysis yielding the lowest value is the best model for that dosage response. A correction for the multiplicity of analyses can be applied. If none of the three analyses are significant at the 0.05 level, the analysis is complete and the high-dosage level is referred to as the "no statistical significance of trend dose", or the NOSTASOT dose. If there is a significant trend through the high-dosage level, the data from the high-dosage level is deleted and the trend test repeated. This process is repeated until a NOSTASOT dose is determined. Effects at dosage levels above the NOSTASOT dose are then considered to be statistically significant.

There are two major benefits of the NOSTASOT method. One is that spurious statistically significant results only at the low- and/or middle-dosage levels are eliminated, resulting in a reduction in false positives. A second benefit is that in some cases there may be real effects at multiple dosage levels that at any single dosage level are not statistically significant but will nevertheless result in a significant trend, thus providing increased sensitivity and reducing false negatives.

### 22.5.9.  Need for Age Adjustment

Where there are marked differences in survival between treated groups, it is widely recognized that there is a need for an age adjustment (i.e., an adjustment for age at death or onset). This is illustrated in Example 22.1, where, because of the greater number of deaths occurring early in the treated group, the true effect of treatment disappears if no adjustment is made. Thus, a major purpose of age adjustment is to avoid bias.

It is not so generally recognized, however, that, even where there are no survial differences, age adjustment can increase the power to detect between-group differences. This is illustrated in this example.

|               | Control | Exposed |
| ------------- | ------- | ------- |
| Early deaths  | 0/20    | 0/20    |
| Middle deaths | 1/10    | 9/10    |
| Late deaths   | 20/20   | 20/20   |
| Total         | 21/50   | 29/50   |

Here treatment results in a somewhat earlier onset of a condition which occurs eventually in all animals. Failure to age-adjust will result in a comparison of 29/50 with 21/50, which is not statistically significant. Age adjustment will essentially ignore the early and late deaths, which contribute no comparative statistical information, and be based on the comparison of 9/10 with 1/10, which is statistically significant. Here age adjustment sharpens the contrast, rather than avoiding bias, by avoiding diluting data capable of detecting treatment effects with data that are of little or no value for this purpose.

### 22.5.10.  Need to Take Context of Observation into Account

It is now widely recognized that age adjustment cannot properly be carried out unless the context of observation is taken into account. There are three relevant contexts, the first two relating to the situation where the condition is only observed at death (e.g., an internal tumor) and the third where it can be observed in life (e.g., a skin tumor).

In the first context the condition is assumed to have caused the death of the animal, that is, to be *fatal*. Here the incidence rate for a time interval and a group is calculated by

(number of animals dying in the interval because of the lesion)/(number of
animals alive at the start of the interval).

In the second context, the animal is assumed to have died of another cause, that
is, the condition is *incidental*. Here the rate is calculated by

(number of animals dying in the interval with the lesion)/(total number of
animals dying in the interval).

In the third context, where the condition is *visible*, the rate is calculated by

(number of animals getting the condition in the interval)/(number of animals
without the condition at the start of the interval).

A problem with the method of Peto et al. (1980), which takes context of
observation into account, is that some pathologists are unwilling or feel unable to
decide whether, in any given case, a condition is fatal or incidental. A number of
points should be made here.

First, where there are marked survival differences, it may not be possible to
conclude reliably whether a treatment is beneficial or harmful unless such a decision
is made. This is well illustrated by the example in Peto et al (1980), where assuming
all pituitary tumors were fatal results in the (false) conclusion that $N$-nitrosodi-
methylamine (NDMA) was carcinogenic, while assuming they were all incidental
resulted in the (false) conclusion that NDMA was protective. Using, correctly, the
pathologist's best opinion as to which were, and which were not, likely to be fatal,
resulted in an analysis which (correctly) concluded NDMA had no effect. If the
pathologist, in this case, had been unwilling to make a judgment as to fatality,
believing it to be unreliable, no conclusion could have been reached. This state of
affairs would, however, be a fact of life, and *not* a position reached because an
inappropriate statistical method was being used.

Although it will normally be a good routine for the pathologist to ascribe "factors
contributory to death" for each animal that was not part of a scheduled sacrifice, it
is in fact not strictly necessary to determine the context of observation for all
conditions at the outset. An alternative strategy is to analyze under differing
assumptions: (1) no cases fatal, (2) all cases occurring in decedents fatal and (3)
all cases of same defined severity occurring in decedents fatal, with, under each
assumption, other cases incidental.

If the conclusion turns out the same under each assumption, or if the pathologist
can say, on general grounds, that one assumption is likely to be a close approximation to the truth, it may not be necessary to know the context of observation for the
condition in question for each individual animal. Using the alternative strategy might
result in a saving of the pathologist's time by only having to make a judgment for a
limited number of conditions where the conclusion seems to hand on correct
knowledge of the context of observation.

Finally, it should be noted that, although many nonneoplastic conditions observed at death are never causes of death, it is, in principle, as necessary to know the context of observation for nonneoplastic conditions as it is for tumors.

### 22.5.11. Experimental and Observational Units

In many situations, the animal is both the "experimental unit" and the "observational unit", but this is not always so. For determining treatment effects by the methods of the next section, it is important that each experimental unit provide only one item of data for analysis, as the methods all assume that individual data items are statistically independent. In many feeding studies, where the cage is assigned to a treatment, it is the cage, rather than the animal, that is the experimental unit. In histopathology, observations for a tissue are often based on multiple sections per animal, so that the section is the observational unit. Multiple observations per experimental unit should be combined in some suitable way into an overall average for that unit before analysis.

### 22.5.12. Missing Data

In many types of analysis, animals with missing data are simply removed from the analysis. There are, however, some situations where this can be an inappropriate thing to do. One situation is when carrying out an analysis of a condition that is assumed to have caused the death of the animal. Although an animal dying at week 83 for which the section was unavailable for microscopic examination cannot contribute to the group comparison at week 83, one knows that it did not die because of any condition in previous weeks, so it should contribute to the denominator of the calculations in all previous weeks.

Another situation is when histopathological examination of a tissue is not carried out unless an abnormality is seen at post mortem. In such an experiment one might have the following data for that tissue:

*Control Group.* 50 animals, 2 abnormal at post mortem, 2 examined microscopically, 2 with tumor of specific type.

*Treated Group.* 50 animals, 15 abnormal at post mortem, 15 examined microscopically, 14 with tumor of specific type.

Ignoring animals with no microscopic sections, one would compare $2/2 = 100\%$ with $14/15 = 93\%$ and conclude that treatment nonsignificantly decreased incidence. This is likely to be a false conclusion, and it would be better here to compare the percentages of animals which had a post mortem abnormality which turned out to be a tumor, that is, $2/50 = 4\%$ with $14/50 = 28\%$. Unless some aspect of treatment made tumors much easier to detect at post mortem, one could then conclude that treatment did have an effect on tumor incidence.

Particular care has to be taken in studies where the procedures for histopathological examination vary by group. In a number of studies conducted in recent years, the protocol demands full microscopic examination of a given tissue list in decedents in all groups, and in terminally killed controls in high-dose animals. In other animals, terminally killed low- and mid-dose animals, microscopic examination of a tissue is only conducted if the tissue is found to be abnormal at post mortem. Such a protocol is designed to save money, but leads to difficulty in commparing the treatment groups validly. Suppose, for example, responses in terminally killed animals are 8/20 in the controls, 3/3 (with 17 unexamined) in the low-dose and 5/6 (with 14 unexamined) in the mid-dose animals. Is one supposed to conclude that treatment at the low- and mid-doses increased response, based on a comparison of the proportions examined microscopically (40%, 100% and 83%), or that it decreased response, bassed on the proportion of animals in the group (40%, 15% and 25%)? It could well be that treatment had no effect but some small tumors were missed at post mortem. In this situation, a valid comparison can only be achieved by ignoring the low- and mid-dose groups when carrying out the comparison for the age stratum "terminal kill". This, of course, seems wasteful of data, but these are data that cannot be usefully used owing to the inappropriate protocol.

### 22.5.13.  Use of Historical Control Data

In some situations, particularly where incidences are low, the results from a single study may suggest an effect of treatment on tumor incidence but be unable to demonstrate it conclusively. The possibility of comparing results in the treated groups with those of control groups from other studies is then often raised. Thus, a non-significant incidence of 2 cases out of 50 in a treated group may seem much more significant if no cases have been seen in, say, 1000 animals representing controls from 20 similar studies. Conversely, a significant incidence of 5 cases out of 50 in a treated group as compared with 0 out of 50 in the study controls may seem far less convincing if many other control groups had incidences around 5 out of 50.

While not understating the importance of looking at historical control data, it must be emphasized that there are a number of reasons why variation between study may be greater than variation within study. Differences in diet, in duration of the study, in intercurrent mortality and in who the study pathologist is may all contribute. Statistical techniques that ignore this and carry out simple statistical tests of treatment incidence against a pooled control incidence may well give results that are seriously in error, and are likely to overstate statistical significance considerably.

### 22.5.14.  Methods for Data Examination and Preparation

The data from toxicology studies should always be examined before any formal analysis Such examinations should be directed to determining if the data are suitable for analysis, and if so what form the analysis should take (see Figure 22.2.) If the data as collected are not suitable for analysis, or if they are only suitable for low-powered analytical techniques, one may wish to use one of many forms of data transformation to change the data characteristics so that they are more amenable to analysis.

The above two objectives, data examination and preparation, are the primary focus of this section. For data examination, two major techniques are presented: the scattergram and Bartlett's test. Likewise, for data preparation (with the issues of rounding and outliers having been addressed in a previous chapter) two techniques are presented: randomization (including a test for randomness in a sample of data) and transformation. Exploratory data analysis (EDA) is presented and briefly reviewed later. This is a broad collection of techniques and approaches to "probe" data, that is, to both examine and to perform some initial, flexible analysis of the data.

### 22.5.15. Scattergram

Two of the major points to be made throughout this chapter are (1) the use of the appropriate statistical tests, and (2) the effects of small sample sizes (as is often the case in toxicology) on our selection of statistical techniques. Frequently, simple examination of the nature and distribution of data collected from a study can also suggest patterns and results which were unanticipated and for which the use of additional or alternative statistical methodology is warranted. It was these three points which caused the author to consider a section on scattergrams and their use essential for toxicologists.

Bartlett's test may be used to determine if the values in groups of data are homogeneous. If they are, this (along with the knowledge that they are from a continuous distribution) demonstrates that parametric methods are applicable. But, if the values in the (continuous data) groups fail Bartlett's test (i.e., are heterogeneous), we cannot be secure in our belief that parametric methods are appropriate until we gain some confidence that the values are normally distributed. With large groups of data, we can compute parameters of the population (kurtosis and skewness, in particular) and from these parameters determine if the population is normal (with a certain level of confidence). If our concern is especially marked, we can use a chi-square goodness-of-fit test for normality. But when each group of data consists of 25 or fewer values, these measures or tests (kurtosis, skewness, and chi-square goodness-of-fit) are not accurate indicators of normality. Instead, in these cases we should prepare a scattergram of the data, then evaluate the scattergram to estimate if the data are normally distributed. This procedure consists of developing a histogram of the data, then examining the histogram to get a visual appreciation of the location and distribution of the data.

The abscissa (or horizontal scale) should be in the same scale as the values, and should be divided so that the entire range of observed values is covered by the scale of the abscissa. Across such a scale we then simply enter symbols for each of our values. Figure 22.2 shows such a plot.

Example 22.2 is a traditional and rather limited form of scatterplot but such plots can reveal significant information about the amount and types of association between the two variables, the existence and nature of outliers, the clustering of data, and a number of other two-dimensional factors (Anscombe, 1973 and Chambers et al. 1983).

Current technology allows us to add significantly more graphical information to scatterplots by means of graphic symbols (letters, faces, different shapes such as squares, colors, etc.) for the plotted data points. One relatively simple example of this approach is shown in Figure 22.5, where the simple case of dose (in a dermal study), dermal irritation, and white blood cell count are presented. This graph quite clearly suggests that as dose (variable $x$) is increased, dermal irritation (variable $y$) also increases; and as irritation becomes more severe, white blood cell count (variable $z$) an indicator of immune system involvement, suggesting infection or persistent inflammation, also increases. There is no direct association of variables $x$ and $z$, however (Cleveland and McGill, 1984; Cleveland, 1985; and Tufte, 1990).

Group 1 can be seen to approximate a normal distribution (bell-shaped curve); we can proceed to perform the appropriate parametric tests with such data. But group 2 clearly does not appear to be normally distributed. In this case, the appropriate nonparametric technique must be used.

**EXAMPLE 22.2.**

---

Suppose we have the two data sets below:

Group 1: 4.5, 5.4, 5.9, 6.0, 6.4, 6.5, 6.9, 7.0, 7.1, 7.0, 7.4, 7.5, 7.5, 7.5, 7.6, 8.0, 8.1, 8.4, 8.5, 8.6, 9.0, 9.4, 9.5 and 10.4.

Group 2: 4.0, 4.5, 5.0, 5.1, 5.4, 5.5, 5.6, 6.5, 6.5, 7.0, 7.4, 7.5, 7.5 8.0, 8.1, 8.5, 8.5, 9.0, 9.1, 9.5, 9.5, 10.1, 10.0 and 10.4.

Both of these groups contain 24 values and cover the same range. From them we can prepare the following scattergrams.

Group 1:

```
                         X
                 X       X
                 X       X               X
             X   X   X   X   X   X               X
     X       X   X   X   X   X   X   X   X               X
 |   |   |   |   |   |   |   |   |   |   |   |   |   |
 _   _   _   _   _   _   _   _   _   _   _   _   _   _
 4       5       6       7       8       9       10
```

Group 2:

```
             X               X
         X   X       X       X   X   X   X   X   X
 X   X   X   X       X   X   X   X   X   X   X   X   X
 |   |   |   |   |   |   |   |   |   |   |   |   |   |
 _   _   _   _   _   _   _   _   _   _   _   _   _   _
 4       5       6       7       8       9       10
```

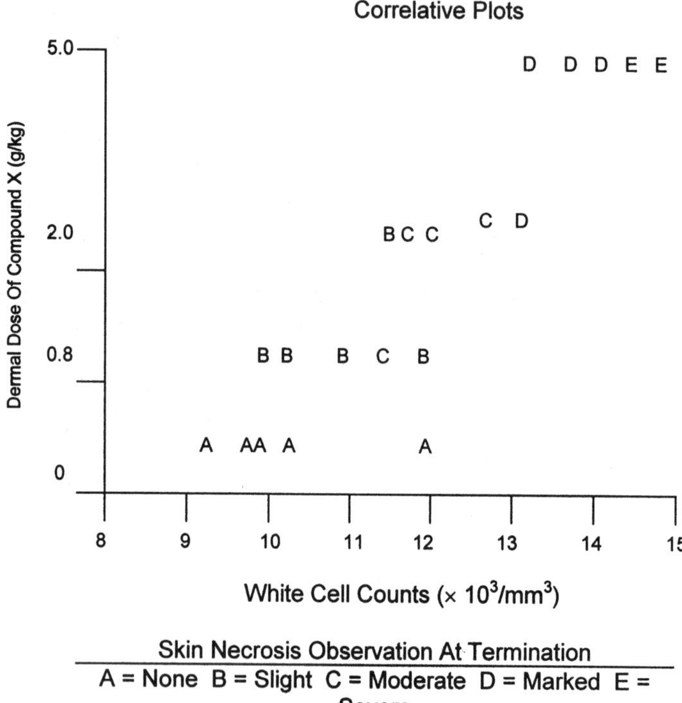


**FIGURE 22.5.** Exploratory data analysis.

## 22.5.16. Bartlett's Test for Homogeneity of Variance

Bartlett's test (Sokal and Rohlf, 1994) is used to compare the variances (values reflecting the degree of variability in data sets) among three or more groups of data, where the data in the groups are continuous sets (such as body weights, organ weights, red blood cell counts, or diet consumption measurements). It is expected that such data will be suitable for parametric methods (normality of data is assumed) and Bartlett's is frequently used as a test for the assumption of equivalent variances.

Bartlett's is based on the calculation of the corrected $\chi^2$ (chi-square) value by the formula

$$\chi^2_{\text{corr}} = 2.3026 \frac{\sum df \left( \log_{10}\left[ \frac{\sum[df(S^2)]}{\sum df} \right] \right) - \sum[df(\log_{10} S^2)]}{1 + \frac{1}{3(K-1)}\left[ \sum \frac{1}{df} - \frac{1}{\sum df} \right]}$$

where $S^2 = \text{variance} = \dfrac{\dfrac{n\sum X^2 - (\sum X)^2}{n}}{n-1}$

$X$ = individual datum within each group.

$n$ = number of data within each group.

$K$ = number of groups being compared.

$D_f$ = degrees of freedom for each group = $(N - 1)$.

The corrected $\chi^2$ value yielded by the above calculations is compared to the values listed in the chi square table according to the numbers of degrees of freedom (Snedecor and Cochran, 1980).

If the calculated value is smaller than the table value at the selected $p$ level (traditionally 0.05) the groups are accepted to be homogeneous and the use of ANOVA is assumed proper. If the calculated $\chi^2$ is greater than the table value, the groups are heterogeneous and other tests (as indicated in Figure 22.2, the decision tree) are necessary.

### *Assumptions and Limitations.*

1. Bartlett's test does not test for normality, but rather homogeneity of variance (also called equality of variances or homoscedasticity).

2. Homoscedasticity is an important assumption for Student's $t$-test, analysis of variance, and analysis of covariance.

3. The $F$-test (covered in the next section) is actually a test for the two sample (that is, control and one test group) case of homoscedasticity. Bartlett's is designed for three or more samples.

4. Bartlett's is very sensitive to departures from normality. As a result, a finding of a significant chi square value in Bartlett's may indicate nonnormality rather than heteroscedasticity. Such a finding can be brought about by outliers, and the sensitivity to such erroneous findings is extreme with small sample sizes.

### 22.5.17. Statistical Goodness-of-Fit Tests

A goodness-of-fit test is a statistical procedure for comparing individual measurements to a specified type of statistical distribution. For example, a normal distribution is completely specified by its arithmetic mean and variance (the square of the standard deviation). The null hypothesis, that the data represent a sample from a single normal distribution, can be tested by a statistical goodness-of-fit test. Various goodness-of-fit tests have been devised to determine if the data deviate significantly from a specified distribution. If a significant departure occurs, it indicates only that the specified distribution can be rejected with some assurance. This does not necessarily mean that the true distribution contains two or more subpopulations. The true distribution may be a single distribution, based upon a different mathematical relationship, for example, log-normal. In the latter case, logarithms of the measurement would not be expected to exhibit by a goodness-of-fit test a statistically significant departure from a log-normal distribution.

Everitt & Hand (1981) recommended use of a sample of 200 or more to conduct a valid analysis of mixtures of populations. Even the maximum likelihood method, the best available method, should be used with extreme caution, or not at all, when separation between the means of the sub-populations is less than 3 SD and sample sizes are less than 300. None of the available methods conclusively establish bimodality, which may, however, occur when separation between the two means (modes) exceeds 2 SD. Conversely, inflections in probits or separations in histograms *less than* 2 SD apart may arise from genetic differences in test subjects.

Mendal et al. (1993) compared eight tests of normality to detect a mixture consisting of two normally distributed components with different means but equal variances. Fisher's skewness statistic was preferable when one component comprised less than 15% of the total distribution. When the two components comprised more nearly equal proportions (35–65%) of the total distribution, the Engelman and Hartigan test (1969) was preferable. For other mixing proportions, the maximum likelihood ratio test was best. Thus, the maximum likelihood ratio test appears to perform very well, with only small loss from optimality, even when it is not the best procedure.

The method of *maximum likelihood* provides estimators which are usually quite satisfactory. They have the desirable properties of being consistent, asymptotically normal, and asymptotically efficient for large samples under quite general conditions. They are often biased, but the bias is frequently removable by a simple adjustment. Other methods of obtaining estimators are also available, but the maximum likelihood method is the most frequently used.

Maximum likelihood estimators also have another desirable property: *invariance*. Let us denote the maximum likelihood estimator of the parameter $\theta$ by $\hat{\sigma}$. Then, if $f(\theta)$ is a single-valued function of $\theta$, the maximum likelihood estimator of $f(\theta)$ is $f(\hat{\sigma})$. Thus, for example, $\hat{\sigma} = (\hat{\sigma}^2)^{1/2}$.

The principle of maximum likelihood tells us that we should use as our estimate that value which maximizes the likelihood of the observed event.

These maximum likelihood methods can be used to obtain *point estimates* of a parameter, but we must remember that a point estimator is a random variable distributed in some way around the true value of the parameter. The true parameter value may be higher or lower than our estimate. It is often useful therefore to obtain an interval within which we are reasonably confident the true value will lie, and the generally accepted method is to construct what are known as *confidence limits*.

The following procedure will yield upper and lower 95% confidence limits with the property that when we say that these limits include the true value of the parameter, 95% of all such statements will be true and 5% will be incorrect.

1. Choose a (test) statistic involving the unknown parameter and no other unknown parameter.
2. Place the appropriate sample values in the statistic.
3. Obtain an equation for the unknown parameter by equating the test statistic to the upper $2\frac{1}{2}\%$ point of the relevant distribution.
4. The solution of the equation gives one limit.
5. Repeat the process with the lower $2\frac{1}{2}\%$ point to obtain the other limit.

One can also construct 95% confidence intervals using unequal tails (for example, using the upper 2% point and the lower 3% point). We usually want our confidence interval to be as short as possible, however, and with a symmetric distribution such as the normal or $t$, this is achieved using equal tails. The same procedure very nearly minimizes the confidence interval with other nonsymmetric distributions (for example, chi-square) and has the advantage of avoiding rather tedious computation.

When the appropriate statistic involves the square of the unknown parameter, both limits are obtained by equating the statistic to the upper 5% point of the relevant distribution. The use of two tails in this situation would result in a pair of nonintersecting intervals. When two or more parameters are involved, it is possible to construct a region within which we are reasonably confident the true parameter values will lie. Such regions are referred to as confidence regions. The implied interval for $p_1$ does not form a 95% confidence interval, however. Nor is it true that an 85.7375% confidence region for $p_1, p_2$, and $p_3$ can be obtained by considering the intersection of the three separate 95% confidence intervals, because the statistics used to obtain the individual confidence intervals are not independent. This problem is obvious with a multiparameter distribution such as the multinomial, but it even occurs with the normal distribution because the statistic that we use to obtain a confidence interval for the mean and the statistic that we use to obtain a confidence interval for the variance are not independent. The problem is not likely to be of great concern unless a large number of parameters is involved.

### 22.5.18. Randomization

Randomization is the act of assigning a number of items (plates of bacteria or test animals, for example) to groups in such a manner that there is an equal chance for any one item to end up in any one group. This is a control against any possible bias in assignment of subjects to test groups. A variation on this is censored randomization, which insures that the groups are equivalent in some aspect after the assignment process is complete. The most common example of a censored randomization is one in which it is insured that the body weights of test animals in each group are not significantly different from those in the other groups. This is done by analyzing group weights both for homogeneity of variance and by analysis of variance after animal assignment, then rerandomizing if there is a significant difference at some nominal level, such as $p \leq 0.10$. The process is repeated until there is no significant difference.

There are several methods for actually performing the randomization process. The three most commonly used are card assignment, use of a random number table, and use of a computerized algorithm.

For the card-based method, individual identification numbers for items (plates or animals, for example) are placed on separate index cards. These cards are then shuffled, placed one at a time in succession into piles corresponding to the required test groups. The results are a random group assignment.

The random number table method requires only that one have unique numbers assigned to test subjects and access to a random number table. One simply sets up a table with a column for each group to which subjects are to be assigned. We start from the head of any one column of numbers in the random table (each time the table is used, a new starting point should be utilized). If our test subjects number less than 100, we utilize only the last two digits in each random number in the table. If they number more than 99 but less than 1000, we use only the last three digits. To generate group assignments, we read down a column, one number at a time. As we come across digits which correspond to a subject number, we assign that subject to a group (enter its identifying number in a column) proceeding to assign subjects to groups from left to right filling one row at a time. After a number is assigned to an animal, any duplication of its unique number is ignored. We use as many successive columns of random numbers as we may need to complete the process.

The third (and now most common) method is to use a random number generator that is built into a calculator or computer program. Procedures for generating these are generally documented in user manuals.

### 22.5.19. Transformations

If our initial inspection of a data set reveals it to have an unusual or undesired set of characteristics (or to lack a desired set of characteristics), we have a choice of three courses of action. We may proceed to select a method or test appropriate to this new set of conditions, abandon the entire exercise, or transform the variable(s) under consideration in such a manner that the resulting transformed variates ($X'$ and $Y'$, for example, as opposed to the original variates $X$ and $Y$) meet the assumptions or have the characteristics that are desired.

The key to all this is that the scale of measurement of most (if not all) variables is arbitrary. Although we are most familiar with a linear scale of measurement, there is nothing which makes this the "correct" scale on its own, as opposed to a logarithmic scale [familiar logarithmic measurements are that of pH values, or earthquake intensity (Richter scale)]. Transforming a set of data (converting $X$ to $X'$) is really as simple as changing a scale of measurement.

There are at least four good reasons to transform data.

1. The first is to normalize the data, making them suitable for analysis by our most common parametric techniques such as analysis of variance ANOVA. A simple test of whether a selected transformation will yield a distribution of data which satisfies the underlying assumptions for ANOVA is to plot the cumulative distribution of samples on probability paper (that is a commercially available paper which has the probability function scale as one axis). One can then alter the scale of the second axis (that is, the axis other than the one which is on a probability scale) from linear to any other (logarithmic, reciprocal, square root, etc.) and see if a previously curved line indicating a skewed distribution becomes linear to indicate normality. The slope of the transformed line gives us an estimate of the standard deviation. If

the slopes of the lines of several samples or groups of data are similar, we accordingly know that the variance of the different groups are homogenous.

2. Another reason is to linearize the relationship between a paired set of data, such as dose and response. This is the most common use in toxicology for transformations and is demonstrated in the section under probit and logit plots.

3. Data transformation adjusts for the influence of another variable. This is an alternative in some situations to the more complicated process of analysis of covariance. A ready example of this usage is the calculation of organ weight to body weight ratios in *in vivo* toxicity studies, with the resulting ratios serving as the raw data for an analysis of variance performed to identify possible target organs. This use is discussed in detail in Section 22.11.1.

4. Finally, transformation makes the relationships between variables clearer by removing or adjusting for interactions with third, fourth, and so on. Uncontrolled variables which influence the pair of variables of interest. This case is discussed in detail under time series analysis.

Common transformations are presented in Table 22.6.

**TABLE 22.6. Common Data Transformations**

| Transformation | How Calculated[a] | Example of Use |
| --- | --- | --- |
| Arithmetic | $x' = \dfrac{x}{y}$ <br> or <br> $x' = x + c$ | Organ weight/body weight |
| Reciprocals | $x' = \dfrac{1}{x}$ | Linearizing data, particularly rate phenomena |
| Arcsine (also called Angular) | $x' = \text{arcsine } \sqrt{x}$ | Normalizing dominant lethal and mutation rate data |
| Logarithmic | $x' = \log x$ | pH values |
| Probability (Probit) | $x' = \text{probability } X$ | Percentage responding |
| Square roots | $x' = \sqrt{x}$ | Surface area of animal from body weights |
| Box Cox | $x' = (x^v - 1)v$: <br> for $v \neq 0$ <br><br><br><br> $x' = \ln x$: for $v = 0$ | A family of transforms <br> For use when one has no prior knowledge of the appropriate transformation to use |
| Rank transformations | Depends on nature of samples | As a bridge between parametric and nonparametric statistics |

[a]$x$ and $y$ are original variables, $x'$ and $y'$ transformed values. "$C$" stands for a constant.
[b]Plotting a double reciprocal (that is, $1/x$ vs. $1/y$) will linearize almost any data set. So will plotting the log transforms of a set of variables.
*Source:* Conover and Iman, (1981).

### 22.5.20. Exploratory Data Analysis

Over the past twenty years, an entirely new approach has been developed to get the most information out of the increasingly larger and more complex data sets that scientists are faced with. This approach involves the use of a very diverse set of fairly simple techniques which comprise exploratory data analysis (EDA). As expounded by Tukey (1977), there are four major ingredients to EDA.

> *Displays.* These visually reveal the behavior of the data and suggest a framework for analysis. The scatterplot (presented as a scattergram) is an example of this approach.
>
> *Residuals.* These are what remain of a set of data after a fitted model (such as a linear regression) or some similar level of analysis has been removed.
>
> *Re-expressions.* These involved questions of what scale would serve to best simplify and improve the analysis of the data. Simple transformations, such as those presented earlier in this chapter, are used to simplify data behavior (for example, linearizing or normalizing) and clarify analysis.
>
> *Resistance.* This is a matter of decreasing the sensitivity of analysis and summary of data to misbehavior, so that the occurrence of a few outliers, for example, will not complicate or invalidate the methods used to analyze the data. For example, in summarizing the location of a set of data, the median (but not the arithmetic mean) is highly resistant.

These four ingredients are utilized in a process falling into two broad phases: an exploratory phase and a confirmatory phase. The exploratory phase isolates patterns in and features of, the data and reveals them, allowing an inspection of the data before any firm choice of actual hypothesis testing or modeling methods has been made.

Confirmatory analysis allows evaluation of the reproducibility of the patterns or effects. Its role is close to that of classical hypothesis testing, but also often includes steps such as (i) incorporating information from an analysis of another, closely related set of data and (ii) validating a result by assembling and analyzing additional data. These techniques are in general beyond the scope of this text. However, Velleman and Hoaglin (1981) and Hoaglin et al. (1983) present a clear overview of the more important methods, along with codes for their execution on a micro-computer (they have also now been incorporated into Minitab). A short examination of a single case of the use of these methods, however, is in order.

Toxicology has long recognized that no population, animal or human, is completely uniform in its response to any particular toxicant. Rather, a population is composed of a (presumably normal) distribution of individuals: some resistant to intoxication (hyporesponders), the bulk that respond close to a central value (such as an $LD_{50}$), and some that are very sensitive to intoxication (hyperresponders). This population distribution can, in fact, result in additional statistical techniques. The sensitivity of techniques such as ANOVA is reduced markedly by the occurrence of outliers (extreme high or low values, including hyper- and hyporesponders), which,

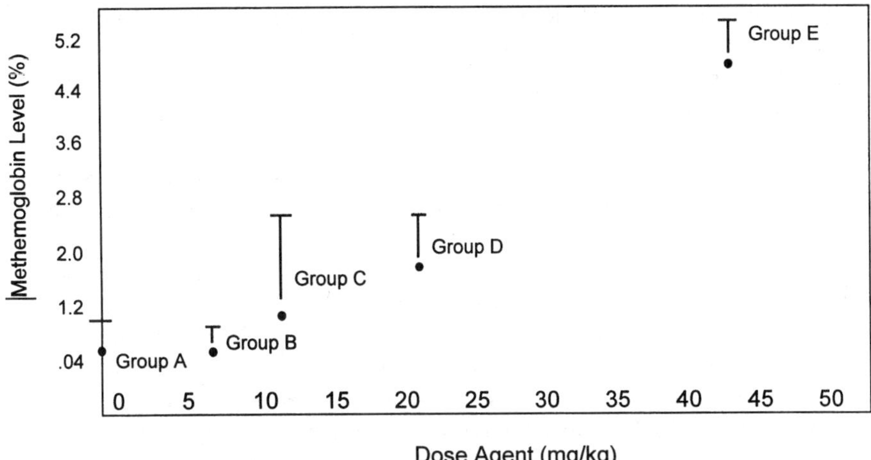



(Points Are Means - Error Bars Are + One Standard Deviation)

**FIGURE 22.6.** Variance inflation.

in fact, serve to markedly inflate the variance (standard deviation) associated with a sample. Such variance inflation is particularly common in small groups that are exposed or dosed at just over or under a threshold level, causing a small number of individuals in the sample (who are more sensitive than the other members) to respond markedly. Such a situation is displayed in Figure 22.6 which plots the mean and standard deviations of methemoglobin levels in a series of groups of animals exposed to successively higher levels of a hemolytic agent.

Though the mean level of methemoglobin in group C is more than double that of the control group (A), no hypothesis test will show this difference to be significant because it has such a large standard deviation associated with it. Yet this "inflated" variance exists because a single individual has such a marked response. The occurrence of the inflation is certainly an indicator that the data need to be examined closely. Indeed, all tabular data in toxicology should be visually inspected for both trend and variance inflation.

A concept related (but not identical) to resistance and exploratory data analysis is that of robustness. Robustness generally implies insensitivity to departures from assumptions surrounding an underlying model, such as normality.

In summarizing the location of data the median, though highly resistant, is not extremely robust. But the mean is both nonresistant and nonrobust.

## 22.6. HYPOTHESIS TESTING OF CATEGORICAL AND RANKED DATA

Categorical (or contingency table) presentations of data can contain any single type of data, but generally the contents are collected and arranged so that they can be classified as belonging to treatment and control groups, with the members of each of these groups then classified as belonging to one of two or more response categories (such as tumor–no tumor or normal–hyperplastic–neoplastic). For these cases, two forms of analysis are presented: Fisher's exact test (for the 2×2 contingency table) and the R×C chi square test (for large tables). It should be noted, however, that there are versions of both of these tests which permit the analysis of any size of contingency table.

The analysis of rank data, what is generally called nonparametric statistical analysis, is an exact parallel of the more traditional (and familiar) parametric methods. There are methods for the single comparison case (just as Student's *t*-test is used) and for the multiple comparison case (just as analysis of variance is used) with appropriate *post hoc* tests for exact identification of the significance with a set of groups. Four tests are presented for evaluating statistical significance in rank data: the Wilcoxon Rank Sum Test, distribution-free multiple comparisons, Mann–Whitney U Test, and the Kruskall–Wallis nonparametric analysis of variance. For each of these tests, tables of distribution values for the evaluations of results can be found in any of a number of reference volumes (Gad, 1998).

It should be clearly understood that for data that do not fulfill the necessary assumptions for parametric analysis, these nonparametric methods are either as powerful or in fact, more powerful than the equivalent parametric test.

### 22.6.1. Fisher's Exact Test

Fisher's exact test should be used to compare two sets of discontinuous, quantal (all or none) data. Small sets of such data can be checked by contingency data tables, such as those of Finney et al. (1963). Larger sets, however, require computation. These include frequency data such as incidences of mortality or certain histopathological findings, and so on. Thus, the data can be expressed as ratios. These data do not fit on a continuous scale of measurement but usually involve numbers of responses classified as either negative or positive; that is, contingency table situation (Sokal and Rohlf, 1994).

The analysis is started by setting up a 2×2 contingency table to summarize the numbers of "positive" and "negative" responses as well as the totals of these, as follows:

|  | Positive | Negative | Total |
|---|---|---|---|
| Group I | A | B | A + B |
| Group II | C | D | C + D |
| Totals | A + C | B + D | $A + B + C + D = N_{total}$ |

Using the above set of symbols, the formula for *P* appears as follows:

$$P = \frac{(A + B)!1(C + D)!(A + C)!(B + D)!\,*}{N!A!B!C!D!}$$

*A! is A factorial. For 4!, as an example this would be (4) (3) (2) (1) = 24.

The exact test produces a probability ($P$) which is the sum of the above calculation repeated for each possible arrangement of the numbers in the above cells (that is, A, B, C, and D) showing an association equal to or stronger than that between the two variables.

The $P$ resulting from these computations will be the exact one- or two-tailed probability depending on which of these two approaches is being employed. This value tells us if the groups differ significantly (with a probability less than 0.05, say) and the degree of significance.

***Assumptions and Limitations.***

1. Tables are available which provide individual exact probabilities for small sample size contingency tables. See Zar, 1974, pp. 518–542.
2. Fisher's exact test must be used in preference to the chi-square test when there are small cell sizes.
3. The probability resulting from a two-tailed test is exactly double that of a one-tailed from the same data.
4. Ghent has developed and proposed a good (though, if performed by hand, laborious) method extending the calculation of exact probabilities to $2 \times 3$, $3 \times 3$, and $R \times C$ contingency tables (Ghent, 1972).
5. Fisher's probabilities are not necessary symmetric. Although some analysts will double the one-tailed $p$ value to obtain the two-tailed result, this method is usually overly conservative.

### 22.6.3. $2 \times 2$ Chi Square

Though Fisher's Exact Test is preferable for analysis of most $2 \times 2$ contingency tables in toxicology, the chi square test is still widely used and is preferable in a few unusual situations (particularly if cell sizes are large yet only limited computational support is available).

The formula is simply

$$\chi^2 = \frac{(0_1 - E_1)^2}{E_1} + \frac{(0_2 - E_2)^2}{E_2}$$

$$= \sum \frac{(0_i - E_i)^2}{E_i}$$

where $0$ are observed numbers (or counts) and $E$ are expected numbers. The common practice in toxicology is for the observed figures to be test or treatment group counts. The expected figure is calculated as

$$E = \frac{(\text{column total})(\text{row total})}{\text{grand total}}$$

for each box or cell in a contingency table.

Our degrees of freedom are $(R - 1)(C - 1) = (2 - 1)(2 - 1) = 1$. Looking at a chi square table for one degree of freedom we see that this is greater than the test statistic at 0.05 (3.84) but less than that at 0.01 (6.64) so that $0.05 > p > 0.01$.

### 22.6.4. Assumptions and Limitations

***Assumptions.***
1. Data are univariate and categorical.
2. Data are from a multinomial population.
3. Data are collected by random, independent sampling.
4. Groups being compared are of approximately same size, particularly for small group sizes.

***When to Use.***
1. When the data are of a categorical (or frequency) nature.
2. When the data fit the assumptions above.
3. To test goodness-to-fit to a known form of distribution.
4. When cell sizes are large.

***When Not to Use.***
1. When the data are continuous rather than categorical.
2. When sample sizes are small and very unequal.
3. When sample sizes are too small (for example, when total $N$ is less than 50 or if any expected value is less than 5)
4. For any $2 \times 2$ comparison (use Fisher's exact test instead).

### 22.6.5. R × C Chi Square

The R×C chi-square test can be used to analyze discontinuous (frequency) data as in the Fisher's exact or $2 \times 2$ chi-square tests. However, in the R×C test (R = row, C = Column) we wish to compare three or more sets of data. An example would be comparison of the incidence of tumors among mice on three or more oral dosage levels. We can consider the data as "positive" (tumors) or "negative" (no tumors). The expected frequency for any box is equal to: (row total)(column total)/($N_{total}$).

As in Fisher's exact test, the initial step is setting up a table (this time a R×C contingency table). This table would appear as follows:

|          | Positive | Negative | Total |
|----------|----------|----------|-------|
| Group I  | $A_1$    | $B_1$    | $A_1 + B_1 = N_1$ |
| Group II | $A_2$    | $B_2$    | $A_2 + B_2 = N_2$ |
|          | $\downarrow$ | $\downarrow$ | |
| Group R  | $A_R$    | $B_R$    | $A_R + B_R = N_R$ |
| Totals   | $N_A$    | $N_B$    | $N_{total}$ |

Using these symbols, the formula for chi-square ($\chi^2$) is

$$\chi^2 = \frac{N_{tot}^2}{N_A N_B N_K} \left( \frac{A_1^2}{N_1} + \frac{A_2^2}{N_2} + \cdots \frac{A_K^2}{N_K} - \frac{N_A^2}{N_{tot}} \right)$$

The resulting $\chi^2$ value is compared to table values (as in Snedecor and Cochran, 1994, pp. 470–471) according to the number of degrees of freedom, which is equal to $(R - 1)(C - 1)$. If $\chi^2$ is smaller than the table value at the 0.05 probability level, the groups are not significantly different. If the calculated $\chi^2$ is larger, there is some difference among the groups and $2 \times R$ chi square or Fisher's exact tests will have to be compared to determine which group(s) differ from which other group(s).

### 22.6.6. Assumptions and Limitations

1. Based on data being organized in a table (such as below) so that there are cells (below, A, B, C and D are "cells").

|  |  | Control | | Treated | | Total |
|---|---|---|---|---|---|---|
|  | No Effect | A | | B | | A + B |
| Rows (R) |  | | | | | |
|  | Effect | C | | D | | C + D |
| Total |  | A + C | | B + D | | A + B + C + D |

Columns (C)

2. None of the "expected" frequency values should be less than 5.0.
3. Chi square test is always one tailed.
4. Without the use of some form of correction, the test becomes less accurate as the differences between group sizes increases.
5. The results from each additional column (group) is approximately additive. Due to this characteristic, chi square can be readily used for evaluating any $R \times C$ combination.
6. The results of the chi square calculation must be a positive number.
7. Test is weak with either small sample sizes or when the expected frequency in any cell is less than 5 (this latter limitation can be overcome by "pooling": combining cells).
8. Test results are independent of order of cells, unlike Kolmogorov–Smirnov.
9. Can be used to test the probability of validity of any distribution.

### 22.6.7. Wilcoxon Rank-Sum Test

The Wilcoxon Rank-Sum test is commonly used for the comparison of two groups of nonparametric (inteval or not normally distributed) data, such as those which are not measured exactly but rather as falling within certain limits (for example, how many animals died during each hour of an acute study.) The test is also used when there is no variability (variance $= 0$) within one or more of the groups we wish to compare (Sokal and Rohlf, 1994).

The data in both groups being compared are initially arranged and listed in order of increasing value. Then each number in the two groups must receive a rank value. Beginning with the smallest number in either group (which is given a rank of 1.0), each number is assigned a rank. If there are duplicate numbers (called "ties"), then each value of equal size will receive the median rank for the entire identically sized group. Thus if the lowest number appears twice, both figures receive a rank of 1.5. This, in turn, means that the ranks of 1.0 and 2.0 have been used and that the next highest number has a rank of 3.0. If the lowest number appears three times, then each is ranked as 2.0 and the next number has a rank of 4.0. Thus, each tied number gets a "median" rank. This process continues until all of the numbers are ranked. Each of the two columns of ranks (one for each group) is totaled giving the "sum of ranks" for each group being compared. As a check, we can calculate the value:

$$\frac{(N)(N+1)}{2}$$

where $N$ is the total number of data in both groups. The result should be equal to the sum of the sum of ranks for both groups.

The sum of rank values are compared to table values (Beyer, 1976, pp. 409–413) to determine the degree of significant differences, if any. These tables include two limits (an upper and a lower) that are dependent upon the probability level. If the number of data is the same in both groups ($N_1 \neq N_2$), then the lesser sum of ranks (smaller $N$) is compared to the table limits to find the degree of significance. Normally the comparison of the two groups ends here and the degree of significant difference can be reported.

### 22.6.8. Distribution-Free Multiple Comparison

The distribution-free multiple comparison test should be used to compare three or more groups of nonparametric data. These groups are then analyzed two at a time for any significant differences (Hollander and Wolfe, 1973, pp. 124–129). The test can be used for data similar to those compared by the rank-sum test. We often employ this test for reproduction and mutagenicity studies (such as comparing survival rates of offspring of rats fed various amounts of test materials in the diet).

Two values must be calculated for each pair of groups; the difference in mean ranks, and the probability level value against which the difference will be compared. To determine the difference in mean ranks we must first arrange the data within each of the groups in order of increasing values. Then we must assign rank values, beginning with the smallest overall figure. Note that this ranking is similar to that in the Wilcoxon test except that it applies to more than two groups.

The ranks are then added for each of the groups. As a check, the sum of these should equal

$$\frac{N_{\text{tot}}(N_{\text{tot}} + 1)}{2}$$

where $N_{\text{tot}}$ is the total number of figures from all groups. Next we can find the mean rank (R) for each group by dividing the sum of ranks by the numbers in the data ($N$) in the group. These mean ranks are then taken in those pairs which we want to compare (usually each test group versus the control) and the differences are found ($|R_1\_R_2|$). This value is expressed as an absolute figure; that is, it is always a positive number.

The second value for each pair of groups (the probability value) is calculated from the expression

$$z\left[\frac{a}{K}(K - 1)\right]\sqrt{\frac{N_{\text{tot}}(N_{\text{tot}} + 1)}{12}}\sqrt{\frac{1}{N_1}\frac{1}{N_2}}$$

where $a$ is the level of significance for the comparison (usually 0.05, 0.01, 0.001, etc.), $K$ is the total number of groups, and $Z$ is a figure obtained from a normal probability table and determining the corresponding "Z-score".

The result of the probability value calculation for each pair of groups is compared to the corresponding mean difference $|R_1 - R_2|$. If $|R_1 - R_2|$ is smaller, there is no significant difference between the groups. If it is larger, the groups are different and $|R_1 - R_2|$ must be compared to the calculated probability values for $a = 0.01$ and $a = 0.001$ to find the degree of significance.

### 22.6.9. Assumptions and Limitations

1. As with the Wilcoxon Rank-Sum, too many tied ranks inflate the false positive.
2. Generally, this test should be used as a *post hoc* comparison after Kruskall–Wallis.

### 22.6.10. Mann–Whitney U Test

This is a nonparametric test in which the data in each group are first ordered from lowest to highest values, then the entire set (both control and treated values) is ranked, with the average rank being assigned to tied values. The ranks are then summed for each group and U is determined according to

$$U_t = n_c n_t + \frac{n_t(n_t + 1)}{2} - R_t$$

$$U_c = n_c n_t + \frac{n_c(n_c + 1)}{2} - R_c$$

where $n_c$, $n_t$ = sample size for control and treated groups; and $R_c$, $R_t$ = sum of ranks for the control and treated groups.

For the level of significance for a comparison of the two groups, the larger value of $U_c$ or $U_t$ is used. This is compared to critical values as found in tables (Siegel, 1956).

The Mann–Whitney U test is employed for the count data, but which test should be employed for the percentage variables should be decided on the same grounds as described later under reproduction studies.

### 22.6.11.  Assumptions and Limitations

1. It does not matter whether the observations are ranked from smallest to largest or vice versa.

2. This test should not be used for paired observations.

3. The test statistics from a Mann–Whitney are linearly related to those of Wilcoxon. The two tests will always yield the same result. The Mann-Whitney is presented here for historical completeness, as it has been much favored in reproductive and developmental toxicology studies. However, it should be noted that the author does not include it in the decision tree for method selection (Figure 22.2).

### 22.6.12.  Kruskal-Wallis Nonparametric ANOVA

The Kruskal-Wallis nonparametric one-way analysis of variance should be the initial analysis performed when we have three or more groups of data which are by nature nonparametric (either not a normally distributed population, or of a discontinuous nature, or all the groups being analyzed are not from the same population) but not a categorical (or quantal) nature. Commonly these will be either rank type evaluation data (such as behavioral toxicity observation scores) or reproduction study data. The analysis is initiated (Pollard, 1977, pp. 170–173) by ranking all the observations from the combined groups to be analyzed. Ties are given the average rank of the tied values (that is, if two values would tie for twelfth rank and therefore would be ranked twelfth and thirteenth, both would be assigned the average rank of 12.5).

The sum of ranks of each group $(r_1, r_2, \ldots, r_k)$ is computed by adding all the rank values for each group. The test value $H$ is then computed as

$$H = \frac{12}{n(n+1)} \sum r_1^2/n_1 + r_2^2/n_2 + \cdots + r_k^2/n_k) - 3(n+1)$$

where $n_1, n_2, \ldots, n_k$ are the number of observations in each group. The test statistic is then compared with a table of $H$ values. If the calculated value of $H$ is greater than the table value for the appropriate number of observations in each group, there is significant difference between the groups, but further testing (using the distribution-free multiple comparisons method) is necessary to determine where the difference lies.

### 22.6.13. Assumptions and Limitations

1. The test statistic $H$ is used for both small and large samples.

2. When we find a significant difference, we do not know which groups are different. It is not correct to then perform a Mann–Whitney U Test on all possible combinations; rather, a multiple comparison method must be used, such as the distribution-free multiple comparisons.

3. Data must be independent for the test to be valid.

4. Too many tied ranks will decrease the power of this test and also lead to increased false-positive levels.

5. When $k = 2$, the Kruskal–Wallis chi-square value has 1 $df$. This test is identical to the normal approximation used for the Wilcoxon Rank-Sum Test. As noted in previous sections, a chi square with 1 df can be represented by the square of a standardized normal random variable. In the case of $k = 2$, the $H$-statistic is the square of the Wilcoxon Rank-Sum $Z$-test (without the continuity correction).

6. The effect of adjusting for tied ranks is to slightly increase the value of the test statistic, $H$. Therefore, omission of this adjustment results in a more conservative test.

### 22.6.14. Log-Rank Test

The Log-Rank Test is a statistical methodology for comparing the distribution of time until the occurrence of the event in independent groups. In toxicology, the most common event of interest is death or occurrence of a tumor, but it could just as well be liver failure, neurotoxicity, or any other event which occurs only once in an individual. The elapsed time from initial treatment or observation until the *event* is the *event time*, often referred to as "survival time", even when the *event* is not "death".

The Log-Rank Test provides a method for comparing "risk-adjusted" event rates, useful when test subjects in a study are subject to varying degrees of opportunity to experience the event. Such situations arise frequently in toxicology studies due to the finite duration of the study, early termination of the animal or interruption of treatment before the event occurs.

Examples where use of the Log-Rank Test might be appropriate include comparing survival times in carcinogenity bioassay animals which are given a new treatment with those in the control group or comparing times to liver failure for several dose levels of a new NSAID where the animals are treated for 10 weeks or until cured, whichever comes first.

If every animal were followed until the event occurrence, the event times could be compared between two groups using the Wilcoxon Rank-Sum Test. However, some animals may die or complete the study before the event occurs. In such cases, the actual time the event is unknown since the event does not occur while under study observation. The event times for these animals are based on the last known time of study observation, and are called "censored" observations since they represent the lower bound of the true, unknown event times. The Wilcoxon Rank-Sum Test can be highly biased in the presence of the censored data.

The null hypothesis tested by the Log-Rank Test is that of equal event time distributions among groups. Equality of the distributions of event times implies similar event rates among groups not only for the clinical trial as a whole, but also for any arbitrary time point during the trial. Rejection of the null hypothesis indicates that the event rates differ among groups at one or more time points during the study.

The idea behind the Log-Rank Test for comparison of two life tables is simple; if there were no difference between the groups, the total deaths occurring at any time should split between the two groups at that time. So if the numbers at risk in the first and second groups in (say) the sixth month were 70 and 30, respectively, and 10 deaths occurred in that month we would expect

$$10 \times \frac{70}{70 + 30} = 7$$

of these deaths to have occurred in the first group, and

$$10 \times \frac{30}{70 + 30} = 3$$

of the deaths to have occurred in the second group.

A similar calculation can be made at each time of death (in either group). By adding together for the first group the results of all such calculations, we obtain a single number, called the extent of exposure $(E_1)$, which represents the "expected" number of deaths in that group if the two groups had the distribution of survival time. An extent of exposure $(E_2)$ can be obtained for the second group in the same way. Let $O_1$ and $O_2$ denote the actual total numbers of deaths in the two groups. A useful arithmetic check is that the total number of deaths $O_1 + O_2$ must equal the sum $E_1 + E_2$ of the extents of exposure.

The discrepancy between the $O$'s and $E$'s can be measured by the quantity

$$x^2 = \frac{(|O_1 - E_1| - 1/2)^2}{E_1} + \frac{(|O_2 - E_2| - 1/2)^2}{E_2}$$

For rather obscure reasons, $x^2$ is known as the log-rank statistic. An approximate significance test of the null hypothesis of identical distributions of survival time in the two groups is obtained by $x^2$ to a chi-square distribution on 1 degree of freedom.

The Log-Rank Test as presented by Peto et al. (1977) uses the product-limit life-table calculations rather than the actuarial estimators shown above. The distinction is unlikely to be of practical importance unless the grouping intervals are very coarse.

Peto and Pike (1973) suggest that the approximation in treating the null distribution of $\chi^2$ as a chi-square is conservative, so that it will tend to understate the degree of statistical significance. In the formula for $\chi^2$ we have used the continuity correction of subtracting $1/2$ from $|O_1 - E_1|$ and $|O_2 - E_2|$ before squaring. This is recommended by Peto et al. (1977) when, as in nonrandomized studies, the permutational argument does not apply. Peto et al. (1977) gives further details of the Log-Rank Test and its extension to comparisons of more than two treatment groups and to tests that control for categorical confounding factors.

### 22.6.15. Assumptions and Limitations

1. The endpoint of concern is or is defined so that it is "right censored", once it happens, it does not reoccur. Examples are death or a minimum or maximum value of an enzyme or physiologic function (such as respiration rate).

2. The method makes no assumptions on distribution.

3. Many variations of the Log-Rank Test for comparing survival distributions exist. The most common variant has the form:

$$X^2 = \frac{(O_1 - E_1)^2}{E_1} + \frac{(O_2 - E_2)^2}{E_2}$$

   where $O_i$ and $E_i$ are computed for each group, as in the formulas given previously. This statistic also has an approximate chi-square distribution with 1 degree-of-freedom under $H_0$.

   A continuity correction can also be used to reduce the numerators by $1/2$ before squaring. Use of such a correction leads to even further conservatism and may be omitted when sample sizes are moderate or large.

4. The Wilcoxon Rank-Sum Test could be used to analyze the event times in the absence of censoring. A "Generalized Wilcoxon" Test, sometimes called the Gehan Test, based on an approximate chi-square distribution, has been developed for use in the presence of censored observations.

   Both the Log-Rank and the Generalized Wilcoxon Tests are nonparametric tests, and require no assumptions regarding the distribution of event times. When the event rate is greater early in the trial than toward the end, the Generalized Wilcoxon Test is the more appropriate test since it gives greater weight to the earlier differences.

5. Survival and failure times often follow the exponential distribution. If such a model can be assumed, a more powerful alternative to the Log-Rank Test is the Likelihood Ratio Test.

   This parametric test assumes that event probabilities are constant over time. That is, the chance that a patient becomes event-positive at time $t$ given that he is event-negative up to time $t$ does not depend on $t$. A plot of the negative log of the event times distribution showing a linear trend through the origin is consistent with exponential event times.

6. Life tables can be constructed to provide estimates of the event time distributions. Estimates commonly used are known as the Kaplan–Meier estimates.

## 22.7. HYPOTHESIS TESTING: UNIVARIATE PARAMETRIC TESTS

Univariate case[†] data from normally distributed populations generally have a higher information value associated with them but the traditional hypothesis testing techniques (which include all the methods described in this section) are generally neither resistant nor robust. All the data analyzed by these methods are also, effectively, continuous; that is, at least for practical purposes, the data may be represented by any number and each such data number has a measurable relationship to other data numbers.

### 22.7.1. Student's *t*-Test (Unpaired *t*-Test)

Pairs of groups of continuous, randomly distributed data are compared via this test. We can use this test to compare three or more groups of data, but they must be intercompared by examination of two groups taken at time and are preferentially compared by analysis of variance (ANOVA). Usually this means comparison of a test group versus a control group, although two test groups may be compared as well. To determine which of the three types of *t*-tests described in this chapter should be employed, the *F*-test is usually performed first. This will tell us if the variances of the data are approximately equal, which is a requirement for the use of the parametric methods. If the *F*-test indicates homogeneous variances and the numbers of data within the groups ($N$) are equal, then the Student's *t*-test is the appropriate procedure (Sokal and Rohlf, 1994). If the $F$ is significant (the data are heterogeneous) and the two groups have equal numbers of data, the modified Student's *t*-test is applicable (Cochran and Cox, 1975).

The value of $t$ for Student's *t*-test is calculated using the formula

$$t = \frac{\overline{X}_1 - \overline{X}_2}{\sum D_1^2 + \sum D_2^2} \sqrt{\frac{N_1 N_2}{N_1 + N_2}(N_1 + N_2 - 2)}$$

where the value of $\sum D^2 = (N \sum X^2 - (\sum X)^2)/N$

The value of $t$ obtained from the above calculations is compared to the values in a *t*-distribution table according to the appropriate number of degrees of freedom ($df$). If the $F$ value is not significant (i.e., variances are homogeneous), then $df = N_1 + N_2 - 2$. If the $F$ was significant and $N_1 = N_2$, then the $df = N - 1$. Although this case indicates a nonrandom distribution, the modified *t*-test is still

---

[†]That is, where each datum is defined by one treatment and one effect variable.

valid. If the calculated value is larger than the table value at $p = 0.05$, it may then be compared to the appropriate other table values in order of decreasing probability to determine the degree of significance between the two groups.

### 22.7.2. Assumptions and Limitations

1. The test assumes that the data are univariate, continuous and normally distributed.
2. Data are collected by random sampling.
3. The test should be used when the assumptions in (1) and (2) are met and there are only two groups to be compared.
4. Do not use when the data are ranked, when the data are not approximately normally distributed, or when there are more than two groups to be compared. Do not use for paired observations.
5. This is the most commonly misused test method, except in those few cases where one is truly only comparing two groups of data and the group sizes are roughly equivalent. Not valid for multiple comparisons (because of resulting additive errors) or where group sizes are very unequal.
6. Test is robust for moderate departures from normality and, when $N_1$ and $N_2$ are approximately equal, robust for moderate departures from homogeneity of variances.
7. The main difference between the $Z$-test and the $t$-test is that the $Z$-statistic is based on a known standard deviation, $\sigma$, while the $t$-statistic uses the sample standard deviation, $s$, as an estimate of $\sigma$. With the assumption of normally distributed data, the variance $\sigma^2$ is more closely estimated by the sample variance $s^2$ as $n$ gets large. It can be shown that the $t$-test is equivalent to the $Z$-test for infinite degrees-of-freedom. In practice, a "large" sample is usually considered $n \geq 30$.

### 22.7.3. Cochran *t*-test

The Cochran test should be used to compare two groups of continuous data when the variances (as indicated by the $F$ test) are heterogeneous and the numbers of data within the groups are not equal ($N_1 \neq N_2$). This is the situation, for example, when the data, though expected to be randomly distributed, were found not to be (Cochran and Cox, 1975, pp. 100–102).

Two $t$ values are calculated for this test, the "observed" $t$ ($t_{\text{obs}}$) and the "expected" $t$ ($t'$). The observed $t$ is obtained by

$$t_{\text{obs}} = \frac{\overline{X}_1 - \overline{X}_2}{\sqrt{W_1 + W_2}}$$

where $W = \text{SEM}^2$ (standard error of the mean squared)

$$= S^2/N$$

where $S$ (variance) can be calculated from

$$S = \frac{\dfrac{n \sum X^2 - (\sum X)^2}{N}}{N - 1}$$

The value for $t'$ is obtained from

$$t' = \frac{t'_1 W_1 + t'_2 W_2}{W_1 + W_2}$$

where $t'_1$ and $t'_2$ are values for the two groups taken from the $t$-distribution table corresponding to $N - 1$ degrees of freedom (for each group) at the 0.05 probability level (or such level as one may select).

The calculated $t_{\text{obs}}$ is compared to the calculated $t'$ value (or values, if $t'$ values were prepared for more than one probability level). If $t_{\text{obs}}$ is smaller than a $t'$, the groups are not considered to be significantly different at that probability level.

### 22.7.4. Assumptions and Limitations

1. The test assumes that the data are univariate, continuous, normally distributed and that group sizes are unequal.
2. The test is robust for moderate departures from normality, and very robust for departures from equality of variances.

### 22.7.5. *F* Test

This is a test of the homogeneity of variances between two groups of data (Sokal and Rohlf, 1994). It is used in two separate cases. The first is when Bartlett's indicates heterogeneity of variances among three or more groups (i.e., it is used to determine which pairs of groups are heterogeneous). Second, the $F$ test is the initial step in comparing two groups of continuous data which we would expect to be parametric (two groups not usually being compared using ANOVA), the results indicating whether the data are from the same population and whether subsequent parametric comparisons would be valid.

The $F$ is calculated by dividing the larger variance ($S_1^2$) by the smaller one ($S_2^2$). $S^2$ is calculated as

$$S^2 = \frac{\dfrac{N \sum X^2 - (\sum X)^2}{N}}{N - 1}$$

where $N$ is the number of data in the group and $X$ represents the individual values within the group. Frequently, $S^2$ values may be obtained from ANOVA calculations.

The calculated $F$ value is compared to the appropriate number in an $F$ value table for the appropriate degrees of freedom ($N - 1$) in the numerator (along the top of the table) and in the denominator (along the side of the table). If the calculated value is smaller, it is not significant and the variances are considered homogeneous (and the Student's $t$-test would be appropriate for further comparison). If the calculated $F$ value is greater, $F$ is significant and the variances are heterogeneous (and the next test would be modified Student's $t$-test if $N_1 = N_2$ or the Cochran $t$-test if $N_1 \neq N_2$; see Figure 22.2 to review the decision tree).

### 22.7.6. Assumptions and Limitations

1. This test could be considered as a two group equivalent of the Bartlett's test.
2. If the test statistic is close to 1.0, the results are (of course) not significant.
3. The test assumes normality and independence of data.

### 22.7.7. Analysis of Variance (ANOVA)

ANOVA is used for comparison of three or more groups of continuous data when the variances are homogeneous and the data are independent and normally distributed.

A series of calculations are required for ANOVA, starting with the values within each group being added ($\sum X$) and then these sums being added ($\sum \sum X$). Each figure within the groups is squared, and these squares are then summed ($\sum X^2$) and these sums added ($\sum \sum X^2$). Next the "correction factor" (CF) can be calculated from the following formula:

$$CF = \frac{\left( \sum\limits_{1}^{K} \sum\limits_{1}^{N} X \right)^2}{N_1 + N_2 + \cdots N_k}$$

where $N$ is the number of values in each group and $K$ is the number of groups. The total sum of squares ($SS$) is then determined as follows:

$$SS_{\text{total}} = \sum\limits_{1}^{K} \sum\limits_{1}^{N} X^2 - CF$$

In turn, the sum of squares between groups (bg) is found from

$$SS_{\text{bg}} = \frac{(\sum X_1)^2}{N_1} + \frac{(\sum X_2)^2}{N_2} + \cdots + \frac{(\sum X_k)^2}{N_k} - CF$$

The sum of squares within group (wg) is then the difference between the last two figures, or

$$SS_{\text{wg}} = SS_{\text{total}} - SS_{\text{bg}}$$

Now, there are three types of degrees of freedom to determine. The first, total $df$, is the total number of data within all groups under analysis minus one

$(N_1 + N_2 + \cdots + N_k - 1)$. The second figure (the *df* between groups) is the number of groups minus one $(K - 1)$. The last figure (the *df* within groups or "error *df*") is the difference between the first two figures $(df_{\text{total}} - df_{\text{bg}})$.

The next set of calculations requires determination of the two mean squares ($MS_{bg}$ and $MS_{wg}$). These are the respective sum of square values divided by the corresponding *df* figures ($MS = SS/df$). The final calculation is that of the $F$ ratio. For this, the MS between groups is divided by the MS within groups ($F = MS_{bg}/MS_{wg}$).

A table of the results of these calculations would appear as

|       | *df* | *SS*    | MS      | *F*  |
|-------|------|---------|---------|------|
| Bg    | 3    | 0.04075 | 0.01358 | 4.94 |
| Wg    | 12   | 0.03305 | 0.00275 |      |
| Total | 15   | 0.07380 |         |      |

For interpretation, the $F$ ratio value obtained in the ANOVA is compared to a table of $F$ values. If $F \leq 1.0$, the results are not significant and comparison with the table values is not necessary. The degrees of freedom $(df)$ for the greater mean square ($MS_{bg}$) are indicated along the top of the table. Then read down the side of the table to the line corresponding to the *df* for the lesser mean square ($MS_{wg}$). The figure shown at the desired significance level (traditionally 0.05) is compared to the calculated $F$ value. If the calculated number is smaller, there is no significant differences among the groups being compared. If the calculated value is larger, there is some difference but further (*post hoc*) testing will be required before we know which groups differ significantly.

### 22.7.8. Assumptions and Limitations

1. What is presented here is the workhorse of toxicology—the one-way analysis of variance. Many other forms exist for more complicated experimental designs.

2. The test is robust for moderate departures from normality if the sample sizes are large enough. Unfortunately, this is rarely the case in toxicology.

3. ANOVA is robust for moderate departures from equality of variances (as determined by Bartlett's test) if the sample sizes are approximately equal.

4. It is not appropriate to use a *t*-test (or a two groups at a time version of ANOVA) to identify where significant differences are within the design group. A multiple-comparison *post hoc* method must be used.

### 22.7.9. *Post Hoc* Tests

There is a wide variety of *post hoc* tests available to analyze data after finding significant result in an ANOVA. Each of these tests has advantages and disadvantages, proponents and critics. Four of the tests are commonly used in toxicology and will be presented or previewed here. These are Dunnett's $t$-test and Williams' $t$-test. Two other tests which are available in many statistical packages are Turkey's method and the Student–Newman–Keuls method (Zar, 1974, 151–161).

If ANOVA reveals no significance it is not appropriate to proceed to perform a *post hoc* test in hope of finding differences. To do so would only be another form of multiple comparisons, increasing the type I error rate beyond the desired level.

### 22.7.10. Duncan's Multiple Range Test

Duncan's (1955) is used to compare groups of continuous and randomly distributed data (such as body weights, organ weights, etc.). The test normally involves three or more groups taken one pair at a time. It should only follow observation of a significant $F$ value in the ANOVA and can serve to determine which group (or groups) differs significantly from which other group (or groups).

There are two alternative methods of calculation. The selection of the proper one is based on whether the number of data ($N$) are equal or unequal in the groups.

### 22.7.11. Groups with Equal Number of Data ($N_1 = N_2$)

Two sets of calculations must be carried out; first, the determination of the difference between the means of pairs of groups; second, the preparation of a probability rate against which each difference in means is compared.

The means (averages) are determined (or taken from the ANOVA calculation) and ranked in either decreasing or increasing order. If two means are the same, they take up two equal positions (thus, for four means we could have ranks of 1, 2, 2, and 4 rather than 1, 2, 3, and 4). The groups are then taken in pairs and the differences between the means ($\bar{\chi}_1 - \bar{\chi}_2$), expressed as positive numbers, are calculated. Usually, each pair consists of a test group and the control group, through multiple tests groups may be intracompared if so desired. The relative rank of the two groups being compared must be considered. If a test group is ranked "2" and the control group is ranked "1", then we say that there are two places between them, while if the test group were ranked "3", then there would be three places between it and the control.

To establish the probability table, the standard error of the mean (SEM) must be calculated as presented earlier or as

$$\sqrt{\frac{\text{error mean square}}{N}} = \sqrt{\frac{\text{mean square within group}}{N}}$$

where $N$ is the number of animals or replications per dose level. The mean square within groups ($MS_{wg}$) can be calculated from the information given in the ANOVA procedure (refer to the earlier section on ANOVA). The SEM is then multiplied by a series of table values (Harter, 1960; Beyer, 1976) to set up a probability table. The table values used for the calculations are chosen according to the probability levels (note that the tables have sections for 0.05, 0.01, and 0.001 levels) and the number of means apart for the groups being compared and the number of "error" degrees of freedom ($df$). The "error" $df$ is the number of $df$ within the groups. This last figure is determined from the ANOVA calculation and can be taken from ANOVA output. For some values of df, the table values are not given and should thus be interpolated.

### 22.7.12. Groups with Unequal Numbers of Data ($N_1 \neq N_2$)

This procedure is very similar to that discussed above. As before, the means are ranked and the differences between the means are determined ($\overline{\chi}_1 - \overline{\chi}_2$). Next, weighing values ("$a_{ij}$" values) are calculated for the pairs of groups being compared in accordance with

$$a_u = \sqrt{2N_i N_j, (N_i + N_j)} = \sqrt{2N_1 N_2/(N_1 + N_2)}$$

This weighting value for each pair of groups is multiplied by ($\overline{\chi}_1 - \overline{\chi}_2$) for each value to arrive at a $t$ value. It is the $t$ that will later be compared to a probability table.

The probability table is set up as before except that instead of multiplying the appropriate table values by SEM, SEM$^2$ is used. This is equal to $\sqrt{\mathrm{MS}_{\mathrm{wg}}}$.

For the desired comparison of two groups at a time, either the ($\overline{\chi}_1 - \overline{\chi}_2$) value (if $N_1 = N_2$) is compared to the appropriate probability table. Each comparison must be made according to the number of places between the means. If the table value is larger at the 0.05 level, the two groups are not considered to be statistically different. If the table value is smaller, the groups are different and the comparison is repeated at lower levels of significance. Thus, the degree of significance may be determined. We might have significant differences at 0.05 but not at 0.01, in which case the probability would be represented at $0.05 > p > 0.01$.

### 22.7.13. Assumptions and Limitations

Duncan's assures a set alpha level or type I error rate for all tests when means are separated by no more than ordered step increases. Preserving this alpha level means that the test is less sensitive than some others, such as the Student–Newman–Keuls. The test is inherently conservative and not resistant or robust.

### 22.7.14. Scheffe's Multiple Comparisons

Scheffe's is another *post hoc* comparison method for groups of continuous and randomly distributed data. It also normally involves three or more groups (Scheffe, 1959; Harris, 1975). It is widely considered a more powerful significance test than Duncan's.

Each *post hoc* comparison is tested by comparing an obtained test value ($F_{\mathrm{contr}}$) with the appropriate critical $F$ value at the selected level of significance (the table $F$

value multiplied by $K - 1$ for an $F$ with $K - 1$ and $N - K$ degrees of freedom[2]). $F_{\text{contr}}$ is computed as follows:

1. Compute the mean for each sample (group);
2. Denote the residual mean square by $\text{MS}_{\text{wg}}$;
3. Compute the test statistic as

$$F_{\text{contr}} = \frac{(C_1\bar{\chi}_1 + C_2\bar{\chi}_2 + \cdots + C_k\bar{\chi}_k^{12})}{(K-1)\text{MS}_{\text{wg}}(C_1^2/n_1 + \cdots + C_k^2/n_k)}$$

where $C_k$ is the comparison number such that the sum of $C_1, C_2 \cdots C_k = 0$.

## 22.7.15. Assumptions and Limitations

1. The Scheffe procedure is robust to moderate violations of the normality and homogeneity of variance assumptions.
2. It is not formulated on the basis of groups with equal numbers (as one of Duncan's procedures is), and if $N_1 \neq N_2$ there is no separate weighing procedure.
3. It tests all linear contrasts among the population means (the other three methods confine themselves to pairwise comparison, except they use a Bonferroni type correlation procedure).
4. The Scheffe procedure is powerful because of it robustness, yet it is very conservative. Type I error (the false positive rate) is held constant at the selected test level for each comparison.

## 22.7.16. Dunnett's $t$-Test

Dunnet's $t$-test (Dunnett, 1955a, b, 1964) has as its starting point the assumption that what is desired is a comparison of each of several means with one other mean and only one other mean; in other words, that one wishes to compare each and every treatment group with the control group, but not compare treatment groups with each other. The problem here is that, in toxicology, one is frequently interested in comparing treatment groups with other treatment groups. However, if one does want only to compare treatment groups versus a control group, Dunnett's is a useful approach. In a study with $K$ groups (one of them being the control) we will wish to make $K - 1$ comparisons. In such a situation, we want to have a $P$ level for the entire set of $K - 1$ decisions (not for each individual decision). The Dunnett's distribution is predicated on this assumption. The parameters for utilizing a Dunnett's table, such as found in his original article, are $K$ (as above) and the number of degrees of freedom for mean square with groups ($\text{MS}_{\text{wg}}$). The test value is calculated as

$$t = \frac{|T_j - T_i|}{\sqrt{2\text{MS}_{\text{wg}/n}}}$$

where $n$ is the number of observation $s$ in each of the groups. The mean square within group ($MS_{wg}$) is as we have defined it previously; $T_j$ is the control group mean and $T_i$ is the mean of, in order, each successive test group observation. Note that one uses the absolute value of the positive number resulting from subtracting $T_i$ from $T_j$. This is to ensure a positive number for our final $t$.

### 22.7.17. Assumptions and Limitations

1. Dunnett's seeks to ensure that the type I error rate will be fixed at the desired level by incorporating correction factors into the design of the test value table.
2. Treated group sizes must be approximately equal.

### 22.7.18. Williams' $t$-Test

Williams' $t$-test (Williams, 1971, 1972) is popular, although its use is quite limited in toxicology. It is designed to detect the highest level (in a set of dose and exposure levels) at which there is no significant effect. It assumes that the response of interest (such as change in body weights) occurs at higher levels, but not at lower levels, and that the responses are monotonically ordered so that $X_0 \leq X_1 \cdots \leq X_k$. This is, however, frequently not the case. The Williams' technique handles the occurrence of such discontinuities in a response series by replacing the offending value and the value immediately preceding it with weighted average values. The test also is adversely affected by any mortality at high-dose levels. Such moralities "impose a severe penalty, reducing the power of detecting an effect not only at level $K$ but also at all lower doses" (Williams, 1972, p. 529). Accordingly, it is not generally applicable in toxicology studies.

### 22.7.19. Analysis of Covariance

Analysis of covariance (ANCOVA) is a method for comparing sets of data that consist of two variables (treatment and effect, with our effect variable being called the "variate"), when a third variable (called the "covariate") exists that can be measured but not controlled and which has a definite effect on the variable of interest. In other words, it provides an indirect type of statistical control, allowing us to increase the precision of a study and to remove a potential source of bias. One common example of this is in the analysis of organ weights in toxicity studies. Our true interest here is the effect of our dose or exposure level on the specific organ weights, but most organ weights also increase (in the young, growing animals most commonly used in such studies) in proportion to increases in animal body weight. As we are not here interested in the effect of this covariate (body weight), we measure it to allow for adjustment. We must be careful before using ANCOVA, however, to ensure that the underlying nature of the correspondence between the variate and covariate is such that we can rely on it as a tool for adjustments (Anderson et al, 1980; Kotz and Johnson, 1982).

Calculation is performed in two steps. The first is a type of linear regression between the variate $Y$ and the covariate $X$.

This regression, performed as described under the linear regression section, gives us the model

$$Y = a_1 + BX + e$$

which in turn allows us to define adjusted means ($\overline{Y}$ and $X$) such that $\overline{Y}_{1a} =_1 -(\overline{\chi}_1 - (\overline{\chi}^*))$.

If we consider the case where $K$ treatments are being compared such that $K = 1, 2, \ldots, K$, and we let $X_{ik}$ and $Y_{ik}$ represent the predictor and predicted values for each individual $i$ in group $k$, we can let $X_k$ and $Y_k$ be the means. Then, we define the between-group (for treatment) sum of squares and cross products as

$$T_{xx} = \sum_{k-1}^{K} n_k(\overline{X}_K - \overline{X})^2$$

$$T_{yy} = \sum_{k-1}^{K} n_k(\overline{Y}_K - \overline{Y})^2$$

$$T_{xy} = \sum_{k-1}^{K} n_k(\overline{X}_k - \overline{X})(\overline{Y}_k - \overline{Y})$$

In a like manner, within-group sums of squares and cross products are calculated as

$$\sum xx = \sum_{k=1}^{k} \sum_i (X_{ik} - X_k)^2$$

$$\sum yy = \sum_{k=1}^{k} \sum_i (Y_{ik} - Y_k)^2$$

$$\sum xy = \sum_{k=1}^{k} \sum_i (X_{ik} - X_k)(Y_{ik} - Y_k)$$

where $i$ indicates the sum from all the individuals within each group; $f = $ total number of subjects minus number of groups,

$$S_{xx} = T_{xx} + \sum\nolimits_{xx}$$
$$S_{yy} = T_{yy} + \sum\nolimits_{xx}$$
$$S_{xy} = T_{xy} + \sum\nolimits_{xy}$$

With these in hand, we can then calculate the residual mean squares of treatments ($St^2$) and error ($Se^2$),

$$St^2 = \frac{T_{yy}(S_{xy}^2/S_{xx}) + \sum_{xy}^2 / \sum_{xx}}{lc - 1}$$

$$Se^2 = \frac{(\sum_{yy}(\sum_y^2 / \sum_{xx}))}{f - 1}$$

These can be used to calculate an $F$ statistic to test the null hypothesis that all treatment effects are equal.

$$F = \frac{St^2}{Se^2}$$

The estimated regression coefficient of $Y$ or $X$ is

$$B = \frac{\sum xy}{\sum xx}$$

The estimated standard error for the adjusted difference between two groups is given by

$$Sd = Se\sqrt{\frac{1}{n_j} + \frac{1}{n_j} + \frac{(X_i - X_j)^2}{\sum xx}}$$

where $n_0$ and $n_1$ are the sample sizes of the two groups. A test of the null hypothesis that the adjusted differences between the groups is zero is provided by

$$t = \frac{Y_1 - Y_0 - B(\chi_1 - \chi_0)}{Sd}$$

The test value for the $t$ is then looked up in the $t$-table with $f - 1$ degrees of freedom.

Computation is markedly simplified if all the groups are of equal size.


### 22.7.20. Assumptions and Limitations

1. The underlying assumptions for ANCOVA are fairly rigid and restrictive. The assumptions include

   a. That the slopes of the regression lines of a $Y$ and $X$ are equal from group to group. This can be examined visually or formally (i.e., by a test). If this condition is not met, ANCOVA cannot be used.

   b. That the relationship between $X$ and $Y$ is linear.

   c. That the covariate $X$ is measured without error. Power of the test declines as error increases.

   d. That there are no unmeasured confounding variables.

   e. That the errors inherent in each variable are independent of each other. Lack of independence effectively (but to an immeasurable degree) reduces sample size.

   f. That the variances of the errors in groups are equivalent between groups.

    g. That the measured data which form the groups are normally distributed. ANCOVA is generally robust to departures from normality.

2. Of the seven assumptions above, the most serious are the first four.


### 22.7.21. Modeling

The mathematical modeling of biological systems, restricted even to the field of toxicology, is an extremely large and vigorously growing area. Broadly speaking, modeling is the principal conceptual tool by which toxicology seeks to develop as a mechanistic science. In an iterative process, models are developed or proposed, tested by experiment, reformulated and so on in a continuous cycle. Such a cycle could also be described as two related types of modeling: explanatory (where the concept is formed) and correlative (where data are organized and relationships derived). An excellent introduction to the broader field of modeling of biological systems can be found in Gold (1977).

In toxicology, modeling is of prime interest in seeking to relate a treatment variable with an effect variable and, from the resulting model, predict effects at exact points where no experiment has been done (but in the range where we have performed experiments, such as "determining" $LD_{50}$'s), to estimate how good our prediction is, and occasionally, simply to determine if a pattern of effects is related to a pattern of treatment.

For use in prediction, the techniques of linear regression, probit–logit analysis (a special case of linear regression), moving averages (an efficient approximation method), and nonlinear regression (for doses where data cannot be made to fit a linear pattern) are presented. For evaluating the predictive value of these models, both the correlations coefficient (for parametric data) and Kendall's rank correlation (for nonparametric data) are given. And finally, the concept of trend analysis is introduced and a method presented.

When we are trying to establish a pattern between several data points (whether this pattern is in the form of a line or a curve), what we are doing is interpolating. It is possible for any given set of points to produce an infinite set of lines or curves which pass near (for lines) or through (for curves) the data points. In most cases, we cannot actually know the "real" pattern. Se we apply a basic principle of science: Occam's razor. We use the simplest explanation (or, in this case, model) which fits the facts (or data). A line is, of course, the simplest pattern to deal with and describe, so fitting the best line (linear regression) is the most common form of model in toxicology.


### 22.7.22. Linear Regression

Foremost among the methods for interpolating within a known data relationship is regression: the fitting of a line or curve to a set of known data points on a graph, and the interpolation ("estimation") of this line or curve in areas where we have no data points. The simplest of these regression models is that of linear regression (valid when increasing the value of one variable changes the value of the related variable in a linear fashion, either positively or negatively). This is the case we will explore here, using the method of least squares.

Given that we have two sets of variables, $x$ (say mg/kg of test material administered) and $y$ (say percentage of animals so dosed that die), what is required is solving for $a$ and $b$ in the equation $Y_i = a + bx_i$ [where the uppercase $Y_i$ is the fitted value of $y_i$ at $x_i$, and we wish to minimize $(y_i - Y_i)^2$]. So we solve the equations

$$b = \frac{\sum x_1 y_1 - nx\bar{y}}{\sum x_1^2 - n\bar{x}^2}$$

and

$$a = \bar{y} - b\bar{x}$$

where $a$ is the $y$ intercept, $b$ is the slope of the time and $n$ is the number of data points.

Note that in actuality, dose-response relationships are often not linear and instead we must use either a transform (to linearlize the data) or a nonlinear regression method (Gallant, 1975).

Note also that we can use the correlation test statistic (described in the correlation coefficient section) to determine if the regression is significant (and, therefore, valid at a defined level of certainty. A more specific test for significance would be the linear regression analysis of variance (Pollard, 1977). To so we start by developing the appropriate ANOVA table.

Finally, we might wish to determine the confidence intervals for our regression line; that is, given a regression line with calculated values for $Y_i$ given $x_i$, within what limits may we be certain (with, say, a 95% probability) what the real value of $Y_i$ is?

If we denote the residual mean square in the ANOVA by $s^2$, the 95% confidence limits for $a$ (denoted by $A$, the notation for the true—as opposed to the estimated—value for this parameter) are calculated as

$$t_{n-2} = \frac{a - A}{\sqrt{\dfrac{s^2(\sum x^2)}{n \sum x_1^2 - n_2 \bar{x}^2}}}$$

$$\frac{9.2 - A}{\sqrt{\dfrac{8.8(51)}{4(51) - (16)(10.562)}}} = \frac{9.2 - A}{\sqrt{\dfrac{448}{35.008}}}$$

$$= \frac{9.2 - A}{3.58} = -4303$$

$$9.2 - A = -15.405$$

$$A = 9.2 - 15.405$$

### 22.7.23. Assumptions and Limitations

1. All the regression methods are for interpolation, not extrapolation. That is, they are valid only in the range that we have data, the experimental region. Not beyond.

2. The method assumes that the data are independent and normally distributed, and it is sensitive to outliers. The $x$-axis (or horizontal) component plays an extremely important part in developing the least square fit. All points have equal weight in determining the height of a regression line, but extreme $x$-axis values unduly influence the slope of the line.

3. A good fit between a line and a set of data (that is, a strong correlation between treatment and response variables) does not imply any casual relationship.

4. It is assumed that the treatment variable can be measured without error, that each data point is independent, that variances are equivalent, and that a linear relationship does not exist between the variables.

5. There are many excellent texts on regression, which is a powerful technique. These include Draper and Smith, 1981 and Montgomery and Smith, 1983, which are not overly rigorous mathematically.

### 22.7.24. Probit–Log Transforms and Regression

As we noted in the preceding section, dose-response problems (among the most common interpolation problems encountered in toxicology) rarely are straightforward enough to make a valid linear regression directly from the raw data. The most common valid interpolation methods are based upon probability ("probit") and logarithmic ("log") value scales, with percentage responses (death, tumor incidence, etc.) being expressed on the probit scale while doses ($Y_i$) are expressed on the log scale. There are two strategies for such an approach. The first is based on transforming the data to these scales, then doing a weighted linear regression on the transformed data (if one does not have access to a computer or a high-powered programmable calculator, the only practical strategy is not to assign weights). The second requires the use of algorithms (approximate calculation techniques) for the probit value and regression process, and is extremely burdensome to perform manually.

Our approach to the first strategy requires that we construct a table with the pairs of values of $x_i$ and $y_i$ listed in order of increasing values of $Y_i$ (percentage response). Beside each of these columns a set of blank columns should be left so that the transformed values may be listed. We then simply add the columns described in the linear regression procedure. Log and probit values may be taken from any of a number of sets of tables and the rest of the table is then developed from these transformed $x_i'$ and $y_i'$ values (denoted as $x_i'$ and $y_i'$). A standard linear regression is then performed.

The second strategy we discussed has been broached by a number of authors (Bliss, 1935; Finney, 1977; Litchfield and Wilcoxon, 1949; and Prentice, 1976). All of these methods, however, are computationally cumbersome. It is possible to approximate the necessary iterative process using the algorithms developed by Abramowitz and Stegun (1964) but even this merely reduces the complexity to a point where the procedure may be readily programmed on a small computer or programmable calculator.

### 22.7.25. Assumptions and Limitations

1. The probit distribution is derived form a common error function, with the mid point (50% point) moved to a score of 5.00.
2. The underlying frequency distribution becomes asymptotic as it approaches the extremes of the range. That is, in the range of 16 to 84%, the corresponding probit values change gradually; the curve is relatively linear. But beyond this range, they change ever more rapidly as they approach either 0% or 100%. In fact, there are no values for either of these numbers.
3. A normally distributed population is assumed, and the results are sensitive to outliers.

### 22.7.26. Nonlinear Regression

More often than not in toxicology we find that our data demonstrate a relationship between two variables (such as age and body weight) which is not linear. That is, a change in one variable (say age) does not produce a directly proportional change in the other (e.g., body weight). But some form of relationship between the variables is apparent. If understanding such a relationship and being able to predict unknown points is of value, we have a pair of options available to us. The first, which was discussed and reviewed earlier, is to use one or more transformations to linearize our data and then to make use of linear regression. This approach, though most commonly used, has a number of drawbacks. Not all data can be suitably transformed; sometimes the transformations necessary to linearize the data require a cumbersome series of calculations, and the resulting linear regression is not always sufficient to account for the differences among sample values; there are significant deviations around the linear regression line (that is, a line may still not give us a good fit to the data or do an adequate job of representing the relationship between the data). In such cases, we have available a second option: the fitting of data to some nonlinear function such as some form of the curve. This is, in general form, nonlinear regression and may involve fitting data to an infinite number of possible functions. But most often we are interested in fitting curves to a polynomial function of the general form.

$$Y = a + bx + cx^2 + dx^3 + \cdots$$

where $x$ is the independent variable. As the number of powers of $x$ increases, the curve becomes increasingly complex and will be able to fit a given set of data increasingly well.

Generally in toxicology, however, if we plot the log of a response (such as body weight) versus a linear scale of our dose or stimulus, we get one of four types of nonlinear curves. These are (Snedecor and Cochran, 1980)

1. Exponential growth, where $\log Y = A(B^x)$, such as the growth curve for the log phase of a bacterial culture.
2. Exponential decay, where $\log Y = A(B^{-x})$, such as a radioactive decay curve.
3. Asymptotic regression, where $\log Y = A - B(p^x)$, such as a first-order reaction curve.
4. Logistic growth curve, where $\log Y = A/(1 + Bp^x)$, such as a population growth curve.

In all these cases, $A$ and $B$ are constant while $p$ is a log transform. These curves are illustrated in Figure 22.7.

All four types of curves are fit by iterative processes; that is, best-guess numbers are initially chosen for each of the constants and, after a fit is attempted, the constants are modified to improve the fit. This process is repeated until an acceptable fit has been generated. Analysis of variance or covariance can be used to objectively

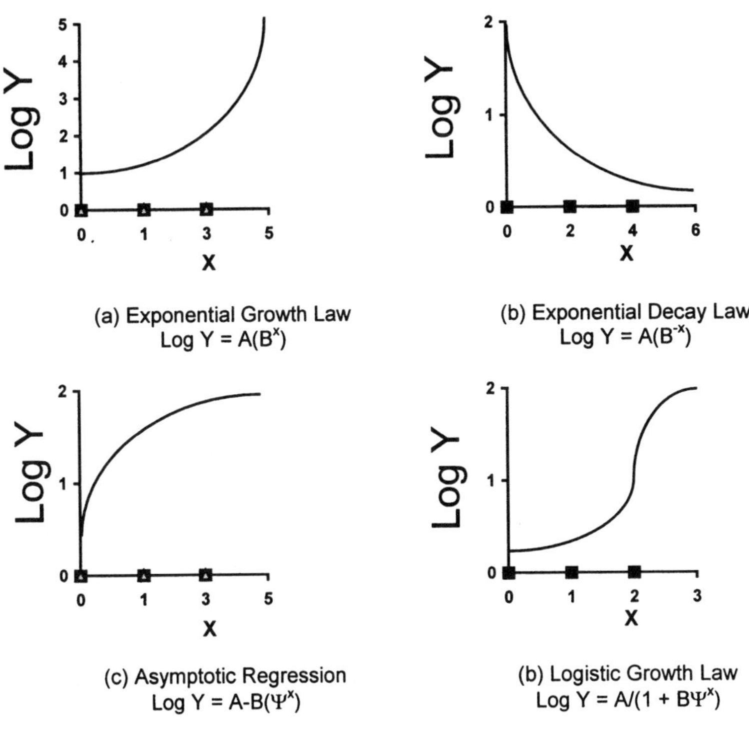



**FIGURE 22.7.** Common curvilinear curves.

evaluate the acceptability of it. Needless to say, the use of a computer generally accelerates such a curve-fitting process.

### 22.7.27. Assumptions and Limitations

1. The principle of using least squares may still be applicable in fitting the best curve, if the assumptions of normality, independence, and reasonably error-free measurement of response are valid.
2. Growth curves are best modeled using a nonlinear method.

### 22.7.28. Correlation Coefficient

The correlation procedure is used to determine the degree of linear correlation (direct relationship) between two groups of continuous (and normally distributed) variables; it will indicate whether there is any statistical relationship between the variables in the two groups. For example, we may wish to determine if the liver weights of dogs on a feeding study are correlated with their body weights. Thus, we will record the body and liver weights at the time of sacrifice and then calculate the correlation coefficient between these pairs of values to determine if there is some relationship.

A formula for calculating the linear correlation coefficient ($r_{xy}$) is

$$r_{xy} = \frac{N \sum XY - (\sum X)(\sum Y)}{\sqrt{N \sum X^2 - (\sum X)^2}\sqrt{N \sum Y^2 - (\sum Y)^2}}$$

where $X$ is each value for one variable (such as the dog body weights in the above example), $Y$ is the matching value for the second variable (the liver weights), and $N$ is the number of pairs of $X$ and $Y$. Once we have obtained $r_{xy}$ it is possible to calculate $t_r$, which can be used for more precise examination of the degree of significant linear relationship between the two groups. This value is calculated as follows

$$t_r = \frac{r_{zy}\sqrt{N-2}}{\sqrt{1 - r_{zy}^2}}$$

This calculation is also equivalent to $r =$ sample covariance$/\ (S_x S_y)$, as was seen earlier under ANCOVA.

The value obtained for $r_{xy}$ can be compared to table values (Snedecor and Cochran, 1980) for the number of pairs of data involved minus two. If the $r_{xy}$ is smaller (at the selected test probability level, such as 0.05), the correlation is not significantly different from zero (no correlation). If $r_{xy}$ is larger than the table value, there is a positive statistical relationship between the groups. Comparisons are then made at lower levels of probability to determine the degree of relationship (note that if $r_{xy}$ = either 1.0 or −1.0, there is complete correlation between the groups). If $r_{xy}$ is a negative number and the absolute is greater than the table value, there is an inverse relationship between the groups; that is, a change in one group is associated with a change in the opposite direction in the second group of variables.

Since the comparison of $r_{xy}$ with the table values may be considered a somewhat weak test, it is perhaps more meaningful to compare the $t_r$ value with values in a $t$-distribution table for N-2 degrees of freedom ($df$), as is done for Student's $t$-test. This will give a more exact determination of the degree of statistical correlation between the two groups.

Note that this method examines only possible linear relationships between sets of continuous, normally distributed data.

### 22.7.29. Assumptions and Limitations

1. A strong correlation does not imply that a treatment causes an effect.
2. The distances of data points from the regression line are the portions of the data not "explained" by the model. These are called residuals. Poor correlation coefficients imply high residuals, which may be due to many small contributions (variations of data from the regression line) or a few large ones. Extreme values (outliers) greatly reduce correlation.
3. $X$ and $Y$ are assumed to be independent.
4. Feinstein (1979) has provided a fine discussion of the difference between correlation (or association of variables) and causation.

### 22.7.30. Kendall's Coefficient of Rank Correlation

Kendall's rank correlation, represented by $\tau$(tau), should be used to evaluate the degree of association between two sets of data when the nature of the data is such that the relationship may not be linear. Most commonly, this is when the data are not continuous and/or normally distributed. An example of such a case is when we are trying to determine if there is a relationship between the length of hydra and their survival time in a test medium in hours. Both of our variables here are discontinuous, yet we suspect a relationship exists. Another common use is in comparing the subjective scoring done by two different observers.

Tau is calculated at $\tau = N/n(n-1)$ where $n$ is the sample size and $N$ is the count of ranks, calculated as $N = 4 \, (^n C_i) - n(n-1)$, with the computing of $^n C_i$ being demonstrated in the example.

If a second variable $Y_2$ is exactly correlated with the first variable $Y_1$, then the variates $Y_2$ should be in the same order as the $Y_1$ variates. However, if the correlation is less than exact, the order of the variates $Y_2$ will not correspond entirely to that of $Y$. The quantity $N$ measures how well the second variable corresponds to the order of the first. It has maximum value of $n(n-1)$ and a minimum value of $-n(n-1)$.

A table of data is set up with each of the two variables being ranked separately. Tied ranks are assigned as demonstrated earlier under the Kruskall Wallis test. From this point, disregard the original variates and deal only with the ranks. Place the ranks of one of the two variables in rank order (from lowest to highest), paired with the rank values assigned for the other variable. If one (but not the other) variable has tied ranks, order the pairs by the variables without ties (Sokal and Rohlf, 1994).

The resulting value of tau will range from $-1$ to $+1$, as does the familiar parametric correlation coefficient, $r$.

### 22.7.31. Assumption and Limitation

This is a very robust estimator which does not assume normality, linearity, or minimal error of measurement.

### 22.7.32. Trend Analysis

Trend analysis is a collection of techniques that have been "discovered" by toxicology since the mid-1970s (Tarone, 1975). The actual methodology dates back to the mid-1950s (Cox and Stuart, 1955).

Trend analysis methods are a variation on the theme of regression testing. In the broadest sense, the methods are used to determine whether a sequence of observations taken over an ordered range of a variable (most commonly time) exhibit some form of pattern of change (either an increase-upward trend or decrease-downward trend) associated with another variable of interest (in toxicology, some form or measure of dosage and exposure).

Trend corresponds to sustained and systematic variations over a long period of time. It is associated with the structural causes of the phenomenon in question, for example, population growth, technological progress, new ways of organization, or capital accumulation.

The identification of trend has always posed a serious statistical problem. The problem is not one of mathematical or analytical complexity but of conceptual complexity. This problem exists because the trend as well as the remaining components of a time series are latent (nonobservables) variables and, therefore, assumptions must be made on their behavioral pattern. The trend is generally thought of as a smooth and slow movement over a long term. The concept of "long" in this connection is relative and what is identified as trend for a given series span might well be part of a long cycle once the series is considerably augmented. Often, a long cycle is treated as a trend because the length of the observed time series is shorter than one complete face of this type of cycle.

The ways in which data are collected in toxicology studies frequently serve to complicate trend analysis, as the length of time for the phenomena underlying a trend to express themselves is frequently artificially censored.

To avoid the complexity of the problem posed by a statistically vague definition, statisticians have resorted to two simple solutions: One consists of estimating trend and cyclical fluctuations together, calling this combined movement *trend-cycle*; the other consists of defining the trend in terms of the series length , denoting it as the longest nonperiodic movement.

Within the large class of models identified for trend, we can distinguish two main categories, deterministic trends and stochastic trends.

Deterministic trend models are based on the assumption that the trend of a time series can be approximated closely by simple mathematical functions of time over the entire span of the series. The most common representation of a deterministic trend is by means of polynomials or of transcendental functions. The time series from which the trend is to be identified is assumed to be generated by a nonstationary process where the nonstationarity results from a deterministic trend. A classical model is the regression or error model (Anderson, 1971) where the observed series is treated as the sum of a systematic part or trend and a random part or irregular. This model can be written as

$$Z_t = Y_t + U_t'$$

where $U_t$ is a purely random process, that is, $U_t \sim$ i.i.d. $(O, 2/u)$ (independent and identically distributed with expected value 0 and variance $\sigma(2/u)$).

Trend tests are generally described as "$k$-sample tests of the null hypothesis of identical distribution against an alternative of linear order"; that is, if sample I has distribution function $F_i$, $i = 1$, then the null hypothesis

$$H- : F_1 = F_2 - \cdots = F_k$$

is tested against the alternative

$$H1 : F_1 \geq F_2 \geq \cdots = F_k$$

(or its reverse), there at least one of the inequalities is strict. These tests can be thought of as special cases of tests of regression or correlation in which association is sought between the observations and its ordered sample index. They are also related to analysis of variance except that the tests are tailored to be powerful against the subset of alternatives $H_1$, instead of the more general set $\{F_1 \neq F_j$, some $i \neq j\}$.

Different tests arise from requiring power against specific elements or subsets of this rather extensive set of alternatives.

The most popular trend test in toxicology is currently that presented by Tarone in 1975 because it is that used by the National Cancer Institute in the analysis of carcinogenicity data. A simple, but efficient alternative is the Cox and Stuart test (Cox and Stuart, 1955) which is a modification of the sign test. For each point at which we have a measure (such as the incidence of animals observed with tumors) we form a pair of observations, one from each of the groups we wish to compare. In a traditional NCI bioassay this would mean pairing control with low dose and low dose with high dose (to explore a dose-related trend) or each time period observation in a dose group (except the first) with its predecessor (to evaluate time-related trend). When the second observation in a pair exceeds the earlier observation, we record a plus sign for that pair. When the first observation is greater than the second, we record a minus sign for that pair. A preponderance of plus signs suggests a downward trend while an excess of minus signs suggests an upward trend. A formal test at a preselected confidence level can then be performed.

More formally put, after having defined what trend we want to test for, we first match pairs as $(X_1 - X_{1+C})$, $(X_2, X_{2+C})$, ..., $(X_{n'-c}, X_{n'})$ where $c = n'/2$ when $n'$ is even and $c = (n' + 1)/2$ when $n'$ is odd (where $n'$ is the number of observations in a set). The hypothesis is then tested by comparing the resulting number of excess positive or negative signs against a sign test table such as is found in Beyer (1976).

We can, of course, combine a number of observations to allow ourselves to actively test for a set of trends, such as the existence of a trend of increasing difference between two groups of animals over a period of time.

### 22.7.33. Assumptions and Limitations

Trend tests seek to evaluate whether there is a monotonic tendency in response to a change in treatment. That is, the dose-response direction is absolute: as dose goes up; the incidence of tumors increases. Thus the test loses power rapidly in response to the occurrences of "reversals", for example, a low dose group with a decreased tumor incidence. There are methods (Dykstra and Robertson, 1983) that "smooth the bumps" of reversals in long data series. In toxicology, however, most data series are short (that is, there are only a few dose levels).

Tarone's trend test is most powerful at detecting dose-related trends when tumor onset hazard functions are proportional to each other. For more power against other dose related group differences, weighted versions of the statistic are also available (Breslow, 1984; and Crowley and Breslow, 1984).

In 1985, the United States *Federal Register* recommended that the analysis of tumor incidence data be carried out with a Cochran–Armitage (Armitage, 1955; Cochran, 1954) trend test. The test statistic of the Cochran–Armitage test is defined:

$$T_{\mathrm{CA}} = \sqrt{\frac{N}{(N-r)r}, \frac{\sum_{i=0}^{k}(R_1 - (n_1/Nr)d_1}{\sqrt{\sum_{i=0}^{k}(n_i/N)d_i^2 - (\sum_{i=0}^{k}(n_i/N)d_1)^2}}}$$

with dose scores $d_i$. Armitage's test statistic is the square of this term ($T_{\mathrm{CA}}^2$. As one-sided tests are carried out for an increase of tumor rates, the square is not considered. Instead, the above-mentioned test statistic which is presented by Portier and Hoel (1984) is used. This test statistic is asymptotically standard normal distributed. The Cochran–Armitage test is asymptotically efficient for all monotone alternatives (Tarone, 1975), but this result only holds asymptotically. And tumors are rare events, so the binominal proportions are small. In this situation approximations may become unreliable.

Therefore, exact tests which can be performed using two different approaches: conditional and unconditional are considered. In the first case, the total number of tumors $r$ is regarded as fixed. As a result the null distribution of the test statistic is independent of the common probability $p$. The exact conditional null distribution is a multivariate hypergeometric distribution.

The unconditional model treats the sum of all tumors as a random variable. Then the exact unconditional null distribution is a multivariate binomial distribution. The distribution depends on the unknown probability.

## 22.8. METHODS FOR THE REDUCTION OF DIMENSIONALITY

Techniques for the reduction of dimensionality are those that simplify the understanding of data, either visually or numerically, while causing only minimal reductions in the amount of information present. These techniques operate primarily by pooling or combining groups of variables into single variables, but may also entail the identification and elimination of low-information-content (or irrelevant) variables.

Descriptive statistics (calculations of means, standard deviations, etc.) are the simplest and most familiar form of reduction of dimensionality. Here we first need to address classification, which provides the general conceptual tools for identifying and quantifying similarities and differences between groups of things which have more than a single linear scale of measurement in common (for example, which have both been determined to have or lack a number of enzyme activities). Then we will consider two collections of methodologies which combine graphic and computational methods, multidimensional and nonmetric scaling and cluster analysis. Multidimensional scaling (MDS) is a set of techniques for quantitatively analyzing similarities, dissimilarities and distances between data in a display-like manner. Nonmetric scaling is an analogous set of methods for displaying and relating data when measurements are non-quantitative (the data are described by attributes or ranks). Cluster analysis is a collection of graphic and numerical methodologies for classifying things based on the relationships between the values of the variables that they share.

The final pair of methods for reduction of dimensionality which will be tackled in this chapter are Fourier analysis and the life table analysis. Fourier analysis seeks to identify cyclic patterns in data and then either analyze the patterns or the residuals after the patterns are taken out. Life table analysis techniques are directed to identifying and quantitating the time course of risks (such as death, or the occurrence of tumors).

### 22.8.1. Classification

Classification is both a basic concept and a collection of techniques which are necessary prerequisites for further analysis of data when the members of a set of data are (or can be) each described by several variables. At least some degree of classification (which is broadly defined as the dividing of the members of a group into smaller groups in accordance with a set of decision rules) is necessary prior to any data collection. Whether formally or informally, an investigator has to decide which things are similar enough to be counted as the same and develop rules for governing collection procedures. Such rules can be as simple as "measure and record body weights only of live animals on study", or as complex as that demonstrated by the expanded weighting classification procedure demonstrated below. Such a classification also demonstrates that the selection of which variables to measure will determine the final classification of data.

### Expanded Weighting Procedure

<table>
<tr><td>I. Is animal of desired species?</td><td align="right">Yes/No</td></tr>
<tr><td>II. Is animal member of study group?</td><td align="right">Yes/No</td></tr>
<tr><td>III. Is animal alive?</td><td align="right">Yes/No</td></tr>
<tr><td>IV. Which group does animal belong to?</td><td></td></tr>
<tr><td>   A. Control</td><td></td></tr>
<tr><td>   B. Low Dose</td><td></td></tr>
<tr><td>   C. Intermediate Dose</td><td></td></tr>
<tr><td>   D. High Dose</td><td></td></tr>
<tr><td>V. What sex is animal?</td><td align="right">Male/Female</td></tr>
<tr><td>VI. Is the measured weight in acceptable range?</td><td align="right">Yes/No</td></tr>
</table>

Classifications of data have two purposes (Hartigan, 1983; Gordon, 1981); data simplification (also called a descriptive function) and prediction. Simplification is necessary because there is a limit to both the volume and complexity of data that the human mind can comprehend and deal with conceptually. Classification allows us to attach a label (or name) to each group of data, to summarize the data (that is, assign individual elements of data to groups and to characterize the population of the group), and to define the relationships between groups (that is, develop a taxonomy).

Prediction, meanwhile, is the use of summaries of data and knowledge of the relationships between groups to develop hypotheses as to what will happen when further data are collected (as when more animals or people are exposed to an agent under defined conditions) and as to the mechanisms which cause such relationships to develop. Indeed, classification is the prime device for the discovery of mechanisms in all of science. A classic example of this was Darwin's realization that there were reasons (the mechanisms of evolution) behind the differences and similarities in species which had caused Linaeus to earlier develop his initial modern classification scheme (or taxonomy) for animals.

To develop a classification, one first sets bounds wide enough to encompass the entire range of data to be considered but not unnecessarily wide. This is typically done by selecting some global variables (variables every piece of data have in common) and limiting the range of each so that it just encompasses all the cases on hand. Then one selects a set of local variables (characteristics that only some of the cases have, say the occurrence of certain tumor types, enzyme activity levels or dietary preferences) and which thus serve to differentiate between groups. Data are then collected, and a system for measuring differences and similarities is developed. Such measurements are based on some form of measurement of distance between two cases ($x$ and $y$) in terms of each single variable scale. If the variable is a continuous one, then the simplest measure of distance between two pieces of data is the Euclidean distance, ($d[x, y]$) defined as

$$d(x, y) = \sqrt{(x_i - y_i)^2}$$

For categorical or discontinuous data, the simplest distance measure is the matching distance, defined as

$$d(x, y) = \text{number of times } x_i \neq y_i.$$

After we have developed a table of such distance measurements for each of the local variables, some weighting factor is assigned to each variable. A weighting factor seeks to give greater importance to those variables which are believed to have more relevance or predictive value. The weighted variables are then used to assign each piece of data to a group. The actual act of developing numerically based classifications and assigning data members to them is the realm of cluster analysis, which will be discussed later in this chapter. Classification of biological data based on qualitative factors has been well discussed (Glass, 1975; Schaper et al., 1985) does an excellent job of introducing the entire field and mathematical concepts.

Relevant examples of the use of classification techniques range from the simple to the complex. Schaper et al. (1985) developed and used a very simple classification of response methodology to identify those airborne chemicals which alter the normal respiratory response induced by $CO_2$. At the other end of the spectrum, Kowalski and Bender (1972) developed a more mathematically based system to classify chemical data (a methodology they termed pattern recognition).

### 22.8.2. Statistical Graphics

The use of graphics in one form or another in statistics is the single most effective and robust statistical tool and at the same time, one of the most poorly understood and improperly used.

Graphs are used for one of four major purposes. Each of the four is a variation on the central theme of making complex data easier to understand and use. These four major functions are exploration, analysis, communication and display of data, and graphical aids. Exploration (which may be simply summarizing data or trying to expose relationships between variables) is determining the characteristics of data sets and deciding on one or more appropriate forms of further analysis, such as the scatter plot. Analysis is the use of graphs to formally evaluate some aspect of the data, such as whether there are outliers present or if an underlying assumption of a population distribution is fulfilled. As long ago as 1960 (Anderson), some 18 graphical methods for analyzing multivariate data relationships were developed and proposed. Table 22.7 presents a summary of major graphical techniques that are available.

Communication and display of data are the most commonly used function of statistical graphics in toxicology, whether used for internal reports, presentations at meetings, or formal publications in the literature. In communicating data, graphs should not be used to duplicate data that are presented in tables, but rather to show important trends and/or relationships in the data. Though such communication is most commonly of a quantitative compilation of actual data, it can be also be used to

**TABLE 22.7. Forms of Statistical Graphics (by Function)**

| | Exploration | |
| Data Summary | Two Variables | Three or More Variables |
| --- | --- | --- |
| Box and whisker plot | Autocorrelation plot | Biplot |
| Histogram | Cross-correlation plot | Cluster trees |
| Dot-array diagram | Scatter plot | Labeled scatter plot |
| Frequently polygon | Sequence plot | Glyphs and metroglyphs |
| Ogive | | Face plots |
| Stem and lead diagram | | Fourier plots |
| | | Similarity and preference maps |
| | | Multidimensional scaling displays |
| | | Weathervane plot |

| | Analysis | |
| Distribution Assessment | Model Evaluation and Assumption Verification | Decision Making |
| --- | --- | --- |
| Probability plot | Average versus standard deviation | Control chart |
| Q-Q plot | | Cusum chart |
| P-P Plot | Component-plus-residual plot | Half-normal plot |
| Hanging histogram | Partial-residual plot | Ridge trace |
| Rootagram | Residual plots | Youden plot |
| Poissonness plot | | |

| | Communication and Display of Data | |
| Quantitative Graphics | Summary of Statistical Analyses | Graphical Aids |
| --- | --- | --- |
| Line chart | Means plot | Confidence limits |
| Pictogram | Sliding reference distribution | Graph paper |
| Pie chart | Notched box plot | Power curves |
| Contour plot | Factor space/response | Nomographs |
| Stereogram | Interaction plot | Sample-size curves |
| Color map | Contour plot | Trilinear coordinates |
| Histogram | Predicted response plot | |
| | Confidence region plot | |

summarize and present the results of statistical analysis. The fourth and final function of graphics is one that is largely becoming outdated as microcomputers become more widely available. Graphical aids to calculation include nomograms (the classic example in toxicology of a nomogram is that presented by Litchfield and Wilcoxon (1949) for determining median effective doses) and extrapolating and interpolating data graphically based on plotted data.

There are many forms of statistical graphics (a partial list, classified by function, is presented in Table 22.7), and a number of these (such as scatter plots and histograms) can be used for each of a number of possible functions. Most of these plots are based on a Cartesian system (that is, they use a set of rectangular coordinates), and our review of construction and use will focus on these forms of graphs.

Construction of a rectangular graph of any form starts with the selection of the appropriate form of graph followed by the laying out of the coordinates (or axes). Even graphs that are going to encompass multivariate data (that is, more than two variables) generally have as their starting point two major coordinates. The vertical axis, or ordinate (also called the $Y$ axis), is used to present an independent variable. Each of these axes is scaled in the units of measure which will most clearly present the trends of interest in the data. The range covered by the scale of each axis is selected to cover the entire region for which data is presented. The actual demarking of the measurement scale along an axis should allow for easy and accurate assessment of the coordinates of any data point, yet should not be cluttered.

Actual data points should be presented by symbols which present the appropriate indicators of location. If they represent a summaries of data from a normal data population, it would be appropriate to present a symbol for the mean and some indication of the variability (or error) associated with that population, commonly by using "error bars" which present the standard deviation (or standard error) from the mean. If, however, the data are not normal or continuous it would be more appropriate to indicate location by the median and present the range or semiquartile distance for variability estimates. The symbols which are used to present data points can also be used to present a significant amount of additional information. At the simplest level a set a clearly distinct symbols (circles, triangles, squares, etc.) are very commonly used to provide a third dimension of data (most commonly treatment group). But by clever use of symbols, all sorts of additional information can be presented. Using a method such as Chernoff's faces (Chernoff, 1973), in which faces are used as symbols of the data points (and various aspects of the faces present additional data, such as the presence or absence of eyes denoting presence or absence of a secondary pathological condition), it is possible to present a large number of different variables on a single graph.

The three other forms of graphs that are commonly used are histograms, pie charts, and contour plots.

Histograms are graphs of simple frequency distribution. Commonly, the abscissa is the variable of interest (such as lifespan or litter size), and is generally shown as classes or intervals or measurements (such as age ranges of 0 to 10, 10 to 20, weeks, etc.). The ordinate, meanwhile, is the incidence or frequency of observations. The result is a set of vertical bars, each of which represents the incidence of a particular set of observations. Measures of error or variability about each incidence are reflected by some form of error bar on top of, or in the frequency bars, as shown in Figure 22.8. The size of class intervals may be unequal (in effect, one can

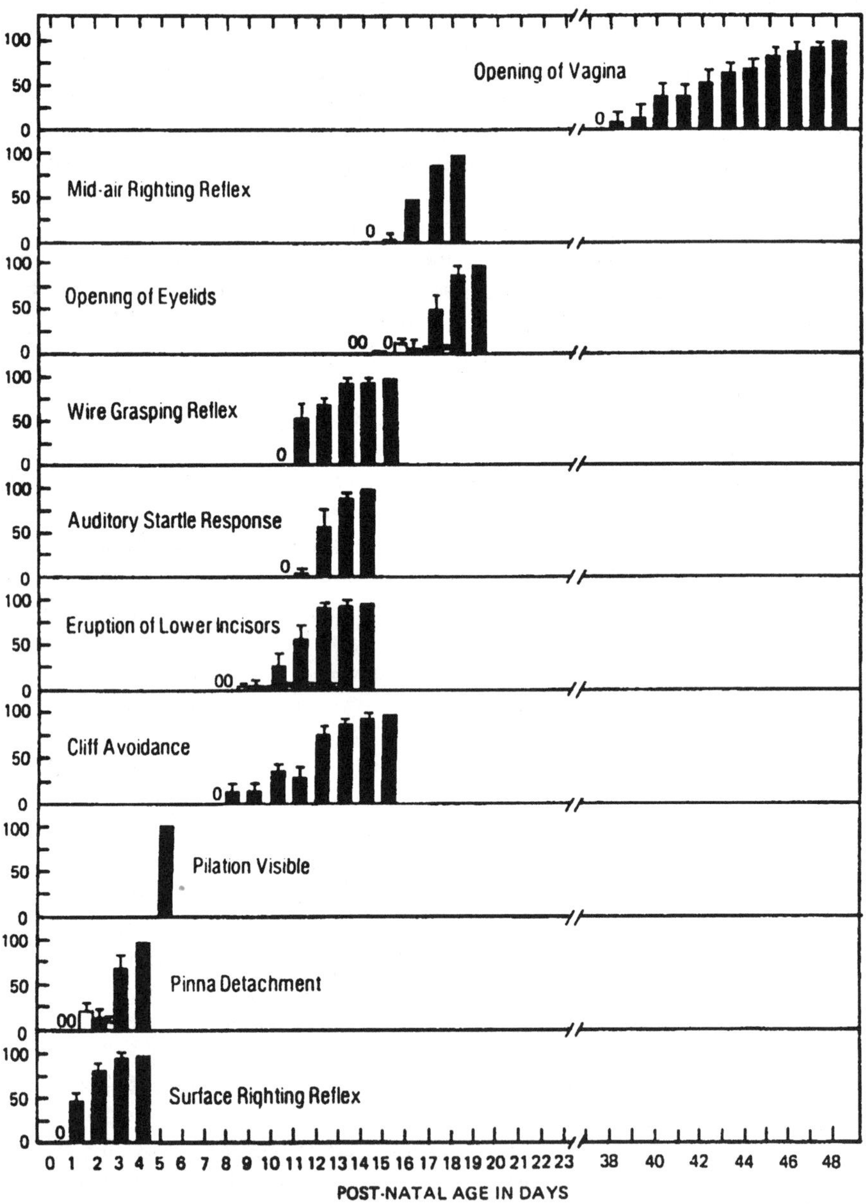


**FIGURE 22.8.** Acquisitions of post-natal development landmarks in rats.

combine or poor several small class intervals), but it is proper in such cases to vary the width of the bars to indicate differences in interval size.

Pie charts are the only common form of quantitative graphic technique that is not rectangular. Rather, the figure is presented as a circle out of which several "slices" are delimited. The only major use of the pie chart is in presenting a breakdown of the components of a group. Typically the entire set of data under consideration (such as total body weight), constitutes the pie while each slice represents a percentage of the whole (such as the percentages represented by each of several organs). The total number of slices in a pie should be small for the presentation to be effective. Variability or error can be readily presented by having a subslice of each sector shaded and labeled accordingly.

Finally, there is the contour plot, which is used to depict the relationships in a three variable, continuous data system. That is, a contour plot visually portrays each contour as a locus of the values of two variables associated with a constant value of the third variable. An example would be a relief map that gives both latitude and longitude of constant altitude using contour lines.

The most common misuse of graphs is to either conceal or exaggerate the extent of the difference by using inappropriately scaled or ranged axis. Tufte (1983) has termed a statistic for evaluating the appropriateness of scale size, the "lie factor", calculated as the ratio of the shown effect size to the range of potential change or effect. An acceptable range for the lie factor is from 0.95 to 1.05. Less means the size of an effect is being understated, more that the effect is being exaggerated.

There are a number of excellent references available for those who would like to pursue statistical graphics more. Anscombe (1973) presents an excellent short overview, while others (Tufte, 1983, 1990, 1997; Schmid, 1983; and Young, 1985) provide a wealth of information.

### 22.8.3. Multidimensional and Nonmetric Scaling

Multidimensional scaling (MDS) is a collection of analysis methods for data sets which have three or more variables making up each data point. MDS displays the relationships of three or more dimensional extensions of the methods of statistical graphics.

MDS presents the structure of a set of objects from data that approximate the distances between pairs of the objects. The data, called similarities, dissimilarities, distances, or proximities, must be in such a form that the degree of similarities and differences between the pairs of the objects (each of which represents a real-life data point) can be measured and handled as a distance (remember the discussion of measures of distances under classifications). Similarity is a matter of degree-small differences between objects cause them to be similar (a high degree of similarity) while large differences cause them to be considered dissimilar (a small degree of similarity).

In addition to the traditional human conceptual or subjective judgments or similarity, data can be an "objective" similarity measure (the difference in weight between a pair of animals) or an index calculated from multivariate data (the proportion of agreement in the results of a number of carcinogenicity studies). However, the data must always represent the degree of similarity of pairs of objects.

Each object or data point is represented by a point in a multidimensional space. These plots or projected points are arranged in this space so that the distances between pairs of points have the strongest possible relation to the degree of similarity among the pairs of objects. That is, two similar objects are represented by two points that are close together, and two dissimilar objects are represented by a pair of points that are far apart. The space is usually a two- or three-dimensional Euclidean space, but may be non-Euclidean and may have more dimensions.

MDS is a general term that includes a number of different types of techniques. However, all seek to allow geometric analysis of multivariate data. The forms of MDS can be classified (Young, 1985) according to the nature of the similarities in the data. It can be qualitative (nonmetric) or quantitative (metric MDS). The types can also be classified by the number of variables involved and by the nature of the model used; for example, classical MDS (there is only one data matrix, and no weighting factors are used on the data), replicated MDS (more than one matrix and no weighting) and weighted MDS (more than one matrix and at least some of the data being weighted).

MDS can be used in toxicology to analyze the similarities and differences between effects produced by different agents, in an attempt to use an understanding of the mechanism underlying the actions of one agent to determine the mechanisms of the other agents. Actual algorithms and a good intermediate level presentation of MDS can be found in Davison (1983).

Nonmetric scaling is a set of graphic techniques closely related to MDS, and definitely useful for the reduction of dimensionality. Its major objective is to arrange a set of objects (each object, for our purposes, consisting of a number of related observations) graphically in a few dimensions, while retaining the maximum possible fidelity to the original relationships between members (that is, values which are most different are portrayed as most distant). It is not a linear technique, it does not preserve linear relationships (i.e., A is not shown as twice as far from C as B, even though its "value difference" may be twice as much). The spacings (interpoint distances) are kept such that if the distance of the original scale between members A and B is greater than that between C and D, the distances on the model scale shall likewise be greater between A and B than between C and D. Figure 22.5, presented earlier, uses a form of this technique in adding a third dimension by using letters to present degrees of effect on the skin.

This technique functions by taking observed measures of similarity or dissimilarity between every pair of M objects, then finding a representation of the objects as points in Euclidean space so that the interpoint distances in some sense "match" the observed similarities or dissimilarities by means of weighting constants.


## 22.8.4. Cluster Analysis

Cluster analysis is a quantitative form of classification. It serves to help develop decision rules and then use these rules to assign a heterogeneous collection of objects to a series of sets. This is almost entirely an applied methodology (as opposed to theoretical). The final result of cluster analysis is one of several forms of graphic displays and a methodology (set of decision classifying rules) for the assignment of new members into the classifications.

The classification procedures used are based on either density of population or distance between members. These methods can serve to generate a basis for the classification of large numbers of dissimilar variables such as behavioral observations and compounds with distinct but related structures and mechanisms (Gad, 1984; Gad et al., 1985), or to separate tumor patterns caused by treatment from those caused by old age (Hammond et al., 1978).

There are five types of clustering techniques (Everitt, 1980; Romesburg, 1984)

1. *Hierarchical Techniques.* Classes are subclassified into groups, with the process being repeated at several levels to produce a tree which gives sufficient definition to groups.

2. *Optimizing Techniques.* Clusters are formed by optimization of a clustering criterion. The resulting classes are mutually exclusive, the objects are partitioned clearly into sets.

3. *Density or Mode-Seeking Techniques.* Clusters are identified and formed by locating regions in a graphic representation which contains concentrations of data points.

4. *Clumping Techniques.* A variation of density-seeking techniques in which assignment to a cluster is weighted on some variables, so that clusters may overlap in graphic projections.

5. *Others.* Methods which do not clearly fall into classes (1)–(4).

Romesburg (1984) provides an excellent step-by-step guide to cluster analysis.

### 22.8.5. Fourier or Time Analysis

Fourier analysis (Bloomfield, 1976) is most frequently a univariate method used for either simplifying data (which is the basis for its inclusion in this chapter) or for modeling. It can, however, also be a multivariate technique for data analysis.

In a sense, it is like trend analysis; it looks at the relationship of sets of data from a different perspective. In the case of Fourier analysis, the approach is by resolving the time dimension variable in the data set. At the most simple level, it assumes that many events are periodic in nature, and if we can remove the variation in other variables because of this periodicity (by using Fourier transforms), we can better analyze the remaining variation from other variables. The complications to this are (1) there may be several overlying cyclic time-based periodicities, and (2) we may be interested in the time cycle events for their own sake.

Fourier analysis allows one to identify, quantitate, and (if we wish) remove the time-based cycles in data (with their amplitudes, phases and frequencies) by use of the Fourier transform,

$$nJ_i = x_i \exp(-iw_i t)$$

where

$n =$ length.

$J =$ The discrete Fourier transform for that case.

$x =$ actual data.

$i =$ increment in the series.

$w =$ frequency.

$t =$ time.

### 22.8.6. Life Tables

Chronic *in vivo* toxicity studies are generally the most complex and expensive studies conducted by a toxicologist. Answers to a number of questions are sought in such a study, notably if a material results in a significant increase in mortality or in the incidence of tumors in those animals exposed to it. But we are also interested in the time course of these adverse effects (or risks). The classic approach to assessing these age-specific hazard rates is by the use of life tables (also called survivorship tables).

It may readily be seen that during any selected period of time $(t_i)$ we have a number of risks competing to affect an animal. There are risks of (i) "natural death", (ii) death induced by a direct or indirect action of the test compound, and (iii) death due to such occurrences of interest of tumors (Hammond et al., 1978 and Salsburg, 1980). We are indeed interested in determining if (and when) the last two of these risks become significantly different than the "natural" risks (defined as what is seen to happen in the control group). Life table methods enable us to make such determinations as the duration of survival (or time until tumors develop) and the probability of survival (or of developing a tumor) during any period of time.

We start by deciding the interval length $(t_i)$ we wish to examine within the study. The information we gain becomes more exact as the interval is shortened. But as interval length is decreased, the number of intervals increases and calculations become more cumbersome and less indicative of time-related trends because random fluctuations become more apparent. For a two-year or lifetime rodent study, an interval length of a month is commonly employed. Some life table methods, such as the Kaplan–Meyer, have each new event (such as a death) define the start of a new interval.

Having established the interval length we can tabulate our data (Cutler and Ederer, 1958). We start by establishing the following columns in each table (a separate table being established for each group of animals, i.e., by sex and dose level).

1. The interval of time selected $(t_i)$;
2. The number of animals in the group that entered that interval of the study alive $(l_i)$;
3. The number of animals withdrawn from study during the interval (such as those taken for an interim sacrifice or that may have been killed by a technician error) $(\omega_i)$;
4. The number of animals that died during the interval $(d_i)$;
5. The number of animals at risk during the interval, $l_i = l_i = \frac{1}{2}\omega_1$, or the number on study at the start of the interval minus one-half of the number withdrawn during the interval;
6. The proportion of animals that died $= D_i = d_i/l_i$;
7. The cumulative probability of an animal surviving until the end of that interval of study, $P_i = 1 - D_i$, or one minus the number of animals that died during that interval divided by the number of animals at risk;
8. The number of animals dying until that interval $(M_i)$;
9. Animals found to have died during the interval $(m_i)$;
10. The probability of dying during the interval of the study $c_i = 1 - (M_i + m_i/l_i)$, or the total number of animals dead until that interval plus the animals discovered to have died during that interval divided by the number of animals at risk through the end of that interval;
11. The cumulative proportion surviving, $p_i$, is equivalent to the cumulative product of the interval probabilities of survival (i.e., $p_i = p_1 \cdot p_2 \cdot p_3 \cdots p_x$);
12. The cumulative probability of dying, $C_i$, equal to the cumulative product of the interval probabilities to that point (i.e., $C_i = c_1 \cdot c_2 \cdot c_3 \cdots c_x$).

With such tables established for each group in a study, we may now proceed to test the hypotheses that each of the treated groups has a significantly shorter duration of survival, or that of the treated groups died more quickly (note that plots of total animals dead and total animals surviving will give one an appreciation of the data, but can lead to no statistical conclusions).

There are a multiplicity of methods for testing significance in life tables, with (as is often the case) the power of the tests increasing as does the difficulty of computation (Salsburg, 1980; Cox, 1972; Haseman, 1977; and Tarone, 1975).

We begin our method of statistical comparison of survival at any point in the study by determining the standard error of the $K$ interval survival rate as (Garrett, 1947)

$$S_K = P_k \sqrt{\sum_{l}^{k}\left(\frac{D_i}{1'_x - d_x}\right)}$$

We may also determine the effective sample size $(l_l)$ in accordance with

$$l_l = \frac{P(l - P)}{S^2}$$

We may now compute the standard error of difference for any two groups (1 and 2) as

$$S_D = \sqrt{S_1^2 + S_2^2}$$

The difference in survival probabilities for the two groups is then calculated as

$$P_D = P_1 - P_2$$

We can then calculate a test statistic as

$$t' = \frac{P_D}{S_D}$$

This is then compared to the $z$ distribution table. If $t' > z$ at the desired probability level, it is significant at that level. With increasing recognition of the effects of time (both as age and length of exposure to unmeasured background risks), life table analysis has become a mainstay in chronic toxicology. An example is the reassessment of the $ED_{01}$ study (SOT, 1981) which radically changed interpretation of the results and understanding of underlying methods when adjustment for time on study was made.

The increased importance and interest in the analysis of survival data has not been restricted to toxicology, but rather has encompassed all the life sciences. Those with further interest should consult Lee (1980) or Elandt-Johnson and Johnson (1980), both general in their approach to the subject.


## 22.9. META-ANALYSIS

Meta-analysis (meaning "analysis among") is being used increasingly in biomedical research to try to obtain a qualitative or quantitative synthesis of the research literature on a particular issue. The technique is usually applied to the synthesis of several separate but comparable studies.


### 22.9.1. Selection of the Studies to Be Analyzed

The issue of study selection is perhaps the most troublesome issue for those doing meta-analysis. Several questions need to be addressed.

1. Should studies be limited to those which are published? It is well known that negative studies that report little or no benefit from following a particular course of action are less likely to be published than are positive studies. Therefore, the published literature may be biased toward studies with positive results, and a synthesis of these studies would give a biased estimate of the impact of pursuing

some courses of action. Unpublished studies, however, may be of lower quality than the published studies, and poor research methods often produce an underestimate of impact. Moreover, the unpublished studies may be difficult to discover.

2. Should studies be limited to those which appear in peer-reviewed publications? Peer review is considered the primary method for quality control in scientific publishing. Some investigators recommend that only those studies that are published in peer-reviewed publications be considered in meta-analysis. Although this may seem an attractive option, it might produce an even more highly biased selection of studies.

3. Should studies be limited those which meet additional quality-control criteria? If investigators impose an additional set of criteria before including a study in meta-analysis, this may further improve the average quality of the studies used, but it introduces still greater concerns about selection bias. Moreover, different investigators might use different criteria for a "valid" study and therefore select a different group of studies for meta-analysis.

4. Should studies be limited to randomized controlled studies? This is a variant of the above question concerning quality control. At one time, rigid quality standards were more likely to be met by randomized controlled studies than by observational studies. Increasingly, however, observational methods have been used to evaluate certain kinds of effects, particularly those that are uncommon. A larger issue may well be that of combining data from studies performed in different laboratories and, even more so, using different strains of a single animal species.

5. Should studies be limited to those using identical methods? For practical purposes, this would mean using only separately published studies from the same lab in a limited time frame, for which the methods were the same for all and the similarity of methods was monitored. This criterion is very difficult to achieve.

### 22.9.2. Pooled (Quantitative) Analysis

Usually, the main purpose of meta-analysis is quantitative. The goal is to develop better overall estimates of the degree of benefit achieved by specific exposure and dosing techniques, based on the combining (pooling) of estimates found in the existing studies of the interventions. This type of meta-analysis is sometimes called a pooled analysis (Gerbarg and Horwitz, 1988) because the analysts pool the observations of many studies and then calculate parameters such as risk ratios or odds ratios from the pooled data.

Because of the many decisions regarding inclusion or exclusion of studies, different meta-analyses might reach very different conclusions on the same topic. Even after the studies are chosen, there are many other methodologic issues in choosing how to combine means and variances (e.g., what weighting methods should be used). Pooled analysis should report both relative risks and risk reductions as well as absolute risks and risk reductions (Sinclair and Bracken, 1994).

### 22.9.3. Methodologic (Qualitative) Analysis

Sometimes the question to be answered is not how much toxicity is induced by the use of a particular exposure but whether there is any biologically significant toxicity at all. In this case, a qualitative meta-analysis may be done, in which the quality of the research is scored according to a list of objective criteria. The meta-analyst then examines the methodologically superior studies to determine whether or not the question of toxicity is answered consistently by them. This qualitative approach has been called methodologic analysis (Gerbarg and Horwitz, 1988) or quality scores analysis (Greenland, 1994). In some cases, the methodologically strongest studies agree with one another and disagree with the weaker studies, which may or may not be consistent with one another.

## 22.10. BAYSIAN INFERENCE

It is useful to know the sensitivity and specificity of a test. Once a researcher decides to use a certain test, two important questions require answers: If the test results are positive, what is the probability that the researcher has the condition of interest? If the test results are negative, what is the probability that the patient does not have the disease? Bayes' theorem provides a way to answer these questions.

Bayes' theorem, which was first described centuries ago by the English clergyman after whom it is named, is one of the most imposing statistical formulas in the biomedical sciences (Lindley, 1971). Put in symbols more meaningful for researchers such as pathologists, the formula is

$$P(D|T+) = \frac{p(T+|D+)p(D+)}{p(T+|D+)p(D+)] + [p(T+|D-)p(D-)]}$$

where $p$ denotes probability; $D+$ means that the animal has the effect in question; $D-$ means that the animal does not have the effect; $T+$ means that a certain diagnostic test for the effect is positive; $T-$ means that the test is negative; and the vertical line ($|$) means "conditional upon" what immediately follows.

Most researchers, even those who can deal with sensitivity, specificity, and predictive values, throw in the towel when it comes to Bayes' theorem. This is odd, because a close look at the equation reveals that Bayes' theorem is merely the formula for the positive predictive value (Box and Tiao, 1973).

The numerator of Bayes' theorem merely describes cell $a$ (the true-positive results). The probability of being in cell $a$ is equal to the prevalence times the sensitivity, where $p(D+)$ is the prevalence (the probability of being in the effected column) and where $p(T+|D+)$ is the sensitivity (the probability of being in the top row, *given the fact of being in the effected column*). The denominator of Bayes' theorem consists of two terms, the first of which once again describes cell $a$ (the true-positive results) and the second of which describes cell $b$ (the false-positive error rate, or $p(T+|D-)$, is multiplied by the prevalence of noneffected animals, or

$p(D-)$). The true-positive results ($a$) divided by the true-positive plus false-positive results ($a + b$) gives $a/(a + b)$, which is the positive predictive value.

In genetics, an even simpler-appearing formula for Bayes' theorem is sometimes used. The numerator is the same, but the denominator is merely $p(T+)$. This makes sense because the denominator in $a/(a + b)$ is equal to all of those who have positive test results, whether they are true-positive or false-positive results.

### 22.10.1. Bayes' Theorem and Evaluation of Safety Assessment Studies

In a population with a low prevalence of a particular toxicity, most of the positive results in a screening program for that lesion or effect would be falsely positive. Although this does not automatically invalidate a study or assessment program, it raises some concerns about cost-effectiveness, and these can be explored using Bayes' theorem (Racine et al., 1986)

A program employing a immunochemical stain based test to screen tissues for a specific effect will be discussed as an example. This test uses small amounts of antibody tissues for a specific effect, and the presence of an immunologically bound stain is considered a positive result. If the sensitivity and specificity of the test and the prevalence of biochemical effect are known, Bayes' theorem can be used to predict what proportion of the tissues with positive test results will have true-positive results (actually be effected).

Example 22.3 shows how the calculations are made. If the test has a sensitivity of 96% and if the true prevalence is 1%, only 13.9% of tissues with a positive test result are predicted actually to be effected.

**EXAMPLE 22.3. Use of Bayes' Theorem or a 2×2 Table to Determine the Positive Predictive Value of a Hypothetical Tuberculin Screening Program**

---

Part 1. Beginning Data

Sensitivity of immunological stain $= 96\% = 0.96$
False-negative error rate of the test $= 4\% = 0.04$
Specificity of the test $= 94\% = 0.94$
False-positive error rate of the test $= 6\% = 0.06$
Prevalence of effect in the tissues $= 1\% = 0.01$

---

Part 2. Use of Bayes' Theorem

$$p(D) + |T+ = \frac{p(T + |D + p(D+)}{[p(T + |D+)p(D+) + [PT + |D-)p(D-)]}$$

$$= \frac{(\text{Sensitivity})(\text{Prevalence})}{[(\text{Sensitivity})(\text{Prevalence}) + (\text{False} - \text{positive error rate})(1 - \text{Prevalence})]}$$

$$= \frac{(0.96)(0.01)}{[(0.96)(0.01)] + [(0.06)(0.99)]} = \frac{0.0096}{0.0096 + 0.0594}$$

$$= \frac{0.0096}{0.0690} = 0.139 - \mathbf{13.9\%}$$

Part 3. Use of a $2 \times 2$ Table, with Numbers Based on the Assumption That 10,000 Tissues are in the Study

| | | True Disease Status | | | | | |
|---|---|---|---|---|---|---|---|
| | | Effected | | Not Effected | | Total | |
| | | Number | (Percentage) | Number | (Percentage) | Number | (Percentage) |
| Test | Positive | 96 | (96) | 594 | (6) | 690 | (7) |
| Result | Negative | 4 | (4) | 9,306 | (94) | 9,310 | (93) |
| | Total | 100 | (100) | 9,900 | (100) | 10,000 | (100) |

Positive predictive value $= 96/690 = 0.139 = \mathbf{13.9\%}$

Pathologists and toxicologists can quickly develop a table that lists different levels of test sensitivity, test specificity, and effect prevalence and shows how these levels affect the proportion of positive results that are likely to be true-positive results. Although this calculation is fairly straightforward and is extremely useful, it has seldom been used in the early stages of planning for large studies or safety assessment programs.

### 22.10.2. Bayes' Theorem and Individual Animal Evaluation

Suppose a pathologist is uncertain about an animal's cause of death and obtains a positive test result for a certain pathology. Even if the pathologist knows the sensitivity and specificity of the test, that does not solve the problem, because to calculate the positive predictive value, it is necessary to know the prevalence of the particular tissue or effect that the test is designed to detect. The prevalence is thought of as the expected prevalence in the population from which the animal comes. The actual prevalence is usually not known, but often a reasonable estimate can be made.

Say, for example, a pathologist evaluates a male primate that was observed to have easy fatigability and has signs of kidney stones but has no other symptoms or signs of parathyroid disease on physical examination. The pathologist considers the probability of hyperparathyroidism and decides that it is now, perhaps 2% (reflecting that in 100 such primates, probably only 2 of them would have the disease). This probability is called the prior probability, reflecting the fact that it is estimated prior to the performance of laboratory tests and is based on the estimated prevalence of a particular pathology among primates with similar signs and symptoms. Although the pathologist believes that the probability of hyperparathyroidism is low, he considers the results of the serum calcium test to "rule out" the diagnosis. Somewhat to his surprise, the results of the test were positive, with an elevated level of 12.2 mg/dL. She could order more special tests or stains for parathyroid disease, but some tests results might come back positive and some negative.

Under the circumstances, Bayes' theorem could be used to make a second estimate of probability, which is called the posterior probability, reflecting the fact that it is made after the test results are known. Calculation of the posterior probability is based on the sensitivity and specificity of the test that was performed, which in this case was the serum calcium test, and on the prior probability, which in this case was 2%. If the serum calcium test had a 90% sensitivity and a 95% specificity, that means it had a false-positve error rate of 5% (specificity plus the false-positive error rate equals 100%). When this information is used in the Bayes' equation, as shown in Example 22.3, the result is a posterior probability of 27%. This means that the patient is now in a group of primates with a significant possibility of parathyroid disease. In Example 22.4, note that the result is the same (i.e., 27%) when a 2×2 table is used. This is true because, as discussed above, the probability based on the Bayes' theorem is identical to the positive predictive value.

**EXAMPLE 22.4. Use of Bayes' Theorem or a 2×2 Table to Determine the Posterior Probability and the Positive Predictive Value**

---

Part 1. Beginnning Data

Sensitivity of the first test $= 90\% = 0.90$
Specificity of the first test $= 95\% = 0.95$
Prior probability of disease $= 2\% = 0.02$

---

Part 2. Use of Bayes' theorem

$$p(D+|T+) = \frac{p(T+|D+)p(D+)}{[p(T+|D+)p(D+)] + [p(T+|D-)p(D-]}$$

$$= \frac{(0.90)(0.02)}{[(0.90)(0.02) + (0.05)(0.98)]}$$

$$= \frac{0.018}{0.018 + 0.049} = \frac{0.018}{0.067} = 0.269 = 27\%$$

---

Part 3. Use of a 2×2 Table

True Disease Status

|  |  | Diseased |  | Nondiseased |  | Total |  |
|---|---|---|---|---|---|---|---|
|  |  | Number | (Percentage) | Number | (Percentage) | Number | (Percentage) |
| Test | Positive | 18 | (90) | 49 | (5) | 67 | (6.7) |
| Result | Negative | 2 | (10) | 931 | (95) | 933 | (93.3) |
|  | Total | 20 | (100) | 980 | (100) | 1000 | (100.0) |

Positive predictive value $= 18/67 = 0.269 = $ **27%**

---

In light of the 27% posterior probability, the pathologist decides to order a parathyroid hormone radioimmunoassay, even though this test is expensive. If the radioimmunoassay had a sensitivity of 95% and a specificity of 98% and the results turned out to be positive, the Bayes' theorem could again be used to calculate the probability of parathyroid disease. This time, however, the posterior probability for the first test (27%) would be used as the prior probability for the second test. The result of the calculation, as shown in Example 22.5, is a new probability of 94%. Thus, the primate in all probability did have hyperparathyroidism.

**EXAMPLE 22.5. Use of Bayes' Theorem or a 2×2 Table to Determine the Second Posterior Probability and the Second Positive Predictive Value**

Part 1. Beginnning Data

Sensitivity of the first test $= 95\% = 0.95$
Specificity of the first test $= 98\% = 0.98$
Prior probability of disease $= 27\% = 0.27$

Part 2. Use of Bayes' theorem

$$p(D+|T+) = \frac{p(T+|D+)p(D+)}{[p(T+|D+)p(D+)] + [p(T+|D-)p(D-)]}$$

$$= \frac{(0.95)(0.27)}{[(0.95)(0.27) + (0.02)(0.73)]}$$

$$= \frac{0.257}{0.257 + 0.0146} = \frac{0.257}{0.272} = 0.9449^{a} = 94\%$$

Part 3. Use of a 2×2 Table

True Disease Status

|  |  | Diseased | | Nondiseased | | Total | |
|---|---|---|---|---|---|---|---|
|  |  | Number | (Percentage) | Number | (Percentage) | Number | (Percentage) |
| Test | Positive | 256 | (95) | 15 | (2) | 271 | (27.1) |
| Result | Negative | 13 | (5) | 716 | (98) | 729 | (72.9) |
| | Total | 269 | (100) | 731 | (100) | 1000 | (100.0) |

Positive predictive value $= 256/271 = 0.9446^{a} = $ **94%**
[a]The slight difference in the results for the two approaches is due to rounding errors. It is not important biologically.

Why did the posterior probability increase so much the second time? One reason was that the prior probability was considerably higher in the second calculation than in the first (27% versus 2%), based on the fact that the first test yielded positive results. Another reason was that the specificity of the second test was quite high (98%), which markedly reduced the false-positive error rate and therefore increased the positive predictive value.

## 22.11. DATA ANALYSIS APPLICATIONS IN SAFETY ASSESSMENT STUDIES

Basic principles have been reviewed and a set of methods provided for statistical handling of data, the remainder of this chapter will address the practical aspects and difficulties encountered in working in safety assessment.

There are now common practices in the analysis of safety data, though they are not necessarily the best. These are discussed in the remainder of this chapter, which seeks to review statistical methods on a use-by-use basis and to provide a foundation for the selection of alternatives in specific situations. Some of the newer available methodologies (meta-analysis and Bayesian approaches) should be kept in mind, however.

### 22.11.1. Body and Organ Weights

Among the sets of data commonly collected in studies where animals are dosed with (or exposed to) a chemical are body weight and the weights of selected organs. In fact, body weight is frequently the most sensitive indication of an adverse effect. How to best analyze this and in what form to analyze the organ weight data (as absolute weights, weight changes, or percentages of body weight) have been the subject of a number of articles (Jackson, 1962; Weil, 1962; Weil and Gad, 1980).

Both absolute body weights and rates of body weight change (calculated as changes from a baseline measurement value which is traditionally the animal's weight immediately prior to the first dosing with or exposure to test material) are almost universally best analyzed by ANOVA followed, if called for, by a *post hoc* test. Even if the groups were randomized properly at the beginning of a study (no group being significantly different in mean body weight from any other group, and all animals in all groups within two standard deviations of the overall mean body weight), there is an advantage to performing the computationally slightly more cumbersome (compared to absolute body weights) changes in body weight analysis. The advantage is an increase in sensitivity, because the adjustment of starting points (the setting of initial weights as a "zero" value) acts to reduce the amount of initial variability. In this case, Bartlett's test is performed first to ensure homogeneity of variance and the appropriate sequence of analysis follows.

With smaller sample sizes, the normality of the data becomes increasingly uncertain and nonparametric methods such as Kruskal–Wallis may be more appropriate (Zar, 1974).

The analysis of relative (to body weight) organ weights is a valuable tool for identifying possible target organs (Lee and Lovell, 1999; Bickis, 1990). How to perform this analysis is still a matter of some disagreement, however. Weil (1962) presented evidence that organ weight data expressed as percentages of body weight should be analyzed separately for each sex. Furthermore, since the conclusions from organ weight data of males differed so often from those of females, data from animals of each sex should be used in this measurement. Others (Grubbs, 1969; Weil, 1973; Bayd and Knight, 1963; Boyd, 1972) have discussed in detail other factors which influence organ weights and must be taken into account.

The two competing approaches to analyzing relative organ weights call for either (1) calculating organ weights as a percentage of total body weight (at the time of necropsy) and analyzing the results by ANOVA, or (2) analyzing results by ANCOVA, with body weights as the covariates as discussed previously by the author (Weil and Gad, 1980).

A number of considerations should be kept in mind when these questions are addressed. First, one must keep a firm grasp on the difference between biological significance and statistical significance. In this particular case, we are especially interested in examining organ weights when an organ weight change is not proportional to changes in whole body weights. Second, we are now required to detect smaller and small changes while still retaining a similar sensitivity (i.e., the $p < 0.05$ level).

There are several devices to attain the desired increase in power. One is to use larger and larger sample sizes (number of animals) and the other is to utilize the most powerful test we can. However, the use of even the currently employed numbers of animals is being vigorously questioned and the power of statistical tests must, therefore, now assume an increased importance in our considerations.

The biological rationale behind analyzing both absolute body weight and the organ weight to body weight ratio (this latter as opposed to a covariance analysis of organ weights) is that in the majority of cases, except for the brain, the organs of interest in the body change weight (except in extreme cases of obesity or starvation) in proportion to total body weight. We are particularly interested in detecting cases where this is not so. Analysis of actual data from several hundred studies (unpublished data) has shown no significant difference in rates of weight change of target organs (other than the brain) compared to total body weight for healthy animals in those species commonly used for repeated dose studies (rats, mice, rabbits, and dogs). Furthermore, it should be noted that analysis of covariance is of questionable validity in analyzing body weight and related organ weight changes, since a primary assumption is the independence of treatment, that the relationship of the two variables is the same for all treatments (Ridgemen, 1975). Plainly, in toxicology this is not true.

In cases where the differences between the error mean squares are much greater, the ratio of $F$ ratios will diverge in precision from the result of the efficiency of covariance adjustment. These cases are where either sample sizes are much larger or where the differences between means themselves are much larger. This latter case is one which does not occur in the designs under discussion in any manner that would leave analysis of covariance as a valid approach, because group means start out being very similar and cannot diverge markedly unless there is a treatment effect. As we have discussed earlier, a treatment effect invalidates a prime underpinning assumption of analysis of covariance.

## 22.11.2. Clinical Chemistry

A number of clinical chemistry parameters are commonly determined on the blood and urine collected from animals in chronic, subchronic, and occasionally, acute toxicity studies. In the past (and still, in some places), the accepted practice has been to evaluate these data using univariate–parametric methods (primarily $t$-tests and/or ANOVA). However, this can be shown to be not the best approach on a number of grounds.

First, such biochemical parameters are rarely independent of each other. Neither is our interest often focused on just one of the parameters. Rather, there are batteries of the parameters associated with toxic actions at particular target organs. For example, increases in creatinine phosphokinase (CPK), $\gamma$-hydroxybutyrate dehydrogenase ($\gamma$-HBDH), and lactate dehydrogenase (LDH), occurring together, are strongly indicative of myocardial damage. In such cases, we are not just interested in a significant increase in one of these, but in all three. Detailed coverage of the interpretation of such clinical laboratory tests can be found in other references (Gad and Chengelis, 1992; Loeb and Quimby, 1999; Harris, 1978; and Martin et al., 1975) or elsewhere in this text.

Similarly, the serum electrolytes (sodium, potassium, and calcium) interact with each other; a decrease in one is frequently tied, for instance, to an increase in one of the others. Furthermore, the nature of the data (in the case of some parameters), either because of the biological nature of the parameter or the way in which it is measured, is frequently either not normally distributed (particularly because of being markedly skewed) or not continuous in nature. This can be seen in some of the reference data for experimental animals in Mitruka and Rawnsley (1957) or Weil (1982) in, for example, creatinine, sodium, potassium, chloride, calcium and blood.

### 22.11.3. Hematology

Much of what we said about clinical chemistry parameters is also true for the hematologic measurements made in toxicology studies. Which test to perform should be evaluated by use of a decision tree until one becomes confident as to the most appropriate methods. Keep in mind that sets of values and (in some cases) population distribution vary not only between species, but also between the commonly used strains of species and that "control" or "standard" values will "drift" over the course of only a few years.

Again, the majority of these parameters are interrelated and highly dependent on the method used to determine them. Red blood cell count (RBC), platelet counts, and mean corpuscular volume (MCV) may be determined using a device such as a Coulter counter to take direct measurements, and the resulting data are usually stable for parametric methods. The hematocrit, however, may actually be a value calculated from the RBC and MCV values and, if so, is dependent on them. If the hematocrit is measured directly, instead of being calculated from the RBC and MCV, it may be compared by parametric methods.

Hemoglobin is directly measured and is an independent and continuous variable However, and probably because at any one time a number of forms and conformations (oxyhemoglobin, deoxyhemoglobin, methemoglobin, etc.) of hemoglobin are actually present the distribution seen is not typically a normal one, but rather may be a multimodal one. Here a nonparametric technique such as the Wilcoxon or multiple rank-sum is called for.

Consideration of the white blood cell (WBC) and differential counts leads to another problem. The total WBC is, typically, a normal population amenable to parametric analysis, but differential counts are normally determined by counting, manually, one or more sets of one hundred cells each. The resulting relative percentages of neutrophils are then reported as either percentages or are multiplied by the total WBC count with the resulting "count" being reported as the "absolute" differential WBC. Such data, particularly in the case of eosinophils (where the distribution does not approach normality), should usually be analyzed by nonparametric methods. It is widely believed that "relative" (%) differential data should not be reported because they are likely to be misleading.

Last, it should always be kept in mind that it is rare for a change in any single hematologic parameter to be meaningful. Rather, because these parameters are so interrelated, patterns of changes in parameters should be expected if a real effect is present, and analysis and interpretation of results should focus on such patterns of changes. Classification analysis techniques often provide the basis for a useful approach to such problems.

### 22.11.4. Histopathologic Lesion Incidence

The last twenty years have seen increasing emphasis placed on histopathological examination of tissues collected from animals in subchronic and chronic toxicity studies. While it is not true that only those lesions which occur at a statistically significantly increased rate in treated or exposed animals are of concern (for there are the cases where a lesion may be of such a rare type that the occurrence of only one or a few such in treated animals "raises a flag"), it is true that, in most cases, a statistical evaluation is the only way to determine if what we see in treated animals is significantly worse than what has been seen in control animals. Although cancer is not our only concern, this category of lesions is that of greatest interest.

Typically, comparison of incidences of any one type of lesion between controls and treated animals are made using the multiple $2 \times 2$ chi square test or Fisher's exact test with a modification of the numbers of animals as the denominators. Too often, experimenters exclude from consideration all those animals (in both groups) that died prior to the first animals being found with a lesion at that site.

An option which should be kept in mind is that, frequently, a pathologist can not only identify a lesion as present, but also grade those present as to severity. This represents a significant increase in the information content of the data which should not be given up by performing an analysis based only on the perceived quantal nature (present–absent) of the data. Quantal data, analyzed by chi-square or Fisher's exact tests, are a subset (the $2 \times 2$ case) of categorical or contingency table data. In this case it also becomes ranked (or "ordinal") data: the categories are naturally ordered (for example, no effect < mild lesion < moderate lesion < severe lesion). This gives a $2 \times R$ table if there are only one treatment and one control group, or an $N \times R$ ("multiway") table if there are three or more groups of animals.

The traditional method of analyzing multiple, cross-classified data has been to collapse the $N \times R$ contingency table over all but two of the variables, and to follow this with the computation of some measure of association between these variables. For an $N$-dimensional table this results in $N$ $(N - 1)/2$ separate analyses. The result is crude, "giving away" information and even (by inappropriate pooling of data) yielding a faulty understanding of the meaning of data. Though computationally more laborious, a multiway (N×R table) analysis should be utilized.

### 22.11.5. Carcinogenesis

In the experimental evaluation of substances for carcinogenesis based on experimental results in a nonhuman species at some relatively high dose or exposure level, an attempt is made to predict the occurrence and level of tumorogenesis in humans at much lower levels. An entire chapter could be devoted to examining the assumptions involved in this undertaking and a review of the aspects of design and interpretation of animal carcinogenicity studies. Such is beyond the scope of this effort. The reader is referred to Gad (1998) for such an examination.

The single most important statistical consideration in the design of carcinogenicity bioassays in the past was based on the point of view that what was being observed and evaluated was a simple quantal response (cancer occurred or it did not), and that a sufficient number of animals needed to be used to have reasonable expectations of detecting such an effect. Though the single fact of whether or not the simple incidence of neoplastic tumors is increased due to an agent of concern is of interest, a much more complex model must now be considered. The time-to-tumor, patterns of tumor incidence, effects on survival rate, and age at first tumor all must now to included in a model.

The rationale behind this assumption is that though humans may be exposed at very low levels, detecting the resulting small increase (over background) in the incidence of tumors would require the use of an impractically large number of test animals per group. This point was illustrated by Table 22.1, where, for instance, while only forty-six animals (per group) are needed to show a 10% increase over a zero background (that is, a rarely occurring tumor type), 770,000 animals (per group) would be needed to detect a tenth of a percent increase above a five percent background. As we increase the dose, however, the incidence of tumors (the response) will also increase until it reaches the point where a modest increase (say 10% over a reasonably small background level (say 1%) could be detected using an acceptably small-sized group of test animals (in Table 22.8 we see that 51 animals would be needed for this example case). There are, however, at least two real limitations to the highest dose level. First, the test rodent population must have a sufficient survival rate after receiving a lifetime (or two years) of regular doses to allow for meaningful statistical analysis. Second, we really want the metabolism and mechanism of action of the chemical at the highest level tested to be the same as at the low levels where human exposure would occur. Unfortunately, toxicologists usually must select the high dose level based only on the information provided by a subchronic or range-finding study (usually 90 days in length), but selection of either too low or too high a dose will make the study invalid for detection of carcinogenicity, and may seriously impair the use of the results for risk assessment.

**TABLE 22.8. Average Number of Animals Needed to Detect a Significant Increase in the Incidence of an Event (tumors, anomalies, etc.) over the Background Incidence (control) at Several Expected Incidence Levels Using the Fisher Exact Probability Test ($p = 0.05$)**

| Background Incidence, % | Expected Increase in Incidence, % | | | | | |
|---|---|---|---|---|---|---|
| | 0.01 | 0.1 | 1 | 3 | 5 | 10 |
| 0 | 46,000,000[a] | 460,000 | 4,600 | 511 | 164 | 46 |
| 0.01 | 46,000,000 | 460,000 | 4,600 | 511 | 164 | 46 |
| 0.1 | 47,000,000 | 470,000 | 4,700 | 520 | 168 | 47 |
| 1 | 51,000,000 | 510,000 | 5,100 | 570 | 204 | 51 |
| 5 | 77,000,000 | 770,000 | 7,700 | 856 | 304 | 77 |
| 10 | 100,000,000 | 1,000,000 | 10,000 | 1,100 | 400 | 100 |
| 20 | 148,000,000 | 1,480,000 | 14,800 | 1,644 | 592 | 148 |
| 25 | 160,000,000 | 1,600,000 | 16,000 | 1,840 | 664 | 166 |

[a]Number of animals needed in each group—controls as well as treated.

There are several solutions to this problem. One of these has been the rather simplistic approach of the NTP Bioassay Program, which is to conduct a three-month range-finding study with sufficient dose levels to establish a level which significantly (10%) decreases the rate of body weight gain. This dose is defined as the maximum tolerated dose (MTD) and is selected as the highest dose. Two other levels, generally one-half MTD and one-quarter MTD, are selected for testing as the intermediate and low-dose levels. In many earlier NCI studies, only one other level was used.

The dose range-finding study is necessary in most cases, but the suppression of body weight gain is a scientifically questionable bench mark when dealing with establishment of safety factors. Physiologic, pharmacologic or metabolic markers generally serve as better indicators of systemic response than body weight. A series of well-defined acute and subchronic studies designed to determine the "chronicity factor" and to study onset of pathology can be more predictive for dose setting than body weight suppression.

Also, the NTPs MTD may well be at a level where the metabolic mechanisms for handling a compound at real-life exposure levels have been saturated or overwhelmed, bringing into play entirely artifactual metabolic and physiologic mechanisms (Gehring and Blau, 1977). The regulatory response to questioning the appropriateness of the MTD as a high dose level (Haseman, 1985) has been to acknowledge that occasionally an excessively high dose is selected, but to counter by saying that using lower doses would seriously decrease the sensitivity of detection.

## REFERENCES

Abramowitz, M. and Stegun, I.A. (1964). *Handbook of Mathematical Functions*. National Bureau of Standards, Washington, D.C., pp. 925–964.

Anderson, E. (1960). A semigraphical method for the analysis of complex problems. *Technomet.* 2: 387–391.

Anderson, S., Auquier, A., Hauck, W.W., Oakes, D., Vandaele, W. and Weisburg, H.I. (1980). *Statistical Methods for Comparative Studies*. Wiley, New York.

Anderson, T.W. (1971). *The Statistical Analysis of Time Series*. Wiley, New York.

Anscombe, F.J. (1973). Graphics in statistical analysis. *Am. Stat.* 27: 17–21.

Antonello, J.M., Clark, R.L. and Heyse, J.F. (1993). Application of Tahey Trend Test procedures to assess developmental and reproductive toxicity. I. Measurement data. *Fundam. Appl. Toxicol.* 21: 52–58.

Armitage, P. (1955). Tests for linear trends in proportions and frequencies. *Biometrics.* 11: 375–386.

Beyer, W.H. (1976). *Handbook of Tables for Probability and Statistics*. CRC Press, Boca Raton, FL.

Bickis, M.G. (1990). Experimental design. In: *Handbook of in Vivo Toxicity Testing* (Arnold, D.L., Grice, H.C. and Krewski, D.R., Eds.) Academic Press, San Diego, CA. pp. 113–166.

Bliss, C.I. (1935). The calculation of the dosage-mortality curve. *Ann. Appl. Biol.* 22: 134–167.

Bloomfield, P. (1976). *Fourier Analysis of Time Series: An Introduction*. Wiley, New York.

Box, G.E.P. and Tiao, G.C. (1973). *Bayesian Inference in Statistical Analysis*. Addison-Wesley, Reading, MA.

Boyd, E.M. (1972). *Predictive Toxicometrics*. Williams and Wilkins, Baltimore.

Boyd, E.M. and Knight, L.M. (1963). Postmortem shifts in the weight and water levels of body organs. *Toxicol. Appl. Pharmacol.* 5: 119–128.

Breslow, N. (1984). Comparison of survival curves. In: *Cancer Clinical Trials: Methods and Practice* (Buse, M.F., Staguet, M.J. and Sylvester, R.F., Eds.) Oxford University Press, pp. 381–406.

Chambers, J.M., Cleveland, W.S., Kleiner, B. and Tukey, P.A. (1983). *Graphical Methods for Data Analysis*. Wadsworth, Belmont, CA.

Chernoff, H. (1973). The use of faces to represent points in K-dimensional space graphically. *J. Am. Stat Assoc.*, 68: 361–368.

Cleveland, W.S. (1985). *The Elements of Graphing Data*. Wadsworth, Monterey, CA.

Cleveland, W.S. and McGill, R. (1984). Graphical perception: Theory, experimentation, and application to the development of graphical methods. *J. Amer. Stat. Assoc.* 79: 531–554.

Cochran, W.F. (1954). Some models for strengthening the common $x^2$ tests. *Biometrics* 10: 417–451.

Cochran, W.G. and Cox, G.M. (1975). *Experimental Designs*. John Wiley, New York.

Conover, J.W. and Inman, R.L. (1981). Rank transformation as a bridge between parametric and nonparametric statistics. *Am. Statistician* 35: 124–129.

Cox, D.R. (1972). Regression models and life-tables. *J. Roy. Stat. Soc.* 34B: 187–220.

Cox, D.R. and Stuart, A. (1955). Some quick tests for trend in location and dispersion. *Biometrics* 42: 80–95.

Crowley, J. and Breslow, N. (1984). Statistical analysis of survival data. *Ann. Rev. Public Health* 5: 385–411.

Cutler, S.J. and Ederer, F. (1958). Maximum utilization of the life table method in analyzing survival. *J. Chron. Dis.* 8: 699–712.

Davison, M.L. (1983). *Multidimensional Scaling.* Wiley, New York.

Diamond, W.J. (1981). *Practical Experimental Designs.* Lifetime Learning, Belmont, CA.

Diem, K. and Lentner, C. (1975). *Documenta Geigy Scientific Tables.* Geigy, New York, pp. 158–159.

Draper, N.R. and Smith, H. (1981). *Applied Regression Analysis.* Wiley, New York.

Duncan, D.B. (1955). Multiple range and multiple *F* tests. *Biometrics* 11: 1–42.

Dunnett, C.W. (1955). A multiple comparison procedure for comparing several treatments with a control. *J. Am. Stat. Assoc.*, 50: 1096–1121.

Dunnett, C.W. (1964). New tables for multiple comparison with a control. Biometrics. 16: 671–685.

Dykstra, R.L. and Robertson, T. (1983). On Testing Monotone Tendencies. *J. Amer. Stat. Assoc.*, 78: 342–350.

Elandt-Johnson, R.C. and Johnson, N.L. (1980). *Survival Models and Data Analysis.* Wiley, New York.

Engelman, L. and Hartigan, J.A. (1969). Percentage points of a test for clusters. *J. Am. Stat. Assoc.* 64: 1647–1648.

Everitt, B. (1980). *Cluster Analysis.* Halsted Press, New York.

Everitt, B.S. and Hand, D.J. (1981). Finite mixture distributions. Chapman and Hall, New York.

*Federal Register* (1985). Vol. 50, No. 50. Washington, D.C.

Federer, W.T. (1955). *Experimental Design.* Macmillan, New York.

Feinstein, A.R. (1979). Scientific standards vs. statistical associations and biological logic in the analysis of causation. *Clin. Pharmacol. Ther.* 25: 481–492.

Finney, D.J., Latscha, R., Bennet, B.M. and Hsu, P. (1963). *Tables for Testing Significance in a $2\times2$ Contingency Table.* Cambridge University Press.

Finney, D.K. (1977). *Probit Analysis*, 3rd ed. Cambridge University Press.

Gad, S.C. (1984). Statistical analysis of behavioral toxicology data and studies. *Arch. Toxicol. Suppl.* 5: 256–266.

Gad, S.C. (1998). *Statistics and Experimental Design for Toxicologists*, 3rd ed. CRC Press, Boca Raton, FL.

Gad, S.C. and Chengelis, C.P. (1992). *Animal Models in Toxicology.* Marcel Dekker, New York.

Gad, S.C. and Taulbee, S.M. (1996). *Handbook of Data Recording, Maintenance and Management for the Biomedical Sciences.* CRC Press, Boca Raton, FL.

Gad, S.C., Reilly, C., Siino, K.M. and Gavigan, F.A. (1985). Thirteen cationic ionophores: Neurobehavioral and membrane effects. *Drug Chemical Toxicol.* 8: (6)451–468.

Gallant, A.R. (1975). Nonlinear regression. *Am. Stat.* 29: 73–81.

Garrett, H.E. (1947). *Statistics in Psychology and Education.* Longmans, Green, New York, pp. 215–218.

Gehring, P.J. and Blau, G.E. (1977). Mechanisms of Carcinogenicity: Dose Response. *J. Environ. Path. Toxicol.* 1:163–179.

Gerbarg, Z.B. and Horwitz, R.I. (1988). Resolving conflicting clinical trials: guidelines for meta-analysis. *J. Clin. Epidem.* 41: 503–509.

Ghent, A.W. (1972). A method for exact testing of $2\times2$, $2\times3$, $3\times3$ and other contingency tables, employing binomiate coefficients. *Am. Midland Naturalist.* 88: 15–27.

Glass, L. (1975). Classification of biological networks by their qualitative dynamics. *J. Theor. Biol.* 54: 85–107.

Gold, H.J. (1977). *Mathematical Modeling of Biological System—An Introductory Guidebook.* Wiley, New York.

Gordon, A.D. (1981). *Classification.* Chapman and Hall, New York.

Greenland, S. (1994). Invited commentary: a critical look at some popular meta-analytic methods. *Am. J. Epidem.* 140: 290–296.

Grubbs, F.E. (1969). Procedure for detecting outlying observations in samples. *Technometrics* 11: 1–21.

Hammond, E.C., Garfinkel, L. and Lew, E.A. (1978). Longevity, selective mortality, and competitive risks in relation to chemical carcinogenesis. *Environ. Res.* 16. 153–173.

Harris, E.K. (1978). Review of statistical methods of analysis of series of biochemical test results. *Ann. Biol. Clin.* 36: 194–197.

Harris, R.J. (1975). *A Primer of Multivariate Statistics.* Academic Press, New York, pp. 96–101.

Harter, A.L. (1960). Critical values for Duncan's new multiple range test. *Biometrics* 16: 671–685.

Hartigan, J.A. (1983). Classification. In: *Encyclopedia of Statistical Sciences*, Vol. 2. (Katz, S. and Johnson, N.L., Eds.).

Haseman, J.K. (1977). Response to use of statistics when examining life time studies in rodents to detect carcinogenicity. *J. Toxicol. Environ. Health.* 3: 633–636.

Haseman, J.K. (1985). Issues in carcinogenicity testing: Dose selection. *Fundam. Appl. Toxicol.* 5: 66–78.

Hicks, C.R. (1982). *Fundamental Concepts in the Design of Experiments.* Holt, Rinehart, and Winston, New York.

Hoaglin, D.C., Mosteller, F. and Tukey, J.W. (1983). *Understanding Robust and Explanatory Data Analysis.* Wiley, New York.

Hollander, M. and Wolfe, D.A. (1973). *Nonparametric Statistical Methods.* Wiley, New York, pp. 124–129.

Jackson, B. (1962). Statistical analysis of body weight data. *Toxicol. Appl. Pharmacol.* 4: 432–443.

Kotz, S. and Johnson, N.L. (1982). *Encyclopedia of Statistical Sciences*, Vol. 1. Wiley, New York, pp. 61–69.

Kowalski, B.R. and Bender, C.F. (1972). Pattern recognition, a powerful approach to interpreting chemical data. *J. Amer. Chem. Soc.* 94: 5632–5639.

Kraemer, H.C. and Thiemann, G. (1987). *How Many Subjects? Statistical Power Analysis in Research.* Sage Publications, Newbury Park, CA.

Lee, E.T. (1980). *Statistical Methods for Survival Data Analysis.* Lifetime Learning, Belmont, CA.

Lee, P.N. and Lovell, D. (1999). Statistics for Toxicology. In: *General and Applied Toxicology*, 2nd ed., (Ballantyne, B., Marrs, T. and Syversen, T., Eds.), Grove's Dictionaries, New York, pp. 291–302.

Lindley, S.V. (1971). *Bayesian Statistics: A Review.* SIAM, Philadelphia.

Litchfield, J.T. and Wilcoxon, F. (1949). A simplified method of evaluating dose effect experiments. *J. Pharmacol. Exp. Ther.* 96: 99–113.

Loeb, W.F. and Quimby, F.W. (1999). *The Clinical Chemistry of Laboratory Animals*, 2nd ed. Taylor and Francis, Philadelphia, PA.

Marriott, F.H.C. (1991). *The Dictionary of Statistical Terms*. Longman Scientific and Technical, Essex, England.

Martin, H.F., Gudzinowicz, B.J. and Fanger, H. (1975). *Normal Values in Clinical Chemistry*. Marcel Dekker, New York.

Mendell, N.R., Finch, S.J. and Thode, H.C., Jr. (1993). Where is the likelihood ratio test powerful for detecting two component normal mixtures? *Biometrics* 49: 907–915.

Mitruka, B.M. and Rawnsley, H.M. (1977). *Clinical Biochemical and Hematological Reference Values in Normal Animals*. Masson, New York.

Montgomery, D.C. and Smith, E.A. (1983). *Introduction to Linear Regression Analysis*. Wiley, New York.

Myers, J.L. (1972). *Fundamentals of Experimental Designs*. Allyn and Bacon, Boston.

Peto, R. and Pike, M.C. (1973). Conservatism of Approximation; $(0 - E)^2/E$ in the Log Rank Test for survival data on tumour incidence data. *Biometrics* 29: 579–584.

Peto, R., Pike, M.C., Armitage, P., Breslow, N.E., Cox. D.R., Howard, S.V., Kantel, N., McPherson, K., Peto, J. and Smith, P.G. (1977). Design and analysis of randomized clinical trials requiring prolonged observations of each patient, II. Analyses and examples. *Br. J. Cancer* 35: 1–39.

Peto, R., Pike, M., Day, N., Gray, R., Lee, P., Parish, S., Peto, J., Richards, S. and Wahrendorf, J. (1980). Guidelines for simple, sensitive significance tests for carcinogenic effects in long-term animal experiments. *IARC Monographs on the Evaluation of the Carcinogenic Risk of Chemicals to Humans, Supplement 2, Long-Term and Short-Term Screening Assays for Carcinogens: A Critical Appraisal.* International Agency for Research in Cancer, Lyon. pp. 311–346.

Pollard, J.H. (1977). *Numerical and Statistical Techniques*. Cambridge University Press, New York.

Portier, C. and Hoel, D. (1984). Type I error of trend tests in proportions and the design of cancer screens. *Comm. Stat. Theory Meth.* A13: 1–14.

Prentice, R.L. (1976). A generalization of the probit and logit methods for dose response curves. *Biometrics* 32: 761–768.

Racine, A., Grieve, A.P. and Fluhler, H. (1986). Bayesian methods in practice: Experiences in the pharmaceutical industry. *Applied Stat.* 35: 93–150.

Ridgemen, W.J. (1975). *Experimentation in Biology*. Wiley, New York, pp. 214–215.

Romesburg, H.C. (1984). *Cluster Analysis for Researchers*. Lifetime Learning, Belmont, CA, 43: 45–58.

Salsburg, D. (1980). The effects of life-time feeding studies on patterns of senile lesions in mice and rats. *Drug Chem. Tox.* 3: 1–33.

Schaper, M., Thompson, R.D. and Alarie, Y. (1985). A method to classify airborne chemicals which alter the normal ventilatory response induced by $CO_2$. *Toxicol Appl Pharmacol.* 79: 332–341.

Scheffe, H. (1959). *The Analysis of Variance*. Wiley, New York.

Schmid, C.F. (1983). *Statistical Graphics*. Wiley, New York.

Siegel, S. (1956). *Nonparametric Statistics for the Behavioral Sciences*. McGraw-Hill, New York.

Sinclair, J.C. and Bracken, M.B. (1994). Clinically useful measures of effect in binary analyses of randomized trials. *J. Clin. Epidem.* 47: 881–889.

Snedecor, G.W. and Cochran, W.G. (1980). *Statistical Methods*, 7th ed. Iowa State University Press, Ames, IA.

Sokal, R.R. and Rohlf, F.J. (1994). *Biometry*, 3rd ed. W.II. Freeman, San Francisco.

SOT $ED_{01}$ Task Force (1981). Reexamination of the $ED_{01}$ study-adjusting for time on study. *Fundam. Appl. Toxicol.* 1: 8–123.

Tarone, R.E. (1975). Tests for trend in life table analysis. *Biometrika* 62: 679–682.

Tufte, E.R. (1983). *The Visual Display of Quantitative Information.* Graphics Press, Cheshire, CT.

Tufte, E.R. (1990). *Envisioning Information.* Graphics Press, Cheshire, CT.

Tufte, E.R. (1997). *Visual Explanations.* Graphics Press, Cheshire, CT.

Tukey, J.W. (1977). *Exploratory Data Analysis.* Addison-Wesley, Reading, MA.

Tukey, J.W., Ciminera, J.L. and Heyes, J.F. (1985). Testing the statistical certainty of a response to increasing doses of a drug. *Biometrics* 41: 295–301.

Velleman, P.F. and Hoaglin, D.C. (1981). *Applications, Basics and Computing of Exploratory Data Analysis.* Duxbury Press, Boston.

Weil, C.S. (1962). Applications of methods of statistical analysis to efficient repeated-dose toxicological tests. I. General considerations and problems involved. Sex differences in rat liver and kidney weights. *Toxicol. Appl. Pharmacol.* 4: 561–571.

Weil, C.S. (1973). Experimental design and interpretation of data from prolonged toxicity studies. In *Proc. Fifth Int. Congr. Pharmacol.* Vol. 2. Beacon Press, San Francisco, pp. 4–12.

Weil, C.S. (1982). Statistical analysis and normality of selected hematologic and clinical chemistry measurements used in toxicologic studies. *Arch. Toxicol.* Suppl. 5: 237–253.

Weil, C.S. and Gad, S.C. (1980). Applications of methods of statistical analysis to efficient repeated-dose toxicologic tests. 2. Methods for analysis of body, liver and kidney weight data. *Toxicol. Appl. Pharmacol.* 52: 214–226.

Williams, D.A. (1971). A test for differences between treatment means when several dose levels are compared with a zero dose control. *Biomet.* 27: 103–117.

Williams, D.A. (1972). The comparison of several dose levels with a zero dose control. *Biomet.* 28: 519–531.

Wilson, J.S. and Holland, L.M. (1982). The effect of application frequency on epidermal carcinogenesis assays. *Toxicology* 24: 45–53.

Young, F.W. (1985). Multidimensional scaling. In: Katz, S. and Johnson, N.L., Eds. *Encyclopedia of Statistical Sciences*, Vol. 5. Wiley, New York, pp. 649–659.

Zar, J.H. (1974). *Biostatistical Analysis.* Prentice-Hall, Englewood Cliffs, NJ, p. 50.

# APPENDIX A

# SELECTED REGULATORY AND TOXICOLOGICAL ACRONYMS

| | |
|---|---|
| 510(k) | Premarket notification for change in a device |
| AALAS | American Association of Laboratory Animal Science |
| AAMI | Association for the Advancement of Medical Instrumentation |
| ABT | American Board of Toxicology |
| ACGIH | American Conference of Governmental Industrial Hygienists |
| ACT | American College of Toxicology |
| ADE | Adverse Drug Event (of drug substances) |
| ADI | Allowable Daily Intake |
| AIDS | Acquired Immune Deficiency Syndrome |
| AIMD | Active Implantable Medical Device |
| ANSI | American National Standards Institute |
| APHIS | Animal and Plant Health Inspection Service |
| ASTM | American Society for Testing and Materials |
| CAS | Chemical Abstract Service |
| CBER | Center for Biologic Evaluation and Research (FDA) |
| CDER | Center for Drug Evaluation and Research (FDA) |
| CDRH | Center for Devices and Radiological Health (FDA) |
| CFAN | Center for Food and Nutrition (FDA) |
| CFR | *Code of Federal Regulations* |
| CIIT | Chemical Industries Institute of Toxicology |
| CPMP | Committee on Proprietary Medicinal Products (U.K.) |
| CSE | Control Standard Endotoxin |
| CSM | Committee on Safety of Medicines (U.K.) |

| | |
|---|---|
| CTC | Clinical Trial Certificate (U.K.) |
| CTX | Clinical Trial Certificate Exemption (U.K.) |
| CVM | Center for Veterinary Medicine (FDA) |
| DART | Development and Reproduction Toxicology |
| DHHS | Department of Health and Human Services |
| DIA | Drug Information Associates |
| DMF | Drug (or Device) Master File |
| DSHEA | Dietrary Supplement Health and Education Act |
| EEC | European Economic Community |
| EFPIA | European Federation of Pharmaceutical Industries Association |
| EM | Electron Microscopy |
| EPA | Environmental Protection Agency |
| EU | European Union |
| FCA | Freund's Complete Adjuvant |
| FDA | Food and Drug Administration |
| FDCA | Food, Drug and Cosmetic Act |
| FDLI | Food and Drug Law Institute |
| FIFRA | Federal Insecticides, Fungicides and Rodenticides Act |
| GCP | Good Clinical Practices |
| GLP | Good Laboratory Practices |
| GMP | Good Manufacturing Practices |
| GPMT | Guinea Pig Maximization Test |
| HEW | Department of Health, Education and Welfare (no longer existent) |
| HIMA | Health Industry Manufacturer's Association |
| HSDB | Hazardous Substances Data Bank |
| IARC | International Agency for Research on Cancer |
| ICH | International Conference on Harmonization |
| ID | Intradermal |
| IDE | Investigational Device Exemption |
| IND(A) | Investigational New Drug Application |
| INN | International Nonproprietary Names |
| IP | Intraperitoneal |
| IRAG | Interagency Regulatory Alternatives Group |
| IRB | Institutional Review Board |
| IRLG | Interagency Regulatory Liaison Group |
| ISO | International Standards Organization |
| IUD | Intrauterine Device |
| IV | Intravenous |
| JECFA | Joint Expert Committee for Food Additives |
| JMAFF | Japanese Ministry of Agriculture, Forestry, and Fishery |
| JPMA | Japanese Pharmaceutical Manufacturers Association |
| LA | Licensing Authority (U.K.) |
| LAL | *Limulus* amebocyte lysate |
| $LD_{50}$ | Lethal dose 50: The dose calculated to kill 50% of a subject population, median lethal dose |

| | |
|---|---|
| LOEL | Lowest observed effect level |
| MAA | Marketing Authorization Application (EEC) |
| MCA | Medicines Control Agency |
| MD | Medical device |
| MedDRA | Medical Dictionary for Regulatory Activities |
| MHW | Ministry of Health and Welfare (Japan) |
| MID | Maximum implantable dose |
| MOE | Margin of Exposure |
| MOU | Memorandum of Understanding |
| MRL | Maximum Residue Limits |
| MSDS | Material Safety Data Sheet |
| MTD | Maximum tolerated dose |
| NAS | National Academy of Science |
| NCTR | National Center for Toxicological Research |
| NDA | New drug application |
| NIH | National Institutes of Health |
| NIOSH | National Institute Occupational Safety and Health |
| NK | Natural killer |
| NLM | National Library of Medicine |
| NOEL | No-observable-effect level |
| NTP | National Toxicology Program |
| ODE | Office of Device Evaluation |
| OECD | Organization for Economic Cooperation and Development |
| PDI | Primary Dermal Irritancy |
| PDN | Product Development Notification |
| PEL | Permissible Exposure Limit |
| PhRMA | Pharmaceutical Research and Manufacturers Association |
| PL | Produce License (U.K.) |
| PLA | Produce License Application |
| PMA | Premarket approval Applications |
| po | Per os (orally) |
| PTC | Points to Consider |
| QAU | Quality Assurance Unit |
| RAC | Recombinant DNA Advisory Committee |
| RCRA | Resources Conservation and Recovery Act |
| RTECS | Registry of Toxic Effects of Chemical Substances |
| SARA | Superfund/Amendments and Reauthorization Act |
| sc | Subcutaneous |
| SCE | Sister chromatic exchange |
| SNUR | Significant New Use Regulations |
| SOP | Standerd Operating Procedure |
| SOT | Society of Toxicology |
| SRM | Standard Reference Materials (Japan) |
| STEL | Short Term Exposure Limit |
| TLV | Threshold limit value |

| | |
|---|---|
| USAN | United States Adopted Name Council |
| USDA | United States Department of Agriculture |
| USEPA | United States Environmental Protection Agency |
| USP | United States Pharmacopoeia |
| VAERS | Vaccine Adverse Event Reporting System |
| VSD | Vaccine Safety Data Link |
| WHO | World Health Organization |

# APPENDIX B

# DEFINITION OF TERMS AND LEXICON OF CLINICAL OBSERVATIONS IN NONCLINICAL (ANIMAL) STUDIES

### Movement

| | |
|---|---|
| Anesthetized | The absence of or reduced response to external stimuli, accompanied with a loss of righting reflex. |
| Ataxia | Incoordination of muscular action involving locomotion, including loss of coordination and unsteady gait. |
| Hyperactivity | An abnormally high level of motor activity. |
| Hypersensitivity | An abnormally strong reaction to external stimuli such as noise or touch. |
| Lethargy | A state of deep and prolonged depression stupor from which it is possible to be aroused, followed by an immediate relapse. |
| Low carriage | The animal's torso is carried very close to the ground during movement. |
| Prostrate | Animal assumes a recumbent position due to loss of strength or exhaustion and may show intermittent uncoordinated movements. |
| Righting reflex | The ability of an animal, when placed on its back, to regain a position on all fours. |
| Unsteady gait | An erratic manner or style of walking. |

| | |
|---|---|
| Catalepsy | A condition characterized by a waxy rigidity of the muscles such that the animal tends to remain in any position in which it is placed. |
| Paralysis | Inhibition or loss of motor function; may be characterized by affected portion of the body. |

## Respiration

| | |
|---|---|
| Audible respiration | An abnormal respiratory sound heard while listening to the breathing of the animal (e.g., wheezing and rales). |
| Bradypnea | An abnormal slowness of the respiration rate. |
| Dyspnea | "Shortness of breath"; difficult or labored breathing. |
| Gasping | Spasmodic breathing with the mouth open, or laborious respiration with the breath caught convulsively. |
| Hyperpnea | Deep and rapid breathing. |
| Cheyne–Stokes respiration | Breathing characterized by rhythmic waning and waxing of the depth of respiration, with regularly recurring periods of apnea: seen especially in coma resulting from affection of the nervous centers. |
| Hypopnea | Shallow and slow breathing. |
| Irregular respiration | No definite cycle or rate of breathing. |
| Labored respiration | Forced or difficult, usually irregular breathing. |
| Tachypnea | An excessive rapidity of the respiration rate. |

## Condition of Skin and Fur

| | |
|---|---|
| Alopecia | Deficiency of hair (baldness). |
| Cyanosis | Visible skin and/or mucous membranes turn dusky blue due to lack of oxygenation of the blood. |
| Necrosis | Actual tissue destruction, masses of dead/destroyed tissue. |

## Urogenital Region

| | |
|---|---|
| Anuria | An absence of or sharp decline in urine excretion. |
| Diarrhea | An abnormal frequency and liquidity of fecal discharge. |
| Polyuria | An abnormally sharp increase in the amount of urine excretion. |

## Convulsions and Tremors

| | |
|---|---|
| Convulsions | Transient, self-sustaining electrical dysrhythmias which have a tendency to recur. Convulsions are generally associated with a finite period of unconsciousness and have a muscular involvement manifested as disorganized limb movements. |
| Clonic | This is often seen as a "paddling" motion of the forelegs of the animal. |

| | |
|---|---|
| Tonic | Muscular contraction, keeping limbs in a fixed position, generally extended to the rear. |
| Torsion | Postural incoordination or rolling. This is generally associated with the vestibular (ear canal) system. |
| Fasciculation | Rapid, often continuous contraction of a bundle of skeletal muscle fibers which does not produce a purposeful movement (twitching). |
| Tremor | Fine oscillating muscular movements which may or may not be rhythmic. |

## Condition of Eyes

| | |
|---|---|
| Blepharospasm | A twitching or spasmodic contraction of the orbicularis occuli muscle. |
| Chemosis | Edema of conjunctiva(e). The conjunctival tissue responds to noxious stimuli by swelling. |
| Chromodacryorrhea | The response of reddish conjunctival exudate; no blood cells present in exudate (i.e., not true "bloody tears"). |
| Conjunctivitis | Inflammation of conjunctiva (mucous membrane which lines the eyelids and is reflected into the eyeball). |
| Exophthalmos | An abnormal protrusion of the eyeball from the orbit. |
| Lacrimation | The secretion of tears. |
| Miosis | Constriction of the pupil. |
| Mydriasis | Dilation of the pupil. |
| Nystagmus | An abnormal involuntary movement of the eyes. It may be rotational or horizontal or vertical plane. |
| Ocular exudate | Secretion (usually transparent and yellow) directly from the eye. |
| Opacity | A loss of transparency of the eyeball. |
| Pinpoint pupils | Ultimate state of miosis. |
| Ptosis | Refers to a dropping of the upper eyelid, thought to be due to impaired conduction in the third cranial nerve. |

## Miscellaneous

| | |
|---|---|
| Analgesia | The absence of (or reduced response to) painful stimuli. |
| Hunched posture | The drawing-in of both ends of the body and extremities with a sharp arching of the back. |
| Kyphosis | Humpback-an abnormal curvature and dorsal prominence of the vertebrae column. |
| Nasal discharge | Fluid secretion from the nostrils. |
| Piloerection | Body hair stands on end; dilation of the pupils usually accompanies piloerection. |
| Salivation | Excessive secretion of saliva from the mouth. |
| Straub tail | Condition, especially in mice, in which the animal carries its tail in an erect (vertical or nearly vertical) position. This |

sign is commonly associated with chemicals (e.g., morphine) that bind to opiate receptors.

## Reflexes

Corneal reflex
: Closure of the eyelids in response to a corneal touch (e.g., with a soft brush bristle).

Grip strength (or Screen Grip)
: Measure of the grip strength of the forelimbs or hindlimbs; may be evaluated quantitatively or by subjective estimate or impairment (rodents only).

Pinna reflex
: Twitch of the outer ear in response to a gentle touch.

Preyer's reflex (auditory startle response)
: Involuntary movement of the outer ears produced by an auditory stimulus (especially in rats).

Pupillary reflex
: Contraction of the pupil in response to light stimulation of the retina.

Righting Reflex
: The ability to land on (when dropped) or regain normal stance on all four limbs.

Startle reflex
: Response to sharp sound, touch, or other startling stimulus; response may range from "absent," to "normal," to "hyperreactive," including exaggerated jerking, jumping, frantic attempts to escape, and even convulsion.

# APPENDIX C

# NOTABLE REGULATORY INTERNET ADDRESSES

| Organization or Publication | Web Address (URL) | Sample Main Topics |
| --- | --- | --- |
| ABPI | http://www.abpi.org.uk/ | |
| Adverse Reactions Bulletin | http://www.thomsonscience.co | |
| Agency for Toxic Substances and Disease Registry | www.atsdr.cdc.gov | |
| Association of Clinical Biochemists | http://www.leeds.ac.uk/acb/ | Items of general medical interest and an assay finder to help researcher find methods or labs to measure a wide variety of hormones, metals, enzymes and drugs in body fluids |
| Australian Therapeutic Goods Administration | http://www.health.gov.au/tga | Medical Devices; GMP Codes; Parliamentary Secretary's Working; Status Document; Party on Complementary medicines; Medical Releases; Publications; Site map; Related Sites |
| BioMedNet | http://www.cursci.co.uk/BioMedNet/biomed.html/ OR http://www.BioMedNet.com | The World Wide Web club for the biological and medical community (free membership) |
| Canadian Health Protection Board | http://www.hwc.ca/hpb | |
| Canadian Health Protection Branch | http://www.hc-sc.gc.ca/hpb | Medical Devices; Chemical Hazards; Food; Product Safety; Science Advisory Board; Diseases; Radiation Protection; Drugs; HPB Transition Policy, Planning and Coordination |
| Centre for Medicines Research | http://www.cmr.org/ | |
| ChemInfo | www.indiana.edu/~cheminfo/ca_csti.html | SirCH: Chemical Safety or Toxicology Information |

| Clinical Pharmacology Drug Monograph Service | http://www.cponline.gsm.com | |
| Clinician's Computer-Assisted Guide to the Choice of Instruments for Quality of Life Assessment in Medicine | http://www.glamm.com/ql/guide.htm | Contains hypertext with references to QoL measurements divided into (a) general diseases, (b) specific diseases and therapies, (c) health organizations, (d) bibliography |
| ClinWeb | http://www.ohsu.edu/clinweb | Oregon Health Sciences University |
| CNN Interactive (Health) | http://www.cnn.com/HEALTH/index.html | Up-to-date information on health issues including drug safety concerns and withdrawals |
| Code of Federal Register | http://www.access.gpo.gov/nara/cfr/index.html OR http://www.access.gpo.gov/su_docs/aces/aces140.html | For proposed rules and regulations |
| Code of Federal Regulations | http://www.access.gpo.gov/nara/cfr/cfr-table-search.html | NARA Code Sections |
| Committee on Safety of Medicines (CSM) | http://www.open.gov.uk/mca/csmhome.htm | |
| Cornell Legal Library | http://www.law.cornell.edu | Code of Federal Regulations; Supreme Court Decisions; U.S. Code; Circuit Courts of Appeal |
| Current Problems in Pharmacovigilance | http://www.opwn.gov.uk/mca/mcahome.htm | |
| Cutaneous Drug Reactions | http://triz.dermatology.uiowa.edu/home.html | |
| DIA Home Page | http://www.diahome.org | Home Page of the Drug Information Association |

(continued)

| Organization or Publication | Web Address (URL) | Sample Main Topics |
| --- | --- | --- |
| Doctor's Guide to the Internet | http://www.psigroup.com | |
| Documents for Clinical Research | http://www.ams.med.unigoettingen.de/~rhilger/Document.html | *Declaration of Helsinki*, other documents and collection of related sites |
| Druginfonet | http://www.druginfonet.com | |
| EC DGXIII Telecommunications | http://.www.ispo.cec.be/ | Information |
| EMBASE | http://www.healthgate.com/healthGate/price/embase.html | |
| EPA | www.epa.gov | |
| Eudra Net: Network Services for the European Union Pharmaceutical Regulatory Sector | http://www.eudra.org | Includes information on the European Agency for the Evaluation of Medicinal Products. |
| EMEA | http://www.eudra.org/emea.html | |
| Europa | http://www.cec.lu | Official website of the European Union |
| European Agency for the Evaluation of Medicinal Products | http://www.eudra.org/en_home.htm | What's New; Documents Forum; Other Sites |
| European Sites | http://www.eucomed.-www.eucomed.-be/eucomed/links/links.htm | European Institutions; Related Sites |
| European Pharmacovigilance Research Group | http://www.ncl.ac.uk/~neprg/ | |
| Food and Drug Administration (FDA) | www.fda.gov | Foods; Human Drugs; Biologics; Animal Drugs; Cosmetics; Medical Devices/Radiological Health |
| FDA: CBER<br>Center for Biologics Evaulation and Research | http://www.fda.gov/cber | |

| CBER What's New | http://www.fda.gov/cber/whatsnew.htm | |
| FDA: CDER | http://www.fda.gov/cder | |
|    Center for Drug Evaluation and Research | | |
| FDA Adverse Events Database | http://www.fda.gov/cder/adr | |
| CDER What's New | http://www.fda.gov/cder/whatsnew.htm | |
| FDA: CDRH | www.fda.gov/cdrh/index.html | Home page |
| Search site | www.fda.gov/cdrh/search.html | Search CDRH site |
| Comment | www.fda.gov/cdrh/comment4.html | Comment on CDRH site |
| Device Advice | www.fda.gov/cdrh/devadvice/32.html | |
| PDF Reader | www.fda.gov/cdrh/acrobat.html | |
| FDA: CFSAN | http://vm.cfsan.fda.gov | |
|    Center for Food Safety and Applied Nutrition | | |
| FDA: Center for Toxicological Research | http://www.fda.gov/nctr | |
| FDA: CVM | http://www.fda.gov/cvm | |
| Center for Veterinary Medicine | | |
| FDA: Bioengineered food | http:www.fda.gov/oc/biotech/default.htm | |
| FDA: Breast Implants | http:www.fda.gov/cdrh/breastimplants/index.html | |
| FDA: Cosmetics | http://vm.cfsan.fda.gov//~lrd/cosmetm.html | |
| FDA: Dietary Supplements | http:vm.cfsan.fda.gov/~dms/supplmt.html | |

(*continued*)

| Organization or Publication | Web Address (URL) | Sample Main Topics |
| --- | --- | --- |
| FDA's Electronic Freedom of Information Act | http:www.fda.gov/foi/foia2.htm | |
| FDA-Field Operations | www.fda.gov/ora/ | What's New; Import Program; Inspectional, Science and Compliance References; Federal/State Relations |
| The Common Technical Document for the Registration of Pharmaceuticals for Human use: 08-24-00 | http://www.fda.gov/cder/guidance/4022dfts.htm | |
| Design Controls | www.fda.gov/ora/inspect_ref/qsreq/dcrpgd.html | Design Control Report and Guidance Text |
| | www.fda.gov/ora/inspect_ref/igs/elec_med_dev/emcl.html | Guide to Inspections of Electromagnetic Compatibility Aspects of Medical Device Quality Systems Text |
| Guide to Inspections of Quality Systems | www.fda.gov/ora/inspect_ref/igs/qsit/qsitguide.htm | QSIT Inspection Handbook Text |
| Guide to Inspections of Quality Systems | www.fda.gov/ora/inspect_ref/igs/qsit/QSITGUIDE.PDF | PDF version of QSIT Inspection Handbook Text |
| Photosafety Testing 07-05-00 | http://www.fda.gov/cder/guidance/3281dft.htm | |
| Skin Irritation and Sensitization Testing of Generic Transdermal Drug Products 06 : 01 : 00 | http://www.fda.gov/cder/guidance/2887fnl.htm | |
| FDA: MedWatch | http://www.fda.gov/medwatch/ | USFDA drug adverse event reporting system |
| FDA: Tampons | http://www.fda.gov/oc/opacpm/topicindexes/tampons.html | |

| | | |
|---|---|---|
| Food and Drug Law Institute | http://www.fdli.org | Special Interest; Publications; Multimedia; Order Products; Academic Programs; Directory of lawyers and Consultants; Contact Us |
| Health Industry and Manufacturers Association (HIMA) | http://www.himanet.com | About HIMA; Newsletter; HIMA Calendar; Industry Resources; Business Opportunities; FDA/EPA/OSHA; Reimbursement/ Payment; Global Year 2000; Government Relations; Public Relations; Small Company; Diagnostics |
| Health on the Net | http://www.hon.ch | |
| Health Information on the Internet | http://www.wellcome.ac.uk.healthinfo/ | New bimonthly newsletter from the Wellcome Trust and the RSM |
| Hyppos Project | http://ifinet.it/hypposnet | Information in Italian and English about the Hyppos Project, which has led to the development of a QoL tool for the measurement of hypertensive patients in Italy. It contains a description of the project, the tool, publications about the development of the tool and its application, plus general references to QoL and hypertension |
| International Classification of Disease (ICD)-10 | http://www.cihi.ca.newinit/scope.htm | |
| International Conference on Harmonization (ICH) 3 Home Page | http://cc.umin.u-tokyo.ac.jp/ich/ich3.html | Official ICH website with documents (needs a password) |

*(continued)*

| Organization or Publication | Web Address (URL) | Sample Main Topics |
| --- | --- | --- |
| ICH documents | http://www.pharmweb.net/pwmirror/pw9/ifpma/ich1/html | |
| International Conference on Harmonization of Technical Requirements for Registration of Pharmaceuticals for Human use | http://www.ifpma.org/ich1.html | |
| International Federation of Pharmaceutical Manufacturers | http://www.ifpharma.com | ICH documents and postings; International Pharmaceutical issues |
| International Regulatory Monitor (Monitor) | http://www.go-nsi.com/pubs | Editorial Portion of Newsletter |
| International Society of Pharmacoepidemiology | http://www.pharmacoepi.org | |
| Internet Grateful Med | www.igm.nlm.nih.gov | |
| InterPharma | http://www.interpharma.co.uk | The latter are vast sites with links to other databases for pharmaceutical support sites—http://www.MedsiteNavigator.com |
| JAMA (J. Am. Med. Assoc.) | http://www.ama-assn.org/jama | Gives many other useful USA sites |
| Japanese Ministry of Health and Welfare | http://www.mhw.go.jp/english/index.html | Organization; Y2K Problem; Statistics; White Paper; Related Sites |
| Library of Congress | http://thomas.loc.gov | Searchable database of federal legislation, Congressional Record and committee information |
| Market and Exploitation of Research | http://www.cordis.lu | |
| Medical Device Link | http://www.devicelink. com | News; Consultants; Bookstore; Links; Discussion; Magazines (MDDI; MPMN; IVD Technology) |

| | | |
|---|---|---|
| Medicines Control Agency (MCA) | http://www.opengov.uk/mcahome.htm | |
| Medical Matrix | http://www.medmatrix.org | |
| Medical Research Council | http://nimr.mcr.ac.uk/MRC/ | |
| MEDLINE (free) | http://www.ncbi.nlm.nih.gov/PubMed | List of free sites |
| | or http://www.medmatrix.org/Spages/medline.asp | |
| MEDLINE | http://www.medmatrix.org/SPAges/medline.asp | A metasite with full and changing MEDLINE search engines; List of free sites |
| | or http://www.medsitenavigator.com/medline/medline.html | |
| Medscape | http://www.medscape.com | |
| Multilingual glossary of medical terms | http://allserv.rug.ac.be/~rvdstich/eugloss/welcome.html | |
| National Archives and Public Records Administration | http://www.access.gpo.gov/su_docs/aces/aces140.html | Code of Federal Regulations; Federal Register; Laws; U.S. Congress Information |
| National Institutes of Health (USA) | http://www.nih.gov | |
| National Library Network | www.toxnet.nlm.nih.gov | TOXNET: Toxicology Data Network, a cluster of databases on toxicology, hazardous chemicals, and related areas |
| National Toxicology Program | http://ntp-server.niehs.nih.gov/ | |
| New Quality System (QS) Regulation | www.fda.gov/bbs/topics/ANSWERS/ANS00763.html | FDA Talk Paper Announcing the GMP Final Rule text |
| Organized Medical Network Information | http://www.omni.ac.uk | |

(*continued*)

987

| Organization or Publication | Web Address (URL) | Sample Main Topics |
| --- | --- | --- |
| Pharmaceutical and Medical Safety Bureau (Japan) | http://www.mhlw.go.jp/english | |
| PharminfoNet | http://www.pharminfo.com or http://www.pharminfo.com/phrm-o.com/phrmlink.html | Independent assessment of therapeutics and advances in new drug development |
| Pharmweb | http://www.pharmweb.net | Information resource for pharmaceutical and health-related information |
| Quality of Life | http://www.glamm.com/ql/guide.htm | The choice of instrument |
| Quality of Life Assessment in Medicine | http://www.glamm.com/q1/ursl.htm | This contains hypertext with references to QoL measurements divided into (a) assessment tools, (b) reference organizations and groups, (c) diseases, symptoms and specific populations, (d) the top ten journals that publish articles of interest to QoL assessment in medicine, (e) methodology, (f) bibliographical research. |
| Regulatory Affairs Professionals Society (RAPS) | http://www.raps.org | Certificates; Resource Center; Publications; Chapters; Related Links; Contacting RAPS |
| Reuters Health Information Services | http://www.reuters health.com | |
| SCRIP: World Pharmaceutical News | http://www.pjbpubs.co.uk/scrip | |
| SNOMED | http://snomed.org | Systemised Nomenclature of Human and Veterinary Medicines |
| Swedish Medical Products Agency | http://www.mpa.Se | |
| U.S. Department of Agriculture (USDA) | http://www.usda.gov | |

| | | |
| --- | --- | --- |
| Food Safety | http://www.foodsafety.gov/ | |
| USDA-FMS Farm Service Agency | http://www.fsa.usda.gov/pas/default.asp | |
| USDA-FSA Food and Nutrition Service | http://www.fns.usda.gov/fns/ | |
| USDA-FSIS Food Safety and Inspection Service | http://www.usda.gov/fsis | |
| U.S. Department of Commerce | http://204.193.246.62 | Bureau of Export Administration; International Trade Association; Patent and Trademark; National Institute of Standards and Technology |
| U.S. Pharmacopoeia | www.usp.org/prn | |
| University of Pittsburgh | www.pitt.edu | |
| World Health Organization | http://www.who.int | Governance; Health Topics; Information Sources; Reports; Director-General; About WHO; International Digest of Health; Legislation (http://www.who.int/pub/dig.html) |
| WHO Collaborating Centre for International Drug Monitoring | http://www.who.ch/ or http://www.who.pharmasoft.se | |

# APPENDIX D

# GLOSSARY OF TERMS USED IN THE CLINICAL EVALUATION OF THERAPEUTIC AGENTS

**Abnormality.** A sign, symptom, or laboratory result not characteristic of normal individuals.

**Adverse event.** Unwanted effects that occur and are detected in populations. The term is used whether there is or is not any attribution to a medicine or other cause. Adverse events may be known parts of a disease that are observed to occur within a period of observation, and they may be analyzed to test for their frequency in a given population or trial. This is done to determine if there is an unexpectedly increased frequency resulting from nondisease factors such as medicine treatment. The term "adverse event" or "adverse experience" is used to encompass adverse reactions plus any injury, toxicity, or hypersensitivity that may be medicine-related, as well as any medical events that are apparently unrelated to medicine that occur during the study (e.g., surgery, illness, and trauma). See definition of **Adverse reaction**.

**Adverse experience.** See **Adverse event**.

**Adverse reaction.** Unwanted effect(s) (i.e., physical and psychological symptoms and signs) resulting from treatment. A less rigid definition of adverse reaction includes the previous definition plus any undesirable effect or problem that is present during the period of treatment and may or may not be a well-known or obvious complication of the disease itself. Thus, many common personality, physical, psychological, and behavioral characteristics that are observed in medicine studies are sometimes characterized as adverse reactions even if they were present during baseline.

990

Synonyms of adverse reactions generally include adverse medical effects, untoward effects, side effects, adverse drug experiences, and adverse drug reactions. Specific distinctions among some of these terms may be defined operationally. For example, the term "adverse reaction" is used to denote those signs and symptoms at least possibly related to a medicine, whereas the term "adverse experience" is used to include nonmedicine-related medical problems in a trial such as those emanating from trauma or concurrent illness. Distinctions among side effects, adverse events, and adverse reactions are illustrated in the definitions of the two former terms.

**Bias.**  (1) A point of view that prevents impartial judgement on issues relating to that point of view. Clinical trials attempt to control this through double blinding. (2) Any tendency for a value to deviate in one direction from the true value. Statisticians attempt to prevent this type of bias by various techniques, including randomization.

**Clinical significance.**  The quality of a study's outcome that convinces physicians to modify or maintain their current practice of medicine. The greater the clinical significance, the greater is the influence on the practice of medicine. The assessment of clinical significance is usually based on the magnitude of the effect observed, the quality of the study that yielded the data, and the probability that the effect is a true one. Although this operational definition is presented from the physician's perspective, the term could operationally be defined from the patient's perspective. Patients are primarily concerned with results that will lead to an improved quality of life or a lengthening of their life. In addition, clinical significance may be applied to either positive data or efficacy or negative safety data such as for adverse reactions. Synonyms include clinical importance, clinical relevance, and clinical meaningfulness.

**Clinical studies.**  The class of all scientific approaches to evaluate medical disease preventions, diagnostic techniques, and treatments. Investigational and marketed prescription medicine evaluations plus over-the-counter medicines are included.

**Clinical trials.**  A subset of those clinical studies that evaluates investigational medicines in Phases I, II, and III. Phase IV evaluations of marketed medicines in formal clinical trials using the same or similar types of protocols to those used in Phases I and III are also referred to as clinical trials.

**Compliance.**  (1) Adherence of patients to following medical advice and prescriptions. Primarily applied to taking medicine as directed, but also applies to following advice on diet, exercise, or other aspects of a patient's life. (2) Adherence of investigators to following a protocol and related administrative and regulatory responsibilities. (3) Adherence of sponsors to following regulatory, legal and other responsibilities and requirements relating to a clinical trial.

**Compound.**  A chemical synthesized or prepared from natural sources that is evaluated for its biological activities in preclinical tests.

**Development of medicines.**  The term "development" as applied to medicines is used in several different contexts, even within the pharmaceutical industry. This often leads to confusion and misunderstanding. No single definition is preferred, but the particular meaning intended should be made clear by all people using the term. Three operational definitions are presented, from the broadest to the narrowest:

1. All stages and processes involved in discovering, evaluating, and formulating a new medicine, until it reaches the market (i.e., commercial sale).

2. All stages involving the evaluation and formulation of a new medicine (after the medicine has been discovered and has gone through preclinical testing), until it reaches the market.

3. Those stages after the preclinical discovery and evaluation that involve technical development. These processes include formulation work, stability testing, scaling-up the compound for larger-scale synthesis, and providing analytical support. Clinical trials are not included in this definition.

**Disease.** Disorders (e.g., anxiety disorders, seizure disorders), conditions (e.g., obesity, menopause), syndromes, specific illnesses, and other medical problems that are an acquired morbid change in a tissue, organ, or organism. Synonyms are illness and sickness.

**Dosage regimen.** (1) The number of doses per given time period (usually days), (2) the time that elapses between doses (e.g., dose to be given every six hours) or the time that the doses are to be given (e.g., dose to be given at 8 A.M., noon, and 4 P.M. each day), or (3) the quantity of a medicine (e.g., number of tablets, capsules, etc.) that is given at each specific time of dosing.

**Efficacy.** A relative concept referring to the ability of a medicine to elicit a beneficial clinical effect. This may be measured or evaluated using objective or subjective parameters, and in terms ranging form global impressions to highly precise measurements. Efficacy is assessed at one or more levels of organization (e.g., subcellular, cellular, tissue, organ, whole body) and may be extrapolated to other levels.

**Endpoint.** An indicator measured in a patient or biological sample to assess safety, efficacy, or another trial objective. Some endpoints are derived from primary endpoints (e.g., cardiac output is derived from stroke volume and heart rate). Synonyms include outcome, variable, parameter, marker, and measure. See surrogate endpoint in the text. Also defined as the final trial objective by some authors.

**Incidence rate.** The rate of occurrence of new cases of a disease, adverse reaction, or other event in a given population at risk (e.g., the incidence of disease $X$ is $Y$ patients per year per 100,000 population).

**Interpretation.** The process whereby one determines the clinical meaning or significance of data after the relevant statistical analyses have been performed. These processes often involve developing an explanation of the data that are being evaluated.

**Medicine.** When a compound or substance is tested for biological and clinical activity in humans, it is considered to be a medicine. Some individuals prefer to define a medicine as a compound that has demonstrated clinically useful properties in patients. This definition, however, would restrict the term to use sometime during or after Phase II. Others use the term loosely and apply it to compounds with biological properties during the preclinical period that suggest medical usefulness in humans. The author has adopted the first definition for use in this book.

**Patient.** The term "patient" is used almost exclusively throughout this book in preference to subject or volunteer. Patient is used to cover those cases in which the term "volunteer" would be appropriate.

**Pharmacodynamics.** The processes of the body's responses resulting from treatment with a medicine or compound. The processes include pharmacological, biochemical, physiological, and therapeutic effects. The pharmacodynamics of a response to treatment are presented with the scientific and/or clinical language of the disciplines involved in detecting, measuring, and describing the effects.

**Pharmacokinetics.** The processes of absorption, distribution, metabolism, and excretion of compounds and medicines.

**Phases of clinical trials and medicine development.** Four phases of clinical trials and medicine development exist and are defined below. Each of these definitions is a functional one and the terms are not defined on a strict chronological basis. An investigational medicine is often evaluated in two or more phases simultaneously in different clinical trials. Also, some clinical trials may overlap two different phases.

**Phase I.** Initial safety trials on a new medicine, usually conducted in normal male volunteers. An attempt is made to establish the dose range tolerated by volunteers for single and for multiple doses. Phase I trials are sometimes conducted in severely ill patients (e.g., in the field of cancer) or in less ill patients when pharmacokinetic issues are addressed (e.g., metabolism of a new antiepileptic medicine in stable epileptic patients whose microsomal liver enzymes have been induced by other antiepileptic medicines). Pharmacokinetic trials are usually considered Phase I trials regardless of when they are conducted during a medicine's development.

**Phase IIa.** Pilot clinical trials to evaluate efficacy (and safety) in selected populations of patients with the disease or condition to be treated, diagnosed, or prevented. Objectives may focus on dose-response, type of patient, frequency of dosing, or numerous other characteristics of safety and efficacy.

**Phase IIb.** Well-controlled trials to evaluate efficacy (and safety) in patients with the disease or condition to be treated, diagnosed, or prevented. These clinical trials usually represent the most rigorous demonstration of a medicine's efficacy. Sometimes referred to as pivotal trials.

**Phase IIIa.** Trials conducted after efficacy of the medicine is demonstrated, but prior to regulatory submission of a New Drug Application (NDA) or other dossier. These clinical trials are conducted in patient populations for which the medicine is eventually intended. Phase IIIa clinical trials generate additional data on both safety and efficacy in relatively large numbers of patients in both controlled and uncontrolled trials. Clinical trials are also conducted in special groups of patients (e.g., renal failure patients), or under special conditions dictated by the nature of the medicine and disease. These trials often provide much of the information needed for the packaging insert and labeling of the medicine.

**Phase IIIb.** Clinical trials conducted after regulatory submission of an NDA or other dossier, but prior to the medicine's approval and launch. These trials may supplement earlier trials, complete earlier trials, or may be directed toward new types of trials (e.g., quality of life, marketing) or Phase IV evaluations. This is the period between submission and approval of a regulatory dossier for marketing authorization.

**Phase IV.** Studies or trials conducted after a medicine is marketed to provide additional details about the medicine's efficacy or safety profile. Different formulations, dosages, durations of treatment, medicine interactions, and other medicine comparisons may be evaluated. New age groups, races, and other types of patients can be studied. Detection and definition of previously unknown or inadequately quantified adverse reactions and related risk factors are an important aspect of many Phase IV studies. If a marketed medicine is to be evaluated for another (i.e., new) indication, then those clinical trials are considered Phase II clinical trials. The term "postmarketing surveillance" is frequently used to describe those clinical studies in Phase IV (i.e., the period following marketing) that are primarily observational or nonexperimental in nature, to distinguish them from well-controlled Phase IV clinical trials or marketing studies.

**Prevalence.** The total number of people in a population that are affected with a particular disease at a given time. This term is expressed as the rate of all cases (e.g., the prevalence of disease $X$ is $Y$ patients per 100,000 population) at a given point or period of time.

**Research (on medicines).** Numerous definitions of research are used both in the literature and among scientists. In the broadest sense, research in the pharmaceutical industry includes all processes of medicine discovery, preclinical and clinical evaluation, and technical development. In a more restricted sense, research concentrates on the preclinical discovery phase, where the basic characteristics of a new medicine are determined. Once a decision is reached to study the medicine in humans to evaluate its therapeutic potential, the compound passes from the research to the development phase.

**Research and development.** When research and development are used together, it refers to the broadest definition for research (see above). Some people use the term "research" colloquially to include most or all of the scientific and medical areas (discovery, evaluation, and development) covered by the single term "research and development." "Medicine development" has several definitions and, in its broadest definition, is exactly the same as the broad definition of research.

**Risk.** A measure of (1) the probability of occurrence of harm to human health or (2) the severity of harm that may occur. Such a measure includes judgment of the acceptability of risk. Assessment of safety involves judgment, and there are numerous perspectives (e.g., patients, physicians, company, regulatory authorities) used for judging it.

**Safety.** A relative concept referring to the freedom from harm or damage resulting from adverse reactions or physical, psychological, or behavioral abnormalities that occur as a result of medicine or nonmedicine use. Safety is usually measured with one or more of the following: physical examination (e.g., vital signs, neurological, ophthalmological, general physical), laboratory evaluations of biological samples (e.g., hematology, clinical chemistry, urinalysis), special tests and procedures (e.g., electrocardiogram, pulmonary function tests), psychiatric tests and evaluations, and determination of clinical signs and symptoms.

**Serious adverse reactions.** Multiple definitions are possible and no single one is correct in all situations. In general usage referring to patients in clinical trials, a serious adverse reaction may be (1) any bad adverse reaction that is observed, (2) any bad adverse reaction that one does not expect to observe, (3) any bad adverse reaction that one does not expect to observe and is not on the label, or (4) any bad adverse reaction that has not been reported with standard therapy. Definitions also may be based on the degree to which an adverse reaction compromises a patient's function or requires treatment.

**Side effect.** Any effect other than the primary intended effect(s) resulting from medicine or nonmedicine treatment or intervention. Side effects may be negative (i.e., an adverse reaction), neutral, or positive (i.e., a beneficial effect) for the patient. This term, therefore, includes all adverse reactions plus other effects of treatment. See definition of **Adverse reaction**.

**Site.** This refers to the place where a clinical trial is conducted. A physician who has offices and sees patients in three separate location is viewed as having one site. A physician who is on the staff of four hospitals could be viewed as having one or four sites, depending on how similar or different the patient populations are and whether the data from these four locations will be pooled and considered a single site. For example, a single physician who enrolls groups of patients at a university hospital, private clinic, community hospital, and Veterans Administration Hospital should generally be viewed as having four sites, since the patient populations would be expected to differ at each site.

**Statistical significance.** This term relates to the probability that an event or difference occurred by chance alone. Thus, it is a measure of whether a difference is likely to be real, but it does not indicate whether the difference is small or large, important or trivial. The level of statistical significance depends on the number of patients studied or observations made, as well as the magnitude of difference observed.

**Therapeutic window.** This term is applied to the difference between the minimum and maximum doses that may be given patients to obtain an adequate clinical response and avoid intolerable toxic effects. The greater the value calculated for the therapeutic window, the greater a medicine's margin of safety. Synonyms are "therapeutic ratio" and "therapeutic index."

**Volunteer.** A normal individual who participates in a clinical trial for reasons other than medical need and who does not receive any direct medical benefit from participating in the trial.

# INDEX